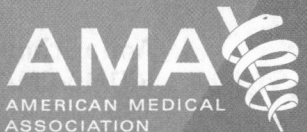

AMA

AMERICAN MEDICAL
ASSOCIATION

W9-BEI-360

ICD-10-PCS 2022
The Complete Official Codebook

AMA publications fund initiatives that drive improvements in patient
health, practice innovation and medical education.

Notice

ICD-10-PCS: The Complete Official Codebook is designed to be an accurate and authoritative source regarding coding and every reasonable effort has been made to ensure accuracy and completeness of the content. However, the American Medical Association (AMA) makes no guarantee, warranty, or representation that this publication is accurate, complete, or without errors. It is understood that the AMA is not rendering any legal or other professional services or advice in this publication and that the AMA bears no liability for any results or consequences that may arise from the use of this book.

Our Commitment to Accuracy

The AMA is committed to producing accurate and reliable materials. To report corrections, please call the AMA Unified Service Center at (800) 621-8335. AMA product updates, errata, and addendum can be found at amaproductupdates.org.

To purchase additional copies, contact the AMA at 612-435-6065 or visit the AMA store at amastore.com. Refer to product number OP201122.

Acknowledgments

Marianne Randall, CPC, *Product Manager*

Anita Schmidt, BS, RHIA, AHIMA-approved ICD-10-CM/PCS Trainer, *Subject Matter Expert*

Karen Krawzik, RHIT, CCS, AHIMA-approved ICD-10-CM/PCS Trainer, *Subject Matter Expert*

LaJuana Green, RHIA, CCS, *Subject Matter Expert*

Stacy Perry, *Manager, Desktop Publishing*

Tracy Betzler, *Senior Desktop Publishing Specialist*

Hope M. Dunn, *Senior Desktop Publishing Specialist*

Katie Russell, *Desktop Publishing Specialist*

Kate Holden, *Editor*

Anita Schmidt, BS, RHIA, AHIMA-approved ICD-10-CM/PCS Trainer

Ms. Schmidt has expertise in ICD-10-CM/PCS, DRG, and CPT with more than 15 years' experience in coding in multiple settings, including inpatient, observation, and same-day surgery. Her experience includes analysis of medical record documentation, assignment of ICD-10-CM and PCS codes, and DRG validation. She has conducted training for ICD-10-CM/PCS and electronic health record. She has also collaborated with clinical documentation specialists to identify documentation needs and potential areas for physician education. Most recently she has been developing content for resource and educational products related to ICD-10-CM, ICD-10-PCS, DRG, and CPT. Ms. Schmidt is an AHIMA-approved ICD-10-CM/PCS trainer and is an active member of the American Health Information Management Association (AHIMA) and the Minnesota Health Information Management Association (MHIMA).

Karen Krawzik, RHIT, CCS, AHIMA-approved ICD-10-CM/PCS Trainer

Ms. Krawzik has expertise in ICD-10-CM, ICD-9-CM, CPT/HCPCS, DRG, and data quality and analytics, with more than 30 years' experience coding in multiple settings, including inpatient, observation, ambulatory surgery, ancillary, and emergency room. She has served as a DRG analyst and auditor of commercial and government payer claims, as a contract administrator, and worked on a team providing enterprise-wide conversion of the ICD-9-CM code set to ICD-10. More recently, she has been developing print and electronic content related to ICD-10-CM and ICD-10-PCS coding systems, MS-DRGs, and HCCs. Ms. Krawzik is credentialed by the American Health Information Management Association (AHIMA) as a Registered Health Information Technician (RHIT) and a Certified Coding Specialist (CCS) and is an AHIMA-approved ICD-10-CM/PCS trainer. She is an active member of AHIMA and the Missouri Health Information Management Association.

Contents

What's New for 2022

The Centers for Medicare and Medicaid Services is the agency charged with maintaining and updating ICD-10-PCS. CMS released the most current revisions, a summary of which may be found on the CMS website at https://www.cms.gov/medicare/icd-10/2022-icd-10-pcs.

Due to the unique structure of ICD-10-PCS, a change in a character value may affect individual codes and several code tables.

Change Summary Table

2021 Total	New Codes	Revised Titles	Deleted Codes	2022 Total
78,136	191	62	107	78,220

ICD-10-PCS Code FY 2022 Totals, By Section

Medical and Surgical	67,754
Obstetrics	304
Placement	861
Administration	1,253
Measurement and Monitoring	422
Extracorporeal or Systemic Assistance and Performance	52
Extracorporeal or Systemic Therapies	46
Osteopathic	100
Other Procedures	78
Chiropractic	90
Imaging	2,977
Nuclear Medicine	463
Radiation Therapy	2,087
Physical Rehabilitation and Diagnostic Audiology	1,380
Mental Health	30
Substance Abuse Treatment	59
New Technology	264
Total	78,220

ICD-10-PCS Table Changes Highlights

- New rows added to root operation table Extraction in the Central Nervous System and Cranial Nerves body system, capturing body part values Brain and Cerebral Hemisphere

- New qualifier Orbital Atherectomy Technique added to root operation table Extirpation in the Heart and Great Vessels body system, Percutaneous approach, for body parts Coronary Artery, One; Coronary Artery, Two; Coronary Artery, Three Arteries; and Coronary Artery, Four or More Arteries

- New row added to root operation table Fragmentation in the Heart and Great Vessels body system, capturing body parts Coronary Artery, One; Coronary Artery, Two; Coronary Artery, Three Arteries; and Coronary Artery, Four or More Arteries

- New rows added to root operation table Replacement in the Heart and Great Vessels body system, adding body part Heart, Open approach, with Devices Biologic with Synthetic Substitute, Autoregulated Electrohydraulic and Synthetic Substitute, Pneumatic, and new rows added to body part Pulmonary Valve, device Zooplastic Tissue, to capture new Device qualifiers In Existing Conduit and Native Site

- New body part value Ventricle, Left, added to root operation table Restriction in the Heart and Great Vessels body system

- Approach value Percutaneous added to body parts Brachial Artery, Left, and Brachial Artery, Right, in the root operation table Bypass in the Upper Arteries body system

- New body part value Intracranial Artery added to root operation table Fragmentation in the Upper Arteries body system

- New approach values Via Natural or Artificial Opening and Via Natural or Artificial Opening Endoscopic added to root operation table Occlusion in the Lower Veins body system, body part Lower Vein

- New body part value Bone Marrow added to root operation table Extraction in the Lymphatic and Hemic Systems body system

- New body part values Liver; Liver, Right Lobe; and Liver, Left Lobe, added to root operation table Division in the Hepatobiliary System and Pancreas body system

- New row added specific to body part Tongue, Palate, Pharynx Muscle, to root operation table Division in the Muscles body system with two new approach values, Via Natural and Artificial Opening and Via Natural and Artificial Opening Endoscopic

- New device value added to body part Skull in the root operation table Insertion in the Head and Facial Bones body system to capture Infusion Device

- New device value for Spinal Stabilization Device, Vertebral Body Tether, added to root operation table Reposition in the Upper Bones body system for body part Thoracic Vertebra and root operation table Reposition in the Lower Bones body system for body part Lumbar Vertebra

- New rows added to root operation table Excision in the Lower Bones body system, specific to body parts Metatarsal, Right, and Metatarsal, Left, adding new qualifier value Sesamoid Bone(s) 1st Toe

- New rows added specific to body parts Shoulder Joint, Right, and Shoulder Joint, Left, adding new qualifier values Humeral Surface and Glenoid Surface to root operation tables Removal and Revision in the Upper Joints body system

- New substance Pathogen Reduced Cryoprecipitated Fibrinogen Complex, with qualifier Nonautologous, added to root operation table Transfusion, Circulatory, in the Administration section

- New approach Percutaneous Endoscopic added to root operation table Irrigation, Physiological Systems and Anatomical Regions, in the Administration section, for body part Peritoneal Cavity

- New row added to root operation table Measurement, Physiological Devices, in the Measurement and Monitory section for body system Central Nervous with Function/Device value Cerebrospinal Fluid Shunt and qualifier Wireless Sensor

- New qualifier Automated added to root operation table Performance, Physiological Systems, for body system Cardiac, Duration Continuous, Function Output

- New rows added for body part Liver to root operation table Fluoroscopy, Hepatobiliary System and Pancreas, in the Imaging section

- New row added to New Technology root operation table Extirpation, Cardiovascular System New Technology Group 7, and deleted rows for New Technology Group 1

- New body part Thoracic Aorta, Arch, added to New Technology root operation table Replacement, Cardiovascular System, with device Branched Synthetic Substitute with Intraluminal Device, New Technology Group 7

- New row added to New Technology root operation table Replacement, Skin, Subcutaneous Tissue, Fascia and Breast, to capture Device/Substance/Technology Bioengineered Allogeneic Construct, New Technology Group 7

- New device value Posterior (Dynamic) Distraction Device added to New Technology root operation table Reposition, Bones, New Technology Group 7

- New device value Interbody Fusion Device, Customizable, added to New Technology root operation table Fusion, Joints, New Technology Group 7

- Multiple Device/Substance/Technology values added to New Technology root operation table Introduction, Anatomical Regions

- New Device/Substance/Technology values Hyperimmune Globulin and High-Dose Intravenous Immune Globulin added to New Technology root operation table Transfusion, Anatomical Regions

- New row added in New Technology root operation table Measurement, Physiological Systems, for body part Central Nervous, Device/Substance/Technology Computer-aided Triage and Notification, New Technology Group 7, and body part Arterial, Device/Substance/Technology Pulmonary Artery Flow, Computer-Aided Triage and Notification, and body part Nose, Device/Substance/Technology Infection, Nasopharyngeal Fluid SARS-CoV-2 Polymerase Chain Reaction

- New row added to New Technology root operation table Introduction, Extracorporeal, for body part Extracorporeal, Device/Substance/Technology Nafamostat Anticoagulant, New Technology Group 7

- Seven new tables in New Technology section:
  - X2J Cardiovascular System, Inspection
  - X2K Cardiovascular System, Bypass
  - X2V Cardiovascular System, Restriction
  - XD2 Gastrointestinal System, Monitoring
  - XDP Gastrointestinal System, Irrigation
  - XFJ Hepatobiliary System and Pancreas, Inspection
  - XWH Anatomical Regions, Insertion
- Two deleted tables in the New Technology Section:
  - XR2 Joints, Monitoring
  - XW2 Anatomical Regions, Transfusion

New Definitions Addenda

Section 0 — Medical and Surgical Body Part Definitions

ICD-10-PCS Value	Definition	
Cervical Spinal Cord	Add	Dorsal root ganglion
Lumbar Spinal Cord	Add	Dorsal root ganglion
Metatarsal, Left	Add	Fibular sesamoid
	Add	Tibial sesamoid
Metatarsal, Right	Add	Fibular sesamoid
	Add	Tibial sesamoid
Neck	Add	Parapharyngeal space
	Add	Retropharyngeal space
Spinal Cord	Add	Dorsal root ganglion
Thoracic Spinal Cord	Add	Dorsal root ganglion

Section 0 — Medical and Surgical Device Definitions

ICD-10-PCS Value		Definition	
Add	Biologic with Synthetic Substitute, Autoregulated Electrohydraulic for Replacement in Heart and Great Vessels	Add	Carmat total artificial heart (TAH)
Add	Other Device	Add	Alfapump® system
	Stimulator Generator, Multiple Array for Insertion in Subcutaneous Tissue and Fascia	Add	PERCEPT™ PC neurostimulator
	Stimulator Generator, Single Array for Insertion in Subcutaneous Tissue and Fascia	Delete	InterStim® Therapy neurostimulator
		Add	InterStim™ II Therapy neurostimulator
	Stimulator Generator, Single Array Rechargeable for Insertion in Subcutaneous Tissue and Fascia	Add	InterStim™ Micro Therapy neurostimulator
	Synthetic Substitute, Pneumatic for Replacement in Heart and Great Vessels	Add	SynCardia (temporary) total artificial heart (TAH)

Section 0 — Medical and Surgical Device Aggregation Table

Specific Device		for Operation		in Body System		General Device	
Add	Spinal Stabilization Device, Vertebral Body Tether	Add	Reposition	Add	Lower Bones	Add	4 Internal Fixation Device
				Add	Upper Bones		

Section 3 - Administration Substance Definitions

ICD-10-PCS Value	Definition
Add Globulin	Add Gammaglobulin Add Hyperimmune globulin Add Immunoglobulin Add Polyclonal hyperimmune globulin
Hematopoietic Stem/Progenitor Cells, Genetically Modified	Add OTL-101 Add OTL-103 Add OTL-200
Add Other Anti-infective	Add AVYCAZ® (ceftazidime-avibactam) Add Ceftazidime-avibactam Add CRESEMBA® (isavuconazonium sulfate) Add Isavuconazole (isavuconazonium sulfate)
Add Other Antineoplastic	Add Blinatumomab Add BLINCYTO® (blinatumomab)
Add Other Therapeutic Substance	Add Idarucizumab, Pradaxa®(dabigatran) reversal agent Add Praxbind® (idarucizumab), Pradaxa®(dabigatran) reversal agent
Add Pathogen Reduced Cryoprecipitated Fibrinogen Complex	Add INTERCEPT Blood System for Plasma Pathogen Reduced Cryoprecipitated Fibrinogen Complex Add INTERCEPT Fibrinogen Complex

Section X — New Technology Root Operation Definitions

ICD-10-PCS Value	Definition
Add Bypass	Add Definition: Altering the route of passage of the contents of a tubular body part.
Add Insertion	Add Definition: Putting in a nonbiological appliance that monitors, assists, performs, or prevents a physiological function but does not physically take the place of a body part.
Add Inspection	Add Definition: Visually and/or manually exploring a body part.
Add Irrigation	Add Definition: Putting in or on a cleansing substance
Add Restriction	Add Definition: Partially closing an orifice or the lumen of a tubular body part.

Section X — New Technology Device/Substance/Technology Definitions

ICD-10-PCS Value	Definition
Add Antibiotic-eluting Bone Void Filler	Add CERAMENT® G
Add Axicabtagene Ciloleucel Immunotherapy	Add Axicabtagene Ciloleucel Add Yescarta®

ICD-10-PCS Value	Definition
Add Bioengineered Allogeneic Construct	Add StrataGraft®
Add Branched Synthetic Substitute with Intraluminal Device in New Technology	Add Thoraflex™ Hybrid device
Brexucabtagene Autoleucel Immunotherapy	Add Tecartus™
Delete Engineered Autologous Chimeric Antigen Receptor T-cell Immunotherapy	Delete Axicabtagene Ciloeucel Delete KYMRIAH Delete Tisagenlecleucel
Add Bromelain-enriched Proteolytic Enzyme	Add NexoBrid™
Add Ciltacabtagene Autoleucel	Add cilta-cel
Add High-Dose Intravenous Immune Globulin	Add GAMUNEX-C, for COVID-19 treatment Add hdIVIG (high-dose intravenous immunoglobulin), for COVID-19 treatment Add High-dose intravenous immunoglobulin (hdIVIG), for COVID-19 treatment Add Octagam 10%, for COVID-19 treatment
Add Hyperimmune Globulin	Add Anti-SARS-CoV-2 hyperimmune globulin Add HIG (hyperimmune globulin), for COVID-19 treatment Add hIVIG (hyperimmune intravenous immunoglobulin), for COVID-19 treatment Add Hyperimmune intravenous immunoglobulin (hIVIG), for COVID-19 treatment Add IGIV-C, for COVID-19 treatment
Add Idecabtagene Vicleucel Immunotherapy	Add ABECMA® Add Ide-cel Add Idecabtagene Vicleucel
Add Interbody Fusion Device, Customizable in New Technology	Add aprevo™
Add Lifileucel Immunotherapy	Add Lifileucel
Add Lurbinectedin	Add ZEPZELCA™
Add Nafamostat Anticoagulant	Add LTX Regional Anticoagulant Add Niyad™
Add Posterior (Dynamic) Distraction Device in New Technology	Add ApiFix® Minimally Invasive Deformity Correction (MID-C) System
Add Reduction Device in New Technology	Add Neovasc Reducer™ Add Reducer™ System
Add REGN-COV2 Monoclonal Antibody	Add Casirivimab (REGN10933) and Imdevimab (REGN10987) Add Imdevimab (REGN10987) and Casirivimab (REGN10933)
Add Satralizumab-mwge	Add ENSPRYNG™
Add Terlipressin	Add TERLIVAZ®
Add Tisagenlecleucel Immunotherapy	Add KYMRIAH® Add Tisagenlecleucel
Add Trilaciclib	Add COSELA™

What's New for 2022 *(side tab)*

List of Updated Files

2022 Official ICD-10-PCS Coding Guidelines
- Guidelines B3.7, B4.1c, B4.8, E.1a, and E.1b revised in response to public comment and internal review
- Downloadable PDF

2022 ICD-10-PCS Code Tables and Index (Zip file)
- Code tables for use beginning October 1, 2021
- Downloadable PDF, file name is pcs_2022.pdf
- Downloadable xml files for developers, file names are icd10pcs_tables_2022.xml, icd10pcs_index_2022.xml, icd10pcs_definitions_2022.xml
- Accompanying schema for developers, file names are icd10pcs_tables.xsd, icd10pcs_index.xsd, icd10pcs_definitions.xsd

2022 ICD-10-PCS Codes File (Zip file)
- ICD-10-PCS codes file is a simple format for nontechnical uses, containing the valid FY 2022 ICD-10-PCS codes and their long titles
- File is in text file format: file name is icd10pcs_codes_2022.txt
- Accompanying documentation for codes file: file name is icd10pcsCodesFile.pdf
- Codes file addenda in text format: file name is codes_addenda_2022.txt

2022 ICD-10-PCS Order File (Long and Abbreviated Titles) (Zip file)
- ICD-10-PCS order file is for developers, provides a unique five-digit "order number" for each ICD-10-PCS table and code, as well as a long and abbreviated code title.
- ICD-10-PCS order file name is icd10pcs_order_2022.txt
- Accompanying documentation for tabular order file: file name is icd10pcsOrderFile.pdf
- Tabular order file addenda in text format: file name is order_addenda_2022.txt

2022 ICD-10-PCS Final Addenda (Zip file)
- Addenda files in downloadable PDF: file names are tables_addenda_2022.pdf, index_addenda_2022.pdf, definitions_addenda_2022.pdf
- Addenda files also in machine readable text format for developers: file names are tables_addenda_2022.txt, index_addenda_2022.txt, definitions_addenda_2022.txt

2022 ICD-10-PCS Conversion Table (Zip file)
- ICD-10-PCS code conversion table is provided to assist users in data retrieval, in downloadable Excel spreadsheet: file name is icd10pcs_conversion_table_2022.xlsx
- Conversion table also in machine readable text format for developers: file name is icd10pcs_conversion_table_2022.txt
- Accompanying documentation for code conversion table: file name is icd10pcsConversionTable.pdf

Introduction

ICD-10-PCS: The Complete Official Code Set is your definitive coding resource for procedure coding in acute inpatient hospitals. In addition to the official ICD-10-PCS Coding System Files, revised and distributed by the Centers for Medicare and Medicaid Services (CMS), Optum360's coding experts have incorporated Medicare-related coding edits and proprietary features, such as coding tools and appendixes, into a comprehensive and easy-to-use reference.

This manual provides the most current information that was available at the time of publication. For updates to official source documents that may have occurred after this manual was published, please refer to the following:

- **CMS International Classification of Disease, 10th Revision, Procedural Coding System (ICD-10-PCS):**

  https://www.cms.gov/medicare/icd-10/2022-icd-10-pcs

- **CMS Inpatient Prospective Payment System Proposed Rule, FY2022**

  https://www.cms.gov/medicare/acute-inpatient-pps/fy-2022-ipps-proposed-rule-home-page

- **CMS Inpatient Prospective Payment System Proposed Rule, FY 2022 - Proposed, version 39, MS-DRG Grouper software, Definitions Manual files and Medicare Code Editor (MCE) files**

  https://www.cms.gov/Medicare/Medicare-Fee-for-Service-Payment/AcuteInpatientPPS/MS-DRG-Classifications-and-Software

- **American Hospital Association (AHA) Coding Clinics**

  https://www.codingclinicadvisor.com/

ICD-10-PCS Code Structure

ICD-10-PCS has a seven-character alphanumeric code structure. Each character contains up to 34 possible values. Each value represents a specific option for the general character definition. The 10 digits Ø–9 and the 24 letters A–H, J–N, and P–Z may be used in each character. The letters O and I are not used so as to avoid confusion with the digits Ø and 1. An ICD-10-PCS code is the result of a process rather than as a single fixed set of digits or alphabetic characters. The process consists of combining semi-independent values from among a selection of values, according to the rules governing the construction of codes.

	Section	Body System	Root Operation	Body Part	Approach	Device	Qualifier
Characters:	1	2	3	4	5	6	7

A code is derived by choosing a specific value for each of the seven characters. Based on details about the procedure performed, values for each character specifying the section, body system, root operation, body part, approach, device, and qualifier are assigned. Because the definition of each character is also a function of its physical position in the code, the same letter or number placed in a different position in the code has a different meaning.

The seven characters that make up a complete code have specific meanings that vary for each of the 17 sections of the manual.

Procedures are then divided into sections that identify the general type of procedure (e.g., Medical and Surgical, Obstetrics, Imaging). The first character of the procedure code always specifies the section. The second through seventh characters have the same meaning within each section, but may mean different things in other sections. In all sections, the third character specifies the general type of procedure performed (e.g., Resection, Transfusion, Fluoroscopy), while the other characters give additional information such as the body part and approach.

In ICD-10-PCS, the term *procedure* refers to the complete specification of the seven characters.

Number of Codes in ICD-10-PCS

The table structure of ICD-10-PCS permits the specification of a large number of codes on a single page. At the time of this publication, there are 78,220 codes in the 2022 ICD-10-PCS.

ICD-10-PCS Manual

Index

Codes may be found in the index based on the general type of procedure (e.g., resection, transfusion, fluoroscopy), or a more commonly used term (e.g., appendectomy). For example, the code for percutaneous intraluminal dilation of the coronary arteries with an intraluminal device can be found in the Index under *Dilation*, or a synonym of *Dilation* (e.g., angioplasty). The Index then specifies the first three or four values of the code or directs the user to see another term.

Example:

> **Dilation**
>   Artery
>   Coronary
>   One Artery Ø27Ø

Based on the first three values of the code provided in the Index, the corresponding table can be located. In the example above, the first three values indicate table Ø27 is to be referenced for code completion.

The tables and characters are arranged first by number and then by letter for each character (tables for ØØ-, Ø1-, Ø2-, etc., are followed by those for ØB-, ØC-, ØD-, etc., followed by ØB1, ØB2, etc., followed by ØBB, ØBC, ØBD, etc.).

Note: The Tables section must be used to construct a complete and valid code by specifying the last three or four values.

Tables

The tables in ICD-10-PCS provide the valid combination of character values needed to build a unique procedure code. Each table is preceded by the first three characters of the code, along with their descriptions. In the Medical and Surgical section, for example, the first three characters contain the name of the section (character 1), the body system (character 2), and the root operation performed (character 3).

Listed underneath the first three characters is a table comprising four columns and one or more rows. The four columns in the table specify the last four characters needed to complete the ICD-10-PCS code. Depending on the section, the labels for each column may be different. In the Medical and Surgical section, they are labeled body part (character 4), approach (character 5), device (character 6), and qualifier (character 7). Each row in the table specifies the valid combination of values for characters 4 through 7.

Table 1: Row from table 027

0   **Medical and Surgical**
2   **Heart and Great Vessels**
7   **Dilation**   Definition: Expanding an orifice or the lumen of a tubular body part

Explanation: The orifice can be a natural orifice or an artificially created orifice. Accomplished by stretching a tubular body part using intraluminal pressure or by cutting part of the orifice or wall of the tubular body part.

Body Part Character 4	Approach Character 5	Device Character 6	Qualifier Character 7
0 Coronary Artery, One Artery 1 Coronary Artery, Two Arteries 2 Coronary Artery, Three Arteries 3 Coronary Artery, Four or More Arteries	0 Open 3 Percutaneous 4 Percutaneous Endoscopic	4 Intraluminal Device, Drug-eluting 5 Intraluminal Device, Drug-eluting, Two 6 Intraluminal Device, Drug-eluting, Three 7 Intraluminal Device, Drug-eluting, Four or More D Intraluminal Device E Intraluminal Device, Two F Intraluminal Device, Three G Intraluminal Device, Four or More T Intraluminal Device, Radioactive Z No Device	6 Bifurcation Z No Qualifier

For instance, table 1 above shows the first row from table 027 in ICD-10-PCS. The values 027 specify the section *Medical and Surgical (0)*, the body system *Heart and Great Vessels (2)*, and the root operation *Dilation (7)*. As shown, the root operation (Dilation) is also accompanied by its corresponding definition and explanation. Note, a definition of the root operation is provided for every table in ICD-10-PCS; however, an explanation may not always be applicable.

In total, this single row can be used to construct 240 unique procedure codes. The valid codes shown in table 2 (below) are constructed using the body part (character 4) value of 0, Coronary artery, one artery, combined with all valid approach (character 5) values, device (character 6) values, and a qualifier (character 7) value of Z, No Qualifier.

Table 2: Code titles for dilation of one coronary artery (0270)

027004Z	Dilation of Coronary Artery, One Artery with Drug-eluting Intraluminal Device, Open Approach
027005Z	Dilation of Coronary Artery, One Artery with Two Drug-eluting Intraluminal Devices, Open Approach
027006Z	Dilation of Coronary Artery, One Artery with Three Drug-eluting Intraluminal Devices, Open Approach
027007Z	Dilation of Coronary Artery, One Artery with Four or More Drug-eluting Intraluminal Devices, Open Approach
02700DZ	Dilation of Coronary Artery, One Artery with Intraluminal Device, Open Approach
02700EZ	Dilation of Coronary Artery, One Artery with Two Intraluminal Devices, Open Approach
02700FZ	Dilation of Coronary Artery, One Artery with Three Intraluminal Devices, Open Approach
02700GZ	Dilation of Coronary Artery, One Artery with Four or More Intraluminal Devices, Open Approach
02700TZ	Dilation of Coronary Artery, One Artery with Radioactive Intraluminal Device, Open Approach
02700ZZ	Dilation of Coronary Artery, One Artery, Open Approach
027034Z	Dilation of Coronary Artery, One Artery with Drug-eluting Intraluminal Device, Percutaneous Approach
027035Z	Dilation of Coronary Artery, One Artery with Two Drug-eluting Intraluminal Devices, Percutaneous Approach
027036Z	Dilation of Coronary Artery, One Artery with Three Drug-eluting Intraluminal Devices, Percutaneous Approach

027037Z	Dilation of Coronary Artery, One Artery with Four or More Drug-eluting Intraluminal Devices, Percutaneous Approach
02703DZ	Dilation of Coronary Artery, One Artery with Intraluminal Device, Percutaneous Approach
02703EZ	Dilation of Coronary Artery, One Artery with Two Intraluminal Devices, Percutaneous Approach
02703FZ	Dilation of Coronary Artery, One Artery with Three Intraluminal Devices, Percutaneous Approach
02703GZ	Dilation of Coronary Artery, One Artery with Four or More Intraluminal Devices, Percutaneous Approach
02703TZ	Dilation of Coronary Artery, One Artery with Radioactive Intraluminal Device, Percutaneous Approach
02703ZZ	Dilation of Coronary Artery, One Artery, Percutaneous Approach
027044Z	Dilation of Coronary Artery, One Artery with Drug-eluting Intraluminal Device, Percutaneous Endoscopic Approach
027045Z	Dilation of Coronary Artery, One Artery with Two Drug-eluting Intraluminal Devices, Percutaneous Endoscopic Approach
027046Z	Dilation of Coronary Artery, One Artery with Three Drug-eluting Intraluminal Devices, Percutaneous Endoscopic Approach
027047Z	Dilation of Coronary Artery, One Artery with Four or More Drug-eluting Intraluminal Devices, Percutaneous Endoscopic Approach
02704DZ	Dilation of Coronary Artery, One Artery with Intraluminal Device, Percutaneous Endoscopic Approach
02704EZ	Dilation of Coronary Artery, One Artery with Two Intraluminal Devices, Percutaneous Endoscopic Approach
02704FZ	Dilation of Coronary Artery, One Artery with Three Intraluminal Devices, Percutaneous Endoscopic Approach
02704GZ	Dilation of Coronary Artery, One Artery with Four or More Intraluminal Devices, Percutaneous Endoscopic Approach
02704TZ	Dilation of Coronary Artery, One Artery with Radioactive Intraluminal Device, Percutaneous Endoscopic Approach
02704ZZ	Dilation of Coronary Artery, One Artery, Percutaneous Endoscopic Approach

Table 3: Rows from table 00H

Ø **Medical and Surgical**
Ø **Central Nervous System and Cranial Nerves**
H **Insertion**   Definition: Putting in a nonbiological appliance that monitors, assists, performs, or prevents a physiological function but does not physically take the place of a body part
Explanation: None

Body Part Character 4		Approach Character 5	Device Character 6	Qualifier Character 7
Ø **Brain** Cerebrum Corpus callosum Encephalon		Ø Open	1 Radioactive Element 2 Monitoring Device 3 Infusion Device 4 Radioactive Element, Cesium-131 Collagen Implant M Neurostimulator Lead Y Other Device	Z No Qualifier
Ø **Brain** Cerebrum Corpus callosum Encephalon		3 Percutaneous 4 Percutaneous Endoscopic	1 Radioactive Element 2 Monitoring Device 3 Infusion Device M Neurostimulator Lead Y Other Device	Z No Qualifier
6 **Cerebral Ventricle** Aqueduct of Sylvius Cerebral aqueduct (Sylvius) Choroid plexus Ependyma Foramen of Monro (intraventricular) Fourth ventricle Interventricular foramen (Monro) Left lateral ventricle Right lateral ventricle Third ventricle	E **Cranial Nerve** U **Spinal Canal** Epidural space, spinal Extradural space, spinal Subarachnoid space, spinal Subdural space, spinal Vertebral canal V **Spinal Cord** Dorsal root ganglion	Ø Open 3 Percutaneous 4 Percutaneous Endoscopic	1 Radioactive Element 2 Monitoring Device 3 Infusion Device M Neurostimulator Lead Y Other Device	Z No Qualifier

Table 3, is split into three rows; values of characters must all be selected from within the same row of the table. Rows 1 and 2 have the same body part (character 4) value of Ø Brain and the same qualifier value (character 7) of Z No Qualifier. However, the approach (character 5) values are not the same for these two rows, and there is one additional device (character 6) value in row 1 that is not included in row 2. As shown in row 1, body part value Brain (Ø) with device value Radioactive Element, Cesium-131 Collagen Implant (4) can only be used with approach value Open (Ø). In other words, code 00H034Z would be invalid as the approach value 3 is only applicable to row 2 and the device value 4 is only applicable to row 1. It would be inappropriate to build a code for body part Ø if all of the values are not contained in its own row.

Note: In this manual, there are instances in which some tables due to length must be continued on the next page. Each section must be used separately and value selection must be made within the same row of the table.

Character Meanings

In each section, each character has a specific meaning, and this character meaning remains constant within that section. Character meaning tables have been provided at the beginning of each body system in the Medical and Surgical section (Ø) and the Obstetric section (1) to help the user identify the character members available within that section. These tables have purple headers, unlike the official code tables that have green headers and **SHOULD NOT** be used to build a PCS code. Following is an excerpt of a character meaning table.

Table 4: Rows from Central Nervous System and Cranial Nerves - Character Meanings Table

Operation–Character 3		Body Part–Character 4		Approach–Character 5		Device–Character 6		Qualifier–Character 7	
1	Bypass	Ø	Brain	Ø	Open	Ø	Drainage Device	Ø	Nasopharynx
2	Change	1	Cerebral Meninges	3	Percutaneous	1	Radioactive Element	1	Mastoid Sinus
5	Destruction	2	Dura Mater	4	Percutaneous Endoscopic	2	Monitoring Device	2	Atrium
7	Dilation	3	Epidural Space, Intracranial	X	External	3	Infusion Device	3	Blood Vessel
8	Division	4	Subdural Space, Intracranial			4	Radioactive Element, Cesium-131 Collagen Implant	4	Pleural Cavity
9	Drainage	5	Subarachnoid Space, Intracranial			7	Autologous Tissue Substitute	5	Intestine
B	Excision	6	Cerebral Ventricle			J	Synthetic Substitute	6	Peritoneal Cavity
C	Extirpation	7	Cerebral Hemisphere			K	Nonautologous Tissue Substitute	7	Urinary Tract
D	Extraction	8	Basal Ganglia			M	Neurostimulator Lead	8	Bone Marrow
F	Fragmentation	9	Thalamus			Y	Other Device	9	Fallopian Tube
H	Insertion	A	Hypothalamus			Z	No Device	A	Subgaleal space
J	Inspection	B	Pons					B	Cerebral Cisterns

Sections

Procedures are divided into sections that identify the general type of procedure (e.g., Medical and Surgical, Obstetrics, Imaging). The first character of the procedure code always specifies the section.

The sections are listed below:

Medical and Surgical section

Ø   Medical and Surgical

Medical and Surgical-related sections

1   Obstetrics

2   Placement

3   Administration

4   Measurement and Monitoring

5   Extracorporeal or Systemic Assistance and Performance

6   Extracorporeal or Systemic Therapies

7   Osteopathic

8   Other Procedures

9   Chiropractic

Ancillary Sections

B   Imaging

C   Nuclear Medicine

D   Radiation Therapy

F   Physical Rehabilitation and Diagnostic Audiology

G   Mental Health

H   Substance Abuse Treatment

New Technology Section

X   New Technology

Medical and Surgical Section (Ø)

Character Meaning

The seven characters for Medical and Surgical procedures have the following meaning:

Character	Meaning
1	Section
2	Body System
3	Root Operation
4	Body Part
5	Approach
6	Device
7	Qualifier

The Medical and Surgical section constitutes the vast majority of procedures reported in an inpatient setting. Medical and Surgical procedure codes all have a first character value of Ø. The second character indicates the general body system (e.g., Mouth and Throat, Gastrointestinal). The third character indicates the root operation, or specific objective, of the procedure (e.g., Excision). The fourth character indicates the specific body part on which the procedure was performed (e.g., Tonsils, Duodenum). The fifth character indicates the approach used to reach the procedure site (e.g., Open). The sixth character indicates whether a device was left in place during the procedure (e.g.,

Synthetic Substitute). The seventh character is qualifier, which has a specific meaning for each root operation. For example, the qualifier can be used to identify the destination site of a *Bypass*. The first through fifth characters are always assigned a specific value, but the device (sixth character) and the qualifier (seventh character) are not applicable to all procedures. The value *Z* is used for the sixth and seventh characters to indicate that a specific device or qualifier does not apply to the procedure.

Section (Character 1)

Medical and Surgical procedure codes all have a first character value of Ø.

Body Systems (Character 2)

Body systems for Medical and Surgical section codes are specified in the second character.

Body Systems

Ø   Central Nervous System and Cranial Nerves

1   Peripheral Nervous System

2   Heart and Great Vessels

3   Upper Arteries

4   Lower Arteries

5   Upper Veins

6   Lower Veins

7   Lymphatic and Hemic Systems

8   Eye

9   Ear, Nose, Sinus

B   Respiratory System

C   Mouth and Throat

D   Gastrointestinal System

F   Hepatobiliary System and Pancreas

G   Endocrine System

H   Skin and Breast

J   Subcutaneous Tissue and Fascia

K   Muscles

L   Tendons

M   Bursae and Ligaments

N   Head and Facial Bones

P   Upper Bones

Q   Lower Bones

R   Upper Joints

S   Lower Joints

T   Urinary System

U   Female Reproductive System

V   Male Reproductive System

W   Anatomical Regions, General

X   Anatomical Regions, Upper Extremities

Y   Anatomical Regions, Lower Extremities

Root Operations (Character 3)

The root operation is specified in the third character. In the Medical and Surgical section there are 31 different root operations. The root operation identifies the objective of the procedure. Each root operation has a precise definition.

- *Alteration:* Modifying the natural anatomic structure of a body part without affecting the function of the body part

- *Bypass:* Altering the route of passage of the contents of a tubular body part

- *Change:* Taking out or off a device from a body part and putting back an identical or similar device in or on the same body part without cutting or puncturing the skin or a mucous membrane

- *Control:* Stopping, or attempting to stop, postprocedural or other acute bleeding

- *Creation:* Putting in or on biological or synthetic material to form a new body part that to the extent possible replicates the anatomic structure or function of an absent body part

- *Destruction:* Physical eradication of all or a portion of a body part by the direct use of energy, force, or a destructive agent

- *Detachment:* Cutting off all or a portion of the upper or lower extremities

- *Dilation:* Expanding an orifice or the lumen of a tubular body part

- *Division:* Cutting into a body part without draining fluids and/or gases from the body part in order to separate or transect a body part

- *Drainage:* Taking or letting out fluids and/or gases from a body part

- *Excision:* Cutting out or off, without replacement, a portion of a body part

- *Extirpation:* Taking or cutting out solid matter from a body part

- *Extraction:* Pulling or stripping out or off all or a portion of a body part by the use of force

- *Fragmentation:* Breaking solid matter in a body part into pieces

- *Fusion:* Joining together portions of an articular body part rendering the articular body part immobile

- *Insertion:* Putting in a nonbiological appliance that monitors, assists, performs, or prevents a physiological function but does not physically take the place of a body part

- *Inspection:* Visually and/or manually exploring a body part

- *Map:* Locating the route of passage of electrical impulses and/or locating functional areas in a body part

- *Occlusion:* Completely closing an orifice or lumen of a tubular body part

- *Reattachment:* Putting back in or on all or a portion of a separated body part to its normal location or other suitable location

- *Release:* Freeing a body part from an abnormal physical constraint by cutting or by use of force

- *Removal:* Taking out or off a device from a body part

- *Repair:* Restoring, to the extent possible, a body part to its normal anatomic structure and function

- *Replacement:* Putting in or on biological or synthetic material that physically takes the place and/or function of all or a portion of a body part

- *Reposition:* Moving to its normal location or other suitable location all or a portion of a body part

- *Resection:* Cutting out or off, without replacement, all of a body part

- *Restriction:* Partially closing an orifice or lumen of a tubular body part

- *Revision:* Correcting, to the extent possible, a portion of a malfunctioning device or the position of a displaced device

- *Supplement:* Putting in or on biological or synthetic material that physically reinforces and/or augments the function of a portion of a body part

- *Transfer:* Moving, without taking out, all or a portion of a body part to another location to take over the function of all or a portion of a body part

- *Transplantation:* Putting in or on all or a portion of a living body part taken from another individual or animal to physically take the place and/or function of all or a portion of a similar body part

The above definitions of root operations illustrate the precision of code values defined in the system. There is a clear distinction between each root operation.

A root operation specifies the objective of the procedure. The term *anastomosis* is not a root operation, because it is a means of joining and is always an integral part of another procedure (e.g., Bypass, Resection) with a specific objective. Similarly, *incision* is not a root operation, since it is always part of the objective of another procedure (e.g., Division, Drainage). The root operation *Repair* in the Medical and Surgical section functions as a "not elsewhere classified" option. *Repair* is used when the procedure performed is not one of the other specific root operations.

Appendix B provides additional explanation and representative examples of the Medical and Surgical root operations. Appendix C groups all root operations in the Medical and Surgical section into subcategories and provides an example of each root operation.

Body Part (Character 4)
The body part is specified in the fourth character. The body part indicates the specific anatomical site of the body system on which the procedure was performed (e.g., Duodenum). Tubular body parts are defined in ICD-10-PCS as those hollow body parts that provide a route of passage for solids, liquids, or gases. They include the cardiovascular system and body parts such as those contained in the gastrointestinal tract, genitourinary tract, biliary tract, and respiratory tract.

Approach (Character 5)
The technique used to reach the site of the procedure is specified in the fifth character. There are seven different approaches:

- *Open*: Cutting through the skin or mucous membrane and any other body layers necessary to expose the site of the procedure

- *Percutaneous*: Entry, by puncture or minor incision, of instrumentation through the skin or mucous membrane and any other body layers necessary to reach the site of the procedure

- *Percutaneous Endoscopic*: Entry, by puncture or minor incision, of instrumentation through the skin or mucous membrane and any other body layers necessary to reach and visualize the site of the procedure

- *Via Natural or Artificial Opening*: Entry of instrumentation through a natural or artificial external opening to reach the site of the procedure

- *Via Natural or Artificial Opening Endoscopic*: Entry of instrumentation through a natural or artificial external opening to reach and visualize the site of the procedure

- *Via Natural or Artificial Opening with Percutaneous Endoscopic Assistance:* Entry of instrumentation through a natural or artificial external opening and entry, by puncture or minor incision, of instrumentation through the skin or mucous membrane and any other body layers necessary to aid in the performance of the procedure

- *External*: Procedures performed directly on the skin or mucous membrane and procedures performed indirectly by the application of external force through the skin or mucous membrane

The approach comprises three components: the access location, method, and type of instrumentation.

Access location: For procedures performed on an internal body part, the access location specifies the external site through which the site of the procedure is reached. There are two general types of access locations: skin or mucous membranes, and external orifices. Every approach value except external includes one of these two access locations. The skin or mucous membrane can be cut or punctured to reach the procedure site. All open and percutaneous approach values use this access location. The site of a procedure can also be reached through an external opening. External openings can be natural (e.g., mouth) or artificial (e.g., colostomy stoma).

Method: For procedures performed on an internal body part, the method specifies how the external access location is entered. An open method specifies cutting through the skin or mucous membrane and any other intervening body layers necessary to expose the site of the procedure. An instrumentation method specifies the entry of instrumentation through the access location to the internal procedure site. Instrumentation can be introduced by puncture or minor incision, or through an external opening. The puncture or minor incision does not constitute an open approach because it does not expose the site of the procedure. An approach can define multiple methods. For example, *Via Natural or Artificial Opening with Percutaneous Endoscopic Assistance* includes both the initial entry of instrumentation to reach the site of the procedure, and the placement of additional percutaneous instrumentation into the body part to visualize and assist in the performance of the procedure.

Type of instrumentation: For procedures performed on an internal body part, instrumentation means that specialized equipment is used to perform the procedure. Instrumentation is used in all internal approaches other than the basic open approach. Instrumentation may or may not include the capacity to visualize the procedure site. For example, the instrumentation used to perform a sigmoidoscopy permits the internal site of the procedure to be visualized, while the instrumentation used to perform a needle biopsy of the liver does not. The term "endoscopic" as used in approach values refers to instrumentation that permits a site to be visualized.

Procedures performed directly on the skin or mucous membrane are identified by the external approach (e.g., skin excision). Procedures performed indirectly by the application of external force are also identified by the external approach (e.g., closed reduction of fracture).

Appendix A compares the components (access location, method, and type of instrumentation) of each approach and provides an example and illustration of each approach.

Device (Character 6)

The device is specified in the sixth character. There are four general types of devices:

- Biological or synthetic material that takes the place of all or a portion of a body part (e.g, skin graft, joint prosthesis).

- Biological or synthetic material that assists or prevents a physiological function (e.g., IUD).

- Therapeutic material that is not absorbed by, eliminated by, or incorporated into a body part (e.g., radioactive implant).

- Mechanical or electronic appliances used to assist, monitor, take the place of or prevent a physiological function (e.g., cardiac pacemaker, orthopedic pin).

Appendix F compares the general device types and provides examples of each.

While all devices can be removed, some cannot be removed without putting in another nonbiological appliance or body-part substitute.

When a specific device value is used to identify the device for a root operation, such as *Insertion* and that same device value is not an option for a more broad range root operation such as *Removal*, select the general device value. For example, in the body system Heart and Great Vessels, the specific device character for Cardiac Lead, Pacemaker in root operation *Insertion* is J. For the root operation *Removal*, the general device character M Cardiac Lead would be selected for the pacemaker lead.

ICD-10-PCS contains a PCS Device Aggregation Table (see appendix G) that crosswalks the *specific* device character values that have been created for specific root operations and specific body part character values to the *general* device character value that would be used for root operations that represent a broad range of procedures and general body part character values, such as Removal and Revision.

Instruments used to visualize the procedure site are specified in the approach, not the device, value.

If the objective of the procedure is to put in the device, then the root operation is *Insertion*. If the device is put in to meet an objective other than *Insertion*, then the root operation defining the underlying objective of the procedure is used, with the device specified in the device character. For example, if a procedure to replace the hip joint is performed, the root operation *Replacement* is coded, and the prosthetic device is specified in the device character. Materials that are incidental to a procedure such as clips, ligatures, and sutures are not specified in the device character. Because new devices can be developed, the value *Other Device* is provided as a temporary option for use until a specific device value is added to the system.

Qualifier (Character 7)

The qualifier is specified in the seventh character. The qualifier contains unique values for individual procedures. For example, the qualifier can be used to identify the destination site in a *Bypass*.

Medical and Surgical Section Principles

In developing the Medical and Surgical procedure codes, several specific principles were followed.

Composite Terms Are Not Root Operations

Composite terms such as colonoscopy, sigmoidectomy, or appendectomy do not describe root operations, but they do specify multiple components of a specific root operation. In ICD-10-PCS, the components of a procedure are defined separately by the characters making up the complete code. The only component of a procedure specified in the root operation is the objective of the procedure. With each complete code the underlying objective of the procedure is specified by the root operation (third character), the precise part is specified by the body part (fourth character), and the method used to reach and visualize the procedure site is specified by the approach (fifth character). While colonoscopy, sigmoidectomy, and appendectomy are included in the Index, they do not constitute root operations in the Tables section. The objective of colonoscopy is the visualization of the colon and the root operation (character 3) is *Inspection*. Character 4 specifies the body part, which in this case is part of the colon. These composite terms, like colonoscopy or appendectomy, are included as cross-reference only. The index provides the correct root operation reference. Examples of other types of composite terms not representative of root operations are *partial* sigmoidectomy, *total* hysterectomy, and *partial* hip replacement. Always refer to the correct root operation in the Index and Tables section.

Root Operation Based on Objective of Procedure

The root operation is based on the objective of the procedure, such as *Resection* of transverse colon or *Dilation* of an artery. The assignment of the root operation is based on the procedure actually performed, which may or may not have been the intended procedure. If the intended procedure is modified or discontinued (e.g., excision instead of resection is performed), the root operation is determined by the procedure actually performed. If the desired result is not attained after completing the procedure (i.e., the artery does not remain expanded after the dilation procedure), the root operation is still determined by the procedure actually performed.

Examples:

- Dilating the urethra is coded as *Dilation* since the objective of the procedure is to dilate the urethra. If dilation of the urethra includes putting in an intraluminal stent, the root operation remains *Dilation* and not *Insertion* of the intraluminal device because the underlying objective of the procedure is dilation of the urethra. The stent is identified by the intraluminal device value in the sixth character of the dilation procedure code.

- If the objective is solely to put a radioactive element in the urethra, then the procedure is coded to the root operation *Insertion*, with the radioactive element identified in the sixth character of the code.

- If the objective of the procedure is to correct a malfunctioning or displaced device, then the procedure is coded to the root operation *Revision*. In the root operation *Revision*, the original device being revised is identified in the device character. *Revision* is typically performed on mechanical appliances (e.g., pacemaker) or materials used in replacement procedures (e.g., synthetic substitute). Typical revision procedures include adjustment of pacemaker position and correction of malfunctioning knee prosthesis.

Combination Procedures Are Coded Separately

If multiple procedures as defined by distinct objectives are performed during an operative episode, then multiple codes are used. For example, obtaining the vein graft used for coronary bypass surgery is coded as a separate procedure from the bypass itself.

Redo of Procedures

The complete or partial redo of the original procedure is coded to the root operation that identifies the procedure performed rather than *Revision*.

Example:

A complete redo of a hip replacement procedure that requires putting in a new prosthesis is coded to the root operation *Replacement* rather than *Revision*.

The correction of complications arising from the original procedure, other than device complications, is coded to the procedure performed. Correction of a malfunctioning or displaced device would be coded to the root operation *Revision*.

Example:

A procedure to control hemorrhage arising from the original procedure is coded to *Control* rather than *Revision*.

Examples of Procedures Coded in the Medical Surgical Section

The following are examples of procedures from the Medical and Surgical section, coded in ICD-10-PCS.

- Suture of skin laceration, left lower arm: ØHQEXZZ

  Medical and Surgical section (Ø), body system *Skin and Breast* (H), root operation *Repair* (Q), body part *Skin, Left Lower Arm* (E), *External* Approach (X) *No device* (Z), and *No qualifier* (Z).

- Laparoscopic appendectomy: ØDTJ4ZZ

  Medical and Surgical section (Ø), body system *Gastrointestinal* (D), root operation *Resection* (T), body part *Appendix* (J), *Percutaneous Endoscopic* approach (4), No Device (Z), and No qualifier (Z).

- Sigmoidoscopy with biopsy: ØDBN8ZX

  Medical and Surgical section (Ø), body system *Gastrointestinal* (D), root operation *Excision* (B), body part *Sigmoid Colon* (N), *Via Natural or Artificial Opening Endoscopic* approach (8), *No Device* (Z), and with qualifier *Diagnostic* (X).

- Tracheostomy with tracheostomy tube: ØB11ØF4

  Medical and Surgical section (Ø), body system *Respiratory* (B), root operation *Bypass* (1), body part *Trachea* (1), *Open* approach (Ø), with *Tracheostomy Device* (F), and qualifier *Cutaneous* (4).

Obstetrics Section (1)

Character Meanings

The seven characters in the Obstetrics section have the same meaning as in the Medical and Surgical section.

Character	Meaning
1	Section
2	Body System
3	Root Operation
4	Body Part
5	Approach
6	Device
7	Qualifier

The Obstetrics section includes procedures performed on the products of conception only. Procedures on the pregnant female are coded in the Medical and Surgical section (e.g., episiotomy). The term "products of conception" refers to all physical components of a pregnancy, including the fetus, amnion, umbilical cord, and placenta. There is no differentiation of the products of conception based on gestational age.

Thus, the specification of the products of conception as a zygote, embryo or fetus, or the trimester of the pregnancy is not part of the procedure code but can be found in the diagnosis code.

Section (Character 1)
Obstetrics procedure codes have a first character value of *1*.

Body System (Character 2)
The second character value for body system is *Pregnancy*.

Root Operation (Character 3)
The root operations *Change, Drainage, Extraction, Insertion, Inspection, Removal, Repair, Reposition, Resection,* and *Transplantation* are used in the obstetrics section and have the same meaning as in the Medical and Surgical section.

The Obstetrics section also includes two additional root operations, *Abortion* and *Delivery*, defined below:

- *Abortion*: Artificially terminating a pregnancy

- *Delivery*: Assisting the passage of the products of conception from the genital canal

A cesarean section is not a separate root operation because the underlying objective is *Extraction* (i.e., pulling out all or a portion of a body part).

Body Part (Character 4)
The body part values in the obstetrics section are:

- *Products of conception*

- *Products of conception, retained*

- *Products of conception, ectopic*

Approach (Character 5)
The fifth character specifies approaches as defined in the Medical and Surgical section.

Device (Character 6)
The sixth character is used for devices such as fetal monitoring electrodes.

Qualifier (Character 7)
Qualifier values are specific to the root operation and are used to capture details of the procedure, such as whether forceps or a vacuum were used during an Extraction, the type of fluid taken out during a Drainage procedure, or the products of conception body system that was repaired.

Placement Section (2)

Character Meanings
The seven characters in the Placement section have the following meaning:

Character	Meaning
1	Section
2	Body System
3	Root Operation
4	Body Region
5	Approach
6	Device
7	Qualifier

Placement section codes represent procedures for putting a device in or on a body region for the purpose of protection, immobilization, stretching, compression, or packing.

Section (Character 1)
Placement procedure codes have a first character value of *2*.

Body System (Character 2)
The second character contains two values specifying either *Anatomical Regions* or *Anatomical Orifices*.

Root Operation (Character 3)
The root operations in the Placement section include only those procedures that are performed without making an incision or a puncture. The root operations *Change* and *Removal* are in the Placement section and have the same meaning as in the Medical and Surgical section.

The Placement section also includes five additional root operations, defined as follows:

- *Compression*: Putting pressure on a body region

- *Dressing*: Putting material on a body region for protection

- *Immobilization*: Limiting or preventing motion of an external body region

- *Packing*: Putting material in a body region or orifice

- *Traction*: Exerting a pulling force on a body region in a distal direction

Body Region (Character 4)
The fourth character values are either body regions (e.g., *Upper Leg*) or natural orifices (e.g., *Ear*).

Approach (Character 5)
Since all placement procedures are performed directly on the skin or mucous membrane, or performed indirectly by applying external force through the skin or mucous membrane, the approach value is always *External*.

Device (Character 6)
The device character is always specified (except in the case of manual traction) and indicates the device placed during the procedure (e.g., cast, splint, bandage, etc.). Except for casts for fractures and dislocations, devices in the Placement section are off the shelf and do not require any extensive design, fabrication, or fitting. Placement of devices that require extensive design, fabrication, or fitting are coded in the Rehabilitation section.

Qualifier (Character 7)

The qualifier character is not specified in the Placement section; the qualifier value is always *No Qualifier*.

Administration Section (3)

Character Meanings

The seven characters in the Administration section have the following meaning:

Character	Meaning
1	Section
2	Body System
3	Root Operation
4	Body System/Region
5	Approach
6	Substance
7	Qualifier

Administration section codes represent procedures for putting in or on a therapeutic, prophylactic, protective, diagnostic, nutritional, or physiological substance. The section includes transfusions, infusions, and injections, along with other similar services such as irrigation and tattooing.

Section (Character 1)

Administration procedure codes have a first character value of *3*.

Body System (Character 2)

The body system character contains only three values: *Indwelling Device, Physiological Systems and Anatomical Regions,* or *Circulatory System*. The *Circulatory System* is used for transfusion procedures.

Root Operation (Character 3)

There are three root operations in the Administration section.

- *Introduction*: Putting in or on a therapeutic, diagnostic, nutritional, physiological, or prophylactic substance except blood or blood products

- *Irrigation*: Putting in or on a cleansing substance

- *Transfusion*: Putting in blood or blood products

Body/System Region (Character 4)

The fourth character specifies the body system/region. The fourth character identifies the site where the substance is administered, not the site where the substance administered takes effect. Sites include *Skin and Mucous Membranes, Subcutaneous Tissue,* and *Muscle*. These differentiate intradermal, subcutaneous, and intramuscular injections, respectively. Other sites include *Eye, Respiratory Tract, Peritoneal Cavity,* and *Epidural Space*.

The body systems/regions for arteries and veins are *Peripheral Artery, Central Artery, Peripheral Vein,* and *Central Vein*. The *Peripheral Artery* or *Vein* is typically used when a substance is introduced locally into an artery or vein. For example, chemotherapy is the introduction of an antineoplastic substance into a peripheral artery or vein by a percutaneous approach. In general, the substance introduced into a peripheral artery or vein has a systemic effect.

The *Central Artery* or *Vein* is typically used when the site where the substance is introduced is distant from the point of entry into the artery or vein. For example, the introduction of a substance directly at the site of a clot within an artery or vein using a catheter is coded as an introduction of a thrombolytic substance into a central artery or vein by a percutaneous approach. In general, the substance introduced into a central artery or vein has a local effect.

Approach (Character 5)

The fifth character specifies approaches as defined in the Medical and Surgical section. The approach for intradermal, subcutaneous, and intramuscular introductions (i.e., injections) is *Percutaneous*. If a catheter is placed to introduce a substance into an internal site within the circulatory system, then the approach is also *Percutaneous*. For example, if a catheter is used to introduce contrast directly into the heart for angiography, then the procedure would be coded as a percutaneous introduction of contrast into the heart.

Substance (Character 6)

The sixth character specifies the substance being introduced. Broad categories of substances are defined, such as anesthetic, contrast, dialysate, and blood products such as platelets.

Qualifier (Character 7)

The seventh character is a qualifier and is used to indicate whether the transfused substance is *Autologous, Nonautologous, or Allogeneic* (related, unrelated, unspecified), or to further specify the substance.

Measurement and Monitoring Section (4)

Character Meanings

The seven characters in the Measurement and Monitoring section have the following meaning:

Character	Meaning
1	Section
2	Body System
3	Root Operation
4	Body System
5	Approach
6	Function/Device
7	Qualifier

Measurement and Monitoring section codes represent procedures for determining the level of a physiological or physical function.

Section (Character 1)

Measurement and Monitoring procedure codes have a first character value of *4*.

Body System (Character 2)

The second character values for body system are A, *Physiological Systems* or B, *Physiological Devices*.

Root Operation (Character 3)

There are two root operations in the Measurement and Monitoring section, as defined below:

- *Measurement*: Determining the level of a physiological or physical function at a point in time

- *Monitoring*: Determining the level of a physiological or physical function repetitively over a period of time

Body System (Character 4)

The fourth character specifies the specific body system measured or monitored.

Approach (Character 5)

The fifth character specifies approaches as defined in the Medical and Surgical section.

Function/Device (Character 6)

The sixth character specifies the physiological or physical function being measured or monitored. Examples of physiological or physical functions are *Conductivity, Metabolism, Pulse, Temperature,* and *Volume.* If a device used to perform the measurement or monitoring is inserted and left in, then insertion of the device is coded as a separate Medical and Surgical procedure.

Qualifier (Character 7)

The seventh character qualifier contains specific values as needed to further specify the body part (e.g., central, portal, pulmonary) or a variation of the procedure performed (e.g., ambulatory, stress). Examples of typical procedures coded in this section are EKG, EEG, and cardiac catheterization. An EKG is the measurement of cardiac electrical activity, while an EEG is the measurement of electrical activity of the central nervous system. A cardiac catheterization performed to measure the pressure in the heart is coded as the measurement of cardiac pressure by percutaneous approach.

Extracorporeal or Systemic Assistance and Performance Section (5)

Character Meanings

The seven characters in the Extracorporeal or Systemic Assistance and Performance section have the following meaning:

Character	Meaning
1	Section
2	Body System
3	Root Operation
4	Body System
5	Duration
6	Function
7	Qualifier

In Extracorporeal or Systemic Assistance and Performance procedures, equipment outside the body is used to assist or perform a physiological function. The section includes procedures performed in a critical care setting, such as mechanical ventilation and cardioversion; it also includes other services such as hyperbaric oxygen treatment and hemodialysis.

Section (Character 1)

Extracorporeal or Systemic Assistance and Performance procedure codes have a first character value of *5*.

Body System (Character 2)

The second character value for body system is A, *Physiological Systems.*

Root Operation (Character 3)

There are three root operations in the Extracorporeal or Systemic Assistance and Performance section, as defined below.

- *Assistance*: Taking over a portion of a physiological function by extracorporeal means

- *Performance*: Completely taking over a physiological function by extracorporeal means

- *Restoration*: Returning, or attempting to return, a physiological function to its natural state by extracorporeal means

The root operation *Restoration* contains a single procedure code that identifies extracorporeal cardioversion.

Body System (Character 4)

The fourth character specifies the body system (e.g., cardiac, respiratory) to which extracorporeal or systemic assistance or performance is applied.

Duration (Character 5)

The fifth character specifies the duration of the procedure.

Function (Character 6)

The sixth character specifies the physiological function assisted or performed (e.g., oxygenation, ventilation) during the procedure.

Qualifier (Character 7)

The seventh character qualifier specifies the type of equipment used, if any.

Extracorporeal or Systemic Therapies Section (6)

Character Meanings

The seven characters in the Extracorporeal or Systemic Therapies section have the following meaning:

Character	Meaning
1	Section
2	Body System
3	Root Operation
4	Body System
5	Duration
6	Qualifier
7	Qualifier

In extracorporeal or systemic therapy, equipment outside the body is used for a therapeutic purpose that does not involve the assistance or performance of a physiological function.

Section (Character 1)

Extracorporeal or Systemic Therapy procedure codes have a first character value of 6.

Body System (Character 2)

The second character value for body system is *Physiological Systems.*

Root Operation (Character 3)

There are 11 root operations in the Extracorporeal or Systemic Therapy section, as defined below.

- *Atmospheric Control*: Extracorporeal control of atmospheric pressure and composition

- *Decompression*: Extracorporeal elimination of undissolved gas from body fluids

   Coding note: The root operation *Decompression* involves only one type of procedure: treatment for decompression sickness (the bends) in a hyperbaric chamber.

- *Electromagnetic Therapy*: Extracorporeal treatment by electromagnetic rays

- *Hyperthermia*: Extracorporeal raising of body temperature

   Coding note: The term hyperthermia is used to describe both a temperature imbalance treatment and also as an adjunct radiation treatment for cancer. When treating the temperature imbalance, it is coded to this section; for the cancer treatment, it is coded in section *D Radiation Therapy*.

- *Hypothermia*: Extracorporeal lowering of body temperature

- *Perfusion*: Extracorporeal treatment by diffusion of therapeutic fluid

- *Pheresis*: Extracorporeal separation of blood products

   Coding note: Pheresis may be used for two main purposes: to treat diseases when too much of a blood component is produced (e.g., leukemia) and to remove a blood product such as platelets from a donor, for transfusion into another patient.

- *Phototherapy*: Extracorporeal treatment by light rays

   Coding note: Phototherapy involves using a machine that exposes the blood to light rays outside the body, recirculates it, and then returns it to the body.

- *Shock Wave Therapy*: Extracorporeal treatment by shock waves

- *Ultrasound Therapy*: Extracorporeal treatment by ultrasound

- *Ultraviolet Light Therapy*: Extracorporeal treatment by ultraviolet light

Body System (Character 4)

The fourth character specifies the body system on which the extracorporeal or systemic therapy is performed (e.g., skin, circulatory).

Duration (Character 5)

The fifth character specifies whether the procedure was performed once (single) or multiple times.

Qualifier (Character 6)

The sixth character for Extracorporeal or Systemic Therapies is *No Qualifier*, except for root operation Perfusion which has a sixth character qualifier of *Donor Organ*.

Qualifier (Character 7)

The seventh character qualifier is used in the root operation *Pheresis* to specify the blood component on which pheresis is performed and in the root operation *Ultrasound Therapy* to specify site of treatment.

Osteopathic Section (7)

Character Meanings

The seven characters in the Osteopathic section have the following meaning:

Character	Meaning
1	Section
2	Body System
3	Root Operation
4	Body Region
5	Approach
6	Method
7	Qualifier

Section (Character 1)

Osteopathic procedure codes have a first character value of *7*.

Body System (Character 2)

The body system character contains the value *Anatomical Regions*.

Root Operation (Character 3)

There is only one root operation in the Osteopathic section.

- *Treatment*: Manual treatment to eliminate or alleviate somatic dysfunction and related disorders

Body Region (Character 4)

The fourth character specifies the body region on which the osteopathic treatment is performed.

Approach (Character 5)

The approach for osteopathic treatment is always *External*.

Method (Character 6)

The sixth character specifies the method by which the treatment is accomplished.

Qualifier (Character 7)

The seventh character is not specified in the Osteopathic section and always has the value *None*.

Other Procedures Section (8)

Character Meanings

The seven characters in the Other Procedures section have the following meaning:

Character	Meaning
1	Section
2	Body System
3	Root Operation
4	Body Region
5	Approach
6	Method
7	Qualifier

The Other Procedures section includes acupuncture, suture removal, and in vitro fertilization.

Section (Character 1)
Other Procedure section codes have a first character value of *8*.

Body System (Character 2)
The second character values for body systems are *Physiological Systems and Anatomical Regions* and *Indwelling Device*.

Root Operation (Character 3)
The Other Procedures section has only one root operation, defined as follows:

- *Other Procedures*: Methodologies that attempt to remediate or cure a disorder or disease.

Body Region (Character 4)
The fourth character contains specified body-region values, and also the body-region value *None*.

Approach (Character 5)
The fifth character specifies approaches as defined in the Medical and Surgical section.

Method (Character 6)
The sixth character specifies the method (e.g., *Acupuncture, Therapeutic Massage*).

Qualifier (Character 7)
The seventh character is a qualifier and contains specific values as needed.

Chiropractic Section (9)

Character Meanings
The seven characters in the Chiropractic section have the following meaning:

Character	Meaning
1	Section
2	Body System
3	Root Operation
4	Body Region
5	Approach
6	Method
7	Qualifier

Section (Character 1)
Chiropractic section procedure codes have a first character value of *9*.

Body System (Character 2)
The second character value for body system is *Anatomical Regions*.

Root Operation (Character 3)
There is only one root operation in the *Chiropractic* section.

- *Manipulation:* Manual procedure that involves a directed thrust to move a joint past the physiological range of motion, without exceeding the anatomical limit.

Body Region (Character 4)
The fourth character specifies the body region on which the chiropractic manipulation is performed.

Approach (Character 5)
The approach for chiropractic manipulation is always *External*.

Method (Character 6)
The sixth character is the method by which the manipulation is accomplished.

Qualifier (Character 7)
The seventh character is not specified in the Chiropractic section and always has the value *None*.

Imaging Section (B)

Character Meanings
The seven characters in Imaging procedures have the following meaning:

Character	Meaning
1	Section
2	Body System
3	Type
4	Body Part
5	Contrast
6	Qualifier
7	Qualifier

Imaging procedures include plain radiography, fluoroscopy, CT, MRI, and ultrasound. Nuclear medicine procedures, including PET, uptakes, and scans, are in the nuclear medicine section. Therapeutic radiation procedure codes are in a separate radiation therapy section.

Section (Character 1)
Imaging procedure codes have a first character value of *B*.

Body System (Character 2)
In the Imaging section, the second character defines the body system, such as *Heart* or *Gastrointestinal System*.

Type (Character 3)
The third character defines the type of imaging procedure (e.g., MRI, ultrasound). The following list includes all types in the *Imaging* section with a definition of each type:

- *Computerized Tomography (CT Scan)*: Computer reformatted digital display of multiplanar images developed from the capture of multiple exposures of external ionizing radiation

- *Fluoroscopy*: Single plane or bi-plane real time display of an image developed from the capture of external ionizing radiation on a fluorescent screen. The image may also be stored by either digital or analog means

- *Magnetic Resonance Imaging (MRI)*: Computer reformatted digital display of multiplanar images developed from the capture of radiofrequency signals emitted by nuclei in a body site excited within a magnetic field

- *Other Imaging:* Other specified modality for visualizing a body part

- *Plain Radiography*: Planar display of an image developed from the capture of external ionizing radiation on photographic or photoconductive plate

- *Ultrasonography*: Real time display of images of anatomy or flow information developed from the capture of reflected and attenuated high frequency sound waves

Body Part (Character 4)

The fourth character defines the body part with different values for each body system (character 2) value.

Contrast (Character 5)

The fifth character specifies whether the contrast material used in the imaging procedure is *High Osmolar, Low Osmolar*, or *Other Contrast* when applicable.

Qualifier (Character 6)

The sixth character qualifier provides further detail regarding the nature of the substance or technologies used, such as *Unenhanced and Enhanced (contrast), Laser, or Intravascular Optical Coherence*.

Qualifier (Character 7)

The seventh character is a qualifier that may be used to specify certain procedural circumstances, the method by which the procedure was performed, or technologies utilized, such as *Intraoperative, Intravascular, or Transesophageal*.

Nuclear Medicine Section (C)

Character Meanings

The seven characters in the Nuclear Medicine section have the following meaning:

Character	Meaning
1	Section
2	Body System
3	Type
4	Body Part
5	Radionuclide
6	Qualifier
7	Qualifier

Nuclear Medicine is the introduction of radioactive material into the body to create an image, to diagnose and treat pathologic conditions, or to assess metabolic functions. The Nuclear Medicine section does not include the introduction of encapsulated radioactive material for the treatment of cancer. These procedures are included in the Radiation Therapy section.

Section (Character 1)

Nuclear Medicine procedure codes have a first character value of *C*.

Body System (Character 2)

The second character specifies the body system on which the nuclear medicine procedure is performed.

Type (Character 3)

The third character indicates the type of nuclear medicine procedure (e.g., planar imaging or nonimaging uptake). The following list includes the types of nuclear medicine procedures with a definition of each type.

- *Nonimaging Nuclear Medicine Assay:* Introduction of radioactive materials into the body for the study of body fluids and blood elements, by the detection of radioactive emissions

- *Nonimaging Nuclear Medicine Probe:* Introduction of radioactive materials into the body for the study of distribution and fate of certain substances by the detection of radioactive emissions; or alternatively, measurement of absorption of radioactive emissions from an external source

- *Nonimaging Nuclear Medicine Uptake:* Introduction of radioactive materials into the body for measurements of organ function, from the detection of radioactive emissions

- *Planar Nuclear Medicine Imaging*: Introduction of radioactive materials into the body for single-plane display of images developed from the capture of radioactive emissions

- *Positron Emission Tomography (PET) Imaging:* Introduction of radioactive materials into the body for three dimensional display of images developed from the simultaneous capture, 180 degrees apart, of radioactive emissions

- *Systemic Nuclear Medicine Therapy:* Introduction of unsealed radioactive materials into the body for treatment

- *Tomographic (Tomo) Nuclear Medicine Imaging*: Introduction of radioactive materials into the body for three dimensional display of images developed from the capture of radioactive emissions

Body Part (Character 4)

The fourth character indicates the body part or body region studied; with regional (e.g., *lower extremity veins*) and combination (e.g., *liver and spleen*) body parts commonly used.

Radionuclide (Character 5)

The fifth character specifies the radionuclide, the radiation source. The option *Other Radionuclide* is provided in the nuclear medicine section for newly approved radionuclides until they can be added to the coding system. If more than one radiopharmaceutical is given to perform the procedure, then more than one code is used.

Qualifier (Character 6 and 7)

The sixth and seventh characters are qualifiers but are not specified in the *Nuclear Medicine* section; the value is always *None*.

Radiation Therapy Section (D)

Character Meanings

The seven characters in the Radiation Therapy section have the following meaning:

Character	Meaning
1	Section
2	Body System
3	Modality
4	Treatment Site
5	Modality Qualifier
6	Isotope
7	Qualifier

Section (Character 1)

Radiation therapy procedure codes have a first character value of *D*.

Body System (Character 2)

The second character specifies the body system (e.g., central nervous system, musculoskeletal) irradiated.

Modality (Character 3)

The third character specifies the general modality used (e.g., beam radiation).

Treatment Site (Character 4)

The fourth character specifies the body part that is the focus of the radiation therapy.

Modality Qualifier (Character 5)

The fifth character further specifies the radiation modality used (e.g., photons, electrons).

Isotope (Character 6)

The sixth character specifies the isotopes introduced into the body, if applicable.

Qualifier (Character 7)

The seventh character may specify whether the procedure was performed intraoperatively.

Physical Rehabilitation and Diagnostic Audiology Section (F)

Character Meanings

The seven characters in the Physical Rehabilitation and Diagnostic Audiology section have the following meaning:

Character	Meaning
1	Section
2	Section Qualifier
3	Type
4	Body System/Region
5	Type Qualifier
6	Equipment
7	Qualifier

Physical rehabilitation procedures include physical therapy, occupational therapy, and speech-language pathology. Osteopathic procedures and chiropractic procedures are in separate sections.

Section (Character 1)

Physical Rehabilitation and Diagnostic Audiology procedure codes have a first character value of *F*.

Section Qualifier (Character 2)

The section qualifier *Rehabilitation* or *Diagnostic Audiology* is specified in the second character.

Type (Character 3)

The third character specifies the type. There are 14 different values, which can be classified into four basic types of rehabilitation and diagnostic audiology procedures, defined as follows:

Assessment: Includes a determination of the patient's diagnosis when appropriate, need for treatment, planning for treatment, periodic assessment, and documentation related to these activities

Assessments are further classified into more than 100 different tests or methods. The majority of these focus on the faculties of hearing and speech, but others focus on various aspects of body function, and on the patient's quality of life, such as muscle performance, neuromotor development, and reintegration skills.

- *Speech Assessment*: Measurement of speech and related functions

- *Motor and/or Nerve Function Assessment*: Measurement of motor, nerve, and related functions

- *Activities of Daily Living Assessment*: Measurement of functional level for activities of daily living

- *Hearing Assessment*: Measurement of hearing and related functions

- *Hearing Aid Assessment*: Measurement of the appropriateness and/or effectiveness of a hearing device

- *Vestibular Assessment*: Measurement of the vestibular system and related functions

Caregiver Training: Educating caregiver with the skills and knowledge used to interact with and assist the patient

Caregiver Training is divided into 18 different broad subjects taught to help a caregiver provide proper patient care.

- *Caregiver Training*: Training in activities to support patient's optimal level of function

Fitting(s): Design, fabrication, modification, selection, and/or application of splint, orthosis, prosthesis, hearing aids, and/or other rehabilitation device

The fifth character used in *Device Fitting* procedures describes the device being fitted rather than the method used to fit the device. Definitions of devices, when provided, are located in the definitions portion of the ICD-10-PCS tables and index, under section F, character 5.

- *Device Fitting*: Fitting of a device designed to facilitate or support achievement of a higher level of function

Treatment: Use of specific activities or methods to develop, improve, and/or restore the performance of necessary functions, compensate for dysfunction and/or minimize debilitation

Treatment procedures include swallowing dysfunction exercises, bathing and showering techniques, wound management, gait training, and a host of activities typically associated with rehabilitation.

- *Speech Treatment*: Application of techniques to improve, augment, or compensate for speech and related functional impairment

- *Motor Treatment*: Exercise or activities to increase or facilitate motor function

- *Activities of Daily Living Treatment*: Exercise or activities to facilitate functional competence for activities of daily living

- *Hearing Treatment*: Application of techniques to improve, augment, or compensate for hearing and related functional impairment

- *Cochlear Implant Treatment*: Application of techniques to improve the communication abilities of individuals with cochlear implant

- *Vestibular Treatment*: Application of techniques to improve, augment, or compensate for vestibular and related functional impairment

The type of treatment includes training as well as activities that restore function.

Body System/Region (Character 4)
The fourth character specifies the body region and/or system on which the procedure is performed.

Type Qualifier (Character 5)
The fifth character is a type qualifier that further specifies the procedure performed. Examples include therapy to improve the range of motion and training for bathing techniques. Refer to appendix J for definitions of these types of procedures.

Equipment (Character 6)
The sixth character specifies the equipment used. Specific equipment is not defined in the equipment value. Instead, broad categories of equipment are specified (e.g., aerobic endurance and conditioning, assistive/adaptive/supportive, etc.)

Qualifier (Character 7)
The seventh character is not specified in the Physical Rehabilitation and Diagnostic Audiology section and always has the value *None*.

Mental Health Section (G)

Character Meanings
The seven characters in the Mental Health section have the following meaning:

Character	Meaning
1	Section
2	Body System
3	Type
4	Qualifier
5	Qualifier
6	Qualifier
7	Qualifier

Section (Character 1)
Mental health procedure codes have a first character value of *G*.

Body System (Character 2)
The second character is used to identify the body system elsewhere in ICD-10-PCS. In this section it always has the value *None*.

Type (Character 3)
The third character specifies the procedure type, such as crisis intervention or counseling. There are 12 types of mental health procedures.

- *Psychological Tests:* The administration and interpretation of standardized psychological tests and measurement instruments for the assessment of psychological function

- *Crisis Intervention:* Treatment of a traumatized, acutely disturbed, or distressed individual for the purpose of short-term stabilization

- *Medication Management:* Monitoring and adjusting the use of medications for the treatment of a mental health disorder

- *Individual Psychotherapy:* Treatment of an individual with a mental health disorder by behavioral, cognitive, psychoanalytic, psychodynamic, or psychophysiological means to improve functioning or well-being

- *Counseling:* The application of psychological methods to treat an individual with normal developmental issues and psychological problems in order to increase function, improve well-being, alleviate distress, maladjustment, or resolve crises

- *Family Psychotherapy:* Treatment that includes one or more family members of an individual with a mental health disorder by behavioral, cognitive, psychoanalytic, psychodynamic, or psychophysiological means to improve functioning or well-being

- *Electroconvulsive Therapy:* The application of controlled electrical voltages to treat a mental health disorder

- *Biofeedback:* Provision of information from the monitoring and regulating of physiological processes in conjunction with cognitive-behavioral techniques to improve patient functioning or well-being

- *Hypnosis:* Induction of a state of heightened suggestibility by auditory, visual, and tactile techniques to elicit an emotional or behavioral response

- *Narcosynthesis:* Administration of intravenous barbiturates in order to release suppressed or repressed thoughts

- *Group Psychotherapy:* Treatment of two or more individuals with a mental health disorder by behavioral, cognitive, psychoanalytic, psychodynamic, or psychophysiological means to improve functioning or well-being

- *Light Therapy:* Application of specialized light treatments to improve functioning or well-being

Qualifier (Character 4)
The fourth character is a qualifier to indicate that counseling was educational or vocational or to indicate type of test or method of therapy.

Qualifier (Character 5, 6 and 7)
The fifth, sixth, and seventh characters are not specified and always have the value *None*.

Substance Abuse Treatment Section (H)

Character Meanings
The seven characters in the Substance Abuse Treatment section have the following meaning:

Character	Meaning
1	Section
2	Body System
3	Type
4	Qualifier
5	Qualifier
6	Qualifier
7	Qualifier

Section (Character 1)

Substance Abuse Treatment codes have a first character value of *H*.

Body System (Character 2)

The second character is used to identify the body system elsewhere in ICD-10-PCS. In this section, it always has the value *None*.

Type (Character 3)

The third character specifies the type of procedure. There are seven values classified in this section, as listed below:

- *Detoxification Services:* Detoxification from alcohol and/or drugs

- *Individual Counseling:* The application of psychological methods to treat an individual with addictive behavior

- *Group Counseling:* The application of psychological methods to treat two or more individuals with addictive behavior

- *Individual Psychotherapy:* Treatment of an individual with addictive behavior by behavioral, cognitive, psychoanalytic, psychodynamic, or psychophysiological means

- *Family Counseling:* The application of psychological methods that includes one or more family members to treat an individual with addictive behavior

- *Medication Management:* Monitoring and adjusting the use of replacement medications for the treatment of addiction

- *Pharmacotherapy:* The use of replacement medications for the treatment of addiction

Qualifier (Character 4)

The fourth character further specifies the procedure type. These qualifier values vary dependent upon the Root Type procedure (Character 3). Root type 2, *Detoxification Services* contains only the value Z, *None* and Root type 6, *Family Counseling* contains only the value 3, *Other Family Counseling*, whereas the remainder Root Type procedures include multiple possible values.

Qualifier (Character 5, 6 and 7)

The fifth through seventh characters are designated as qualifiers but are never specified, so they always have the value *None*.

New Technology Section (X)

General Information

Section X New Technology is a section added to ICD-10-PCS beginning October 1, 2015. The new section provides a place for codes that uniquely identify procedures requested via the New Technology Application Process or that capture other new technologies not currently classified in ICD-10-PCS.

Section X does not introduce any new coding concepts or unusual guidelines for correct coding. In fact, Section X codes maintain continuity with the other sections in ICD-10-PCS by using the same root operation and body part values as their closest counterparts in other sections of ICD-10-PCS. For example, the codes for the infusion of ceftazidime-avibactam, use the same root operation (Introduction) and body part values (Central Vein and Peripheral Vein) in section X as the infusion codes in section 3 Administration, which are their closest counterparts in the other sections of ICD-10-PCS.

Character Meanings

The seven characters in the new technology section have the following meaning:

Character	Meaning
1	Section
2	Body System
3	Root Operation
4	Body Part
5	Approach
6	Device/Substance/Technology
7	Qualifier

Section (Character 1)

New technology procedure codes have a first character value of *X*.

Body System (Character 2)

The second character values for body system combine the uses of body system, body region, and physiological system as specified in other sections in ICD-10-PCS.

Root Operation (Character 3)

The third character utilizes the same root operation values as their counterparts in other sections of ICD-10-PCS.

Body Part (Character 4)

The fourth character specifies the same body part values as their closest counterparts in other sections of ICD-10-PCS.

Approach (Character 5)

The fifth character specifies approaches as defined in the Medical and Surgical section.

Device/Substance/Technology (Character 6)

The sixth character specifies the key feature of the new technology procedure. It may be specified as a new device, a new substance, or other new technology. Examples of sixth character values are *blinatumomab antineoplastic immunotherapy, orbital atherectomy technology,* and *intraoperative knee replacement sensor.*

Qualifier (Character 7)

The seventh character qualifier is used exclusively to specify the new technology group, a number or letter that changes each year that new technology codes are added to the system. For example, Section X codes added for the first year have the seventh character value 1, *New Technology Group 1*, and the next year that Section X codes are added have the seventh character value 2, *New Technology Group 2*, and so on. Changing the seventh character value to a unique letter or number every year that there are new codes in the new technology section allows the ICD-10-PCS to "recycle" the values in the third, fourth, and sixth characters as needed.

New Technology Coding Instruction

Section X codes are standalone codes. They are not supplemental codes. Section X codes fully represent the specific procedure described in the code title, and do not require any additional codes from other sections of ICD-10-PCS. When section X contains a code title which describes a specific new technology procedure, only that X code is reported for the procedure. There is no need to report a broader, non-specific code in another section of ICD-10-PCS.

For example, code XW033G5 Introduction of Sarilumab into Peripheral Vein, Percutaneous Approach, New Technology Group 5, would be reported to indicate that Sarilumab was administered via peripheral vein. A separate code from table 3EØ in the Administration section of ICD-10-PCS would not be reported in addition to this code. The X section code fully identifies the administration of the sarilumab, and no additional code is needed.

The New Technology section codes are easily found by looking in the ICD-10-PCS Index or the Tables. In the Index, the name of the new technology device, substance or technology for a section X code is included as a main term. In addition, all codes in section X are listed under the main term New Technology. The new technology code index entry for sarilumab is shown below.

Sarilumab XWØ

New Technology
Sarilumab XWØ

ICD-10-PCS Index and Tabular Format

The *ICD-10-PCS: The Complete Official Code Set* is based on the official version of the International Classification of Diseases, 10th Revision, Procedure Classification System, issued by the U.S. Department of Health and Human Services, Centers for Medicare and Medicaid Services. This book is consistent with the content of the government's version of ICD-10-PCS and follows their official format.

Index

The Alphabetic Index can be used to locate the appropriate table containing all the information necessary to construct a procedure code, however, the PCS tables should always be consulted to find the most appropriate valid code. Users may choose a valid code directly from the tables—he or she need not consult the index before proceeding to the tables to complete the code.

Main Terms

The Alphabetic Index reflects the structure of the tables. Therefore, the index is organized as an alphabetic listing. The index:

- Is based on the value of the third character
- Contains common procedure terms
- Lists anatomic sites
- Uses device terms

The main terms in the Alphabetic Index are root operations, root procedure types, or common procedure names. In addition, anatomic sites from the Body Part Key and device terms from the Device Key have been added for ease of use.

Examples:

> *Resection* (root operation)
>
> *Fluoroscopy* (root type)
>
> *Prostatectomy* (common procedure name)
>
> *Brachiocephalic artery* (body part)
>
> *Bard® Dulex™ mesh* (device)

The index provides at least the first three or four values of the code, and some entries may provide complete valid codes. However, the user should always consult the appropriate table to verify that the most appropriate valid code has been selected.

Root Operation and Procedure Type Main Terms

For the *Medical and Surgical* and related sections, the root operation values are used as main terms in the index. The subterms under the root operation main terms are body parts. For the Ancillary section of the tables, the main terms in the index are the general type of procedure performed.

Examples:

Biofeedback GZC9ZZZ
Destruction
    Acetabulum
        Left ØQ55
        Right ØQ54
    Adenoids ØC5Q
    Ampulla of Vater ØF5C
Planar Nuclear Medicine Imaging
    Abdomen CW1Ø

See Reference

The second type of term in the index uses common procedure names, such as "appendectomy" or "fundoplication." These common terms are listed as main terms with a "see" reference noting the PCS root operations that are possible valid code tables based on the objective of the procedure.

Examples:

Tendonectomy
    see Excision, Tendons ØLB
    see Resection, Tendons ØLT

Use Reference

The index also lists anatomic sites from the Body Part Key and device terms from the Device Key. These terms are listed with a "use" reference. The purpose of these references is to act as an additional reference to the terms located in the Appendix Keys. The term provided is the Body Part value or Device value to be selected when constructing a procedure code using the code tables. This type of index reference is not intended to direct the user to another term in the index, but to provide guidance regarding character value selection. Therefore, "use" references generally do not refer to specific valid code tables.

Examples:

CoAxia NeuroFlo catheter
    use Intraluminal Device
Epitrochlear lymph node
    use Lymphatic, Left Upper Extremity
    use Lymphatic, Right Upper Extremity
SynCardia Total Artificial Heart
    use Synthetic Substitute

Code Tables

ICD-10-PCS contains 17 sections of Code Tables organized by general type of procedure. The first three characters of a procedure code define each table. The tables consist of columns providing the possible last four characters of codes and rows providing valid values for each character. Within a PCS table, valid codes include all combinations of choices in characters 4 through 7 contained in the same row of the table. All seven characters must be specified to form a valid code.

There are three main sections of tables:

- Medical and Surgical section:
  - *Medical and Surgical* (Ø)
- Medical and Surgical-related sections:
  - *Obstetrics* (1)
  - *Placement* (2)
  - *Administration* (3)
  - *Measurement and Monitoring* (4)
  - *Extracorporeal or Systemic Assistance and Performance* (5)
  - *Extracorporeal or Systemic Therapies* (6)
  - *Osteopathic* (7)
  - *Other Procedures* (8)
  - *Chiropractic* (9)

- Ancillary sections:
  - — *Imaging* (B)
  - — *Nuclear Medicine* (C)
  - — *Radiation Therapy* (D)
  - — *Physical Rehabilitation and Diagnostic Audiology* (F)
  - — *Mental Health* (G)
  - — *Substance Abuse Treatment* (H)
- New Technology section:
  - — *New Technology* (X)

The first three character values define each table. The root operation or root type designated for each table is accompanied by its official definition.

Example:

Table 00F provides codes for procedures on the central nervous system that involve breaking up of solid matter into pieces:

Character 1, Section	0: Medical and Surgical
Character 2, Body System	0: Central Nervous System and Cranial Nerves
Character 3, Root Operation	F: Fragmentation: Breaking solid matter in a body part into pieces

Tables are arranged numerically, then alphabetically.

When reviewing tables, the user should keep in mind that:

- Some tables may cover multiple pages in the code book—to ensure maximum clarity about character choices, valid entries do not split rows between pages. For instance, the entire table of valid characters completing a code beginning with 4A1 is split between two pages, but the split is between, not within, rows. This means that all the valid sixth and seventh characters for, say, body system *Arterial* (3) and approach *External* (X) are contained on one page.
- Individual entries may be listed in several horizontal "selection" lines.
- When a table is continued onto another page, a note to this effect has been added in red.

Body Part Definitions:

An exclusive Optum360 feature in the tables is the incorporation of the body part definitions provided in appendix E into the Medical and Surgical section (0) tables under their appropriate body part characters in the first column (character 4). This provides the user a direct reference to all anatomical descriptions, terms, and sites that could be coded to that particular body part value.

Paired body parts typically have values for the right and left side and in some cases a value for bilateral. These paired body parts often have the same list of inclusive body part definitions. When there are paired body parts with the same body part definitions, the first listed body part (usually the right side) contains the list of body part definitions while the second listed body part (usually the left side) contains a **See** instruction. This **See** instruction references the body part value that contains the body part definitions. In the table below, body part value P – Upper Eyelid, Left is followed by a **See** instruction that states **See** N Upper Eyelid, Right. All body part descriptions under value N also apply to body part value P.

Example:

0 Medical and Surgical
8 Eye
M Reattachment Definition: Putting back in or on all or a portion of a separated body part to its normal location or other suitable location
Explanation: Vascular circulation and nervous pathways may or may not be reestablished

Body Part Character 4	Approach Character 5	Device Character 6	Qualifier Character 7
N Upper Eyelid, Right Lateral canthus Levator palpebrae superioris muscle Orbicularis oculi muscle Superior tarsal plate **P Upper Eyelid, Left** *See N Upper Eyelid, Right* **Q Lower Eyelid, Right** Inferior tarsal plate Medial canthus **R Lower Eyelid, Left** *See Q Lower Eyelid, Right*	**X External**	**Z No Device**	**Z No Qualifier**

ICD-10-PCS Additional Features

Use of Official Sources

Color-coding, symbol, and other annotations in this manual that identify coding and reimbursement issues are derived from various official federal government sources, including the *Federal Register*, volume 86, number 88, May 10, 2021 ("Hospital Inpatient Prospective Payment Systems for Acute Care Hospitals and the Long Term Care Hospital Prospective Payment System and Proposed Policy Changes and Fiscal Year 2022 Rates; Proposed Rule") and the proposed, version 39, MS-DRG Grouper software, Definitions Manual files and Medicare Code Editor (MCE) files published with the fiscal 2022 IPPS proposed rule. For the most current files related to IPPS, please refer to the following:

- FY2022 IPPS Final Rule
  https://www.cms.gov/Medicare/Medicare-Fee-for-Service-Payment/AcuteInpatientPPS/IPPS-Regulations-and-Notices

- FY2022 Final Version 39, MS-DRG Grouper software
  https://www.cms.gov/Medicare/Medicare-Fee-for-Service-Payment/AcuteInpatientPPS/MS-DRG-Classifications-and-Software

Table Notations

Many tables in ICD-10-PCS contain color or symbol annotations that may aid in code selection, provide clinical or coding information, or alert the coder to reimbursement issues affected by the PCS code assignment. These annotations may be displayed on or next to a character 4, character 6, or character 7 value. Please note that some values may have more than one annotation; this is true most often with the character 4 value.

Refer to the color/symbol legend at the bottom of each page in the tables section for an abridged description of each color and symbol.

Annotation Box

An annotation box has been appended to all tables that contain color-coding or symbol annotations. The color bar or symbol attached to a character value is provided in the box, as well as a list of the valid PCS code(s) to which that edit applies. The box may also list conditional criteria that must be met to satisfy the edit.

For example, see Table 00F. Four character 4 body part values have a gray color bar. In the annotation box below the table, the gray color bar is defined as "Non-OR," or a nonoperating room procedure edit. Following the Non-OR annotation are the PCS codes that are considered nonoperating room procedures from that row of Table 00F.

Bracketed Code Notation

The use of bracketed codes is an efficient convention to provide all valid character value alternatives for a specific set of circumstances. The character values in the brackets correspond to the valid values for the character in the position the bracket appears.

Examples:

In the annotation box for Table 00F the Noncovered Procedure edit (NC) applies to codes represented in the bracketed code 00F[3,4,5,6]XZZ.

    00F[3,4,5,6]XZZ Fragmentation in (Central Nervous System and Cranial Nerves), External Approach

---

The valid fourth character values (body part) that may be selected for this specific circumstance are as follows:

    3   Epidural Space, Intracranial

    4   Subdural Space, Intracranial

    5   Subarachnoid Space, Intracranial

    6   Cerebral Ventricle

The fragmentation of matter in the spinal canal, Body Part value U, is not included in the noncovered procedure code edit.

Color-Coding/Symbols

New and Revised Text

To highlight changes to the PCS tables for the current year, the new and revised text is provided in green font.

Medicare Code Edits

Medicare administrative contractors (MACs) and many payers use Medicare code edits to check the coding accuracy on claims. The coding edits provided in this manual include only those directly related to ICD-10-PCS codes used for acute care hospital inpatient admissions. These edits are based on the proposed, version 39, Medicare Code Editor (MCE) files published with the fiscal 2022 IPPS proposed rule.

The PCS related Medicare code edits are listed below:

- Invalid procedure code

- *Sex conflict

- *Questionable obstetric admission

- *Noncovered procedure

- *Limited coverage procedure

Starred edits above that are related to PCS issues are identified in this manual by symbols as described below.

Sex Edit Symbols

The sex edit symbols below are used to detect inconsistencies between the patient's sex and the procedure. The symbols below most often appear to the right of the body part (character 4) value but may also be found to the right of the qualifier (character 7) value:

    ♂   Male procedure only

    ♀   Female procedure only

🆀🅰 Questionable Obstetric Admission

An inpatient admission is considered questionable when a vaginal or cesarean delivery code is assigned without a corresponding secondary diagnosis code describing the outcome of delivery. Both a delivery (ICD-10-PCS) code and an outcome-of-delivery (ICD-10-CM) code must be present to avoid errors in MS-DRG assignment. This symbol is found only in the Obstetrics Section, appearing to the right of the body part (character 4) value.

🅽🅲 Noncovered Procedure

Medicare does not cover all procedures. However, some noncovered procedures, due to the presence of certain diagnoses, are reimbursed.

ICD-10-PCS Additional Features

LC Limited Coverage

For certain procedures whose medical complexity and serious nature incur extraordinary associated costs, Medicare limits coverage to a portion of the cost. The limited coverage edit indicates the type of limited coverage.

ICD-10 MS-DRG Definitions Manual Edits

An MS-DRG is assigned based on specific patient attributes, such as principal diagnosis, secondary diagnoses, procedures, and discharge status. The attributes (edits) provided in this manual include only those directly related to ICD-10-PCS codes used for acute care hospital inpatient admissions. These edits are based on the proposed, version 39, MS-DRG Grouper software and Definitions Manual published with the fiscal 2022 IPPS proposed rule.

Non-Operating Room Procedures Not Affecting MS-DRG Assignment

In the Medical and Surgical section (ØØ1–ØYW) and the Obstetric section (1Ø2–1ØY) tables **only,** ICD-10-PCS procedures codes that DO NOT affect MS-DRG assignment are identified by a gray color bar over the body part (character 4) value and are considered non-operating room (non-OR) procedures.

NOTE: The majority of the ICD-10-PCS codes in the Medical and Surgical-Related, Ancillary and New Technology section tables are non-operating room procedures that do not typically affect MS-DRG assignment. Only the Valid Operating Room and DRG Non-Operating Room procedures are highlighted in these sections, *see* Non-Operating Room Procedures Affecting MS-DRG Assignment and Valid OR Procedure description below.

Non-Operating Room Procedures Affecting MS-DRG Assignment

Some ICD-10-PCS procedure codes, although considered non-operating room procedures, may still affect MS-DRG assignment. In all sections of the ICD-10-PCS book, these procedures are identified by a **purple color bar** over the body part (character 4) value.

Valid OR Procedure

In the Medical and Surgical-Related (2WØ–9WB), Ancillary (BØØ–HZ9) and New Technology (X2A–XYØ) section tables **only**, any codes that are considered a valid operating room procedure are identified with a blue color bar over the body part (character 4) value and will affect MS-DRG assignment. All codes without a color bar (blue or purple) are considered non-operating room procedures.

Hospital-Acquired Condition Related Procedures

Procedures associated with hospital-acquired conditions (HAC) are identified with the yellow color bar over the body part (character 4) value. Appendix K provides each specific HAC category and its associated ICD-10-CM and ICD-10-PCS codes.

Combination Only

Some ICD-10-PCS procedure codes that describe non-operating room procedures can group to a specific MS-DRG but only when used in combination with certain other ICD-10-PCS procedure codes. Such codes are designated by a red color bar over the body part (character 4) value.

⊞ Combination Member

A combination member, which can be either a valid operating room procedure or a non-operating room procedure, is an ICD-10-PCS procedure code that can influence MS-DRG assignment either on its own or in combination with other specific ICD-10-PCS procedure codes. Combination member codes are designated by a plus sign (⊞) to the right of the body part (character 4) value.

Note: In the few instances when a code is both a combination member and a non-operating room procedure affecting the MS-DRG assignment, the body part (character 4) value will have a purple color bar and the combination member icon.

See Appendix L for Procedure Combinations

Under certain circumstances, more than one procedure code is needed in order to group to a specific MS-DRG. When codes within a table have been identified as a Combination Only (**red color bar**) or Combination Member (⊞) code, there is also a footnote instructing the coder to *see Appendix L*. Appendix L contains tables that identify the other procedure codes needed in the combination and the title and number of the MS-DRG to which the combination will group.

Other Table Notations

AHA Coding Clinic:

Official citations from AHA's *Coding Clinic for ICD-10-CM/PCS* have been provided at the beginning of each section, when applicable. Each specific citation is listed below a header identifying the table to which that particular *Coding Clinic* citation applies. The citations appear in purple type with the year, quarter, and page of the reference as well as the title of the question as it appears in that *Coding Clinic's* table of contents. *Coding Clinic* citations included in this edition have been updated through second quarter 2021.

NT New Technology Add-on Payment

This symbol identifies procedure codes that involve new technologies or medical services that have qualified for a new technology add-on payment (NTAP). CMS provides incremental payment, in addition to the DRG payment, for technologies that have received the NTAP designation. This symbol appears to the right of the sixth character value.

Note: Only specific brand or trade named devices, substances, or technologies receive NTAP approval. The sixth character value in the PCS table provides a generalized description that may be applicable to several brand or trade names. Unless otherwise specified in the annotation box, refer to appendix H or I to determine the specific brand or trade name of the device, substance, or technology that is applicable to the new technology add-on payment. New technology add-on payments are not exclusive to the New Technology (X) section.

Appendixes

The resources described below have been included as appendixes for *ICD-10-PCS The Complete Official Code Set*. These resources further instruct the coder on the appropriate application of the ICD-10-PCS code set.

Appendix A: Components of the Medical and Surgical Approach Definitions

This resource further defines the approach characters used in the Medical and Surgical (Ø) section. Complementing the detailed definition of the approach, additional information includes whether or not instrumentation is a part of the approach, the typical access location, the method used to initiate the approach, related procedural examples, and illustrations all of which will help the user determine the appropriate approach value.

Appendix B: Root Operation Definitions

This resource is a compilation of all root operations found in the Medical and Surgical-related sections (0-9) of this PCS manual. It provides a definition and in some cases a more detailed explanation of the root operation, to better reflect the purpose or objective. Examples of related procedure(s) may also be provided.

Appendix C: Comparison of Medical and Surgical Root Operations

The Medical and Surgical (0) section root operations are divided into groups that share similar attributes. These groups, and the root operations in each group, are listed in this resource along with information identifying the target of the root operation, the action used to perform the root operation, any clarification or further explanation on the objective of the root operation, and procedure examples.

Appendix D: Body Part Key

When an anatomical term or description is provided in the documentation but does not have a specific body part character within a table, the user can reference this resource to search for the anatomical description or site noted in the documentation to determine if there is a specific PCS body part character (character 4) to which the anatomical description or site could be coded.

Appendix E: Body Part Definitions

This resource is the reverse look-up of the Body Part Key. Each table in the Medical and Surgical section (0) of the PCS manual contains anatomical terms linked to a body part character or value, for example, in Table 0BB the Body Part (character 4) of 1 is Trachea. The body part Trachea may have anatomical structures or descriptions that may be used in procedure documentation instead of the term trachea. The Body Part Definitions list other anatomical structures or synonyms that are included in specific ICD-10-PCS body part values. According to the body part definitions, in the example above, cricoid cartilage is included in the Trachea (character 1) body part.

Appendix F: Device Classification

This resource provides an explanation of how a device is defined in the ICD-10-PCS classification along with two tables. The first table groups devices used in the ICD-10-PCS tables into general categories, including a definition of each device type and related examples. The second table provides definitions of transplant and grafting tissue types and associated terminology that may be found in the documentation.

Appendix G: Device Key and Aggregation Table

The Device Key helps users code the appropriate PCS sixth character for device. Devices are listed alphabetically by brand name or commonly used medical terminology and are translated to the appropriate PCS language or value. The key also reflects the body system where the device is located. For example, a SAPIEN valve used for transaortic valve replacement translates to Zooplastic Tissue in Heart and Great Vessels.

The following symbol **NT** has been placed next to those devices that have received an NTAP (new technology add-on payment) designation. When the code for this device is applied to an inpatient encounter, CMS provides incremental payment in addition to the DRG payment.

The Aggregation Table crosswalks specific device character value definitions for specific root operations in a specific body system to the more general device character value to be used when the root operation covers a wide range of body parts and the device character represents an entire family of devices.

Appendix H: Device Definitions

This resource is a reverse look-up to the Device Key. The user may reference this resource to see all the specific devices that may be grouped to a particular device character (character 6).

Example:

The operative report states, "An internal fixation device was used to repair a fractured femur. Kirschner wire, bone screws and neutralization plate all used and left in the bone at the end of the procedure. "

Although PCS requires all devices left in the body to be coded and the operative report lists three different devices, a check in the device definitions shows that all of these devices are included in the PCS value "Internal Fixation Device" and require only one code.

The following symbol **NT** has been placed next to those devices that have received an NTAP (new technology add-on payment) designation. When the code for this device is applied to an inpatient encounter, CMS provides incremental payment in addition to the DRG payment.

Appendix I: Substance Key/Substance Definitions

The Substance Key lists substances by trade name or synonym and relates them to a PCS character in the Administration (3) or New Technology (X) section in the Substance (sixth character) or Qualifier (seventh character) column.

The Substance Definitions table is the reverse look-up of the substance key, relating all substance categories, the sixth- or seventh character values, to all trade name or synonyms that may be classified to that particular character.

The following symbol **NT** has been placed next to those substances/technologies that have received an NTAP (new technology add-on payment) designation. When the code for this substance/technology is applied to an inpatient encounter, CMS provides incremental payment in addition to the DRG payment.

Appendix J: Sections B-H Character Definitions

In each ancillary section (B-H) the characters in a particular column may have different meanings depending on which section the user is working from. This resource provides the values for the characters in these sections as well as a definition of the character value.

Appendix K: Hospital Acquired Conditions

Hospital acquired conditions (HACs) are conditions that are considered reasonably preventable when occurring during the hospital admission and may prevent a case from grouping to a higher-paying MS-DRG. In certain instances the HACs are conditional, requiring a specific ICD-10-CM diagnosis code in combination with a specific ICD-10-PCS procedure code. This resource identifies these conditional HACs, listing the diagnosis and procedure codes that, in combination, may trigger a HAC edit. All codes, ICD-10-CM and ICD-10-PCS, are listed with their full descriptions.

Appendix L: Procedure Combination Tables

The procedure combination tables provided in this resource illustrate certain procedure combinations that must occur in order to assign a specific MS-DRG.

Appendix M: Coding Exercises and Answers

This resource provides the coding exercises with answers, and in some cases a brief explanation as to the reason that particular code was used.

ICD-10-PCS Official Guidelines for Coding and Reporting 2022

Narrative changes appear in **bold** text.

The Centers for Medicare and Medicaid Services (CMS) and the National Center for Health Statistics (NCHS), two departments within the U.S. Federal Government's Department of Health and Human Services (DHHS) provide the following guidelines for coding and reporting using the International Classification of Diseases, 10th Revision, Procedure Coding System (ICD-10-PCS). These guidelines should be used as a companion document to the official version of the ICD-10-PCS as published on the CMS website. The ICD-10-PCS is a procedure classification published by the United States for classifying procedures performed in hospital inpatient health care settings.

These guidelines have been approved by the four organizations that make up the Cooperating Parties for the ICD-10-PCS: the American Hospital Association (AHA), the American Health Information Management Association (AHIMA), CMS, and NCHS.

These guidelines are a set of rules that have been developed to accompany and complement the official conventions and instructions provided within the ICD-10-PCS itself. They are intended to provide direction that is applicable in most circumstances. However, there may be unique circumstances where exceptions are applied. The instructions and conventions of the classification take precedence over guidelines. These guidelines are based on the coding and sequencing instructions in the Tables, Index and Definitions of ICD-10-PCS, but provide additional instruction. Adherence to these guidelines when assigning ICD-10-PCS procedure codes is required under the Health Insurance Portability and Accountability Act (HIPAA). The procedure codes have been adopted under HIPAA for hospital inpatient healthcare settings. A joint effort between the healthcare provider and the coder is essential to achieve complete and accurate documentation, code assignment, and reporting of diagnoses and procedures. These guidelines have been developed to assist both the healthcare provider and the coder in identifying those procedures that are to be reported. The importance of consistent, complete documentation in the medical record cannot be overemphasized. Without such documentation accurate coding cannot be achieved.

Conventions

A1. ICD-10-PCS codes are composed of seven characters. Each character is an axis of classification that specifies information about the procedure performed. Within a defined code range, a character specifies the same type of information in that axis of classification.

Example:
The fifth axis of classification specifies the approach in sections Ø through 4 and 7 through 9 of the system.

A2. One of 34 possible values can be assigned to each axis of classification in the seven-character code: they are the numbers Ø through 9 and the alphabet (except I and O because they are easily confused with the numbers 1 and Ø). The number of unique values used in an axis of classification differs as needed.

Example:
Where the fifth axis of classification specifies the approach, seven different approach values are currently used to specify the approach.

A3. The valid values for an axis of classification can be added to as needed.

Example:
If a significantly distinct type of device is used in a new procedure, a new device value can be added to the system.

A4. As with words in their context, the meaning of any single value is a combination of its axis of classification and any preceding values on which it may be dependent.

Example:
The meaning of a body part value in the Medical and Surgical section is always dependent on the body system value. The body part value Ø in the Central Nervous body system specifies Brain and the body part value Ø in the Peripheral Nervous body system specifies Cervical Plexus.

A5. As the system is expanded to become increasingly detailed, over time more values will depend on preceding values for their meaning.

Example:
In the Lower Joints body system, the device value 3 in the root operation Insertion specifies Infusion Device and the device value 3 in the root operation Replacement specifies Ceramic Synthetic Substitute.

A6. The purpose of the alphabetic index is to locate the appropriate table that contains all information necessary to construct a procedure code. The PCS Tables should always be consulted to find the most appropriate valid code.

A7. It is not required to consult the index first before proceeding to the tables to complete the code. A valid code may be chosen directly from the tables.

A8. All seven characters must be specified to be a valid code. If the documentation is incomplete for coding purposes, the physician should be queried for the necessary information.

A9. Within a PCS table, valid codes include all combinations of choices in characters 4 through 7 contained in the same row of the table. In the example below, ØJHT3VZ is a valid code, and ØJHW3VZ is *not* a valid code.

Section:	Ø	**Medical and Surgical**
Body System:	J	**Subcutaneous Tissue and Fascia**
Operation:	H	**Insertion** Putting in a nonbiological appliance that monitors, assists, performs, or prevents a physiological function but does not physically take the place of a body part

Body Part		Approach		Device		Qualifier	
S Subcutaneous Tissue and Fascia, Head and Neck **V** Subcutaneous Tissue and Fascia, Upper Extremity **W** Subcutaneous Tissue and Fascia, Lower Extremity		**Ø** Open **3** Percutaneous		**1** Radioactive Element **3** Infusion Device **Y** Other Device		**Z** No Qualifier	
T Subcutaneous Tissue and Fascia, Trunk		**Ø** Open **3** Percutaneous		**1** Radioactive Element **3** Infusion Device **V** Infusion Pump **Y** Other Device		**Z** No Qualifier	

A10. "And," when used in a code description, means "and/or," except when used to describe a combination of multiple body parts for which separate values exist for each body part (e.g., Skin and Subcutaneous Tissue used as a qualifier, where there are separate body part values for "Skin" and "Subcutaneous Tissue").

Example:
Lower Arm and Wrist Muscle means lower arm and/or wrist muscle.

A11. Many of the terms used to construct PCS codes are defined within the system. It is the coder's responsibility to determine what the documentation in the medical record equates to in the PCS definitions. The physician is not expected to use the terms used in PCS code descriptions, nor is the coder required to query the physician when the correlation between the documentation and the defined PCS terms is clear.

Example:
When the physician documents "partial resection" the coder can independently correlate "partial resection" to the root operation Excision without querying the physician for clarification.

Medical and Surgical Section Guidelines (section Ø)

B2. Body System

General guidelines

B2.1a. The procedure codes in Anatomical Regions, General, Anatomical Regions, Upper Extremities and Anatomical Regions, Lower Extremities can be used when the procedure is performed on an anatomical region rather than a specific body part, or on the rare occasion when no information is available to support assignment of a code to a specific body part.

Examples:
Chest tube drainage of the pleural cavity is coded to the root operation Drainage found in the body system Anatomical Regions, General.

Suture repair of the abdominal wall is coded to the root operation Repair in the body system Anatomical Regions, General.

Amputation of the foot is coded to the root operation Detachment in the body system Anatomical Regions, Lower Extremities.

B2.1b. Where the general body part values "upper" and "lower" are provided as an option in the Upper Arteries, Lower Arteries, Upper Veins, Lower Veins, Muscles and Tendons body systems, "upper" or "lower" specifies body parts located above or below the diaphragm respectively.

Example:
Vein body parts above the diaphragm are found in the Upper Veins body system; vein body parts below the diaphragm are found in the Lower Veins body system.

B3. Root Operation

General guidelines

B3.1a. In order to determine the appropriate root operation, the full definition of the root operation as contained in the PCS Tables must be applied.

B3.1b. Components of a procedure specified in the root operation definition or explanation as integral to that root operation are not coded separately. Procedural steps necessary to reach the operative site

and close the operative site, including anastomosis of a tubular body part, are also not coded separately.

Examples:
Resection of a joint as part of a joint replacement procedure is included in the root operation definition of Replacement and is not coded separately.

Laparotomy performed to reach the site of an open liver biopsy is not coded separately.

In a resection of sigmoid colon with anastomosis of descending colon to rectum, the anastomosis is not coded separately.

Multiple procedures

B3.2. During the same operative episode, multiple procedures are coded if:

a. The same root operation is performed on different body parts as defined by distinct values of the body part character.

   Examples:
   Diagnostic excision of liver and pancreas are coded separately.

   Excision of lesion in the ascending colon and excision of lesion in the transverse colon are coded separately.

b. The same root operation is repeated in multiple body parts, and those body parts are separate and distinct body parts classified to a single ICD-10-PCS body part value.

   Examples:
   Excision of the sartorius muscle and excision of the gracilis muscle are both included in the upper leg muscle body part value, and multiple procedures are coded.

   Extraction of multiple toenails are coded separately.

c. Multiple root operations with distinct objectives are performed on the same body part.

   Example:
   Destruction of sigmoid lesion and bypass of sigmoid colon are coded separately.

d. The intended root operation is attempted using one approach but is converted to a different approach.

   Example:
   Laparoscopic cholecystectomy converted to an open cholecystectomy is coded as percutaneous endoscopic Inspection and open Resection.

Discontinued or incomplete procedures

B3.3. If the intended procedure is discontinued or otherwise not completed, code the procedure to the root operation performed. If a procedure is discontinued before any other root operation is performed, code the root operation Inspection of the body part or anatomical region inspected.

Example:
A planned aortic valve replacement procedure is discontinued after the initial thoracotomy and before any incision is made in the heart muscle, when the patient becomes hemodynamically unstable. This procedure is coded as an open Inspection of the mediastinum.

Biopsy procedures

B3.4a. Biopsy procedures are coded using the root operations Excision, Extraction, or Drainage and the qualifier Diagnostic.

Examples:
Fine needle aspiration biopsy of fluid in the lung is coded to the root operation Drainage with the qualifier Diagnostic.

Biopsy of bone marrow is coded to the root operation Extraction with the qualifier Diagnostic.

Lymph node sampling for biopsy is coded to the root operation Excision with the qualifier Diagnostic.

Biopsy followed by more definitive treatment

B3.4b. If a diagnostic Excision, Extraction, or Drainage procedure (biopsy) is followed by a more definitive procedure, such as Destruction, Excision or Resection at the same procedure site, both the biopsy and the more definitive treatment are coded.

Example:
Biopsy of breast followed by partial mastectomy at the same procedure site, both the biopsy and the partial mastectomy procedure are coded.

Overlapping body layers

B3.5. If root operations such as Excision, Extraction, Repair or Inspection are performed on overlapping layers of the musculoskeletal system, the body part specifying the deepest layer is coded.

Example:
Excisional debridement that includes skin and subcutaneous tissue and muscle is coded to the muscle body part.

Bypass procedures

B3.6a. Bypass procedures are coded by identifying the body part bypassed "from" and the body part bypassed "to." The fourth character body part specifies the body part bypassed from, and the qualifier specifies the body part bypassed to.

Example:
Bypass from stomach to jejunum, stomach is the body part and jejunum is the qualifier.

B3.6b. Coronary artery bypass procedures are coded differently than other bypass procedures as described in the previous guideline. Rather than identifying the body part bypassed from, the body part identifies the number of coronary arteries bypassed to, and the qualifier specifies the vessel bypassed from.

Example:
Aortocoronary artery bypass of the left anterior descending coronary artery and the obtuse marginal coronary artery is classified in the body part axis of classification as two coronary arteries, and the qualifier specifies the aorta as the body part bypassed from.

B3.6c. If multiple coronary arteries are bypassed, a separate procedure is coded for each coronary artery that uses a different device and/or qualifier.

Example:
Aortocoronary artery bypass and internal mammary coronary artery bypass are coded separately.

Control vs. more **specific** root operations

B3.7. The root operation Control is defined as, "Stopping, or attempting to stop, postprocedural or other acute bleeding." **Control is the root operation coded when the procedure performed to achieve hemostasis, beyond what would be considered integral to a procedure, utilizes techniques (e.g. cautery, application of substances or pressure, suturing or ligation or clipping of bleeding points at the site) that are not described by a more specific root operation definition, such as Bypass, Detachment, Excision, Extraction, Reposition, Replacement, or Resection. If a more specific root operation definition applies to the procedure performed, then the more specific root operation is coded instead of Control.**

Example:
Silver nitrate cautery to treat acute nasal bleeding is coded to the root operation Control.

Example:
Liquid embolization of the right internal iliac artery to treat acute hematoma by stopping blood flow is coded to the root operation Occlusion.

Example:
Suctioning of residual blood to achieve hemostasis during a transbronchial cryobiopsy is considered integral to the cryobiopsy procedure and is not coded separately.

Excision vs. Resection

B3.8. PCS contains specific body parts for anatomical subdivisions of a body part, such as lobes of the lungs or liver and regions of the intestine. Resection of the specific body part is coded whenever all of the body part is cut out or off, rather than coding Excision of a less specific body part.

Example:
Left upper lung lobectomy is coded to Resection of Upper Lung Lobe, Left rather than Excision of Lung, Left.

Excision for graft

B3.9. If an autograft is obtained from a different procedure site in order to complete the objective of the procedure, a separate procedure is coded, except when the seventh character qualifier value in the ICD-10-PCS table fully specifies the site from which the autograft was obtained.

Examples:
Coronary bypass with excision of saphenous vein graft, excision of saphenous vein is coded separately.

Replacement of breast with autologous deep inferior epigastric artery perforator (DIEP) flap, excision of the DIEP flap is not coded separately. The seventh character qualifier value Deep Inferior Epigastric Artery Perforator Flap in the Replacement table fully specifies the site of the autograft harvest.

Fusion procedures of the spine

B3.10a. The body part coded for a spinal vertebral joint(s) rendered immobile by a spinal fusion procedure is classified by the level of the spine (e.g. thoracic). There are distinct body part values for a single vertebral joint and for multiple vertebral joints at each spinal level.

Example:
Body part values specify Lumbar Vertebral Joint, Lumbar Vertebral Joints, 2 or More and Lumbosacral Vertebral Joint.

B3.10b. If multiple vertebral joints are fused, a separate procedure is coded for each vertebral joint that uses a different device and/or qualifier.

Example:
Fusion of lumbar vertebral joint, posterior approach, anterior column and fusion of lumbar vertebral joint, posterior approach, posterior column are coded separately.

B3.10c. Combinations of devices and materials are often used on a vertebral joint to render the joint immobile. When combinations of devices are used on the same vertebral joint, the device value coded for the procedure is as follows:

- If an interbody fusion device is used to render the joint immobile (containing bone graft or bone graft substitute), the procedure is coded with the device value Interbody Fusion Device
- If bone graft is the *only* device used to render the joint immobile, the procedure is coded with the device value Nonautologous Tissue Substitute or Autologous Tissue Substitute

- If a mixture of autologous and nonautologous bone graft (with or without biological or synthetic extenders or binders) is used to render the joint immobile, code the procedure with the device value Autologous Tissue Substitute

Examples:

Fusion of a vertebral joint using a cage style interbody fusion device containing morsellized bone graft is coded to the device Interbody Fusion Device.

Fusion of a vertebral joint using a bone dowel interbody fusion device made of cadaver bone and packed with a mixture of local morsellized bone and demineralized bone matrix is coded to the device Interbody Fusion Device.

Fusion of a vertebral joint using both autologous bone graft and bone bank bone graft is coded to the device Autologous Tissue Substitute.

Inspection procedures

B3.11a. Inspection of a body part(s) performed in order to achieve the objective of a procedure is not coded separately.

Example:

Fiberoptic bronchoscopy performed for irrigation of bronchus, only the irrigation procedure is coded.

B3.11b. If multiple tubular body parts are inspected, the most distal body part (the body part furthest from the starting point of the inspection) is coded. If multiple non-tubular body parts in a region are inspected, the body part that specifies the entire area inspected is coded.

Examples:

Cystoureteroscopy with inspection of bladder and ureters is coded to the ureter body part value.

Exploratory laparotomy with general inspection of abdominal contents is coded to the peritoneal cavity body part value.

B3.11c. When both an Inspection procedure and another procedure are performed on the same body part during the same episode, if the Inspection procedure is performed using a different approach than the other procedure, the Inspection procedure is coded separately.

Example:

Endoscopic Inspection of the duodenum is coded separately when open Excision of the duodenum is performed during the same procedural episode.

Occlusion vs. Restriction for vessel embolization procedures

B3.12. If the objective of an embolization procedure is to completely close a vessel, the root operation Occlusion is coded. If the objective of an embolization procedure is to narrow the lumen of a vessel, the root operation Restriction is coded.

Examples:

Tumor embolization is coded to the root operation Occlusion, because the objective of the procedure is to cut off the blood supply to the vessel.

Embolization of a cerebral aneurysm is coded to the root operation Restriction, because the objective of the procedure is not to close off the vessel entirely, but to narrow the lumen of the vessel at the site of the aneurysm where it is abnormally wide.

Release procedures

B3.13. In the root operation Release, the body part value coded is the body part being freed and not the tissue being manipulated or cut to free the body part.

Example:

Lysis of intestinal adhesions is coded to the specific intestine body part value.

Release vs. Division

B3.14. If the sole objective of the procedure is freeing a body part without cutting the body part, the root operation is Release. If the sole objective of the procedure is separating or transecting a body part, the root operation is Division.

Examples:

Freeing a nerve root from surrounding scar tissue to relieve pain is coded to the root operation Release.

Severing a nerve root to relieve pain is coded to the root operation Division.

Reposition for fracture treatment

B3.15. Reduction of a displaced fracture is coded to the root operation Reposition and the application of a cast or splint in conjunction with the Reposition procedure is not coded separately. Treatment of a nondisplaced fracture is coded to the procedure performed.

Examples:

Casting of a nondisplaced fracture is coded to the root operation Immobilization in the Placement section.

Putting a pin in a nondisplaced fracture is coded to the root operation Insertion.

Transplantation vs. Administration

B3.16. Putting in a mature and functioning living body part taken from another individual or animal is coded to the root operation Transplantation. Putting in autologous or nonautologous cells is coded to the Administration section.

Example:

Putting in autologous or nonautologous bone marrow, pancreatic islet cells or stem cells is coded to the Administration section.

Transfer procedures using multiple tissue layers

B3.17. The root operation Transfer contains qualifiers that can be used to specify when a transfer flap is composed of more than one tissue layer, such as a musculocutaneous flap. For procedures involving transfer of multiple tissue layers including skin, subcutaneous tissue, fascia or muscle, the procedure is coded to the body part value that describes the deepest tissue layer in the flap, and the qualifier can be used to describe the other tissue layer(s) in the transfer flap.

Example:

A musculocutaneous flap transfer is coded to the appropriate body part value in the body system Muscles, and the qualifier is used to describe the additional tissue layer(s) in the transfer flap.

Excision/Resection followed by replacement

B3.18. If an excision or resection of a body part is followed by a replacement procedure, code both procedures to identify each distinct objective, except when the excision or resection is considered integral and preparatory for the replacement procedure.

Examples:

Mastectomy followed by reconstruction, both resection and replacement of the breast are coded to fully capture the distinct objectives of the procedures performed.

Maxillectomy with obturator reconstruction, both excision and replacement of the maxilla are coded to fully capture the distinct objectives of the procedures performed.

Excisional debridement of tendon with skin graft, both the excision of the tendon and the replacement of the skin with a graft are coded to fully capture the distinct objectives of the procedures performed.

Esophagectomy followed by reconstruction with colonic interposition, both the resection and the transfer of the large intestine to function as the esophagus are coded to fully capture the distinct objectives of the procedures performed.

Examples:
Resection of a joint as part of a joint replacement procedure is considered integral and preparatory for the replacement of the joint and the resection is not coded separately.

Resection of a valve as part of a valve replacement procedure is considered integral and preparatory for the valve replacement and the resection is not coded separately.

B4. Body Part

General guidelines
B4.1a. If a procedure is performed on a portion of a body part that does not have a separate body part value, code the body part value corresponding to the whole body part.

Example:
A procedure performed on the alveolar process of the mandible is coded to the mandible body part.

B4.1b. If the prefix "peri" is combined with a body part to identify the site of the procedure, and the site of the procedure is not further specified, then the procedure is coded to the body part named. This guideline applies only when a more specific body part value is not available.

Examples:
A procedure site identified as perirenal is coded to the kidney body part when the site of the procedure is not further specified.

A procedure site described in the documentation as peri-urethral, and the documentation also indicates that it is the vulvar tissue and not the urethral tissue that is the site of the procedure, then the procedure is coded to the vulva body part.

A procedure site documented as involving the periosteum is coded to the corresponding bone body part.

B4.1c. If a procedure is performed on a continuous section of a tubular body part, code the body part value corresponding to the **anatomically most proximal (closest to the heart) portion of the tubular body part.**

Example:
A procedure performed on a continuous section of artery from the femoral artery to the external iliac artery with the point of entry at the femoral artery is coded to the external iliac body part.

A procedure performed on a continuous section of artery from the femoral artery to the external iliac artery with the point of entry at the external iliac artery is also coded to the external iliac artery body part.

Branches of body parts
B4.2. Where a specific branch of a body part does not have its own body part value in PCS, the body part is typically coded to the closest proximal branch that has a specific body part value. In the cardiovascular body systems, if a general body part is available in the correct root operation table, and coding to a proximal branch would require assigning a code in a different body system, the procedure is coded using the general body part value.

Examples:
A procedure performed on the mandibular branch of the trigeminal nerve is coded to the trigeminal nerve body part value.

Occlusion of the bronchial artery is coded to the body part value Upper Artery in the body system Upper Arteries, and not to the body part value Thoracic Aorta, Descending in the body system Heart and Great Vessels.

Bilateral body part values
B4.3. Bilateral body part values are available for a limited number of body parts. If the identical procedure is performed on contralateral body parts, and a bilateral body part value exists for that body part, a single procedure is coded using the bilateral body part value. If no bilateral body part value exists, each procedure is coded separately using the appropriate body part value.

Examples:
The identical procedure performed on both fallopian tubes is coded once using the body part value Fallopian Tube, Bilateral.

The identical procedure performed on both knee joints is coded twice using the body part values Knee Joint, Right and Knee Joint, Left.

Coronary arteries
B4.4. The coronary arteries are classified as a single body part that is further specified by number of arteries treated. One procedure code specifying multiple arteries is used when the same procedure is performed, including the same device and qualifier values.

Examples:
Angioplasty of two distinct coronary arteries with placement of two stents is coded as Dilation of Coronary Artery, Two Arteries with Two Intraluminal Devices.

Angioplasty of two distinct coronary arteries, one with stent placed and one without, is coded separately as Dilation of Coronary Artery, One Artery with Intraluminal Device, and Dilation of Coronary Artery, One Artery with no device.

Tendons, ligaments, bursae and fascia near a joint
B4.5. Procedures performed on tendons, ligaments, bursae and fascia supporting a joint are coded to the body part in the respective body system that is the focus of the procedure. Procedures performed on joint structures themselves are coded to the body part in the joint body systems.

Examples:
Repair of the anterior cruciate ligament of the knee is coded to the knee bursa and ligament body part in the bursae and ligaments body system.

Knee arthroscopy with shaving of articular cartilage is coded to the knee joint body part in the Lower Joints body system.

Skin, subcutaneous tissue and fascia overlying a joint
B4.6. If a procedure is performed on the skin, subcutaneous tissue or fascia overlying a joint, the procedure is coded to the following body part:

- Shoulder is coded to Upper Arm
- Elbow is coded to Lower Arm
- Wrist is coded to Lower Arm
- Hip is coded to Upper Leg
- Knee is coded to Lower Leg
- Ankle is coded to Foot

Fingers and toes

B4.7. If a body system does not contain a separate body part value for fingers, procedures performed on the fingers are coded to the body part value for the hand. If a body system does not contain a separate body part value for toes, procedures performed on the toes are coded to the body part value for the foot.

> *Example:*
> Excision of finger muscle is coded to one of the hand muscle body part values in the Muscles body system.

Upper and lower intestinal tract

B4.8. In the Gastrointestinal body system, the general body part values Upper Intestinal Tract and Lower Intestinal Tract are provided as an option for the root operations **such as** Change, **Insertion,** Inspection, Removal and Revision. Upper Intestinal Tract includes the portion of the gastrointestinal tract from the esophagus down to and including the duodenum, and Lower Intestinal Tract includes the portion of the gastrointestinal tract from the jejunum down to and including the rectum and anus.

> *Example:*
> In the root operation Change table, change of a device in the jejunum is coded using the body part Lower Intestinal Tract.

B5. Approach

Open approach with percutaneous endoscopic assistance

B5.2a. Procedures performed using the open approach with percutaneous endoscopic assistance are coded to the approach Open.

> *Example:*
> Laparoscopic-assisted sigmoidectomy is coded to the approach Open.

Percutaneous endoscopic approach with extension of incision

B5.2b. Procedures performed using the percutaneous endoscopic approach, with incision or extension of an incision to assist in the removal of all or a portion of a body part or to anastomose a tubular body part to complete the procedure, are coded to the approach value Percutaneous Endoscopic.

> *Examples:*
> Laparoscopic sigmoid colectomy with extension of stapling port for removal of specimen and direct anastomosis is coded to the approach value percutaneous endoscopic.
>
> Laparoscopic nephrectomy with midline incision for removing the resected kidney is coded to the approach value percutaneous endoscopic.
>
> Robotic-assisted laparoscopic prostatectomy with extension of incision for removal of the resected prostate is coded to the approach value percutaneous endoscopic.

External approach

B5.3a. Procedures performed within an orifice on structures that are visible without the aid of any instrumentation are coded to the approach External.

> *Example:*
> Resection of tonsils is coded to the approach External.

B5.3b. Procedures performed indirectly by the application of external force through the intervening body layers are coded to the approach External.

> *Example:*
> Closed reduction of fracture is coded to the approach External.

Percutaneous procedure via device

B5.4. Procedures performed percutaneously via a device placed for the procedure are coded to the approach Percutaneous.

> *Example:*
> Fragmentation of kidney stone performed via percutaneous nephrostomy is coded to the approach Percutaneous.

B6. Device

General guidelines

B6.1a. A device is coded only if a device remains after the procedure is completed. If no device remains, the device value No Device is coded. In limited root operations, the classification provides the qualifier values Temporary and Intraoperative, for specific procedures involving clinically significant devices, where the purpose of the device is to be utilized for a brief duration during the procedure or current inpatient stay. If a device that is intended to remain after the procedure is completed requires removal before the end of the operative episode in which it was inserted (for example, the device size is inadequate or a complication occurs), both the insertion and removal of the device should be coded.

B6.1b. Materials such as sutures, ligatures, radiological markers and temporary post-operative wound drains are considered integral to the performance of a procedure and are not coded as devices.

B6.1c. Procedures performed on a device only and not on a body part are specified in the root operations Change, Irrigation, Removal and Revision, and are coded to the procedure performed.

> *Example:*
> Irrigation of percutaneous nephrostomy tube is coded to the root operation Irrigation of indwelling device in the Administration section.

Drainage device

B6.2. A separate procedure to put in a drainage device is coded to the root operation Drainage with the device value Drainage Device.

Obstetric Section Guidelines (section 1)

C. Obstetrics Section

Products of conception

C1. Procedures performed on the products of conception are coded to the Obstetrics section. Procedures performed on the pregnant female other than the products of conception are coded to the appropriate root operation in the Medical and Surgical section.

> *Examples:*
> Amniocentesis is coded to the products of conception body part in the Obstetrics section.
>
> Repair of obstetric urethral laceration is coded to the urethra body part in the Medical and Surgical section.

Procedures following delivery or abortion

C2. Procedures performed following a delivery or abortion for curettage of the endometrium or evacuation of retained products of conception are all coded in the Obstetrics section, to the root operation Extraction and the body part Products of Conception, Retained.

Diagnostic or therapeutic dilation and curettage performed during times other than the postpartum or post-abortion period are all coded in the Medical and Surgical section, to the root operation Extraction and the body part Endometrium.

Radiation Therapy Section Guidelines (section D)

D. Radiation Therapy Section

Brachytherapy

D1.a. Brachytherapy is coded to the modality Brachytherapy in the Radiation Therapy section. When a radioactive brachytherapy source is left in the body at the end of the procedure, it is coded separately to the root operation Insertion with the device value Radioactive Element.

Example:
Brachytherapy with implantation of a low dose rate brachytherapy source left in the body at the end of the procedure is coded to the applicable treatment site in section D, Radiation Therapy, with the modality Brachytherapy, the modality qualifier value Low Dose Rate, and the applicable isotope value and qualifier value. The implantation of the brachytherapy source is coded separately to the device value Radioactive Element in the appropriate Insertion table of the Medical and Surgical section. The Radiation Therapy section code identifies the specific modality and isotope of the brachytherapy, and the root operation Insertion code identifies the implantation of the brachytherapy source that remains in the body at the end of the procedure.

Exception:
Implantation of Cesium-131 brachytherapy seeds embedded in a collagen matrix to the treatment site after resection of brain tumor is coded to the root operation Insertion with the device value Radioactive Element, Cesium-131 Collagen Implant. The procedure is coded to the root operation Insertion only, because the device value identifies both the implantation of the radioactive element and a specific brachytherapy isotope that is not included in the Radiation Therapy section tables.

D1.b. A separate procedure to place a temporary applicator for delivering the brachytherapy is coded to the root operation Insertion and the device value Other Device.

Examples:
Intrauterine brachytherapy applicator placed as a separate procedure from the brachytherapy procedure is coded to Insertion of Other Device, and the brachytherapy is coded separately using the modality Brachytherapy in the Radiation Therapy section.

Intrauterine brachytherapy applicator placed concomitantly with delivery of the brachytherapy dose is coded with a single code using the modality Brachytherapy in the Radiation Therapy section.

New Technology Section Guidelines (section X)

E. New Technology Section

General guidelines

E1.a. Section X codes fully represent the specific procedure described in the code title, and do not require additional codes from other sections of ICD-10-PCS. When section X contains a code title which fully describes a specific new technology procedure, and it is the only procedure performed, only the section X code is reported for the procedure. There is no need to report an additional code in another section of ICD-10-PCS.

Example:
XW043A6 Introduction of **Cefiderocol** Anti-infective into Central Vein, Percutaneous Approach, New Technology Group **6**, can be coded to indicate that **Cefiderocol** Anti-infective was administered via a central vein. A separate code from table 3E0 in the Administration section of ICD-10-PCS is not coded in addition to this code.

E1.b. When multiple procedures are performed, New Technology section X codes are coded following the multiple procedures guideline.

Examples:
Dual filter cerebral embolic filtration used during transcatheter aortic valve replacement (TAVR), X2A5312 Cerebral Embolic Filtration, Dual Filter in Innominate Artery and Left Common Carotid Artery, Percutaneous Approach, New Technology Group 2, is coded for the cerebral embolic filtration, along with an ICD-10-PCS code for the TAVR procedure.

An extracorporeal flow reversal circuit for embolic neuroprotection placed during a transcarotid arterial revascularization procedure, a code from table X2A, Assistance of the Cardiovascular System is coded for the use of the extracorporeal flow reversal circuit, along with an ICD-10-PCS code for the transcarotid arterial revascularization procedure.

F. Selection of Principal Procedure

The following instructions should be applied in the selection of principal procedure and clarification on the importance of the relation to the principal diagnosis when more than one procedure is performed:

1. Procedure performed for definitive treatment of both principal diagnosis and secondary diagnosis

   a. Sequence procedure performed for definitive treatment most related to principal diagnosis as principal procedure.

2. Procedure performed for definitive treatment and diagnostic procedures performed for both principal diagnosis and secondary diagnosis.

   a. Sequence procedure performed for definitive treatment most related to principal diagnosis as principal procedure

3. A diagnostic procedure was performed for the principal diagnosis and a procedure is performed for definitive treatment of a secondary diagnosis.

   a. Sequence diagnostic procedure as principal procedure, since the procedure most related to the principal diagnosis takes precedence.

4. No procedures performed that are related to principal diagnosis; procedures performed for definitive treatment and diagnostic procedures were performed for secondary diagnosis

   a. Sequence procedure performed for definitive treatment of secondary diagnosis as principal procedure, since there are no procedures (definitive or nondefinitive treatment) related to principal diagnosis.

# #

3f (Aortic) Bioprosthesis valve *use* Zooplastic Tissue in Heart and Great Vessels

A

Abdominal aortic plexus *use* Abdominal Sympathetic Nerve
Abdominal esophagus *use* Esophagus, Lower
Abdominohysterectomy *see* Resection, Uterus ØUT9
Abdominoplasty
  see Alteration, Abdominal Wall ØWØF
  see Repair, Abdominal Wall ØWQF
  see Supplement, Abdominal Wall ØWUF
Abductor hallucis muscle
  use Foot Muscle, Left
  use Foot Muscle, Right
ABECMA® *use* Idecabtagene Vicleucel Immunotherapy
AbioCor® Total Replacement Heart *use* Synthetic Substitute
Ablation
  see Control bleeding in
  see Destruction
Abortion
  Abortifacient 10A07ZX
  Laminaria 10A07ZW
  Products of Conception 10A0
  Vacuum 10A07Z6
Abrasion *see* Extraction
Absolute Pro Vascular (OTW) Self-Expanding Stent System *use* Intraluminal Device
Accelerate PhenoTest™ BC XXE5XN6
Accessory cephalic vein
  use Cephalic Vein, Left
  use Cephalic Vein, Right
Accessory obturator nerve *use* Lumbar Plexus
Accessory phrenic nerve *use* Phrenic Nerve
Accessory spleen *use* Spleen
Acculink (RX) Carotid Stent System *use* Intraluminal Device
Acellular Hydrated Dermis *use* Nonautologous Tissue Substitute
Acetabular cup *use* Liner in Lower Joints
Acetabulectomy
  see Excision, Lower Bones ØQB
  see Resection, Lower Bones ØQT
Acetabulofemoral joint
  use Hip Joint, Left
  use Hip Joint, Right
Acetabuloplasty
  see Repair, Lower Bones ØQQ
  see Replacement, Lower Bones ØQR
  see Supplement, Lower Bones ØQU
Achilles tendon
  use Lower Leg Tendon, Left
  use Lower Leg Tendon, Right
Achillorrhaphy *see* Repair, Tendons ØLQ
Achillotenotomy, achillotomy
  see Division, Tendons ØL8
  see Drainage, Tendons ØL9
Acoustic Pulse Thrombolysis *see* Fragmentation, Artery
Acromioclavicular ligament
  use Shoulder Bursa and Ligament, Left
  use Shoulder Bursa and Ligament, Right
Acromion (process)
  use Scapula, Left
  use Scapula, Right
Acromionectomy
  see Excision, Upper Joints ØRB
  see Resection, Upper Joints ØRT
Acromioplasty
  see Repair, Upper Joints ØRQ
  see Replacement, Upper Joints ØRR
  see Supplement, Upper Joints ØRU
ACTEMRA® *use* Tocilizumab
Activa PC neurostimulator *use* Stimulator Generator, Multiple Array in ØJH
Activa RC neurostimulator *use* Stimulator Generator, Multiple Array Rechargeable in ØJH
Activa SC neurostimulator *use* Stimulator Generator, Single Array in ØJH
Activities of Daily Living Assessment F02
Activities of Daily Living Treatment F08

ACUITY™ Steerable Lead
  use Cardiac Lead, Defibrillator in 02H
  use Cardiac Lead, Pacemaker in 02H
Acupuncture
  Breast
    Anesthesia 8E0H300
    No Qualifier 8E0H30Z
  Integumentary System
    Anesthesia 8E0H300
    No Qualifier 8E0H30Z
Adductor brevis muscle
  use Upper Leg Muscle, Left
  use Upper Leg Muscle, Right
Adductor hallucis muscle
  use Foot Muscle, Left
  use Foot Muscle, Right
Adductor longus muscle
  use Upper Leg Muscle, Left
  use Upper Leg Muscle, Right
Adductor magnus muscle
  use Upper Leg Muscle, Left
  use Upper Leg Muscle, Right
Adenohypophysis *use* Pituitary Gland
Adenoidectomy
  see Excision, Adenoids ØCBQ
  see Resection, Adenoids ØCTQ
Adenoidotomy *see* Drainage, Adenoids ØC9Q
Adhesiolysis *see* Release
Administration
  Blood products *see* Transfusion
  Other substance *see* Introduction of substance in or on
Adrenalectomy
  see Excision, Endocrine System ØGB
  see Resection, Endocrine System ØGT
Adrenalorrhaphy *see* Repair, Endocrine System ØGQ
Adrenalotomy *see* Drainage, Endocrine System ØG9
Advancement
  see Reposition
  see Transfer
Advisa (MRI) *use* Pacemaker, Dual Chamber in ØJH
AFX® Endovascular AAA System *use* Intraluminal Device
Aidoc Briefcase for PE (pulmonary embolism) XXE3X27
AIGISRx Antibacterial Envelope *use* Anti-Infective Envelope
Alar ligament of axis *use* Head and Neck Bursa and Ligament
Alfapump® system *use* Other Device
Alfieri Stitch Valvuloplasty *see* Restriction, Valve, Mitral 02VG
Alimentation *see* Introduction of substance in or on
ALPPS (Associating liver partition and portal vein ligation)
  see Division, Hepatobiliary System and Pancreas ØF8
  see Resection, Hepatobiliary System and Pancreas ØFT
Alteration
  Abdominal Wall ØWØF
  Ankle Region
    Left ØYØL
    Right ØYØK
  Arm
    Lower
      Left ØXØF
      Right ØXØD
    Upper
      Left ØXØ9
      Right ØXØ8
  Axilla
    Left ØXØ5
    Right ØXØ4
  Back
    Lower ØWØL
    Upper ØWØK
  Breast
    Bilateral ØHØV
    Left ØHØU
    Right ØHØT
  Buttock
    Left ØYØ1
    Right ØYØ0
  Chest Wall ØWØ8
  Ear
    Bilateral Ø9Ø2

Alteration — *continued*
  Ear — *continued*
    Left Ø9Ø1
    Right Ø9Ø0
  Elbow Region
    Left ØXØC
    Right ØXØB
  Extremity
    Lower
      Left ØYØB
      Right ØYØ9
    Upper
      Left ØXØ7
      Right ØXØ6
  Eyelid
    Lower
      Left Ø8ØR
      Right Ø8ØQ
    Upper
      Left Ø8ØP
      Right Ø8ØN
  Face ØWØ2
  Head ØWØ0
  Jaw
    Lower ØWØ5
    Upper ØWØ4
  Knee Region
    Left ØYØG
    Right ØYØF
  Leg
    Lower
      Left ØYØJ
      Right ØYØH
    Upper
      Left ØYØD
      Right ØYØC
  Lip
    Lower ØCØ1X
    Upper ØCØ0X
  Nasal Mucosa and Soft Tissue Ø9ØK
  Neck ØWØ6
  Perineum
    Female ØWØN
    Male ØWØM
  Shoulder Region
    Left ØXØ3
    Right ØXØ2
  Subcutaneous Tissue and Fascia
    Abdomen ØJØ8
    Back ØJØ7
    Buttock ØJØ9
    Chest ØJØ6
    Face ØJØ1
    Lower Arm
      Left ØJØH
      Right ØJØG
    Lower Leg
      Left ØJØP
      Right ØJØN
    Neck
      Left ØJØ5
      Right ØJØ4
    Upper Arm
      Left ØJØF
      Right ØJØD
    Upper Leg
      Left ØJØM
      Right ØJØL
  Wrist Region
    Left ØXØH
    Right ØXØG
Alveolar process of mandible
  use Mandible, Left
  use Mandible, Right
Alveolar process of maxilla *use* Maxilla
Alveolectomy
  see Excision, Head and Facial Bones ØNB
  see Resection, Head and Facial Bones ØNT
Alveoloplasty
  see Repair, Head and Facial Bones ØNQ
  see Replacement, Head and Facial Bones ØNR
  see Supplement, Head and Facial Bones ØNU
Alveolotomy
  see Division, Head and Facial Bones ØN8
  see Drainage, Head and Facial Bones ØN9
Ambulatory cardiac monitoring 4A12X45
Amivantamab Monoclonal Antibody XWØ

Amniocentesis see Drainage, Products of Conception 10Q0
Amnioinfusion see Introduction of substance in or on, Products of Conception 3E0E
Amnioscopy 10J08ZZ
Amniotomy see Drainage, Products of Conception 10Q0
AMPLATZER® Muscular VSD Occluder use Synthetic Substitute
Amputation see Detachment
AMS 800® Urinary Control System use Artificial Sphincter in Urinary System
Anal orifice use Anus
Analog radiography see Plain Radiography
Analog radiology see Plain Radiography
Anastomosis see Bypass
Anatomical snuffbox
　use Lower Arm and Wrist Muscle, Left
　use Lower Arm and Wrist Muscle, Right
Andexanet Alfa, Factor Xa Inhibitor Reversal Agent
　use Coagulation Factor Xa, Inactivated
Andexxa use Coagulation Factor Xa, Inactivated
AneuRx® AAA Advantage® use Intraluminal Device
Angiectomy
　see Excision, Heart and Great Vessels 02B
　see Excision, Lower Arteries 04B
　see Excision, Lower Veins 06B
　see Excision, Upper Arteries 03B
　see Excision, Upper Veins 05B
Angiocardiography
　Combined right and left heart see Fluoroscopy, Heart, Right and Left B216
　Left Heart see Fluoroscopy, Heart, Left B215
　Right Heart see Fluoroscopy, Heart, Right B214
　SPY system intravascular fluorescence see Monitoring, Physiological Systems 4A1
Angiography
　see Computerized Tomography (CT Scan), Artery
　see Fluoroscopy, Artery
　see Magnetic Resonance Imaging (MRI), Artery
　see Plain Radiography, Artery
Angioplasty
　see Dilation, Heart and Great Vessels 027
　see Dilation, Lower Arteries 047
　see Dilation, Upper Arteries 037
　see Repair, Heart and Great Vessels 02Q
　see Repair, Lower Arteries 04Q
　see Repair, Upper Arteries 03Q
　see Replacement, Heart and Great Vessels 02R
　see Replacement, Lower Arteries 04R
　see Replacement, Upper Arteries 03R
　see Supplement, Heart and Great Vessels 02U
　see Supplement, Lower Arteries 04U
　see Supplement, Upper Arteries 03U
Angiorrhaphy
　see Repair, Heart and Great Vessels 02Q
　see Repair, Lower Arteries 04Q
　see Repair, Upper Arteries 03Q
Angioscopy 02JY4ZZ, 03JY4ZZ, 04JY4ZZ
Angiotensin II use Synthetic Human Angiotensin II
Angiotripsy
　see Occlusion, Lower Arteries 04L
　see Occlusion, Upper Arteries 03L
Angular artery use Face Artery
Angular vein
　use Face Vein, Left
　use Face Vein, Right
Annular ligament
　use Elbow Bursa and Ligament, Left
　use Elbow Bursa and Ligament, Right
Annuloplasty
　see Repair, Heart and Great Vessels 02Q
　see Supplement, Heart and Great Vessels 02U
Annuloplasty ring use Synthetic Substitute
Anoplasty
　see Repair, Anus 0DQQ
　see Supplement, Anus 0DUQ
Anorectal junction use Rectum
Anoscopy 0DJD8ZZ
Ansa cervicalis use Cervical Plexus
Antabuse therapy HZ93ZZZ
Antebrachial fascia
　use Subcutaneous Tissue and Fascia, Left Lower Arm
　use Subcutaneous Tissue and Fascia, Right Lower Arm
Anterior cerebral artery use Intracranial Artery

Anterior cerebral vein use Intracranial Vein
Anterior choroidal artery use Intracranial Artery
Anterior circumflex humeral artery
　use Axillary Artery, Left
　use Axillary Artery, Right
Anterior communicating artery use Intracranial Artery
Anterior cruciate ligament (ACL)
　use Knee Bursa and Ligament, Left
　use Knee Bursa and Ligament, Right
Anterior crural nerve use Femoral Nerve
Anterior facial vein
　use Face Vein, Left
　use Face Vein, Right
Anterior intercostal artery
　use Internal Mammary Artery, Left
　use Internal Mammary Artery, Right
Anterior interosseous nerve use Median Nerve
Anterior lateral malleolar artery
　use Anterior Tibial Artery, Left
　use Anterior Tibial Artery, Right
Anterior lingual gland use Minor Salivary Gland
Anterior (pectoral) lymph node
　use Lymphatic, Left Axillary
　use Lymphatic, Right Axillary
Anterior medial malleolar artery
　use Anterior Tibial Artery, Left
　use Anterior Tibial Artery, Right
Anterior spinal artery
　use Vertebral Artery, Left
　use Vertebral Artery, Right
Anterior tibial recurrent artery
　use Anterior Tibial Artery, Left
　use Anterior Tibial Artery, Right
Anterior ulnar recurrent artery
　use Ulnar Artery, Left
　use Ulnar Artery, Right
Anterior vagal trunk use Vagus Nerve
Anterior vertebral muscle
　use Neck Muscle, Left
　use Neck Muscle, Right
Antibacterial Envelope (TYRX) (AIGISRx) use Anti-Infective Envelope
Antibiotic-eluting Bone Void Filler XW0V0P7
Antigen-free air conditioning see Atmospheric Control, Physiological Systems 6A0
Antihelix
　use External Ear, Bilateral
　use External Ear, Left
　use External Ear, Right
Antimicrobial envelope use Anti-Infective Envelope
Anti-SARS-CoV-2 hyperimmune globulin use Hyperimmune Globulin
Antitragus
　use External Ear, Bilateral
　use External Ear, Left
　use External Ear, Right
Antrostomy see Drainage, Ear, Nose, Sinus 099
Antrotomy see Drainage, Ear, Nose, Sinus 099
Antrum of Highmore
　use Maxillary Sinus, Left
　use Maxillary Sinus, Right
Aortic annulus use Aortic Valve
Aortic arch use Thoracic Aorta, Ascending/Arch
Aortic intercostal artery use Upper Artery
Aortography
　see Fluoroscopy, Lower Arteries B41
　see Fluoroscopy, Upper Arteries B31
　see Plain Radiography, Lower Arteries B40
　see Plain Radiography, Upper Arteries B30
Aortoplasty
　see Repair, Aorta, Abdominal 04Q0
　see Repair, Aorta, Thoracic, Ascending/Arch 02QX
　see Repair, Aorta, Thoracic, Descending 02QW
　see Replacement, Aorta, Abdominal 04R0
　see Replacement, Aorta, Thoracic, Ascending/Arch 02RX
　see Replacement, Aorta, Thoracic, Descending 02RW
　see Supplement, Aorta, Abdominal 04U0
　see Supplement, Aorta, Thoracic, Ascending/Arch 02UX
　see Supplement, Aorta, Thoracic, Descending 02UW
Apalutamide Antineoplastic XW0DXJ5

Apical (subclavicular) lymph node
　use Lymphatic, Left Axillary
　use Lymphatic, Right Axillary
ApiFix® Minimally Invasive Deformity Correction (MID-C) System use Posterior (Dynamic) Distraction Device in New Technology
Apneustic center use Pons
Appendectomy
　see Excision, Appendix 0DBJ
　see Resection, Appendix 0DTJ
Appendicolysis see Release, Appendix 0DNJ
Appendicotomy see Drainage, Appendix 0D9J
Application see Introduction of substance in or on
aprevo™ use Interbody Fusion Device, Customizable in New Technology
Aquablation therapy, prostate XV508A4
Aquapheresis 6A550Z3
Aqueduct of Sylvius use Cerebral Ventricle
Aqueous humour
　use Anterior Chamber, Left
　use Anterior Chamber, Right
Arachnoid mater, intracranial use Cerebral Meninges
Arachnoid mater, spinal use Spinal Meninges
Arcuate artery
　use Foot Artery, Left
　use Foot Artery, Right
Areola
　use Nipple, Left
　use Nipple, Right
AROM (artificial rupture of membranes) 10907ZC
Arterial canal (duct) use Pulmonary Artery, Left
Arterial pulse tracing see Measurement, Arterial 4A03
Arteriectomy
　see Excision, Heart and Great Vessels 02B
　see Excision, Lower Arteries 04B
　see Excision, Upper Arteries 03B
Arteriography
　see Fluoroscopy, Heart B21
　see Fluoroscopy, Lower Arteries B41
　see Fluoroscopy, Upper Arteries B31
　see Plain Radiography, Heart B20
　see Plain Radiography, Lower Arteries B40
　see Plain Radiography, Upper Arteries B30
Arterioplasty
　see Repair, Heart and Great Vessels 02Q
　see Repair, Lower Arteries 04Q
　see Repair, Upper Arteries 03Q
　see Replacement, Heart and Great Vessels 02R
　see Replacement, Lower Arteries 04R
　see Replacement, Upper Arteries 03R
　see Supplement, Heart and Great Vessels 02U
　see Supplement, Lower Arteries 04U
　see Supplement, Upper Arteries 03U
Arteriorrhaphy
　see Repair, Heart and Great Vessels 02Q
　see Repair, Lower Arteries 04Q
　see Repair, Upper Arteries 03Q
Arterioscopy
　see Inspection, Artery, Lower 04JY
　see Inspection, Artery, Upper 03JY
　see Inspection, Great Vessel 02JY
Arthrectomy
　see Excision, Lower Joints 0SB
　see Excision, Upper Joints 0RB
　see Resection, Lower Joints 0ST
　see Resection, Upper Joints 0RT
Arthrocentesis
　see Drainage, Lower Joints 0S9
　see Drainage, Upper Joints 0R9
Arthrodesis
　see Fusion, Lower Joints 0SG
　see Fusion, Upper Joints 0RG
Arthrography
　see Plain Radiography, Non-Axial Lower Bones BQ0
　see Plain Radiography, Non-Axial Upper Bones BP0
　see Plain Radiography, Skull and Facial Bones BN0
Arthrolysis
　see Release, Lower Joints 0SN
　see Release, Upper Joints 0RN
Arthropexy
　see Repair, Lower Joints 0SQ
　see Repair, Upper Joints 0RQ
　see Reposition, Lower Joints 0SS
　see Reposition, Upper Joints 0RS
Arthroplasty
　see Repair, Lower Joints 0SQ

　▽ Subterms under main terms may continue to next column or page

Arthroplasty — *continued*
  see Repair, Upper Joints ØRQ
  see Replacement, Lower Joints ØSR
  see Replacement, Upper Joints ØRR
  see Supplement, Lower Joints ØSU
  see Supplement, Upper Joints ØRU
Arthroplasty, radial head
  see Replacement, Radius, Left ØPRJ
  see Replacement, Radius, Right ØPRH
Arthroscopy
  see Inspection, Lower Joints ØSJ
  see Inspection, Upper Joints ØRJ
Arthrotomy
  see Drainage, Lower Joints ØS9
  see Drainage, Upper Joints ØR9
Articulating Spacer (Antibiotic) *use* Articulating Spacer in Lower Joints
Artificial anal sphincter (AAS) *use* Artificial Sphincter in Gastrointestinal System
Artificial bowel sphincter (neosphincter) *use* Artificial Sphincter in Gastrointestinal System
Artificial Sphincter
  Insertion of device in
    Anus ØDHQ
    Bladder ØTHB
    Bladder Neck ØTHC
    Urethra ØTHD
  Removal of device from
    Anus ØDPQ
    Bladder ØTPB
    Urethra ØTPD
  Revision of device in
    Anus ØDWQ
    Bladder ØTWB
    Urethra ØTWD
Artificial urinary sphincter (AUS) *use* Artificial Sphincter in Urinary System
Aryepiglottic fold *use* Larynx
Arytenoid cartilage *use* Larynx
Arytenoid muscle
  use Neck Muscle, Left
  use Neck Muscle, Right
Arytenoidectomy *see* Excision, Larynx ØCBS
Arytenoidopexy *see* Repair, Larynx ØCQS
Ascenda Intrathecal Catheter *use* Infusion Device
Ascending aorta *use* Thoracic Aorta, Ascending/Arch
Ascending palatine artery *use* Face Artery
Ascending pharyngeal artery
  use External Carotid Artery, Left
  use External Carotid Artery, Right
aScope™ Duodeno *see* New Technology, Hepatobiliary System and Pancreas XFJ
Aspiration, fine needle
  Fluid or gas *see* Drainage
  Tissue biopsy
    see Excision
    see Extraction
Assessment
  Activities of daily living *see* Activities of Daily Living Assessment, Rehabilitation FØ2
  Hearing *see* Hearing Assessment, Diagnostic Audiology F13
  Hearing aid *see* Hearing Aid Assessment, Diagnostic Audiology F14
  Intravascular perfusion, using indocyanine green (ICG) dye *see* Monitoring, Physiological Systems 4A1
  Motor function *see* Motor Function Assessment, Rehabilitation FØ1
  Nerve function *see* Motor Function Assessment, Rehabilitation FØ1
  Speech *see* Speech Assessment, Rehabilitation FØØ
  Vestibular *see* Vestibular Assessment, Diagnostic Audiology F15
  Vocational *see* Activities of Daily Living Treatment, Rehabilitation FØ8
Assistance
  Cardiac
    Continuous
      Balloon Pump 5AØ221Ø
      Impeller Pump 5AØ221D
      Other Pump 5AØ2216
      Pulsatile Compression 5AØ2215
    Intermittent
      Balloon Pump 5AØ211Ø
      Impeller Pump 5AØ211D
      Other Pump 5AØ2116

Assistance — *continued*
  Cardiac — *continued*
    Intermittent — *continued*
      Pulsatile Compression 5AØ2115
  Circulatory
    Continuous
      Hyperbaric 5AØ5221
      Supersaturated 5AØ522C
    Intermittent
      Hyperbaric 5AØ5121
      Supersaturated 5AØ512C
  Respiratory
    24-96 Consecutive Hours
      Continuous Negative Airway Pressure 5AØ9459
      Continuous Positive Airway Pressure 5AØ9457
      High Nasal Flow/Velocity 5AØ945A
      Intermittent Negative Airway Pressure 5AØ945B
      Intermittent Positive Airway Pressure 5AØ9458
      No Qualifier 5AØ945Z
    Continuous, Filtration 5AØ920Z
    Greater than 96 Consecutive Hours
      Continuous Negative Airway Pressure 5AØ9559
      Continuous Positive Airway Pressure 5AØ9557
      High Nasal Flow/Velocity 5AØ955A
      Intermittent Negative Airway Pressure 5AØ955B
      Intermittent Positive Airway Pressure 5AØ9558
      No Qualifier 5AØ955Z
    Less than 24 Consecutive Hours
      Continuous Negative Airway Pressure 5AØ9359
      Continuous Positive Airway Pressure 5AØ9357
      High Nasal Flow/Velocity 5AØ935A
      Intermittent Negative Airway Pressure 5AØ935B
      Intermittent Positive Airway Pressure 5AØ9358
      No Qualifier 5AØ935Z
Associating liver partition and portal vein ligation (ALPPS)
  see Division, Hepatobiliary System and Pancreas ØF8
  see Resection, Hepatobiliary System and Pancreas ØFT
Assurant (Cobalt) stent *use* Intraluminal Device
Atezolizumab Antineoplastic XWØ
Atherectomy
  see Extirpation, Heart and Great Vessels Ø2C
  see Extirpation, Lower Arteries Ø4C
  see Extirpation, Upper Arteries Ø3C
Atlantoaxial joint *use* Cervical Vertebral Joint
Atmospheric Control 6AØZ
AtriClip LAA Exclusion System *use* Extraluminal Device
Atrioseptoplasty
  see Repair, Heart and Great Vessels Ø2Q
  see Replacement, Heart and Great Vessels Ø2R
  see Supplement, Heart and Great Vessels Ø2U
Atrioventricular node *use* Conduction Mechanism
Atrium dextrum cordis *use* Atrium, Right
Atrium pulmonale *use* Atrium, Left
Attain Ability® lead Ø2H
  use Cardiac Lead, Defibrillator in Ø2H
  use Cardiac Lead, Pacemaker in Ø2H
Attain Starfix® (OTW) lead
  use Cardiac Lead, Defibrillator in Ø2H
  use Cardiac Lead, Pacemaker in Ø2H
Audiology, diagnostic
  see Hearing Aid Assessment, Diagnostic Audiology F14
  see Hearing Assessment, Diagnostic Audiology F13
  see Vestibular Assessment, Diagnostic Audiology F15
Audiometry *see* Hearing Assessment, Diagnostic Audiology F13
Auditory tube
  use Eustachian Tube, Left
  use Eustachian Tube, Right

Auerbach's (myenteric) plexus *use* Abdominal Sympathetic Nerve
Auricle
  use External Ear, Bilateral
  use External Ear, Left
  use External Ear, Right
Auricularis muscle *use* Head Muscle
Autograft *use* Autologous Tissue Substitute
Autologous artery graft
  use Autologous Arterial Tissue in Heart and Great Vessels
  use Autologous Arterial Tissue in Lower Arteries
  use Autologous Arterial Tissue in Lower Veins
  use Autologous Arterial Tissue in Upper Arteries
  use Autologous Arterial Tissue in Upper Veins
Autologous vein graft
  use Autologous Venous Tissue in Heart and Great Vessels
  use Autologous Venous Tissue in Lower Arteries
  use Autologous Venous Tissue in Lower Veins
  use Autologous Venous Tissue in Upper Arteries
  use Autologous Venous Tissue in Upper Veins
Automated Chest Compression (ACC) 5A1221J
AutoPulse® Resuscitation System 5A1221J
Autotransfusion *see* Transfusion
Autotransplant
  Adrenal tissue *see* Reposition, Endocrine System ØGS
  Kidney *see* Reposition, Urinary System ØTS
  Pancreatic tissue *see* Reposition, Pancreas ØFSG
  Parathyroid tissue *see* Reposition, Endocrine System ØGS
  Thyroid tissue *see* Reposition, Endocrine System ØGS
  Tooth *see* Reattachment, Mouth and Throat ØCM
Avulsion *see* Extraction
AVYCAZ® (ceftazidime-avibactam) *use* Other Anti-infective
Axial Lumbar Interbody Fusion System *use* Interbody Fusion Device in Lower Joints
AxiaLIF® System *use* Interbody Fusion Device in Lower Joints
Axicabtagene Ciloleucel *use* Axicabtagene Ciloleucel Immunotherapy
Axicabtagene Ciloleucel Immunotherapy XWØ
Axillary fascia
  use Subcutaneous Tissue and Fascia, Left Upper Arm
  use Subcutaneous Tissue and Fascia, Right Upper Arm
Axillary nerve *use* Brachial Plexus
AZEDRA® *use* Iobenguane I-131 Antineoplastic

B

BAK/C® Interbody Cervical Fusion System *use* Interbody Fusion Device in Upper Joints
BAL (bronchial alveolar lavage), diagnostic *see* Drainage, Respiratory System ØB9
Balanoplasty
  see Repair, Penis ØVQS
  see Supplement, Penis ØVUS
Balloon atrial septostomy (BAS) Ø2163Z7
Balloon Pump
  Continuous, Output 5AØ221Ø
  Intermittent, Output 5AØ211Ø
Bamlanivimab Monoclonal Antibody XWØ
Bandage, Elastic *see* Compression
Banding
  see Occlusion
  see Restriction
Banding, esophageal varices *see* Occlusion, Vein, Esophageal Ø6L3
Banding, laparoscopic (adjustable) gastric
  Initial procedure ØDV64CZ
  Surgical correction *see* Revision of device in, Stomach ØDW6
Bard® Composix® Kugel® patch *use* Synthetic Substitute
Bard® Composix® (E/X) (LP) mesh *use* Synthetic Substitute
Bard® Dulex™ mesh *use* Synthetic Substitute
Bard® Ventralex™ hernia patch *use* Synthetic Substitute
Baricitinib XWØ

Barium swallow see Fluoroscopy, Gastrointestinal System BD1
Baroreflex Activation Therapy® (BAT®)
  use Stimulator Generator in Subcutaneous Tissue and Fascia
  use Stimulator Lead in Upper Arteries
Barricaid® Annular Closure Device (ACD) *use* Synthetic Substitute
Bartholin's (greater vestibular) gland *use* Vestibular Gland
Basal (internal) cerebral vein *use* Intracranial Vein
Basal metabolic rate (BMR) *see* Measurement, Physiological Systems 4A0Z
Basal nuclei *use* Basal Ganglia
Base of Tongue *use* Pharynx
Basilar artery *use* Intracranial Artery
Basis pontis *use* Pons
Beam Radiation
  Abdomen DW03
    Intraoperative DW033Z0
  Adrenal Gland DG02
    Intraoperative DG023Z0
  Bile Ducts DF02
    Intraoperative DF023Z0
  Bladder DT02
    Intraoperative DT023Z0
  Bone
    Intraoperative DP0C3Z0
    Other DP0C
  Bone Marrow D700
    Intraoperative D7003Z0
  Brain D000
    Intraoperative D0003Z0
  Brain Stem D001
    Intraoperative D0013Z0
  Breast
    Left DM00
      Intraoperative DM003Z0
    Right DM01
      Intraoperative DM013Z0
  Bronchus DB01
    Intraoperative DB013Z0
  Cervix DU01
    Intraoperative DU013Z0
  Chest DW02
    Intraoperative DW023Z0
  Chest Wall DB07
    Intraoperative DB073Z0
  Colon DD05
    Intraoperative DD053Z0
  Diaphragm DB08
    Intraoperative DB083Z0
  Duodenum DD02
    Intraoperative DD023Z0
  Ear D900
    Intraoperative D9003Z0
  Esophagus DD00
    Intraoperative DD003Z0
  Eye D800
    Intraoperative D8003Z0
  Femur DP09
    Intraoperative DP093Z0
  Fibula DP0B
    Intraoperative DP0B3Z0
  Gallbladder DF01
    Intraoperative DF013Z0
  Gland
    Adrenal DG02
      Intraoperative DG023Z0
    Parathyroid DG04
      Intraoperative DG043Z0
    Pituitary DG00
      Intraoperative DG003Z0
    Thyroid DG05
      Intraoperative DG053Z0
  Glands
    Intraoperative D9063Z0
    Salivary D906
  Head and Neck DW01
    Intraoperative DW013Z0
  Hemibody DW04
    Intraoperative DW043Z0
  Humerus DP06
    Intraoperative DP063Z0
  Hypopharynx D903
    Intraoperative D9033Z0
  Ileum DD04
    Intraoperative DD043Z0

Beam Radiation — *continued*
  Jejunum DD03
    Intraoperative DD033Z0
  Kidney DT00
    Intraoperative DT003Z0
  Larynx D90B
    Intraoperative D90B3Z0
  Liver DF00
    Intraoperative DF003Z0
  Lung DB02
    Intraoperative DB023Z0
  Lymphatics
    Abdomen D706
      Intraoperative D7063Z0
    Axillary D704
      Intraoperative D7043Z0
    Inguinal D708
      Intraoperative D7083Z0
    Neck D703
      Intraoperative D7033Z0
    Pelvis D707
      Intraoperative D7073Z0
    Thorax D705
      Intraoperative D7053Z0
  Mandible DP03
    Intraoperative DP033Z0
  Maxilla DP02
    Intraoperative DP023Z0
  Mediastinum DB06
    Intraoperative DB063Z0
  Mouth D904
    Intraoperative D9043Z0
  Nasopharynx D90D
    Intraoperative D90D3Z0
  Neck and Head DW01
    Intraoperative DW013Z0
  Nerve
    Intraoperative D0073Z0
    Peripheral D007
  Nose D901
    Intraoperative D9013Z0
  Oropharynx D90F
    Intraoperative D90F3Z0
  Ovary DU00
    Intraoperative DU003Z0
  Palate
    Hard D908
      Intraoperative D9083Z0
    Soft D909
      Intraoperative D9093Z0
  Pancreas DF03
    Intraoperative DF033Z0
  Parathyroid Gland DG04
    Intraoperative DG043Z0
  Pelvic Bones DP08
    Intraoperative DP083Z0
  Pelvic Region DW06
    Intraoperative DW063Z0
  Pineal Body DG01
    Intraoperative DG013Z0
  Pituitary Gland DG00
    Intraoperative DG003Z0
  Pleura DB05
    Intraoperative DB053Z0
  Prostate DV00
    Intraoperative DV003Z0
  Radius DP07
    Intraoperative DP073Z0
  Rectum DD07
    Intraoperative DD073Z0
  Rib DP05
    Intraoperative DP053Z0
  Sinuses D907
    Intraoperative D9073Z0
  Skin
    Abdomen DH08
      Intraoperative DH083Z0
    Arm DH04
      Intraoperative DH043Z0
    Back DH07
      Intraoperative DH073Z0
    Buttock DH09
      Intraoperative DH093Z0
    Chest DH06
      Intraoperative DH063Z0
    Face DH02
      Intraoperative DH023Z0
    Leg DH0B
      Intraoperative DH0B3Z0

Beam Radiation — *continued*
  Skin — *continued*
    Neck DH03
      Intraoperative DH033Z0
  Skull DP00
    Intraoperative DP003Z0
  Spinal Cord D006
    Intraoperative D0063Z0
  Spleen D702
    Intraoperative D7023Z0
  Sternum DP04
    Intraoperative DP043Z0
  Stomach DD01
    Intraoperative DD013Z0
  Testis DV01
    Intraoperative DV013Z0
  Thymus D701
    Intraoperative D7013Z0
  Thyroid Gland DG05
    Intraoperative DG053Z0
  Tibia DP0B
    Intraoperative DP0B3Z0
  Tongue D905
    Intraoperative D9053Z0
  Trachea DB00
    Intraoperative DB003Z0
  Ulna DP07
    Intraoperative DP073Z0
  Ureter DT01
    Intraoperative DT013Z0
  Urethra DT03
    Intraoperative DT033Z0
  Uterus DU02
    Intraoperative DU023Z0
  Whole Body DW05
    Intraoperative DW053Z0
Bedside swallow F00ZJWZ
Berlin Heart Ventricular Assist Device *use* Implantable Heart Assist System in Heart and Great Vessels
Bezlotoxumab Monoclonal Antibody XW0
Biceps brachii muscle
  use Upper Arm Muscle, Left
  use Upper Arm Muscle, Right
Biceps femoris muscle
  use Upper Leg Muscle, Left
  use Upper Leg Muscle, Right
Bicipital aponeurosis
  use Subcutaneous Tissue and Fascia, Left Lower Arm
  use Subcutaneous Tissue and Fascia, Right Lower Arm
Bicuspid valve *use* Mitral Valve
Bili light therapy *see* Phototherapy, Skin 6A60
Bioactive embolization coil(s) *use* Intraluminal Device, Bioactive in Upper Arteries
Bioengineered Allogeneic Construct, Skin XHRPXF7
Biofeedback GZC9ZZZ
BioFire® FilmArray® Pneumonia Panel XXEBXQ6
Biopsy
  see Drainage with qualifier Diagnostic
  see Excision with qualifier Diagnostic
  see Extraction with qualifier Diagnostic
BiPAP *see* Assistance, Respiratory 5A09
Bisection *see* Division
Biventricular external heart assist system *use* Short-term External Heart Assist System in Heart and Great Vessels
Blepharectomy
  see Excision, Eye 08B
  see Resection, Eye 08T
Blepharoplasty
  see Repair, Eye 08Q
  see Replacement, Eye 08R
  see Reposition, Eye 08S
  see Supplement, Eye 08U
Blepharorrhaphy *see* Repair, Eye 08Q
Blepharotomy *see* Drainage, Eye 089
Blinatumomab *use* Other Antineoplastic
BLINCYTO® (blinatumomab) *use* Other Antineoplastic
Block, Nerve, anesthetic injection 3E0T3BZ
Blood glucose monitoring system *use* Monitoring Device
Blood pressure *see* Measurement, Arterial 4A03
BMR (basal metabolic rate) *see* Measurement, Physiological Systems 4A0Z

Body of femur
   use Femoral Shaft, Left
   use Femoral Shaft, Right
Body of fibula
   use Fibula, Left
   use Fibula, Right
Bone anchored hearing device
   use Hearing Device, Bone Conduction in Ø9H
   use Hearing Device in Head and Facial Bones
Bone bank bone graft *use* Nonautologous Tissue
   Substitute
Bone Growth Stimulator
   Insertion of device in
     Bone
       Facial ØNHW
       Lower ØQHY
       Nasal ØNHB
       Upper ØPHY
     Skull ØNHØ
   Removal of device from
     Bone
       Facial ØNPW
       Lower ØQPY
       Nasal ØNPB
       Upper ØPPY
     Skull ØNPØ
   Revision of device in
     Bone
       Facial ØNWW
       Lower ØQWY
       Nasal ØNWB
       Upper ØPWY
     Skull ØNWØ
Bone marrow transplant *see* Transfusion, Circulatory
   3Ø2
Bone morphogenetic protein 2 (BMP 2) *use* Recombinant Bone Morphogenetic Protein
Bone screw (interlocking) (lag) (pedicle) (recessed)
   use Internal Fixation Device in Head and Facial
     Bones
   use Internal Fixation Device in Lower Bones
   use Internal Fixation Device in Upper Bones
Bony labyrinth
   use Inner Ear, Left
   use Inner Ear, Right
Bony orbit
   use Orbit, Left
   use Orbit, Right
Bony vestibule
   use Inner Ear, Left
   use Inner Ear, Right
Botallo's duct *use* Pulmonary Artery, Left
Bovine pericardial valve *use* Zooplastic Tissue in Heart
   and Great Vessels
Bovine pericardium graft *use* Zooplastic Tissue in
   Heart and Great Vessels
BP (blood pressure) *see* Measurement, Arterial 4AØ3
Brachial (lateral) lymph node
   use Lymphatic, Left Axillary
   use Lymphatic, Right Axillary
Brachialis muscle
   use Upper Arm Muscle, Left
   use Upper Arm Muscle, Right
Brachiocephalic artery *use* Innominate Artery
Brachiocephalic trunk *use* Innominate Artery
Brachiocephalic vein
   use Innominate Vein, Left
   use Innominate Vein, Right
Brachioradialis muscle
   use Lower Arm and Wrist Muscle, Left
   use Lower Arm and Wrist Muscle, Right
Brachytherapy
   Abdomen DW13
   Adrenal Gland DG12
   Back
     Lower DW1LBB
     Upper DW1KBB
   Bile Ducts DF12
   Bladder DT12
   Bone Marrow D71Ø
   Brain DØ1Ø
   Brain Stem DØ11
   Breast
     Left DM1Ø
     Right DM11
   Bronchus DB11
   Cervix DU11

Brachytherapy — *continued*
   Chest DW12
   Chest Wall DB17
   Colon DD15
   Cranial Cavity DW1ØBB
   Diaphragm DB18
   Duodenum DD12
   Ear D91Ø
   Esophagus DD1Ø
   Extremity
     Lower DW1YBB
     Upper DW1XBB
   Eye D81Ø
   Gallbladder DF11
   Gastrointestinal Tract DW1PBB
   Genitourinary Tract DW1RBB
   Gland
     Adrenal DG12
     Parathyroid DG14
     Pituitary DG1Ø
     Thyroid DG15
   Glands, Salivary D916
   Head and Neck DW11
   Hypopharynx D913
   Ileum DD14
   Jejunum DD13
   Kidney DT1Ø
   Larynx D91B
   Liver DF1Ø
   Lung DB12
   Lymphatics
     Abdomen D716
     Axillary D714
     Inguinal D718
     Neck D713
     Pelvis D717
     Thorax D715
   Mediastinum DB16
   Mouth D914
   Nasopharynx D91D
   Neck and Head DW11
   Nerve, Peripheral DØ17
   Nose D911
   Oropharynx D91F
   Ovary DU1Ø
   Palate
     Hard D918
     Soft D919
   Pancreas DF13
   Parathyroid Gland DG14
   Pelvic Region DW16
   Pineal Body DG11
   Pituitary Gland DG1Ø
   Pleura DB15
   Prostate DV1Ø
   Rectum DD17
   Respiratory Tract DW1QBB
   Sinuses D917
   Spinal Cord DØ16
   Spleen D712
   Stomach DD11
   Testis DV11
   Thymus D711
   Thyroid Gland DG15
   Tongue D915
   Trachea DB1Ø
   Ureter DT11
   Urethra DT13
   Uterus DU12
Brachytherapy, CivaSheet®
   see Brachytherapy with qualifier Unidirectional
     Source
   see Insertion with device Radioactive Element
Brachytherapy seeds *use* Radioactive Element
Breast procedures, skin only *use* Skin, Chest
Brexanolone XWØ
Brexucabtagene Autoleucel *use* Brexucabtagene
   Autoleucel Immunotherapy
Brexucabtagene Autoleucel Immunotherapy XWØ
Broad ligament *use* Uterine Supporting Structure
Bromelain-enriched Proteolytic Enzyme XWØ
Bronchial artery *use* Upper Artery
Bronchography
   see Fluoroscopy, Respiratory System BB1
   see Plain Radiography, Respiratory System BBØ
Bronchoplasty
   see Repair, Respiratory System ØBQ
   see Supplement, Respiratory System ØBU

Bronchorrhaphy *see* Repair, Respiratory System ØBQ
Bronchoscopy ØBJØ8ZZ
Bronchotomy *see* Drainage, Respiratory System ØB9
Bronchus Intermedius *use* Main Bronchus, Right
BRYAN® Cervical Disc System *use* Synthetic Substitute
Buccal gland *use* Buccal Mucosa
Buccinator lymph node *use* Lymphatic, Head
Buccinator muscle *use* Facial Muscle
Buckling, scleral with implant *see* Supplement, Eye
   Ø8U
Bulbospongiosus muscle *use* Perineum Muscle
Bulbourethral (Cowper's) gland *use* Urethra
Bundle of His *use* Conduction Mechanism
Bundle of Kent *use* Conduction Mechanism
Bunionectomy *see* Excision, Lower Bones ØQB
Bursectomy
   see Excision, Bursae and Ligaments ØMB
   see Resection, Bursae and Ligaments ØMT
Bursocentesis *see* Drainage, Bursae and Ligaments
   ØM9
Bursography
   see Plain Radiography, Non-Axial Lower Bones BQØ
   see Plain Radiography, Non-Axial Upper Bones BPØ
Bursotomy
   see Division, Bursae and Ligaments ØM8
   see Drainage, Bursae and Ligaments ØM9
BVS 5ØØØ Ventricular Assist Device *use* Short-term
   External Heart Assist System in Heart and Great
   Vessels
Bypass
   Anterior Chamber
     Left Ø8133
     Right Ø8123
   Aorta
     Abdominal Ø41Ø
     Thoracic
       Ascending/Arch Ø21X
       Descending Ø21W
   Artery
     Anterior Tibial
       Left Ø41Q
       Right Ø41P
     Axillary
       Left Ø316Ø
       Right Ø315Ø
     Brachial
       Left Ø318
       Right Ø317
     Common Carotid
       Left Ø31JØ
       Right Ø31HØ
     Common Iliac
       Left Ø41D
       Right Ø41C
     Coronary
       Four or More Arteries Ø213
       One Artery Ø21Ø
       Three Arteries Ø212
       Two Arteries Ø211
     External Carotid
       Left Ø31NØ
       Right Ø31MØ
     External Iliac
       Left Ø41J
       Right Ø41H
     Femoral
       Left Ø41L
       Right Ø41K
     Foot
       Left Ø41W
       Right Ø41V
     Hepatic Ø413
     Innominate Ø312Ø
     Internal Carotid
       Left Ø31LØ
       Right Ø31KØ
     Internal Iliac
       Left Ø41F
       Right Ø41E
     Intracranial Ø31GØ
     Peroneal
       Left Ø41U
       Right Ø41T
     Popliteal
       Left Ø41N
       Right Ø41M
     Posterior Tibial
       Left Ø41S

Bypass — *continued*
  Artery — *continued*
    Posterior Tibial — *continued*
      Right Ø41R
    Pulmonary
      Left Ø21R
      Right Ø21Q
    Pulmonary Trunk Ø21P
    Radial
      Left Ø31C
      Right Ø31B
    Splenic Ø414
    Subclavian
      Left Ø314Ø
      Right Ø313Ø
    Temporal
      Left Ø31TØ
      Right Ø31SØ
    Ulnar
      Left Ø31A
      Right Ø319
  Atrium
    Left Ø217
    Right Ø216
  Bladder ØT1B
  Cavity, Cranial ØW11ØJ
  Cecum ØD1H
  Cerebral Ventricle ØØ16
  Colon
    Ascending ØD1K
    Descending ØD1M
    Sigmoid ØD1N
    Transverse ØD1L
  Duct
    Common Bile ØF19
    Cystic ØF18
    Hepatic
      Common ØF17
      Left ØF16
      Right ØF15
    Lacrimal
      Left Ø81Y
      Right Ø81X
    Pancreatic ØF1D
      Accessory ØF1F
  Duodenum ØD19
  Ear
    Left Ø91EØ
    Right Ø91DØ
  Esophagus ØD15
    Lower ØD13
    Middle ØD12
    Upper ØD11
  Fallopian Tube
    Left ØU16
    Right ØU15
  Gallbladder ØF14
  Ileum ØD1B
  Intestine
    Large ØD1E
    Small ØD18
  Jejunum ØD1A
  Kidney Pelvis
    Left ØT14
    Right ØT13
  Pancreas ØF1G
  Pelvic Cavity ØW1J
  Peritoneal Cavity ØW1G
  Pleural Cavity
    Left ØW1B
    Right ØW19
  Spinal Canal ØØ1U
  Stomach ØD16
  Trachea ØB11
  Ureter
    Left ØT17
    Right ØT16
  Ureters, Bilateral ØT18
  Vas Deferens
    Bilateral ØV1Q
    Left ØV1P
    Right ØV1N
  Vein
    Axillary
      Left Ø518
      Right Ø517
    Azygos Ø51Ø
    Basilic
      Left Ø51C

Bypass — *continued*
  Vein — *continued*
    Basilic — *continued*
      Right Ø51B
    Brachial
      Left Ø51A
      Right Ø519
    Cephalic
      Left Ø51F
      Right Ø51D
    Colic Ø617
    Common Iliac
      Left Ø61D
      Right Ø61C
    Esophageal Ø613
    External Iliac
      Left Ø61G
      Right Ø61F
    External Jugular
      Left Ø51Q
      Right Ø51P
    Face
      Left Ø51V
      Right Ø51T
    Femoral
      Left Ø61N
      Right Ø61M
    Foot
      Left Ø61V
      Right Ø61T
    Gastric Ø612
    Hand
      Left Ø51H
      Right Ø51G
    Hemiazygos Ø511
    Hepatic Ø614
    Hypogastric
      Left Ø61J
      Right Ø61H
    Inferior Mesenteric Ø616
    Innominate
      Left Ø514
      Right Ø513
    Internal Jugular
      Left Ø51N
      Right Ø51M
    Intracranial Ø51L
    Portal Ø618
    Renal
      Left Ø61B
      Right Ø619
    Saphenous
      Left Ø61Q
      Right Ø61P
    Splenic Ø611
    Subclavian
      Left Ø516
      Right Ø515
    Superior Mesenteric Ø615
    Vertebral
      Left Ø51S
      Right Ø51R
    Vena Cava
      Inferior Ø61Ø
      Superior Ø21V
    Ventricle
      Left Ø21L
      Right Ø21K
Bypass, cardiopulmonary 5A1221Z

C

Caesarean section *see* Extraction, Products of Conception 1ØDØ
Calcaneocuboid joint
  use Tarsal Joint, Left
  use Tarsal Joint, Right
Calcaneocuboid ligament
  use Foot Bursa and Ligament, Left
  use Foot Bursa and Ligament, Right
Calcaneofibular ligament
  use Ankle Bursa and Ligament, Left
  use Ankle Bursa and Ligament, Right
Calcaneus
  use Tarsal, Left
  use Tarsal, Right

Cannulation
  see Bypass
  see Dilation
  see Drainage
  see Irrigation
Canthorrhaphy *see* Repair, Eye Ø8Q
Canthotomy *see* Release, Eye Ø8N
Capitate bone
  use Carpal, Left
  use Carpal, Right
Caplacizumab XWØ
Capsulectomy, lens *see* Excision, Eye Ø8B
Capsulorrhaphy, joint
  see Repair, Lower Joints ØSQ
  see Repair, Upper Joints ØRQ
Caption Guidance system X2JAX47
Cardia *use* Esophagogastric Junction
Cardiac contractility modulation lead *use* Cardiac
  Lead in Heart and Great Vessels
Cardiac event recorder *use* Monitoring Device
Cardiac Lead
  Defibrillator
    Atrium
      Left Ø2H7
      Right Ø2H6
    Pericardium Ø2HN
    Vein, Coronary Ø2H4
    Ventricle
      Left Ø2HL
      Right Ø2HK
  Insertion of device in
    Atrium
      Left Ø2H7
      Right Ø2H6
    Pericardium Ø2HN
    Vein, Coronary Ø2H4
    Ventricle
      Left Ø2HL
      Right Ø2HK
  Pacemaker
    Atrium
      Left Ø2H7
      Right Ø2H6
    Pericardium Ø2HN
    Vein, Coronary Ø2H4
    Ventricle
      Left Ø2HL
      Right Ø2HK
  Removal of device from, Heart Ø2PA
  Revision of device in, Heart Ø2WA
Cardiac plexus *use* Thoracic Sympathetic Nerve
Cardiac Resynchronization Defibrillator Pulse
  Generator
  Abdomen ØJH8
  Chest ØJH6
Cardiac Resynchronization Pacemaker Pulse Generator
  Abdomen ØJH8
  Chest ØJH6
Cardiac resynchronization therapy (CRT) lead
  use Cardiac Lead, Defibrillator in Ø2H
  use Cardiac Lead, Pacemaker in Ø2H
Cardiac Rhythm Related Device
  Insertion of device in
    Abdomen ØJH8
    Chest ØJH6
  Removal of device from, Subcutaneous Tissue and
    Fascia, Trunk ØJPT
  Revision of device in, Subcutaneous Tissue and
    Fascia, Trunk ØJWT
Cardiocentesis *see* Drainage, Pericardial Cavity ØW9D
Cardioesophageal junction *use* Esophagogastric
  Junction
Cardiolysis *see* Release, Heart and Great Vessels Ø2N
CardioMEMS® pressure sensor *use* Monitoring Device,
  Pressure Sensor in Ø2H
Cardiomyotomy *see* Division, Esophagogastric Junction ØD84
Cardioplegia *see* Introduction of substance in or on,
  Heart 3EØ8
Cardiorrhaphy *see* Repair, Heart and Great Vessels Ø2Q
Cardioversion 5A22Ø4Z
Caregiver Training FØFZ
Carmat total artificial heart (TAH) *use* Biologic with
  Synthetic Substitute, Autoregulated Electrohydraulic in Ø2R

Caroticotympanic artery
 use Internal Carotid Artery, Left
 use Internal Carotid Artery, Right
Carotid glomus
 use Carotid Bodies, Bilateral
 use Carotid Body, Left
 use Carotid Body, Right
Carotid sinus
 use Internal Carotid Artery, Left
 use Internal Carotid Artery, Right
Carotid (artery) sinus (baroreceptor) lead *use*
 Stimulator Lead in Upper Arteries
Carotid sinus nerve *use* Glossopharyngeal Nerve
Carotid WALLSTENT® Monorail® Endoprosthesis
 use Intraluminal Device
Carpectomy
 see Excision, Upper Bones ØPB
 see Resection, Upper Bones ØPT
Carpometacarpal ligament
 use Hand Bursa and Ligament, Left
 use Hand Bursa and Ligament, Right
**Casirivimab (REGN10933) and Imdevimab
 (REGN10987)** *use* REGN-COV2 Monoclonal Antibody
Casting *see* Immobilization
CAT scan *see* Computerized Tomography (CT Scan)
Catheterization
 see Dilation
 see Drainage
 see Insertion of device in
 see Irrigation
 Heart *see* Measurement, Cardiac 4A02
 Umbilical vein, for infusion 06H033T
Cauda equina *use* Lumbar Spinal Cord
Cauterization
 see Destruction
 see Repair
Cavernous plexus *use* Head and Neck Sympathetic
 Nerve
CBMA (Concentrated Bone Marrow Aspirate) *use*
 Concentrated Bone Marrow Aspirate
CBMA (Concentrated Bone Marrow Aspirate) injection, intramuscular XK02303
CD24Fc Immunomodulator XW0
Cecectomy
 see Excision, Cecum ØDBH
 see Resection, Cecum ØDTH
Cecocolostomy
 see Bypass, Gastrointestinal System ØD1
 see Drainage, Gastrointestinal System ØD9
Cecopexy
 see Repair, Cecum ØDQH
 see Reposition, Cecum ØDSH
Cecoplication *see* Restriction, Cecum ØDVH
Cecorrhaphy *see* Repair, Cecum ØDQH
Cecostomy
 see Bypass, Cecum ØD1H
 see Drainage, Cecum ØD9H
Cecotomy *see* Drainage, Cecum ØD9H
Cefiderocol Anti-infective XW0
Ceftazidime-avibactam *use* Other Anti-infective
Ceftolozane/Tazobactam Anti-infective XW0
Celiac ganglion *use* Abdominal Sympathetic Nerve
Celiac lymph node *use* Lymphatic, Aortic
Celiac (solar) plexus *use* Abdominal Sympathetic
 Nerve
Celiac trunk *use* Celiac Artery
Central axillary lymph node
 use Lymphatic, Left Axillary
 use Lymphatic, Right Axillary
Central venous pressure *see* Measurement, Venous
 4A04
Centrimag® Blood Pump *use* Short-term External
 Heart Assist System in Heart and Great Vessels
Cephalogram BN00ZZZ
CERAMENT® G *use* Antibiotic-eluting Bone Void Filler
Ceramic on ceramic bearing surface *use* Synthetic
 Substitute, Ceramic in ØSR
Cerclage *see* Restriction
Cerebral aqueduct (Sylvius) *use* Cerebral Ventricle
Cerebral Embolic Filtration
 Dual Filter X2A5312
 Extracorporeal Flow Reversal Circuit X2A
 Single Deflection Filter X2A6325
Cerebrum *use* Brain
Cervical esophagus *use* Esophagus, Upper

Cervical facet joint
 use Cervical Vertebral Joint
 use Cervical Vertebral Joint, 2 or more
Cervical ganglion *use* Head and Neck Sympathetic
 Nerve
Cervical interspinous ligament *use* Head and Neck
 Bursa and Ligament
Cervical intertransverse ligament *use* Head and
 Neck Bursa and Ligament
Cervical Ligamentum Flavum *use* Head and Neck
 Bursa and Ligament
Cervical Lymph Node
 use Lymphatic, Left Neck
 use Lymphatic, Right Neck
Cervicectomy
 see Excision, Cervix ØUBC
 see Resection, Cervix ØUTC
Cervicothoracic facet joint *use* Cervicothoracic Vertebral Joint
Cesarean section *see* Extraction, Products of Conception 10D0
Cesium-131 Collagen Implant *use* Radioactive Element, Cesium-131 Collagen Implant in 00H
Change Device in
 Abdominal Wall ØW2FX
 Back
  Lower ØW2LX
  Upper ØW2KX
 Bladder ØT2BX
 Bone
  Facial ØN2WX
  Lower ØQ2YX
  Nasal ØN2BX
  Upper ØP2YX
 Bone Marrow Ø72TX
 Brain ØØ2ØX
 Breast
  Left ØH2UX
  Right ØH2TX
 Bursa and Ligament
  Lower ØM2YX
  Upper ØM2XX
 Cavity, Cranial ØW21X
 Chest Wall ØW28X
 Cisterna Chyli Ø72LX
 Diaphragm ØB2TX
 Duct
  Hepatobiliary ØF2BX
  Pancreatic ØF2DX
 Ear
  Left Ø92JX
  Right Ø92HX
 Epididymis and Spermatic Cord ØV2MX
 Extremity
  Lower
   Left ØY2BX
   Right ØY29X
  Upper
   Left ØX27X
   Right ØX26X
 Eye
  Left Ø821X
  Right Ø820X
 Face ØW22X
 Fallopian Tube ØU28X
 Gallbladder ØF24X
 Gland
  Adrenal ØG25X
  Endocrine ØG2SX
  Pituitary ØG20X
  Salivary ØC2AX
 Head ØW20X
 Intestinal Tract
  Lower ØD2DXUZ
  Upper ØD2ØXUZ
 Jaw
  Lower ØW25X
  Upper ØW24X
 Joint
  Lower ØS2YX
  Upper ØR2YX
 Kidney ØT25X
 Larynx ØC2SX
 Liver ØF2ØX
 Lung
  Left ØB2LX
  Right ØB2KX
 Lymphatic Ø72NX

Change Device in — *continued*
 Lymphatic — *continued*
  Thoracic Duct Ø72KX
 Mediastinum ØW2CX
 Mesentery ØD2VX
 Mouth and Throat ØC2YX
 Muscle
  Lower ØK2YX
  Upper ØK2XX
 Nasal Mucosa and Soft Tissue Ø92KX
 Neck ØW26X
 Nerve
  Cranial ØØ2EX
  Peripheral Ø12YX
 Omentum ØD2UX
 Ovary ØU23X
 Pancreas ØF2GX
 Parathyroid Gland ØG2RX
 Pelvic Cavity ØW2JX
 Penis ØV2SX
 Pericardial Cavity ØW2DX
 Perineum
  Female ØW2NX
  Male ØW2MX
 Peritoneal Cavity ØW2GX
 Peritoneum ØD2WX
 Pineal Body ØG21X
 Pleura ØB2QX
 Pleural Cavity
  Left ØW2BX
  Right ØW29X
 Products of Conception 10207
 Prostate and Seminal Vesicles ØV24X
 Retroperitoneum ØW2HX
 Scrotum and Tunica Vaginalis ØV28X
 Sinus Ø92YX
 Skin ØH2PX
 Skull ØN2ØX
 Spinal Canal ØØ2UX
 Spleen Ø72PX
 Subcutaneous Tissue and Fascia
  Head and Neck ØJ2SX
  Lower Extremity ØJ2WX
  Trunk ØJ2TX
  Upper Extremity ØJ2VX
 Tendon
  Lower ØL2YX
  Upper ØL2XX
 Testis ØV2DX
 Thymus Ø72MX
 Thyroid Gland ØG2KX
 Trachea ØB21
 Tracheobronchial Tree ØB20X
 Ureter ØT29X
 Urethra ØT2DX
 Uterus and Cervix ØU2DXHZ
 Vagina and Cul-de-sac ØU2HXGZ
 Vas Deferens ØV2RX
 Vulva ØU2MX
Change Device in or on
 Abdominal Wall 2WØ3X
 Anorectal 2YØ3X5Z
 Arm
  Lower
   Left 2WØDX
   Right 2WØCX
  Upper
   Left 2WØBX
   Right 2WØAX
 Back 2WØ5X
 Chest Wall 2WØ4X
 Ear 2YØ2X5Z
 Extremity
  Lower
   Left 2WØMX
   Right 2WØLX
  Upper
   Left 2WØ9X
   Right 2WØ8X
 Face 2WØ1X
 Finger
  Left 2WØKX
  Right 2WØJX
 Foot
  Left 2WØTX
  Right 2WØSX
 Genital Tract, Female 2YØ4X5Z
 Hand
  Left 2WØFX

Change Device in or on — *continued*
Hand — *continued*
    Right 2W0EX
  Head 2W00X
  Inguinal Region
    Left 2W07X
    Right 2W06X
  Leg
    Lower
      Left 2W0RX
      Right 2W0QX
    Upper
      Left 2W0PX
      Right 2W0NX
  Mouth and Pharynx 2Y00X5Z
  Nasal 2Y01X5Z
  Neck 2W02X
  Thumb
    Left 2W0HX
    Right 2W0GX
  Toe
    Left 2W0VX
    Right 2W0UX
  Urethra 2Y05X5Z
Chemoembolization *see* Introduction of substance in or on
Chemosurgery, Skin 3E00XTZ
Chemothalamectomy *see* Destruction, Thalamus 0059
Chemotherapy, Infusion for Cancer *see* Introduction of substance in or on
Chest compression (CPR), external
  Manual 5A12012
  Mechanical 5A1221J
Chest x-ray *see* Plain Radiography, Chest BW03
Chiropractic Manipulation
  Abdomen 9WB9X
  Cervical 9WB1X
  Extremities
    Lower 9WB6X
    Upper 9WB7X
  Head 9WB0X
  Lumbar 9WB3X
  Pelvis 9WB5X
  Rib Cage 9WB8X
  Sacrum 9WB4X
  Thoracic 9WB2X
Choana *use* Nasopharynx
Cholangiogram
  see Fluoroscopy, Hepatobiliary System and Pancreas BF1
  see Plain Radiography, Hepatobiliary System and Pancreas BF0
Cholecystectomy
  see Excision, Gallbladder 0FB4
  see Resection, Gallbladder 0FT4
Cholecystojejunostomy
  see Bypass, Hepatobiliary System and Pancreas 0F1
  see Drainage, Hepatobiliary System and Pancreas 0F9
Cholecystopexy
  see Repair, Gallbladder 0FQ4
  see Reposition, Gallbladder 0FS4
Cholecystoscopy 0FJ44ZZ
Cholecystostomy
  see Bypass, Gallbladder 0F14
  see Drainage, Gallbladder 0F94
Cholecystotomy *see* Drainage, Gallbladder 0F94
Choledochectomy
  see Excision, Hepatobiliary System and Pancreas 0FB
  see Resection, Hepatobiliary System and Pancreas 0FT
Choledocholithotomy *see* Extirpation, Duct, Common Bile 0FC9
Choledochoplasty
  see Repair, Hepatobiliary System and Pancreas 0FQ
  see Replacement, Hepatobiliary System and Pancreas 0FR
  see Supplement, Hepatobiliary System and Pancreas 0FU
Choledochoscopy 0FJB8ZZ
Choledochotomy *see* Drainage, Hepatobiliary System and Pancreas 0F9
Cholelithotomy *see* Extirpation, Hepatobiliary System and Pancreas 0FC
Chondrectomy
  see Excision, Lower Joints 0SB

Chondrectomy — *continued*
  see Excision, Upper Joints 0RB
  Knee *see* Excision, Lower Joints 0SB
  Semilunar cartilage *see* Excision, Lower Joints 0SB
Chondroglossus muscle *use* Tongue, Palate, Pharynx Muscle
Chorda tympani *use* Facial Nerve
Chordotomy *see* Division, Central Nervous System and Cranial Nerves 008
Choroid plexus *use* Cerebral Ventricle
Choroidectomy
  see Excision, Eye 08B
  see Resection, Eye 08T
Ciliary body
  use Eye, Left
  use Eye, Right
Ciliary ganglion *use* Head and Neck Sympathetic Nerve
Ciltacabtagene Autoleucel XW0
cilta-cel *use* Ciltacabtagene Autoleucel
Circle of Willis *use* Intracranial Artery
Circumcision 0VTTXZZ
Circumflex iliac artery
  use Femoral Artery, Left
  use Femoral Artery, Right
CivaSheet® *use* Radioactive Element
CivaSheet® Brachytherapy
  see Brachytherapy with qualifier Unidirectional Source
  see Insertion with device Radioactive Element
Clamp and rod internal fixation system (CRIF)
  use Internal Fixation Device in Lower Bones
  use Internal Fixation Device in Upper Bones
Clamping *see* Occlusion
Claustrum *use* Basal Ganglia
Claviculectomy
  see Excision, Upper Bones 0PB
  see Resection, Upper Bones 0PT
Claviculotomy
  see Division, Upper Bones 0P8
  see Drainage, Upper Bones 0P9
Clipping, aneurysm
  see Occlusion using Extraluminal Device
  see Restriction using Extraluminal Device
Clitorectomy, clitoridectomy
  see Excision, Clitoris 0UBJ
  see Resection, Clitoris 0UTJ
Clolar *use* Clofarabine
Closure
  see Occlusion
  see Repair
Clysis *see* Introduction of substance in or on
Coagulation *see* Destruction
Coagulation Factor Xa, Inactivated XW0
Coagulation Factor Xa, (Recombinant) Inactivated *use* Coagulation Factor Xa, Inactivated
COALESCE® radiolucent interbody fusion device *use* Interbody Fusion Device, Radiolucent Porous in New Technology
CoAxia NeuroFlo catheter *use* Intraluminal Device
Cobalt/chromium head and polyethylene socket *use* Synthetic Substitute, Metal on Polyethylene in 0SR
Cobalt/chromium head and socket *use* Synthetic Substitute, Metal in 0SR
Coccygeal body *use* Coccygeal Glomus
Coccygeus muscle
  use Trunk Muscle, Left
  use Trunk Muscle, Right
Cochlea
  use Inner Ear, Left
  use Inner Ear, Right
Cochlear implant (CI), multiple channel (electrode) *use* Hearing Device, Multiple Channel Cochlear Prosthesis in 09H
Cochlear implant (CI), single channel (electrode) *use* Hearing Device, Single Channel Cochlear Prosthesis in 09H
Cochlear Implant Treatment F0BZ0
Cochlear nerve *use* Acoustic Nerve
COGNIS® CRT-D *use* Cardiac Resynchronization Defibrillator Pulse Generator in 0JH
COHERE® radiolucent interbody fusion device *use* Interbody Fusion Device, Radiolucent Porous in New Technology
Colectomy
  see Excision, Gastrointestinal System 0DB

Colectomy — *continued*
  see Resection, Gastrointestinal System 0DT
Collapse *see* Occlusion
Collection from
  Breast, Breast Milk 8E0HX62
  Indwelling Device
    Circulatory System
      Blood 8C02X6K
      Other Fluid 8C02X6L
    Nervous System
      Cerebrospinal Fluid 8C01X6J
      Other Fluid 8C01X6L
  Integumentary System, Breast Milk 8E0HX62
  Reproductive System, Male, Sperm 8E0VX63
Colocentesis *see* Drainage, Gastrointestinal System 0D9
Colofixation
  see Repair, Gastrointestinal System 0DQ
  see Reposition, Gastrointestinal System 0DS
Cololysis *see* Release, Gastrointestinal System 0DN
Colonic Z-Stent® *use* Intraluminal Device
Colonoscopy 0DJD8ZZ
Colopexy
  see Repair, Gastrointestinal System 0DQ
  see Reposition, Gastrointestinal System 0DS
Coloplication *see* Restriction, Gastrointestinal System 0DV
Coloproctectomy
  see Excision, Gastrointestinal System 0DB
  see Resection, Gastrointestinal System 0DT
Coloproctostomy
  see Bypass, Gastrointestinal System 0D1
  see Drainage, Gastrointestinal System 0D9
Colopuncture *see* Drainage, Gastrointestinal System 0D9
Colorrhaphy *see* Repair, Gastrointestinal System 0DQ
Colostomy
  see Bypass, Gastrointestinal System 0D1
  see Drainage, Gastrointestinal System 0D9
Colpectomy
  see Excision, Vagina 0UBG
  see Resection, Vagina 0UTG
Colpocentesis *see* Drainage, Vagina 0U9G
Colpopexy
  see Repair, Vagina 0UQG
  see Reposition, Vagina 0USG
Colpoplasty
  see Repair, Vagina 0UQG
  see Supplement, Vagina 0UUG
Colporrhaphy *see* Repair, Vagina 0UQG
Colposcopy 0UJH8ZZ
Columella *use* Nasal Mucosa and Soft Tissue
Common digital vein
  use Foot Vein, Left
  use Foot Vein, Right
Common facial vein
  use Face Vein, Left
  use Face Vein, Right
Common fibular nerve *use* Peroneal Nerve
Common hepatic artery *use* Hepatic Artery
Common iliac (subaortic) lymph node *use* Lymphatic, Pelvis
Common interosseous artery
  use Ulnar Artery, Left
  use Ulnar Artery, Right
Common peroneal nerve *use* Peroneal Nerve
Complete (SE) stent *use* Intraluminal Device
Compression
  see Restriction
  Abdominal Wall 2W13X
  Arm
    Lower
      Left 2W1DX
      Right 2W1CX
    Upper
      Left 2W1BX
      Right 2W1AX
  Back 2W15X
  Chest Wall 2W14X
  Extremity
    Lower
      Left 2W1MX
      Right 2W1LX
    Upper
      Left 2W19X
      Right 2W18X
  Face 2W11X

Compression — *continued*
Finger
 Left 2W1KX
 Right 2W1JX
Foot
 Left 2W1TX
 Right 2W1SX
Hand
 Left 2W1FX
 Right 2W1EX
Head 2W10X
Inguinal Region
 Left 2W17X
 Right 2W16X
Leg
 Lower
  Left 2W1RX
  Right 2W1QX
 Upper
  Left 2W1PX
  Right 2W1NX
Neck 2W12X
Thumb
 Left 2W1HX
 Right 2W1GX
Toe
 Left 2W1VX
 Right 2W1UX
Computer Assisted Procedure
Extremity
 Lower
  No Qualifier 8E0YXBZ
  With Computerized Tomography
   8E0YXBG
  With Fluoroscopy 8E0YXBF
  With Magnetic Resonance Imaging
   8E0YXBH
 Upper
  No Qualifier 8E0XXBZ
  With Computerized Tomography
   8E0XXBG
  With Fluoroscopy 8E0XXBF
  With Magnetic Resonance Imaging
   8E0XXBH
Head and Neck Region
 No Qualifier 8E09XBZ
 With Computerized Tomography 8E09XBG
 With Fluoroscopy 8E09XBF
 With Magnetic Resonance Imaging 8E09XBH
Trunk Region
 No Qualifier 8E0WXBZ
 With Computerized Tomography 8E0WXBG
 With Fluoroscopy 8E0WXBF
 With Magnetic Resonance Imaging 8E0WXBH
Computer-aided Assessment, Intracranial Vascular Activity XXE0X07
Computer-aided Guidance, Transthoracic Echocardiography X2JAX47
Computer-aided Mechanical Aspiration X2C
Computer-aided Triage and Notification, Pulmonary Artery Flow XXE3X27
Computer-assisted Intermittent Aspiration *see* New Technology, Cardiovascular System X2C
Computerized Tomography (CT Scan)
Abdomen BW20
 Chest and Pelvis BW25
Abdomen and Chest BW24
Abdomen and Pelvis BW21
Airway, Trachea BB2F
Ankle
 Left BQ2H
 Right BQ2G
Aorta
 Abdominal B420
  Intravascular Optical Coherence
   B420Z2Z
 Thoracic B320
  Intravascular Optical Coherence
   B320Z2Z
Arm
 Left BP2F
 Right BP2E
Artery
 Celiac B421
  Intravascular Optical Coherence
   B421Z2Z
 Common Carotid
  Bilateral B325

Computerized Tomography (CT Scan) — *continued*
Artery — *continued*
 Common Carotid — *continued*
  Intravascular Optical Coherence
   B325Z2Z
 Coronary
  Bypass Graft
   Intravascular Optical Coherence
    B223Z2Z
   Multiple B223
  Multiple B221
   Intravascular Optical Coherence
    B221Z2Z
 Internal Carotid
  Bilateral B328
  Intravascular Optical Coherence
   B328Z2Z
 Intracranial B32R
  Intravascular Optical Coherence
   B32RZ2Z
 Lower Extremity
  Bilateral B42H
   Intravascular Optical Coherence
    B42HZ2Z
  Left B42G
   Intravascular Optical Coherence
    B42GZ2Z
  Right B42F
   Intravascular Optical Coherence
    B42FZ2Z
 Pelvic B42C
  Intravascular Optical Coherence
   B42CZ2Z
 Pulmonary
  Left B32T
   Intravascular Optical Coherence
    B32TZ2Z
  Right B32S
   Intravascular Optical Coherence
    B32SZ2Z
 Renal
  Bilateral B428
   Intravascular Optical Coherence
    B428Z2Z
  Transplant B42M
   Intravascular Optical Coherence
    B42MZ2Z
 Superior Mesenteric B424
  Intravascular Optical Coherence
   B424Z2Z
 Vertebral
  Bilateral B32G
   Intravascular Optical Coherence
    B32GZ2Z
Bladder BT20
Bone
 Facial BN25
 Temporal BN2F
Brain B020
Calcaneus
 Left BQ2K
 Right BQ2J
Cerebral Ventricle B028
Chest, Abdomen and Pelvis BW25
Chest and Abdomen BW24
Cisterna B027
Clavicle
 Left BP25
 Right BP24
Coccyx BR2F
Colon BD24
Ear B920
Elbow
 Left BP2H
 Right BP2G
Extremity
 Lower
  Left BQ2S
  Right BQ2R
 Upper
  Bilateral BP2V
  Left BP2U
  Right BP2T
Eye
 Bilateral B827
 Left B826
 Right B825
Femur
 Left BQ24

Computerized Tomography (CT Scan) — *continued*
Femur — *continued*
 Right BQ23
Fibula
 Left BQ2C
 Right BQ2B
Finger
 Left BP2S
 Right BP2R
Foot
 Left BQ2M
 Right BQ2L
Forearm
 Left BP2K
 Right BP2J
Gland
 Adrenal, Bilateral BG22
 Parathyroid BG23
 Parotid, Bilateral B926
 Salivary, Bilateral B92D
 Submandibular, Bilateral B929
 Thyroid BG24
Hand
 Left BP2P
 Right BP2N
Hands and Wrists, Bilateral BP2Q
Head BW28
Head and Neck BW29
Heart
 Intravascular Optical Coherence B226Z2Z
 Right and Left B226
Hepatobiliary System, All BF2C
Hip
 Left BQ21
 Right BQ20
Humerus
 Left BP2B
 Right BP2A
Intracranial Sinus B522
 Intravascular Optical Coherence B522Z2Z
Joint
 Acromioclavicular, Bilateral BP23
 Finger
  Left BP2DZZZ
  Right BP2CZZZ
 Foot
  Left BQ2Y
  Right BQ2X
 Hand
  Left BP2DZZZ
  Right BP2CZZZ
 Sacroiliac BR2D
 Sternoclavicular
  Bilateral BP22
  Left BP21
  Right BP20
 Temporomandibular, Bilateral BN29
 Toe
  Left BQ2Y
  Right BQ2X
Kidney
 Bilateral BT23
 Left BT22
 Right BT21
 Transplant BT29
Knee
 Left BQ28
 Right BQ27
Larynx B92J
Leg
 Left BQ2F
 Right BQ2D
Liver BF25
Liver and Spleen BF26
Lung, Bilateral BB24
Mandible BN26
Nasopharynx B92F
Neck BW2F
Neck and Head BW29
Orbit, Bilateral BN23
Oropharynx B92F
Pancreas BF27
Patella
 Left BQ2W
 Right BQ2V
Pelvic Region BW2G
Pelvis BR2C
 Chest and Abdomen BW25
Pelvis and Abdomen BW21

Compression — Computerized Tomography (CT Scan)

Computerized Tomography (CT Scan) — *continued*
Pituitary Gland B029
Prostate BV23
Ribs
Left BP2Y
Right BP2X
Sacrum BR2F
Scapula
Left BP27
Right BP26
Sella Turcica B029
Shoulder
Left BP29
Right BP28
Sinus
Intracranial B522
Intravascular Optical Coherence B522Z2Z
Paranasal B922
Skull BN20
Spinal Cord B02B
Spine
Cervical BR20
Lumbar BR29
Thoracic BR27
Spleen and Liver BF26
Thorax BP2W
Tibia
Left BQ2C
Right BQ2B
Toe
Left BQ2Q
Right BQ2P
Trachea BB2F
Tracheobronchial Tree
Bilateral BB29
Left BB28
Right BB27
Vein
Pelvic (Iliac)
Left B52G
Intravascular Optical Coherence B52GZ2Z
Right B52F
Intravascular Optical Coherence B52FZ2Z
Pelvic (Iliac) Bilateral B52H
Intravascular Optical Coherence B52HZ2Z
Portal B52T
Intravascular Optical Coherence B52TZ2Z
Pulmonary
Bilateral B52S
Intravascular Optical Coherence B52SZ2Z
Left B52R
Intravascular Optical Coherence B52RZ2Z
Right B52Q
Intravascular Optical Coherence B52QZ2Z
Renal
Bilateral B52L
Intravascular Optical Coherence B52LZ2Z
Left B52K
Intravascular Optical Coherence B52KZ2Z
Right B52J
Intravascular Optical Coherence B52JZ2Z
Spanchnic B52T
Intravascular Optical Coherence B52TZ2Z
Vena Cava
Inferior B529
Intravascular Optical Coherence B529Z2Z
Superior B528
Intravascular Optical Coherence B528Z2Z
Ventricle, Cerebral B028
Wrist
Left BP2M
Right BP2L

Concentrated Bone Marrow Aspirate (CBMA) injection, intramuscular XK02303

Concerto II CRT-D *use* Cardiac Resynchronization Defibrillator Pulse Generator in 0JH
Condylectomy
see Excision, Head and Facial Bones 0NB
see Excision, Lower Bones 0QB
see Excision, Upper Bones 0PB
Condyloid process
use Mandible, Left
use Mandible, Right
Condylotomy
see Division, Head and Facial Bones 0N8
see Division, Lower Bones 0Q8
see Division, Upper Bones 0P8
see Drainage, Head and Facial Bones 0N9
see Drainage, Lower Bones 0Q9
see Drainage, Upper Bones 0P9
Condylysis
see Release, Head and Facial Bones 0NN
see Release, Lower Bones 0QN
see Release, Upper Bones 0PN
Conization, cervix *see* Excision, Cervix 0UBC
Conjunctivoplasty
see Repair, Eye 08Q
see Replacement, Eye 08R
CONSERVE® PLUS Total Resurfacing Hip System
use Resurfacing Device in Lower Joints
Construction
Auricle, ear *see* Replacement, Ear, Nose, Sinus 09R
Ileal conduit *see* Bypass, Urinary System 0T1
Consulta CRT-D *use* Cardiac Resynchronization Defibrillator Pulse Generator in 0JH
Consulta CRT-P *use* Cardiac Resynchronization Pacemaker Pulse Generator in 0JH
Contact Radiation
Abdomen DWY37ZZ
Adrenal Gland DGY27ZZ
Bile Ducts DFY27ZZ
Bladder DTY27ZZ
Bone, Other DPYC7ZZ
Brain D0Y07ZZ
Brain Stem D0Y17ZZ
Breast
Left DMY07ZZ
Right DMY17ZZ
Bronchus DBY17ZZ
Cervix DUY17ZZ
Chest DWY27ZZ
Chest Wall DBY77ZZ
Colon DDY57ZZ
Diaphragm DBY87ZZ
Duodenum DDY27ZZ
Ear D9Y07ZZ
Esophagus DDY07ZZ
Eye D8Y07ZZ
Femur DPY97ZZ
Fibula DPYB7ZZ
Gallbladder DFY17ZZ
Gland
Adrenal DGY27ZZ
Parathyroid DGY47ZZ
Pituitary DGY07ZZ
Thyroid DGY57ZZ
Glands, Salivary D9Y67ZZ
Head and Neck DWY17ZZ
Hemibody DWY47ZZ
Humerus DPY67ZZ
Hypopharynx D9Y37ZZ
Ileum DDY47ZZ
Jejunum DDY37ZZ
Kidney DTY07ZZ
Larynx D9YB7ZZ
Liver DFY07ZZ
Lung DBY27ZZ
Mandible DPY37ZZ
Maxilla DPY27ZZ
Mediastinum DBY67ZZ
Mouth D9Y47ZZ
Nasopharynx D9YD7ZZ
Neck and Head DWY17ZZ
Nerve, Peripheral D0Y77ZZ
Nose D9Y17ZZ
Oropharynx D9YF7ZZ
Ovary DUY07ZZ
Palate
Hard D9Y87ZZ
Soft D9Y97ZZ
Pancreas DFY37ZZ
Parathyroid Gland DGY47ZZ

Contact Radiation — *continued*
Pelvic Bones DPY87ZZ
Pelvic Region DWY67ZZ
Pineal Body DGY17ZZ
Pituitary Gland DGY07ZZ
Pleura DBY57ZZ
Prostate DVY07ZZ
Radius DPY77ZZ
Rectum DDY77ZZ
Rib DPY57ZZ
Sinuses D9Y77ZZ
Skin
Abdomen DHY87ZZ
Arm DHY47ZZ
Back DHY77ZZ
Buttock DHY97ZZ
Chest DHY67ZZ
Face DHY27ZZ
Leg DHYB7ZZ
Neck DHY37ZZ
Skull DPY07ZZ
Spinal Cord D0Y67ZZ
Sternum DPY47ZZ
Stomach DDY17ZZ
Testis DVY17ZZ
Thyroid Gland DGY57ZZ
Tibia DPYB7ZZ
Tongue D9Y57ZZ
Trachea DBY07ZZ
Ulna DPY77ZZ
Ureter DTY17ZZ
Urethra DTY37ZZ
Uterus DUY27ZZ
Whole Body DWY57ZZ
ContaCT software (Measurement of intracranial arterial flow) 4A03X5D
CONTAK RENEWAL® 3 RF (HE) CRT-D *use* Cardiac Resynchronization Defibrillator Pulse Generator in 0JH
Contegra Pulmonary Valved Conduit *use* Zooplastic Tissue in Heart and Great Vessels
CONTEPO™ *use* Fosfomycin Anti-Infective
Continuous Glucose Monitoring (CGM) device *use* Monitoring Device
Continuous Negative Airway Pressure
24-96 Consecutive Hours, Ventilation 5A09459
Greater than 96 Consecutive Hours, Ventilation 5A09559
Less than 24 Consecutive Hours, Ventilation 5A09359
Continuous Positive Airway Pressure
24-96 Consecutive Hours, Ventilation 5A09457
Greater than 96 Consecutive Hours, Ventilation 5A09557
Less than 24 Consecutive Hours, Ventilation 5A09357
Continuous renal replacement therapy (CRRT) 5A1D90Z
Contraceptive Device
Change device in, Uterus and Cervix 0U2DXHZ
Insertion of device in
Cervix 0UHC
Subcutaneous Tissue and Fascia
Abdomen 0JH8
Chest 0JH6
Lower Arm
Left 0JHH
Right 0JHG
Lower Leg
Left 0JHP
Right 0JHN
Upper Arm
Left 0JHF
Right 0JHD
Upper Leg
Left 0JHM
Right 0JHL
Uterus 0UH9
Removal of device from
Subcutaneous Tissue and Fascia
Lower Extremity 0JPW
Trunk 0JPT
Upper Extremity 0JPV
Uterus and Cervix 0UPD
Revision of device in
Subcutaneous Tissue and Fascia
Lower Extremity 0JWW
Trunk 0JWT

⏷ **Subterms under main terms may continue to next column or page**

Contraceptive Device — *continued*
　　Revision of device in — *continued*
　　　　Subcutaneous Tissue and Fascia — *continued*
　　　　　　Upper Extremity ØJWV
　　　　Uterus and Cervix ØUWD
Contractility Modulation Device
　　Abdomen ØJH8
　　Chest ØJH6
Control bleeding in
　　Abdominal Wall ØW3F
　　Ankle Region
　　　　Left ØY3L
　　　　Right ØY3K
　　Arm
　　　　Lower
　　　　　　Left ØX3F
　　　　　　Right ØX3D
　　　　Upper
　　　　　　Left ØX39
　　　　　　Right ØX38
　　Axilla
　　　　Left ØX35
　　　　Right ØX34
　　Back
　　　　Lower ØW3L
　　　　Upper ØW3K
　　Buttock
　　　　Left ØY31
　　　　Right ØY30
　　Cavity, Cranial ØW31
　　Chest Wall ØW38
　　Elbow Region
　　　　Left ØX3C
　　　　Right ØX3B
　　Extremity
　　　　Lower
　　　　　　Left ØY3B
　　　　　　Right ØY39
　　　　Upper
　　　　　　Left ØX37
　　　　　　Right ØX36
　　Face ØW32
　　Femoral Region
　　　　Left ØY38
　　　　Right ØY37
　　Foot
　　　　Left ØY3N
　　　　Right ØY3M
　　Gastrointestinal Tract ØW3P
　　Genitourinary Tract ØW3R
　　Hand
　　　　Left ØX3K
　　　　Right ØX3J
　　Head ØW30
　　Inguinal Region
　　　　Left ØY36
　　　　Right ØY35
　　Jaw
　　　　Lower ØW35
　　　　Upper ØW34
　　Knee Region
　　　　Left ØY3G
　　　　Right ØY3F
　　Leg
　　　　Lower
　　　　　　Left ØY3J
　　　　　　Right ØY3H
　　　　Upper
　　　　　　Left ØY3D
　　　　　　Right ØY3C
　　Mediastinum ØW3C
　　Nasal Mucosa and Soft Tissue Ø93K
　　Neck ØW36
　　Oral Cavity and Throat ØW33
　　Pelvic Cavity ØW3J
　　Pericardial Cavity ØW3D
　　Perineum
　　　　Female ØW3N
　　　　Male ØW3M
　　Peritoneal Cavity ØW3G
　　Pleural Cavity
　　　　Left ØW3B
　　　　Right ØW39
　　Respiratory Tract ØW3Q
　　Retroperitoneum ØW3H
　　Shoulder Region
　　　　Left ØX33
　　　　Right ØX32

Control bleeding in — *continued*
　　Wrist Region
　　　　Left ØX3H
　　　　Right ØX3G
Control bleeding using Tourniquet, External *see* Compression, Anatomical Regions 2W1
Control, Epistaxis *see* Control bleeding in, Nasal Mucosa and Soft Tissue Ø93K
Conus arteriosus *use* Ventricle, Right
Conus medullaris *use* Lumbar Spinal Cord
Convalescent Plasma (Nonautologous) *see* New Technology, Anatomical Regions XW1
Conversion
　　Cardiac rhythm 5A22Ø4Z
　　Gastrostomy to jejunostomy feeding device *see* Insertion of device in, Jejunum ØDHA
Cook Biodesign® Fistula Plug(s) *use* Nonautologous Tissue Substitute
Cook Biodesign® Hernia Graft(s) *use* Nonautologous Tissue Substitute
Cook Biodesign® Layered Graft(s) *use* Nonautologous Tissue Substitute
Cook Zenaprom™ Layered Graft(s) *use* Nonautologous Tissue Substitute
Cook Zenith AAA Endovascular Graft *use* Intraluminal Device
Cook Zenith® Fenestrated AAA Endovascular Graft
　　use Intraluminal Device, Branched or Fenestrated, One or Two Arteries in Ø4V
　　use Intraluminal Device, Branched or Fenestrated, Three or More Arteries in Ø4V
Coracoacromial ligament
　　use Shoulder Bursa and Ligament, Left
　　use Shoulder Bursa and Ligament, Right
Coracobrachialis muscle
　　use Upper Arm Muscle, Left
　　use Upper Arm Muscle, Right
Coracoclavicular ligament
　　use Shoulder Bursa and Ligament, Left
　　use Shoulder Bursa and Ligament, Right
Coracohumeral ligament
　　use Shoulder Bursa and Ligament, Left
　　use Shoulder Bursa and Ligament, Right
Coracoid process
　　use Scapula, Left
　　use Scapula, Right
Cordotomy *see* Division, Central Nervous System and Cranial Nerves ØØ8
Core needle biopsy *see* Excision with qualifier Diagnostic
CoreValve transcatheter aortic valve *use* Zooplastic Tissue in Heart and Great Vessels
Cormet Hip Resurfacing System *use* Resurfacing Device in Lower Joints
Corniculate cartilage *use* Larynx
CoRoent® XL *use* Interbody Fusion Device in Lower Joints
Coronary arteriography
　　see Fluoroscopy, Heart B21
　　see Plain Radiography, Heart B2Ø
Corox (OTW) Bipolar Lead
　　use Cardiac Lead, Defibrillator in Ø2H
　　use Cardiac Lead, Pacemaker in Ø2H
Corpus callosum *use* Brain
Corpus cavernosum *use* Penis
Corpus spongiosum *use* Penis
Corpus striatum *use* Basal Ganglia
Corrugator supercilii muscle *use* Facial Muscle
Cortical strip neurostimulator lead *use* Neurostimulator Lead in Central Nervous System and Cranial Nerves
Corvia IASD® *use* Synthetic Substitute
COSELA™ *use* Trilaciclib
Costatectomy
　　see Excision, Upper Bones ØPB
　　see Resection, Upper Bones ØPT
Costectomy
　　see Excision, Upper Bones ØPB
　　see Resection, Upper Bones ØPT
Costocervical trunk
　　use Subclavian Artery, Left
　　use Subclavian Artery, Right
Costochondrectomy
　　see Excision, Upper Bones ØPB
　　see Resection, Upper Bones ØPT
Costoclavicular ligament
　　use Shoulder Bursa and Ligament, Left

Costoclavicular ligament — *continued*
　　use Shoulder Bursa and Ligament, Right
Costosternoplasty
　　see Repair, Upper Bones ØPQ
　　see Replacement, Upper Bones ØPR
　　see Supplement, Upper Bones ØPU
Costotomy
　　see Division, Upper Bones ØP8
　　see Drainage, Upper Bones ØP9
Costotransverse joint *use* Thoracic Vertebral Joint
Costotransverse ligament *use* Rib(s) Bursa and Ligament
Costovertebral joint *use* Thoracic Vertebral Joint
Costoxiphoid ligament *use* Sternum Bursa and Ligament
Counseling
　　Family, for substance abuse, Other Family Counseling HZ63ZZZ
　　Group
　　　　12-Step HZ43ZZZ
　　　　Behavioral HZ41ZZZ
　　　　Cognitive HZ40ZZZ
　　　　Cognitive-Behavioral HZ42ZZZ
　　　　Confrontational HZ48ZZZ
　　　　Continuing Care HZ49ZZZ
　　　　Infectious Disease
　　　　　　Post-Test HZ4CZZZ
　　　　　　Pre-Test HZ4CZZZ
　　　　Interpersonal HZ44ZZZ
　　　　Motivational Enhancement HZ47ZZZ
　　　　Psychoeducation HZ46ZZZ
　　　　Spiritual HZ4BZZZ
　　　　Vocational HZ45ZZZ
　　Individual
　　　　12-Step HZ33ZZZ
　　　　Behavioral HZ31ZZZ
　　　　Cognitive HZ30ZZZ
　　　　Cognitive-Behavioral HZ32ZZZ
　　　　Confrontational HZ38ZZZ
　　　　Continuing Care HZ39ZZZ
　　　　Infectious Disease
　　　　　　Post-Test HZ3CZZZ
　　　　　　Pre-Test HZ3CZZZ
　　　　Interpersonal HZ34ZZZ
　　　　Motivational Enhancement HZ37ZZZ
　　　　Psychoeducation HZ36ZZZ
　　　　Spiritual HZ3BZZZ
　　　　Vocational HZ35ZZZ
　　Mental Health Services
　　　　Educational GZ60ZZZ
　　　　Other Counseling GZ63ZZZ
　　　　Vocational GZ61ZZZ
Countershock, cardiac 5A22Ø4Z
COVID-19 Vaccine XWØ
COVID-19 Vaccine Dose 1 XWØ
COVID-19 Vaccine Dose 2 XWØ
Cowper's (bulbourethral) gland *use* Urethra
CPAP (continuous positive airway pressure) *see* Assistance, Respiratory 5AØ9
Craniectomy
　　see Excision, Head and Facial Bones ØNB
　　see Resection, Head and Facial Bones ØNT
Cranioplasty
　　see Repair, Head and Facial Bones ØNQ
　　see Replacement, Head and Facial Bones ØNR
　　see Supplement, Head and Facial Bones ØNU
Craniotomy
　　see Division, Head and Facial Bones ØN8
　　see Drainage, Central Nervous System and Cranial Nerves ØØ9
　　see Drainage, Head and Facial Bones ØN9
Creation
　　Perineum
　　　　Female ØW4NØ
　　　　Male ØW4MØ
　　Valve
　　　　Aortic Ø24FØ
　　　　Mitral Ø24GØ
　　　　Tricuspid Ø24JØ
Cremaster muscle *use* Perineum Muscle
CRESEMBA® (isavuconazonium sulfate) *use* Other Anti-infective
Cribriform plate
　　use Ethmoid Bone, Left
　　use Ethmoid Bone, Right
Cricoid cartilage *use* Trachea
Cricoidectomy *see* Excision, Larynx ØCBS

Cricothyroid artery
  use Thyroid Artery, Left
  use Thyroid Artery, Right
Cricothyroid muscle
  use Neck Muscle, Left
  use Neck Muscle, Right
Crisis Intervention GZ2ZZZZ
CRRT (Continuous renal replacement therapy)
  5A1D90Z
Crural fascia
  use Subcutaneous Tissue and Fascia, Left Upper
    Leg
  use Subcutaneous Tissue and Fascia, Right Upper
    Leg
Crushing, nerve
  Cranial *see* Destruction, Central Nervous System
    and Cranial Nerves 005
  Peripheral *see* Destruction, Peripheral Nervous
    System 015
Cryoablation *see* Destruction
Cryotherapy *see* Destruction
Cryptorchidectomy
  see Excision, Male Reproductive System 0VB
  see Resection, Male Reproductive System 0VT
Cryptorchiectomy
  see Excision, Male Reproductive System 0VB
  see Resection, Male Reproductive System 0VT
Cryptotomy
  see Division, Gastrointestinal System 0D8
  see Drainage, Gastrointestinal System 0D9
CT scan *see* Computerized Tomography (CT Scan)
CT sialogram *see* Computerized Tomography (CT Scan),
  Ear, Nose, Mouth and Throat B92
Cubital lymph node
  use Lymphatic, Left Upper Extremity
  use Lymphatic, Right Upper Extremity
Cubital nerve *use* Ulnar Nerve
Cuboid bone
  use Tarsal, Left
  use Tarsal, Right
Cuboideonavicular joint
  use Tarsal Joint, Left
  use Tarsal Joint, Right
Culdocentesis *see* Drainage, Cul-de-sac 0U9F
Culdoplasty
  see Repair, Cul-de-sac 0UQF
  see Supplement, Cul-de-sac 0UUF
Culdoscopy 0UJH8ZZ
Culdotomy *see* Drainage, Cul-de-sac 0U9F
Culmen *use* Cerebellum
Cultured epidermal cell autograft *use* Autologous
  Tissue Substitute
Cuneiform cartilage *use* Larynx
Cuneonavicular joint
  use Joint, Tarsal, Left
  use Joint, Tarsal, Right
Cuneonavicular ligament
  use Foot Bursa and Ligament, Left
  use Foot Bursa and Ligament, Right
Curettage
  see Excision
  see Extraction
Cutaneous (transverse) cervical nerve *use* Cervical
  Plexus
CVP (central venous pressure) *see* Measurement,
  Venous 4A04
Cyclodiathermy *see* Destruction, Eye 085
Cyclophotocoagulation *see* Destruction, Eye 085
CYPHER® Stent *use* Intraluminal Device, Drug-eluting
  in Heart and Great Vessels
Cystectomy
  see Excision, Bladder 0TBB
  see Resection, Bladder 0TTB
Cystocele repair *see* Repair, Subcutaneous Tissue and
  Fascia, Pelvic Region 0JQC
Cystography
  see Fluoroscopy, Urinary System BT1
  see Plain Radiography, Urinary System BT0
Cystolithotomy *see* Extirpation, Bladder 0TCB
Cystopexy
  see Repair, Bladder 0TQB
  see Reposition, Bladder 0TSB
Cystoplasty
  see Repair, Bladder 0TQB
  see Replacement, Bladder 0TRB
  see Supplement, Bladder 0TUB

Cystorrhaphy *see* Repair, Bladder 0TQB
Cystoscopy 0TJB8ZZ
Cystostomy *see* Bypass, Bladder 0T1B
Cystostomy Tube *use* Drainage Device
Cystotomy *see* Drainage, Bladder 0T9B
Cystourethrography
  see Fluoroscopy, Urinary System BT1
  see Plain Radiography, Urinary System BT0
Cystourethroplasty
  see Repair, Urinary System 0TQ
  see Replacement, Urinary System 0TR
  see Supplement, Urinary System 0TU
Cytarabine and Daunorubicin Liposome Antineo-
  plastic XW0

D

DBS lead *use* Neurostimulator Lead in Central Nervous
  System and Cranial Nerves
DeBakey Left Ventricular Assist Device *use* Im-
  plantable Heart Assist System in Heart and Great
  Vessels
Debridement
  Excisional *see* Excision
  Non-excisional *see* Extraction
Decompression, Circulatory 6A15
Decortication, lung
  see Extirpation, Respiratory System 0BC
  see Release, Respiratory System 0BN
Deep brain neurostimulator lead *use* Neurostimula-
  tor Lead in Central Nervous System and Cranial
  Nerves
Deep cervical fascia
  use Subcutaneous Tissue and Fascia, Left Neck
  use Subcutaneous Tissue and Fascia, Right Neck
Deep cervical vein
  use Vertebral Vein, Left
  use Vertebral Vein, Right
Deep circumflex iliac artery
  use External Iliac Artery, Left
  use External Iliac Artery, Right
Deep facial vein
  use Face Vein, Left
  use Face Vein, Right
Deep femoral artery
  use Femoral Artery, Left
  use Femoral Artery, Right
Deep femoral (profunda femoris) vein
  use Femoral Vein, Left
  use Femoral Vein, Right
Deep Inferior Epigastric Artery Perforator Flap
  Replacement
    Bilateral 0HRV077
    Left 0HRU077
    Right 0HRT077
  Transfer
    Left 0KXG
    Right 0KXF
Deep palmar arch
  use Hand Artery, Left
  use Hand Artery, Right
Deep transverse perineal muscle *use* Perineum
  Muscle
Deferential artery
  use Internal Iliac Artery, Left
  use Internal Iliac Artery, Right
Defibrillator Generator
  Abdomen 0JH8
  Chest 0JH6
Defibrotide Sodium Anticoagulant XW0
Defibtech Automated Chest Compression (ACC)
  device 5A1221J
Defitelio *use* Defibrotide Sodium Anticoagulant
Delivery
  Cesarean *see* Extraction, Products of Conception
    10D0
  Forceps *see* Extraction, Products of Conception
    10D0
  Manually assisted 10E0XZZ
  Products of Conception 10E0XZZ
  Vacuum assisted *see* Extraction, Products of Con-
    ception 10D0
Delta frame external fixator
  use External Fixation Device, Hybrid in 0PH
  use External Fixation Device, Hybrid in 0PS
  use External Fixation Device, Hybrid in 0QH

Delta frame external fixator — *continued*
  use External Fixation Device, Hybrid in 0QS
Delta III Reverse shoulder prosthesis *use* Synthetic
  Substitute, Reverse Ball and Socket in 0RR
Deltoid fascia
  use Subcutaneous Tissue and Fascia, Left Upper
    Arm
  use Subcutaneous Tissue and Fascia, Right Upper
    Arm
Deltoid ligament
  use Ankle Bursa and Ligament, Left
  use Ankle Bursa and Ligament, Right
Deltoid muscle
  use Shoulder Muscle, Left
  use Shoulder Muscle, Right
Deltopectoral (infraclavicular) lymph node
  use Lymphatic, Left Upper Extremity
  use Lymphatic, Right Upper Extremity
Denervation
  Cranial nerve *see* Destruction, Central Nervous
    System and Cranial Nerves 005
  Peripheral nerve *see* Destruction, Peripheral Ner-
    vous System 015
Dens *use* Cervical Vertebra
Densitometry
  Plain Radiography
    Femur
      Left BQ04ZZ1
      Right BQ03ZZ1
    Hip
      Left BQ01ZZ1
      Right BQ00ZZ1
    Spine
      Cervical BR00ZZ1
      Lumbar BR09ZZ1
      Thoracic BR07ZZ1
      Whole BR0GZZ1
  Ultrasonography
    Elbow
      Left BP4HZZ1
      Right BP4GZZ1
    Hand
      Left BP4PZZ1
      Right BP4NZZ1
    Shoulder
      Left BP49ZZ1
      Right BP48ZZ1
    Wrist
      Left BP4MZZ1
      Right BP4LZZ1
Denticulate (dentate) ligament *use* Spinal Meninges
Depressor anguli oris muscle *use* Facial Muscle
Depressor labii inferioris muscle *use* Facial Muscle
Depressor septi nasi muscle *use* Facial Muscle
Depressor supercilii muscle *use* Facial Muscle
Dermabrasion *see* Extraction, Skin and Breast 0HD
Dermis *use* Skin
Descending genicular artery
  use Femoral Artery, Left
  use Femoral Artery, Right
Destruction
  Acetabulum
    Left 0Q55
    Right 0Q54
  Adenoids 0C5Q
  Ampulla of Vater 0F5C
  Anal Sphincter 0D5R
  Anterior Chamber
    Left 08533ZZ
    Right 08523ZZ
  Anus 0D5Q
  Aorta
    Abdominal
    Thoracic
      Ascending/Arch 025X
      Descending 025W
  Aortic Body 0G5D
  Appendix 0D5J
  Artery
    Anterior Tibial
      Left 045Q
      Right 045P
    Axillary
      Left 0356
      Right 0355
    Brachial
      Left 0358
      Right 0357

🔻 Subterms under main terms may continue to next column or page

Destruction — *continued*
  Artery — *continued*
    Celiac 0451
    Colic
      Left 0457
      Middle 0458
      Right 0456
    Common Carotid
      Left 035J
      Right 035H
    Common Iliac
      Left 045D
      Right 045C
    External Carotid
      Left 035N
      Right 035M
    External Iliac
      Left 045J
      Right 045H
    Face 035R
    Femoral
      Left 045L
      Right 045K
    Foot
      Left 045W
      Right 045V
    Gastric 0452
    Hand
      Left 035F
      Right 035D
    Hepatic 0453
    Inferior Mesenteric 045B
    Innominate 0352
    Internal Carotid
      Left 035L
      Right 035K
    Internal Iliac
      Left 045F
      Right 045E
    Internal Mammary
      Left 0351
      Right 0350
    Intracranial 035G
    Lower 045Y
    Peroneal
      Left 045U
      Right 045T
    Popliteal
      Left 045N
      Right 045M
    Posterior Tibial
      Left 045S
      Right 045R
    Pulmonary
      Left 025R
      Right 025Q
    Pulmonary Trunk 025P
    Radial
      Left 035C
      Right 035B
    Renal
      Left 045A
      Right 0459
    Splenic 0454
    Subclavian
      Left 0354
      Right 0353
    Superior Mesenteric 0455
    Temporal
      Left 035T
      Right 035S
    Thyroid
      Left 035V
      Right 035U
    Ulnar
      Left 035A
      Right 0359
    Upper 035Y
    Vertebral
      Left 035Q
      Right 035P
  Atrium
    Left 0257
    Right 0256
  Auditory Ossicle
    Left 095A
    Right 0959
  Basal Ganglia 0058
  Bladder 0T5B

Destruction — *continued*
  Bladder Neck 0T5C
  Bone
    Ethmoid
      Left 0N5G
      Right 0N5F
    Frontal 0N51
    Hyoid 0N5X
    Lacrimal
      Left 0N5J
      Right 0N5H
    Nasal 0N5B
    Occipital 0N57
    Palatine
      Left 0N5L
      Right 0N5K
    Parietal
      Left 0N54
      Right 0N53
    Pelvic
      Left 0Q53
      Right 0Q52
    Sphenoid 0N5C
    Temporal
      Left 0N56
      Right 0N55
    Zygomatic
      Left 0N5N
      Right 0N5M
  Brain 0050
  Breast
    Bilateral 0H5V
    Left 0H5U
    Right 0H5T
  Bronchus
    Lingula 0B59
    Lower Lobe
      Left 0B5B
      Right 0B56
    Main
      Left 0B57
      Right 0B53
    Middle Lobe, Right 0B55
    Upper Lobe
      Left 0B58
      Right 0B54
  Buccal Mucosa 0C54
  Bursa and Ligament
    Abdomen
      Left 0M5J
      Right 0M5H
    Ankle
      Left 0M5R
      Right 0M5Q
    Elbow
      Left 0M54
      Right 0M53
    Foot
      Left 0M5T
      Right 0M5S
    Hand
      Left 0M58
      Right 0M57
    Head and Neck 0M50
    Hip
      Left 0M5M
      Right 0M5L
    Knee
      Left 0M5P
      Right 0M5N
    Lower Extremity
      Left 0M5W
      Right 0M5V
    Perineum 0M5K
    Rib(s) 0M5G
    Shoulder
      Left 0M52
      Right 0M51
    Spine
      Lower 0M5D
      Upper 0M5C
    Sternum 0M5F
    Upper Extremity
      Left 0M5B
      Right 0M59
    Wrist
      Left 0M56
      Right 0M55
  Carina 0B52

Destruction — *continued*
  Carotid Bodies, Bilateral 0G58
  Carotid Body
    Left 0G56
    Right 0G57
  Carpal
    Left 0P5N
    Right 0P5M
  Cecum 0D5H
  Cerebellum 005C
  Cerebral Hemisphere 0057
  Cerebral Meninges 0051
  Cerebral Ventricle 0056
  Cervix 0U5C
  Chordae Tendineae 0259
  Choroid
    Left 085B
    Right 085A
  Cisterna Chyli 075L
  Clavicle
    Left 0P5B
    Right 0P59
  Clitoris 0U5J
  Coccygeal Glomus 0G5B
  Coccyx 0Q5S
  Colon
    Ascending 0D5K
    Descending 0D5M
    Sigmoid 0D5N
    Transverse 0D5L
  Conduction Mechanism 0258
  Conjunctiva
    Left 085TXZZ
    Right 085SXZZ
  Cord
    Bilateral 0V5H
    Left 0V5G
    Right 0V5F
  Cornea
    Left 0859XZZ
    Right 0858XZZ
  Cul-de-sac 0U5F
  Diaphragm 0B5T
  Disc
    Cervical Vertebral 0R53
    Cervicothoracic Vertebral 0R55
    Lumbar Vertebral 0S52
    Lumbosacral 0S54
    Thoracic Vertebral 0R59
    Thoracolumbar Vertebral 0R5B
  Duct
    Common Bile 0F59
    Cystic 0F58
    Hepatic
      Common 0F57
      Left 0F56
      Right 0F55
    Lacrimal
      Left 085Y
      Right 085X
    Pancreatic 0F5D
      Accessory 0F5F
    Parotid
      Left 0C5C
      Right 0C5B
  Duodenum 0D59
  Dura Mater 0052
  Ear
    External
      Left 0951
      Right 0950
    External Auditory Canal
      Left 0954
      Right 0953
    Inner
      Left 095E
      Right 095D
    Middle
      Left 0956
      Right 0955
  Endometrium 0U5B
  Epididymis
    Bilateral 0V5L
    Left 0V5K
    Right 0V5J
  Epiglottis 0C5R
  Esophagogastric Junction 0D54
  Esophagus 0D55
    Lower 0D53

Destruction — *continued*
  Nerve — *continued*
    Brachial Plexus Ø153
    Cervical Ø151
    Cervical Plexus Ø15Ø
    Facial ØØ5M
    Femoral Ø15D
    Glossopharyngeal ØØ5P
    Head and Neck Sympathetic Ø15K
    Hypoglossal ØØ5S
    Lumbar Ø15B
    Lumbar Plexus Ø159
    Lumbar Sympathetic Ø15N
    Lumbosacral Plexus Ø15A
    Median Ø155
    Oculomotor ØØ5H
    Olfactory ØØ5F
    Optic ØØ5G
    Peroneal Ø15H
    Phrenic Ø152
    Pudendal Ø15C
    Radial Ø156
    Sacral Ø15R
    Sacral Plexus Ø15Q
    Sacral Sympathetic Ø15P
    Sciatic Ø15F
    Thoracic Ø158
    Thoracic Sympathetic Ø15L
    Tibial Ø15G
    Trigeminal ØØ5K
    Trochlear ØØ5J
    Ulnar Ø154
    Vagus ØØ5Q
  Nipple
    Left ØH5X
    Right ØH5W
  Omentum ØD5U
  Orbit
    Left ØN5Q
    Right ØN5P
  Ovary
    Bilateral ØU52
    Left ØU51
    Right ØU5Ø
  Palate
    Hard ØC52
    Soft ØC53
  Pancreas ØF5G
  Para-aortic Body ØG59
  Paraganglion Extremity ØG5F
  Parathyroid Gland ØG5R
    Inferior
      Left ØG5P
      Right ØG5N
    Multiple ØG5Q
    Superior
      Left ØG5M
      Right ØG5L
  Patella
    Left ØQ5F
    Right ØQ5D
  Penis ØV5S
  Pericardium Ø25N
  Peritoneum ØD5W
  Phalanx
    Finger
      Left ØP5V
      Right ØP5T
    Thumb
      Left ØP5S
      Right ØP5R
    Toe
      Left ØQ5R
      Right ØQ5Q
  Pharynx ØC5M
  Pineal Body ØG51
  Pleura
    Left ØB5P
    Right ØB5N
  Pons ØØ5B
  Prepuce ØV5T
  Prostate ØV5Ø
    Robotic Waterjet Ablation XV5Ø8A4
  Radius
    Left ØP5J
    Right ØP5H
  Rectum ØD5P
  Retina
    Left Ø85F3ZZ

Destruction — *continued*
  Retina — *continued*
    Right Ø85E3ZZ
  Retinal Vessel
    Left Ø85H3ZZ
    Right Ø85G3ZZ
  Ribs
    1 to 2 ØP51
    3 or More ØP52
  Sacrum ØQ51
  Scapula
    Left ØP56
    Right ØP55
  Sclera
    Left Ø857XZZ
    Right Ø856XZZ
  Scrotum ØV55
  Septum
    Atrial Ø255
    Nasal Ø95M
    Ventricular Ø25M
  Sinus
    Accessory Ø95P
    Ethmoid
      Left Ø95V
      Right Ø95U
    Frontal
      Left Ø95T
      Right Ø95S
    Mastoid
      Left Ø95C
      Right Ø95B
    Maxillary
      Left Ø95R
      Right Ø95Q
    Sphenoid
      Left Ø95X
      Right Ø95W
  Skin
    Abdomen ØH57XZ
    Back ØH56XZ
    Buttock ØH58XZ
    Chest ØH55XZ
    Ear
      Left ØH53XZ
      Right ØH52XZ
    Face ØH51XZ
    Foot
      Left ØH5NXZ
      Right ØH5MXZ
    Hand
      Left ØH5GXZ
      Right ØH5FXZ
    Inguinal ØH5AXZ
    Lower Arm
      Left ØH5EXZ
      Right ØH5DXZ
    Lower Leg
      Left ØH5LXZ
      Right ØH5KXZ
    Neck ØH54XZ
    Perineum ØH59XZ
    Scalp ØH5ØXZ
    Upper Arm
      Left ØH5CXZ
      Right ØH5BXZ
    Upper Leg
      Left ØH5JXZ
      Right ØH5HXZ
  Skull ØN5Ø
  Spinal Cord
    Cervical ØØ5W
    Lumbar ØØ5Y
    Thoracic ØØ5X
  Spinal Meninges ØØ5T
  Spleen Ø75P
  Sternum ØP5Ø
  Stomach ØD56
    Pylorus ØD57
  Subcutaneous Tissue and Fascia
    Abdomen ØJ58
    Back ØJ57
    Buttock ØJ59
    Chest ØJ56
    Face ØJ51
    Foot
      Left ØJ5R
      Right ØJ5Q

Destruction — *continued*
  Subcutaneous Tissue and Fascia — *continued*
    Hand
      Left ØJ5K
      Right ØJ5J
    Lower Arm
      Left ØJ5H
      Right ØJ5G
    Lower Leg
      Left ØJ5P
      Right ØJ5N
    Neck
      Left ØJ55
      Right ØJ54
    Pelvic Region ØJ5C
    Perineum ØJ5B
    Scalp ØJ5Ø
    Upper Arm
      Left ØJ5F
      Right ØJ5D
    Upper Leg
      Left ØJ5M
      Right ØJ5L
  Tarsal
    Left ØQ5M
    Right ØQ5L
  Tendon
    Abdomen
      Left ØL5G
      Right ØL5F
    Ankle
      Left ØL5T
      Right ØL5S
    Foot
      Left ØL5W
      Right ØL5V
    Hand
      Left ØL58
      Right ØL57
    Head and Neck ØL5Ø
    Hip
      Left ØL5K
      Right ØL5J
    Knee
      Left ØL5R
      Right ØL5Q
    Lower Arm and Wrist
      Left ØL56
      Right ØL55
    Lower Leg
      Left ØL5P
      Right ØL5N
    Perineum ØL5H
    Shoulder
      Left ØL52
      Right ØL51
    Thorax
      Left ØL5D
      Right ØL5C
    Trunk
      Left ØL5B
      Right ØL59
    Upper Arm
      Left ØL54
      Right ØL53
    Upper Leg
      Left ØL5M
      Right ØL5L
  Testis
    Bilateral ØV5C
    Left ØV5B
    Right ØV59
  Thalamus ØØ59
  Thymus Ø75M
  Thyroid Gland ØG5K
    Left Lobe ØG5G
    Right Lobe ØG5H
  Tibia
    Left ØQ5H
    Right ØQ5G
  Toe Nail ØH5RXZZ
  Tongue ØC57
  Tonsils ØC5P
  Tooth
    Lower ØC5X
    Upper ØC5W
  Trachea ØB51
  Tunica Vaginalis
    Left ØV57

▽ **Subterms under main terms may continue to next column or page**

Dilation — *continued*
  Artery — *continued*
    External Carotid — *continued*
      Right 037M
    External Iliac
      Left 047J
      Right 047H
    Face 037R
    Femoral
      Left 047L
        Sustained Release Drug-eluting
          Intraluminal Device
          X27J385
          Four or More X27J3C5
          Three X27J3B5
          Two X27J395
      Right 047K
        Sustained Release Drug-eluting
          Intraluminal Device
          X27H385
          Four or More X27H3C5
          Three X27H3B5
          Two X27H395
    Foot
      Left 047W
      Right 047V
    Gastric 0472
    Hand
      Left 037F
      Right 037D
    Hepatic 0473
    Inferior Mesenteric 047B
    Innominate 0372
    Internal Carotid
      Left 037L
      Right 037K
    Internal Iliac
      Left 047F
      Right 047E
    Internal Mammary
      Left 0371
      Right 0370
    Intracranial 037G
    Lower 047Y
    Peroneal
      Left 047U
        Sustained Release Drug-eluting
          Intraluminal Device
          X27U385
          Four or More X27U3C5
          Three X27U3B5
          Two X27U395
      Right 047T
        Sustained Release Drug-eluting
          Intraluminal Device
          X27T385
          Four or More X27T3C5
          Three X27T3B5
          Two X27T395
    Popliteal
      Left 047N
      Left Distal
        Sustained Release Drug-eluting
          Intraluminal Device
          X27N385
          Four or More X27N3C5
          Three X27N3B5
          Two X27N395
      Left Proximal
        Sustained Release Drug-eluting
          Intraluminal Device
          X27L385
          Four or More X27L3C5
          Three X27L3B5
          Two X27L395
      Right 047M
      Right Distal
        Sustained Release Drug-eluting
          Intraluminal Device
          X27M385
          Four or More X27M3C5
          Three X27M3B5
          Two X27M395
      Right Proximal
        Sustained Release Drug-eluting
          Intraluminal Device
          X27K385
          Four or More X27K3C5
          Three X27K3B5

Dilation — *continued*
  Artery — *continued*
    Popliteal — *continued*
      Right Proximal — *continued*
        Sustained Release Drug-eluting In-
          traluminal Device — *contin-*
          ued
          Two X27K395
    Posterior Tibial
      Left 047S
        Sustained Release Drug-eluting
          Intraluminal Device
          X27S385
          Four or More X27S3C5
          Three X27S3B5
          Two X27S395
      Right 047R
        Sustained Release Drug-eluting
          Intraluminal Device
          X27R385
          Four or More X27R3C5
          Three X27R3B5
          Two X27R395
    Pulmonary
      Left 027R
      Right 027Q
    Pulmonary Trunk 027P
    Radial
      Left 037C
      Right 037B
    Renal
      Left 047A
      Right 0479
    Splenic 0474
    Subclavian
      Left 0374
      Right 0373
    Superior Mesenteric 0475
    Temporal
      Left 037T
      Right 037S
    Thyroid
      Left 037V
      Right 037U
    Ulnar
      Left 037A
      Right 0379
    Upper 037Y
    Vertebral
      Left 037Q
      Right 037P
  Bladder 0T7B
  Bladder Neck 0T7C
  Bronchus
    Lingula 0B79
    Lower Lobe
      Left 0B7B
      Right 0B76
    Main
      Left 0B77
      Right 0B73
    Middle Lobe, Right 0B75
    Upper Lobe
      Left 0B78
      Right 0B74
  Carina 0B72
  Cecum 0D7H
  Cerebral Ventricle 0076
  Cervix 0U7C
  Colon
    Ascending 0D7K
    Descending 0D7M
    Sigmoid 0D7N
    Transverse 0D7L
  Duct
    Common Bile 0F79
    Cystic 0F78
    Hepatic
      Common 0F77
      Left 0F76
      Right 0F75
    Lacrimal
      Left 087Y
      Right 087X
    Pancreatic 0F7D
      Accessory 0F7F
    Parotid
      Left 0C7C
      Right 0C7B

Dilation — *continued*
  Duodenum 0D79
  Esophagogastric Junction 0D74
  Esophagus 0D75
    Lower 0D73
    Middle 0D72
    Upper 0D71
  Eustachian Tube
    Left 097G
    Right 097F
  Fallopian Tube
    Left 0U76
    Right 0U75
  Fallopian Tubes, Bilateral 0U77
  Hymen 0U7K
  Ileocecal Valve 0D7C
  Ileum 0D7B
  Intestine
    Large 0D7E
      Left 0D7G
      Right 0D7F
    Small 0D78
  Jejunum 0D7A
  Kidney Pelvis
    Left 0T74
    Right 0T73
  Larynx 0C7S
  Pharynx 0C7M
  Rectum 0D7P
  Stomach 0D76
    Pylorus 0D77
  Trachea 0B71
  Ureter
    Left 0T77
    Right 0T76
  Ureters, Bilateral 0T78
  Urethra 0T7D
  Uterus 0U79
  Vagina 0U7G
  Valve
    Aortic 027F
    Mitral 027G
    Pulmonary 027H
    Tricuspid 027J
  Vas Deferens
    Bilateral 0V7Q
    Left 0V7P
    Right 0V7N
  Vein
    Axillary
      Left 0578
      Right 0577
    Azygos 0570
    Basilic
      Left 057C
      Right 057B
    Brachial
      Left 057A
      Right 0579
    Cephalic
      Left 057F
      Right 057D
    Colic 0677
    Common Iliac
      Left 067D
      Right 067C
    Esophageal 0673
    External Iliac
      Left 067G
      Right 067F
    External Jugular
      Left 057Q
      Right 057P
    Face
      Left 057V
      Right 057T
    Femoral
      Left 067N
      Right 067M
    Foot
      Left 067V
      Right 067T
    Gastric 0672
    Hand
      Left 057H
      Right 057G
    Hemiazygos 0571
    Hepatic 0674

Dilation — *continued*
  Vein — *continued*
    Hypogastric
      Left 067J
      Right 067H
    Inferior Mesenteric 0676
    Innominate
      Left 0574
      Right 0573
    Internal Jugular
      Left 057N
      Right 057M
    Intracranial 057L
    Lower 067Y
    Portal 0678
    Pulmonary
      Left 027T
      Right 027S
    Renal
      Left 067B
      Right 0679
    Saphenous
      Left 067Q
      Right 067P
    Splenic 0671
    Subclavian
      Left 0576
      Right 0575
    Superior Mesenteric 0675
    Upper 057Y
    Vertebral
      Left 057S
      Right 057R
  Vena Cava
    Inferior 0670
    Superior 027V
  Ventricle
    Left 027L
    Right 027K
Direct Lateral Interbody Fusion (DLIF) device *use*
  Interbody Fusion Device in Lower Joints
Disarticulation *see* Detachment
Discectomy, diskectomy
  see Excision, Lower Joints 0SB
  see Excision, Upper Joints 0RB
  see Resection, Lower Joints 0ST
  see Resection, Upper Joints 0RT
Discography
  see Fluoroscopy, Axial Skeleton, Except Skull and
    Facial Bones BR1
  see Plain Radiography, Axial Skeleton, Except Skull
    and Facial Bones BR0
Dismembered pyeloplasty *see* Repair, Kidney Pelvis
Distal humerus
  use Humeral Shaft, Left
  use Humeral Shaft, Right
Distal humerus, involving joint
  use Elbow Joint, Left
  use Elbow Joint, Right
Distal radioulnar joint
  use Wrist Joint, Left
  use Wrist Joint, Right
Diversion *see* Bypass
Diverticulectomy *see* Excision, Gastrointestinal System
  0DB
Division
  Acetabulum
    Left 0Q85
    Right 0Q84
  Anal Sphincter 0D8R
  Basal Ganglia 0088
  Bladder Neck 0T8C
  Bone
    Ethmoid
      Left 0N8G
      Right 0N8F
    Frontal 0N81
    Hyoid 0N8X
    Lacrimal
      Left 0N8J
      Right 0N8H
    Nasal 0N8B
    Occipital 0N87
    Palatine
      Left 0N8L
      Right 0N8K
    Parietal
      Left 0N84

Division — *continued*
  Bone — *continued*
    Parietal — *continued*
      Right 0N83
    Pelvic
      Left 0Q83
      Right 0Q82
    Sphenoid 0N8C
    Temporal
      Left 0N86
      Right 0N85
    Zygomatic
      Left 0N8N
      Right 0N8M
  Brain 0080
  Bursa and Ligament
    Abdomen
      Left 0M8J
      Right 0M8H
    Ankle
      Left 0M8R
      Right 0M8Q
    Elbow
      Left 0M84
      Right 0M83
    Foot
      Left 0M8T
      Right 0M8S
    Hand
      Left 0M88
      Right 0M87
    Head and Neck 0M80
    Hip
      Left 0M8M
      Right 0M8L
    Knee
      Left 0M8P
      Right 0M8N
    Lower Extremity
      Left 0M8W
      Right 0M8V
    Perineum 0M8K
    Rib(s) 0M8G
    Shoulder
      Left 0M82
      Right 0M81
    Spine
      Lower 0M8D
      Upper 0M8C
    Sternum 0M8F
    Upper Extremity
      Left 0M8B
      Right 0M89
    Wrist
      Left 0M86
      Right 0M85
  Carpal
    Left 0P8N
    Right 0P8M
  Cerebral Hemisphere 0087
  Chordae Tendineae 0289
  Clavicle
    Left 0P8B
    Right 0P89
  Coccyx 0Q8S
  Conduction Mechanism 0288
  Esophagogastric Junction 0D84
  Femoral Shaft
    Left 0Q89
    Right 0Q88
  Femur
    Lower
      Left 0Q8C
      Right 0Q8B
    Upper
      Left 0Q87
      Right 0Q86
  Fibula
    Left 0Q8K
    Right 0Q8J
  Gland, Pituitary 0G80
  Glenoid Cavity
    Left 0P88
    Right 0P87
  Humeral Head
    Left 0P8D
    Right 0P8C
  Humeral Shaft
    Left 0P8G

Division — *continued*
  Humeral Shaft — *continued*
    Right 0P8F
  Hymen 0U8K
  Kidneys, Bilateral 0T82
  Liver 0F80
    Left Lobe 0F82
    Right Lobe 0F81
  Mandible
    Left 0N8V
    Right 0N8T
  Maxilla 0N8R
  Metacarpal
    Left 0P8Q
    Right 0P8P
  Metatarsal
    Left 0Q8P
    Right 0Q8N
  Muscle
    Abdomen
      Left 0K8L
      Right 0K8K
    Facial 0K81
    Foot
      Left 0K8W
      Right 0K8V
    Hand
      Left 0K8D
      Right 0K8C
    Head 0K80
    Hip
      Left 0K8P
      Right 0K8N
    Lower Arm and Wrist
      Left 0K8B
      Right 0K89
    Lower Leg
      Left 0K8T
      Right 0K8S
    Neck
      Left 0K83
      Right 0K82
    Papillary 028D
    Perineum 0K8M
    Shoulder
      Left 0K86
      Right 0K85
    Thorax
      Left 0K8J
      Right 0K8H
    Tongue, Palate, Pharynx 0K84
    Trunk
      Left 0K8G
      Right 0K8F
    Upper Arm
      Left 0K88
      Right 0K87
    Upper Leg
      Left 0K8R
      Right 0K8Q
  Nerve
    Abdominal Sympathetic 018M
    Abducens 008L
    Accessory 008R
    Acoustic 008N
    Brachial Plexus 0183
    Cervical 0181
    Cervical Plexus 0180
    Facial 008M
    Femoral 018D
    Glossopharyngeal 008P
    Head and Neck Sympathetic 018K
    Hypoglossal 008S
    Lumbar 018B
    Lumbar Plexus 0189
    Lumbar Sympathetic 018N
    Lumbosacral Plexus 018A
    Median 0185
    Oculomotor 008H
    Olfactory 008F
    Optic 008G
    Peroneal 018H
    Phrenic 0182
    Pudendal 018C
    Radial 0186
    Sacral 018R
    Sacral Plexus 018Q
    Sacral Sympathetic 018P
    Sciatic 018F

▽ **Subterms under main terms may continue to next column or page**

Drainage — continued

Artery — continued
Inferior Mesenteric Ø49B
Innominate Ø392
Internal Carotid
  Left Ø39L
  Right Ø39K
Internal Iliac
  Left Ø49F
  Right Ø49E
Internal Mammary
  Left Ø391
  Right Ø390
Intracranial Ø39G
Lower Ø49Y
Peroneal
  Left Ø49U
  Right Ø49T
Popliteal
  Left Ø49N
  Right Ø49M
Posterior Tibial
  Left Ø49S
  Right Ø49R
Radial
  Left Ø39C
  Right Ø39B
Renal
  Left Ø49A
  Right Ø499
Splenic Ø494
Subclavian
  Left Ø394
  Right Ø393
Superior Mesenteric Ø495
Temporal
  Left Ø39T
  Right Ø39S
Thyroid
  Left Ø39V
  Right Ø39U
Ulnar
  Left Ø39A
  Right Ø399
Upper Ø39Y
Vertebral
  Left Ø39Q
  Right Ø39P
Auditory Ossicle
Left Ø99A
Right Ø999
Axilla
Left ØX95
Right ØX94
Back
Lower ØW9L
Upper ØW9K
Basal Ganglia ØØ98
Bladder ØT9B
Bladder Neck ØT9C
Bone
Ethmoid
  Left ØN9G
  Right ØN9F
Frontal ØN91
Hyoid ØN9X
Lacrimal
  Left ØN9J
  Right ØN9H
Nasal ØN9B
Occipital ØN97
Palatine
  Left ØN9L
  Right ØN9K
Parietal
  Left ØN94
  Right ØN93
Pelvic
  Left ØQ93
  Right ØQ92
Sphenoid ØN9C
Temporal
  Left ØN96
  Right ØN95
Zygomatic
  Left ØN9N
  Right ØN9M
Bone Marrow Ø79T
Brain ØØ9Ø

Drainage — continued

Breast
Bilateral ØH9V
Left ØH9U
Right ØH9T
Bronchus
Lingula ØB99
Lower Lobe
  Left ØB9B
  Right ØB96
Main
  Left ØB97
  Right ØB93
Middle Lobe, Right ØB95
Upper Lobe
  Left ØB98
  Right ØB94
Buccal Mucosa ØC94
Bursa and Ligament
Abdomen
  Left ØM9J
  Right ØM9H
Ankle
  Left ØM9R
  Right ØM9Q
Elbow
  Left ØM94
  Right ØM93
Foot
  Left ØM9T
  Right ØM9S
Hand
  Left ØM98
  Right ØM97
Head and Neck ØM9Ø
Hip
  Left ØM9M
  Right ØM9L
Knee
  Left ØM9P
  Right ØM9N
Lower Extremity
  Left ØM9W
  Right ØM9V
Perineum ØM9K
Rib(s) ØM9G
Shoulder
  Left ØM92
  Right ØM91
Spine
  Lower ØM9D
  Upper ØM9C
Sternum ØM9F
Upper Extremity
  Left ØM9B
  Right ØM99
Wrist
  Left ØM96
  Right ØM95
Buttock
Left ØY91
Right ØY9Ø
Carina ØB92
Carotid Bodies, Bilateral ØG98
Carotid Body
Left ØG96
Right ØG97
Carpal
Left ØP9N
Right ØP9M
Cavity, Cranial ØW91
Cecum ØD9H
Cerebellum ØØ9C
Cerebral Hemisphere ØØ97
Cerebral Meninges ØØ91
Cerebral Ventricle ØØ96
Cervix ØU9C
Chest Wall ØW98
Choroid
Left Ø89B
Right Ø89A
Cisterna Chyli Ø79L
Clavicle
Left ØP9B
Right ØP99
Clitoris ØU9J
Coccygeal Glomus ØG9B
Coccyx ØQ9S

Drainage — continued

Colon
Ascending ØD9K
Descending ØD9M
Sigmoid ØD9N
Transverse ØD9L
Conjunctiva
Left Ø89T
Right Ø89S
Cord
Bilateral ØV9H
Left ØV9G
Right ØV9F
Cornea
Left Ø899
Right Ø898
Cul-de-sac ØU9F
Diaphragm ØB9T
Disc
Cervical Vertebral ØR93
Cervicothoracic Vertebral ØR95
Lumbar Vertebral ØS92
Lumbosacral ØS94
Thoracic Vertebral ØR99
Thoracolumbar Vertebral ØR9B
Duct
Common Bile ØF99
Cystic ØF98
Hepatic
  Common ØF97
  Left ØF96
  Right ØF95
Lacrimal
  Left Ø89Y
  Right Ø89X
Pancreatic ØF9D
  Accessory ØF9F
Parotid
  Left ØC9C
  Right ØC9B
Duodenum ØD99
Dura Mater ØØ92
Ear
External
  Left Ø991
  Right Ø990
External Auditory Canal
  Left Ø994
  Right Ø993
Inner
  Left Ø99E
  Right Ø99D
Middle
  Left Ø996
  Right Ø995
Elbow Region
Left ØX9C
Right ØX9B
Epididymis
Bilateral ØV9L
Left ØV9K
Right ØV9J
Epidural Space, Intracranial ØØ93
Epiglottis ØC9R
Esophagogastric Junction ØD94
Esophagus ØD95
Lower ØD93
Middle ØD92
Upper ØD91
Eustachian Tube
Left Ø99G
Right Ø99F
Extremity
Lower
  Left ØY9B
  Right ØY99
Upper
  Left ØX97
  Right ØX96
Eye
Left Ø891
Right Ø890
Eyelid
Lower
  Left Ø89R
  Right Ø89Q
Upper
  Left Ø89P
  Right Ø89N

Drainage — *continued*
  Face ØW92
  Fallopian Tube
    Left ØU96
    Right ØU95
  Fallopian Tubes, Bilateral ØU97
  Femoral Region
    Left ØY98
    Right ØY97
  Femoral Shaft
    Left ØQ99
    Right ØQ98
  Femur
    Lower
      Left ØQ9C
      Right ØQ9B
    Upper
      Left ØQ97
      Right ØQ96
  Fibula
    Left ØQ9K
    Right ØQ9J
  Finger Nail ØH9Q
  Foot
    Left ØY9N
    Right ØY9M
  Gallbladder ØF94
  Gingiva
    Lower ØC96
    Upper ØC95
  Gland
    Adrenal
      Bilateral ØG94
      Left ØG92
      Right ØG93
    Lacrimal
      Left Ø89W
      Right Ø89V
    Minor Salivary ØC9J
    Parotid
      Left ØC99
      Right ØC98
    Pituitary ØG90
    Sublingual
      Left ØC9F
      Right ØC9D
    Submaxillary
      Left ØC9H
      Right ØC9G
    Vestibular ØU9L
  Glenoid Cavity
    Left ØP98
    Right ØP97
  Glomus Jugulare ØG9C
  Hand
    Left ØX9K
    Right ØX9J
  Head ØW90
  Humeral Head
    Left ØP9D
    Right ØP9C
  Humeral Shaft
    Left ØP9G
    Right ØP9F
  Hymen ØU9K
  Hypothalamus ØØ9A
  Ileocecal Valve ØD9C
  Ileum ØD9B
  Inguinal Region
    Left ØY96
    Right ØY95
  Intestine
    Large ØD9E
      Left ØD9G
      Right ØD9F
    Small ØD98
  Iris
    Left Ø89D
    Right Ø89C
  Jaw
    Lower ØW95
    Upper ØW94
  Jejunum ØD9A
  Joint
    Acromioclavicular
      Left ØR9H
      Right ØR9G
    Ankle
      Left ØS9G

Drainage — *continued*
  Joint — *continued*
    Ankle — *continued*
      Right ØS9F
    Carpal
      Left ØR9R
      Right ØR9Q
    Carpometacarpal
      Left ØR9T
      Right ØR9S
    Cervical Vertebral ØR91
    Cervicothoracic Vertebral ØR94
    Coccygeal ØS96
    Elbow
      Left ØR9M
      Right ØR9L
    Finger Phalangeal
      Left ØR9X
      Right ØR9W
    Hip
      Left ØS9B
      Right ØS99
    Knee
      Left ØS9D
      Right ØS9C
    Lumbar Vertebral ØS90
    Lumbosacral ØS93
    Metacarpophalangeal
      Left ØR9V
      Right ØR9U
    Metatarsal-Phalangeal
      Left ØS9N
      Right ØS9M
    Occipital-cervical ØR90
    Sacrococcygeal ØS95
    Sacroiliac
      Left ØS98
      Right ØS97
    Shoulder
      Left ØR9K
      Right ØR9J
    Sternoclavicular
      Left ØR9F
      Right ØR9E
    Tarsal
      Left ØS9J
      Right ØS9H
    Tarsometatarsal
      Left ØS9L
      Right ØS9K
    Temporomandibular
      Left ØR9D
      Right ØR9C
    Thoracic Vertebral ØR96
    Thoracolumbar Vertebral ØR9A
    Toe Phalangeal
      Left ØS9Q
      Right ØS9P
    Wrist
      Left ØR9P
      Right ØR9N
  Kidney
    Left ØT91
    Right ØT90
  Kidney Pelvis
    Left ØT94
    Right ØT93
  Knee Region
    Left ØY9G
    Right ØY9F
  Larynx ØC9S
  Leg
    Lower
      Left ØY9J
      Right ØY9H
    Upper
      Left ØY9D
      Right ØY9C
  Lens
    Left Ø89K
    Right Ø89J
  Lip
    Lower ØC91
    Upper ØC90
  Liver ØF90
    Left Lobe ØF92
    Right Lobe ØF91
  Lung
    Bilateral ØB9M

Drainage — *continued*
  Lung — *continued*
    Left ØB9L
    ·Lower Lobe
      Left ØB9J
      Right ØB9F
    Middle Lobe, Right ØB9D
    Right ØB9K
    Upper Lobe
      Left ØB9G
      Right ØB9C
  Lung Lingula ØB9H
  Lymphatic
    Aortic Ø79D
    Axillary
      Left Ø796
      Right Ø795
    Head Ø790
    Inguinal
      Left Ø79J
      Right Ø79H
    Internal Mammary
      Left Ø799
      Right Ø798
    Lower Extremity
      Left Ø79G
      Right Ø79F
    Mesenteric Ø79B
    Neck
      Left Ø792
      Right Ø791
    Pelvis Ø79C
    Thoracic Duct Ø79K
    Thorax Ø797
    Upper Extremity
      Left Ø794
      Right Ø793
  Mandible
    Left ØN9V
    Right ØN9T
  Maxilla ØN9R
  Mediastinum ØW9C
  Medulla Oblongata ØØ9D
  Mesentery ØD9V
  Metacarpal
    Left ØP9Q
    Right ØP9P
  Metatarsal
    Left ØQ9P
    Right ØQ9N
  Muscle
    Abdomen
      Left ØK9L
      Right ØK9K
    Extraocular
      Left Ø89M
      Right Ø89L
    Facial ØK91
    Foot
      Left ØK9W
      Right ØK9V
    Hand
      Left ØK9D
      Right ØK9C
    Head ØK90
    Hip
      Left ØK9P
      Right ØK9N
    Lower Arm and Wrist
      Left ØK9B
      Right ØK99
    Lower Leg
      Left ØK9T
      Right ØK9S
    Neck
      Left ØK93
      Right ØK92
    Perineum ØK9M
    Shoulder
      Left ØK96
      Right ØK95
    Thorax
      Left ØK9J
      Right ØK9H
    Tongue, Palate, Pharynx ØK94
    Trunk
      Left ØK9G
      Right ØK9F

Drainage — *continued*
  Muscle — *continued*
    Upper Arm
      Left ØK98
      Right ØK97
    Upper Leg
      Left ØK9R
      Right ØK9Q
  Nasal Mucosa and Soft Tissue Ø99K
  Nasopharynx Ø99N
  Neck ØW96
  Nerve
    Abdominal Sympathetic Ø19M
    Abducens ØØ9L
    Accessory ØØ9R
    Acoustic ØØ9N
    Brachial Plexus Ø193
    Cervical Ø191
    Cervical Plexus Ø19Ø
    Facial ØØ9M
    Femoral Ø19D
    Glossopharyngeal ØØ9P
    Head and Neck Sympathetic Ø19K
    Hypoglossal ØØ9S
    Lumbar Ø19B
    Lumbar Plexus Ø199
    Lumbar Sympathetic Ø19N
    Lumbosacral Plexus Ø19A
    Median Ø195
    Oculomotor ØØ9H
    Olfactory ØØ9F
    Optic ØØ9G
    Peroneal Ø19H
    Phrenic Ø192
    Pudendal Ø19C
    Radial Ø196
    Sacral Ø19R
    Sacral Plexus Ø19Q
    Sacral Sympathetic Ø19P
    Sciatic Ø19F
    Thoracic Ø198
    Thoracic Sympathetic Ø19L
    Tibial Ø19G
    Trigeminal ØØ9K
    Trochlear ØØ9J
    Ulnar Ø194
    Vagus ØØ9Q
  Nipple
    Left ØH9X
    Right ØH9W
  Omentum ØD9U
  Oral Cavity and Throat ØW93
  Orbit
    Left ØN9Q
    Right ØN9P
  Ovary
    Bilateral ØU92
    Left ØU91
    Right ØU9Ø
  Palate
    Hard ØC92
    Soft ØC93
  Pancreas ØF9G
  Para-aortic Body ØG99
  Paraganglion Extremity ØG9F
  Parathyroid Gland ØG9R
    Inferior
      Left ØG9P
      Right ØG9N
    Multiple ØG9Q
    Superior
      Left ØG9M
      Right ØG9L
  Patella
    Left ØQ9F
    Right ØQ9D
  Pelvic Cavity ØW9J
  Penis ØV9S
  Pericardial Cavity ØW9D
  Perineum
    Female ØW9N
    Male ØW9M
  Peritoneal Cavity ØW9G
  Peritoneum ØD9W
  Phalanx
    Finger
      Left ØP9V
      Right ØP9T

Drainage — *continued*
  Phalanx — *continued*
    Thumb
      Left ØP9S
      Right ØP9R
    Toe
      Left ØQ9R
      Right ØQ9Q
  Pharynx ØC9M
  Pineal Body ØG91
  Pleura
    Left ØB9P
    Right ØB9N
  Pleural Cavity
    Left ØW9B
    Right ØW99
  Pons ØØ9B
  Prepuce ØV9T
  Products of Conception
    Amniotic Fluid
      Diagnostic 1Ø9Ø
      Therapeutic 1Ø9Ø
    Fetal Blood 1Ø9Ø
    Fetal Cerebrospinal Fluid 1Ø9Ø
    Fetal Fluid, Other 1Ø9Ø
    Fluid, Other 1Ø9Ø
  Prostate ØV9Ø
  Radius
    Left ØP9J
    Right ØP9H
  Rectum ØD9P
  Retina
    Left Ø89F
    Right Ø89E
  Retinal Vessel
    Left Ø89H
    Right Ø89G
  Retroperitoneum ØW9H
  Ribs
    1 to 2 ØP91
    3 or More ØP92
  Sacrum ØQ91
  Scapula
    Left ØP96
    Right ØP95
  Sclera
    Left Ø897
    Right Ø896
  Scrotum ØV95
  Septum, Nasal Ø99M
  Shoulder Region
    Left ØX93
    Right ØX92
  Sinus
    Accessory Ø99P
    Ethmoid
      Left Ø99V
      Right Ø99U
    Frontal
      Left Ø99T
      Right Ø99S
    Mastoid
      Left Ø99C
      Right Ø99B
    Maxillary
      Left Ø99R
      Right Ø99Q
    Sphenoid
      Left Ø99X
      Right Ø99W
  Skin
    Abdomen ØH97
    Back ØH96
    Buttock ØH98
    Chest ØH95
    Ear
      Left ØH93
      Right ØH92
    Face ØH91
    Foot
      Left ØH9N
      Right ØH9M
    Hand
      Left ØH9G
      Right ØH9F
    Inguinal ØH9A
    Lower Arm
      Left ØH9E
      Right ØH9D

Drainage — *continued*
  Skin — *continued*
    Lower Leg
      Left ØH9L
      Right ØH9K
    Neck ØH94
    Perineum ØH99
    Scalp ØH9Ø
    Upper Arm
      Left ØH9C
      Right ØH9B
    Upper Leg
      Left ØH9J
      Right ØH9H
  Skull ØN9Ø
  Spinal Canal ØØ9U
  Spinal Cord
    Cervical ØØ9W
    Lumbar ØØ9Y
    Thoracic ØØ9X
  Spinal Meninges ØØ9T
  Spleen Ø79P
  Sternum ØP9Ø
  Stomach ØD96
    Pylorus ØD97
  Subarachnoid Space, Intracranial ØØ95
  Subcutaneous Tissue and Fascia
    Abdomen ØJ98
    Back ØJ97
    Buttock ØJ99
    Chest ØJ96
    Face ØJ91
    Foot
      Left ØJ9R
      Right ØJ9Q
    Hand
      Left ØJ9K
      Right ØJ9J
    Lower Arm
      Left ØJ9H
      Right ØJ9G
    Lower Leg
      Left ØJ9P
      Right ØJ9N
    Neck
      Left ØJ95
      Right ØJ94
    Pelvic Region ØJ9C
    Perineum ØJ9B
    Scalp ØJ9Ø
    Upper Arm
      Left ØJ9F
      Right ØJ9D
    Upper Leg
      Left ØJ9M
      Right ØJ9L
  Subdural Space, Intracranial ØØ94
  Tarsal
    Left ØQ9M
    Right ØQ9L
  Tendon
    Abdomen
      Left ØL9G
      Right ØL9F
    Ankle
      Left ØL9T
      Right ØL9S
    Foot
      Left ØL9W
      Right ØL9V
    Hand
      Left ØL98
      Right ØL97
    Head and Neck ØL9Ø
    Hip
      Left ØL9K
      Right ØL9J
    Knee
      Left ØL9R
      Right ØL9Q
    Lower Arm and Wrist
      Left ØL96
      Right ØL95
    Lower Leg
      Left ØL9P
      Right ØL9N
    Perineum ØL9H
    Shoulder
      Left ØL92

Subterms under main terms may continue to next column or page

Drainage — *continued*
  Tendon — *continued*
    Shoulder — *continued*
      Right ØL91
    Thorax
      Left ØL9D
      Right ØL9C
    Trunk
      Left ØL9B
      Right ØL99
    Upper Arm
      Left ØL94
      Right ØL93
    Upper Leg
      Left ØL9M
      Right ØL9L
  Testis
    Bilateral ØV9C
    Left ØV9B
    Right ØV99
  Thalamus ØØ99
  Thymus Ø79M
  Thyroid Gland ØG9K
    Left Lobe ØG9G
    Right Lobe ØG9H
  Tibia
    Left ØQ9H
    Right ØQ9G
  Toe Nail ØH9R
  Tongue ØC97
  Tonsils ØC9P
  Tooth
    Lower ØC9X
    Upper ØC9W
  Trachea ØB91
  Tunica Vaginalis
    Left ØV97
    Right ØV96
  Turbinate, Nasal Ø99L
  Tympanic Membrane
    Left Ø998
    Right Ø997
  Ulna
    Left ØP9L
    Right ØP9K
  Ureter
    Left ØT97
    Right ØT96
  Ureters, Bilateral ØT98
  Urethra ØT9D
  Uterine Supporting Structure ØU94
  Uterus ØU99
  Uvula ØC9N
  Vagina ØU9G
  Vas Deferens
    Bilateral ØV9Q
    Left ØV9P
    Right ØV9N
  Vein
    Axillary
      Left Ø598
      Right Ø597
    Azygos Ø590
    Basilic
      Left Ø59C
      Right Ø59B
    Brachial
      Left Ø59A
      Right Ø599
    Cephalic
      Left Ø59F
      Right Ø59D
    Colic Ø697
    Common Iliac
      Left Ø69D
      Right Ø69C
    Esophageal Ø693
    External Iliac
      Left Ø69G
      Right Ø69F
    External Jugular
      Left Ø59Q
      Right Ø59P
    Face
      Left Ø59V
      Right Ø59T
    Femoral
      Left Ø69N
      Right Ø69M

Drainage — *continued*
  Vein — *continued*
    Foot
      Left Ø69V
      Right Ø69T
    Gastric Ø692
    Hand
      Left Ø59H
      Right Ø59G
    Hemiazygos Ø591
    Hepatic Ø694
    Hypogastric
      Left Ø69J
      Right Ø69H
    Inferior Mesenteric Ø696
    Innominate
      Left Ø594
      Right Ø593
    Internal Jugular
      Left Ø59N
      Right Ø59M
    Intracranial Ø59L
    Lower Ø69Y
    Portal Ø698
    Renal
      Left Ø69B
      Right Ø699
    Saphenous
      Left Ø69Q
      Right Ø69P
    Splenic Ø691
    Subclavian
      Left Ø596
      Right Ø595
    Superior Mesenteric Ø695
    Upper Ø59Y
    Vertebral
      Left Ø59S
      Right Ø59R
  Vena Cava, Inferior Ø690
  Vertebra
    Cervical ØP93
    Lumbar ØQ90
    Thoracic ØP94
  Vesicle
    Bilateral ØV93
    Left ØV92
    Right ØV91
  Vitreous
    Left Ø895
    Right Ø894
  Vocal Cord
    Left ØC9V
    Right ØC9T
  Vulva ØU9M
  Wrist Region
    Left ØX9H
    Right ØX9G
Dressing
  Abdominal Wall 2W23X4Z
  Arm
    Lower
      Left 2W2DX4Z
      Right 2W2CX4Z
    Upper
      Left 2W2BX4Z
      Right 2W2AX4Z
  Back 2W25X4Z
  Chest Wall 2W24X4Z
  Extremity
    Lower
      Left 2W2MX4Z
      Right 2W2LX4Z
    Upper
      Left 2W29X4Z
      Right 2W28X4Z
  Face 2W21X4Z
  Finger
    Left 2W2KX4Z
    Right 2W2JX4Z
  Foot
    Left 2W2TX4Z
    Right 2W2SX4Z
  Hand
    Left 2W2FX4Z
    Right 2W2EX4Z
  Head 2W20X4Z
  Inguinal Region
    Left 2W27X4Z

Dressing — *continued*
  Inguinal Region — *continued*
    Right 2W26X4Z
  Leg
    Lower
      Left 2W2RX4Z
      Right 2W2QX4Z
    Upper
      Left 2W2PX4Z
      Right 2W2NX4Z
  Neck 2W22X4Z
  Thumb
    Left 2W2HX4Z
    Right 2W2GX4Z
  Toe
    Left 2W2VX4Z
    Right 2W2UX4Z
Driver stent (RX) (OTW) *use* Intraluminal Device
Drotrecogin alfa, infusion *see* Introduction of Recombinant Human-activated Protein C
Duct of Santorini *use* Pancreatic Duct, Accessory
Duct of Wirsung *use* Pancreatic Duct
Ductogram, mammary *see* Plain Radiography, Skin, Subcutaneous Tissue and Breast BHØ
Ductography, mammary *see* Plain Radiography, Skin, Subcutaneous Tissue and Breast BHØ
Ductus deferens
  use Vas Deferens
  use Vas Deferens, Bilateral
  use Vas Deferens, Left
  use Vas Deferens, Right
Duodenal ampulla *use* Ampulla of Vater
Duodenectomy
  see Excision, Duodenum ØDB9
  see Resection, Duodenum ØDT9
Duodenocholedochotomy *see* Drainage, Gallbladder ØF94
Duodenocystostomy
  see Bypass, Gallbladder ØF14
  see Drainage, Gallbladder ØF94
Duodenoenterostomy
  see Bypass, Gastrointestinal System ØD1
  see Drainage, Gastrointestinal System ØD9
Duodenojejunal flexure *use* Jejunum
Duodenolysis *see* Release, Duodenum ØDN9
Duodenorrhaphy *see* Repair, Duodenum ØDQ9
Duodenoscopy, single-use (aScope™ Duodeno) (EXALT™ Model D) *see* New Technology, Hepatobiliary System and Pancreas XFJ
Duodenostomy
  see Bypass, Duodenum ØD19
  see Drainage, Duodenum ØD99
Duodenotomy *see* Drainage, Duodenum ØD99
Dura mater, intracranial *use* Dura Mater
Dura mater, spinal *use* Spinal Meninges
DuraGraft® Endothelial Damage Inhibitor *use* Endothelial Damage Inhibitor
DuraHeart Left Ventricular Assist System *use* Implantable Heart Assist System in Heart and Great Vessels
Dural venous sinus *use* Intracranial Vein
Durata® Defibrillation Lead *use* Cardiac Lead, Defibrillator in Ø2H
Durvalumab Antineoplastic XWØ
DynaNail Mini®
  use Internal Fixation Device, Sustained Compression in ØRG
  use Internal Fixation Device, Sustained Compression in ØSG
DynaNail®
  use Internal Fixation Device, Sustained Compression in ØRG
  use Internal Fixation Device, Sustained Compression in ØSG
Dynesys® Dynamic Stabilization System
  use Spinal Stabilization Device, Pedicle-Based in ØRH
  use Spinal Stabilization Device, Pedicle-Based in ØSH

E

Earlobe
  use Ear, External, Bilateral
  use Ear, External, Left
  use Ear, External, Right

ECCO2R (Extracorporeal Carbon Dioxide Removal) 5A0920Z
Echocardiogram *see* Ultrasonography, Heart B24
Echography *see* Ultrasonography
EchoTip® Insight™ Portosystemic Pressure Gradient Measurement System 4A044B2
ECMO *see* Performance, Circulatory 5A15
ECMO, intraoperative *see* Performance, Circulatory 5A15A
Eculizumab XW0
EDWARDS INTUITY Elite valve system *use* Zooplastic Tissue, Rapid Deployment Technique in New Technology
EEG (electroencephalogram) *see* Measurement, Central Nervous 4A00
EGD (esophagogastroduodenoscopy) 0DJ08ZZ
Eighth cranial nerve *use* Acoustic Nerve
Ejaculatory duct
　use Vas Deferens
　use Vas Deferens, Bilateral
　use Vas Deferens, Left
　use Vas Deferens, Right
EKG (electrocardiogram) *see* Measurement, Cardiac 4A02
EKOS™ EkoSonic® Endovascular System *see* Fragmentation, Artery
Eladocagene exuparvovec XW0Q316
Electrical bone growth stimulator (EBGS)
　use Bone Growth Stimulator in Head and Facial Bones
　use Bone Growth Stimulator in Lower Bones
　use Bone Growth Stimulator in Upper Bones
Electrical muscle stimulation (EMS) lead *use* Stimulator Lead in Muscles
Electrocautery
　Destruction *see* Destruction
　Repair *see* Repair
Electroconvulsive Therapy
　Bilateral-Multiple Seizure GZB3ZZZ
　Bilateral-Single Seizure GZB2ZZZ
　Electroconvulsive Therapy, Other GZB4ZZZ
　Unilateral-Multiple Seizure GZB1ZZZ
　Unilateral-Single Seizure GZB0ZZZ
Electroencephalogram (EEG) *see* Measurement, Central Nervous 4A00
Electromagnetic Therapy
　Central Nervous 6A22
　Urinary 6A21
Electronic muscle stimulator lead *use* Stimulator Lead in Muscles
Electrophysiologic stimulation (EPS) *see* Measurement, Cardiac 4A02
Electroshock therapy *see* Electroconvulsive Therapy
Elevation, bone fragments, skull *see* Reposition, Head and Facial Bones 0NS
Eleventh cranial nerve *use* Accessory Nerve
Ellipsys® vascular access system *see* New Technology, Cardiovascular System X2K
E-Luminexx™ (Biliary) (Vascular) Stent *use* Intraluminal Device
Eluvia™ Drug-Eluting Vascular Stent System
　use Intraluminal Device, Sustained Release Drug-eluting in New Technology
　use Intraluminal Device, Sustained Release Drug-eluting, Two in New Technology
　use Intraluminal Device, Sustained Release Drug-eluting, Three in New Technology
　use Intraluminal Device, Sustained Release Drug-eluting, Four or More in New Technology
ELZONRIS™ *use* Tagraxofusp-erzs Antineoplastic
Embolectomy *see* Extirpation
Embolization
　see Occlusion
　see Restriction
Embolization coil(s) *use* Intraluminal Device
EMG (electromyogram) *see* Measurement, Musculoskeletal 4A0F
Encephalon *use* Brain
Endarterectomy
　see Extirpation, Lower Arteries 04C
　see Extirpation, Upper Arteries 03C
Endeavor® (III) (IV) (Sprint) Zotarolimus-eluting Coronary Stent System *use* Intraluminal Device, Drug-eluting in Heart and Great Vessels
EndoAVF procedure, using magnetic-guided radiofrequency *see* Bypass, Upper Arteries 031

EndoAVF procedure, using thermal resistance energy *see* New Technology, Cardiovascular System X2K
Endologix AFX® Endovascular AAA System *use* Intraluminal Device
EndoSure® sensor *use* Monitoring Device, Pressure Sensor in 02H
ENDOTAK RELIANCE® (G) Defibrillation Lead *use* Cardiac Lead, Defibrillator in 02H
Endothelial damage inhibitor, applied to vein graft XY0VX83
Endotracheal tube (cuffed) (double-lumen) *use* Intraluminal Device, Endotracheal Airway in Respiratory System
Endovascular fistula creation, using magnetic-guided radiofrequency *see* Bypass, Upper Arteries 031
Endovascular fistula creation, using thermal resistance energy *see* New Technology, Cardiovascular System X2K
Endurant® Endovascular Stent Graft *use* Intraluminal Device
Endurant® II AAA Stent Graft System *use* Intraluminal Device
Engineered Chimeric Antigen Receptor T-cell Immunotherapy
　Allogeneic XW0
　Autologous XW0
Enlargement
　see Dilation
　see Repair
EnRhythm *use* Pacemaker, Dual Chamber in 0JH
ENROUTE® Transcarotid Neuroprotection System *see* New Technology, Cardiovascular System X2A
ENSPRYNG™ *use* Satralizumab-mwge
Enterorrhaphy *see* Repair, Gastrointestinal System 0DQ
Enterra gastric neurostimulator *use* Stimulator Generator, Multiple Array in 0JH
Enucleation
　Eyeball *see* Resection, Eye 08T
　Eyeball with prosthetic implant *see* Replacement, Eye 08R
Ependyma *use* Cerebral Ventricle
Epicel® cultured epidermal autograft *use* Autologous Tissue Substitute
Epic™ Stented Tissue Valve (aortic) *use* Zooplastic Tissue in Heart and Great Vessels
Epidermis *use* Skin
Epididymectomy
　see Excision, Male Reproductive System 0VB
　see Resection, Male Reproductive System 0VT
Epididymoplasty
　see Repair, Male Reproductive System 0VQ
　see Supplement, Male Reproductive System 0VU
Epididymorrhaphy *see* Repair, Male Reproductive System 0VQ
Epididymotomy *see* Drainage, Male Reproductive System 0V9
Epidural space, spinal *use* Spinal Canal
Epiphysiodesis
　see Insertion of device in, Lower Bones 0QH
　see Insertion of device in, Upper Bones 0PH
　see Repair, Lower Bones 0QQ
　see Repair, Upper Bones 0PQ
Epiploic foramen *use* Peritoneum
Epiretinal Visual Prosthesis
　Left 08H105Z
　Right 08H005Z
Episiorrhaphy *see* Repair, Perineum, Female 0WQN
Episiotomy *see* Division, Perineum, Female 0W8N
Epithalamus *use* Thalamus
Epitrochlear lymph node
　use Lymphatic, Left Upper Extremity
　use Lymphatic, Right Upper Extremity
EPS (electrophysiologic stimulation) *see* Measurement, Cardiac 4A02
Eptifibatide, infusion *see* Introduction of Platelet Inhibitor
ERCP (endoscopic retrograde cholangiopancreatography) *see* Fluoroscopy, Hepatobiliary System and Pancreas BF1
Erdafitinib Antineoplastic XW0DXL5
Erector spinae muscle
　use Trunk Muscle, Left
　use Trunk Muscle, Right
ERLEADA™ *use* Apalutamide Antineoplastic

Esketamine Hydrochloride XW097M5
Esophageal artery *use* Upper Artery
Esophageal obturator airway (EOA) *use* Intraluminal Device, Airway in Gastrointestinal System
Esophageal plexus *use* Thoracic Sympathetic Nerve
Esophagectomy
　see Excision, Gastrointestinal System 0DB
　see Resection, Gastrointestinal System 0DT
Esophagocoloplasty
　see Repair, Gastrointestinal System 0DQ
　see Supplement, Gastrointestinal System 0DU
Esophagoenterostomy
　see Bypass, Gastrointestinal System 0D1
　see Drainage, Gastrointestinal System 0D9
Esophagoesophagostomy
　see Bypass, Gastrointestinal System 0D1
　see Drainage, Gastrointestinal System 0D9
Esophagogastrectomy
　see Excision, Gastrointestinal System 0DB
　see Resection, Gastrointestinal System 0DT
Esophagogastroduodenoscopy (EGD) 0DJ08ZZ
Esophagogastroplasty
　see Repair, Gastrointestinal System 0DQ
　see Supplement, Gastrointestinal System 0DU
Esophagogastroscopy 0DJ68ZZ
Esophagogastrostomy
　see Bypass, Gastrointestinal System 0D1
　see Drainage, Gastrointestinal System 0D9
Esophagojejunoplasty *see* Supplement, Gastrointestinal System 0DU
Esophagojejunostomy
　see Bypass, Gastrointestinal System 0D1
　see Drainage, Gastrointestinal System 0D9
Esophagomyotomy *see* Division, Esophagogastric Junction 0D84
Esophagoplasty
　see Repair, Gastrointestinal System 0DQ
　see Replacement, Esophagus 0DR5
　see Supplement, Gastrointestinal System 0DU
Esophagoplication *see* Restriction, Gastrointestinal System 0DV
Esophagorrhaphy *see* Repair, Gastrointestinal System 0DQ
Esophagoscopy 0DJ08ZZ
Esophagotomy *see* Drainage, Gastrointestinal System 0D9
Esteem® implantable hearing system *use* Hearing Device in Ear, Nose, Sinus
ESWL (extracorporeal shock wave lithotripsy) *see* Fragmentation
Etesevimab Monoclonal Antibody XW0
Ethmoidal air cell
　use Ethmoid Sinus, Left
　use Ethmoid Sinus, Right
Ethmoidectomy
　see Excision, Ear, Nose, Sinus 09B
　see Excision, Head and Facial Bones 0NB
　see Resection, Ear, Nose, Sinus 09T
　see Resection, Head and Facial Bones 0NT
Ethmoidotomy *see* Drainage, Ear, Nose, Sinus 099
Evacuation
　Hematoma *see* Extirpation
　Other Fluid *see* Drainage
Evera (XT) (S) (DR/VR) *use* Defibrillator Generator in 0JH
Everolimus-eluting coronary stent *use* Intraluminal Device, Drug-eluting in Heart and Great Vessels
Evisceration
　Eyeball *see* Resection, Eye 08T
　Eyeball with prosthetic implant *see* Replacement, Eye 08R
EXALT™ Model D Single-Use Duodenoscope *see* New Technology, Hepatobiliary System and Pancreas XFJ
Examination *see* Inspection
Exchange *see* Change device in
Excision
　Abdominal Wall 0WBF
　Acetabulum
　　Left 0QB5
　　Right 0QB4
　Adenoids 0CBQ
　Ampulla of Vater 0FBC
　Anal Sphincter 0DBR
　Ankle Region
　　Left 0YBL
　　Right 0YBK

▽ **Subterms under main terms may continue to next column or page**

Excision — *continued*
Anus ØDBQ
Aorta
  Abdominal
  Thoracic
    Ascending/Arch Ø2BX
    Descending Ø2BW
Aortic Body ØGBD
Appendix ØDBJ
Arm
  Lower
    Left ØXBF
    Right ØXBD
  Upper
    Left ØXB9
    Right ØXB8
Artery
  Anterior Tibial
    Left Ø4BQ
    Right Ø4BP
  Axillary
    Left Ø3B6
    Right Ø3B5
  Brachial
    Left Ø3B8
    Right Ø3B7
  Celiac Ø4B1
  Colic
    Left Ø4B7
    Middle Ø4B8
    Right Ø4B6
  Common Carotid
    Left Ø3BJ
    Right Ø3BH
  Common Iliac
    Left Ø4BD
    Right Ø4BC
  External Carotid
    Left Ø3BN
    Right Ø3BM
  External Iliac
    Left Ø4BJ
    Right Ø4BH
  Face Ø3BR
  Femoral
    Left Ø4BL
    Right Ø4BK
  Foot
    Left Ø4BW
    Right Ø4BV
  Gastric Ø4B2
  Hand
    Left Ø3BF
    Right Ø3BD
  Hepatic Ø4B3
  Inferior Mesenteric Ø4BB
  Innominate Ø3B2
  Internal Carotid
    Left Ø3BL
    Right Ø3BK
  Internal Iliac
    Left Ø4BF
    Right Ø4BE
  Internal Mammary
    Left Ø3B1
    Right Ø3BØ
  Intracranial Ø3BG
  Lower Ø4BY
  Peroneal
    Left Ø4BU
    Right Ø4BT
  Popliteal
    Left Ø4BN
    Right Ø4BM
  Posterior Tibial
    Left Ø4BS
    Right Ø4BR
  Pulmonary
    Left Ø2BR
    Right Ø2BQ
  Pulmonary Trunk Ø2BP
  Radial
    Left Ø3BC
    Right Ø3BB
  Renal
    Left Ø4BA
    Right Ø4B9
  Splenic Ø4B4

Excision — *continued*
Artery — *continued*
  Subclavian
    Left Ø3B4
    Right Ø3B3
  Superior Mesenteric Ø4B5
  Temporal
    Left Ø3BT
    Right Ø3BS
  Thyroid
    Left Ø3BV
    Right Ø3BU
  Ulnar
    Left Ø3BA
    Right Ø3B9
  Upper Ø3BY
  Vertebral
    Left Ø3BQ
    Right Ø3BP
Atrium
  Left Ø2B7
  Right Ø2B6
Auditory Ossicle
  Left Ø9BA
  Right Ø9B9
Axilla
  Left ØXB5
  Right ØXB4
Back
  Lower ØWBL
  Upper ØWBK
Basal Ganglia ØØB8
Bladder ØTBB
Bladder Neck ØTBC
Bone
  Ethmoid
    Left ØNBG
    Right ØNBF
  Frontal ØNB1
  Hyoid ØNBX
  Lacrimal
    Left ØNBJ
    Right ØNBH
  Nasal ØNBB
  Occipital ØNB7
  Palatine
    Left ØNBL
    Right ØNBK
  Parietal
    Left ØNB4
    Right ØNB3
  Pelvic
    Left ØQB3
    Right ØQB2
  Sphenoid ØNBC
  Temporal
    Left ØNB6
    Right ØNB5
  Zygomatic
    Left ØNBN
    Right ØNBM
Brain ØØBØ
Breast
  Bilateral ØHBV
  Left ØHBU
  Right ØHBT
  Supernumerary ØHBY
Bronchus
  Lingula ØBB9
  Lower Lobe
    Left ØBBB
    Right ØBB6
  Main
    Left ØBB7
    Right ØBB3
  Middle Lobe, Right ØBB5
  Upper Lobe
    Left ØBB8
    Right ØBB4
Buccal Mucosa ØCB4
Bursa and Ligament
  Abdomen
    Left ØMBJ
    Right ØMBH
  Ankle
    Left ØMBR
    Right ØMBQ
  Elbow
    Left ØMB4

Excision — *continued*
Bursa and Ligament — *continued*
  Elbow — *continued*
    Right ØMB3
  Foot
    Left ØMBT
    Right ØMBS
  Hand
    Left ØMB8
    Right ØMB7
  Head and Neck ØMBØ
  Hip
    Left ØMBM
    Right ØMBL
  Knee
    Left ØMBP
    Right ØMBN
  Lower Extremity
    Left ØMBW
    Right ØMBV
  Perineum ØMBK
  Rib(s) ØMBG
  Shoulder
    Left ØMB2
    Right ØMB1
  Spine
    Lower ØMBD
    Upper ØMBC
  Sternum ØMBF
  Upper Extremity
    Left ØMBB
    Right ØMB9
  Wrist
    Left ØMB6
    Right ØMB5
Buttock
  Left ØYB1
  Right ØYBØ
Carina ØBB2
Carotid Bodies, Bilateral ØGB8
Carotid Body
  Left ØGB6
  Right ØGB7
Carpal
  Left ØPBN
  Right ØPBM
Cecum ØDBH
Cerebellum ØØBC
Cerebral Hemisphere ØØB7
Cerebral Meninges ØØB1
Cerebral Ventricle ØØB6
Cervix ØUBC
Chest Wall ØWB8
Chordae Tendineae Ø2B9
Choroid
  Left Ø8BB
  Right Ø8BA
Cisterna Chyli Ø7BL
Clavicle
  Left ØPBB
  Right ØPB9
Clitoris ØUBJ
Coccygeal Glomus ØGBB
Coccyx ØQBS
Colon
  Ascending ØDBK
  Descending ØDBM
  Sigmoid ØDBN
  Transverse ØDBL
Conduction Mechanism Ø2B8
Conjunctiva
  Left Ø8BTXZ
  Right Ø8BSXZ
Cord
  Bilateral ØVBH
  Left ØVBG
  Right ØVBF
Cornea
  Left Ø8B9XZ
  Right Ø8B8XZ
Cul-de-sac ØUBF
Diaphragm ØBBT
Disc
  Cervical Vertebral ØRB3
  Cervicothoracic Vertebral ØRB5
  Lumbar Vertebral ØSB2
  Lumbosacral ØSB4
  Thoracic Vertebral ØRB9
  Thoracolumbar Vertebral ØRBB

Excision — *continued*
- Duct
  - Common Bile ØFB9
  - Cystic ØFB8
  - Hepatic
    - Common ØFB7
    - Left ØFB6
    - Right ØFB5
  - Lacrimal
    - Left Ø8BY
    - Right Ø8BX
  - Pancreatic ØFBD
    - Accessory ØFBF
  - Parotid
    - Left ØCBC
    - Right ØCBB
- Duodenum ØDB9
- Dura Mater ØØB2
- Ear
  - External
    - Left Ø9B1
    - Right Ø9BØ
  - External Auditory Canal
    - Left Ø9B4
    - Right Ø9B3
  - Inner
    - Left Ø9BE
    - Right Ø9BD
  - Middle
    - Left Ø9B6
    - Right Ø9B5
- Elbow Region
  - Left ØXBC
  - Right ØXBB
- Epididymis
  - Bilateral ØVBL
  - Left ØVBK
  - Right ØVBJ
- Epiglottis ØCBR
- Esophagogastric Junction ØDB4
- Esophagus ØDB5
  - Lower ØDB3
  - Middle ØDB2
  - Upper ØDB1
- Eustachian Tube
  - Left Ø9BG
  - Right Ø9BF
- Extremity
  - Lower
    - Left ØYBB
    - Right ØYB9
  - Upper
    - Left ØXB7
    - Right ØXB6
- Eye
  - Left Ø8B1
  - Right Ø8BØ
- Eyelid
  - Lower
    - Left Ø8BR
    - Right Ø8BQ
  - Upper
    - Left Ø8BP
    - Right Ø8BN
- Face ØWB2
- Fallopian Tube
  - Left ØUB6
  - Right ØUB5
- Fallopian Tubes, Bilateral ØUB7
- Femoral Region
  - Left ØYB8
  - Right ØYB7
- Femoral Shaft
  - Left ØQB9
  - Right ØQB8
- Femur
  - Lower
    - Left ØQBC
    - Right ØQBB
  - Upper
    - Left ØQB7
    - Right ØQB6
- Fibula
  - Left ØQBK
  - Right ØQBJ
- Finger Nail ØHBQXZ
- Floor of mouth *see* Excision, Oral Cavity and Throat ØWB3

Excision — *continued*
- Foot
  - Left ØYBN
  - Right ØYBM
- Gallbladder ØFB4
- Gingiva
  - Lower ØCB6
  - Upper ØCB5
- Gland
  - Adrenal
    - Bilateral ØGB4
    - Left ØGB2
    - Right ØGB3
  - Lacrimal
    - Left Ø8BW
    - Right Ø8BV
  - Minor Salivary ØCBJ
  - Parotid
    - Left ØCB9
    - Right ØCB8
  - Pituitary ØGBØ
  - Sublingual
    - Left ØCBF
    - Right ØCBD
  - Submaxillary
    - Left ØCBH
    - Right ØCBG
  - Vestibular ØUBL
- Glenoid Cavity
  - Left ØPB8
  - Right ØPB7
- Glomus Jugulare ØGBC
- Hand
  - Left ØXBK
  - Right ØXBJ
- Head ØWBØ
- Humeral Head
  - Left ØPBD
  - Right ØPBC
- Humeral Shaft
  - Left ØPBG
  - Right ØPBF
- Hymen ØUBK
- Hypothalamus ØØBA
- Ileocecal Valve ØDBC
- Ileum ØDBB
- Inguinal Region
  - Left ØYB6
  - Right ØYB5
- Intestine
  - Large ØDBE
    - Left ØDBG
    - Right ØDBF
  - Small ØDB8
- Iris
  - Left Ø8BD3Z
  - Right Ø8BC3Z
- Jaw
  - Lower ØWB5
  - Upper ØWB4
- Jejunum ØDBA
- Joint
  - Acromioclavicular
    - Left ØRBH
    - Right ØRBG
  - Ankle
    - Left ØSBG
    - Right ØSBF
  - Carpal
    - Left ØRBR
    - Right ØRBQ
  - Carpometacarpal
    - Left ØRBT
    - Right ØRBS
  - Cervical Vertebral ØRB1
  - Cervicothoracic Vertebral ØRB4
  - Coccygeal ØSB6
  - Elbow
    - Left ØRBM
    - Right ØRBL
  - Finger Phalangeal
    - Left ØRBX
    - Right ØRBW
  - Hip
    - Left ØSBB
    - Right ØSB9
  - Knee
    - Left ØSBD
    - Right ØSBC

Excision — *continued*
- Joint — *continued*
  - Lumbar Vertebral ØSBØ
  - Lumbosacral ØSB3
  - Metacarpophalangeal
    - Left ØRBV
    - Right ØRBU
  - Metatarsal-Phalangeal
    - Left ØSBN
    - Right ØSBM
  - Occipital-cervical ØRBØ
  - Sacrococcygeal ØSB5
  - Sacroiliac
    - Left ØSB8
    - Right ØSB7
  - Shoulder
    - Left ØRBK
    - Right ØRBJ
  - Sternoclavicular
    - Left ØRBF
    - Right ØRBE
  - Tarsal
    - Left ØSBJ
    - Right ØSBH
  - Tarsometatarsal
    - Left ØSBL
    - Right ØSBK
  - Temporomandibular
    - Left ØRBD
    - Right ØRBC
  - Thoracic Vertebral ØRB6
  - Thoracolumbar Vertebral ØRBA
  - Toe Phalangeal
    - Left ØSBQ
    - Right ØSBP
  - Wrist
    - Left ØRBP
    - Right ØRBN
- Kidney
  - Left ØTB1
  - Right ØTBØ
- Kidney Pelvis
  - Left ØTB4
  - Right ØTB3
- Knee Region
  - Left ØYBG
  - Right ØYBF
- Larynx ØCBS
- Leg
  - Lower
    - Left ØYBJ
    - Right ØYBH
  - Upper
    - Left ØYBD
    - Right ØYBC
- Lens
  - Left Ø8BK3Z
  - Right Ø8BJ3Z
- Lip
  - Lower ØCB1
  - Upper ØCBØ
- Liver ØFBØ
  - Left Lobe ØFB2
  - Right Lobe ØFB1
- Lung
  - Bilateral ØBBM
  - Left ØBBL
  - Lower Lobe
    - Left ØBBJ
    - Right ØBBF
  - Middle Lobe, Right ØBBD
  - Right ØBBK
  - Upper Lobe
    - Left ØBBG
    - Right ØBBC
- Lung Lingula ØBBH
- Lymphatic
  - Aortic Ø7BD
  - Axillary
    - Left Ø7B6
    - Right Ø7B5
  - Head Ø7BØ
  - Inguinal
    - Left Ø7BJ
    - Right Ø7BH
  - Internal Mammary
    - Left Ø7B9
    - Right Ø7B8

Excision — continued
  Lymphatic — continued
    Lower Extremity
      Left 07BG
      Right 07BF
    Mesenteric 07BB
    Neck
      Left 07B2
      Right 07B1
    Pelvis 07BC
    Thoracic Duct 07BK
    Thorax 07B7
    Upper Extremity
      Left 07B4
      Right 07B3
  Mandible
    Left 0NBV
    Right 0NBT
  Maxilla 0NBR
  Mediastinum 0WBC
  Medulla Oblongata 00BD
  Mesentery 0DBV
  Metacarpal
    Left 0PBQ
    Right 0PBP
  Metatarsal
    Left 0QBP
    Right 0QBN
  Muscle
    Abdomen
      Left 0KBL
      Right 0KBK
    Extraocular
      Left 08BM
      Right 08BL
    Facial 0KB1
    Foot
      Left 0KBW
      Right 0KBV
    Hand
      Left 0KBD
      Right 0KBC
    Head 0KB0
    Hip
      Left 0KBP
      Right 0KBN
    Lower Arm and Wrist
      Left 0KBB
      Right 0KB9
    Lower Leg
      Left 0KBT
      Right 0KBS
    Neck
      Left 0KB3
      Right 0KB2
    Papillary 02BD
    Perineum 0KBM
    Shoulder
      Left 0KB6
      Right 0KB5
    Thorax
      Left 0KBJ
      Right 0KBH
    Tongue, Palate, Pharynx 0KB4
    Trunk
      Left 0KBG
      Right 0KBF
    Upper Arm
      Left 0KB8
      Right 0KB7
    Upper Leg
      Left 0KBR
      Right 0KBQ
  Nasal Mucosa and Soft Tissue 09BK
  Nasopharynx 09BN
  Neck 0WB6
  Nerve
    Abdominal Sympathetic 01BM
    Abducens 00BL
    Accessory 00BR
    Acoustic 00BN
    Brachial Plexus 01B3
    Cervical 01B1
    Cervical Plexus 01B0
    Facial 00BM
    Femoral 01BD
    Glossopharyngeal 00BP
    Head and Neck Sympathetic 01BK
    Hypoglossal 00BS

Excision — continued
  Nerve — continued
    Lumbar 01BB
    Lumbar Plexus 01B9
    Lumbar Sympathetic 01BN
    Lumbosacral Plexus 01BA
    Median 01B5
    Oculomotor 00BH
    Olfactory 00BF
    Optic 00BG
    Peroneal 01BH
    Phrenic 01B2
    Pudendal 01BC
    Radial 01B6
    Sacral 01BR
    Sacral Plexus 01BQ
    Sacral Sympathetic 01BP
    Sciatic 01BF
    Thoracic 01B8
    Thoracic Sympathetic 01BL
    Tibial 01BG
    Trigeminal 00BK
    Trochlear 00BJ
    Ulnar 01B4
    Vagus 00BQ
  Nipple
    Left 0HBX
    Right 0HBW
  Omentum 0DBU
  Oral Cavity and Throat 0WB3
  Orbit
    Left 0NBQ
    Right 0NBP
  Ovary
    Bilateral 0UB2
    Left 0UB1
    Right 0UB0
  Palate
    Hard 0CB2
    Soft 0CB3
  Pancreas 0FBG
  Para-aortic Body 0GB9
  Paraganglion Extremity 0GBF
  Parathyroid Gland 0GBR
    Inferior
      Left 0GBP
      Right 0GBN
    Multiple 0GBQ
    Superior
      Left 0GBM
      Right 0GBL
  Patella
    Left 0QBF
    Right 0QBD
  Penis 0VBS
  Pericardium 02BN
  Perineum
    Female 0WBN
    Male 0WBM
  Peritoneum 0DBW
  Phalanx
    Finger
      Left 0PBV
      Right 0PBT
    Thumb
      Left 0PBS
      Right 0PBR
    Toe
      Left 0QBR
      Right 0QBQ
  Pharynx 0CBM
  Pineal Body 0GB1
  Pleura
    Left 0BBP
    Right 0BBN
  Pons 00BB
  Prepuce 0VBT
  Prostate 0VB0
  Radius
    Left 0PBJ
    Right 0PBH
  Rectum 0DBP
  Retina
    Left 08BF3Z
    Right 08BE3Z
  Retroperitoneum 0WBH
  Ribs
    1 to 2 0PB1
    3 or More 0PB2

Excision — continued
  Sacrum 0QB1
  Scapula
    Left 0PB6
    Right 0PB5
  Sclera
    Left 08B7XZ
    Right 08B6XZ
  Scrotum 0VB5
  Septum
    Atrial 02B5
    Nasal 09BM
    Ventricular 02BM
  Shoulder Region
    Left 0XB3
    Right 0XB2
  Sinus
    Accessory 09BP
    Ethmoid
      Left 09BV
      Right 09BU
    Frontal
      Left 09BT
      Right 09BS
    Mastoid
      Left 09BC
      Right 09BB
    Maxillary
      Left 09BR
      Right 09BQ
    Sphenoid
      Left 09BX
      Right 09BW
  Skin
    Abdomen 0HB7XZ
    Back 0HB6XZ
    Buttock 0HB8XZ
    Chest 0HB5XZ
    Ear
      Left 0HB3XZ
      Right 0HB2XZ
    Face 0HB1XZ
    Foot
      Left 0HBNXZ
      Right 0HBMXZ
    Hand
      Left 0HBGXZ
      Right 0HBFXZ
    Inguinal 0HBAXZ
    Lower Arm
      Left 0HBEXZ
      Right 0HBDXZ
    Lower Leg
      Left 0HBLXZ
      Right 0HBKXZ
    Neck 0HB4XZ
    Perineum 0HB9XZ
    Scalp 0HB0XZ
    Upper Arm
      Left 0HBCXZ
      Right 0HBBXZ
    Upper Leg
      Left 0HBJXZ
      Right 0HBHXZ
  Skull 0NB0
  Spinal Cord
    Cervical 00BW
    Lumbar 00BY
    Thoracic 00BX
  Spinal Meninges 00BT
  Spleen 07BP
  Sternum 0PB0
  Stomach 0DB6
    Pylorus 0DB7
  Subcutaneous Tissue and Fascia
    Abdomen 0JB8
    Back 0JB7
    Buttock 0JB9
    Chest 0JB6
    Face 0JB1
    Foot
      Left 0JBR
      Right 0JBQ
    Hand
      Left 0JBK
      Right 0JBJ
    Lower Arm
      Left 0JBH
      Right 0JBG

Excision — *continued*
Subcutaneous Tissue and Fascia — *continued*
Lower Leg
Left ØJBP
Right ØJBN
Neck
Left ØJB5
Right ØJB4
Pelvic Region ØJBC
Perineum ØJBB
Scalp ØJBØ
Upper Arm
Left ØJBF
Right ØJBD
Upper Leg
Left ØJBM
Right ØJBL
Tarsal
Left ØQBM
Right ØQBL
Tendon
Abdomen
Left ØLBG
Right ØLBF
Ankle
Left ØLBT
Right ØLBS
Foot
Left ØLBW
Right ØLBV
Hand
Left ØLB8
Right ØLB7
Head and Neck ØLBØ
Hip
Left ØLBK
Right ØLBJ
Knee
Left ØLBR
Right ØLBQ
Lower Arm and Wrist
Left ØLB6
Right ØLB5
Lower Leg
Left ØLBP
Right ØLBN
Perineum ØLBH
Shoulder
Left ØLB2
Right ØLB1
Thorax
Left ØLBD
Right ØLBC
Trunk
Left ØLBB
Right ØLB9
Upper Arm
Left ØLB4
Right ØLB3
Upper Leg
Left ØLBM
Right ØLBL
Testis
Bilateral ØVBC
Left ØVBB
Right ØVB9
Thalamus ØØB9
Thymus Ø7BM
Thyroid Gland
Left Lobe ØGBG
Right Lobe ØGBH
Thyroid Gland Isthmus ØGBJ
Tibia
Left ØQBH
Right ØQBG
Toe Nail ØHBRXZ
Tongue ØCB7
Tonsils ØCBP
Tooth
Lower ØCBX
Upper ØCBW
Trachea ØBB1
Tunica Vaginalis
Left ØVB7
Right ØVB6
Turbinate, Nasal Ø9BL
Tympanic Membrane
Left Ø9B8
Right Ø9B7

Excision — *continued*
Ulna
Left ØPBL
Right ØPBK
Ureter
Left ØTB7
Right ØTB6
Urethra ØTBD
Uterine Supporting Structure ØUB4
Uterus ØUB9
Uvula ØCBN
Vagina ØUBG
Valve
Aortic Ø2BF
Mitral Ø2BG
Pulmonary Ø2BH
Tricuspid Ø2BJ
Vas Deferens
Bilateral ØVBQ
Left ØVBP
Right ØVBN
Vein
Axillary
Left Ø5B8
Right Ø5B7
Azygos Ø5BØ
Basilic
Left Ø5BC
Right Ø5BB
Brachial
Left Ø5BA
Right Ø5B9
Cephalic
Left Ø5BF
Right Ø5BD
Colic Ø6B7
Common Iliac
Left Ø6BD
Right Ø6BC
Coronary Ø2B4
Esophageal Ø6B3
External Iliac
Left Ø6BG
Right Ø6BF
External Jugular
Left Ø5BQ
Right Ø5BP
Face
Left Ø5BV
Right Ø5BT
Femoral
Left Ø6BN
Right Ø6BM
Foot
Left Ø6BV
Right Ø6BT
Gastric Ø6B2
Hand
Left Ø5BH
Right Ø5BG
Hemiazygos Ø5B1
Hepatic Ø6B4
Hypogastric
Left Ø6BJ
Right Ø6BH
Inferior Mesenteric Ø6B6
Innominate
Left Ø5B4
Right Ø5B3
Internal Jugular
Left Ø5BN
Right Ø5BM
Intracranial Ø5BL
Lower Ø6BY
Portal Ø6B8
Pulmonary
Left Ø2BT
Right Ø2BS
Renal
Left Ø6BB
Right Ø6B9
Saphenous
Left Ø6BQ
Right Ø6BP
Splenic Ø6B1
Subclavian
Left Ø5B6
Right Ø5B5
Superior Mesenteric Ø6B5

Excision — *continued*
Vein — *continued*
Upper Ø5BY
Vertebral
Left Ø5BS
Right Ø5BR
Vena Cava
Inferior Ø6BØ
Superior Ø2BV
Ventricle
Left Ø2BL
Right Ø2BK
Vertebra
Cervical ØPB3
Lumbar ØQBØ
Thoracic ØPB4
Vesicle
Bilateral ØVB3
Left ØVB2
Right ØVB1
Vitreous
Left Ø8B53Z
Right Ø8B43Z
Vocal Cord
Left ØCBV
Right ØCBT
Vulva ØUBM
Wrist Region
Left ØXBH
Right ØXBG
EXCLUDER® AAA Endoprosthesis
use Intraluminal Device
use Intraluminal Device, Branched or Fenestrated, One or Two Arteries in Ø4V
use Intraluminal Device, Branched or Fenestrated, Three or More Arteries in Ø4V
EXCLUDER® IBE Endoprosthesis *use* Intraluminal Device, Branched or Fenestrated, One or Two Arteries in Ø4V
Exclusion, Left atrial appendage (LAA) *see* Occlusion, Atrium, Left Ø2L7
Exercise, rehabilitation *see* Motor Treatment, Rehabilitation FØ7
Exploration *see* Inspection
Express® Biliary SD Monorail® Premounted Stent System *use* Intraluminal Device
Express® (LD) Premounted Stent System *use* Intraluminal Device
Express® SD Renal Monorail® Premounted Stent System *use* Intraluminal Device
Ex-PRESS™ mini glaucoma shunt *use* Synthetic Substitute
Extensor carpi radialis muscle
use Lower Arm and Wrist Muscle, Left
use Lower Arm and Wrist Muscle, Right
Extensor carpi ulnaris muscle
use Lower Arm and Wrist Muscle, Left
use Lower Arm and Wrist Muscle, Right
Extensor digitorum brevis muscle
use Foot Muscle, Left
use Foot Muscle, Right
Extensor digitorum longus muscle
use Lower Leg Muscle, Left
use Lower Leg Muscle, Right
Extensor hallucis brevis muscle
use Foot Muscle, Left
use Foot Muscle, Right
Extensor hallucis longus muscle
use Lower Leg Muscle, Left
use Lower Leg Muscle, Right
External anal sphincter *use* Anal Sphincter
External auditory meatus
use External Auditory Canal, Left
use External Auditory Canal, Right
External fixator
use External Fixation Device in Head and Facial Bones
use External Fixation Device in Lower Bones
use External Fixation Device in Lower Joints
use External Fixation Device in Upper Bones
use External Fixation Device in Upper Joints
External maxillary artery *use* Face Artery
External naris *use* Nasal Mucosa and Soft Tissue
External oblique aponeurosis *use* Subcutaneous Tissue and Fascia, Trunk
External oblique muscle
use Abdomen Muscle, Left

External oblique muscle — *continued*
   use Abdomen Muscle, Right
External popliteal nerve *use* Peroneal Nerve
External pudendal artery
   use Femoral Artery, Left
   use Femoral Artery, Right
External pudendal vein
   use Saphenous Vein, Left
   use Saphenous Vein, Right
External urethral sphincter *use* Urethra
Extirpation
  Acetabulum
    Left ØQC5
    Right ØQC4
  Adenoids ØCCQ
  Ampulla of Vater ØFCC
  Anal Sphincter ØDCR
  Anterior Chamber
    Left Ø8C3
    Right Ø8C2
  Anus ØDCQ
  Aorta
    Abdominal Ø4CØ
    Thoracic
      Ascending/Arch Ø2CX
      Descending Ø2CW
  Aortic Body ØGCD
  Appendix ØDCJ
  Artery
    Anterior Tibial
      Left Ø4CQ
      Right Ø4CP
    Axillary
      Left Ø3C6
      Right Ø3C5
    Brachial
      Left Ø3C8
      Right Ø3C7
    Celiac Ø4C1
    Colic
      Left Ø4C7
      Middle Ø4C8
      Right Ø4C6
    Common Carotid
      Left Ø3CJ
      Right Ø3CH
    Common Iliac
      Left Ø4CD
      Right Ø4CC
    Coronary
      Four or More Arteries Ø2C3
      One Artery Ø2CØ
      Three Arteries Ø2C2
      Two Arteries Ø2C1
    External Carotid
      Left Ø3CN
      Right Ø3CM
    External Iliac
      Left Ø4CJ
      Right Ø4CH
    Face Ø3CR
    Femoral
      Left Ø4CL
      Right Ø4CK
    Foot
      Left Ø4CW
      Right Ø4CV
    Gastric Ø4C2
    Hand
      Left Ø3CF
      Right Ø3CD
    Hepatic Ø4C3
    Inferior Mesenteric Ø4CB
    Innominate Ø3C2
    Internal Carotid
      Left Ø3CL
      Right Ø3CK
    Internal Iliac
      Left Ø4CF
      Right Ø4CE
    Internal Mammary
      Left Ø3C1
      Right Ø3CØ
    Intracranial Ø3CG
    Lower Ø4CY
    Peroneal
      Left Ø4CU
      Right Ø4CT

Extirpation — *continued*
  Artery — *continued*
    Popliteal
      Left Ø4CN
      Right Ø4CM
    Posterior Tibial
      Left Ø4CS
      Right Ø4CR
    Pulmonary
      Left Ø2CR
      Right Ø2CQ
    Pulmonary Trunk Ø2CP
    Radial
      Left Ø3CC
      Right Ø3CB
    Renal
      Left Ø4CA
      Right Ø4C9
    Splenic Ø4C4
    Subclavian
      Left Ø3C4
      Right Ø3C3
    Superior Mesenteric Ø4C5
    Temporal
      Left Ø3CT
      Right Ø3CS
    Thyroid
      Left Ø3CV
      Right Ø3CU
    Ulnar
      Left Ø3CA
      Right Ø3C9
    Upper Ø3CY
    Vertebral
      Left Ø3CQ
      Right Ø3CP
  Atrium
    Left Ø2C7
    Right Ø2C6
  Auditory Ossicle
    Left Ø9CA
    Right Ø9C9
  Basal Ganglia ØØC8
  Bladder ØTCB
  Bladder Neck ØTCC
  Bone
    Ethmoid
      Left ØNCG
      Right ØNCF
    Frontal ØNC1
    Hyoid ØNCX
    Lacrimal
      Left ØNCJ
      Right ØNCH
    Nasal ØNCB
    Occipital ØNC7
    Palatine
      Left ØNCL
      Right ØNCK
    Parietal
      Left ØNC4
      Right ØNC3
    Pelvic
      Left ØQC3
      Right ØQC2
    Sphenoid ØNCC
    Temporal
      Left ØNC6
      Right ØNC5
    Zygomatic
      Left ØNCN
      Right ØNCM
  Brain ØØCØ
  Breast
    Bilateral ØHCV
    Left ØHCU
    Right ØHCT
  Bronchus
    Lingula ØBC9
    Lower Lobe
      Left ØBCB
      Right ØBC6
    Main
      Left ØBC7
      Right ØBC3
    Middle Lobe, Right ØBC5
    Upper Lobe
      Left ØBC8
      Right ØBC4

Extirpation — *continued*
  Buccal Mucosa ØCC4
  Bursa and Ligament
    Abdomen
      Left ØMCJ
      Right ØMCH
    Ankle
      Left ØMCR
      Right ØMCQ
    Elbow
      Left ØMC4
      Right ØMC3
    Foot
      Left ØMCT
      Right ØMCS
    Hand
      Left ØMC8
      Right ØMC7
    Head and Neck ØMCØ
    Hip
      Left ØMCM
      Right ØMCL
    Knee
      Left ØMCP
      Right ØMCN
    Lower Extremity
      Left ØMCW
      Right ØMCV
    Perineum ØMCK
    Rib(s) ØMCG
    Shoulder
      Left ØMC2
      Right ØMC1
    Spine
      Lower ØMCD
      Upper ØMCC
    Sternum ØMCF
    Upper Extremity
      Left ØMCB
      Right ØMC9
    Wrist
      Left ØMC6
      Right ØMC5
  Carina ØBC2
  Carotid Bodies, Bilateral ØGC8
  Carotid Body
    Left ØGC6
    Right ØGC7
  Carpal
    Left ØPCN
    Right ØPCM
  Cavity, Cranial ØWC1
  Cecum ØDCH
  Cerebellum ØØCC
  Cerebral Hemisphere ØØC7
  Cerebral Meninges ØØC1
  Cerebral Ventricle ØØC6
  Cervix ØUCC
  Chordae Tendineae Ø2C9
  Choroid
    Left Ø8CB
    Right Ø8CA
  Cisterna Chyli Ø7CL
  Clavicle
    Left ØPCB
    Right ØPC9
  Clitoris ØUCJ
  Coccygeal Glomus ØGCB
  Coccyx ØQCS
  Colon
    Ascending ØDCK
    Descending ØDCM
    Sigmoid ØDCN
    Transverse ØDCL
  Computer-aided Mechanical Aspiration X2C
  Conduction Mechanism Ø2C8
  Conjunctiva
    Left Ø8CTXZZ
    Right Ø8CSXZZ
  Cord
    Bilateral ØVCH
    Left ØVCG
    Right ØVCF
  Cornea
    Left Ø8C9XZZ
    Right Ø8C8XZZ
  Cul-de-sac ØUCF
  Diaphragm ØBCT

Extirpation — *continued*
- Disc
  - Cervical Vertebral ØRC3
  - Cervicothoracic Vertebral ØRC5
  - Lumbar Vertebral ØSC2
  - Lumbosacral ØSC4
  - Thoracic Vertebral ØRC9
  - Thoracolumbar Vertebral ØRCB
- Duct
  - Common Bile ØFC9
  - Cystic ØFC8
  - Hepatic
    - Common ØFC7
    - Left ØFC6
    - Right ØFC5
  - Lacrimal
    - Left Ø8CY
    - Right Ø8CX
  - Pancreatic ØFCD
    - Accessory ØFCF
  - Parotid
    - Left ØCCC
    - Right ØCCB
- Duodenum ØDC9
- Dura Mater ØØC2
- Ear
  - External
    - Left Ø9C1
    - Right Ø9CØ
  - External Auditory Canal
    - Left Ø9C4
    - Right Ø9C3
  - Inner
    - Left Ø9CE
    - Right Ø9CD
  - Middle
    - Left Ø9C6
    - Right Ø9C5
- Endometrium ØUCB
- Epididymis
  - Bilateral ØVCL
  - Left ØVCK
  - Right ØVCJ
- Epidural Space, Intracranial ØØC3
- Epiglottis ØCCR
- Esophagogastric Junction ØDC4
- Esophagus ØDC5
  - Lower ØDC3
  - Middle ØDC2
  - Upper ØDC1
- Eustachian Tube
  - Left Ø9CG
  - Right Ø9CF
- Eye
  - Left Ø8C1XZZ
  - Right Ø8CØXZZ
- Eyelid
  - Lower
    - Left Ø8CR
    - Right Ø8CQ
  - Upper
    - Left Ø8CP
    - Right Ø8CN
- Fallopian Tube
  - Left ØUC6
  - Right ØUC5
- Fallopian Tubes, Bilateral ØUC7
- Femoral Shaft
  - Left ØQC9
  - Right ØQC8
- Femur
  - Lower
    - Left ØQCC
    - Right ØQCB
  - Upper
    - Left ØQC7
    - Right ØQC6
- Fibula
  - Left ØQCK
  - Right ØQCJ
- Finger Nail ØHCQXZZ
- Gallbladder ØFC4
- Gastrointestinal Tract ØWCP
- Genitourinary Tract ØWCR
- Gingiva
  - Lower ØCC6
  - Upper ØCC5

Extirpation — *continued*
- Gland
  - Adrenal
    - Bilateral ØGC4
    - Left ØGC2
    - Right ØGC3
  - Lacrimal
    - Left Ø8CW
    - Right Ø8CV
  - Minor Salivary ØCCJ
  - Parotid
    - Left ØCC9
    - Right ØCC8
  - Pituitary ØGCØ
  - Sublingual
    - Left ØCCF
    - Right ØCCD
  - Submaxillary
    - Left ØCCH
    - Right ØCCG
  - Vestibular ØUCL
- Glenoid Cavity
  - Left ØPC8
  - Right ØPC7
- Glomus Jugulare ØGCC
- Humeral Head
  - Left ØPCD
  - Right ØPCC
- Humeral Shaft
  - Left ØPCG
  - Right ØPCF
- Hymen ØUCK
- Hypothalamus ØØCA
- Ileocecal Valve ØDCC
- Ileum ØDCB
- Intestine
  - Large ØDCE
    - Left ØDCG
    - Right ØDCF
  - Small ØDC8
- Iris
  - Left Ø8CD
  - Right Ø8CC
- Jaw
  - Lower ØWC5
  - Upper ØWC4
- Jejunum ØDCA
- Joint
  - Acromioclavicular
    - Left ØRCH
    - Right ØRCG
  - Ankle
    - Left ØSCG
    - Right ØSCF
  - Carpal
    - Left ØRCR
    - Right ØRCQ
  - Carpometacarpal
    - Left ØRCT
    - Right ØRCS
  - Cervical Vertebral ØRC1
  - Cervicothoracic Vertebral ØRC4
  - Coccygeal ØSC6
  - Elbow
    - Left ØRCM
    - Right ØRCL
  - Finger Phalangeal
    - Left ØRCX
    - Right ØRCW
  - Hip
    - Left ØSCB
    - Right ØSC9
  - Knee
    - Left ØSCD
    - Right ØSCC
  - Lumbar Vertebral ØSCØ
  - Lumbosacral ØSC3
  - Metacarpophalangeal
    - Left ØRCV
    - Right ØRCU
  - Metatarsal-Phalangeal
    - Left ØSCN
    - Right ØSCM
  - Occipital-cervical ØRCØ
  - Sacrococcygeal ØSC5
  - Sacroiliac
    - Left ØSC8
    - Right ØSC7

Extirpation — *continued*
- Joint — *continued*
  - Shoulder
    - Left ØRCK
    - Right ØRCJ
  - Sternoclavicular
    - Left ØRCF
    - Right ØRCE
  - Tarsal
    - Left ØSCJ
    - Right ØSCH
  - Tarsometatarsal
    - Left ØSCL
    - Right ØSCK
  - Temporomandibular
    - Left ØRCD
    - Right ØRCC
  - Thoracic Vertebral ØRC6
  - Thoracolumbar Vertebral ØRCA
  - Toe Phalangeal
    - Left ØSCQ
    - Right ØSCP
  - Wrist
    - Left ØRCP
    - Right ØRCN
- Kidney
  - Left ØTC1
  - Right ØTCØ
- Kidney Pelvis
  - Left ØTC4
  - Right ØTC3
- Larynx ØCCS
- Lens
  - Left Ø8CK
  - Right Ø8CJ
- Lip
  - Lower ØCC1
  - Upper ØCCØ
- Liver ØFCØ
  - Left Lobe ØFC2
  - Right Lobe ØFC1
- Lung
  - Bilateral ØBCM
  - Left ØBCL
  - Lower Lobe
    - Left ØBCJ
    - Right ØBCF
  - Middle Lobe, Right ØBCD
  - Right ØBCK
  - Upper Lobe
    - Left ØBCG
    - Right ØBCC
- Lung Lingula ØBCH
- Lymphatic
  - Aortic Ø7CD
  - Axillary
    - Left Ø7C6
    - Right Ø7C5
  - Head Ø7CØ
  - Inguinal
    - Left Ø7CJ
    - Right Ø7CH
  - Internal Mammary
    - Left Ø7C9
    - Right Ø7C8
  - Lower Extremity
    - Left Ø7CG
    - Right Ø7CF
  - Mesenteric Ø7CB
  - Neck
    - Left Ø7C2
    - Right Ø7C1
  - Pelvis Ø7CC
  - Thoracic Duct Ø7CK
  - Thorax Ø7C7
  - Upper Extremity
    - Left Ø7C4
    - Right Ø7C3
- Mandible
  - Left ØNCV
  - Right ØNCT
- Maxilla ØNCR
- Mediastinum ØWCC
- Medulla Oblongata ØØCD
- Mesentery ØDCV
- Metacarpal
  - Left ØPCQ
  - Right ØPCP

Extirpation — *continued*
Metatarsal
  Left ØQCP
  Right ØQCN
Muscle
  Abdomen
    Left ØKCL
    Right ØKCK
  Extraocular
    Left Ø8CM
    Right Ø8CL
  Facial ØKC1
  Foot
    Left ØKCW
    Right ØKCV
  Hand
    Left ØKCD
    Right ØKCC
  Head ØKCØ
  Hip
    Left ØKCP
    Right ØKCN
  Lower Arm and Wrist
    Left ØKCB
    Right ØKC9
  Lower Leg
    Left ØKCT
    Right ØKCS
  Neck
    Left ØKC3
    Right ØKC2
  Papillary Ø2CD
  Perineum ØKCM
  Shoulder
    Left ØKC6
    Right ØKC5
  Thorax
    Left ØKCJ
    Right ØKCH
  Tongue, Palate, Pharynx ØKC4
  Trunk
    Left ØKCG
    Right ØKCF
  Upper Arm
    Left ØKC8
    Right ØKC7
  Upper Leg
    Left ØKCR
    Right ØKCQ
Nasal Mucosa and Soft Tissue Ø9CK
Nasopharynx Ø9CN
Nerve
  Abdominal Sympathetic Ø1CM
  Abducens ØØCL
  Accessory ØØCR
  Acoustic ØØCN
  Brachial Plexus Ø1C3
  Cervical Ø1C1
  Cervical Plexus Ø1CØ
  Facial ØØCM
  Femoral Ø1CD
  Glossopharyngeal ØØCP
  Head and Neck Sympathetic Ø1CK
  Hypoglossal ØØCS
  Lumbar Ø1CB
  Lumbar Plexus Ø1C9
  Lumbar Sympathetic Ø1CN
  Lumbosacral Plexus Ø1CA
  Median Ø1C5
  Oculomotor ØØCH
  Olfactory ØØCF
  Optic ØØCG
  Peroneal Ø1CH
  Phrenic Ø1C2
  Pudendal Ø1CC
  Radial Ø1C6
  Sacral Ø1CR
  Sacral Plexus Ø1CQ
  Sacral Sympathetic Ø1CP
  Sciatic Ø1CF
  Thoracic Ø1C8
  Thoracic Sympathetic Ø1CL
  Tibial Ø1CG
  Trigeminal ØØCK
  Trochlear ØØCJ
  Ulnar Ø1C4
  Vagus ØØCQ
Nipple
  Left ØHCX

Extirpation — *continued*
Nipple — *continued*
  Right ØHCW
Omentum ØDCU
Oral Cavity and Throat ØWC3
Orbit
  Left ØNCQ
  Right ØNCP
Orbital Atherectomy *see* Extirpation, Heart and
    Great Vessels Ø2C
Ovary
  Bilateral ØUC2
  Left ØUC1
  Right ØUCØ
Palate
  Hard ØCC2
  Soft ØCC3
Pancreas ØFCG
Para-aortic Body ØGC9
Paraganglion Extremity ØGCF
Parathyroid Gland ØGCR
  Inferior
    Left ØGCP
    Right ØGCN
  Multiple ØGCQ
  Superior
    Left ØGCM
    Right ØGCL
Patella
  Left ØQCF
  Right ØQCD
Pelvic Cavity ØWCJ
Penis ØVCS
Pericardial Cavity ØWCD
Pericardium Ø2CN
Peritoneal Cavity ØWCG
Peritoneum ØDCW
Phalanx
  Finger
    Left ØPCV
    Right ØPCT
  Thumb
    Left ØPCS
    Right ØPCR
  Toe
    Left ØQCR
    Right ØQCQ
Pharynx ØCCM
Pineal Body ØGC1
Pleura
  Left ØBCP
  Right ØBCN
Pleural Cavity
  Left ØWCB
  Right ØWC9
Pons ØØCB
Prepuce ØVCT
Prostate ØVCØ
Radius
  Left ØPCJ
  Right ØPCH
Rectum ØDCP
Respiratory Tract ØWCQ
Retina
  Left Ø8CF
  Right Ø8CE
Retinal Vessel
  Left Ø8CH
  Right Ø8CG
Retroperitoneum ØWCH
Ribs
  1 to 2 ØPC1
  3 or More ØPC2
Sacrum ØQC1
Scapula
  Left ØPC6
  Right ØPC5
Sclera
  Left Ø8C7XZZ
  Right Ø8C6XZZ
Scrotum ØVC5
Septum
  Atrial Ø2C5
  Nasal Ø9CM
  Ventricular Ø2CM
Sinus
  Accessory Ø9CP
  Ethmoid
    Left Ø9CV

Extirpation — *continued*
Sinus — *continued*
  Ethmoid — *continued*
    Right Ø9CU
  Frontal
    Left Ø9CT
    Right Ø9CS
  Mastoid
    Left Ø9CC
    Right Ø9CB
  Maxillary
    Left Ø9CR
    Right Ø9CQ
  Sphenoid
    Left Ø9CX
    Right Ø9CW
Skin
  Abdomen ØHC7XZZ
  Back ØHC6XZZ
  Buttock ØHC8XZZ
  Chest ØHC5XZZ
  Ear
    Left ØHC3XZZ
    Right ØHC2XZZ
  Face ØHC1XZZ
  Foot
    Left ØHCNXZZ
    Right ØHCMXZZ
  Hand
    Left ØHCGXZZ
    Right ØHCFXZZ
  Inguinal ØHCAXZZ
  Lower Arm
    Left ØHCEXZZ
    Right ØHCDXZZ
  Lower Leg
    Left ØHCLXZZ
    Right ØHCKXZZ
  Neck ØHC4XZZ
  Perineum ØHC9XZZ
  Scalp ØHCØXZZ
  Upper Arm
    Left ØHCCXZZ
    Right ØHCBXZZ
  Upper Leg
    Left ØHCJXZZ
    Right ØHCHXZZ
Spinal Canal ØØCU
Spinal Cord
  Cervical ØØCW
  Lumbar ØØCY
  Thoracic ØØCX
Spinal Meninges ØØCT
Spleen Ø7CP
Sternum ØPCØ
Stomach ØDC6
  Pylorus ØDC7
Subarachnoid Space, Intracranial ØØC5
Subcutaneous Tissue and Fascia
  Abdomen ØJC8
  Back ØJC7
  Buttock ØJC9
  Chest ØJC6
  Face ØJC1
  Foot
    Left ØJCR
    Right ØJCQ
  Hand
    Left ØJCK
    Right ØJCJ
  Lower Arm
    Left ØJCH
    Right ØJCG
  Lower Leg
    Left ØJCP
    Right ØJCN
  Neck
    Left ØJC5
    Right ØJC4
  Pelvic Region ØJCC
  Perineum ØJCB
  Scalp ØJCØ
  Upper Arm
    Left ØJCF
    Right ØJCD
  Upper Leg
    Left ØJCM
    Right ØJCL
Subdural Space, Intracranial ØØC4

Extirpation — *continued*
Tarsal
Left ØQCM
Right ØQCL
Tendon
Abdomen
Left ØLCG
Right ØLCF
Ankle
Left ØLCT
Right ØLCS
Foot
Left ØLCW
Right ØLCV
Hand
Left ØLC8
Right ØLC7
Head and Neck ØLCØ
Hip
Left ØLCK
Right ØLCJ
Knee
Left ØLCR
Right ØLCQ
Lower Arm and Wrist
Left ØLC6
Right ØLC5
Lower Leg
Left ØLCP
Right ØLCN
Perineum ØLCH
Shoulder
Left ØLC2
Right ØLC1
Thorax
Left ØLCD
Right ØLCC
Trunk
Left ØLCB
Right ØLC9
Upper Arm
Left ØLC4
Right ØLC3
Upper Leg
Left ØLCM
Right ØLCL
Testis
Bilateral ØVCC
Left ØVCB
Right ØVC9
Thalamus ØØC9
Thymus Ø7CM
Thyroid Gland ØGCK
Left Lobe ØGCG
Right Lobe ØGCH
Tibia
Left ØQCH
Right ØQCG
Toe Nail ØHCRXZZ
Tongue ØCC7
Tonsils ØCCP
Tooth
Lower ØCCX
Upper ØCCW
Trachea ØBC1
Tunica Vaginalis
Left ØVC7
Right ØVC6
Turbinate, Nasal Ø9CL
Tympanic Membrane
Left Ø9C8
Right Ø9C7
Ulna
Left ØPCL
Right ØPCK
Ureter
Left ØTC7
Right ØTC6
Urethra ØTCD
Uterine Supporting Structure ØUC4
Uterus ØUC9
Uvula ØCCN
Vagina ØUCG
Valve
Aortic Ø2CF
Mitral Ø2CG
Pulmonary Ø2CH
Tricuspid Ø2CJ

Extirpation — *continued*
Vas Deferens
Bilateral ØVCQ
Left ØVCP
Right ØVCN
Vein
Axillary
Left Ø5C8
Right Ø5C7
Azygos Ø5CØ
Basilic
Left Ø5CC
Right Ø5CB
Brachial
Left Ø5CA
Right Ø5C9
Cephalic
Left Ø5CF
Right Ø5CD
Colic Ø6C7
Common Iliac
Left Ø6CD
Right Ø6CC
Coronary Ø2C4
Esophageal Ø6C3
External Iliac
Left Ø6CG
Right Ø6CF
External Jugular
Left Ø5CQ
Right Ø5CP
Face
Left Ø5CV
Right Ø5CT
Femoral
Left Ø6CN
Right Ø6CM
Foot
Left Ø6CV
Right Ø6CT
Gastric Ø6C2
Hand
Left Ø5CH
Right Ø5CG
Hemiazygos Ø5C1
Hepatic Ø6C4
Hypogastric
Left Ø6CJ
Right Ø6CH
Inferior Mesenteric Ø6C6
Innominate
Left Ø5C4
Right Ø5C3
Internal Jugular
Left Ø5CN
Right Ø5CM
Intracranial Ø5CL
Lower Ø6CY
Portal Ø6C8
Pulmonary
Left Ø2CT
Right Ø2CS
Renal
Left Ø6CB
Right Ø6C9
Saphenous
Left Ø6CQ
Right Ø6CP
Splenic Ø6C1
Subclavian
Left Ø5C6
Right Ø5C5
Superior Mesenteric Ø6C5
Upper Ø5CY
Vertebral
Left Ø5CS
Right Ø5CR
Vena Cava
Inferior Ø6CØ
Superior Ø2CV
Ventricle
Left Ø2CL
Right Ø2CK
Vertebra
Cervical ØPC3
Lumbar ØQCØ
Thoracic ØPC4
Vesicle
Bilateral ØVC3

Extirpation — *continued*
Vesicle — *continued*
Left ØVC2
Right ØVC1
Vitreous
Left Ø8C5
Right Ø8C4
Vocal Cord
Left ØCCV
Right ØCCT
Vulva ØUCM
Extracorporeal Carbon Dioxide Removal (ECCO2R)
5AØ92ØZ
Extracorporeal shock wave lithotripsy *see* Fragmentation
Extracranial-intracranial bypass (EC-IC) *see* Bypass, Upper Arteries Ø31
Extraction
Acetabulum
Left ØQD5ØZZ
Right ØQD4ØZZ
Ampulla of Vater ØFDC
Anus ØDDQ
Appendix ØDDJ
Auditory Ossicle
Left Ø9DAØZZ
Right Ø9D9ØZZ
Bone
Ethmoid
Left ØNDGØZZ
Right ØNDFØZZ
Frontal ØND1ØZZ
Hyoid ØNDXØZZ
Lacrimal
Left ØNDJØZZ
Right ØNDHØZZ
Nasal ØNDBØZZ
Occipital ØND7ØZZ
Palatine
Left ØNDLØZZ
Right ØNDKØZZ
Parietal
Left ØND4ØZZ
Right ØND3ØZZ
Pelvic
Left ØQD3ØZZ
Right ØQD2ØZZ
Sphenoid ØNDCØZZ
Temporal
Left ØND6ØZZ
Right ØND5ØZZ
Zygomatic
Left ØNDNØZZ
Right ØNDMØZZ
Bone Marrow Ø7DT
Iliac Ø7DR
Sternum Ø7DQ
Vertebral Ø7DS
Brain ØØDØ
Breast
Bilateral ØHDVØZZ
Left ØHDUØZZ
Right ØHDTØZZ
Supernumerary ØHDYØZZ
Bronchus
Lingula ØBD9
Lower Lobe
Left ØBDB
Right ØBD6
Main
Left ØBD7
Right ØBD3
Middle Lobe, Right ØBD5
Upper Lobe
Left ØBD8
Right ØBD4
Bursa and Ligament
Abdomen
Left ØMDJ
Right ØMDH
Ankle
Left ØMDR
Right ØMDQ
Elbow
Left ØMD4
Right ØMD3
Foot
Left ØMDT
Right ØMDS

Extraction — *continued*
  Products of Conception — *continued*
    Retained 10D1
    Vacuum 10D07Z6
  Radius
    Left ØPDJØZZ
    Right ØPDHØZZ
  Rectum ØDDP
  Ribs
    1 to 2 ØPD1ØZZ
    3 or More ØPD2ØZZ
  Sacrum ØQD1ØZZ
  Scapula
    Left ØPD6ØZZ
    Right ØPD5ØZZ
  Septum, Nasal Ø9DM
  Sinus
    Accessory Ø9DP
    Ethmoid
      Left Ø9DV
      Right Ø9DU
    Frontal
      Left Ø9DT
      Right Ø9DS
    Mastoid
      Left Ø9DC
      Right Ø9DB
    Maxillary
      Left Ø9DR
      Right Ø9DQ
    Sphenoid
      Left Ø9DX
      Right Ø9DW
  Skin
    Abdomen ØHD7XZZ
    Back ØHD6XZZ
    Buttock ØHD8XZZ
    Chest ØHD5XZZ
    Ear
      Left ØHD3XZZ
      Right ØHD2XZZ
    Face ØHD1XZZ
    Foot
      Left ØHDNXZZ
      Right ØHDMXZZ
    Hand
      Left ØHDGXZZ
      Right ØHDFXZZ
    Inguinal ØHDAXZZ
    Lower Arm
      Left ØHDEXZZ
      Right ØHDDXZZ
    Lower Leg
      Left ØHDLXZZ
      Right ØHDKXZZ
    Neck ØHD4XZZ
    Perineum ØHD9XZZ
    Scalp ØHDØXZZ
    Upper Arm
      Left ØHDCXZZ
      Right ØHDBXZZ
    Upper Leg
      Left ØHDJXZZ
      Right ØHDHXZZ
  Skull ØNDØØZZ
  Spinal Meninges ØØDT
  Spleen Ø7DP
  Sternum ØPDØØZZ
  Stomach ØDD6
    Pylorus ØDD7
  Subcutaneous Tissue and Fascia
    Abdomen ØJD8
    Back ØJD7
    Buttock ØJD9
    Chest ØJD6
    Face ØJD1
    Foot
      Left ØJDR
      Right ØJDQ
    Hand
      Left ØJDK
      Right ØJDJ
    Lower Arm
      Left ØJDH
      Right ØJDG
    Lower Leg
      Left ØJDP
      Right ØJDN

Extraction — *continued*
  Subcutaneous Tissue and Fascia — *continued*
    Neck
      Left ØJD5
      Right ØJD4
    Pelvic Region ØJDC
    Perineum ØJDB
    Scalp ØJDØ
    Upper Arm
      Left ØJDF
      Right ØJDD
    Upper Leg
      Left ØJDM
      Right ØJDL
  Tarsal
    Left ØQDMØZZ
    Right ØQDLØZZ
  Tendon
    Abdomen
      Left ØLDGØZZ
      Right ØLDFØZZ
    Ankle
      Left ØLDTØZZ
      Right ØLDSØZZ
    Foot
      Left ØLDWØZZ
      Right ØLDVØZZ
    Hand
      Left ØLD8ØZZ
      Right ØLD7ØZZ
    Head and Neck ØLDØØZZ
    Hip
      Left ØLDKØZZ
      Right ØLDJØZZ
    Knee
      Left ØLDRØZZ
      Right ØLDQØZZ
    Lower Arm and Wrist
      Left ØLD6ØZZ
      Right ØLD5ØZZ
    Lower Leg
      Left ØLDPØZZ
      Right ØLDNØZZ
    Perineum ØLDHØZZ
    Shoulder
      Left ØLD2ØZZ
      Right ØLD1ØZZ
    Thorax
      Left ØLDDØZZ
      Right ØLDCØZZ
    Trunk
      Left ØLDBØZZ
      Right ØLD9ØZZ
    Upper Arm
      Left ØLD4ØZZ
      Right ØLD3ØZZ
    Upper Leg
      Left ØLDMØZZ
      Right ØDLLØZZ
  Thymus Ø7DM
  Tibia
    Left ØQDHØZZ
    Right ØQDGØZZ
  Toe Nail ØHDRXZZ
  Tooth
    Lower ØCDXXZ
    Upper ØCDWXZ
  Trachea ØBD1
  Turbinate, Nasal Ø9DL
  Tympanic Membrane
    Left Ø9D8
    Right Ø9D7
  Ulna
    Left ØPDLØZZ
    Right ØPDKØZZ
  Vein
    Basilic
      Left Ø5DC
      Right Ø5DB
    Brachial
      Left Ø5DA
      Right Ø5D9
    Cephalic
      Left Ø5DF
      Right Ø5DD
    Femoral
      Left Ø6DN
      Right Ø6DM

Extraction — *continued*
  Vein — *continued*
    Foot
      Left Ø6DV
      Right Ø6DT
    Hand
      Left Ø5DH
      Right Ø5DG
    Lower Ø6DY
    Saphenous
      Left Ø6DQ
      Right Ø6DP
    Upper Ø5DY
  Vertebra
    Cervical ØPD3ØZZ
    Lumbar ØQDØØZZ
    Thoracic ØPD4ØZZ
  Vocal Cord
    Left ØCDV
    Right ØCDT
Extradural space, intracranial *use* Epidural Space, Intracranial
Extradural space, spinal *use* Spinal Canal
EXtreme Lateral Interbody Fusion (XLIF) device
    use Interbody Fusion Device in Lower Joints

F

Face lift *see* Alteration, Face ØWØ2
Facet replacement spinal stabilization device
    use Spinal Stabilization Device, Facet Replacement in ØRH
    use Spinal Stabilization Device, Facet Replacement in ØSH
Facial artery *use* Face Artery
Factor Xa Inhibitor Reversal Agent, Andexanet Alfa *use* Coagulation Factor Xa, Inactivated
False vocal cord *use* Larynx
Falx cerebri *use* Dura Mater
Fascia lata
    use Subcutaneous Tissue and Fascia, Left Upper Leg
    use Subcutaneous Tissue and Fascia, Right Upper Leg
Fasciaplasty, fascioplasty
    see Repair, Subcutaneous Tissue and Fascia ØJQ
    see Replacement, Subcutaneous Tissue and Fascia ØJR
Fasciectomy *see* Excision, Subcutaneous Tissue and Fascia ØJB
Fasciorrhaphy *see* Repair, Subcutaneous Tissue and Fascia ØJQ
Fasciotomy
    see Division, Subcutaneous Tissue and Fascia ØJ8
    see Drainage, Subcutaneous Tissue and Fascia ØJ9
    see Release
Feeding Device
  Change device in
    Lower ØD2DXUZ
    Upper ØD2ØXUZ
  Insertion of device in
    Duodenum ØDH9
    Esophagus ØDH5
    Ileum ØDHB
    Intestine, Small ØDH8
    Jejunum ØDHA
    Stomach ØDH6
  Removal of device from
    Esophagus ØDP5
    Intestinal Tract
      Lower ØDPD
      Upper ØDPØ
    Stomach ØDP6
  Revision of device in
    Intestinal Tract
      Lower ØDWD
      Upper ØDWØ
    Stomach ØDW6
Femoral head
    use Upper Femur, Left
    use Upper Femur, Right
Femoral lymph node
    use Lymphatic, Left Lower Extremity
    use Lymphatic, Right Lower Extremity
Femoropatellar joint
    use Knee Joint, Left
    use Knee Joint, Left, Tibial Surface

Femoropatellar joint — *continued*
use Knee Joint, Right
use Knee Joint, Right, Femoral Surface

Femorotibial joint
use Knee Joint, Left
use Knee Joint, Left, Tibial Surface
use Knee Joint, Right
use Knee Joint, Right, Tibial Surface

FETROJA® *use* Cefiderocol Anti-infective

FGS (fluoroscopy-guided surgery) *see* Fluorescence Guided Procedure

Fibular artery
use Peroneal Artery, Left
use Peroneal Artery, Right

Fibular sesamoid
use Metatarsal, Left
use Metatarsal, Right

Fibularis brevis muscle
use Lower Leg Muscle, Left
use Lower Leg Muscle, Right

Fibularis longus muscle
use Lower Leg Muscle, Left
use Lower Leg Muscle, Right

Fifth cranial nerve *use* Trigeminal Nerve

Filum terminale *use* Spinal Meninges

Fimbriectomy
see Excision, Female Reproductive System 0UB
see Resection, Female Reproductive System 0UT

Fine needle aspiration
Fluid or gas *see* Drainage
Tissue biopsy
see Excision
see Extraction

First cranial nerve *use* Olfactory Nerve

First intercostal nerve *use* Brachial Plexus

Fistulization
see Bypass
see Drainage
see Repair

Fitting
Arch bars, for fracture reduction *see* Reposition, Mouth and Throat 0CS
Arch bars, for immobilization *see* Immobilization, Face 2W31
Artificial limb *see* Device Fitting, Rehabilitation F0D
Hearing aid *see* Device Fitting, Rehabilitation F0D
Ocular prosthesis F0DZ8UZ
Prosthesis, limb *see* Device Fitting, Rehabilitation F0D
Prosthesis, ocular F0DZ8UZ

Fixation, bone
External, with fracture reduction *see* Reposition
External, without fracture reduction *see* Insertion
Internal, with fracture reduction *see* Reposition
Internal, without fracture reduction *see* Insertion

FLAIR® Endovascular Stent Graft *use* Intraluminal Device

Flexible Composite Mesh *use* Synthetic Substitute

Flexor carpi radialis muscle
use Lower Arm and Wrist Muscle, Left
use Lower Arm and Wrist Muscle, Right

Flexor carpi ulnaris muscle
use Lower Arm and Wrist Muscle, Left
use Lower Arm and Wrist Muscle, Right

Flexor digitorum brevis muscle
use Foot Muscle, Left
use Foot Muscle, Right

Flexor digitorum longus muscle
use Lower Leg Muscle, Left
use Lower Leg Muscle, Right

Flexor hallucis brevis muscle
use Foot Muscle, Left
use Foot Muscle, Right

Flexor hallucis longus muscle
use Lower Leg Muscle, Left
use Lower Leg Muscle, Right

Flexor pollicis longus muscle
use Lower Arm and Wrist Muscle, Left
use Lower Arm and Wrist Muscle, Right

Flow Diverter embolization device *use* Intraluminal Device, Flow Diverter in 03V

FlowSense Noninvasive Thermal Sensor *see* Measurement, Central Nervous Cerebrospinal Fluid Shunt

Fluorescence Guided Procedure
Extremity
Lower 8E0Y
Upper 8E0X
Head and Neck Region 8E09
Aminolevulinic Acid 8E090EM
No Qualifier 8E090EZ
Trunk Region 8E0W

Fluorescent Pyrazine, Kidney XT25XE5

Fluoroscopy
Abdomen and Pelvis BW11
Airway, Upper BB1DZZZ
Ankle
Left BQ1H
Right BQ1G
Aorta
Abdominal B410
Laser, Intraoperative B410
Thoracic B310
Laser, Intraoperative B310
Thoraco-Abdominal B31P
Laser, Intraoperative B31P
Aorta and Bilateral Lower Extremity Arteries B41D
Laser, Intraoperative B41D
Arm
Left BP1FZZZ
Right BP1EZZZ
Artery
Brachiocephalic-Subclavian
Laser, Intraoperative B311
Right B311
Bronchial B31L
Laser, Intraoperative B31L
Bypass Graft, Other B21F
Cervico-Cerebral Arch B31Q
Laser, Intraoperative B31Q
Common Carotid
Bilateral B315
Laser, Intraoperative B315
Left B314
Laser, Intraoperative B314
Right B313
Laser, Intraoperative B313
Coronary
Bypass Graft
Multiple B213
Laser, Intraoperative B213
Single B212
Laser, Intraoperative B212
Multiple B211
Laser, Intraoperative B211
Single B210
Laser, Intraoperative B210
External Carotid
Bilateral B31C
Laser, Intraoperative B31C
Left B31B
Laser, Intraoperative B31B
Right B319
Laser, Intraoperative B319
Hepatic B412
Laser, Intraoperative B412
Inferior Mesenteric B415
Laser, Intraoperative B415
Intercostal B31L
Laser, Intraoperative B31L
Internal Carotid
Bilateral B318
Laser, Intraoperative B318
Left B317
Laser, Intraoperative B317
Right B316
Laser, Intraoperative B316
Internal Mammary Bypass Graft
Left B218
Right B217
Intra-Abdominal
Laser, Intraoperative B41B
Other B41B
Intracranial B31R
Laser, Intraoperative B31R
Lower
Laser, Intraoperative B41J
Other B41J
Lower Extremity
Bilateral and Aorta B41D
Laser, Intraoperative B41D
Left B41G
Laser, Intraoperative B41G

Fluoroscopy — *continued*
Artery — *continued*
Lower Extremity — *continued*
Right B41F
Laser, Intraoperative B41F
Lumbar B419
Laser, Intraoperative B419
Pelvic B41C
Laser, Intraoperative B41C
Pulmonary
Left B31T
Laser, Intraoperative B31T
Right B31S
Laser, Intraoperative B31S
Pulmonary Trunk B31U
Laser, Intraoperative B31U
Renal
Bilateral B418
Laser, Intraoperative B418
Left B417
Laser, Intraoperative B417
Right B416
Laser, Intraoperative B416
Spinal B31M
Laser, Intraoperative B31M
Splenic B413
Laser, Intraoperative B413
Subclavian
Laser, Intraoperative B312
Left B312
Superior Mesenteric B414
Laser, Intraoperative B414
Upper
Laser, Intraoperative B31N
Other B31N
Upper Extremity
Bilateral B31K
Laser, Intraoperative B31K
Left B31J
Laser, Intraoperative B31J
Right B31H
Laser, Intraoperative B31H
Vertebral
Bilateral B31G
Laser, Intraoperative B31G
Left B31F
Laser, Intraoperative B31F
Right B31D
Laser, Intraoperative B31D
Bile Duct BF10
Pancreatic Duct and Gallbladder BF14
Bile Duct and Gallbladder BF13
Biliary Duct BF11
Bladder BT10
Kidney and Ureter BT14
Left BT1F
Right BT1D
Bladder and Urethra BT1B
Bowel, Small BD1
Calcaneus
Left BQ1KZZZ
Right BQ1JZZZ
Clavicle
Left BP15ZZZ
Right BP14ZZZ
Coccyx BR1F
Colon BD14
Corpora Cavernosa BV10
Dialysis Fistula B51W
Dialysis Shunt B51W
Diaphragm BB16ZZZ
Disc
Cervical BR11
Lumbar BR13
Thoracic BR12
Duodenum BD19
Elbow
Left BP1H
Right BP1G
Epiglottis B91G
Esophagus BD11
Extremity
Lower BW1C
Upper BW1J
Facet Joint
Cervical BR14
Lumbar BR16
Thoracic BR15

Fluoroscopy — *continued*
Fallopian Tube
  Bilateral BU12
  Left BU11
  Right BU10
Fallopian Tube and Uterus BU18
Femur
  Left BQ14ZZZ
  Right BQ13ZZZ
Finger
  Left BP1SZZZ
  Right BP1RZZZ
Foot
  Left BQ1MZZZ
  Right BQ1LZZZ
Forearm
  Left BP1KZZZ
  Right BP1JZZZ
Gallbladder BF12
  Bile Duct and Pancreatic Duct BF14
Gallbladder and Bile Duct BF13
Gastrointestinal, Upper BD1
Hand
  Left BP1PZZZ
  Right BP1NZZZ
Head and Neck BW19
Heart
  Left B215
  Right B214
  Right and Left B216
Hip
  Left BQ11
  Right BQ10
Humerus
  Left BP1BZZZ
  Right BP1AZZZ
Ileal Diversion Loop BT1C
Ileal Loop, Ureters and Kidney BT1G
Intracranial Sinus B512
Joint
  Acromioclavicular, Bilateral BP13ZZZ
  Finger
    Left BP1D
    Right BP1C
  Foot
    Left BQ1Y
    Right BQ1X
  Hand
    Left BP1D
    Right BP1C
  Lumbosacral BR1B
  Sacroiliac BR1D
  Sternoclavicular
    Bilateral BP12ZZZ
    Left BP11ZZZ
    Right BP10ZZZ
  Temporomandibular
    Bilateral BN19
    Left BN18
    Right BN17
  Thoracolumbar BR18
  Toe
    Left BQ1Y
    Right BQ1X
Kidney
  Bilateral BT13
  Ileal Loop and Ureter BT1G
  Left BT12
  Right BT11
  Ureter and Bladder BT14
    Left BT1F
    Right BT1D
Knee
  Left BQ18
  Right BQ17
Larynx B91J
Leg
  Left BQ1FZZZ
  Right BQ1DZZZ
Liver BF15
Lung
  Bilateral BB14ZZZ
  Left BB13ZZZ
  Right BB12ZZZ
Mediastinum BB1CZZZ
Mouth BD1B
Neck and Head BW19
Oropharynx BD1B
Pancreatic Duct BF1

Fluoroscopy — *continued*
Pancreatic Duct — *continued*
  Gallbladder and Bile Buct BF14
Patella
  Left BQ1WZZZ
  Right BQ1VZZZ
Pelvis BR1C
Pelvis and Abdomen BW11
Pharynx B91G
Ribs
  Left BP1YZZZ
  Right BP1XZZZ
Sacrum BR1F
Scapula
  Left BP17ZZZ
  Right BP16ZZZ
Shoulder
  Left BP19
  Right BP18
Sinus, Intracranial B512
Spinal Cord B01B
Spine
  Cervical BR10
  Lumbar BR19
  Thoracic BR17
  Whole BR1G
Sternum BR1H
Stomach BD12
Toe
  Left BQ1QZZZ
  Right BQ1PZZZ
Tracheobronchial Tree
  Bilateral BB19YZZ
  Left BB18YZZ
  Right BB17YZZ
Ureter
  Ileal Loop and Kidney BT1G
  Kidney and Bladder BT14
    Left BT1F
    Right BT1D
  Left BT17
  Right BT16
Urethra BT15
Urethra and Bladder BT1B
Uterus BU16
Uterus and Fallopian Tube BU18
Vagina BU19
Vasa Vasorum BV18
Vein
  Cerebellar B511
  Cerebral B511
  Epidural B510
  Jugular
    Bilateral B515
    Left B514
    Right B513
  Lower Extremity
    Bilateral B51D
    Left B51C
    Right B51B
  Other B51V
  Pelvic (Iliac)
    Left B51G
    Right B51F
  Pelvic (Iliac) Bilateral B51H
  Portal B51T
  Pulmonary
    Bilateral B51S
    Left B51R
    Right B51Q
  Renal
    Bilateral B51L
    Left B51K
    Right B51J
  Spanchnic B51T
  Subclavian
    Left B517
    Right B516
  Upper Extremity
    Bilateral B51P
    Left B51N
    Right B51M
Vena Cava
  Inferior B519
  Superior B518
Wrist
  Left BP1M
  Right BP1L

Fluoroscopy, laser intraoperative
  see Fluoroscopy, Heart B21
  see Fluoroscopy, Lower Arteries B41
  see Fluoroscopy, Upper Arteries B31
Flushing *see* Irrigation
Foley catheter *use* Drainage Device
Fontan completion procedure Stage II *see* Bypass, Vena Cava, Inferior 0610
Foramen magnum *use* Occipital Bone
Foramen of Monro (intraventricular) *use* Cerebral Ventricle
Foreskin *use* Prepuce
Formula™ Balloon-Expandable Renal Stent System *use* Intraluminal Device
Fosfomycin Anti-infective XW0
Fosfomycin injection *use* Fosfomycin Anti-infective
Fossa of Rosenmuller *use* Nasopharynx
Fourth cranial nerve *use* Trochlear Nerve
Fourth ventricle *use* Cerebral Ventricle
Fovea
  use Retina, Left
  use Retina, Right
Fragmentation
Ampulla of Vater 0FFC
Anus 0DFQ
Appendix 0DFJ
Artery
  Anterior Tibial
    Left 04FQ3Z
    Right 04FP3Z
  Axillary
    Left 03F63Z
    Right 03F53Z
  Brachial
    Left 03F83Z
    Right 03F73Z
  Common Iliac
    Left 04FD3Z
    Right 04FC3Z
  Coronary
    Four or More Arteries 02F33ZZ
    One Artery 02F03ZZ
    Three Arteries 02F23ZZ
    Two Arteries 02F13ZZ
  External Iliac
    Left 04FJ3Z
    Right 04FH3Z
  Femoral
    Left 04FL3Z
    Right 04FK3Z
  Innominate 03F23Z
  Internal Iliac
    Left 04FF3Z
    Right 04FE3Z
  Intracranial 03FG3Z
  Lower 04FY3Z
  Peroneal
    Left 04FU3Z
    Right 04FT3Z
  Popliteal
    Left 04FN3Z
    Right 04FM3Z
  Posterior Tibial
    Left 04FS3Z
    Right 04FR3Z
  Pulmonary
    Left 02FR3Z
    Right 02FQ3Z
  Pulmonary Trunk 02FP3Z
  Radial
    Left 03FC3Z
    Right 03FB3Z
  Subclavian
    Left 03F43Z
    Right 03F33Z
  Ulnar
    Left 03FA3Z
    Right 03F93Z
  Upper 03FY3Z
Bladder 0TFB
Bladder Neck 0TFC
Bronchus
  Lingula 0BF9
  Lower Lobe
    Left 0BFB
    Right 0BF6
  Main
    Left 0BF7

▽ Subterms under main terms may continue to next column or page

Fragmentation — *continued*
  Bronchus — *continued*
    Main — *continued*
      Right ØBF3
    Middle Lobe, Right ØBF5
    Upper Lobe
      Left ØBF8
      Right ØBF4
  Carina ØBF2
  Cavity, Cranial ØWF1
  Cecum ØDFH
  Cerebral Ventricle ØØF6
  Colon
    Ascending ØDFK
    Descending ØDFM
    Sigmoid ØDFN
    Transverse ØDFL
  Duct
    Common Bile ØFF9
    Cystic ØFF8
    Hepatic
      Common ØFF7
      Left ØFF6
      Right ØFF5
    Pancreatic ØFFD
      Accessory ØFFF
    Parotid
      Left ØCFC
      Right ØCFB
  Duodenum ØDF9
  Epidural Space, Intracranial ØØF3
  Esophagus ØDF5
  Fallopian Tube
    Left ØUF6
    Right ØUF5
  Fallopian Tubes, Bilateral ØUF7
  Gallbladder ØFF4
  Gastrointestinal Tract ØWFP
  Genitourinary Tract ØWFR
  Ileum ØDFB
  Intestine
    Large ØDFE
      Left ØDFG
      Right ØDFF
    Small ØDF8
  Jejunum ØDFA
  Kidney Pelvis
    Left ØTF4
    Right ØTF3
  Mediastinum ØWFC
  Oral Cavity and Throat ØWF3
  Pelvic Cavity ØWFJ
  Pericardial Cavity ØWFD
  Pericardium Ø2FN
  Peritoneal Cavity ØWFG
  Pleural Cavity
    Left ØWFB
    Right ØWF9
  Rectum ØDFP
  Respiratory Tract ØWFQ
  Spinal Canal ØØFU
  Stomach ØDF6
  Subarachnoid Space, Intracranial ØØF5
  Subdural Space, Intracranial ØØF4
  Trachea ØBF1
  Ureter
    Left ØTF7
    Right ØTF6
  Urethra ØTFD
  Uterus ØUF9
  Vein
    Axillary
      Left Ø5F83Z
      Right Ø5F73Z
    Basilic
      Left Ø5FC3Z
      Right Ø5FB3Z
    Brachial
      Left Ø5FA3Z
      Right Ø5F93Z
    Cephalic
      Left Ø5FF3Z
      Right Ø5FD3Z
    Common Iliac
      Left Ø6FD3Z
      Right Ø6FC3Z
    External Iliac
      Left Ø6FG3Z
      Right Ø6FF3Z

Fragmentation — *continued*
  Vein — *continued*
    Femoral
      Left Ø6FN3Z
      Right Ø6FM3Z
    Hypogastric
      Left Ø6FJ3Z
      Right Ø6FH3Z
    Innominate
      Left Ø5F43Z
      Right Ø5F33Z
    Lower Ø6FY3Z
    Pulmonary
      Left Ø2FT3Z
      Right Ø2FS3Z
    Saphenous
      Left Ø6FQ3Z
      Right Ø6FP3Z
    Subclavian
      Left Ø5F63Z
      Right Ø5F53Z
    Upper Ø5FY3Z
  Vitreous
    Left Ø8F5
    Right Ø8F4
Fragmentation, Ultrasonic *see* Fragmentation, Artery
Freestyle (Stentless) Aortic Root Bioprosthesis *use* Zooplastic Tissue in Heart and Great Vessels
Frenectomy
  see Excision, Mouth and Throat ØCB
  see Resection, Mouth and Throat ØCT
Frenoplasty, frenuloplasty
  see Repair, Mouth and Throat ØCQ
  see Replacement, Mouth and Throat ØCR
  see Supplement, Mouth and Throat ØCU
Frenotomy
  see Drainage, Mouth and Throat ØC9
  see Release, Mouth and Throat ØCN
Frenulotomy
  see Drainage, Mouth and Throat ØC9
  see Release, Mouth and Throat ØCN
Frenulum labii inferioris *use* Lower Lip
Frenulum labii superioris *use* Upper Lip
Frenulum linguae *use* Tongue
Frenulumectomy
  see Excision, Mouth and Throat ØCB
  see Resection, Mouth and Throat ØCT
Frontal lobe *use* Cerebral Hemisphere
Frontal vein
  use Face Vein, Left
  use Face Vein, Right
Frozen elephant trunk (FET) technique, aortic arch replacement
  see New Technology, Cardiovascular System X2R
  see Replacement, Heart and Great Vessels Ø2R
Frozen elephant trunk (FET) technique, thoracic aorta restriction
  see New Technology, Cardiovascular System X2V
  see Restriction, Heart and Great Vessels Ø2V
FUJIFILM EP-7ØØØX System for Oxygen Saturation Endoscopic Imaging (OXEI) *see* New Technology, Gastrointestinal System XD2
Fulguration *see* Destruction
Fundoplication, gastroesophageal *see* Restriction, Esophagogastric Junction ØDV4
Fundus uteri *use* Uterus
Fusion
  Acromioclavicular
    Left ØRGH
    Right ØRGG
  Ankle
    Left ØSGG
    Right ØSGF
  Carpal
    Left ØRGR
    Right ØRGQ
  Carpometacarpal
    Left ØRGT
    Right ØRGS
  Cervical Vertebral ØRG1
    2 or more ØRG2
      Interbody Fusion Device
        Nanotextured Surface XRG2Ø92
        Radiolucent Porous XRG2ØF3
    Interbody Fusion Device
      Nanotextured Surface XRG1Ø92
      Radiolucent Porous XRG1ØF3

Fusion — *continued*
  Cervicothoracic Vertebral ØRG4
    Interbody Fusion Device
      Nanotextured Surface XRG4Ø92
      Radiolucent Porous XRG4ØF3
  Coccygeal ØSG6
  Elbow
    Left ØRGM
    Right ØRGL
  Finger Phalangeal
    Left ØRGX
    Right ØRGW
  Hip
    Left ØSGB
    Right ØSG9
  Knee
    Left ØSGD
    Right ØSGC
  Lumbar Vertebral ØSGØ
    2 or more ØSG1
      Interbody Fusion Device
        Customizable XRGC
        Nanotextured Surface XRGCØ92
        Radiolucent Porous XRGCØF3
    Interbody Fusion Device
      Customizable XRGB
      Nanotextured Surface XRGBØ92
      Radiolucent Porous XRGBØF3
  Lumbosacral ØSG3
    Interbody Fusion Device
      Customizable XRGD
      Nanotextured Surface XRGDØ92
      Radiolucent Porous XRGDØF3
  Metacarpophalangeal
    Left ØRGV
    Right ØRGU
  Metatarsal-Phalangeal
    Left ØSGN
    Right ØSGM
  Occipital-cervical ØRGØ
    Interbody Fusion Device
      Nanotextured Surface XRGØØ92
      Radiolucent Porous XRGØØF3
  Sacrococcygeal ØSG5
  Sacroiliac
    Left ØSG8
    Right ØSG7
  Shoulder
    Left ØRGK
    Right ØRGJ
  Sternoclavicular
    Left ØRGF
    Right ØRGE
  Tarsal
    Left ØSGJ
    Right ØSGH
  Tarsometatarsal
    Left ØSGL
    Right ØSGK
  Temporomandibular
    Left ØRGD
    Right ØRGC
  Thoracic Vertebral ØRG6
    2 to 7 ØRG7
      Interbody Fusion Device
        Nanotextured Surface XRG7Ø92
        Radiolucent Porous XRG7ØF3
    8 or more ØRG8
      Interbody Fusion Device
        Nanotextured Surface XRG8Ø92
        Radiolucent Porous XRG8ØF3
    Interbody Fusion Device
      Nanotextured Surface XRG6Ø92
      Radiolucent Porous XRG6ØF3
  Thoracolumbar Vertebral ØRGA
    Interbody Fusion Device
      Customizable XRGA
      Nanotextured Surface XRGAØ92
      Radiolucent Porous XRGAØF3
  Toe Phalangeal
    Left ØSGQ
    Right ØSGP
  Wrist
    Left ØRGP
    Right ØRGN
Fusion screw (compression) (lag) (locking)
  use Internal Fixation Device in Lower Joints
  use Internal Fixation Device in Upper Joints

G

Gait training *see* Motor Treatment, Rehabilitation F07
Galea aponeurotica *use* Subcutaneous Tissue and Fascia, Scalp
Gammaglobulin *use* Globulin
GammaTile™ *use* Radioactive Element, Cesium-131 Collagen Implant in 00H
GAMUNEX-C, for COVID-19 treatment *use* High-Dose Intravenous Immune Globulin
Ganglion impar (ganglion of Walther) *use* Sacral Sympathetic Nerve
Ganglionectomy
  Destruction of lesion *see* Destruction
  Excision of lesion *see* Excision
Gasserian ganglion *use* Trigeminal Nerve
Gastrectomy
  Partial *see* Excision, Stomach 0DB6
  Total *see* Resection, Stomach 0DT6
  Vertical (sleeve) *see* Excision, Stomach 0DB6
Gastric electrical stimulation (GES) lead *use* Stimulator Lead in Gastrointestinal System
Gastric lymph node *use* Lymphatic, Aortic
Gastric pacemaker lead *use* Stimulator Lead in Gastrointestinal System
Gastric plexus *use* Abdominal Sympathetic Nerve
Gastrocnemius muscle
  use Lower Leg Muscle, Left
  use Lower Leg Muscle, Right
Gastrocolic ligament *use* Omentum
Gastrocolic omentum *use* Omentum
Gastrocolostomy
  see Bypass, Gastrointestinal System 0D1
  see Drainage, Gastrointestinal System 0D9
Gastroduodenal artery *use* Hepatic Artery
Gastroduodenectomy
  see Excision, Gastrointestinal System 0DB
  see Resection, Gastrointestinal System 0DT
Gastroduodenoscopy 0DJ08ZZ
Gastroenteroplasty
  see Repair, Gastrointestinal System 0DQ
  see Supplement, Gastrointestinal System 0DU
Gastroenterostomy
  see Bypass, Gastrointestinal System 0D1
  see Drainage, Gastrointestinal System 0D9
Gastroesophageal (GE) junction *use* Esophagogastric Junction
Gastrogastrostomy
  see Bypass, Stomach 0D16
  see Drainage, Stomach 0D96
Gastrohepatic omentum *use* Omentum
Gastrojejunostomy
  see Bypass, Stomach 0D16
  see Drainage, Stomach 0D96
Gastrolysis *see* Release, Stomach 0DN6
Gastropexy
  see Repair, Stomach 0DQ6
  see Reposition, Stomach 0DS6
Gastrophrenic ligament *use* Omentum
Gastroplasty
  see Repair, Stomach 0DQ6
  see Supplement, Stomach 0DU6
Gastroplication *see* Restriction, Stomach 0DV6
Gastropylorectomy *see* Excision, Gastrointestinal System 0DB
Gastrorrhaphy *see* Repair, Stomach 0DQ6
Gastroscopy 0DJ68ZZ
Gastrosplenic ligament *use* Omentum
Gastrostomy
  see Bypass, Stomach 0D16
  see Drainage, Stomach 0D96
Gastrotomy *see* Drainage, Stomach 0D96
Gemellus muscle
  use Hip Muscle, Left
  use Hip Muscle, Right
Geniculate ganglion *use* Facial Nerve
Geniculate nucleus *use* Thalamus
Genioglossus muscle *use* Tongue, Palate, Pharynx Muscle
Genioplasty *see* Alteration, Jaw, Lower 0W05
Genitofemoral nerve *use* Lumbar Plexus
GIAPREZA™ *use* Synthetic Human Angiotensin II
Gilteritinib Antineoplastic XW0DXV5
Gingivectomy *see* Excision, Mouth and Throat 0CB

Gingivoplasty
  see Repair, Mouth and Throat 0CQ
  see Replacement, Mouth and Throat 0CR
  see Supplement, Mouth and Throat 0CU
Glans penis *use* Prepuce
Glenohumeral joint
  use Shoulder Joint, Left
  use Shoulder Joint, Right
Glenohumeral ligament
  use Shoulder Bursa and Ligament, Left
  use Shoulder Bursa and Ligament, Right
Glenoid fossa (of scapula)
  use Glenoid Cavity, Left
  use Glenoid Cavity, Right
Glenoid ligament (labrum)
  use Shoulder Joint, Left
  use Shoulder Joint, Right
Globus pallidus *use* Basal Ganglia
Glomectomy
  see Excision, Endocrine System 0GB
  see Resection, Endocrine System 0GT
Glossectomy
  see Excision, Tongue 0CB7
  see Resection, Tongue 0CT7
Glossoepiglottic fold *use* Epiglottis
Glossopexy
  see Repair, Tongue 0CQ7
  see Reposition, Tongue 0CS7
Glossoplasty
  see Repair, Tongue 0CQ7
  see Replacement, Tongue 0CR7
  see Supplement, Tongue 0CU7
Glossorrhaphy *see* Repair, Tongue 0CQ7
Glossotomy *see* Drainage, Tongue 0C97
Glottis *use* Larynx
Gluteal Artery Perforator Flap
  Replacement
    Bilateral 0HRV079
    Left 0HRU079
    Right 0HRT079
  Transfer
    Left 0KXG
    Right 0KXF
Gluteal lymph node *use* Lymphatic, Pelvis
Gluteal vein
  use Hypogastric Vein, Left
  use Hypogastric Vein, Right
Gluteus maximus muscle
  use Hip Muscle, Left
  use Hip Muscle, Right
Gluteus medius muscle
  use Hip Muscle, Left
  use Hip Muscle, Right
Gluteus minimus muscle
  use Hip Muscle, Left
  use Hip Muscle, Right
GORE EXCLUDER® AAA Endoprosthesis
  use Intraluminal Device
  use Intraluminal Device, Branched or Fenestrated, One or Two Arteries in 04V
  use Intraluminal Device, Branched or Fenestrated, Three or More Arteries in 04V
GORE EXCLUDER® IBE Endoprosthesis *use* Intraluminal Device, Branched or Fenestrated, One or Two Arteries in 04V
GORE TAG® Thoracic Endoprosthesis *use* Intraluminal Device
GORE® DUALMESH® *use* Synthetic Substitute
Gracilis muscle
  use Upper Leg Muscle, Left
  use Upper Leg Muscle, Right
Graft
  see Replacement
  see Supplement
Great auricular nerve *use* Cervical Plexus
Great cerebral vein *use* Intracranial Vein
Great(er) saphenous vein
  use Saphenous Vein, Left
  use Saphenous Vein, Right
Greater alar cartilage *use* Nasal Mucosa and Soft Tissue
Greater occipital nerve *use* Cervical Nerve
Greater Omentum *use* Omentum
Greater splanchnic nerve *use* Thoracic Sympathetic Nerve
Greater superficial petrosal nerve *use* Facial Nerve

Greater trochanter
  use Upper Femur, Left
  use Upper Femur, Right
Greater tuberosity
  use Humeral Head, Left
  use Humeral Head, Right
Greater vestibular (Bartholin's) gland *use* Vestibular Gland
Greater wing *use* Sphenoid Bone
GS-5734 *use* Remdesivir Anti-infective
Guedel airway *use* Intraluminal Device, Airway in Mouth and Throat
Guidance, catheter placement
  EKG *see* Measurement, Physiological Systems 4A0
  Fluoroscopy *see* Fluoroscopy, Veins B51
  Ultrasound *see* Ultrasonography, Veins B54

H

Hallux
  use 1st Toe, Left
  use 1st Toe, Right
Hamate bone
  use Carpal, Left
  use Carpal, Right
Hancock Bioprosthesis (aortic) (mitral) valve *use* Zooplastic Tissue in Heart and Great Vessels
Hancock Bioprosthetic Valved Conduit *use* Zooplastic Tissue in Heart and Great Vessels
Harmony™ transcatheter pulmonary valve (TPV) placement 02RH38M
Harvesting, Stem Cells *see* Pheresis, Circulatory 6A55
hdIVIG (high-dose intravenous immunoglobulin), for COVID-19 treatment *use* High-Dose Intravenous Immune Globulin
Head of fibula
  use Fibula, Left
  use Fibula, Right
Hearing Aid Assessment F14Z
Hearing Assessment F13Z
Hearing Device
  Bone Conduction
    Left 09HE
    Right 09HD
  Insertion of device in
    Left 0NH6
    Right 0NH5
  Multiple Channel Cochlear Prosthesis
    Left 09HE
    Right 09HD
  Removal of device from, Skull 0NP0
  Revision of device in, Skull 0NW0
  Single Channel Cochlear Prosthesis
    Left 09HE
    Right 09HD
Hearing Treatment F09Z
Heart Assist System
  Implantable
    Insertion of device in, Heart 02HA
    Removal of device from, Heart 02PA
    Revision of device in, Heart 02WA
  Short-term External
    Insertion of device in, Heart 02HA
    Removal of device from, Heart 02PA
    Revision of device in, Heart 02WA
HeartMate 3™ LVAS *use* Implantable Heart Assist System in Heart and Great Vessels
HeartMate II® Left Ventricular Assist Device (LVAD) *use* Implantable Heart Assist System in Heart and Great Vessels
HeartMate XVE® Left Ventricular Assist Device (LVAD) *use* Implantable Heart Assist System in Heart and Great Vessels
HeartMate® implantable heart assist system *see* Insertion of device in, Heart 02HA
Helix
  use Ear, External, Bilateral
  use Ear, External, Left
  use Ear, External, Right
Hematopoietic cell transplant (HCT) *see* Transfusion, Circulatory 302
Hemicolectomy *see* Resection, Gastrointestinal System 0DT
Hemicystectomy *see* Excision, Urinary System 0TB
Hemigastrectomy *see* Excision, Gastrointestinal System 0DB

▽ **Subterms under main terms may continue to next column or page**

Hemiglossectomy *see* Excision, Mouth and Throat 0CB
Hemilaminectomy
　see Excision, Lower Bones 0QB
　see Excision, Upper Bones 0PB
Hemilaminotomy
　see Drainage, Lower Bones 0Q9
　see Drainage, Upper Bones 0P9
　see Excision, Lower Bones 0QB
　see Excision, Upper Bones 0PB
　see Release, Central Nervous System and Cranial
　　Nerves 00N
　see Release, Lower Bones 0QN
　see Release, Peripheral Nervous System 01N
　see Release, Upper Bones 0PN
Hemilaryngectomy *see* Excision, Larynx 0CBS
Hemimandibulectomy *see* Excision, Head and Facial
　Bones 0NB
Hemimaxillectomy *see* Excision, Head and Facial Bones
　0NB
Hemipylorectomy *see* Excision, Gastrointestinal System 0DB
Hemispherectomy
　see Excision, Central Nervous System and Cranial
　　Nerves 00B
　see Resection, Central Nervous System and Cranial
　　Nerves 00T
Hemithyroidectomy
　see Excision, Endocrine System 0GB
　see Resection, Endocrine System 0GT
Hemodialysis *see* Performance, Urinary 5A1D
Hemolung® Respiratory Assist System (RAS)
　5A0920Z
Hemospray® Endoscopic Hemostat *use* Mineral-
　based Topical Hemostatic Agent
Hepatectomy
　see Excision, Hepatobiliary System and Pancreas
　　0FB
　see Resection, Hepatobiliary System and Pancreas
　　0FT
Hepatic artery proper *use* Hepatic Artery
Hepatic flexure *use* Transverse Colon
Hepatic lymph node *use* Lymphatic, Aortic
Hepatic plexus *use* Abdominal Sympathetic Nerve
Hepatic portal vein *use* Portal Vein
Hepaticoduodenostomy
　see Bypass, Hepatobiliary System and Pancreas
　　0F1
　see Drainage, Hepatobiliary System and Pancreas
　　0F9
Hepaticotomy *see* Drainage, Hepatobiliary System and
　Pancreas 0F9
Hepatocholedochostomy *see* Drainage, Duct, Com-
　mon Bile 0F99
Hepatogastric ligament *use* Omentum
Hepatopancreatic ampulla *use* Ampulla of Vater
Hepatopexy
　see Repair, Hepatobiliary System and Pancreas 0FQ
　see Reposition, Hepatobiliary System and Pancreas
　　0FS
Hepatorrhaphy *see* Repair, Hepatobiliary System and
　Pancreas 0FQ
Hepatotomy *see* Drainage, Hepatobiliary System and
　Pancreas 0F9
Herculink (RX) Elite Renal Stent System *use* Intralu-
　minal Device
Herniorrhaphy
　see Repair, Anatomical Regions, General 0WQ
　see Repair, Anatomical Regions, Lower Extremities
　　0YQ
　With synthetic substitute
　　see Supplement, Anatomical Regions, Gener-
　　　al 0WU
　　see Supplement, Anatomical Regions, Lower
　　　Extremities 0YU
HIG (hyperimmune globulin), for COVID-19 treat-
　ment *use* Hyperimmune Globulin
High-Dose Intravenous Immune Globulin, for
　COVID-19 treatment XW1
High-dose intravenous immunoglobulin (hdIVIG),
　for COVID-19 treatment *use* High-Dose Intra-
　venous Immune Globulin
Hip (joint) liner *use* Liner in Lower Joints
HIPEC (hyperthermic intraperitoneal chemother-
　apy) 3E0M30Y
hIVIG (hyperimmune intravenous immunoglobu-
　lin), for COVID-19 treatment *use* Hyperimmune
　Globulin

Holter Monitoring 4A12X45
Holter valve ventricular shunt *use* Synthetic Substi-
　tute
Human angiotensin II, synthetic *use* Synthetic Hu-
　man Angiotensin II
Humeroradial joint
　use Elbow Joint, Left
　use Elbow Joint, Right
Humeroulnar joint
　use Elbow Joint, Left
　use Elbow Joint, Right
Humerus, distal
　use Humeral Shaft, Left
　use Humeral Shaft, Right
Hydrocelectomy *see* Excision, Male Reproductive Sys-
　tem 0VB
Hydrotherapy
　Assisted exercise in pool *see* Motor Treatment,
　　Rehabilitation F07
　Whirlpool *see* Activities of Daily Living Treatment,
　　Rehabilitation F08
Hymenectomy
　see Excision, Hymen 0UBK
　see Resection, Hymen 0UTK
Hymenoplasty
　see Repair, Hymen 0UQK
　see Supplement, Hymen 0UUK
Hymenorrhaphy *see* Repair, Hymen 0UQK
Hymenotomy
　see Division, Hymen 0U8K
　see Drainage, Hymen 0U9K
Hyoglossus muscle *use* Tongue, Palate, Pharynx
　Muscle
Hyoid artery
　use Thyroid Artery, Left
　use Thyroid Artery, Right
Hyperalimentation *see* Introduction of substance in
　or on
Hyperbaric oxygenation
　Decompression sickness treatment *see* Decompres-
　　sion, Circulatory 6A15
　Wound treatment *see* Assistance, Circulatory 5A05
Hyperimmune globulin *use* Globulin
Hyperimmune Globulin, for COVID-19 treatment
　XW1
Hyperimmune intravenous immunoglobulin
　(hIVIG), for COVID-19 treatment *use* Hyperim-
　mune Globulin
Hyperthermia
　Radiation Therapy
　　Abdomen DWY38ZZ
　　Adrenal Gland DGY28ZZ
　　Bile Ducts DFY28ZZ
　　Bladder DTY28ZZ
　　Bone Marrow D7Y08ZZ
　　Bone, Other DPYC8ZZ
　　Brain D0Y08ZZ
　　Brain Stem D0Y18ZZ
　　Breast
　　　Left DMY08ZZ
　　　Right DMY18ZZ
　　Bronchus DBY18ZZ
　　Cervix DUY18ZZ
　　Chest DWY28ZZ
　　Chest Wall DBY78ZZ
　　Colon DDY58ZZ
　　Diaphragm DBY88ZZ
　　Duodenum DDY28ZZ
　　Ear D9Y08ZZ
　　Esophagus DDY08ZZ
　　Eye D8Y08ZZ
　　Femur DPY98ZZ
　　Fibula DPYB8ZZ
　　Gallbladder DFY18ZZ
　　Gland
　　　Adrenal DGY28ZZ
　　　Parathyroid DGY48ZZ
　　　Pituitary DGY08ZZ
　　　Thyroid DGY58ZZ
　　Glands, Salivary D9Y68ZZ
　　Head and Neck DWY18ZZ
　　Hemibody DWY48ZZ
　　Humerus DPY68ZZ
　　Hypopharynx D9Y38ZZ
　　Ileum DDY48ZZ
　　Jejunum DDY38ZZ
　　Kidney DTY08ZZ
　　Larynx D9YB8ZZ

Hyperthermia — *continued*
　Radiation Therapy — *continued*
　　Liver DFY08ZZ
　　Lung DBY28ZZ
　　Lymphatics
　　　Abdomen D7Y68ZZ
　　　Axillary D7Y48ZZ
　　　Inguinal D7Y88ZZ
　　　Neck D7Y38ZZ
　　　Pelvis D7Y78ZZ
　　　Thorax D7Y58ZZ
　　Mandible DPY38ZZ
　　Maxilla DPY28ZZ
　　Mediastinum DBY68ZZ
　　Mouth D9Y48ZZ
　　Nasopharynx D9YD8ZZ
　　Neck and Head DWY18ZZ
　　Nerve, Peripheral D0Y78ZZ
　　Nose D9Y18ZZ
　　Oropharynx D9YF8ZZ
　　Ovary DUY08ZZ
　　Palate
　　　Hard D9Y88ZZ
　　　Soft D9Y98ZZ
　　Pancreas DFY38ZZ
　　Parathyroid Gland DGY48ZZ
　　Pelvic Bones DPY88ZZ
　　Pelvic Region DWY68ZZ
　　Pineal Body DGY18ZZ
　　Pituitary Gland DGY08ZZ
　　Pleura DBY58ZZ
　　Prostate DVY08ZZ
　　Radius DPY78ZZ
　　Rectum DDY78ZZ
　　Rib DPY58ZZ
　　Sinuses D9Y78ZZ
　　Skin
　　　Abdomen DHY88ZZ
　　　Arm DHY48ZZ
　　　Back DHY78ZZ
　　　Buttock DHY98ZZ
　　　Chest DHY68ZZ
　　　Face DHY28ZZ
　　　Leg DHYB8ZZ
　　　Neck DHY38ZZ
　　Skull DPY08ZZ
　　Spinal Cord D0Y68ZZ
　　Spleen D7Y28ZZ
　　Sternum DPY48ZZ
　　Stomach DDY18ZZ
　　Testis DVY18ZZ
　　Thymus D7Y18ZZ
　　Thyroid Gland DGY58ZZ
　　Tibia DPYB8ZZ
　　Tongue D9Y58ZZ
　　Trachea DBY08ZZ
　　Ulna DPY78ZZ
　　Ureter DTY18ZZ
　　Urethra DTY38ZZ
　　Uterus DUY28ZZ
　　Whole Body DWY58ZZ
　Whole Body 6A3Z
Hyperthermic Intraperitoneal Chemotherapy
　(HIPEC) 3E0M30Y
Hypnosis GZFZZZZ
Hypogastric artery
　use Internal Iliac Artery, Left
　use Internal Iliac Artery, Right
Hypopharynx *use* Pharynx
Hypophysectomy
　see Excision, Gland, Pituitary 0GB0
　see Resection, Gland, Pituitary 0GT0
Hypophysis *use* Pituitary Gland
Hypothalamotomy *see* Destruction, Thalamus 0059
Hypothenar muscle
　use Hand Muscle, Left
　use Hand Muscle, Right
Hypothermia, Whole Body 6A4Z
Hysterectomy
　Supracervical *see* Resection, Uterus 0UT9
　Total *see* Resection, Uterus 0UT9
Hysterolysis *see* Release, Uterus 0UN9
Hysteropexy
　see Repair, Uterus 0UQ9
　see Reposition, Uterus 0US9
Hysteroplasty *see* Repair, Uterus 0UQ9
Hysterorrhaphy *see* Repair, Uterus 0UQ9
Hysteroscopy 0UJD8ZZ

Hysterotomy *see* Drainage, Uterus ØU99
Hysterotrachelectomy
  see Resection, Cervix ØUTC
  see Resection, Uterus ØUT9
Hysterotracheloplasty *see* Repair, Uterus ØUQ9
Hysterotrachelorrhaphy *see* Repair, Uterus ØUQ9

I

IABP (Intra-aortic balloon pump) *see* Assistance, Cardiac 5AØ2
IAEMT (Intraoperative anesthetic effect monitoring and titration) *see* Monitoring, Central Nervous 4A1Ø
IASD® (InterAtrial Shunt Device), Corvia *use* Synthetic Substitute
Idarucizumab, Pradaxa® (dabigatran) reversal agent *use* Other Therapeutic Substance
Idecabtagene Vicleucel *use* Idecabtagene Vicleucel Immunotherapy
Idecabtagene Vicleucel Immunotherapy XWØ
Ide-cel *use* Idecabtagene Vicleucel Immunotherapy
IGIV-C, for COVID-19 treatment *use* Hyperimmune Globulin
IHD (Intermittent hemodialysis) 5A1D7ØZ
Ileal artery *use* Superior Mesenteric Artery
Ileectomy
  see Excision, Ileum ØDBB
  see Resection, Ileum ØDTB
Ileocolic artery *use* Superior Mesenteric Artery
Ileocolic vein *use* Colic Vein
Ileopexy
  see Repair, Ileum ØDQB
  see Reposition, Ileum ØDSB
Ileorrhaphy *see* Repair, Ileum ØDQB
Ileoscopy ØDJD8ZZ
Ileostomy
  see Bypass, Ileum ØD1B
  see Drainage, Ileum ØD9B
Ileotomy *see* Drainage, Ileum ØD9B
Ileoureterostomy *see* Bypass, Urinary System ØT1
Iliac crest
  use Pelvic Bone, Left
  use Pelvic Bone, Right
Iliac fascia
  use Subcutaneous Tissue and Fascia, Left Upper Leg
  use Subcutaneous Tissue and Fascia, Right Upper Leg
Iliac lymph node *use* Lymphatic, Pelvis
Iliacus muscle
  use Hip Muscle, Left
  use Hip Muscle, Right
Iliofemoral ligament
  use Hip Bursa and Ligament, Left
  use Hip Bursa and Ligament, Right
Iliohypogastric nerve *use* Lumbar Plexus
Ilioinguinal nerve *use* Lumbar Plexus
Iliolumbar artery
  use Internal Iliac Artery, Left
  use Internal Iliac Artery, Right
Iliolumbar ligament *use* Lower Spine Bursa and Ligament
Iliotibial tract (band)
  use Subcutaneous Tissue and Fascia, Left Upper Leg
  use Subcutaneous Tissue and Fascia, Right Upper Leg
Ilium
  use Pelvic Bone, Left
  use Pelvic Bone, Right
Ilizarov external fixator
  use External Fixation Device, Ring in ØPH
  use External Fixation Device, Ring in ØPS
  use External Fixation Device, Ring in ØQH
  use External Fixation Device, Ring in ØQS
Ilizarov-Vecklich device
  use External Fixation Device, Limb Lengthening in ØPH
  use External Fixation Device, Limb Lengthening in ØQH
Imaging, diagnostic
  see Computerized Tomography (CT Scan)
  see Fluoroscopy
  see Magnetic Resonance Imaging (MRI)
  see Plain Radiography

Imaging, diagnostic — *continued*
  see Ultrasonography
Imdevimab (REGN1Ø987) and Casirivimab (REGN1Ø933) *use* REGN-COV2 Monoclonal Antibody
IMFINZI® *use* Durvalumab Antineoplastic
Imipenem-cilastatin-relebactam Anti-infective XWØ
IMI/REL *use* Imipenem-cilastatin-relebactam Anti-infective
Immobilization
  Abdominal Wall 2W33X
  Arm
    Lower
      Left 2W3DX
      Right 2W3CX
    Upper
      Left 2W3BX
      Right 2W3AX
  Back 2W35X
  Chest Wall 2W34X
  Extremity
    Lower
      Left 2W3MX
      Right 2W3LX
    Upper
      Left 2W39X
      Right 2W38X
  Face 2W31X
  Finger
    Left 2W3KX
    Right 2W3JX
  Foot
    Left 2W3TX
    Right 2W3SX
  Hand
    Left 2W3FX
    Right 2W3EX
  Head 2W30X
  Inguinal Region
    Left 2W37X
    Right 2W36X
  Leg
    Lower
      Left 2W3RX
      Right 2W3QX
    Upper
      Left 2W3PX
      Right 2W3NX
  Neck 2W32X
  Thumb
    Left 2W3HX
    Right 2W3GX
  Toe
    Left 2W3VX
    Right 2W3UX
Immunization *see* Introduction of Serum, Toxoid, and Vaccine
Immunoglobulin *use* Globulin
Immunotherapy *see* Introduction of Immunotherapeutic Substance
Immunotherapy, antineoplastic
  Interferon *see* Introduction of Low-dose Interleukin-2
  Interleukin-2, high-dose *see* Introduction of High-dose Interleukin-2
  Interleukin-2, low-dose *see* Introduction of Low-dose Interleukin-2
  Monoclonal antibody *see* Introduction of Monoclonal Antibody
  Proleukin, high-dose *see* Introduction of High-dose Interleukin-2
  Proleukin, low-dose *see* Introduction of Low-dose Interleukin-2
Impella® heart pump *use* Short-term External Heart Assist System in Heart and Great Vessels
Impeller Pump
  Continuous, Output 5AØ221D
  Intermittent, Output 5AØ211D
Implantable cardioverter-defibrillator (ICD) *use* Defibrillator Generator in ØJH
Implantable drug infusion pump (anti-spasmodic) (chemotherapy) (pain) *use* Infusion Device, Pump in Subcutaneous Tissue and Fascia
Implantable glucose monitoring device *use* Monitoring Device
Implantable hemodynamic monitor (IHM) *use* Monitoring Device, Hemodynamic in ØJH

Implantable hemodynamic monitoring system (IHMS) *use* Monitoring Device, Hemodynamic in ØJH
Implantable Miniature Telescope™ (IMT) *use* Synthetic Substitute, Intraocular Telescope in Ø8R
Implantation
  see Insertion
  see Replacement
Implanted (venous)(access) port *use* Vascular Access Device, Totally Implantable in Subcutaneous Tissue and Fascia
IMV (intermittent mandatory ventilation) *see* Assistance, Respiratory 5AØ9
In Vitro Fertilization 8EØZXY1
Incision, abscess *see* Drainage
Incudectomy
  see Excision, Ear, Nose, Sinus Ø9B
  see Resection, Ear, Nose, Sinus Ø9T
Incudopexy
  see Repair, Ear, Nose, Sinus Ø9Q
  see Reposition, Ear, Nose, Sinus Ø9S
Incus
  use Auditory Ossicle, Left
  use Auditory Ossicle, Right
Induction of labor
  Artificial rupture of membranes *see* Drainage, Pregnancy 1Ø9
  Oxytocin *see* Introduction of Hormone
InDura, intrathecal catheter (1P) (spinal) *use* Infusion Device
Inferior cardiac nerve *use* Thoracic Sympathetic Nerve
Inferior cerebellar vein *use* Intracranial Vein
Inferior cerebral vein *use* Intracranial Vein
Inferior epigastric artery
  use External Iliac Artery, Left
  use External Iliac Artery, Right
Inferior epigastric lymph node *use* Lymphatic, Pelvis
Inferior genicular artery
  use Popliteal Artery, Left
  use Popliteal Artery, Right
Inferior gluteal artery
  use Internal Iliac Artery, Left
  use Internal Iliac Artery, Right
Inferior gluteal nerve *use* Sacral Plexus
Inferior hypogastric plexus *use* Abdominal Sympathetic Nerve
Inferior labial artery *use* Face Artery
Inferior longitudinal muscle *use* Tongue, Palate, Pharynx Muscle
Inferior mesenteric ganglion *use* Abdominal Sympathetic Nerve
Inferior mesenteric lymph node *use* Lymphatic, Mesenteric
Inferior mesenteric plexus *use* Abdominal Sympathetic Nerve
Inferior oblique muscle
  use Extraocular Muscle, Left
  use Extraocular Muscle, Right
Inferior pancreaticoduodenal artery *use* Superior Mesenteric Artery
Inferior phrenic artery *use* Abdominal Aorta
Inferior rectus muscle
  use Extraocular Muscle, Left
  use Extraocular Muscle, Right
Inferior suprarenal artery
  use Renal Artery, Left
  use Renal Artery, Right
Inferior tarsal plate
  use Lower Eyelid, Left
  use Lower Eyelid, Right
Inferior thyroid vein
  use Innominate Vein, Left
  use Innominate Vein, Right
Inferior tibiofibular joint
  use Ankle Joint, Left
  use Ankle Joint, Right
Inferior turbinate *use* Nasal Turbinate
Inferior ulnar collateral artery
  use Brachial Artery, Left
  use Brachial Artery, Right
Inferior vesical artery
  use Internal Iliac Artery, Left
  use Internal Iliac Artery, Right
Infraauricular lymph node *use* Lymphatic, Head
Infraclavicular (deltopectoral) lymph node
  use Lymphatic, Left Upper Extremity

Infraclavicular (deltopectoral) lymph node —
continued
  use Lymphatic, Right Upper Extremity
Infrahyoid muscle
  use Neck Muscle, Left
  use Neck Muscle, Right
Infraparotid lymph node *use* Lymphatic, Head
Infraspinatus fascia
  use Subcutaneous Tissue and Fascia, Left Upper
    Arm
  use Subcutaneous Tissue and Fascia, Right Upper
    Arm
Infraspinatus muscle
  use Shoulder Muscle, Left
  use Shoulder Muscle, Right
Infundibulopelvic ligament *use* Uterine Supporting
    Structure
Infusion *see* Introduction of substance in or on
Infusion Device, Pump
  Insertion of device in
    Abdomen ØJH8
    Back ØJH7
    Chest ØJH6
    Lower Arm
      Left ØJHH
      Right ØJHG
    Lower Leg
      Left ØJHP
      Right ØJHN
    Trunk ØJHT
    Upper Arm
      Left ØJHF
      Right ØJHD
    Upper Leg
      Left ØJHM
      Right ØJHL
  Removal of device from
    Lower Extremity ØJPW
    Trunk ØJPT
    Upper Extremity ØJPV
  Revision of device in
    Lower Extremity ØJWW
    Trunk ØJWT
    Upper Extremity ØJWV
Infusion, glucarpidase
  Central Vein 3EØ43GQ
  Peripheral Vein 3EØ33GQ
Inguinal canal
  use Inguinal Region, Bilateral
  use Inguinal Region, Left
  use Inguinal Region, Right
Inguinal triangle
  use Inguinal Region, Bilateral
  use Inguinal Region, Left
  use Inguinal Region, Right
Injection *see* Introduction of substance in or on
Injection, Concentrated Bone Marrow Aspirate
    (CBMA), intramuscular XKØ23Ø3
Injection reservoir, port *use* Vascular Access Device,
    Totally Implantable in Subcutaneous Tissue and
    Fascia
Injection reservoir, pump *use* Infusion Device, Pump
    in Subcutaneous Tissue and Fascia
Insemination, artificial 3EØP7LZ
Insertion
  Antimicrobial envelope *see* Introduction of Anti-
    infective
  Aqueous drainage shunt
    see Bypass, Eye Ø81
    see Drainage, Eye Ø89
  Products of Conception 1ØHØ
  Spinal Stabilization Device
    see Insertion of device in, Lower Joints ØSH
    see Insertion of device in, Upper Joints ØRH
Insertion of device in
  Abdominal Wall ØWHF
  Acetabulum
    Left ØQH5
    Right ØQH4
  Anal Sphincter ØDHR
  Ankle Region
    Left ØYHL
    Right ØYHK
  Anus ØDHQ
  Aorta
    Abdominal Ø4HØ
    Thoracic
      Ascending/Arch Ø2HX

Insertion of device in — *continued*
  Aorta — *continued*
    Thoracic — *continued*
      Descending Ø2HW
  Arm
    Lower
      Left ØXHF
      Right ØXHD
    Upper
      Left ØXH9
      Right ØXH8
  Artery
    Anterior Tibial
      Left Ø4HQ
      Right Ø4HP
    Axillary
      Left Ø3H6
      Right Ø3H5
    Brachial
      Left Ø3H8
      Right Ø3H7
    Celiac Ø4H1
    Colic
      Left Ø4H7
      Middle Ø4H8
      Right Ø4H6
    Common Carotid
      Left Ø3HJ
      Right Ø3HH
    Common Iliac
      Left Ø4HD
      Right Ø4HC
    Coronary
      Four or More Arteries Ø2H3
      One Artery Ø2HØ
      Three Arteries Ø2H2
      Two Arteries Ø2H1
    External Carotid
      Left Ø3HN
      Right Ø3HM
    External Iliac
      Left Ø4HJ
      Right Ø4HH
    Face Ø3HR
    Femoral
      Left Ø4HL
      Right Ø4HK
    Foot
      Left Ø4HW
      Right Ø4HV
    Gastric Ø4H2
    Hand
      Left Ø3HF
      Right Ø3HD
    Hepatic Ø4H3
    Inferior Mesenteric Ø4HB
    Innominate Ø3H2
    Internal Carotid
      Left Ø3HL
      Right Ø3HK
    Internal Iliac
      Left Ø4HF
      Right Ø4HE
    Internal Mammary
      Left Ø3H1
      Right Ø3HØ
    Intracranial Ø3HG
    Lower Ø4HY
    Peroneal
      Left Ø4HU
      Right Ø4HT
    Popliteal
      Left Ø4HN
      Right Ø4HM
    Posterior Tibial
      Left Ø4HS
      Right Ø4HR
    Pulmonary
      Left Ø2HR
      Right Ø2HQ
    Pulmonary Trunk Ø2HP
    Radial
      Left Ø3HC
      Right Ø3HB
    Renal
      Left Ø4HA
      Right Ø4H9
    Splenic Ø4H4

Insertion of device in — *continued*
  Artery — *continued*
    Subclavian
      Left Ø3H4
      Right Ø3H3
    Superior Mesenteric Ø4H5
    Temporal
      Left Ø3HT
      Right Ø3HS
    Thyroid
      Left Ø3HV
      Right Ø3HU
    Ulnar
      Left Ø3HA
      Right Ø3H9
    Upper Ø3HY
    Vertebral
      Left Ø3HQ
      Right Ø3HP
  Atrium
    Left Ø2H7
    Right Ø2H6
  Axilla
    Left ØXH5
    Right ØXH4
  Back
    Lower ØWHL
    Upper ØWHK
  Bladder ØTHB
  Bladder Neck ØTHC
  Bone
    Ethmoid
      Left ØNHG
      Right ØNHF
    Facial ØNHW
    Frontal ØNH1
    Hyoid ØNHX
    Lacrimal
      Left ØNHJ
      Right ØNHH
    Lower ØQHY
    Nasal ØNHB
    Occipital ØNH7
    Palatine
      Left ØNHL
      Right ØNHK
    Parietal
      Left ØNH4
      Right ØNH3
    Pelvic
      Left ØQH3
      Right ØQH2
    Sphenoid ØNHC
    Temporal
      Left ØNH6
      Right ØNH5
    Upper ØPHY
    Zygomatic
      Left ØNHN
      Right ØNHM
  Bone Marrow Ø7HT
  Brain ØØHØ
  Breast
    Bilateral ØHHV
    Left ØHHU
    Right ØHHT
  Bronchus
    Lingula ØBH9
    Lower Lobe
      Left ØBHB
      Right ØBH6
    Main
      Left ØBH7
      Right ØBH3
    Middle Lobe, Right ØBH5
    Upper Lobe
      Left ØBH8
      Right ØBH4
  Bursa and Ligament
    Lower ØMHY
    Upper ØMHX
  Buttock
    Left ØYH1
    Right ØYHØ
  Carpal
    Left ØPHN
    Right ØPHM
  Cavity, Cranial ØWH1
  Cerebral Ventricle ØØH6

⛛ **Subterms under main terms may continue to next column or page**   73

Insertion of device in — *continued*

Cervix ØUHC
Chest Wall ØWH8
Cisterna Chyli Ø7HL
Clavicle
    Left ØPHB
    Right ØPH9
Coccyx ØQHS
Cul-de-sac ØUHF
Diaphragm ØBHT
Disc
    Cervical Vertebral ØRH3
    Cervicothoracic Vertebral ØRH5
    Lumbar Vertebral ØSH2
    Lumbosacral ØSH4
    Thoracic Vertebral ØRH9
    Thoracolumbar Vertebral ØRHB
Duct
    Hepatobiliary ØFHB
    Pancreatic ØFHD
Duodenum ØDH9
Ear
    Inner
        Left Ø9HE
        Right Ø9HD
    Left Ø9HJ
    Right Ø9HH
Elbow Region
    Left ØXHC
    Right ØXHB
Epididymis and Spermatic Cord ØVHM
Esophagus ØDH5
Extremity
    Lower
        Left ØYHB
        Right ØYH9
    Upper
        Left ØXH7
        Right ØXH6
Eye
    Left Ø8H1
    Right Ø8HØ
Face ØWH2
Fallopian Tube ØUH8
Femoral Region
    Left ØYH8
    Right ØYH7
Femoral Shaft
    Left ØQH9
    Right ØQH8
Femur
    Lower
        Left ØQHC
        Right ØQHB
    Upper
        Left ØQH7
        Right ØQH6
Fibula
    Left ØQHK
    Right ØQHJ
Foot
    Left ØYHN
    Right ØYHM
Gallbladder ØFH4
Gastrointestinal Tract ØWHP
Genitourinary Tract ØWHR
Gland
    Endocrine ØGHS
    Salivary ØCHA
Glenoid Cavity
    Left ØPH8
    Right ØPH7
Hand
    Left ØXHK
    Right ØXHJ
Head ØWHØ
Heart Ø2HA
Humeral Head
    Left ØPHD
    Right ØPHC
Humeral Shaft
    Left ØPHG
    Right ØPHF
Ileum ØDHB
Inguinal Region
    Left ØYH6
    Right ØYH5
Intestinal Tract
    Lower ØDHD

Insertion of device in — *continued*

Intestinal Tract — *continued*
    Upper ØDHØ
Intestine
    Large ØDHE
    Small ØDH8
Jaw
    Lower ØWH5
    Upper ØWH4
Jejunum ØDHA
Joint
    Acromioclavicular
        Left ØRHH
        Right ØRHG
    Ankle
        Left ØSHG
        Right ØSHF
    Carpal
        Left ØRHR
        Right ØRHQ
    Carpometacarpal
        Left ØRHT
        Right ØRHS
    Cervical Vertebral ØRH1
    Cervicothoracic Vertebral ØRH4
    Coccygeal ØSH6
    Elbow
        Left ØRHM
        Right ØRHL
    Finger Phalangeal
        Left ØRHX
        Right ØRHW
    Hip
        Left ØSHB
        Right ØSH9
    Knee
        Left ØSHD
        Right ØSHC
    Lumbar Vertebral ØSHØ
    Lumbosacral ØSH3
    Metacarpophalangeal
        Left ØRHV
        Right ØRHU
    Metatarsal-Phalangeal
        Left ØSHN
        Right ØSHM
    Occipital-cervical ØRHØ
    Sacrococcygeal ØSH5
    Sacroiliac
        Left ØSH8
        Right ØSH7
    Shoulder
        Left ØRHK
        Right ØRHJ
    Sternoclavicular
        Left ØRHF
        Right ØRHE
    Tarsal
        Left ØSHJ
        Right ØSHH
    Tarsometatarsal
        Left ØSHL
        Right ØSHK
    Temporomandibular
        Left ØRHD
        Right ØRHC
    Thoracic Vertebral ØRH6
    Thoracolumbar Vertebral ØRHA
    Toe Phalangeal
        Left ØSHQ
        Right ØSHP
    Wrist
        Left ØRHP
        Right ØRHN
Kidney ØTH5
Knee Region
    Left ØYHG
    Right ØYHF
Larynx ØCHS
Leg
    Lower
        Left ØYHJ
        Right ØYHH
    Upper
        Left ØYHD
        Right ØYHC
Liver ØFHØ
    Left Lobe ØFH2
    Right Lobe ØFH1

Insertion of device in — *continued*

Lung
    Left ØBHL
    Right ØBHK
Lymphatic Ø7HN
    Thoracic Duct Ø7HK
Mandible
    Left ØNHV
    Right ØNHT
Maxilla ØNHR
Mediastinum ØWHC
Metacarpal
    Left ØPHQ
    Right ØPHP
Metatarsal
    Left ØQHP
    Right ØQHN
Mouth and Throat ØCHY
Muscle
    Lower ØKHY
    Upper ØKHX
Nasal Mucosa and Soft Tissue Ø9HK
Nasopharynx Ø9HN
Neck ØWH6
Nerve
    Cranial ØØHE
    Peripheral Ø1HY
Nipple
    Left ØHHX
    Right ØHHW
Oral Cavity and Throat ØWH3
Orbit
    Left ØNHQ
    Right ØNHP
Ovary ØUH3
Pancreas ØFHG
Patella
    Left ØQHF
    Right ØQHD
Pelvic Cavity ØWHJ
Penis ØVHS
Pericardial Cavity ØWHD
Pericardium Ø2HN
Perineum
    Female ØWHN
    Male ØWHM
Peritoneal Cavity ØWHG
Phalanx
    Finger
        Left ØPHV
        Right ØPHT
    Thumb
        Left ØPHS
        Right ØPHR
    Toe
        Left ØQHR
        Right ØQHQ
Pleura ØBHQ
Pleural Cavity
    Left ØWHB
    Right ØWH9
Prostate ØVHØ
Prostate and Seminal Vesicles ØVH4
Radius
    Left ØPHJ
    Right ØPHH
Rectum ØDHP
Respiratory Tract ØWHQ
Retroperitoneum ØWHH
Ribs
    1 to 2 ØPH1
    3 or More ØPH2
Sacrum ØQH1
Scapula
    Left ØPH6
    Right ØPH5
Scrotum and Tunica Vaginalis ØVH8
Shoulder Region
    Left ØXH3
    Right ØXH2
Sinus Ø9HY
Skin ØHHPXYZ
Skull ØNHØ
Spinal Canal ØØHU
Spinal Cord ØØHV
Spleen Ø7HP
Sternum ØPHØ
Stomach ØDH6

▼ **Subterms under main terms may continue to next column or page**

Insertion of device in — *continued*
  Subcutaneous Tissue and Fascia
    Abdomen ØJH8
    Back ØJH7
    Buttock ØJH9
    Chest ØJH6
    Face ØJH1
    Foot
      Left ØJHR
      Right ØJHQ
    Hand
      Left ØJHK
      Right ØJHJ
    Head and Neck ØJHS
    Lower Arm
      Left ØJHH
      Right ØJHG
    Lower Extremity ØJHW
    Lower Leg
      Left ØJHP
      Right ØJHN
    Neck
      Left ØJH5
      Right ØJH4
    Pelvic Region ØJHC
    Perineum ØJHB
    Scalp ØJHØ
    Trunk ØJHT
    Upper Arm
      Left ØJHF
      Right ØJHD
    Upper Extremity ØJHV
    Upper Leg
      Left ØJHM
      Right ØJHL
  Tarsal
    Left ØQHM
    Right ØQHL
  Tendon
    Lower ØLHY
    Upper ØLHX
  Testis ØVHD
  Thymus Ø7HM
  Tibia
    Left ØQHH
    Right ØQHG
  Tongue ØCH7
  Trachea ØBH1
  Tracheobronchial Tree ØBHØ
  Ulna
    Left ØPHL
    Right ØPHK
  Ureter ØTH9
  Urethra ØTHD
  Uterus ØUH9
  Uterus and Cervix ØUHD
  Vagina ØUHG
  Vagina and Cul-de-sac ØUHH
  Vas Deferens ØVHR
  Vein
    Axillary
      Left Ø5H8
      Right Ø5H7
    Azygos Ø5HØ
    Basilic
      Left Ø5HC
      Right Ø5HB
    Brachial
      Left Ø5HA
      Right Ø5H9
    Cephalic
      Left Ø5HF
      Right Ø5HD
    Colic Ø6H7
    Common Iliac
      Left Ø6HD
      Right Ø6HC
    Coronary Ø2H4
    Esophageal Ø6H3
    External Iliac
      Left Ø6HG
      Right Ø6HF
    External Jugular
      Left Ø5HQ
      Right Ø5HP
    Face
      Left Ø5HV
      Right Ø5HT

Insertion of device in — *continued*
  Vein — *continued*
    Femoral
      Left Ø6HN
      Right Ø6HM
    Foot
      Left Ø6HV
      Right Ø6HT
    Gastric Ø6H2
    Hand
      Left Ø5HH
      Right Ø5HG
    Hemiazygos Ø5H1
    Hepatic Ø6H4
    Hypogastric
      Left Ø6HJ
      Right Ø6HH
    Inferior Mesenteric Ø6H6
    Innominate
      Left Ø5H4
      Right Ø5H3
    Internal Jugular
      Left Ø5HN
      Right Ø5HM
    Intracranial Ø5HL
    Lower Ø6HY
    Portal Ø6H8
    Pulmonary
      Left Ø2HT
      Right Ø2HS
    Renal
      Left Ø6HB
      Right Ø6H9
    Saphenous
      Left Ø6HQ
      Right Ø6HP
    Splenic Ø6H1
    Subclavian
      Left Ø5H6
      Right Ø5H5
    Superior Mesenteric Ø6H5
    Upper Ø5HY
    Vertebral
      Left Ø5HS
      Right Ø5HR
  Vena Cava
    Inferior Ø6HØ
    Superior Ø2HV
  Ventricle
    Left Ø2HL
    Right Ø2HK
  Vertebra
    Cervical ØPH3
    Lumbar ØQHØ
    Thoracic ØPH4
  Wrist Region
    Left ØXHH
    Right ØXHG

Inspection
  Abdominal Wall ØWJF
  Ankle Region
    Left ØYJL
    Right ØYJK
  Arm
    Lower
      Left ØXJF
      Right ØXJD
    Upper
      Left ØXJ9
      Right ØXJ8
  Artery
    Lower Ø4JY
    Upper Ø3JY
  Axilla
    Left ØXJ5
    Right ØXJ4
  Back
    Lower ØWJL
    Upper ØWJK
  Bladder ØTJB
  Bone
    Facial ØNJW
    Lower ØQJY
    Nasal ØNJB
    Upper ØPJY
  Bone Marrow Ø7JT
  Brain ØØJØ
  Breast
    Left ØHJU

Inspection — *continued*
  Breast — *continued*
    Right ØHJT
  Bursa and Ligament
    Lower ØMJY
    Upper ØMJX
  Buttock
    Left ØYJ1
    Right ØYJØ
  Cavity, Cranial ØWJ1
  Chest Wall ØWJ8
  Cisterna Chyli Ø7JL
  Diaphragm ØBJT
  Disc
    Cervical Vertebral ØRJ3
    Cervicothoracic Vertebral ØRJ5
    Lumbar Vertebral ØSJ2
    Lumbosacral ØSJ4
    Thoracic Vertebral ØRJ9
    Thoracolumbar Vertebral ØRJB
  Duct
    Hepatobiliary ØFJB
    Pancreatic ØFJD
  Ear
    Inner
      Left Ø9JE
      Right Ø9JD
    Left Ø9JJ
    Right Ø9JH
  Elbow Region
    Left ØXJC
    Right ØXJB
  Epididymis and Spermatic Cord ØVJM
  Extremity
    Lower
      Left ØYJB
      Right ØYJ9
    Upper
      Left ØXJ7
      Right ØXJ6
  Eye
    Left Ø8J1XZZ
    Right Ø8JØXZZ
  Face ØWJ2
  Fallopian Tube ØUJ8
  Femoral Region
    Bilateral ØYJE
    Left ØYJ8
    Right ØYJ7
  Finger Nail ØHJQXZZ
  Foot
    Left ØYJN
    Right ØYJM
  Gallbladder ØFJ4
  Gastrointestinal Tract ØWJP
  Genitourinary Tract ØWJR
  Gland
    Adrenal ØGJ5
    Endocrine ØGJS
    Pituitary ØGJØ
    Salivary ØCJA
  Great Vessel Ø2JY
  Hand
    Left ØXJK
    Right ØXJJ
  Head ØWJØ
  Heart Ø2JA
  Inguinal Region
    Bilateral ØYJA
    Left ØYJ6
    Right ØYJ5
  Intestinal Tract
    Lower ØDJD
    Upper ØDJØ
  Jaw
    Lower ØWJ5
    Upper ØWJ4
  Joint
    Acromioclavicular
      Left ØRJH
      Right ØRJG
    Ankle
      Left ØSJG
      Right ØSJF
    Carpal
      Left ØRJR
      Right ØRJQ
    Carpometacarpal
      Left ØRJT

Inspection — *continued*
 Joint — *continued*
  Carpometacarpal — *continued*
   Right ØRJS
  Cervical Vertebral ØRJ1
  Cervicothoracic Vertebral ØRJ4
  Coccygeal ØSJ6
  Elbow
   Left ØRJM
   Right ØRJL
  Finger Phalangeal
   Left ØRJX
   Right ØRJW
  Hip
   Left ØSJB
   Right ØSJ9
  Knee
   Left ØSJD
   Right ØSJC
  Lumbar Vertebral ØSJØ
  Lumbosacral ØSJ3
  Metacarpophalangeal
   Left ØRJV
   Right ØRJU
  Metatarsal-Phalangeal
   Left ØSJN
   Right ØSJM
  Occipital-cervical ØRJØ
  Sacrococcygeal ØSJ5
  Sacroiliac
   Left ØSJ8
   Right ØSJ7
  Shoulder
   Left ØRJK
   Right ØRJJ
  Sternoclavicular
   Left ØRJF
   Right ØRJE
  Tarsal
   Left ØSJJ
   Right ØSJH
  Tarsometatarsal
   Left ØSJL
   Right ØSJK
  Temporomandibular
   Left ØRJD
   Right ØRJC
  Thoracic Vertebral ØRJ6
  Thoracolumbar Vertebral ØRJA
  Toe Phalangeal
   Left ØSJQ
   Right ØSJP
  Wrist
   Left ØRJP
   Right ØRJN
 Kidney ØTJ5
 Knee Region
  Left ØYJG
  Right ØYJF
 Larynx ØCJS
 Leg
  Lower
   Left ØYJJ
   Right ØYJH
  Upper
   Left ØYJD
   Right ØYJC
 Lens
  Left Ø8JKXZZ
  Right Ø8JJXZZ
 Liver ØFJØ
 Lung
  Left ØBJL
  Right ØBJK
 Lymphatic Ø7JN
  Thoracic Duct Ø7JK
 Mediastinum ØWJC
 Mesentery ØDJV
 Mouth and Throat ØCJY
 Muscle
  Extraocular
   Left Ø8JM
   Right Ø8JL
  Lower ØKJY
  Upper ØKJX
 Nasal Mucosa and Soft Tissue Ø9JK
 Neck ØWJ6
 Nerve
  Cranial ØØJE

Inspection — *continued*
 Nerve — *continued*
  Peripheral Ø1JY
 Omentum ØDJU
 Oral Cavity and Throat ØWJ3
 Ovary ØUJ3
 Pancreas ØFJG
 Parathyroid Gland ØGJR
 Pelvic Cavity ØWJJ
 Penis ØVJS
 Pericardial Cavity ØWJD
 Perineum
  Female ØWJN
  Male ØWJM
 Peritoneal Cavity ØWJG
 Peritoneum ØDJW
 Pineal Body ØGJ1
 Pleura ØBJQ
 Pleural Cavity
  Left ØWJB
  Right ØWJ9
 Products of Conception 1ØJØ
  Ectopic 1ØJ2
  Retained 1ØJ1
 Prostate and Seminal Vesicles ØVJ4
 Respiratory Tract ØWJQ
 Retroperitoneum ØWJH
 Scrotum and Tunica Vaginalis ØVJ8
 Shoulder Region
  Left ØXJ3
  Right ØXJ2
 Sinus Ø9JY
 Skin ØHJPXZZ
 Skull ØNJØ
 Spinal Canal ØØJU
 Spinal Cord ØØJV
 Spleen Ø7JP
 Stomach ØDJ6
 Subcutaneous Tissue and Fascia
  Head and Neck ØJJS
  Lower Extremity ØJJW
  Trunk ØJJT
  Upper Extremity ØJJV
 Tendon
  Lower ØLJY
  Upper ØLJX
 Testis ØVJD
 Thymus Ø7JM
 Thyroid Gland ØGJK
 Toe Nail ØHJRXZZ
 Trachea ØBJ1
 Tracheobronchial Tree ØBJØ
 Tympanic Membrane
  Left Ø9J8
  Right Ø9J7
 Ureter ØTJ9
 Urethra ØTJD
 Uterus and Cervix ØUJD
 Vagina and Cul-de-sac ØUJH
 Vas Deferens ØVJR
 Vein
  Lower Ø6JY
  Upper Ø5JY
 Vulva ØUJM
 Wrist Region
  Left ØXJH
  Right ØXJG
Instillation *see* Introduction of substance in or on
Insufflation *see* Introduction of substance in or on
Interatrial septum *use* Atrial Septum
InterAtrial Shunt Device IASD®, Corvia *use* Synthetic Substitute
Interbody fusion (spine) cage
 use Interbody Fusion Device in Lower Joints
 use Interbody Fusion Device in Upper Joints
Interbody Fusion Device
 Customizable
  Lumbar Vertebral XRGB
   2 or more XRGC
  Lumbosacral XRGD
  Thoracolumbar Vertebral XRGA
 Nanotextured Surface
  Cervical Vertebral XRG1Ø92
   2 or more XRG2Ø92
  Cervicothoracic Vertebral XRG4Ø92
  Lumbar Vertebral XRGBØ92
   2 or more XRGCØ92
  Lumbosacral XRGDØ92

Interbody Fusion Device — *continued*
 Nanotextured Surface — *continued*
  Occipital-cervical XRGØØ92
  Thoracic Vertebral XRG6Ø92
   2 to 7 XRG7Ø92
   8 or more XRG8Ø92
  Thoracolumbar Vertebral XRGAØ92
 Radiolucent Porous
  Cervical Vertebral XRG1ØF3
   2 or more XRG2ØF3
  Cervicothoracic Vertebral XRG4ØF3
  Lumbar Vertebral XRGBØF3
   2 or more XRGCØF3
  Lumbosacral XRGDØF3
  Occipital-cervical XRGØØF3
  Thoracic Vertebral XRG6ØF3
   2 to 7 XRG7ØF3
   8 or more XRG8ØF3
  Thoracolumbar Vertebral XRGAØF3
Intercarpal joint
 use Carpal Joint, Left
 use Carpal Joint, Right
Intercarpal ligament
 use Hand Bursa and Ligament, Left
 use Hand Bursa and Ligament, Right
INTERCEPT Blood System for Plasma Pathogen Reduced Cryoprecipitated Fibrinogen Complex *use* Pathogen Reduced Cryoprecipitated Fibrinogen Complex
INTERCEPT Fibrinogen Complex *use* Pathogen Reduced Cryoprecipitated Fibrinogen Complex
Interclavicular ligament
 use Shoulder Bursa and Ligament, Left
 use Shoulder Bursa and Ligament, Right
Intercostal lymph node *use* Lymphatic, Thorax
Intercostal muscle
 use Thorax Muscle, Left
 use Thorax Muscle, Right
Intercostal nerve *use* Thoracic Nerve
Intercostobrachial nerve *use* Thoracic Nerve
Intercuneiform joint
 use Tarsal Joint, Left
 use Tarsal Joint, Right
Intercuneiform ligament
 use Foot Bursa and Ligament, Left
 use Foot Bursa and Ligament, Right
Intermediate bronchus *use* Main Bronchus, Right
Intermediate cuneiform bone
 use Tarsal, Left
 use Tarsal, Right
Intermittent hemodialysis (IHD) 5A1D7ØZ
Intermittent mandatory ventilation *see* Assistance, Respiratory 5AØ9
Intermittent Negative Airway Pressure
 24-96 Consecutive Hours, Ventilation 5AØ945B
 Greater than 96 Consecutive Hours, Ventilation 5AØ955B
 Less than 24 Consecutive Hours, Ventilation 5AØ935B
Intermittent Positive Airway Pressure
 24-96 Consecutive Hours, Ventilation 5AØ9458
 Greater than 96 Consecutive Hours, Ventilation 5AØ9558
 Less than 24 Consecutive Hours, Ventilation 5AØ9358
Intermittent positive pressure breathing *see* Assistance, Respiratory 5AØ9
Internal anal sphincter *use* Anal Sphincter
Internal carotid artery, intracranial portion *use* Intracranial Artery
Internal carotid plexus *use* Head and Neck Sympathetic Nerve
Internal (basal) cerebral vein *use* Intracranial Vein
Internal iliac vein
 use Hypogastric Vein, Left
 use Hypogastric Vein, Right
Internal maxillary artery
 use External Carotid Artery, Left
 use External Carotid Artery, Right
Internal naris *use* Nasal Mucosa and Soft Tissue
Internal oblique muscle
 use Abdomen Muscle, Left
 use Abdomen Muscle, Right
Internal pudendal artery
 use Internal Iliac Artery, Left
 use Internal Iliac Artery, Right

Introduction of substance in or on — *continued*
Brain — *continued*
Hypnotics 3E0Q
Nutritional Substance 3E0Q
Radioactive Substance 3E0Q
Sedatives 3E0Q
Stem Cells
Embryonic 3E0Q
Somatic 3E0Q
Water Balance Substance 3E0Q
Cranial Cavity 3E0Q
Analgesics 3E0Q
Anesthetic Agent 3E0Q
Anti-infective 3E0Q
Anti-inflammatory 3E0Q
Antineoplastic 3E0Q
Destructive Agent 3E0Q
Diagnostic Substance, Other 3E0Q
Electrolytic Substance 3E0Q
Gas 3E0Q
Hypnotics 3E0Q
Nutritional Substance 3E0Q
Radioactive Substance 3E0Q
Sedatives 3E0Q
Stem Cells
Embryonic 3E0Q
Somatic 3E0Q
Water Balance Substance 3E0Q
Ear 3E0B
Analgesics 3E0B
Anesthetic Agent 3E0B
Anti-infective 3E0B
Anti-inflammatory 3E0B
Antineoplastic 3E0B
Destructive Agent 3E0B
Diagnostic Substance, Other 3E0B
Hypnotics 3E0B
Radioactive Substance 3E0B
Sedatives 3E0B
Epidural Space 3E0S3GC
Analgesics 3E0S3NZ
Anesthetic Agent 3E0S3BZ
Anti-infective 3E0S32
Anti-inflammatory 3E0S33Z
Antineoplastic 3E0S30
Destructive Agent 3E0S3TZ
Diagnostic Substance, Other 3E0S3KZ
Electrolytic Substance 3E0S37Z
Gas 3E0S
Hypnotics 3E0S3NZ
Nutritional Substance 3E0S36Z
Radioactive Substance 3E0S3HZ
Sedatives 3E0S3NZ
Water Balance Substance 3E0S37Z
Eye 3E0C
Analgesics 3E0C
Anesthetic Agent 3E0C
Anti-infective 3E0C
Anti-inflammatory 3E0C
Antineoplastic 3E0C
Destructive Agent 3E0C
Diagnostic Substance, Other 3E0C
Gas 3E0C
Hypnotics 3E0C
Pigment 3E0C
Radioactive Substance 3E0C
Sedatives 3E0C
Gastrointestinal Tract
Lower 3E0H
Analgesics 3E0H
Anesthetic Agent 3E0H
Anti-infective 3E0H
Anti-inflammatory 3E0H
Antineoplastic 3E0H
Destructive Agent 3E0H
Diagnostic Substance, Other 3E0H
Electrolytic Substance 3E0H
Gas 3E0H
Hypnotics 3E0H
Nutritional Substance 3E0H
Radioactive Substance 3E0H
Sedatives 3E0H
Water Balance Substance 3E0H
Upper 3E0G
Analgesics 3E0G
Anesthetic Agent 3E0G
Anti-infective 3E0G
Anti-inflammatory 3E0G
Antineoplastic 3E0G

Introduction of substance in or on — *continued*
Gastrointestinal Tract — *continued*
Upper — *continued*
Destructive Agent 3E0G
Diagnostic Substance, Other 3E0G
Electrolytic Substance 3E0G
Gas 3E0G
Hypnotics 3E0G
Nutritional Substance 3E0G
Radioactive Substance 3E0G
Sedatives 3E0G
Water Balance Substance 3E0G
Genitourinary Tract 3E0K
Analgesics 3E0K
Anesthetic Agent 3E0K
Anti-infective 3E0K
Anti-inflammatory 3E0K
Antineoplastic 3E0K
Destructive Agent 3E0K
Diagnostic Substance, Other 3E0K
Electrolytic Substance 3E0K
Gas 3E0K
Hypnotics 3E0K
Nutritional Substance 3E0K
Radioactive Substance 3E0K
Sedatives 3E0K
Water Balance Substance 3E0K
Heart 3E08
Diagnostic Substance, Other 3E08
Platelet Inhibitor 3E08
Thrombolytic 3E08
Joint 3E0U
Analgesics 3E0U3NZ
Anesthetic Agent 3E0U3BZ
Anti-infective 3E0U
Anti-inflammatory 3E0U33Z
Antineoplastic 3E0U30
Destructive Agent 3E0U3TZ
Diagnostic Substance, Other 3E0U3KZ
Electrolytic Substance 3E0U37Z
Gas 3E0U3SF
Hypnotics 3E0U3NZ
Nutritional Substance 3E0U36Z
Radioactive Substance 3E0U3HZ
Sedatives 3E0U3NZ
Water Balance Substance 3E0U37Z
Lymphatic 3E0W3GC
Analgesics 3E0W3NZ
Anesthetic Agent 3E0W3BZ
Anti-infective 3E0W32
Anti-inflammatory 3E0W33Z
Antineoplastic 3E0W30
Destructive Agent 3E0W3TZ
Diagnostic Substance, Other 3E0W3KZ
Electrolytic Substance 3E0W37Z
Hypnotics 3E0W3NZ
Nutritional Substance 3E0W36Z
Radioactive Substance 3E0W3HZ
Sedatives 3E0W3NZ
Water Balance Substance 3E0W37Z
Mouth 3E0D
Analgesics 3E0D
Anesthetic Agent 3E0D
Antiarrhythmic 3E0D
Anti-infective 3E0D
Anti-inflammatory 3E0D
Antineoplastic 3E0D
Destructive Agent 3E0D
Diagnostic Substance, Other 3E0D
Electrolytic Substance 3E0D
Hypnotics 3E0D
Nutritional Substance 3E0D
Radioactive Substance 3E0D
Sedatives 3E0D
Serum 3E0D
Toxoid 3E0D
Vaccine 3E0D
Water Balance Substance 3E0D
Mucous Membrane 3E00XGC
Analgesics 3E00XNZ
Anesthetic Agent 3E00XBZ
Anti-infective 3E00X2
Anti-inflammatory 3E00X3Z
Antineoplastic 3E00X0
Destructive Agent 3E00XTZ
Diagnostic Substance, Other 3E00XKZ
Hypnotics 3E00XNZ
Pigment 3E00XMZ
Sedatives 3E00XNZ

Introduction of substance in or on — *continued*
Mucous Membrane — *continued*
Serum 3E00X4Z
Toxoid 3E00X4Z
Vaccine 3E00X4Z
Muscle 3E023GC
Analgesics 3E023NZ
Anesthetic Agent 3E023BZ
Anti-infective 3E0232
Anti-inflammatory 3E0233Z
Antineoplastic 3E0230
Destructive Agent 3E023TZ
Diagnostic Substance, Other 3E023KZ
Electrolytic Substance 3E0237Z
Hypnotics 3E023NZ
Nutritional Substance 3E0236Z
Radioactive Substance 3E023HZ
Sedatives 3E023NZ
Serum 3E0234Z
Toxoid 3E0234Z
Vaccine 3E0234Z
Water Balance Substance 3E0237Z
Nerve
Cranial 3E0X3GC
Anesthetic Agent 3E0X3BZ
Anti-inflammatory 3E0X33Z
Destructive Agent 3E0X3TZ
Peripheral 3E0T3GC
Anesthetic Agent 3E0T3BZ
Anti-inflammatory 3E0T33Z
Destructive Agent 3E0T3TZ
Plexus 3E0T3GC
Anesthetic Agent 3E0T3BZ
Anti-inflammatory 3E0T33Z
Destructive Agent 3E0T3TZ
Nose 3E09
Analgesics 3E09
Anesthetic Agent 3E09
Anti-infective 3E09
Anti-inflammatory 3E09
Antineoplastic 3E09
Destructive Agent 3E09
Diagnostic Substance, Other 3E09
Hypnotics 3E09
Radioactive Substance 3E09
Sedatives 3E09
Serum 3E09
Toxoid 3E09
Vaccine 3E09
Pancreatic Tract 3E0J
Analgesics 3E0J
Anesthetic Agent 3E0J
Anti-infective 3E0J
Anti-inflammatory 3E0J
Antineoplastic 3E0J
Destructive Agent 3E0J
Diagnostic Substance, Other 3E0J
Electrolytic Substance 3E0J
Gas 3E0J
Hypnotics 3E0J
Islet Cells, Pancreatic 3E0J
Nutritional Substance 3E0J
Radioactive Substance 3E0J
Sedatives 3E0J
Water Balance Substance 3E0J
Pericardial Cavity 3E0Y
Analgesics 3E0Y3NZ
Anesthetic Agent 3E0Y3BZ
Anti-infective 3E0Y32
Anti-inflammatory 3E0Y33Z
Antineoplastic 3E0Y
Destructive Agent 3E0Y3TZ
Diagnostic Substance, Other 3E0Y3KZ
Electrolytic Substance 3E0Y37Z
Gas 3E0Y
Hypnotics 3E0Y3NZ
Nutritional Substance 3E0Y36Z
Radioactive Substance 3E0Y3HZ
Sedatives 3E0Y3NZ
Water Balance Substance 3E0Y37Z
Peritoneal Cavity 3E0M
Adhesion Barrier 3E0M
Analgesics 3E0M3NZ
Anesthetic Agent 3E0M3BZ
Anti-infective 3E0M32
Anti-inflammatory 3E0M33Z
Antineoplastic 3E0M
Destructive Agent 3E0M3TZ
Diagnostic Substance, Other 3E0M3KZ

Intubation
  Airway
    see Insertion of device in, Esophagus 0DH5
    see Insertion of device in, Mouth and Throat
      0CHY
    see Insertion of device in, Trachea 0BH1
  Drainage device *see* Drainage
  Feeding Device *see* Insertion of device in, Gastroin-
    testinal System 0DH

INTUITY Elite valve system, EDWARDS *use*
  Zooplastic Tissue, Rapid Deployment Technique
  in New Technology

Iobenguane I-131 Antineoplastic XW0

Iobenguane I-131, High Specific Activity (HSA) *use*
  Iobenguane I-131 Antineoplastic

IPPB (intermittent positive pressure breathing)
  see Assistance, Respiratory 5A09

IRE (Irreversible Electroporation) *see* Destruction,
  Hepatobiliary System and Pancreas 0F5

Iridectomy
  see Excision, Eye 08B
  see Resection, Eye 08T

Iridoplasty
  see Repair, Eye 08Q
  see Replacement, Eye 08R
  see Supplement, Eye 08U

Iridotomy *see* Drainage, Eye 089

Irreversible Electroporation (IRE) *see* Destruction,
  Hepatobiliary System and Pancreas 0F5

Irrigation
  Biliary Tract, Irrigating Substance 3E1J
  Brain, Irrigating Substance 3E1Q38Z
  Cranial Cavity, Irrigating Substance 3E1Q38Z
  Ear, Irrigating Substance 3E1B
  Epidural Space, Irrigating Substance 3E1S38Z
  Eye, Irrigating Substance 3E1C
  Gastrointestinal Tract
    Lower, Irrigating Substance 3E1H
    Upper, Irrigating Substance 3E1G
  Genitourinary Tract, Irrigating Substance 3E1K
  Irrigating Substance 3C1ZX8Z
  Joint, Irrigating Substance 3E1U
  Mucous Membrane, Irrigating Substance 3E10
  Nose, Irrigating Substance 3E19
  Pancreatic Tract, Irrigating Substance 3E1J
  Pericardial Cavity, Irrigating Substance 3E1Y38Z
  Peritoneal Cavity
    Dialysate 3E1M39Z
    Irrigating Substance 3E1M
  Pleural Cavity, Irrigating Substance 3E1L38Z
  Reproductive
    Female, Irrigating Substance 3E1P
    Male, Irrigating Substance 3E1N
  Respiratory Tract, Irrigating Substance 3E1F

Irrigation — *continued*
  Skin, Irrigating Substance 3E1Ø
  Spinal Canal, Irrigating Substance 3E1R38Z
Isavuconazole (isavuconazonium sulfate) *use* Other Anti-infective
Ischiatic nerve *use* Sciatic Nerve
Ischiocavernosus muscle *use* Perineum Muscle
Ischiofemoral ligament
  use Hip Bursa and Ligament, Left
  use Hip Bursa and Ligament, Right
Ischium
  use Pelvic Bone, Left
  use Pelvic Bone, Right
ISC-REST kit
  ISCDx XXE5XT7
  QIAGEN Access Anti-SARS-CoV-2 Total Test XXE5XV7
  QIAstat-Dx Respiratory SARS-CoV-2 Panel XXE97U7
Isolation 8EØZXY6
Isotope Administration, Other Radiation, Whole Body DWY5G
Itrel (3) (4) neurostimulator *use* Stimulator Generator, Single Array in ØJH

J

Jakafi® *use* Ruxolitinib
Jejunal artery *use* Superior Mesenteric Artery
Jejunectomy
  see Excision, Jejunum ØDBA
  see Resection, Jejunum ØDTA
Jejunocolostomy
  see Bypass, Gastrointestinal System ØD1
  see Drainage, Gastrointestinal System ØD9
Jejunopexy
  see Repair, Jejunum ØDQA
  see Reposition, Jejunum ØDSA
Jejunostomy
  see Bypass, Jejunum ØD1A
  see Drainage, Jejunum ØD9A
Jejunotomy *see* Drainage, Jejunum ØD9A
Joint fixation plate
  use Internal Fixation Device in Lower Joints
  use Internal Fixation Device in Upper Joints
Joint liner (insert) *use* Liner in Lower Joints
Joint spacer (antibiotic)
  use Spacer in Lower Joints
  use Spacer in Upper Joints
Jugular body *use* Glomus Jugulare
Jugular lymph node
  use Lymphatic, Left Neck
  use Lymphatic, Right Neck

K

Kappa *use* Pacemaker, Dual Chamber in ØJH
Kcentra *use* 4-Factor Prothrombin Complex Concentrate
Keratectomy, kerectomy
  see Excision, Eye Ø8B
  see Resection, Eye Ø8T
Keratocentesis *see* Drainage, Eye Ø89
Keratoplasty
  see Repair, Eye Ø8Q
  see Replacement, Eye Ø8R
  see Supplement, Eye Ø8U
Keratotomy
  see Drainage, Eye Ø89
  see Repair, Eye Ø8Q
KEVZARA® *use* Sarilumab
Keystone Heart TriGuard 3™ CEPD (cerebral embolic protection device) X2A6325
Kirschner wire (K-wire)
  use Internal Fixation Device in Head and Facial Bones
  use Internal Fixation Device in Lower Bones
  use Internal Fixation Device in Lower Joints
  use Internal Fixation Device in Upper Bones
  use Internal Fixation Device in Upper Joints
Knee (implant) insert *use* Liner in Lower Joints
KUB x-ray *see* Plain Radiography, Kidney, Ureter and Bladder BTØ4
Kuntscher nail
  use Internal Fixation Device, Intramedullary in Lower Bones

Kuntscher nail — *continued*
  use Internal Fixation Device, Intramedullary in Upper Bones
KYMRIAH® *use* Tisagenlecleucel Immunotherapy

L

Labia majora *use* Vulva
Labia minora *use* Vulva
Labial gland
  use Lower Lip
  use Upper Lip
Labiectomy
  see Excision, Female Reproductive System ØUB
  see Resection, Female Reproductive System ØUT
Lacrimal canaliculus
  use Lacrimal Duct, Left
  use Lacrimal Duct, Right
Lacrimal punctum
  use Lacrimal Duct, Left
  use Lacrimal Duct, Right
Lacrimal sac
  use Lacrimal Duct, Left
  use Lacrimal Duct, Right
LAGB (laparoscopic adjustable gastric banding)
  Initial procedure ØDV64CZ
  Surgical correction *see* Revision of device in, Stomach ØDW6
Laminectomy
  see Excision, Lower Bones ØQB
  see Excision, Upper Bones ØPB
  see Release, Central Nervous System and Cranial Nerves ØØN
  see Release, Peripheral Nervous System Ø1N
Laminotomy
  see Drainage, Lower Bones ØQ9
  see Drainage, Upper Bones ØP9
  see Excision, Lower Bones ØQB
  see Excision, Upper Bones ØPB
  see Release, Central Nervous System and Cranial Nerves ØØN
  see Release, Lower Bones ØQN
  see Release, Peripheral Nervous System Ø1N
  see Release, Upper Bones ØPN
Laparoscopic-assisted transanal pull-through
  see Excision, Gastrointestinal System ØDB
  see Resection, Gastrointestinal System ØDT
Laparoscopy *see* Inspection
Laparotomy
  Drainage *see* Drainage, Peritoneal Cavity ØW9G
  Exploratory *see* Inspection, Peritoneal Cavity ØWJG
LAP-BAND® adjustable gastric banding system *use* Extraluminal Device
Laryngectomy
  see Excision, Larynx ØCBS
  see Resection, Larynx ØCTS
Laryngocentesis *see* Drainage, Larynx ØC9S
Laryngogram *see* Fluoroscopy, Larynx B91J
Laryngopexy *see* Repair, Larynx ØCQS
Laryngopharynx *use* Pharynx
Laryngoplasty
  see Repair, Larynx ØCQS
  see Replacement, Larynx ØCRS
  see Supplement, Larynx ØCUS
Laryngorrhaphy *see* Repair, Larynx ØCQS
Laryngoscopy ØCJS8ZZ
Laryngotomy *see* Drainage, Larynx ØC9S
Laser Interstitial Thermal Therapy
  Adrenal Gland DGY2KZZ
  Anus DDY8KZZ
  Bile Ducts DFY2KZZ
  Brain DØYØKZZ
  Brain Stem DØY1KZZ
  Breast
    Left DMYØKZZ
    Right DMY1KZZ
  Bronchus DBY1KZZ
  Chest Wall DBY7KZZ
  Colon DDY5KZZ
  Diaphragm DBY8KZZ
  Duodenum DDY2KZZ
  Esophagus DDYØKZZ
  Gallbladder DFY1KZZ
  Gland
    Adrenal DGY2KZZ
    Parathyroid DGY4KZZ

Laser Interstitial Thermal Therapy — *continued*
  Gland — *continued*
    Pituitary DGYØKZZ
    Thyroid DGY5KZZ
  Ileum DDY4KZZ
  Jejunum DDY3KZZ
  Liver DFYØKZZ
  Lung DBY2KZZ
  Mediastinum DBY6KZZ
  Nerve, Peripheral DØY7KZZ
  Pancreas DFY3KZZ
  Parathyroid Gland DGY4KZZ
  Pineal Body DGY1KZZ
  Pituitary Gland DGYØKZZ
  Pleura DBY5KZZ
  Prostate DVYØKZZ
  Rectum DDY7KZZ
  Spinal Cord DØY6KZZ
  Stomach DDY1KZZ
  Thyroid Gland DGY5KZZ
  Trachea DBYØKZZ
Lateral canthus
  use Upper Eyelid, Left
  use Upper Eyelid, Right
Lateral collateral ligament (LCL)
  use Knee Bursa and Ligament, Left
  use Knee Bursa and Ligament, Right
Lateral condyle of femur
  use Lower Femur, Left
  use Lower Femur, Right
Lateral condyle of tibia
  use Tibia, Left
  use Tibia, Right
Lateral cuneiform bone
  use Tarsal, Left
  use Tarsal, Right
Lateral epicondyle of femur
  use Lower Femur, Left
  use Lower Femur, Right
Lateral epicondyle of humerus
  use Humeral Shaft, Left
  use Humeral Shaft, Right
Lateral femoral cutaneous nerve *use* Lumbar Plexus
Lateral (brachial) lymph node
  use Lymphatic, Left Axillary
  use Lymphatic, Right Axillary
Lateral malleolus
  use Fibula, Left
  use Fibula, Right
Lateral meniscus
  use Knee Joint, Left
  use Knee Joint, Right
Lateral nasal cartilage *use* Nasal Mucosa and Soft Tissue
Lateral plantar artery
  use Foot Artery, Left
  use Foot Artery, Right
Lateral plantar nerve *use* Tibial Nerve
Lateral rectus muscle
  use Extraocular Muscle, Left
  use Extraocular Muscle, Right
Lateral sacral artery
  use Internal Iliac Artery, Left
  use Internal Iliac Artery, Right
Lateral sacral vein
  use Hypogastric Vein, Left
  use Hypogastric Vein, Right
Lateral sural cutaneous nerve *use* Peroneal Nerve
Lateral tarsal artery
  use Foot Artery, Left
  use Foot Artery, Right
Lateral temporomandibular ligament *use* Head and Neck Bursa and Ligament
Lateral thoracic artery
  use Axillary Artery, Left
  use Axillary Artery, Right
Latissimus dorsi muscle
  use Trunk Muscle, Left
  use Trunk Muscle, Right
Latissimus Dorsi Myocutaneous Flap
  Replacement
    Bilateral ØHRVØ75
    Left ØHRUØ75
    Right ØHRTØ75
  Transfer
    Left ØKXG
    Right ØKXF

Lavage

see Irrigation
Bronchial alveolar, diagnostic see Drainage, Respiratory System 0B9

Least splanchnic nerve use Thoracic Sympathetic Nerve
Lefamulin Anti-infective XW0
Left ascending lumbar vein use Hemiazygos Vein
Left atrioventricular valve use Mitral Valve
Left auricular appendix use Atrium, Left
Left colic vein use Colic Vein
Left coronary sulcus use Heart, Left
Left gastric artery use Gastric Artery
Left gastroepiploic artery use Splenic Artery
Left gastroepiploic vein use Splenic Vein
Left inferior phrenic vein use Renal Vein, Left
Left inferior pulmonary vein use Pulmonary Vein, Left
Left jugular trunk use Thoracic Duct
Left lateral ventricle use Cerebral Ventricle
Left ovarian vein use Renal Vein, Left
Left second lumbar vein use Renal Vein, Left
Left subclavian trunk use Thoracic Duct
Left subcostal vein use Hemiazygos Vein
Left superior pulmonary vein use Pulmonary Vein, Left
Left suprarenal vein use Renal Vein, Left
Left testicular vein use Renal Vein, Left

Lengthening
Bone, with device see Insertion of Limb Lengthening Device
Muscle, by incision see Division, Muscles 0K8
Tendon, by incision see Division, Tendons 0L8

Leptomeninges, intracranial use Cerebral Meninges
Leptomeninges, spinal use Spinal Meninges
Leronlimab Monoclonal Antibody XW013K6
Lesser alar cartilage use Nasal Mucosa and Soft Tissue
Lesser occipital nerve use Cervical Plexus
Lesser Omentum use Omentum
Lesser saphenous vein
use Saphenous Vein, Left
use Saphenous Vein, Right
Lesser splanchnic nerve use Thoracic Sympathetic Nerve
Lesser trochanter
use Upper Femur, Left
use Upper Femur, Right
Lesser tuberosity
use Humeral Head, Left
use Humeral Head, Right
Lesser wing use Sphenoid Bone
Leukopheresis, therapeutic see Pheresis, Circulatory 6A55
Levator anguli oris muscle use Facial Muscle
Levator ani muscle use Perineum Muscle
Levator labii superioris alaeque nasi muscle use Facial Muscle
Levator labii superioris muscle use Facial Muscle
Levator palpebrae superioris muscle
use Upper Eyelid, Left
use Upper Eyelid, Right
Levator scapulae muscle
use Neck Muscle, Left
use Neck Muscle, Right
Levator veli palatini muscle use Tongue, Palate, Pharynx Muscle
Levatores costarum muscle
use Thorax Muscle, Left
use Thorax Muscle, Right
Lifeline ARM Automated Chest Compression (ACC) device 5A1221J
LifeStent® (Flexstar) (XL) Vascular Stent System use Intraluminal Device
Lifileucel use Lifileucel Immunotherapy
Lifileucel Immunotherapy XW0
Ligament of head of fibula
use Knee Bursa and Ligament, Left
use Knee Bursa and Ligament, Right
Ligament of the lateral malleolus
use Ankle Bursa and Ligament, Left
use Ankle Bursa and Ligament, Right
Ligamentum flavum, cervical use Head and Neck Bursa and Ligament
Ligamentum flavum, lumbar use Lower Spine Bursa and Ligament

Ligamentum flavum, thoracic use Upper Spine Bursa and Ligament
Ligation see Occlusion
Ligation, hemorrhoid see Occlusion, Lower Veins, Hemorrhoidal Plexus
Light Therapy GZJZZZZ
Liner
Removal of device from
Hip
Left 0SPB09Z
Right 0SP909Z
Knee
Left 0SPD09Z
Right 0SPC09Z
Revision of device in
Hip
Left 0SWB09Z
Right 0SW909Z
Knee
Left 0SWD09Z
Right 0SWC09Z
Supplement
Hip
Left 0SUB09Z
Acetabular Surface 0SUE09Z
Femoral Surface 0SUS09Z
Right 0SU909Z
Acetabular Surface 0SUA09Z
Femoral Surface 0SUR09Z
Knee
Left 0SUD09
Femoral Surface 0SUU09Z
Tibial Surface 0SUW09Z
Right 0SUC09
Femoral Surface 0SUT09Z
Tibial Surface 0SUV09Z
Lingual artery
use External Carotid Artery, Left
use External Carotid Artery, Right
Lingual tonsil use Pharynx
Lingulectomy, lung
see Excision, Lung Lingula 0BBH
see Resection, Lung Lingula 0BTH
Lisocabtagene Maraleucel use Lisocabtagene Maraleucel Immunotherapy
Lisocabtagene Maraleucel Immunotherapy XW0
Lithoplasty see Fragmentation
Lithotripsy
see Fragmentation
With removal of fragments see Extirpation
LITT (laser interstitial thermal therapy) see Laser Interstitial Thermal Therapy
LIVIAN™ CRT-D use Cardiac Resynchronization Defibrillator Pulse Generator in 0JH
Lobectomy
see Excision, Central Nervous System and Cranial Nerves 00B
see Excision, Endocrine System 0GB
see Excision, Hepatobiliary System and Pancreas 0FB
see Excision, Respiratory System 0BB
see Resection, Endocrine System 0GT
see Resection, Hepatobiliary System and Pancreas 0FT
see Resection, Respiratory System 0BT
Lobotomy see Division, Brain 0080
Localization
see Imaging
see Map
Locus ceruleus use Pons
Long thoracic nerve use Brachial Plexus
Loop ileostomy see Bypass, Ileum 0D1B
Loop recorder, implantable use Monitoring Device
Lower GI series see Fluoroscopy, Colon BD14
Lower Respiratory Fluid Nucleic Acid-base Microbial Detection XXEBXQ6
LTX Regional Anticoagulant use Nafamostat Anticoagulant
LUCAS® Chest Compression System 5A1221J
Lumbar artery use Abdominal Aorta
Lumbar facet joint use Lumbar Vertebral Joint
Lumbar ganglion use Lumbar Sympathetic Nerve
Lumbar lymph node use Lymphatic, Aortic
Lumbar lymphatic trunk use Cisterna Chyli
Lumbar splanchnic nerve use Lumbar Sympathetic Nerve
Lumbosacral facet joint use Lumbosacral Joint

Lumbosacral trunk use Lumbar Nerve
Lumpectomy see Excision
Lunate bone
use Carpal, Left
use Carpal, Right
Lunotriquetral ligament
use Hand Bursa and Ligament, Left
use Hand Bursa and Ligament, Right
Lurbinectedin XW0
Lymphadenectomy
see Excision, Lymphatic and Hemic Systems 07B
see Resection, Lymphatic and Hemic Systems 07T
Lymphadenotomy see Drainage, Lymphatic and Hemic Systems 079
Lymphangiectomy
see Excision, Lymphatic and Hemic Systems 07B
see Resection, Lymphatic and Hemic Systems 07T
Lymphangiogram see Plain Radiography, Lymphatic System B70
Lymphangioplasty
see Repair, Lymphatic and Hemic Systems 07Q
see Supplement, Lymphatic and Hemic Systems 07U
Lymphangiorrhaphy see Repair, Lymphatic and Hemic Systems 07Q
Lymphangiotomy see Drainage, Lymphatic and Hemic Systems 079
Lysis see Release

M

Macula XXE5XR7
use Retina, Left
use Retina, Right
MAGEC® Spinal Bracing and Distraction System
use Magnetically Controlled Growth Rod(s) in New Technology
Magnet extraction, ocular foreign body see Extirpation, Eye 08C
Magnetic Resonance Imaging (MRI)
Abdomen BW30
Ankle
Left BQ3H
Right BQ3G
Aorta
Abdominal B430
Thoracic B330
Arm
Left BP3F
Right BP3E
Artery
Celiac B431
Cervico-Cerebral Arch B33Q
Common Carotid, Bilateral B335
Coronary
Bypass Graft, Multiple B233
Multiple B231
Internal Carotid, Bilateral B338
Intracranial B33R
Lower Extremity
Bilateral B43H
Left B43G
Right B43F
Pelvic B43C
Renal, Bilateral B438
Spinal B33M
Superior Mesenteric B434
Upper Extremity
Bilateral B33K
Left B33J
Right B33H
Vertebral, Bilateral B33G
Bladder BT30
Brachial Plexus BW3P
Brain B030
Breast
Bilateral BH32
Left BH31
Right BH30
Calcaneus
Left BQ3K
Right BQ3J
Chest BW33Y
Coccyx BR3F
Connective Tissue
Lower Extremity BL31
Upper Extremity BL30

Magnetic Resonance Imaging (MRI) — *continued*
Corpora Cavernosa BV3Ø
Disc
    Cervical BR31
    Lumbar BR33
    Thoracic BR32
Ear B93Ø
Elbow
    Left BP3H
    Right BP3G
Eye
    Bilateral B837
    Left B836
    Right B835
Femur
    Left BQ34
    Right BQ33
Fetal Abdomen BY33
Fetal Extremity BY35
Fetal Head BY3Ø
Fetal Heart BY31
Fetal Spine BY34
Fetal Thorax BY32
Fetus, Whole BY36
Foot
    Left BQ3M
    Right BQ3L
Forearm
    Left BP3K
    Right BP3J
Gland
    Adrenal, Bilateral BG32
    Parathyroid BG33
    Parotid, Bilateral B936
    Salivary, Bilateral B93D
    Submandibular, Bilateral B939
    Thyroid BG34
Head BW38
Heart, Right and Left B236
Hip
    Left BQ31
    Right BQ3Ø
Intracranial Sinus B532
Joint
    Finger
        Left BP3D
        Right BP3C
    Hand
        Left BP3D
        Right BP3C
    Temporomandibular, Bilateral BN39
Kidney
    Bilateral BT33
    Left BT32
    Right BT31
    Transplant BT39
Knee
    Left BQ38
    Right BQ37
Larynx B93J
Leg
    Left BQ3F
    Right BQ3D
Liver BF35
Liver and Spleen BF36
Lung Apices BB3G
Nasopharynx B93F
Neck BW3F
Nerve
    Acoustic BØ3C
    Brachial Plexus BW3P
Oropharynx B93F
Ovary
    Bilateral BU35
    Left BU34
    Right BU33
Ovary and Uterus BU3C
Pancreas BF37
Patella
    Left BQ3W
    Right BQ3V
Pelvic Region BW3G
Pelvis BR3C
Pituitary Gland BØ39
Plexus, Brachial BW3P
Prostate BV33
Retroperitoneum BW3H
Sacrum BR3F
Scrotum BV34

Magnetic Resonance Imaging (MRI) — *continued*
Sella Turcica BØ39
Shoulder
    Left BP39
    Right BP38
Sinus
    Intracranial B532
    Paranasal B932
Spinal Cord BØ3B
Spine
    Cervical BR3Ø
    Lumbar BR39
    Thoracic BR37
Spleen and Liver BF36
Subcutaneous Tissue
    Abdomen BH3H
    Extremity
        Lower BH3J
        Upper BH3F
    Head BH3D
    Neck BH3D
    Pelvis BH3H
    Thorax BH3G
Tendon
    Lower Extremity BL33
    Upper Extremity BL32
Testicle
    Bilateral BV37
    Left BV36
    Right BV35
Toe
    Left BQ3Q
    Right BQ3P
Uterus BU36
    Pregnant BU3B
Uterus and Ovary BU3C
Vagina BU39
Vein
    Cerebellar B531
    Cerebral B531
    Jugular, Bilateral B535
    Lower Extremity
        Bilateral B53D
        Left B53C
        Right B53B
    Other B53V
    Pelvic (Iliac) Bilateral B53H
    Portal B53T
    Pulmonary, Bilateral B53S
    Renal, Bilateral B53L
    Spanchnic B53T
    Upper Extremity
        Bilateral B53P
        Left B53N
        Right B53M
Vena Cava
    Inferior B539
    Superior B538
Wrist
    Left BP3M
    Right BP3L
Magnetically Controlled Growth Rod(s)
Cervical XNS3
Lumbar XNSØ
Thoracic XNS4
Magnetic-guided radiofrequency endovascular fistula
Radial Artery, Left Ø31C3ZF
Radial Artery, Right Ø31B3ZF
Ulnar Artery, Left Ø31A3ZF
Ulnar Artery, Right Ø3193ZF
Malleotomy *see* Drainage, Ear, Nose, Sinus Ø99
Malleus
use Auditory Ossicle, Left
use Auditory Ossicle, Right
Mammaplasty, mammoplasty
see Alteration, Skin and Breast ØHØ
see Repair, Skin and Breast ØHQ
see Replacement, Skin and Breast ØHR
see Supplement, Skin and Breast ØHU
Mammary duct
use Breast, Bilateral
use Breast, Left
use Breast, Right
Mammary gland
use Breast, Bilateral
use Breast, Left
use Breast, Right

Mammectomy
see Excision, Skin and Breast ØHB
see Resection, Skin and Breast ØHT
Mammillary body *use* Hypothalamus
Mammography *see* Plain Radiography, Skin, Subcutaneous Tissue and Breast BHØ
Mammotomy *see* Drainage, Skin and Breast ØH9
Mandibular nerve *use* Trigeminal Nerve
Mandibular notch
use Mandible, Left
use Mandible, Right
Mandibulectomy
see Excision, Head and Facial Bones ØNB
see Resection, Head and Facial Bones ØNT
Manipulation
Adhesions *see* Release
Chiropractic *see* Chiropractic Manipulation
Manual removal, retained placenta *see* Extraction, Products of Conception, Retained 10D1
Manubrium *use* Sternum
Map
Basal Ganglia ØØK8
Brain ØØKØ
Cerebellum ØØKC
Cerebral Hemisphere ØØK7
Conduction Mechanism Ø2K8
Hypothalamus ØØKA
Medulla Oblongata ØØKD
Pons ØØKB
Thalamus ØØK9
Mapping
Doppler ultrasound *see* Ultrasonography
Electrocardiogram only *see* Measurement, Cardiac 4AØ2
Mark IV Breathing Pacemaker System *use* Stimulator Generator in Subcutaneous Tissue and Fascia
Marsupialization
see Drainage
see Excision
Massage, cardiac
External 5A12012
Open Ø2QAØZZ
Masseter muscle *use* Head Muscle
Masseteric fascia *use* Subcutaneous Tissue and Fascia, Face
Mastectomy
see Excision, Skin and Breast ØHB
see Resection, Skin and Breast ØHT
Mastoid air cells
use Mastoid Sinus, Left
use Mastoid Sinus, Right
Mastoid (postauricular) lymph node
use Lymphatic, Left Neck
use Lymphatic, Right Neck
Mastoid process
use Temporal Bone, Left
use Temporal Bone, Right
Mastoidectomy
see Excision, Ear, Nose, Sinus Ø9B
see Resection, Ear, Nose, Sinus Ø9T
Mastoidotomy *see* Drainage, Ear, Nose, Sinus Ø99
Mastopexy
see Repair, Skin and Breast ØHQ
see Reposition, Skin and Breast ØHS
Mastorrhaphy *see* Repair, Skin and Breast ØHQ
Mastotomy *see* Drainage, Skin and Breast ØH9
Maxillary artery
use External Carotid Artery, Left
use External Carotid Artery, Right
Maxillary nerve *use* Trigeminal Nerve
Maximo II DR (VR) *use* Defibrillator Generator in ØJH
Maximo II DR CRT-D *use* Cardiac Resynchronization Defibrillator Pulse Generator in ØJH
Measurement
Arterial
    Flow
        Coronary 4AØ3
        Intracranial 4AØ3X5D
        Peripheral 4AØ3
        Pulmonary 4AØ3
    Pressure
        Coronary 4AØ3
        Peripheral 4AØ3
        Pulmonary 4AØ3
        Thoracic, Other 4AØ3
    Pulse
        Coronary 4AØ3

Measurement — continued
- Arterial — continued
  - Pulse — continued
    - Peripheral 4A03
    - Pulmonary 4A03
  - Saturation, Peripheral 4A03
  - Sound, Peripheral 4A03
- Biliary
  - Flow 4A0C
  - Pressure 4A0C
- Cardiac
  - Action Currents 4A02
  - Defibrillator 4B02XTZ
  - Electrical Activity 4A02
    - Guidance 4A02X4A
    - No Qualifier 4A02X4Z
  - Output 4A02
  - Pacemaker 4B02XSZ
  - Rate 4A02
  - Rhythm 4A02
  - Sampling and Pressure
    - Bilateral 4A02
    - Left Heart 4A02
    - Right Heart 4A02
  - Sound 4A02
  - Total Activity, Stress 4A02XM4
- Central Nervous
  - Cerebrospinal Fluid Shunt, Wireless Sensor 4B00XW0
  - Conductivity 4A00
  - Electrical Activity 4A00
  - Pressure 4A000BZ
    - Intracranial 4A00
  - Saturation, Intracranial 4A00
  - Stimulator 4B00XVZ
  - Temperature, Intracranial 4A00
- Circulatory, Volume 4A05XLZ
- Gastrointestinal
  - Motility 4A0B
  - Pressure 4A0B
  - Secretion 4A0B
- Lower Respiratory Fluid Nucleic Acid-base Microbial Detection XXEBXQ6
- Lymphatic
  - Flow 4A06
  - Pressure 4A06
- Metabolism 4A0Z
- Musculoskeletal
  - Contractility 4A0F
  - Pressure 4A0F3BE
  - Stimulator 4B0FXVZ
- Olfactory, Acuity 4A08X0Z
- Peripheral Nervous
  - Conductivity
    - Motor 4A01
    - Sensory 4A01
  - Electrical Activity 4A01
  - Stimulator 4B01XVZ
- Positive Blood Culture Fluorescence Hybridization for Organism Identification, Concentration and Susceptibility XXE5XN6
- Products of Conception
  - Cardiac
    - Electrical Activity 4A0H
    - Rate 4A0H
    - Rhythm 4A0H
    - Sound 4A0H
  - Nervous
    - Conductivity 4A0J
    - Electrical Activity 4A0J
    - Pressure 4A0J
- Respiratory
  - Capacity 4A09
  - Flow 4A09
  - Pacemaker 4B09XSZ
  - Rate 4A09
  - Resistance 4A09
  - Total Activity 4A09
  - Volume 4A09
- Sleep 4A0ZXQZ
- Temperature 4A0Z
- Urinary
  - Contractility 4A0D
  - Flow 4A0D
  - Pressure 4A0D
  - Resistance 4A0D
  - Volume 4A0D

Measurement — continued
- Venous
  - Flow
    - Central 4A04
    - Peripheral 4A04
    - Portal 4A04
    - Pulmonary 4A04
  - Pressure
    - Central 4A04
    - Peripheral 4A04
    - Portal 4A04
    - Pulmonary 4A04
  - Pulse
    - Central 4A04
    - Peripheral 4A04
    - Portal 4A04
    - Pulmonary 4A04
  - Saturation, Peripheral 4A04
- Visual
  - Acuity 4A07X0Z
  - Mobility 4A07X7Z
  - Pressure 4A07XBZ
- Whole Blood Nucleic Acid-base Microbial Detection XXE5XM5

Meatoplasty, urethra see Repair, Urethra 0TQD
Meatotomy see Drainage, Urinary System 0T9
Mechanical chest compression (mCPR) 5A1221J
Mechanical Initial Specimen Diversion Technique Using Active Negative Pressure (blood collection) XXE5XR7
Mechanical ventilation see Performance, Respiratory 5A19
Medial canthus
- use Lower Eyelid, Left
- use Lower Eyelid, Right

Medial collateral ligament (MCL)
- use Knee Bursa and Ligament, Left
- use Knee Bursa and Ligament, Right

Medial condyle of femur
- use Lower Femur, Left
- use Lower Femur, Right

Medial condyle of tibia
- use Tibia, Left
- use Tibia, Right

Medial cuneiform bone
- use Tarsal, Left
- use Tarsal, Right

Medial epicondyle of femur
- use Lower Femur, Left
- use Lower Femur, Right

Medial epicondyle of humerus
- use Humeral Shaft, Left
- use Humeral Shaft, Right

Medial malleolus
- use Tibia, Left
- use Tibia, Right

Medial meniscus
- use Knee Joint, Left
- use Knee Joint, Right

Medial plantar artery
- use Foot Artery, Left
- use Foot Artery, Right

Medial plantar nerve use Tibial Nerve
Medial popliteal nerve use Tibial Nerve
Medial rectus muscle
- use Extraocular Muscle, Left
- use Extraocular Muscle, Right

Medial sural cutaneous nerve use Tibial Nerve
Median antebrachial vein
- use Basilic Vein, Left
- use Basilic Vein, Right

Median cubital vein
- use Basilic Vein, Left
- use Basilic Vein, Right

Median sacral artery use Abdominal Aorta
Mediastinal cavity use Mediastinum
Mediastinal lymph node use Lymphatic, Thorax
Mediastinal space use Mediastinum
Mediastinoscopy 0WJC4ZZ
Medication Management GZ3ZZZZ
- for substance abuse
  - Antabuse HZ83ZZZ
  - Bupropion HZ87ZZZ
  - Clonidine HZ86ZZZ
  - Levo-alpha-acetyl-methadol (LAAM) HZ82ZZZ
  - Methadone Maintenance HZ81ZZZ

Medication Management — continued
- for substance abuse — continued
  - Naloxone HZ85ZZZ
  - Naltrexone HZ84ZZZ
  - Nicotine Replacement HZ80ZZZ
  - Other Replacement Medication HZ89ZZZ
  - Psychiatric Medication HZ88ZZZ

Meditation 8E0ZXY5
Medtronic Endurant® II AAA stent graft system use Intraluminal Device
Meissner's (submucous) plexus use Abdominal Sympathetic Nerve
Melody® transcatheter pulmonary valve use Zooplastic Tissue in Heart and Great Vessels
Membranous urethra use Urethra
Meningeorrhaphy
- see Repair, Cerebral Meninges 00Q1
- see Repair, Spinal Meninges 00QT

Meniscectomy, knee
- see Excision, Joint, Knee, Left 0SBD
- see Excision, Joint, Knee, Right 0SBC

Mental foramen
- use Mandible, Left
- use Mandible, Right

Mentalis muscle use Facial Muscle
Mentoplasty see Alteration, Jaw, Lower 0W05
Meropenem-vaborbactam Anti-infective XW0
Mesenterectomy see Excision, Mesentery 0DBV
Mesenteriorrhaphy, mesenterorrhaphy see Repair, Mesentery 0DQV
Mesenteriplication see Repair, Mesentery 0DQV
Mesoappendix use Mesentery
Mesocolon use Mesentery
Metacarpal ligament
- use Hand Bursa and Ligament, Left
- use Hand Bursa and Ligament, Right

Metacarpophalangeal ligament
- use Hand Bursa and Ligament, Left
- use Hand Bursa and Ligament, Right

Metal on metal bearing surface use Synthetic Substitute, Metal in 0SR
Metatarsal ligament
- use Foot Bursa and Ligament, Left
- use Foot Bursa and Ligament, Right

Metatarsectomy
- see Excision, Lower Bones 0QB
- see Resection, Lower Bones 0QT

Metatarsophalangeal (MTP) joint
- use Metatarsal-Phalangeal Joint, Left
- use Metatarsal-Phalangeal Joint, Right

Metatarsophalangeal ligament
- use Foot Bursa and Ligament, Left
- use Foot Bursa and Ligament, Right

Metathalamus use Thalamus
Micro-Driver stent (RX) (OTW) use Intraluminal Device
MicroMed HeartAssist use Implantable Heart Assist System in Heart and Great Vessels
Micrus CERECYTE Microcoil use Intraluminal Device, Bioactive in Upper Arteries
Midcarpal joint
- use Carpal Joint, Left
- use Carpal Joint, Right

Middle cardiac nerve use Thoracic Sympathetic Nerve
Middle cerebral artery use Intracranial Artery
Middle cerebral vein use Intracranial Vein
Middle colic vein use Colic Vein
Middle genicular artery
- use Popliteal Artery, Left
- use Popliteal Artery, Right

Middle hemorrhoidal vein
- use Hypogastric Vein, Left
- use Hypogastric Vein, Right

Middle rectal artery
- use Internal Iliac Artery, Left
- use Internal Iliac Artery, Right

Middle suprarenal artery use Abdominal Aorta
Middle temporal artery
- use Temporal Artery, Left
- use Temporal Artery, Right

Middle turbinate use Nasal Turbinate
Mineral-based Topical Hemostatic Agent XW0
MIRODERM™ Biologic Wound Matrix use Skin Substitute, Porcine Liver Derived in New Technology
MitraClip valve repair system use Synthetic Substitute
Mitral annulus use Mitral Valve

Mitroflow® Aortic Pericardial Heart Valve *use*
Zooplastic Tissue in Heart and Great Vessels
Mobilization, adhesions *see* Release
Molar gland *use* Buccal Mucosa
MolecuLight i:X® wound imaging *see* Other Imaging,
Anatomical Regions BW5
Monitoring
Arterial
Flow
Coronary 4A13
Peripheral 4A13
Pulmonary 4A13
Pressure
Coronary 4A13
Peripheral 4A13
Pulmonary 4A13
Pulse
Coronary 4A13
Peripheral 4A13
Pulmonary 4A13
Saturation, Peripheral 4A13
Sound, Peripheral 4A13
Cardiac
Electrical Activity 4A12
Ambulatory 4A12X45
No Qualifier 4A12X4Z
Output 4A12
Rate 4A12
Rhythm 4A12
Sound 4A12
Total Activity, Stress 4A12XM4
Vascular Perfusion, Indocyanine Green Dye
4A12XSH
Central Nervous
Conductivity 4A10
Electrical Activity
Intraoperative 4A10
No Qualifier 4A10
Pressure 4A100BZ
Intracranial 4A10
Saturation, Intracranial 4A10
Temperature, Intracranial 4A10
Gastrointestinal
Motility 4A1B
Pressure 4A1B
Secretion 4A1B
Vascular Perfusion, Indocyanine Green Dye
4A1BXSH
Kidney, Fluorescent Pyrazine XT25XE5
Lymphatic
Flow
Indocyanine Green Dye 4A16
No Qualifier 4A16
Pressure 4A16
Oxygen Saturation Endoscopic Imaging (OXEI) XD2
Peripheral Nervous
Conductivity
Motor 4A11
Sensory 4A11
Electrical Activity
Intraoperative 4A11
No Qualifier 4A11
Products of Conception
Cardiac
Electrical Activity 4A1H
Rate 4A1H
Rhythm 4A1H
Sound 4A1H
Nervous
Conductivity 4A1J
Electrical Activity 4A1J
Pressure 4A1J
Respiratory
Capacity 4A19
Flow 4A19
Rate 4A19
Resistance 4A19
Volume 4A19
Skin and Breast, Vascular Perfusion, Indocyanine
Green Dye 4A1GXSH
Sleep 4A1ZXQZ
Temperature 4A1Z
Urinary
Contractility 4A1D
Flow 4A1D
Pressure 4A1D
Resistance 4A1D
Volume 4A1D

Monitoring — *continued*
Venous
Flow
Central 4A14
Peripheral 4A14
Portal 4A14
Pulmonary 4A14
Pressure
Central 4A14
Peripheral 4A14
Portal 4A14
Pulmonary 4A14
Pulse
Central 4A14
Peripheral 4A14
Portal 4A14
Pulmonary 4A14
Saturation
Central 4A14
Portal 4A14
Pulmonary 4A14
Monitoring Device, Hemodynamic
Abdomen 0JH8
Chest 0JH6
Mosaic Bioprosthesis (aortic) (mitral) valve *use*
Zooplastic Tissue in Heart and Great Vessels
Motor Function Assessment F01
Motor Treatment F07
MR Angiography
see Magnetic Resonance Imaging (MRI), Heart B23
see Magnetic Resonance Imaging (MRI), Lower
Arteries B43
see Magnetic Resonance Imaging (MRI), Upper
Arteries B33
**MULTI-LINK (VISION) (MINI-VISION) (ULTRA)
Coronary Stent System** *use* Intraluminal Device
Multiple sleep latency test 4A0ZXQZ
Musculocutaneous nerve *use* Brachial Plexus
Musculopexy
see Repair, Muscles 0KQ
see Reposition, Muscles 0KS
Musculophrenic artery
use Internal Mammary Artery, Left
use Internal Mammary Artery, Right
Musculoplasty
see Repair, Muscles 0KQ
see Supplement, Muscles 0KU
Musculorrhaphy *see* Repair, Muscles 0KQ
Musculospiral nerve *use* Radial Nerve
Myectomy
see Excision, Muscles 0KB
see Resection, Muscles 0KT
Myelencephalon *use* Medulla Oblongata
Myelogram
CT *see* Computerized Tomography (CT Scan),
Central Nervous System B02
MRI *see* Magnetic Resonance Imaging (MRI), Cen-
tral Nervous System B03
Myenteric (Auerbach's) plexus *use* Abdominal Sym-
pathetic Nerve
Myocardial Bridge Release *see* Release, Artery,
Coronary
Myomectomy *see* Excision, Female Reproductive Sys-
tem 0UB
Myometrium *use* Uterus
Myopexy
see Repair, Muscles 0KQ
see Reposition, Muscles 0KS
Myoplasty
see Repair, Muscles 0KQ
see Supplement, Muscles 0KU
Myorrhaphy *see* Repair, Muscles 0KQ
Myoscopy *see* Inspection, Muscles 0KJ
Myotomy
see Division, Muscles 0K8
see Drainage, Muscles 0K9
Myringectomy
see Excision, Ear, Nose, Sinus 09B
see Resection, Ear, Nose, Sinus 09T
Myringoplasty
see Repair, Ear, Nose, Sinus 09Q
see Replacement, Ear, Nose, Sinus 09R
see Supplement, Ear, Nose, Sinus 09U
Myringostomy *see* Drainage, Ear, Nose, Sinus 099
Myringotomy *see* Drainage, Ear, Nose, Sinus 099

N

NA-1 (Nerinitide) *use* Nerinitide
Nafamostat Anticoagulant XY0YX37
Nail bed
use Finger Nail
use Toe Nail
Nail plate
use Finger Nail
use Toe Nail
nanoLOCK™ interbody fusion device *use* Interbody
Fusion Device, Nanotextured Surface in New
Technology
Narcosynthesis GZGZZZZ
Narsoplimab Monoclonal Antibody XW0
Nasal cavity *use* Nasal Mucosa and Soft Tissue
Nasal concha *use* Nasal Turbinate
Nasalis muscle *use* Facial Muscle
Nasolacrimal duct
use Lacrimal Duct, Left
use Lacrimal Duct, Right
Nasopharyngeal airway (NPA) *use* Intraluminal De-
vice, Airway in Ear, Nose, Sinus
Navicular bone
use Tarsal, Left
use Tarsal, Right
Near Infrared Spectroscopy, Circulatory System
8E02
Neck of femur
use Upper Femur, Left
use Upper Femur, Right
Neck of humerus (anatomical) (surgical)
use Humeral Head, Left
use Humeral Head, Right
Neovasc Reducer™ *use* Reduction Device in New
Technology
Nephrectomy
see Excision, Urinary System 0TB
see Resection, Urinary System 0TT
Nephrolithotomy *see* Extirpation, Urinary System 0TC
Nephrolysis *see* Release, Urinary System 0TN
Nephropexy
see Repair, Urinary System 0TQ
see Reposition, Urinary System 0TS
Nephroplasty
see Repair, Urinary System 0TQ
see Supplement, Urinary System 0TU
Nephropyeloureterostomy
see Bypass, Urinary System 0T1
see Drainage, Urinary System 0T9
Nephrorrhaphy *see* Repair, Urinary System 0TQ
Nephroscopy, transurethral 0TJ58ZZ
Nephrostomy
see Bypass, Urinary System 0T1
see Drainage, Urinary System 0T9
Nephrotomography
see Fluoroscopy, Urinary System BT1
see Plain Radiography, Urinary System BT0
Nephrotomy
see Division, Urinary System 0T8
see Drainage, Urinary System 0T9
Nerinitide XW0
Nerve conduction study
see Measurement, Central Nervous 4A00
see Measurement, Peripheral Nervous 4A01
Nerve Function Assessment F01
Nerve to the stapedius *use* Facial Nerve
Nesiritide *use* Human B-Type Natriuretic Peptide
Neurectomy
see Excision, Central Nervous System and Cranial
Nerves 00B
see Excision, Peripheral Nervous System 01B
Neurexeresis
see Extraction, Central Nervous System and Cranial
Nerves 00D
see Extraction, Peripheral Nervous System 01D
Neurohypophysis *use* Pituitary Gland
Neurolysis
see Release, Central Nervous System and Cranial
Nerves 00N
see Release, Peripheral Nervous System 01N
Neuromuscular electrical stimulation (NEMS) lead
use Stimulator Lead in Muscles
Neurophysiologic monitoring *see* Monitoring, Central
Nervous 4A10

Neuroplasty
see Repair, Central Nervous System and Cranial
　　Nerves 00Q
see Repair, Peripheral Nervous System 01Q
see Supplement, Central Nervous System and
　　Cranial Nerves 00U
see Supplement, Peripheral Nervous System 01U

Neurorrhaphy
see Repair, Central Nervous System and Cranial
　　Nerves 00Q
see Repair, Peripheral Nervous System 01Q

Neurostimulator Generator
Insertion of device in, Skull 0NH00NZ
Removal of device from, Skull 0NP00NZ
Revision of device in, Skull 0NW00NZ

Neurostimulator generator, multiple channel use
　Stimulator Generator, Multiple Array in 0JH

**Neurostimulator generator, multiple channel
　rechargeable** use Stimulator Generator, Multiple
　Array Rechargeable in 0JH

Neurostimulator generator, single channel use
　Stimulator Generator, Single Array in 0JH

**Neurostimulator generator, single channel
　rechargeable** use Stimulator Generator, Single
　Array Rechargeable in 0JH

Neurostimulator Lead
Insertion of device in
　Brain 00H0
　Cerebral Ventricle 00H6
　Nerve
　　Cranial 00HE
　　Peripheral 01HY
　Spinal Canal 00HU
　Spinal Cord 00HV
　Vein
　　Azygos 05H0
　　Innominate
　　　Left 05H4
　　　Right 05H3
Removal of device from
　Brain 00P0
　Cerebral Ventricle 00P6
　Nerve
　　Cranial 00PE
　　Peripheral 01PY
　Spinal Canal 00PU
　Spinal Cord 00PV
　Vein
　　Azygos 05P0
　　Innominate
　　　Left 05P4
　　　Right 05P3
Revision of device in
　Brain 00W0
　Cerebral Ventricle 00W6
　Nerve
　　Cranial 00WE
　　Peripheral 01WY
　Spinal Canal 00WU
　Spinal Cord 00WV
　Vein
　　Azygos 05W0
　　Innominate
　　　Left 05W4
　　　Right 05W3

Neurostimulator Lead in Oropharynx XWHD7Q7
Neurotomy
see Division, Central Nervous System and Cranial
　　Nerves 008
see Division, Peripheral Nervous System 018

Neurotripsy
see Destruction, Central Nervous System and Cra-
　　nial Nerves 005
see Destruction, Peripheral Nervous System 015

Neutralization plate
use Internal Fixation Device in Head and Facial
　　Bones
use Internal Fixation Device in Lower Bones
use Internal Fixation Device in Upper Bones

New Technology
Amivantamab Monoclonal Antibody XW0
Antibiotic-eluting Bone Void Filler XW0V0P7
Aorta
　Thoracic Arch using Branched Synthetic
　　Substitute with Intraluminal Device
　　X2RX0N7

New Technology — continued
Aorta — continued
　Thoracic Descending using Branched Synthet-
　　ic Substitute with Intraluminal Device
　　X2VW0N7
Apalutamide Antineoplastic XW0DXJ5
Atezolizumab Antineoplastic XW0
Axicabtagene Ciloleucel Immunotherapy XW0
Bamlanivimab Monoclonal Antibody XW0
Baricitinib XW0
Bezlotoxumab Monoclonal Antibody XW0
Bioengineered Allogeneic Construct, Skin XHRPXF7
Brexanolone XW0
Brexucabtagene Autoleucel Immunotherapy XW0
Bromelain-enriched Proteolytic Enzyme XW0
Caplacizumab XW0
CD24Fc Immunomodulator XW0
Cefiderocol Anti-infective XW0
Ceftolozane/Tazobactam Anti-infective XW0
Cerebral Embolic Filtration
　Dual Filter X2A5312
　Extracorporeal Flow Reversal Circuit X2A
　Single Deflection Filter X2A6325
Ciltacabtagene Autoleucel XW0
Coagulation Factor Xa, Inactivated XW0
Computer-aided Assessment, Intracranial Vascular
　　Activity XXE0X07
Computer-aided Guidance, Transthoracic
　　Echocardiography X2JAX47
Computer-aided Mechanical Aspiration X2C
Computer-aided Triage and Notification, Pul-
　　monary Artery Flow XXE3X27
Concentrated Bone Marrow Aspirate XK02303
Coronary Sinus, Reduction Device X2V73Q7
COVID-19 Vaccine XW0
COVID-19 Vaccine Dose 1 XW0
COVID-19 Vaccine Dose 2 XW0
Cytarabine and Daunorubicin Liposome Antineo-
　　plastic XW0
Defibrotide Sodium Anticoagulant XW0
Destruction, Prostate, Robotic Waterjet Ablation
　　XV508A4
Dilation
　Anterior Tibial
　　Left
　　　Sustained Release Drug-eluting
　　　　Intraluminal Device
　　　　X27Q385
　　　Four or More X27Q3C5
　　　Three X27Q3B5
　　　Two X27Q395
　　Right
　　　Sustained Release Drug-eluting
　　　　Intraluminal Device
　　　　X27P385
　　　Four or More X27P3C5
　　　Three X27P3B5
　　　Two X27P395
　Femoral
　　Left
　　　Sustained Release Drug-eluting
　　　　Intraluminal Device
　　　　X27J385
　　　Four or More X27J3C5
　　　Three X27J3B5
　　　Two X27J395
　　Right
　　　Sustained Release Drug-eluting
　　　　Intraluminal Device
　　　　X27H385
　　　Four or More X27H3C5
　　　Three X27H3B5
　　　Two X27H395
　Peroneal
　　Left
　　　Sustained Release Drug-eluting
　　　　Intraluminal Device
　　　　X27U385
　　　Four or More X27U3C5
　　　Three X27U3B5
　　　Two X27U395
　　Right
　　　Sustained Release Drug-eluting
　　　　Intraluminal Device
　　　　X27T385
　　　Four or More X27T3C5
　　　Three X27T3B5
　　　Two X27T395

New Technology — continued
Dilation — continued
　Popliteal
　　Left Distal
　　　Sustained Release Drug-eluting
　　　　Intraluminal Device
　　　　X27N385
　　　Four or More X27N3C5
　　　Three X27N3B5
　　　Two X27N395
　　Left Proximal
　　　Sustained Release Drug-eluting
　　　　Intraluminal Device
　　　　X27L385
　　　Four or More X27L3C5
　　　Three X27L3B5
　　　Two X27L395
　　Right Distal
　　　Sustained Release Drug-eluting
　　　　Intraluminal Device
　　　　X27M385
　　　Four or More X27M3C5
　　　Three X27M3B5
　　　Two X27M395
　　Right Proximal
　　　Sustained Release Drug-eluting
　　　　Intraluminal Device
　　　　X27K385
　　　Four or More X27K3C5
　　　Three X27K3B5
　　　Two X27K395
　Posterior Tibial
　　Left
　　　Sustained Release Drug-eluting
　　　　Intraluminal Device
　　　　X27S385
　　　Four or More X27S3C5
　　　Three X27S3B5
　　　Two X27S395
　　Right
　　　Sustained Release Drug-eluting
　　　　Intraluminal Device
　　　　X27R385
　　　Four or More X27R3C5
　　　Three X27R3B5
　　　Two X27R395
Durvalumab Antineoplastic XW0
Eculizumab XW0
Eladocagene exuparvovec XW0Q316
Endothelial Damage Inhibitor XY0VX83
Engineered Chimeric Antigen Receptor T-cell Im-
　　munotherapy
　Allogeneic XW0
　Autologous XW0
Erdafitinib Antineoplastic XW0DXL5
Esketamine Hydrochloride XW097M5
Etesevimab Monoclonal Antibody XW0
Fosfomycin Anti-infective XW0
Fusion
　Cervical Vertebral
　　2 or more
　　　Nanotextured Surface XRG2092
　　　Radiolucent Porous XRG20F3
　　Interbody Fusion Device
　　　Nanotextured Surface XRG1092
　　　Radiolucent Porous XRG10F3
　Cervicothoracic Vertebral
　　Nanotextured Surface XRG4092
　　Radiolucent Porous XRG40F3
　Lumbar Vertebral
　　2 or more
　　　Customizable XRGC
　　　Nanotextured Surface XRGC092
　　　Radiolucent Porous XRGC0F3
　　Interbody Fusion Device
　　　Customizable XRGB
　　　Nanotextured Surface XRGB092
　　　Radiolucent Porous XRGB0F3
　Lumbosacral
　　Customizable XRGD
　　Nanotextured Surface XRGD092
　　Radiolucent Porous XRGD0F3
　Occipital-cervical
　　Nanotextured Surface XRG0092
　　Radiolucent Porous XRG00F3
　Thoracic Vertebral
　　2 to 7
　　　Nanotextured Surface XRG7092
　　　Radiolucent Porous XRG70F3

Occlusion — *continued*
  Artery — *continued*
    Pulmonary — *continued*
      Right 02LQ
    Pulmonary Trunk 02LP
    Radial
      Left 03LC
      Right 03LB
    Renal
      Left 04LA
      Right 04L9
    Splenic 04L4
    Subclavian
      Left 03L4
      Right 03L3
    Superior Mesenteric 04L5
    Temporal
      Left 03LT
      Right 03LS
    Thyroid
      Left 03LV
      Right 03LU
    Ulnar
      Left 03LA
      Right 03L9
    Upper 03LY
    Vertebral
      Left 03LQ
      Right 03LP
  Atrium, Left 02L7
  Bladder 0TLB
  Bladder Neck 0TLC
  Bronchus
    Lingula 0BL9
    Lower Lobe
      Left 0BLB
      Right 0BL6
    Main
      Left 0BL7
      Right 0BL3
    Middle Lobe, Right 0BL5
    Upper Lobe
      Left 0BL8
      Right 0BL4
  Carina 0BL2
  Cecum 0DLH
  Cisterna Chyli 07LL
  Colon
    Ascending 0DLK
    Descending 0DLM
    Sigmoid 0DLN
    Transverse 0DLL
  Cord
    Bilateral 0VLH
    Left 0VLG
    Right 0VLF
  Cul-de-sac 0ULF
  Duct
    Common Bile 0FL9
    Cystic 0FL8
    Hepatic
      Common 0FL7
      Left 0FL6
      Right 0FL5
    Lacrimal
      Left 08LY
      Right 08LX
    Pancreatic 0FLD
      Accessory 0FLF
    Parotid
      Left 0CLC
      Right 0CLB
  Duodenum 0DL9
  Esophagogastric Junction 0DL4
  Esophagus 0DL5
    Lower 0DL3
    Middle 0DL2
    Upper 0DL1
  Fallopian Tube
    Left 0UL6
    Right 0UL5
  Fallopian Tubes, Bilateral 0UL7
  Ileocecal Valve 0DLC
  Ileum 0DLB
  Intestine
    Large 0DLE
      Left 0DLG
      Right 0DLF
    Small 0DL8

Occlusion — *continued*
  Jejunum 0DLA
  Kidney Pelvis
    Left 0TL4
    Right 0TL3
  Left atrial appendage (LAA) *see* Occlusion, Atrium, Left 02L7
  Lymphatic
    Aortic 07LD
    Axillary
      Left 07L6
      Right 07L5
    Head 07L0
    Inguinal
      Left 07LJ
      Right 07LH
    Internal Mammary
      Left 07L9
      Right 07L8
    Lower Extremity
      Left 07LG
      Right 07LF
    Mesenteric 07LB
    Neck
      Left 07L2
      Right 07L1
    Pelvis 07LC
    Thoracic Duct 07LK
    Thorax 07L7
    Upper Extremity
      Left 07L4
      Right 07L3
  Rectum 0DLP
  Stomach 0DL6
    Pylorus 0DL7
  Trachea 0BL1
  Ureter
    Left 0TL7
    Right 0TL6
  Urethra 0TLD
  Vagina 0ULG
  Valve, Pulmonary 02LH
  Vas Deferens
    Bilateral 0VLQ
    Left 0VLP
    Right 0VLN
  Vein
    Axillary
      Left 05L8
      Right 05L7
    Azygos 05L0
    Basilic
      Left 05LC
      Right 05LB
    Brachial
      Left 05LA
      Right 05L9
    Cephalic
      Left 05LF
      Right 05LD
    Colic 06L7
    Common Iliac
      Left 06LD
      Right 06LC
    Esophageal 06L3
    External Iliac
      Left 06LG
      Right 06LF
    External Jugular
      Left 05LQ
      Right 05LP
    Face
      Left 05LV
      Right 05LT
    Femoral
      Left 06LN
      Right 06LM
    Foot
      Left 06LV
      Right 06LT
    Gastric 06L2
    Hand
      Left 05LH
      Right 05LG
    Hemiazygos 05L1
    Hepatic 06L4
    Hypogastric
      Left 06LJ
      Right 06LH

Occlusion — *continued*
  Vein — *continued*
    Inferior Mesenteric 06L6
    Innominate
      Left 05L4
      Right 05L3
    Internal Jugular
      Left 05LN
      Right 05LM
    Intracranial 05LL
    Lower 06LY
    Portal 06L8
    Pulmonary
      Left 02LT
      Right 02LS
    Renal
      Left 06LB
      Right 06L9
    Saphenous
      Left 06LQ
      Right 06LP
    Splenic 06L1
    Subclavian
      Left 05L6
      Right 05L5
    Superior Mesenteric 06L5
    Upper 05LY
    Vertebral
      Left 05LS
      Right 05LR
  Vena Cava
    Inferior 06L0
    Superior 02LV

Occlusion, REBOA (resuscitative endovascular balloon occlusion of the aorta)
  02LW3DJ
  04L03DJ

Occupational therapy *see* Activities of Daily Living Treatment, Rehabilitation F08

Octagam 10%, for COVID-19 treatment *use* High-Dose Intravenous Immune Globulin

Odentectomy
  see Excision, Mouth and Throat 0CB
  see Resection, Mouth and Throat 0CT

Odontoid process *use* Cervical Vertebra

Olecranon bursa
  use Elbow Bursa and Ligament, Left
  use Elbow Bursa and Ligament, Right

Olecranon process
  use Ulna, Left
  use Ulna, Right

Olfactory bulb *use* Olfactory Nerve

Olumiant® *use* Baricitinib

Omadacycline Anti-infective XW0

Omentectomy, omentumectomy
  see Excision, Gastrointestinal System 0DB
  see Resection, Gastrointestinal System 0DT

Omentofixation *see* Repair, Gastrointestinal System 0DQ

Omentoplasty
  see Repair, Gastrointestinal System 0DQ
  see Replacement, Gastrointestinal System 0DR
  see Supplement, Gastrointestinal System 0DU

Omentorrhaphy *see* Repair, Gastrointestinal System 0DQ

Omentotomy *see* Drainage, Gastrointestinal System 0D9

Omnilink Elite Vascular Balloon Expandable Stent System *use* Intraluminal Device

Onychectomy
  see Excision, Skin and Breast 0HB
  see Resection, Skin and Breast 0HT

Onychoplasty
  see Repair, Skin and Breast 0HQ
  see Replacement, Skin and Breast 0HR

Onychotomy *see* Drainage, Skin and Breast 0H9

Oophorectomy
  see Excision, Female Reproductive System 0UB
  see Resection, Female Reproductive System 0UT

Oophoropexy
  see Repair, Female Reproductive System 0UQ
  see Reposition, Female Reproductive System 0US

Oophoroplasty
  see Repair, Female Reproductive System 0UQ
  see Supplement, Female Reproductive System 0UU

Oophorrhaphy *see* Repair, Female Reproductive System 0UQ

Oophorostomy *see* Drainage, Female Reproductive System 0U9
Oophorotomy
　see Division, Female Reproductive System 0U8
　see Drainage, Female Reproductive System 0U9
Oophorrhaphy *see* Repair, Female Reproductive System 0UQ
Open Pivot Aortic Valve Graft (AVG) *use* Synthetic Substitute
Open Pivot (mechanical) Valve *use* Synthetic Substitute
Ophthalmic artery *use* Intracranial Artery
Ophthalmic nerve *use* Trigeminal Nerve
Ophthalmic vein *use* Intracranial Vein
Opponensplasty
　Tendon replacement *see* Replacement, Tendons 0LR
　Tendon transfer *see* Transfer, Tendons 0LX
Optic chiasma *use* Optic Nerve
Optic disc
　use Retina, Left
　use Retina, Right
Optic foramen *use* Sphenoid Bone
Optical coherence tomography, intravascular *see* Computerized Tomography (CT Scan)
Optimizer™ III implantable pulse generator *use* Contractility Modulation Device in 0JH
Orbicularis oculi muscle
　use Upper Eyelid, Left
　use Upper Eyelid, Right
Orbicularis oris muscle *use* Facial Muscle
Orbital Atherectomy *see* Extirpation, Heart and Great Vessels 02C
Orbital fascia *use* Subcutaneous Tissue and Fascia, Face
Orbital portion of ethmoid bone
　use Orbit, Left
　use Orbit, Right
Orbital portion of frontal bone
　use Orbit, Left
　use Orbit, Right
Orbital portion of lacrimal bone
　use Orbit, Left
　use Orbit, Right
Orbital portion of maxilla
　use Orbit, Left
　use Orbit, Right
Orbital portion of palatine bone
　use Orbit, Left
　use Orbit, Right
Orbital portion of sphenoid bone
　use Orbit, Left
　use Orbit, Right
Orbital portion of zygomatic bone
　use Orbit, Left
　use Orbit, Right
Orchectomy, orchidectomy, orchiectomy
　see Excision, Male Reproductive System 0VB
　see Resection, Male Reproductive System 0VT
Orchidoplasty, orchioplasty
　see Repair, Male Reproductive System 0VQ
　see Replacement, Male Reproductive System 0VR
　see Supplement, Male Reproductive System 0VU
Orchidorrhaphy, orchiorrhaphy *see* Repair, Male Reproductive System 0VQ
Orchidotomy, orchiotomy, orchotomy *see* Drainage, Male Reproductive System 0V9
Orchiopexy
　see Repair, Male Reproductive System 0VQ
　see Reposition, Male Reproductive System 0VS
Oropharyngeal airway (OPA) *use* Intraluminal Device, Airway in Mouth and Throat
Oropharynx *use* Pharynx
Ossiculectomy
　see Excision, Ear, Nose, Sinus 09B
　see Resection, Ear, Nose, Sinus 09T
Ossiculotomy *see* Drainage, Ear, Nose, Sinus 099
Ostectomy
　see Excision, Head and Facial Bones 0NB
　see Excision, Lower Bones 0QB
　see Excision, Upper Bones 0PB
　see Resection, Head and Facial Bones 0NT
　see Resection, Lower Bones 0QT
　see Resection, Upper Bones 0PT
Osteoclasis
　see Division, Head and Facial Bones 0N8

Osteoclasis — *continued*
　see Division, Lower Bones 0Q8
　see Division, Upper Bones 0P8
Osteolysis
　see Release, Head and Facial Bones 0NN
　see Release, Lower Bones 0QN
　see Release, Upper Bones 0PN
Osteopathic Treatment
　Abdomen 7W09X
　Cervical 7W01X
　Extremity
　　Lower 7W06X
　　Upper 7W07X
　Head 7W00X
　Lumbar 7W03X
　Pelvis 7W05X
　Rib Cage 7W08X
　Sacrum 7W04X
　Thoracic 7W02X
Osteopexy
　see Repair, Head and Facial Bones 0NQ
　see Repair, Lower Bones 0QQ
　see Repair, Upper Bones 0PQ
　see Reposition, Head and Facial Bones 0NS
　see Reposition, Lower Bones 0QS
　see Reposition, Upper Bones 0PS
Osteoplasty
　see Repair, Head and Facial Bones 0NQ
　see Repair, Lower Bones 0QQ
　see Repair, Upper Bones 0PQ
　see Replacement, Head and Facial Bones 0NR
　see Replacement, Lower Bones 0QR
　see Replacement, Upper Bones 0PR
　see Supplement, Head and Facial Bones 0NU
　see Supplement, Lower Bones 0QU
　see Supplement, Upper Bones 0PU
Osteorrhaphy
　see Repair, Head and Facial Bones 0NQ
　see Repair, Lower Bones 0QQ
　see Repair, Upper Bones 0PQ
Osteotomy, ostotomy
　see Division, Head and Facial Bones 0N8
　see Division, Lower Bones 0Q8
　see Division, Upper Bones 0P8
　see Drainage, Head and Facial Bones 0N9
　see Drainage, Lower Bones 0Q9
　see Drainage, Upper Bones 0P9
Other Imaging
　Bile Duct and Gallbladder, Indocyanine Green Dye, Intraoperative BF53200
　Bile Duct, Indocyanine Green Dye, Intraoperative BF50200
　Extremity
　　Lower BW5CZ1Z
　　Upper BW5JZ1Z
　Gallbladder and Bile Duct, Indocyanine Green Dye, Intraoperative BF53200
　Gallbladder, Indocyanine Green Dye, Intraoperative BF52200
　Head and Neck BW59Z1Z
　Hepatobiliary System, All, Indocyanine Green Dye, Intraoperative BF5C200
　Liver and Spleen, Indocyanine Green Dye, Intraoperative BF56200
　Liver, Indocyanine Green Dye, Intraoperative BF55200
　Neck and Head BW59Z1Z
　Pancreas, Indocyanine Green Dye, Intraoperative BF57200
　Spleen and Liver, Indocyanine Green Dye, Intraoperative BF56200
　Trunk BW52Z1Z
Other New Technology Monoclonal Antibody XW0
Other New Technology Therapeutic Substance XW0
Otic ganglion *use* Head and Neck Sympathetic Nerve
OTL-101 *use* Hematopoietic Stem/Progenitor Cells, Genetically Modified
OTL-103 *use* Hematopoietic Stem/Progenitor Cells, Genetically Modified
OTL-200 *use* Hematopoietic Stem/Progenitor Cells, Genetically Modified
Otoplasty
　see Repair, Ear, Nose, Sinus 09Q
　see Replacement, Ear, Nose, Sinus 09R
　see Supplement, Ear, Nose, Sinus 09U
Otoscopy *see* Inspection, Ear, Nose, Sinus 09J

Oval window
　use Middle Ear, Left
　use Middle Ear, Right
Ovarian artery *use* Abdominal Aorta
Ovarian ligament *use* Uterine Supporting Structure
Ovariectomy
　see Excision, Female Reproductive System 0UB
　see Resection, Female Reproductive System 0UT
Ovariocentesis *see* Drainage, Female Reproductive System 0U9
Ovariopexy
　see Repair, Female Reproductive System 0UQ
　see Reposition, Female Reproductive System 0US
Ovariotomy
　see Division, Female Reproductive System 0U8
　see Drainage, Female Reproductive System 0U9
Ovatio™ CRT-D *use* Cardiac Resynchronization Defibrillator Pulse Generator in 0JH
Oversewing
　Gastrointestinal ulcer *see* Repair, Gastrointestinal System 0DQ
　Pleural bleb *see* Repair, Respiratory System 0BQ
Oviduct
　use Fallopian Tube, Left
　use Fallopian Tube, Right
Oximetry, Fetal pulse 10H073Z
OXINIUM *use* Synthetic Substitute, Oxidized Zirconium on Polyethylene in 0SR
Oxygen Saturation Endoscopic Imaging (OXEI) XD2
Oxygenation
　Extracorporeal membrane (ECMO) *see* Performance, Circulatory 5A15
　Hyperbaric *see* Assistance, Circulatory 5A05
　Supersaturated *see* Assistance, Circulatory 5A05

P

Pacemaker
　Dual Chamber
　　Abdomen 0JH8
　　Chest 0JH6
　Intracardiac
　　Insertion of device in
　　　Atrium
　　　　Left 02H7
　　　　Right 02H6
　　　Vein, Coronary 02H4
　　　Ventricle
　　　　Left 02HL
　　　　Right 02HK
　　Removal of device from, Heart 02PA
　　Revision of device in, Heart 02WA
　Single Chamber
　　Abdomen 0JH8
　　Chest 0JH6
　Single Chamber Rate Responsive
　　Abdomen 0JH8
　　Chest 0JH6
Packing
　Abdominal Wall 2W43X5Z
　Anorectal 2Y43X5Z
　Arm
　　Lower
　　　Left 2W4DX5Z
　　　Right 2W4CX5Z
　　Upper
　　　Left 2W4BX5Z
　　　Right 2W4AX5Z
　Back 2W45X5Z
　Chest Wall 2W44X5Z
　Ear 2Y42X5Z
　Extremity
　　Lower
　　　Left 2W4MX5Z
　　　Right 2W4LX5Z
　　Upper
　　　Left 2W49X5Z
　　　Right 2W48X5Z
　Face 2W41X5Z
　Finger
　　Left 2W4KX5Z
　　Right 2W4JX5Z
　Foot
　　Left 2W4TX5Z
　　Right 2W4SX5Z
　Genital Tract, Female 2Y44X5Z

Packing — *continued*
Hand
Left 2W4FX5Z
Right 2W4EX5Z
Head 2W40X5Z
Inguinal Region
Left 2W47X5Z
Right 2W46X5Z
Leg
Lower
Left 2W4RX5Z
Right 2W4QX5Z
Upper
Left 2W4PX5Z
Right 2W4NX5Z
Mouth and Pharynx 2Y40X5Z
Nasal 2Y41X5Z
Neck 2W42X5Z
Thumb
Left 2W4HX5Z
Right 2W4GX5Z
Toe
Left 2W4VX5Z
Right 2W4UX5Z
Urethra 2Y45X5Z
Paclitaxel-eluting coronary stent *use* Intraluminal Device, Drug-eluting in Heart and Great Vessels
Paclitaxel-eluting peripheral stent
use Intraluminal Device, Drug-eluting in Lower Arteries
use Intraluminal Device, Drug-eluting in Upper Arteries
Palatine gland *use* Buccal Mucosa
Palatine tonsil *use* Tonsils
Palatine uvula *use* Uvula
Palatoglossal muscle *use* Tongue, Palate, Pharynx Muscle
Palatopharyngeal muscle *use* Tongue, Palate, Pharynx Muscle
Palatoplasty
see Repair, Mouth and Throat 0CQ
see Replacement, Mouth and Throat 0CR
see Supplement, Mouth and Throat 0CU
Palatorrhaphy *see* Repair, Mouth and Throat 0CQ
Palmar cutaneous nerve
use Median Nerve
use Radial Nerve
Palmar (volar) digital vein
use Hand Vein, Left
use Hand Vein, Right
Palmar fascia (aponeurosis)
use Subcutaneous Tissue and Fascia, Left Hand
use Subcutaneous Tissue and Fascia, Right Hand
Palmar interosseous muscle
use Hand Muscle, Left
use Hand Muscle, Right
Palmar (volar) metacarpal vein
use Hand Vein, Left
use Hand Vein, Right
Palmar ulnocarpal ligament
use Wrist Bursa and Ligament, Left
use Wrist Bursa and Ligament, Right
Palmaris longus muscle
use Lower Arm and Wrist Muscle, Left
use Lower Arm and Wrist Muscle, Right
Pancreatectomy
see Excision, Pancreas 0FBG
see Resection, Pancreas 0FTG
Pancreatic artery *use* Splenic Artery
Pancreatic plexus *use* Abdominal Sympathetic Nerve
Pancreatic vein *use* Splenic Vein
Pancreaticoduodenostomy *see* Bypass, Hepatobiliary System and Pancreas 0F1
Pancreaticosplenic lymph node *use* Lymphatic, Aortic
Pancreatogram, endoscopic retrograde *see* Fluoroscopy, Pancreatic Duct BF18
Pancreatolithotomy *see* Extirpation, Pancreas 0FCG
Pancreatotomy
see Division, Pancreas 0F8G
see Drainage, Pancreas 0F9G
Panniculectomy
see Excision, Skin, Abdomen 0HB7
see Excision, Subcutaneous Tissue and Fascia, Abdomen 0JB8
Paraaortic lymph node *use* Lymphatic, Aortic

Paracentesis
Eye *see* Drainage, Eye 089
Peritoneal Cavity *see* Drainage, Peritoneal Cavity 0W9G
Tympanum *see* Drainage, Ear, Nose, Sinus 099
Parapharyngeal space *use* Neck
Pararectal lymph node *use* Lymphatic, Mesenteric
Parasternal lymph node *use* Lymphatic, Thorax
Parathyroidectomy
see Excision, Endocrine System 0GB
see Resection, Endocrine System 0GT
Paratracheal lymph node *use* Lymphatic, Thorax
Paraurethral (Skene's) gland *use* Vestibular Gland
Parenteral nutrition, total *see* Introduction of Nutritional Substance
Parietal lobe *use* Cerebral Hemisphere
Parotid lymph node *use* Lymphatic, Head
Parotid plexus *use* Facial Nerve
Parotidectomy
see Excision, Mouth and Throat 0CB
see Resection, Mouth and Throat 0CT
Pars flaccida
use Tympanic Membrane, Left
use Tympanic Membrane, Right
Partial joint replacement
Hip *see* Replacement, Lower Joints 0SR
Knee *see* Replacement, Lower Joints 0SR
Shoulder *see* Replacement, Upper Joints 0RR
Partially absorbable mesh *use* Synthetic Substitute
Patch, blood, spinal 3E0R3GC
Patellapexy
see Repair, Lower Bones 0QQ
see Reposition, Lower Bones 0QS
Patellaplasty
see Repair, Lower Bones 0QQ
see Replacement, Lower Bones 0QR
see Supplement, Lower Bones 0QU
Patellar ligament
use Knee Bursa and Ligament, Left
use Knee Bursa and Ligament, Right
Patellar tendon
use Knee Tendon, Left
use Knee Tendon, Right
Patellectomy
see Excision, Lower Bones 0QB
see Resection, Lower Bones 0QT
Patellofemoral joint
use Knee Joint, Left
use Knee Joint, Left, Femoral Surface
use Knee Joint, Right
use Knee Joint, Right, Femoral Surface
pAVF (percutaneous arteriovenous fistula), using magnetic-guided radiofrequency *see* Bypass, Upper Arteries 031
pAVF (percutaneous arteriovenous fistula), using thermal resistance energy *see* New Technology, Cardiovascular System X2K
Pectineus muscle
use Upper Leg Muscle, Left
use Upper Leg Muscle, Right
Pectoral fascia *use* Subcutaneous Tissue and Fascia, Chest
Pectoral (anterior) lymph node
use Lymphatic Left, Axillary
use Lymphatic Right, Axillary
Pectoralis major muscle
use Thorax Muscle, Left
use Thorax Muscle, Right
Pectoralis minor muscle
use Thorax Muscle, Left
use Thorax Muscle, Right
Pedicle-based dynamic stabilization device
use Spinal Stabilization Device, Pedicle-Based in 0SH
use Spinal Stabilization Device, Pedicle-Based in 0RH
PEEP (positive end expiratory pressure) *see* Assistance, Respiratory 5A09
PEG (percutaneous endoscopic gastrostomy) 0DH63UZ
PEJ (percutaneous endoscopic jejunostomy) 0DHA3UZ
Pelvic splanchnic nerve
use Abdominal Sympathetic Nerve
use Sacral Sympathetic Nerve

Penectomy
see Excision, Male Reproductive System 0VB
see Resection, Male Reproductive System 0VT
Penile urethra *use* Urethra
Penumbra Indigo® Aspiration System *see* New Technology, Cardiovascular System X2C
PERCEPT™ PC neurostimulator *use* Stimulator Generator, Multiple Array in 0JH
Perceval sutureless valve *use* Zooplastic Tissue, Rapid Deployment Technique in New Technology
Percutaneous endoscopic gastrojejunostomy (PEG/J) tube *use* Feeding Device in Gastrointestinal System
Percutaneous endoscopic gastrostomy (PEG) tube *use* Feeding Device in Gastrointestinal System
Percutaneous nephrostomy catheter *use* Drainage Device
Percutaneous transluminal coronary angioplasty (PTCA) *see* Dilation, Heart and Great Vessels 027
Performance
Biliary
Multiple, Filtration 5A1C60Z
Single, Filtration 5A1C00Z
Cardiac
Continuous
Output 5A1221Z
Pacing 5A1223Z
Intermittent, Pacing 5A1213Z
Single, Output, Manual 5A12012
Circulatory
Continuous
Central Membrane 5A1522F
Peripheral Veno-arterial Membrane 5A1522G
Peripheral Veno-venous Membrane 5A1522H
Intraoperative
Central Membrane 5A15A2F
Peripheral Veno-arterial Membrane 5A15A2G
Peripheral Veno-venous Membrane 5A15A2H
Respiratory
24-96 Consecutive Hours, Ventilation 5A1945Z
Greater than 96 Consecutive Hours, Ventilation 5A1955Z
Less than 24 Consecutive Hours, Ventilation 5A1935Z
Single, Ventilation, Nonmechanical 5A19054
Urinary
Continuous, Greater than 18 hours per day, Filtration 5A1D90Z
Intermittent, Less than 6 Hours Per Day, Filtration 5A1D70Z
Prolonged Intermittent, 6-18 hours per day, Filtration 5A1D80Z
Perfusion *see* Introduction of substance in or on
Perfusion, donor organ
Heart 6AB50BZ
Kidney(s) 6ABT0BZ
Liver 6ABF0BZ
Lung(s) 6ABB0BZ
Pericardiectomy
see Excision, Pericardium 02BN
see Resection, Pericardium 02TN
Pericardiocentesis *see* Drainage, Pericardial Cavity 0W9D
Pericardiolysis *see* Release, Pericardium 02NN
Pericardiophrenic artery
use Internal Mammary Artery, Left
use Internal Mammary Artery, Right
Pericardioplasty
see Repair, Pericardium 02QN
see Replacement, Pericardium 02RN
see Supplement, Pericardium 02UN
Pericardiorrhaphy *see* Repair, Pericardium 02QN
Pericardiostomy *see* Drainage, Pericardial Cavity 0W9D
Pericardiotomy *see* Drainage, Pericardial Cavity 0W9D
Perimetrium *use* Uterus
Peripheral Intravascular Lithotripsy (Peripheral IVL) *see* Fragmentation
Peripheral parenteral nutrition *see* Introduction of Nutritional Substance
Peripherally inserted central catheter (PICC) *use* Infusion Device
Peritoneal dialysis 3E1M39Z

Peritoneocentesis
  see Drainage, Peritoneal Cavity ØW9G
  see Drainage, Peritoneum ØD9W
Peritoneoplasty
  see Repair, Peritoneum ØDQW
  see Replacement, Peritoneum ØDRW
  see Supplement, Peritoneum ØDUW
Peritoneoscopy ØDJW4ZZ
Peritoneotomy see Drainage, Peritoneum ØD9W
Peritoneumectomy see Excision, Peritoneum ØDBW
Peroneus brevis muscle
  use Lower Leg Muscle, Left
  use Lower Leg Muscle, Right
Peroneus longus muscle
  use Lower Leg Muscle, Left
  use Lower Leg Muscle, Right
Pessary ring use Intraluminal Device, Pessary in Female
  Reproductive System
PET scan see Positron Emission Tomographic (PET)
  Imaging
Petrous part of temoporal bone
  use Temporal Bone, Left
  use Temporal Bone, Right
Phacoemulsification, lens
  With IOL implant see Replacement, Eye Ø8R
  Without IOL implant see Extraction, Eye Ø8D
Phagenyx® System XWHD7Q7
Phalangectomy
  see Excision, Lower Bones ØQB
  see Excision, Upper Bones ØPB
  see Resection, Lower Bones ØQT
  see Resection, Upper Bones ØPT
Phallectomy
  see Excision, Penis ØVBS
  see Resection, Penis ØVTS
Phalloplasty
  see Repair, Penis ØVQS
  see Supplement, Penis ØVUS
Phallotomy see Drainage, Penis ØV9S
Pharmacotherapy, for substance abuse
  Antabuse HZ93ZZZ
  Bupropion HZ97ZZZ
  Clonidine HZ96ZZZ
  Levo-alpha-acetyl-methadol (LAAM) HZ92ZZZ
  Methadone Maintenance HZ91ZZZ
  Naloxone HZ95ZZZ
  Naltrexone HZ94ZZZ
  Nicotine Replacement HZ90ZZZ
  Psychiatric Medication HZ98ZZZ
  Replacement Medication, Other HZ99ZZZ
Pharyngeal constrictor muscle use Tongue, Palate,
  Pharynx Muscle
Pharyngeal plexus use Vagus Nerve
Pharyngeal recess use Nasopharynx
Pharyngeal tonsil use Adenoids
Pharyngogram see Fluoroscopy, Pharynix B91G
Pharyngoplasty
  see Repair, Mouth and Throat ØCQ
  see Replacement, Mouth and Throat ØCR
  see Supplement, Mouth and Throat ØCU
Pharyngorrhaphy see Repair, Mouth and Throat ØCQ
Pharyngotomy see Drainage, Mouth and Throat ØC9
Pharyngotympanic tube
  use Eustachian Tube, Left
  use Eustachian Tube, Right
Pheresis
  Erythrocytes 6A55
  Leukocytes 6A55
  Plasma 6A55
  Platelets 6A55
  Stem Cells
    Cord Blood 6A55
    Hematopoietic 6A55
Phlebectomy
  see Excision, Lower Veins Ø6B
  see Excision, Upper Veins Ø5B
  see Extraction, Lower Veins Ø6D
  see Extraction, Upper Veins Ø5D
Phlebography
  see Plain Radiography, Veins B5Ø
  Impedance 4AØ4X51
Phleborrhaphy
  see Repair, Lower Veins Ø6Q
  see Repair, Upper Veins Ø5Q
Phlebotomy
  see Drainage, Lower Veins Ø69
  see Drainage, Upper Veins Ø59

Photocoagulation
  For Destruction see Destruction
  For Repair see Repair
Photopheresis, therapeutic see Phototherapy, Circu-
  latory 6A65
Phototherapy
  Circulatory 6A65
  Skin 6A6Ø
  Ultraviolet light see Ultraviolet Light Therapy,
    Physiological Systems 6A8
Phrenectomy, phrenoneurectomy see Excision,
  Nerve, Phrenic Ø1B2
Phrenemphraxis see Destruction, Nerve, Phrenic Ø152
Phrenic nerve stimulator generator use Stimulator
  Generator in Subcutaneous Tissue and Fascia
Phrenic nerve stimulator lead use Diaphragmatic
  Pacemaker Lead in Respiratory System
Phreniclasis see Destruction, Nerve, Phrenic Ø152
Phrenicoexeresis see Extraction, Nerve, Phrenic Ø1D2
Phrenicotomy see Division, Nerve, Phrenic Ø182
Phrenicotripsy see Destruction, Nerve, Phrenic Ø152
Phrenoplasty
  see Repair, Respiratory System ØBQ
  see Supplement, Respiratory System ØBU
Phrenotomy see Drainage, Respiratory System ØB9
Physiatry see Motor Treatment, Rehabilitation FØ7
Physical medicine see Motor Treatment, Rehabilitation
  FØ7
Physical therapy see Motor Treatment, Rehabilitation
  FØ7
PHYSIOMESH™ Flexible Composite Mesh use Syn-
  thetic Substitute
Pia mater, intracranial use Cerebral Meninges
Pia mater, spinal use Spinal Meninges
Pinealectomy
  see Excision, Pineal Body ØGB1
  see Resection, Pineal Body ØGT1
Pinealoscopy ØGJ14ZZ
Pinealotomy see Drainage, Pineal Body ØG91
Pinna
  use External Ear, Bilateral
  use External Ear, Left
  use External Ear, Right
Pipeline™ (Flex) embolization device use Intraluminal Device, Flow Diverter in Ø3V
Piriform recess (sinus) use Pharynx
Piriformis muscle
  use Hip Muscle, Left
  use Hip Muscle, Right
**PIRRT (Prolonged intermittent renal replacement
  therapy)** 5A1D8ØZ
Pisiform bone
  use Carpal, Left
  use Carpal, Right
Pisohamate ligament
  use Hand Bursa and Ligament, Left
  use Hand Bursa and Ligament, Right
Pisometacarpal ligament
  use Hand Bursa and Ligament, Left
  use Hand Bursa and Ligament, Right
Pituitectomy
  see Excision, Gland, Pituitary ØGBØ
  see Resection, Gland, Pituitary ØGTØ
Plain film radiology see Plain Radiography
Plain Radiography
  Abdomen BWØØZZZ
  Abdomen and Pelvis BWØ1ZZZ
  Abdominal Lymphatic
    Bilateral B7Ø1
    Unilateral B7ØØ
  Airway, Upper BBØDZZZ
  Ankle
    Left BQØH
    Right BQØG
  Aorta
    Abdominal B4ØØ
    Thoracic B3ØØ
    Thoraco-Abdominal B3ØP
  Aorta and Bilateral Lower Extremity Arteries B4ØD
  Arch
    Bilateral BNØDZZZ
    Left BNØCZZZ
    Right BNØBZZZ
  Arm
    Left BPØFZZZ
    Right BPØEZZZ

Plain Radiography — continued
  Artery
    Brachiocephalic-Subclavian, Right B3Ø1
    Bronchial B3ØL
    Bypass Graft, Other B2ØF
    Cervico-Cerebral Arch B3ØQ
    Common Carotid
      Bilateral B3Ø5
      Left B3Ø4
      Right B3Ø3
    Coronary
      Bypass Graft
        Multiple B2Ø3
        Single B2Ø2
      Multiple B2Ø1
      Single B2ØØ
    External Carotid
      Bilateral B3ØC
      Left B3ØB
      Right B3Ø9
    Hepatic B4Ø2
    Inferior Mesenteric B4Ø5
    Intercostal B3ØL
    Internal Carotid
      Bilateral B3Ø8
      Left B3Ø7
      Right B3Ø6
    Internal Mammary Bypass Graft
      Left B2Ø8
      Right B2Ø7
    Intra-Abdominal, Other B4ØB
    Intracranial B3ØR
    Lower Extremity
      Bilateral and Aorta B4ØD
      Left B4ØG
      Right B4ØF
    Lower, Other B4ØJ
    Lumbar B4Ø9
    Pelvic B4ØC
    Pulmonary
      Left B3ØT
      Right B3ØS
    Renal
      Bilateral B4Ø8
      Left B4Ø7
      Right B4Ø6
      Transplant B4ØM
    Spinal B3ØM
    Splenic B4Ø3
    Subclavian, Left B3Ø2
    Superior Mesenteric B4Ø4
    Upper Extremity
      Bilateral B3ØK
      Left B3ØJ
      Right B3ØH
    Upper, Other B3ØN
    Vertebral
      Bilateral B3ØG
      Left B3ØF
      Right B3ØD
  Bile Duct BFØØ
  Bile Duct and Gallbladder BFØ3
  Bladder BTØØ
    Kidney and Ureter BTØ4
  Bladder and Urethra BTØB
  Bone
    Facial BNØ5ZZZ
    Nasal BNØ4ZZZ
  Bones, Long, All BWØBZZZ
  Breast
    Bilateral BHØ2ZZZ
    Left BHØ1ZZZ
    Right BHØØZZZ
  Calcaneus
    Left BQØKZZZ
    Right BQØJZZZ
  Chest BWØ3ZZZ
  Clavicle
    Left BPØ5ZZZ
    Right BPØ4ZZZ
  Coccyx BRØFZZZ
  Corpora Cavernosa BVØØ
  Dialysis Fistula B5ØW
  Dialysis Shunt B5ØW
  Disc
    Cervical BRØ1
    Lumbar BRØ3
    Thoracic BRØ2

Plain Radiography — *continued*
  Duct
    Lacrimal
      Bilateral B8Ø2
      Left B8Ø1
      Right B8ØØ
    Mammary
      Multiple
        Left BHØ6
        Right BHØ5
      Single
        Left BHØ4
        Right BHØ3
  Elbow
    Left BPØH
    Right BPØG
  Epididymis
    Left BVØ2
    Right BVØ1
  Extremity
    Lower BWØCZZZ
    Upper BWØJZZZ
  Eye
    Bilateral B8Ø7ZZZ
    Left B8Ø6ZZZ
    Right B8Ø5ZZZ
  Facet Joint
    Cervical BRØ4
    Lumbar BRØ6
    Thoracic BRØ5
  Fallopian Tube
    Bilateral BUØ2
    Left BUØ1
    Right BUØØ
  Fallopian Tube and Uterus BUØ8
  Femur
    Left, Densitometry BQØ4ZZ1
    Right, Densitometry BQØ3ZZ1
  Finger
    Left BPØSZZZ
    Right BPØRZZZ
  Foot
    Left BQØMZZZ
    Right BQØLZZZ
  Forearm
    Left BPØKZZZ
    Right BPØJZZZ
  Gallbladder and Bile Duct BFØ3
  Gland
    Parotid
      Bilateral B9Ø6
      Left B9Ø5
      Right B9Ø4
    Salivary
      Bilateral B9ØD
      Left B9ØC
      Right B9ØB
    Submandibular
      Bilateral B9Ø9
      Left B9Ø8
      Right B9Ø7
  Hand
    Left BPØPZZZ
    Right BPØNZZZ
  Heart
    Left B2Ø5
    Right B2Ø4
    Right and Left B2Ø6
  Hepatobiliary System, All BFØC
  Hip
    Left BQØ1
      Densitometry BQØ1ZZ1
    Right BQØØ
      Densitometry BQØØZZ1
  Humerus
    Left BPØBZZZ
    Right BPØAZZZ
  Ileal Diversion Loop BTØC
  Intracranial Sinus B5Ø2
  Joint
    Acromioclavicular, Bilateral BPØ3ZZZ
    Finger
      Left BPØD
      Right BPØC
    Foot
      Left BQØY
      Right BQØX
    Hand
      Left BPØD

Plain Radiography — *continued*
  Joint — *continued*
    Hand — *continued*
      Right BPØC
    Lumbosacral BRØBZZZ
    Sacroiliac BRØD
    Sternoclavicular
      Bilateral BPØ2ZZZ
      Left BPØ1ZZZ
      Right BPØØZZZ
    Temporomandibular
      Bilateral BNØ9
      Left BNØ8
      Right BNØ7
    Thoracolumbar BRØ8ZZZ
    Toe
      Left BQØY
      Right BQØX
  Kidney
    Bilateral BTØ3
    Left BTØ2
    Right BTØ1
    Ureter and Bladder BTØ4
  Knee
    Left BQØ8
    Right BQØ7
  Leg
    Left BQØFZZZ
    Right BQØDZZZ
  Lymphatic
    Head B7Ø4
    Lower Extremity
      Bilateral B7ØB
      Left B7Ø9
      Right B7Ø8
    Neck B7Ø4
    Pelvic B7ØC
    Upper Extremity
      Bilateral B7Ø7
      Left B7Ø6
      Right B7Ø5
  Mandible BNØ6ZZZ
  Mastoid B9ØHZZZ
  Nasopharynx B9ØFZZZ
  Optic Foramina
    Left B8Ø4ZZZ
    Right B8Ø3ZZZ
  Orbit
    Bilateral BNØ3ZZZ
    Left BNØ2ZZZ
    Right BNØ1ZZZ
  Oropharynx B9ØFZZZ
  Patella
    Left BQØWZZZ
    Right BQØVZZZ
  Pelvis BRØCZZZ
  Pelvis and Abdomen BWØ1ZZZ
  Prostate BVØ3
  Retroperitoneal Lymphatic
    Bilateral B7Ø1
    Unilateral B7ØØ
  Ribs
    Left BPØYZZZ
    Right BPØXZZZ
  Sacrum BRØFZZZ
  Scapula
    Left BPØ7ZZZ
    Right BPØ6ZZZ
  Shoulder
    Left BPØ9
    Right BPØ8
  Sinus
    Intracranial B5Ø2
    Paranasal B9Ø2ZZZ
  Skull BNØØZZZ
  Spinal Cord BØØB
  Spine
    Cervical, Densitometry BRØØZZ1
    Lumbar, Densitometry BRØ9ZZ1
    Thoracic, Densitometry BRØ7ZZ1
    Whole, Densitometry BRØGZZ1
  Sternum BRØHZZZ
  Teeth
    All BNØJZZZ
    Multiple BNØHZZZ
  Testicle
    Left BVØ6
    Right BVØ5

Plain Radiography — *continued*
  Toe
    Left BQØQZZZ
    Right BQØPZZZ
  Tooth, Single BNØGZZZ
  Tracheobronchial Tree
    Bilateral BBØ9YZZ
    Left BBØ8YZZ
    Right BBØ7YZZ
  Ureter
    Bilateral BTØ8
    Kidney and Bladder BTØ4
    Left BTØ7
    Right BTØ6
  Urethra BTØ5
  Urethra and Bladder BTØB
  Uterus BUØ6
  Uterus and Fallopian Tube BUØ8
  Vagina BUØ9
  Vasa Vasorum BVØ8
  Vein
    Cerebellar B5Ø1
    Cerebral B5Ø1
    Epidural B5ØØ
    Jugular
      Bilateral B5Ø5
      Left B5Ø4
      Right B5Ø3
    Lower Extremity
      Bilateral B5ØD
      Left B5ØC
      Right B5ØB
    Other B5ØV
    Pelvic (Iliac)
      Left B5ØG
      Right B5ØF
    Pelvic (Iliac) Bilateral B5ØH
    Portal B5ØT
    Pulmonary
      Bilateral B5ØS
      Left B5ØR
      Right B5ØQ
    Renal
      Bilateral B5ØL
      Left B5ØK
      Right B5ØJ
    Spanchnic B5ØT
    Subclavian
      Left B5Ø7
      Right B5Ø6
    Upper Extremity
      Bilateral B5ØP
      Left B5ØN
      Right B5ØM
  Vena Cava
    Inferior B5Ø9
    Superior B5Ø8
  Whole Body BWØKZZZ
    Infant BWØMZZZ
  Whole Skeleton BWØLZZZ
  Wrist
    Left BPØM
    Right BPØL

Planar Nuclear Medicine Imaging
  Abdomen CW1Ø
  Abdomen and Chest CW14
  Abdomen and Pelvis CW11
  Anatomical Region, Other CW1ZZZZ
  Anatomical Regions, Multiple CW1YYZZ
  Bladder and Ureters CT1H
  Bladder, Kidneys and Ureters CT13
  Blood C713
  Bone Marrow C71Ø
  Brain CØ1Ø
  Breast CH1YYZZ
    Bilateral CH12
    Left CH11
    Right CH1Ø
  Bronchi and Lungs CB12
  Central Nervous System CØ1YYZZ
  Cerebrospinal Fluid CØ15
  Chest CW13
  Chest and Abdomen CW14
  Chest and Neck CW16
  Digestive System CD1YYZZ
  Ducts, Lacrimal, Bilateral C819
  Ear, Nose, Mouth and Throat C91YYZZ
  Endocrine System CG1YYZZ

Planar Nuclear Medicine Imaging — continued
    Extremity
      Lower CW1D
        Bilateral CP1F
        Left CP1D
        Right CP1C
      Upper CW1M
        Bilateral CP1B
        Left CP19
        Right CP18
    Eye C81YYZZ
    Gallbladder CF14
    Gastrointestinal Tract CD17
      Upper CD15
    Gland
      Adrenal, Bilateral CG14
      Parathyroid CG11
      Thyroid CG12
    Glands, Salivary, Bilateral C91B
    Head and Neck CW1B
    Heart C21YYZZ
      Right and Left C216
    Hepatobiliary System, All CF1C
    Hepatobiliary System and Pancreas CF1YYZZ
    Kidneys, Ureters and Bladder CT13
    Liver CF15
    Liver and Spleen CF16
    Lungs and Bronchi CB12
    Lymphatics
      Head C71J
      Head and Neck C715
      Lower Extremity C71P
      Neck C71K
      Pelvic C71D
      Trunk C71M
      Upper Chest C71L
      Upper Extremity C71N
    Lymphatics and Hematologic System C71YYZZ
    Musculoskeletal System
      All CP1Z
      Other CP1YYZZ
    Myocardium C21G
    Neck and Chest CW16
    Neck and Head CW1B
    Pancreas and Hepatobiliary System CF1YYZZ
    Pelvic Region CW1J
    Pelvis CP16
    Pelvis and Abdomen CW11
    Pelvis and Spine CP17
    Reproductive System, Male CV1YYZZ
    Respiratory System CB1YYZZ
    Skin CH1YYZZ
    Skull CP11
    Spine CP15
    Spine and Pelvis CP17
    Spleen C712
    Spleen and Liver CF16
    Subcutaneous Tissue CH1YYZZ
    Testicles, Bilateral CV19
    Thorax CP14
    Ureters and Bladder CT1H
    Ureters, Kidneys and Bladder CT13
    Urinary System CT1YYZZ
    Veins C51YYZZ
      Central C51R
      Lower Extremity
        Bilateral C51D
        Left C51C
        Right C51B
      Upper Extremity
        Bilateral C51Q
        Left C51P
        Right C51N
    Whole Body CW1N
Plantar digital vein
    use Foot Vein, Left
    use Foot Vein, Right
Plantar fascia (aponeurosis)
    use Subcutaneous Tissue and Fascia, Left Foot
    use Subcutaneous Tissue and Fascia, Right Foot
Plantar metatarsal vein
    use Foot Vein, Left
    use Foot Vein, Right
Plantar venous arch
    use Foot Vein, Left
    use Foot Vein, Right
Plaque Radiation
    Abdomen DWY3FZZ

Plaque Radiation — continued
    Adrenal Gland DGY2FZZ
    Anus DDY8FZZ
    Bile Ducts DFY2FZZ
    Bladder DTY2FZZ
    Bone Marrow D7Y0FZZ
    Bone, Other DPYCFZZ
    Brain D0Y0FZZ
    Brain Stem D0Y1FZZ
    Breast
      Left DMY0FZZ
      Right DMY1FZZ
    Bronchus DBY1FZZ
    Cervix DUY1FZZ
    Chest DWY2FZZ
    Chest Wall DBY7FZZ
    Colon DDY5FZZ
    Diaphragm DBY8FZZ
    Duodenum DDY2FZZ
    Ear D9Y0FZZ
    Esophagus DDY0FZZ
    Eye D8Y0FZZ
    Femur DPY9FZZ
    Fibula DPYBFZZ
    Gallbladder DFY1FZZ
    Gland
      Adrenal DGY2FZZ
      Parathyroid DGY4FZZ
      Pituitary DGY0FZZ
      Thyroid DGY5FZZ
    Glands, Salivary D9Y6FZZ
    Head and Neck DWY1FZZ
    Hemibody DWY4FZZ
    Humerus DPY6FZZ
    Ileum DDY4FZZ
    Jejunum DDY3FZZ
    Kidney DTY0FZZ
    Larynx D9YBFZZ
    Liver DFY0FZZ
    Lung DBY2FZZ
    Lymphatics
      Abdomen D7Y6FZZ
      Axillary D7Y4FZZ
      Inguinal D7Y8FZZ
      Neck D7Y3FZZ
      Pelvis D7Y7FZZ
      Thorax D7Y5FZZ
    Mandible DPY3FZZ
    Maxilla DPY2FZZ
    Mediastinum DBY6FZZ
    Mouth D9Y4FZZ
    Nasopharynx D9YDFZZ
    Neck and Head DWY1FZZ
    Nerve, Peripheral D0Y7FZZ
    Nose D9Y1FZZ
    Ovary DUY0FZZ
    Palate
      Hard D9Y8FZZ
      Soft D9Y9FZZ
    Pancreas DFY3FZZ
    Parathyroid Gland DGY4FZZ
    Pelvic Bones DPY8FZZ
    Pelvic Region DWY6FZZ
    Pharynx D9YCFZZ
    Pineal Body DGY1FZZ
    Pituitary Gland DGY0FZZ
    Pleura DBY5FZZ
    Prostate DVY0FZZ
    Radius DPY7FZZ
    Rectum DDY7FZZ
    Rib DPY5FZZ
    Sinuses D9Y7FZZ
    Skin
      Abdomen DHY8FZZ
      Arm DHY4FZZ
      Back DHY7FZZ
      Buttock DHY9FZZ
      Chest DHY6FZZ
      Face DHY2FZZ
      Foot DHYCFZZ
      Hand DHY5FZZ
      Leg DHYBFZZ
      Neck DHY3FZZ
    Skull DPY0FZZ
    Spinal Cord D0Y6FZZ
    Spleen D7Y2FZZ
    Sternum DPY4FZZ
    Stomach DDY1FZZ
    Testis DVY1FZZ

Plaque Radiation — continued
    Thymus D7Y1FZZ
    Thyroid Gland DGY5FZZ
    Tibia DPYBFZZ
    Tongue D9Y5FZZ
    Trachea DBY0FZZ
    Ulna DPY7FZZ
    Ureter DTY1FZZ
    Urethra DTY3FZZ
    Uterus DUY2FZZ
    Whole Body DWY5FZZ
Plasma, Convalescent (Nonautologous) XW1
Plasmapheresis, therapeutic see Pheresis, Physiological Systems 6A5
Plateletpheresis, therapeutic see Pheresis, Physiological Systems 6A5
Platysma muscle
    use Neck Muscle, Left
    use Neck Muscle, Right
Plazomicin Anti-infective XW0
Pleurectomy
    see Excision, Respiratory System 0BB
    see Resection, Respiratory System 0BT
Pleurocentesis see Drainage, Anatomical Regions, General 0W9
Pleurodesis, pleurosclerosis
    Chemical injection see Introduction of Substance in or on, Pleural Cavity 3E0L
    Surgical see Destruction, Respiratory System 0B5
Pleurolysis see Release, Respiratory System 0BN
Pleuroscopy 0BJQ4ZZ
Pleurotomy see Drainage, Respiratory System 0B9
Plica semilunaris
    use Conjunctiva, Left
    use Conjunctiva, Right
Plication see Restriction
Pneumectomy
    see Excision, Respiratory System 0BB
    see Resection, Respiratory System 0BT
Pneumocentesis see Drainage, Respiratory System 0B9
Pneumogastric nerve use Vagus Nerve
Pneumolysis see Release, Respiratory System 0BN
Pneumonectomy see Resection, Respiratory System 0BT
Pneumonolysis see Release, Respiratory System 0BN
Pneumonopexy
    see Repair, Respiratory System 0BQ
    see Reposition, Respiratory System 0BS
Pneumonorrhaphy see Repair, Respiratory System 0BQ
Pneumonotomy see Drainage, Respiratory System 0B9
Pneumotaxic center use Pons
Pneumotomy see Drainage, Respiratory System 0B9
Pollicization see Transfer, Anatomical Regions, Upper Extremities 0XX
Polyclonal hyperimmune globulin use Globulin
Polyethylene socket use Synthetic Substitute, Polyethylene in 0SR
Polymethylmethacrylate (PMMA) use Synthetic Substitute
Polypectomy, gastrointestinal see Excision, Gastrointestinal System 0DB
Polypropylene mesh use Synthetic Substitute
Polysomnogram 4A1ZXQZ
Pontine tegmentum use Pons
Popliteal ligament
    use Knee Bursa and Ligament, Left
    use Knee Bursa and Ligament, Right
Popliteal lymph node
    use Lymphatic, Left Lower Extremity
    use Lymphatic, Right Lower Extremity
Popliteal vein
    use Femoral Vein, Left
    use Femoral Vein, Right
Popliteus muscle
    use Lower Leg Muscle, Left
    use Lower Leg Muscle, Right
Porcine (bioprosthetic) valve use Zooplastic Tissue in Heart and Great Vessels
Positive Blood Culture Fluorescence Hybridization for Organism Identification, Concentration and Susceptibility XXE5XN6
Positive end expiratory pressure see Performance, Respiratory 5A19
Positron Emission Tomographic (PET) Imaging
    Brain C030

▽ Subterms under main terms may continue to next column or page

Positron Emission Tomographic (PET) Imaging —
continued
  Bronchi and Lungs CB32
  Central Nervous System C03YYZZ
  Heart C23YYZZ
  Lungs and Bronchi CB32
  Myocardium C23G
  Respiratory System CB3YYZZ
  Whole Body CW3NYZZ
Positron emission tomography *see* Positron Emission Tomographic (PET) Imaging
Postauricular (mastoid) lymph node
  use Lymphatic, Left Neck
  use Lymphatic, Right Neck
Postcava *use* Inferior Vena Cava
Posterior auricular artery
  use External Carotid Artery, Left
  use External Carotid Artery, Right
Posterior auricular nerve *use* Facial Nerve
Posterior auricular vein
  use External Jugular Vein, Left
  use External Jugular Vein, Right
Posterior cerebral artery *use* Intracranial Artery
Posterior chamber
  use Eye, Left
  use Eye, Right
Posterior circumflex humeral artery
  use Axillary Artery, Left
  use Axillary Artery, Right
Posterior communicating artery *use* Intracranial Artery
Posterior cruciate ligament (PCL)
  use Knee Bursa and Ligament, Left
  use Knee Bursa and Ligament, Right
Posterior (Dynamic) Distraction Device
  Lumbar XNS0
  Thoracic XNS4
Posterior facial (retromandibular) vein
  use Face Vein, Left
  use Face Vein, Right
Posterior femoral cutaneous nerve *use* Sacral Plexus
Posterior inferior cerebellar artery (PICA) *use* Intracranial Artery
Posterior interosseous nerve *use* Radial Nerve
Posterior labial nerve *use* Pudendal Nerve
Posterior (subscapular) lymph node
  use Lymphatic, Left Axillary
  use Lymphatic, Right Axillary
Posterior scrotal nerve *use* Pudendal Nerve
Posterior spinal artery
  use Vertebral Artery, Left
  use Vertebral Artery, Right
Posterior tibial recurrent artery
  use Anterior Tibial Artery, Left
  use Anterior Tibial Artery, Right
Posterior ulnar recurrent artery
  use Ulnar Artery, Left
  use Ulnar Artery, Right
Posterior vagal trunk *use* Vagus Nerve
PPN (peripheral parenteral nutrition) *see* Introduction of Nutritional Substance
Praxbind® (idarucizumab), Pradaxa® (dabigatran) reversal agent *use* Other Therapeutic Substance
Preauricular lymph node *use* Lymphatic, Head
Precava *use* Superior Vena Cava
PRECICE intramedullary limb lengthening system
  use Internal Fixation Device, Intramedullary Limb Lengthening in 0PH
  use Internal Fixation Device, Intramedullary Limb Lengthening in 0QH
Prepatellar bursa
  use Knee Bursa and Ligament, Left
  use Knee Bursa and Ligament, Right
Preputiotomy *see* Drainage, Male Reproductive System 0V9
Pressure support ventilation *see* Performance, Respiratory 5A19
PRESTIGE® Cervical Disc *use* Synthetic Substitute
Pretracheal fascia
  use Subcutaneous Tissue and Fascia, Left Neck
  use Subcutaneous Tissue and Fascia, Right Neck
Prevertebral fascia
  use Subcutaneous Tissue and Fascia, Left Neck
  use Subcutaneous Tissue and Fascia, Right Neck
PrimeAdvanced neurostimulator (SureScan) (MRI Safe) *use* Stimulator Generator, Multiple Array in 0JH

Princeps pollicis artery
  use Hand Artery, Left
  use Hand Artery, Right
Probing, duct
  Diagnostic *see* Inspection
  Dilation *see* Dilation
PROCEED™ Ventral Patch *use* Synthetic Substitute
Procerus muscle *use* Facial Muscle
Proctectomy
  see Excision, Rectum 0DBP
  see Resection, Rectum 0DTP
Proctoclysis *see* Introduction of substance in or on, Gastrointestinal Tract, Lower 3E0H
Proctocolectomy
  see Excision, Gastrointestinal System 0DB
  see Resection, Gastrointestinal System 0DT
Proctocolpoplasty
  see Repair, Gastrointestinal System 0DQ
  see Supplement, Gastrointestinal System 0DU
Proctoperineoplasty
  see Repair, Gastrointestinal System 0DQ
  see Supplement, Gastrointestinal System 0DU
Proctoperineorrhaphy *see* Repair, Gastrointestinal System 0DQ
Proctopexy
  see Repair, Rectum 0DQP
  see Reposition, Rectum 0DSP
Proctoplasty
  see Repair, Rectum 0DQP
  see Supplement, Rectum 0DUP
Proctorrhaphy *see* Repair, Rectum 0DQP
Proctoscopy 0DJD8ZZ
Proctosigmoidectomy
  see Excision, Gastrointestinal System 0DB
  see Resection, Gastrointestinal System 0DT
Proctosigmoidoscopy 0DJD8ZZ
Proctostomy *see* Drainage, Rectum 0D9P
Proctotomy *see* Drainage, Rectum 0D9P
Prodisc-C *use* Synthetic Substitute
Prodisc-L *use* Synthetic Substitute
Production, atrial septal defect *see* Excision, Septum, Atrial 02B5
Profunda brachii
  use Brachial Artery, Left
  use Brachial Artery, Right
Profunda femoris (deep femoral) vein
  use Femoral Vein, Left
  use Femoral Vein, Right
PROLENE Polypropylene Hernia System (PHS) *use* Synthetic Substitute
Prolonged intermittent renal replacement therapy (PIRRT) 5A1D80Z
Pronator quadratus muscle
  use Lower Arm and Wrist Muscle, Left
  use Lower Arm and Wrist Muscle, Right
Pronator teres muscle
  use Lower Arm and Wrist Muscle, Left
  use Lower Arm and Wrist Muscle, Right
Prostatectomy
  see Excision, Prostate 0VB0
  see Resection, Prostate 0VT0
Prostatic urethra *use* Urethra
Prostatomy, prostatotomy *see* Drainage, Prostate 0V90
Protecta XT CRT-D *use* Cardiac Resynchronization Defibrillator Pulse Generator in 0JH
Protecta XT DR (XT VR) *use* Defibrillator Generator in 0JH
Protege® RX Carotid Stent System *use* Intraluminal Device
Proximal radioulnar joint
  use Elbow Joint, Left
  use Elbow Joint, Right
Psoas muscle
  use Hip Muscle, Left
  use Hip Muscle, Right
PSV (pressure support ventilation) *see* Performance, Respiratory 5A19
Psychoanalysis GZ54ZZZ
Psychological Tests
  Cognitive Status GZ14ZZZ
  Developmental GZ10ZZZ
  Intellectual and Psychoeducational GZ12ZZZ
  Neurobehavioral Status GZ14ZZZ
  Neuropsychological GZ13ZZZ
  Personality and Behavioral GZ11ZZZ

Psychotherapy
  Family, Mental Health Services GZ72ZZZ
  Group GZHZZZZ
    Mental Health Services GZHZZZZ
  Individual
    see Psychotherapy, Individual, Mental Health Services
  for substance abuse
    12-Step HZ53ZZZ
    Behavioral HZ51ZZZ
    Cognitive HZ50ZZZ
    Cognitive-Behavioral HZ52ZZZ
    Confrontational HZ58ZZZ
    Interactive HZ55ZZZ
    Interpersonal HZ54ZZZ
    Motivational Enhancement HZ57ZZZ
    Psychoanalysis HZ5BZZZ
    Psychodynamic HZ5CZZZ
    Psychoeducation HZ56ZZZ
    Psychophysiological HZ5DZZZ
    Supportive HZ59ZZZ
  Mental Health Services
    Behavioral GZ51ZZZ
    Cognitive GZ52ZZZ
    Cognitive-Behavioral GZ58ZZZ
    Interactive GZ50ZZZ
    Interpersonal GZ53ZZZ
    Psychoanalysis GZ54ZZZ
    Psychodynamic GZ55ZZZ
    Psychophysiological GZ59ZZZ
    Supportive GZ56ZZZ
PTCA (percutaneous transluminal coronary angioplasty) *see* Dilation, Heart and Great Vessels 027
Pterygoid muscle *use* Head Muscle
Pterygoid process *use* Sphenoid Bone
Pterygopalatine (sphenopalatine) ganglion *use* Head and Neck Sympathetic Nerve
Pubis
  use Pelvic Bone, Left
  use Pelvic Bone, Right
Pubofemoral ligament
  use Hip Bursa and Ligament, Left
  use Hip Bursa and Ligament, Right
Pudendal nerve *use* Sacral Plexus
Pull-through, laparoscopic-assisted transanal
  see Excision, Gastrointestinal System 0DB
  see Resection, Gastrointestinal System 0DT
Pull-through, rectal *see* Resection, Rectum 0DTP
Pulmoaortic canal *use* Pulmonary Artery, Left
Pulmonary annulus *use* Pulmonary Valve
Pulmonary artery wedge monitoring *see* Monitoring, Arterial 4A13
Pulmonary plexus
  use Thoracic Sympathetic Nerve
  use Vagus Nerve
Pulmonic valve *use* Pulmonary Valve
Pulpectomy *see* Excision, Mouth and Throat 0CB
Pulverization *see* Fragmentation
Pulvinar *use* Thalamus
Pump reservoir *use* Infusion Device, Pump in Subcutaneous Tissue and Fascia
Punch biopsy *see* Excision with qualifier Diagnostic
Puncture *see* Drainage
Puncture, lumbar *see* Drainage, Spinal Canal 009U
Pure-Vu® System XDPH8K7
Pyelography
  see Fluoroscopy, Urinary System BT1
  see Plain Radiography, Urinary System BT0
Pyeloileostomy, urinary diversion *see* Bypass, Urinary System 0T1
Pyeloplasty
  see Repair, Urinary System 0TQ
  see Replacement, Urinary System 0TR
  see Supplement, Urinary System 0TU
Pyeloplasty, dismembered *see* Repair, Kidney Pelvis
Pyelorrhaphy *see* Repair, Urinary System 0TQ
Pyeloscopy 0TJ58ZZ
Pyelostomy
  see Bypass, Urinary System 0T1
  see Drainage, Urinary System 0T9
Pyelotomy *see* Drainage, Urinary System 0T9
Pylorectomy
  see Excision, Stomach, Pylorus 0DB7
  see Resection, Stomach, Pylorus 0DT7
Pyloric antrum *use* Stomach, Pylorus
Pyloric canal *use* Stomach, Pylorus
Pyloric sphincter *use* Stomach, Pylorus

Pylorodiosis *see* Dilation, Stomach, Pylorus ØD77
Pylorogastrectomy
   see Excision, Gastrointestinal System ØDB
   see Resection, Gastrointestinal System ØDT
Pyloroplasty
   see Repair, Stomach, Pylorus ØDQ7
   see Supplement, Stomach, Pylorus ØDU7
Pyloroscopy ØDJ68ZZ
Pylorotomy *see* Drainage, Stomach, Pylorus ØD97
Pyramidalis muscle
   use Abdomen Muscle, Left
   use Abdomen Muscle, Right

Q

Quadrangular cartilage *use* Nasal Septum
Quadrant resection of breast *see* Excision, Skin and
   Breast ØHB
Quadrate lobe *use* Liver
Quadratus femoris muscle
   use Hip Muscle, Left
   use Hip Muscle, Right
Quadratus lumborum muscle
   use Trunk Muscle, Left
   use Trunk Muscle, Right
Quadratus plantae muscle
   use Foot Muscle, Left
   use Foot Muscle, Right
Quadriceps (femoris)
   use Upper Leg Muscle, Left
   use Upper Leg Muscle, Right
Quarantine 8EØZXY6

R

Radial artery arteriovenous fistula, using Thermal
   Resistance Energy X2K
Radial collateral carpal ligament
   use Wrist Bursa and Ligament, Left
   use Wrist Bursa and Ligament, Right
Radial collateral ligament
   use Elbow Bursa and Ligament, Left
   use Elbow Bursa and Ligament, Right
Radial notch
   use Ulna, Left
   use Ulna, Right
Radial recurrent artery
   use Radial Artery, Left
   use Radial Artery, Right
Radial vein
   use Brachial Vein, Left
   use Brachial Vein, Right
Radialis indicis
   use Hand Artery, Left
   use Hand Artery, Right
Radiation Therapy
   see Beam Radiation
   see Brachytherapy
   see Other Radiation
   see Stereotactic Radiosurgery
Radiation treatment *see* Radiation Therapy
Radiocarpal joint
   use Wrist Joint, Left
   use Wrist Joint, Right
Radiocarpal ligament
   use Wrist Bursa and Ligament, Left
   use Wrist Bursa and Ligament, Right
Radiography *see* Plain Radiography
Radiology, analog *see* Plain Radiography
Radiology, diagnostic *see* Imaging, Diagnostic
Radioulnar ligament
   use Wrist Bursa and Ligament, Left
   use Wrist Bursa and Ligament, Right
Range of motion testing *see* Motor Function Assess-
   ment, Rehabilitation FØ1
Rapid ASPECTS XXEØXØ7
REALIZE® Adjustable Gastric Band *use* Extraluminal
   Device
Reattachment
   Abdominal Wall ØWMFØZZ
   Ampulla of Vater ØFMC
   Ankle Region
     Left ØYMLØZZ
     Right ØYMKØZZ

Reattachment — *continued*
   Arm
     Lower
       Left ØXMFØZZ
       Right ØXMDØZZ
     Upper
       Left ØXM9ØZZ
       Right ØXM8ØZZ
   Axilla
     Left ØXM5ØZZ
     Right ØXM4ØZZ
   Back
     Lower ØWMLØZZ
     Upper ØWMKØZZ
   Bladder ØTMB
   Bladder Neck ØTMC
   Breast
     Bilateral ØHMVXZZ
     Left ØHMUXZZ
     Right ØHMTXZZ
   Bronchus
     Lingula ØBM9ØZZ
     Lower Lobe
       Left ØBMBØZZ
       Right ØBM6ØZZ
     Main
       Left ØBM7ØZZ
       Right ØBM3ØZZ
     Middle Lobe, Right ØBM5ØZZ
     Upper Lobe
       Left ØBM8ØZZ
       Right ØBM4ØZZ
   Bursa and Ligament
     Abdomen
       Left ØMMJ
       Right ØMMH
     Ankle
       Left ØMMR
       Right ØMMQ
     Elbow
       Left ØMM4
       Right ØMM3
     Foot
       Left ØMMT
       Right ØMMS
     Hand
       Left ØMM8
       Right ØMM7
     Head and Neck ØMMØ
     Hip
       Left ØMMM
       Right ØMML
     Knee
       Left ØMMP
       Right ØMMN
     Lower Extremity
       Left ØMMW
       Right ØMMV
     Perineum ØMMK
     Rib(s) ØMMG
     Shoulder
       Left ØMM2
       Right ØMM1
     Spine
       Lower ØMMD
       Upper ØMMC
     Sternum ØMMF
     Upper Extremity
       Left ØMMB
       Right ØMM9
     Wrist
       Left ØMM6
       Right ØMM5
   Buttock
     Left ØYM1ØZZ
     Right ØYMØØZZ
   Carina ØBM2ØZZ
   Cecum ØDMH
   Cervix ØUMC
   Chest Wall ØWM8ØZZ
   Clitoris ØUMJXZZ
   Colon
     Ascending ØDMK
     Descending ØDMM
     Sigmoid ØDMN
     Transverse ØDML
   Cord
     Bilateral ØVMH
     Left ØVMG

Reattachment — *continued*
   Cord — *continued*
     Right ØVMF
   Cul-de-sac ØUMF
   Diaphragm ØBMTØZZ
   Duct
     Common Bile ØFM9
     Cystic ØFM8
     Hepatic
       Common ØFM7
       Left ØFM6
       Right ØFM5
     Pancreatic ØFMD
       Accessory ØFMF
   Duodenum ØDM9
   Ear
     Left Ø9M1XZZ
     Right Ø9MØXZZ
   Elbow Region
     Left ØXMCØZZ
     Right ØXMBØZZ
   Esophagus ØDM5
   Extremity
     Lower
       Left ØYMBØZZ
       Right ØYM9ØZZ
     Upper
       Left ØXM7ØZZ
       Right ØXM6ØZZ
   Eyelid
     Lower
       Left Ø8MRXZZ
       Right Ø8MQXZZ
     Upper
       Left Ø8MPXZZ
       Right Ø8MNXZZ
   Face ØWM2ØZZ
   Fallopian Tube
     Left ØUM6
     Right ØUM5
   Fallopian Tubes, Bilateral ØUM7
   Femoral Region
     Left ØYM8ØZZ
     Right ØYM7ØZZ
   Finger
     Index
       Left ØXMPØZZ
       Right ØXMNØZZ
     Little
       Left ØXMWØZZ
       Right ØXMVØZZ
     Middle
       Left ØXMRØZZ
       Right ØXMQØZZ
     Ring
       Left ØXMTØZZ
       Right ØXMSØZZ
   Foot
     Left ØYMNØZZ
     Right ØYMMØZZ
   Forequarter
     Left ØXM1ØZZ
     Right ØXMØØZZ
   Gallbladder ØFM4
   Gland
     Left ØGM2
     Right ØGM3
   Hand
     Left ØXMKØZZ
     Right ØXMJØZZ
   Hindquarter
     Bilateral ØYM4ØZZ
     Left ØYM3ØZZ
     Right ØYM2ØZZ
   Hymen ØUMK
   Ileum ØDMB
   Inguinal Region
     Left ØYM6ØZZ
     Right ØYM5ØZZ
   Intestine
     Large ØDME
       Left ØDMG
       Right ØDMF
     Small ØDM8
   Jaw
     Lower ØWM5ØZZ
     Upper ØWM4ØZZ
   Jejunum ØDMA

Reattachment — *continued*
  Kidney
    Left ØTM1
    Right ØTMØ
  Kidney Pelvis
    Left ØTM4
    Right ØTM3
  Kidneys, Bilateral ØTM2
  Knee Region
    Left ØYMGØZZ
    Right ØYMFØZZ
  Leg
    Lower
      Left ØYMJØZZ
      Right ØYMHØZZ
    Upper
      Left ØYMDØZZ
      Right ØYMCØZZ
  Lip
    Lower ØCM1ØZZ
    Upper ØCMØØZZ
  Liver ØFMØ
    Left Lobe ØFM2
    Right Lobe ØFM1
  Lung
    Left ØBMLØZZ
    Lower Lobe
      Left ØBMJØZZ
      Right ØBMFØZZ
    Middle Lobe, Right ØBMDØZZ
    Right ØBMKØZZ
    Upper Lobe
      Left ØBMGØZZ
      Right ØBMCØZZ
  Lung Lingula ØBMHØZZ
  Muscle
    Abdomen
      Left ØKML
      Right ØKMK
    Facial ØKM1
    Foot
      Left ØKMW
      Right ØKMV
    Hand
      Left ØKMD
      Right ØKMC
    Head ØKMØ
    Hip
      Left ØKMP
      Right ØKMN
    Lower Arm and Wrist
      Left ØKMB
      Right ØKM9
    Lower Leg
      Left ØKMT
      Right ØKMS
    Neck
      Left ØKM3
      Right ØKM2
    Perineum ØKMM
    Shoulder
      Left ØKM6
      Right ØKM5
    Thorax
      Left ØKMJ
      Right ØKMH
    Tongue, Palate, Pharynx ØKM4
    Trunk
      Left ØKMG
      Right ØKMF
    Upper Arm
      Left ØKM8
      Right ØKM7
    Upper Leg
      Left ØKMR
      Right ØKMQ
  Nasal Mucosa and Soft Tissue Ø9MKXZZ
  Neck ØWM6ØZZ
  Nipple
    Left ØHMXXZZ
    Right ØHMWXZZ
  Ovary
    Bilateral ØUM2
    Left ØUM1
    Right ØUMØ
  Palate, Soft ØCM3ØZZ
  Pancreas ØFMG
  Parathyroid Gland ØGMR

Reattachment — *continued*
  Parathyroid Gland — *continued*
    Inferior
      Left ØGMP
      Right ØGMN
    Multiple ØGMQ
    Superior
      Left ØGMM
      Right ØGML
  Penis ØVMSXZZ
  Perineum
    Female ØWMNØZZ
    Male ØWMMØZZ
  Rectum ØDMP
  Scrotum ØVM5XZZ
  Shoulder Region
    Left ØXM3ØZZ
    Right ØXM2ØZZ
  Skin
    Abdomen ØHM7XZZ
    Back ØHM6XZZ
    Buttock ØHM8XZZ
    Chest ØHM5XZZ
    Ear
      Left ØHM3XZZ
      Right ØHM2XZZ
    Face ØHM1XZZ
    Foot
      Left ØHMNXZZ
      Right ØHMMXZZ
    Hand
      Left ØHMGXZZ
      Right ØHMFXZZ
    Inguinal ØHMAXZZ
    Lower Arm
      Left ØHMEXZZ
      Right ØHMDXZZ
    Lower Leg
      Left ØHMLXZZ
      Right ØHMKXZZ
    Neck ØHM4XZZ
    Perineum ØHM9XZZ
    Scalp ØHMØXZZ
    Upper Arm
      Left ØHMCXZZ
      Right ØHMBXZZ
    Upper Leg
      Left ØHMJXZZ
      Right ØHMHXZZ
  Stomach ØDM6
  Tendon
    Abdomen
      Left ØLMG
      Right ØLMF
    Ankle
      Left ØLMT
      Right ØLMS
    Foot
      Left ØLMW
      Right ØLMV
    Hand
      Left ØLM8
      Right ØLM7
    Head and Neck ØLMØ
    Hip
      Left ØLMK
      Right ØLMJ
    Knee
      Left ØLMR
      Right ØLMQ
    Lower Arm and Wrist
      Left ØLM6
      Right ØLM5
    Lower Leg
      Left ØLMP
      Right ØLMN
    Perineum ØLMH
    Shoulder
      Left ØLM2
      Right ØLM1
    Thorax
      Left ØLMD
      Right ØLMC
    Trunk
      Left ØLMB
      Right ØLM9
    Upper Arm
      Left ØLM4
      Right ØLM3

Reattachment — *continued*
  Tendon — *continued*
    Upper Leg
      Left ØLMM
      Right ØLML
  Testis
    Bilateral ØVMC
    Left ØVMB
    Right ØVM9
  Thumb
    Left ØXMMØZZ
    Right ØXMLØZZ
  Thyroid Gland
    Left Lobe ØGMG
    Right Lobe ØGMH
  Toe
    1st
      Left ØYMQØZZ
      Right ØYMPØZZ
    2nd
      Left ØYMSØZZ
      Right ØYMRØZZ
    3rd
      Left ØYMUØZZ
      Right ØYMTØZZ
    4th
      Left ØYMWØZZ
      Right ØYMVØZZ
    5th
      Left ØYMYØZZ
      Right ØYMXØZZ
  Tongue ØCM7ØZZ
  Tooth
    Lower ØCMX
    Upper ØCMW
  Trachea ØBM1ØZZ
  Tunica Vaginalis
    Left ØVM7
    Right ØVM6
  Ureter
    Left ØTM7
    Right ØTM6
  Ureters, Bilateral ØTM8
  Urethra ØTMD
  Uterine Supporting Structure ØUM4
  Uterus ØUM9
  Uvula ØCMNØZZ
  Vagina ØUMG
  Vulva ØUMMXZZ
  Wrist Region
    Left ØXMHØZZ
    Right ØXMGØZZ
REBOA (resuscitative endovascular balloon occlusion of the aorta)
  Ø2LW3DJ
  Ø4LØ3DJ
Rebound HRD® (Hernia Repair Device) *use* Synthetic
  Substitute
RECELL® cell suspension autograft *see* Replacement,
  Skin and Breast ØHR
Recession
  see Repair
  see Reposition
Reclosure, disrupted abdominal wall ØWQFXZZ
Reconstruction
  see Repair
  see Replacement
  see Supplement
Rectectomy
  see Excision, Rectum ØDBP
  see Resection, Rectum ØDTP
Rectocele repair *see* Repair, Subcutaneous Tissue and
  Fascia, Pelvic Region ØJQC
Rectopexy
  see Repair, Gastrointestinal System ØDQ
  see Reposition, Gastrointestinal System ØDS
Rectoplasty
  see Repair, Gastrointestinal System ØDQ
  see Supplement, Gastrointestinal System ØDU
Rectorrhaphy *see* Repair, Gastrointestinal System ØDQ
Rectoscopy ØDJD8ZZ
Rectosigmoid junction *use* Sigmoid Colon
Rectosigmoidectomy
  see Excision, Gastrointestinal System ØDB
  see Resection, Gastrointestinal System ØDT
Rectostomy *see* Drainage, Rectum ØD9P
Rectotomy *see* Drainage, Rectum ØD9P

Rectus abdominis muscle
  use Abdomen Muscle, Left
  use Abdomen Muscle, Right
Rectus femoris muscle
  use Upper Leg Muscle, Left
  use Upper Leg Muscle, Right
Recurrent laryngeal nerve use Vagus Nerve
Reducer™ System use Reduction Device in New Technology
Reduction
  Dislocation see Reposition
  Fracture see Reposition
  Intussusception, intestinal see Reposition, Gastrointestinal System ØDS
  Mammoplasty see Excision, Skin and Breast ØHB
  Prolapse see Reposition
  Torsion see Reposition
  Volvulus, gastrointestinal see Reposition, Gastrointestinal System ØDS
Reduction Device, Coronary Sinus X2V73Q7
Refusion see Fusion
REGN-COV2 Monoclonal Antibody XWØ
Rehabilitation
  see Activities of Daily Living Assessment, Rehabilitation FØ2
  see Activities of Daily Living Treatment, Rehabilitation FØ8
  see Caregiver Training, Rehabilitation FØF
  see Cochlear Implant Treatment, Rehabilitation FØB
  see Device Fitting, Rehabilitation FØD
  see Hearing Treatment, Rehabilitation FØ9
  see Motor Function Assessment, Rehabilitation FØ1
  see Motor Treatment, Rehabilitation FØ7
  see Speech Assessment, Rehabilitation FØØ
  see Speech Treatment, Rehabilitation FØ6
  see Vestibular Treatment, Rehabilitation FØC
Reimplantation
  see Reattachment
  see Reposition
  see Transfer
Reinforcement
  see Repair
  see Supplement
Relaxation, scar tissue see Release
Release
  Acetabulum
    Left ØQN5
    Right ØQN4
  Adenoids ØCNQ
  Ampulla of Vater ØFNC
  Anal Sphincter ØDNR
  Anterior Chamber
    Left Ø8N33ZZ
    Right Ø8N23ZZ
  Anus ØDNQ
  Aorta
    Abdominal Ø4NØ
    Thoracic
      Ascending/Arch Ø2NX
      Descending Ø2NW
  Aortic Body ØGND
  Appendix ØDNJ
  Artery
    Anterior Tibial
      Left Ø4NQ
      Right Ø4NP
    Axillary
      Left Ø3N6
      Right Ø3N5
    Brachial
      Left Ø3N8
      Right Ø3N7
    Celiac Ø4N1
    Colic
      Left Ø4N7
      Middle Ø4N8
      Right Ø4N6
    Common Carotid
      Left Ø3NJ
      Right Ø3NH
    Common Iliac
      Left Ø4ND
      Right Ø4NC
    Coronary
      Four or More Arteries Ø2N3

Release — continued
  Artery — continued
    Coronary — continued
      One Artery Ø2NØ
      Three Arteries Ø2N2
      Two Arteries Ø2N1
    External Carotid
      Left Ø3NN
      Right Ø3NM
    External Iliac
      Left Ø4NJ
      Right Ø4NH
    Face Ø3NR
    Femoral
      Left Ø4NL
      Right Ø4NK
    Foot
      Left Ø4NW
      Right Ø4NV
    Gastric Ø4N2
    Hand
      Left Ø3NF
      Right Ø3ND
    Hepatic Ø4N3
    Inferior Mesenteric Ø4NB
    Innominate Ø3N2
    Internal Carotid
      Left Ø3NL
      Right Ø3NK
    Internal Iliac
      Left Ø4NF
      Right Ø4NE
    Internal Mammary
      Left Ø3N1
      Right Ø3NØ
    Intracranial Ø3NG
    Lower Ø4NY
    Peroneal
      Left Ø4NU
      Right Ø4NT
    Popliteal
      Left Ø4NN
      Right Ø4NM
    Posterior Tibial
      Left Ø4NS
      Right Ø4NR
    Pulmonary
      Left Ø2NR
      Right Ø2NQ
    Pulmonary Trunk Ø2NP
    Radial
      Left Ø3NC
      Right Ø3NB
    Renal
      Left Ø4NA
      Right Ø4N9
    Splenic Ø4N4
    Subclavian
      Left Ø3N4
      Right Ø3N3
    Superior Mesenteric Ø4N5
    Temporal
      Left Ø3NT
      Right Ø3NS
    Thyroid
      Left Ø3NV
      Right Ø3NU
    Ulnar
      Left Ø3NA
      Right Ø3N9
    Upper Ø3NY
    Vertebral
      Left Ø3NQ
      Right Ø3NP
  Atrium
    Left Ø2N7
    Right Ø2N6
  Auditory Ossicle
    Left Ø9NA
    Right Ø9N9
  Basal Ganglia ØØN8
  Bladder ØTNB
  Bladder Neck ØTNC
  Bone
    Ethmoid
      Left ØNNG
      Right ØNNF
    Frontal ØNN1
    Hyoid ØNNX

Release — continued
  Bone — continued
    Lacrimal
      Left ØNNJ
      Right ØNNH
    Nasal ØNNB
    Occipital ØNN7
    Palatine
      Left ØNNL
      Right ØNNK
    Parietal
      Left ØNN4
      Right ØNN3
    Pelvic
      Left ØQN3
      Right ØQN2
    Sphenoid ØNNC
    Temporal
      Left ØNN6
      Right ØNN5
    Zygomatic
      Left ØNNN
      Right ØNNM
  Brain ØØNØ
  Breast
    Bilateral ØHNV
    Left ØHNU
    Right ØHNT
  Bronchus
    Lingula ØBN9
    Lower Lobe
      Left ØBNB
      Right ØBN6
    Main
      Left ØBN7
      Right ØBN3
    Middle Lobe, Right ØBN5
    Upper Lobe
      Left ØBN8
      Right ØBN4
  Buccal Mucosa ØCN4
  Bursa and Ligament
    Abdomen
      Left ØMNJ
      Right ØMNH
    Ankle
      Left ØMNR
      Right ØMNQ
    Elbow
      Left ØMN4
      Right ØMN3
    Foot
      Left ØMNT
      Right ØMNS
    Hand
      Left ØMN8
      Right ØMN7
    Head and Neck ØMNØ
    Hip
      Left ØMNM
      Right ØMNL
    Knee
      Left ØMNP
      Right ØMNN
    Lower Extremity
      Left ØMNW
      Right ØMNV
    Perineum ØMNK
    Rib(s) ØMNG
    Shoulder
      Left ØMN2
      Right ØMN1
    Spine
      Lower ØMND
      Upper ØMNC
    Sternum ØMNF
    Upper Extremity
      Left ØMNB
      Right ØMN9
    Wrist
      Left ØMN6
      Right ØMN5
  Carina ØBN2
  Carotid Bodies, Bilateral ØGN8
  Carotid Body
    Left ØGN6
    Right ØGN7
  Carpal
    Left ØPNN

Release — continued
  Carpal — continued
    Right ØPNM
  Cecum ØDNH
  Cerebellum ØØNC
  Cerebral Hemisphere ØØN7
  Cerebral Meninges ØØN1
  Cerebral Ventricle ØØN6
  Cervix ØUNC
  Chordae Tendineae Ø2N9
  Choroid
    Left Ø8NB
    Right Ø8NA
  Cisterna Chyli Ø7NL
  Clavicle
    Left ØPNB
    Right ØPN9
  Clitoris ØUNJ
  Coccygeal Glomus ØGNB
  Coccyx ØQNS
  Colon
    Ascending ØDNK
    Descending ØDNM
    Sigmoid ØDNN
    Transverse ØDNL
  Conduction Mechanism Ø2N8
  Conjunctiva
    Left Ø8NTXZZ
    Right Ø8NSXZZ
  Cord
    Bilateral ØVNH
    Left ØVNG
    Right ØVNF
  Cornea
    Left Ø8N9XZZ
    Right Ø8N8XZZ
  Cul-de-sac ØUNF
  Diaphragm ØBNT
  Disc
    Cervical Vertebral ØRN3
    Cervicothoracic Vertebral ØRN5
    Lumbar Vertebral ØSN2
    Lumbosacral ØSN4
    Thoracic Vertebral ØRN9
    Thoracolumbar Vertebral ØRNB
  Duct
    Common Bile ØFN9
    Cystic ØFN8
    Hepatic
      Common ØFN7
      Left ØFN6
      Right ØFN5
    Lacrimal
      Left Ø8NY
      Right Ø8NX
    Pancreatic ØFND
      Accessory ØFNF
    Parotid
      Left ØCNC
      Right ØCNB
  Duodenum ØDN9
  Dura Mater ØØN2
  Ear
    External
      Left Ø9N1
      Right Ø9NØ
    External Auditory Canal
      Left Ø9N4
      Right Ø9N3
    Inner
      Left Ø9NE
      Right Ø9ND
    Middle
      Left Ø9N6
      Right Ø9N5
  Epididymis
    Bilateral ØVNL
    Left ØVNK
    Right ØVNJ
  Epiglottis ØCNR
  Esophagogastric Junction ØDN4
  Esophagus ØDN5
    Lower ØDN3
    Middle ØDN2
    Upper ØDN1
  Eustachian Tube
    Left Ø9NG
    Right Ø9NF

Release — continued
  Eye
    Left Ø8N1XZZ
    Right Ø8NØXZZ
  Eyelid
    Lower
      Left Ø8NR
      Right Ø8NQ
    Upper
      Left Ø8NP
      Right Ø8NN
  Fallopian Tube
    Left ØUN6
    Right ØUN5
  Fallopian Tubes, Bilateral ØUN7
  Femoral Shaft
    Left ØQN7
    Right ØQN8
  Femur
    Lower
      Left ØQNC
      Right ØQNB
    Upper
      Left ØQN7
      Right ØQN6
  Fibula
    Left ØQNK
    Right ØQNJ
  Finger Nail ØHNQXZZ
  Gallbladder ØFN4
  Gingiva
    Lower ØCN6
    Upper ØCN5
  Gland
    Adrenal
      Bilateral ØGN4
      Left ØGN2
      Right ØGN3
    Lacrimal
      Left Ø8NW
      Right Ø8NV
    Minor Salivary ØCNJ
    Parotid
      Left ØCN9
      Right ØCN8
    Pituitary ØGNØ
    Sublingual
      Left ØCNF
      Right ØCND
    Submaxillary
      Left ØCNH
      Right ØCNG
    Vestibular ØUNL
  Glenoid Cavity
    Left ØPN8
    Right ØPN7
  Glomus Jugulare ØGNC
  Humeral Head
    Left ØPND
    Right ØPNC
  Humeral Shaft
    Left ØPNG
    Right ØPNF
  Hymen ØUNK
  Hypothalamus ØØNA
  Ileocecal Valve ØDNC
  Ileum ØDNB
  Intestine
    Large ØDNE
      Left ØDNG
      Right ØDNF
    Small ØDN8
  Iris
    Left Ø8ND3ZZ
    Right Ø8NC3ZZ
  Jejunum ØDNA
  Joint
    Acromioclavicular
      Left ØRNH
      Right ØRNG
    Ankle
      Left ØSNG
      Right ØSNF
    Carpal
      Left ØRNR
      Right ØRNQ
    Carpometacarpal
      Left ØRNT
      Right ØRNS

Release — continued
  Joint — continued
    Cervical Vertebral ØRN1
    Cervicothoracic Vertebral ØRN4
    Coccygeal ØSN6
    Elbow
      Left ØRNM
      Right ØRNL
    Finger Phalangeal
      Left ØRNX
      Right ØRNW
    Hip
      Left ØSNB
      Right ØSN9
    Knee
      Left ØSND
      Right ØSNC
    Lumbar Vertebral ØSNØ
    Lumbosacral ØSN3
    Metacarpophalangeal
      Left ØRNV
      Right ØRNU
    Metatarsal-Phalangeal
      Left ØSNN
      Right ØSNM
    Occipital-cervical ØRNØ
    Sacrococcygeal ØSN5
    Sacroiliac
      Left ØSN8
      Right ØSN7
    Shoulder
      Left ØRNK
      Right ØRNJ
    Sternoclavicular
      Left ØRNF
      Right ØRNE
    Tarsal
      Left ØSNJ
      Right ØSNH
    Tarsometatarsal
      Left ØSNL
      Right ØSNK
    Temporomandibular
      Left ØRND
      Right ØRNC
    Thoracic Vertebral ØRN6
    Thoracolumbar Vertebral ØRNA
    Toe Phalangeal
      Left ØSNQ
      Right ØSNP
    Wrist
      Left ØRNP
      Right ØRNN
  Kidney
    Left ØTN1
    Right ØTNØ
  Kidney Pelvis
    Left ØTN4
    Right ØTN3
  Larynx ØCNS
  Lens
    Left Ø8NK3ZZ
    Right Ø8NJ3ZZ
  Lip
    Lower ØCN1
    Upper ØCNØ
  Liver ØFNØ
    Left Lobe ØFN2
    Right Lobe ØFN1
  Lung
    Bilateral ØBNM
    Left ØBNL
    Lower Lobe
      Left ØBNJ
      Right ØBNF
    Middle Lobe, Right ØBND
    Right ØBNK
    Upper Lobe
      Left ØBNG
      Right ØBNC
  Lung Lingula ØBNH
  Lymphatic
    Aortic Ø7ND
    Axillary
      Left Ø7N6
      Right Ø7N5
    Head Ø7NØ
    Inguinal
      Left Ø7NJ

Release — continued
  Lymphatic — continued
    Inguinal — continued
      Right 07NH
    Internal Mammary
      Left 07N9
      Right 07N8
    Lower Extremity
      Left 07NG
      Right 07NF
    Mesenteric 07NB
    Neck
      Left 07N2
      Right 07N1
    Pelvis 07NC
    Thoracic Duct 07NK
    Thorax 07N7
    Upper Extremity
      Left 07N4
      Right 07N3
  Mandible
    Left 0NNV
    Right 0NNT
  Maxilla 0NNR
  Medulla Oblongata 00ND
  Mesentery 0DNV
  Metacarpal
    Left 0PNQ
    Right 0PNP
  Metatarsal
    Left 0QNP
    Right 0QNN
  Muscle
    Abdomen
      Left 0KNL
      Right 0KNK
    Extraocular
      Left 08NM
      Right 08NL
    Facial 0KN1
    Foot
      Left 0KNW
      Right 0KNV
    Hand
      Left 0KND
      Right 0KNC
    Head 0KN0
    Hip
      Left 0KNP
      Right 0KNN
    Lower Arm and Wrist
      Left 0KNB
      Right 0KN9
    Lower Leg
      Left 0KNT
      Right 0KNS
    Neck
      Left 0KN3
      Right 0KN2
    Papillary 02ND
    Perineum 0KNM
    Shoulder
      Left 0KN6
      Right 0KN5
    Thorax
      Left 0KNJ
      Right 0KNH
    Tongue, Palate, Pharynx 0KN4
    Trunk
      Left 0KNG
      Right 0KNF
    Upper Arm
      Left 0KN8
      Right 0KN7
    Upper Leg
      Left 0KNR
      Right 0KNQ
  Myocardial Bridge see Release, Artery, Coronary
  Nasal Mucosa and Soft Tissue 09NK
  Nasopharynx 09NN
  Nerve
    Abdominal Sympathetic 01NM
    Abducens 00NL
    Accessory 00NR
    Acoustic 00NN
    Brachial Plexus 01N3
    Cervical 01N1
    Cervical Plexus 01N0
    Facial 00NM

Release — continued
  Nerve — continued
    Femoral 01ND
    Glossopharyngeal 00NP
    Head and Neck Sympathetic 01NK
    Hypoglossal 00NS
    Lumbar 01NB
    Lumbar Plexus 01N9
    Lumbar Sympathetic 01NN
    Lumbosacral Plexus 01NA
    Median 01N5
    Oculomotor 00NH
    Olfactory 00NF
    Optic 00NG
    Peroneal 01NH
    Phrenic 01N2
    Pudendal 01NC
    Radial 01N6
    Sacral 01NR
    Sacral Plexus 01NQ
    Sacral Sympathetic 01NP
    Sciatic 01NF
    Thoracic 01N8
    Thoracic Sympathetic 01NL
    Tibial 01NG
    Trigeminal 00NK
    Trochlear 00NJ
    Ulnar 01N4
    Vagus 00NQ
  Nipple
    Left 0HNX
    Right 0HNW
  Omentum 0DNU
  Orbit
    Left 0NNQ
    Right 0NNP
  Ovary
    Bilateral 0UN2
    Left 0UN1
    Right 0UN0
  Palate
    Hard 0CN2
    Soft 0CN3
  Pancreas 0FNG
  Para-aortic Body 0GN9
  Paraganglion Extremity 0GNF
  Parathyroid Gland 0GNR
    Inferior
      Left 0GNP
      Right 0GNN
    Multiple 0GNQ
    Superior
      Left 0GNM
      Right 0GNL
  Patella
    Left 0QNF
    Right 0QND
  Penis 0VNS
  Pericardium 02NN
  Peritoneum 0DNW
  Phalanx
    Finger
      Left 0PNV
      Right 0PNT
    Thumb
      Left 0PNS
      Right 0PNR
    Toe
      Left 0QNR
      Right 0QNQ
  Pharynx 0CNM
  Pineal Body 0GN1
  Pleura
    Left 0BNP
    Right 0BNN
  Pons 00NB
  Prepuce 0VNT
  Prostate 0VN0
  Radius
    Left 0PNJ
    Right 0PNH
  Rectum 0DNP
  Retina
    Left 08NF3ZZ
    Right 08NE3ZZ
  Retinal Vessel
    Left 08NH3ZZ
    Right 08NG3ZZ

Release — continued
  Ribs
    1 to 2 0PN1
    3 or More 0PN2
  Sacrum 0QN1
  Scapula
    Left 0PN6
    Right 0PN5
  Sclera
    Left 08N7XZZ
    Right 08N6XZZ
  Scrotum 0VN5
  Septum
    Atrial 02N5
    Nasal 09NM
    Ventricular 02NM
  Sinus
    Accessory 09NP
    Ethmoid
      Left 09NV
      Right 09NU
    Frontal
      Left 09NT
      Right 09NS
    Mastoid
      Left 09NC
      Right 09NB
    Maxillary
      Left 09NR
      Right 09NQ
    Sphenoid
      Left 09NX
      Right 09NW
  Skin
    Abdomen 0HN7XZZ
    Back 0HN6XZZ
    Buttock 0HN8XZZ
    Chest 0HN5XZZ
    Ear
      Left 0HN3XZZ
      Right 0HN2XZZ
    Face 0HN1XZZ
    Foot
      Left 0HNNXZZ
      Right 0HNMXZZ
    Hand
      Left 0HNGXZZ
      Right 0HNFXZZ
    Inguinal 0HNAXZZ
    Lower Arm
      Left 0HNEXZZ
      Right 0HNDXZZ
    Lower Leg
      Left 0HNLXZZ
      Right 0HNKXZZ
    Neck 0HN4XZZ
    Perineum 0HN9XZZ
    Scalp 0HN0XZZ
    Upper Arm
      Left 0HNCXZZ
      Right 0HNBXZZ
    Upper Leg
      Left 0HNJXZZ
      Right 0HNHXZZ
  Spinal Cord
    Cervical 00NW
    Lumbar 00NY
    Thoracic 00NX
  Spinal Meninges 00NT
  Spleen 07NP
  Sternum 0PN0
  Stomach 0DN6
    Pylorus 0DN7
  Subcutaneous Tissue and Fascia
    Abdomen 0JN8
    Back 0JN7
    Buttock 0JN9
    Chest 0JN6
    Face 0JN1
    Foot
      Left 0JNR
      Right 0JNQ
    Hand
      Left 0JNK
      Right 0JNJ
    Lower Arm
      Left 0JNH
      Right 0JNG

▼ **Subterms under main terms may continue to next column or page**

Release — *continued*
  Subcutaneous Tissue and Fascia — *continued*
    Lower Leg
      Left ØJNP
      Right ØJNN
    Neck
      Left ØJN5
      Right ØJN4
    Pelvic Region ØJNC
    Perineum ØJNB
    Scalp ØJNØ
    Upper Arm
      Left ØJNF
      Right ØJND
    Upper Leg
      Left ØJNM
      Right ØJNL
  Tarsal
    Left ØQNM
    Right ØQNL
  Tendon
    Abdomen
      Left ØLNG
      Right ØLNF
    Ankle
      Left ØLNT
      Right ØLNS
    Foot
      Left ØLNW
      Right ØLNV
    Hand
      Left ØLN8
      Right ØLN7
    Head and Neck ØLNØ
    Hip
      Left ØLNK
      Right ØLNJ
    Knee
      Left ØLNR
      Right ØLNQ
    Lower Arm and Wrist
      Left ØLN6
      Right ØLN5
    Lower Leg
      Left ØLNP
      Right ØLNN
    Perineum ØLNH
    Shoulder
      Left ØLN2
      Right ØLN1
    Thorax
      Left ØLND
      Right ØLNC
    Trunk
      Left ØLNB
      Right ØLN9
    Upper Arm
      Left ØLN4
      Right ØLN3
    Upper Leg
      Left ØLNM
      Right ØLNL
  Testis
    Bilateral ØVNC
    Left ØVNB
    Right ØVN9
  Thalamus ØØN9
  Thymus Ø7NM
  Thyroid Gland ØGNK
    Left Lobe ØGNG
    Right Lobe ØGNH
  Tibia
    Left ØQNH
    Right ØQNG
  Toe Nail ØHNRXZZ
  Tongue ØCN7
  Tonsils ØCNP
  Tooth
    Lower ØCNX
    Upper ØCNW
  Trachea ØBN1
  Tunica Vaginalis
    Left ØVN7
    Right ØVN6
  Turbinate, Nasal Ø9NL
  Tympanic Membrane
    Left Ø9N8
    Right Ø9N7

Release — *continued*
  Ulna
    Left ØPNL
    Right ØPNK
  Ureter
    Left ØTN7
    Right ØTN6
  Urethra ØTND
  Uterine Supporting Structure ØUN4
  Uterus ØUN9
  Uvula ØCNN
  Vagina ØUNG
  Valve
    Aortic Ø2NF
    Mitral Ø2NG
    Pulmonary Ø2NH
    Tricuspid Ø2NJ
  Vas Deferens
    Bilateral ØVNQ
    Left ØVNP
    Right ØVNN
  Vein
    Axillary
      Left Ø5N8
      Right Ø5N7
    Azygos Ø5NØ
    Basilic
      Left Ø5NC
      Right Ø5NB
    Brachial
      Left Ø5NA
      Right Ø5N9
    Cephalic
      Left Ø5NF
      Right Ø5ND
    Colic Ø6N7
    Common Iliac
      Left Ø6ND
      Right Ø6NC
    Coronary Ø2N4
    Esophageal Ø6N3
    External Iliac
      Left Ø6NG
      Right Ø6NF
    External Jugular
      Left Ø5NQ
      Right Ø5NP
    Face
      Left Ø5NV
      Right Ø5NT
    Femoral
      Left Ø6NN
      Right Ø6NM
    Foot
      Left Ø6NV
      Right Ø6NT
    Gastric Ø6N2
    Hand
      Left Ø5NH
      Right Ø5NG
    Hemiazygos Ø5N1
    Hepatic Ø6N4
    Hypogastric
      Left Ø6NJ
      Right Ø6NH
    Inferior Mesenteric Ø6N6
    Innominate
      Left Ø5N4
      Right Ø5N3
    Internal Jugular
      Left Ø5NN
      Right Ø5NM
    Intracranial Ø5NL
    Lower Ø6NY
    Portal Ø6N8
    Pulmonary
      Left Ø2NT
      Right Ø2NS
    Renal
      Left Ø6NB
      Right Ø6N9
    Saphenous
      Left Ø6NQ
      Right Ø6NP
    Splenic Ø6N1
    Subclavian
      Left Ø5N6
      Right Ø5N5
    Superior Mesenteric Ø6N5

Release — *continued*
  Vein — *continued*
    Upper Ø5NY
    Vertebral
      Left Ø5NS
      Right Ø5NR
  Vena Cava
    Inferior Ø6NØ
    Superior Ø2NV
  Ventricle
    Left Ø2NL
    Right Ø2NK
  Vertebra
    Cervical ØPN3
    Lumbar ØQNØ
    Thoracic ØPN4
  Vesicle
    Bilateral ØVN3
    Left ØVN2
    Right ØVN1
  Vitreous
    Left Ø8N53ZZ
    Right Ø8N43ZZ
  Vocal Cord
    Left ØCNV
    Right ØCNT
  Vulva ØUNM
Relocation *see* Reposition
Remdesivir Anti-infective XWØ
Removal
  Abdominal Wall 2W53X
  Anorectal 2Y53X5Z
  Arm
    Lower
      Left 2W5DX
      Right 2W5CX
    Upper
      Left 2W5BX
      Right 2W5AX
  Back 2W55X
  Chest Wall 2W54X
  Ear 2Y52X5Z
  Extremity
    Lower
      Left 2W5MX
      Right 2W5LX
    Upper
      Left 2W59X
      Right 2W58X
  Face 2W51X
  Finger
    Left 2W5KX
    Right 2W5JX
  Foot
    Left 2W5TX
    Right 2W5SX
  Genital Tract, Female 2Y54X5Z
  Hand
    Left 2W5FX
    Right 2W5EX
  Head 2W50X
  Inguinal Region
    Left 2W57X
    Right 2W56X
  Leg
    Lower
      Left 2W5RX
      Right 2W5QX
    Upper
      Left 2W5PX
      Right 2W5NX
  Mouth and Pharynx 2Y50X5Z
  Nasal 2Y51X5Z
  Neck 2W52X
  Thumb
    Left 2W5HX
    Right 2W5GX
  Toe
    Left 2W5VX
    Right 2W5UX
  Urethra 2Y55X5Z
Removal of device from
  Abdominal Wall ØWPF
  Acetabulum
    Left ØQP5
    Right ØQP4
  Anal Sphincter ØDPR
  Anus ØDPQ

Removal of device from — continued

Artery
- Lower 04PY
- Upper 03PY

Back
- Lower 0WPL
- Upper 0WPK

Bladder 0TPB

Bone
- Facial 0NPW
- Lower 0QPY
- Nasal 0NPB
- Pelvic
  - Left 0QP3
  - Right 0QP2
- Upper 0PPY

Bone Marrow 07PT

Brain 00P0

Breast
- Left 0HPU
- Right 0HPT

Bursa and Ligament
- Lower 0MPY
- Upper 0MPX

Carpal
- Left 0PPN
- Right 0PPM

Cavity, Cranial 0WP1

Cerebral Ventricle 00P6

Chest Wall 0WP8

Cisterna Chyli 07PL

Clavicle
- Left 0PPB
- Right 0PP9

Coccyx 0QPS

Diaphragm 0BPT

Disc
- Cervical Vertebral 0RP3
- Cervicothoracic Vertebral 0RP5
- Lumbar Vertebral 0SP2
- Lumbosacral 0SP4
- Thoracic Vertebral 0RP9
- Thoracolumbar Vertebral 0RPB

Duct
- Hepatobiliary 0FPB
- Pancreatic 0FPD

Ear
- Inner
  - Left 09PJ
  - Right 09PD
- Left 09PJ
- Right 09PH

Epididymis and Spermatic Cord 0VPM

Esophagus 0DP5

Extremity
- Lower
  - Left 0YPB
  - Right 0YP9
- Upper
  - Left 0XP7
  - Right 0XP6

Eye
- Left 08P1
- Right 08P0

Face 0WP2

Fallopian Tube 0UP8

Femoral Shaft
- Left 0QP9
- Right 0QP8

Femur
- Lower
  - Left 0QPC
  - Right 0QPB
- Upper
  - Left 0QP7
  - Right 0QP6

Fibula
- Left 0QPK
- Right 0QPJ

Finger Nail 0HPQX

Gallbladder 0FP4

Gastrointestinal Tract 0WPP

Genitourinary Tract 0WPR

Gland
- Adrenal 0GP5
- Endocrine 0GPS
- Pituitary 0GP0
- Salivary 0CPA

Removal of device from — continued

Glenoid Cavity
- Left 0PP8
- Right 0PP7

Great Vessel 02PY

Hair 0HPSX

Head 0WP0

Heart 02PA

Humeral Head
- Left 0PPD
- Right 0PPC

Humeral Shaft
- Left 0PPG
- Right 0PPF

Intestinal Tract
- Lower 0DPD
- Upper 0DP0

Jaw
- Lower 0WP5
- Upper 0WP4

Joint
- Acromioclavicular
  - Left 0RPH
  - Right 0RPG
- Ankle
  - Left 0SPG
  - Right 0SPF
- Carpal
  - Left 0RPR
  - Right 0RPQ
- Carpometacarpal
  - Left 0RPT
  - Right 0RPS
- Cervical Vertebral 0RP1
- Cervicothoracic Vertebral 0RP4
- Coccygeal 0SP6
- Elbow
  - Left 0RPM
  - Right 0RPL
- Finger Phalangeal
  - Left 0RPX
  - Right 0RPW
- Hip
  - Left 0SPB
    - Acetabular Surface 0SPE
    - Femoral Surface 0SPS
  - Right 0SP9
    - Acetabular Surface 0SPA
    - Femoral Surface 0SPR
- Knee
  - Left 0SPD
    - Femoral Surface 0SPU
    - Tibial Surface 0SPW
  - Right 0SPC
    - Femoral Surface 0SPT
    - Tibial Surface 0SPV
- Lumbar Vertebral 0SP0
- Lumbosacral 0SP3
- Metacarpophalangeal
  - Left 0RPV
  - Right 0RPU
- Metatarsal-Phalangeal
  - Left 0SPN
  - Right 0SPM
- Occipital-cervical 0RP0
- Sacrococcygeal 0SP5
- Sacroiliac
  - Left 0SP8
  - Right 0SP7
- Shoulder
  - Left 0RPK
  - Right 0RPJ
- Sternoclavicular
  - Left 0RPF
  - Right 0RPE
- Tarsal
  - Left 0SPJ
  - Right 0SPH
- Tarsometatarsal
  - Left 0SPL
  - Right 0SPK
- Temporomandibular
  - Left 0RPD
  - Right 0RPC
- Thoracic Vertebral 0RP6
- Thoracolumbar Vertebral 0RPA
- Toe Phalangeal
  - Left 0SPQ
  - Right 0SPP

Removal of device from — continued

Joint — continued
- Wrist
  - Left 0RPP
  - Right 0RPN

Kidney 0TP5

Larynx 0CPS

Lens
- Left 08PK3
- Right 08PJ3

Liver 0FP0

Lung
- Left 0BPL
- Right 0BPK

Lymphatic 07PN
- Thoracic Duct 07PK

Mediastinum 0WPC

Mesentery 0DPV

Metacarpal
- Left 0PPQ
- Right 0PPP

Metatarsal
- Left 0QPP
- Right 0QPN

Mouth and Throat 0CPY

Muscle
- Extraocular
  - Left 08PM
  - Right 08PL
- Lower 0KPY
- Upper 0KPX

Nasal Mucosa and Soft Tissue 09PK

Neck 0WP6

Nerve
- Cranial 00PE
- Peripheral 01PY

Omentum 0DPU

Ovary 0UP3

Pancreas 0FPG

Parathyroid Gland 0GPR

Patella
- Left 0QPF
- Right 0QPD

Pelvic Cavity 0WPJ

Penis 0VPS

Pericardial Cavity 0WPD

Perineum
- Female 0WPN
- Male 0WPM

Peritoneal Cavity 0WPG

Peritoneum 0DPW

Phalanx
- Finger
  - Left 0PPV
  - Right 0PPT
- Thumb
  - Left 0PPS
  - Right 0PPR
- Toe
  - Left 0QPR
  - Right 0QPQ

Pineal Body 0GP1

Pleura 0BPQ

Pleural Cavity
- Left 0WPB
- Right 0WP9

Products of Conception 10P0

Prostate and Seminal Vesicles 0VP4

Radius
- Left 0PPJ
- Right 0PPH

Rectum 0DPP

Respiratory Tract 0WPQ

Retroperitoneum 0WPH

Ribs
- 1 to 2 0PP1
- 3 or More 0PP2

Sacrum 0QP1

Scapula
- Left 0PP6
- Right 0PP5

Scrotum and Tunica Vaginalis 0VP8

Sinus 09PY

Skin 0HPPX

Skull 0NP0

Spinal Canal 00PU

Spinal Cord 00PV

Spleen 07PP

Sternum 0PP0

▽ Subterms under main terms may continue to next column or page

Removal of device from — *continued*
  Stomach ØDP6
  Subcutaneous Tissue and Fascia
    Head and Neck ØJPS
    Lower Extremity ØJPW
    Trunk ØJPT
    Upper Extremity ØJPV
  Tarsal
    Left ØQPM
    Right ØQPL
  Tendon
    Lower ØLPY
    Upper ØLPX
  Testis ØVPD
  Thymus Ø7PM
  Thyroid Gland ØGPK
  Tibia
    Left ØQPH
    Right ØQPG
  Toe Nail ØHPRX
  Trachea ØBP1
  Tracheobronchial Tree ØBPØ
  Tympanic Membrane
    Left Ø9P8
    Right Ø9P7
  Ulna
    Left ØPPL
    Right ØPPK
  Ureter ØTP9
  Urethra ØTPD
  Uterus and Cervix ØUPD
  Vagina and Cul-de-sac ØUPH
  Vas Deferens ØVPR
  Vein
    Azygos Ø5PØ
    Innominate
      Left Ø5P4
      Right Ø5P3
    Lower Ø6PY
    Upper Ø5PY
  Vertebra
    Cervical ØPP3
    Lumbar ØQPØ
    Thoracic ØPP4
  Vulva ØUPM
Renal calyx
  use Kidney
  use Kidney, Left
  use Kidney, Right
  use Kidneys, Bilateral
Renal capsule
  use Kidney
  use Kidney, Left
  use Kidney, Right
  use Kidneys, Bilateral
Renal cortex
  use Kidney
  use Kidney, Left
  use Kidney, Right
  use Kidneys, Bilateral
Renal dialysis *see* Performance, Urinary 5A1D
Renal nerve *use* Abdominal Sympathetic Nerve
Renal plexus *use* Abdominal Sympathetic Nerve
Renal segment
  use Kidney
  use Kidney, Left
  use Kidney, Right
  use Kidneys, Bilateral
Renal segmental artery
  use Renal Artery, Left
  use Renal Artery, Right
Reopening, operative site
  Control of bleeding *see* Control bleeding in
  Inspection only *see* Inspection
Repair
  Abdominal Wall ØWQF
  Acetabulum
    Left ØQQ5
    Right ØQQ4
  Adenoids ØCQQ
  Ampulla of Vater ØFQC
  Anal Sphincter ØDQR
  Ankle Region
    Left ØYQL
    Right ØYQK
  Anterior Chamber
    Left Ø8Q33ZZ
    Right Ø8Q23ZZ

Repair — *continued*
  Anus ØDQQ
  Aorta
    Abdominal Ø4QØ
    Thoracic
      Ascending/Arch Ø2QX
      Descending Ø2QW
  Aortic Body ØGQD
  Appendix ØDQJ
  Arm
    Lower
      Left ØXQF
      Right ØXQD
    Upper
      Left ØXQ9
      Right ØXQ8
  Artery
    Anterior Tibial
      Left Ø4QQ
      Right Ø4QP
    Axillary
      Left Ø3Q6
      Right Ø3Q5
    Brachial
      Left Ø3Q8
      Right Ø3Q7
    Celiac Ø4Q1
    Colic
      Left Ø4Q7
      Middle Ø4Q8
      Right Ø4Q6
    Common Carotid
      Left Ø3QJ
      Right Ø3QH
    Common Iliac
      Left Ø4QD
      Right Ø4QC
    Coronary
      Four or More Arteries Ø2Q3
      One Artery Ø2QØ
      Three Arteries Ø2Q2
      Two Arteries Ø2Q1
    External Carotid
      Left Ø3QN
      Right Ø3QM
    External Iliac
      Left Ø4QJ
      Right Ø4QH
    Face Ø3QR
    Femoral
      Left Ø4QL
      Right Ø4QK
    Foot
      Left Ø4QW
      Right Ø4QV
    Gastric Ø4Q2
    Hand
      Left Ø3QF
      Right Ø3QD
    Hepatic Ø4Q3
    Inferior Mesenteric Ø4QB
    Innominate Ø3Q2
    Internal Carotid
      Left Ø3QL
      Right Ø3QK
    Internal Iliac
      Left Ø4QF
      Right Ø4QE
    Internal Mammary
      Left Ø3Q1
      Right Ø3QØ
    Intracranial Ø3QG
    Lower Ø4QY
    Peroneal
      Left Ø4QU
      Right Ø4QT
    Popliteal
      Left Ø4QN
      Right Ø4QM
    Posterior Tibial
      Left Ø4QS
      Right Ø4QR
    Pulmonary
      Left Ø2QR
      Right Ø2QQ
    Pulmonary Trunk Ø2QP
    Radial
      Left Ø3QC
      Right Ø3QB

Repair — *continued*
  Artery — *continued*
    Renal
      Left Ø4QA
      Right Ø4Q9
    Splenic Ø4Q4
    Subclavian
      Left Ø3Q4
      Right Ø3Q3
    Superior Mesenteric Ø4Q5
    Temporal
      Left Ø3QT
      Right Ø3QS
    Thyroid
      Left Ø3QV
      Right Ø3QU
    Ulnar
      Left Ø3QA
      Right Ø3Q9
    Upper Ø3QY
    Vertebral
      Left Ø3QQ
      Right Ø3QP
  Atrium
    Left Ø2Q7
    Right Ø2Q6
  Auditory Ossicle
    Left Ø9QA
    Right Ø9Q9
  Axilla
    Left ØXQ5
    Right ØXQ4
  Back
    Lower ØWQL
    Upper ØWQK
  Basal Ganglia ØØQ8
  Bladder ØTQB
  Bladder Neck ØTQC
  Bone
    Ethmoid
      Left ØNQG
      Right ØNQF
    Frontal ØNQ1
    Hyoid ØNQX
    Lacrimal
      Left ØNQJ
      Right ØNQH
    Nasal ØNQB
    Occipital ØNQ7
    Palatine
      Left ØNQL
      Right ØNQK
    Parietal
      Left ØNQ4
      Right ØNQ3
    Pelvic
      Left ØQQ3
      Right ØQQ2
    Sphenoid ØNQC
    Temporal
      Left ØNQ6
      Right ØNQ5
    Zygomatic
      Left ØNQN
      Right ØNQM
  Brain ØØQØ
  Breast
    Bilateral ØHQV
    Left ØHQU
    Right ØHQT
    Supernumerary ØHQY
  Bronchus
    Lingula ØBQ9
    Lower Lobe
      Left ØBQB
      Right ØBQ6
    Main
      Left ØBQ7
      Right ØBQ3
    Middle Lobe, Right ØBQ5
    Upper Lobe
      Left ØBQ8
      Right ØBQ4
  Buccal Mucosa ØCQ4
  Bursa and Ligament
    Abdomen
      Left ØMQJ
      Right ØMQH

Repair — continued
- Bursa and Ligament — continued
  - Ankle
    - Left ØMQR
    - Right ØMQQ
  - Elbow
    - Left ØMQ4
    - Right ØMQ3
  - Foot
    - Left ØMQT
    - Right ØMQS
  - Hand
    - Left ØMQ8
    - Right ØMQ7
  - Head and Neck ØMQØ
  - Hip
    - Left ØMQM
    - Right ØMQL
  - Knee
    - Left ØMQP
    - Right ØMQN
  - Lower Extremity
    - Left ØMQW
    - Right ØMQV
  - Perineum ØMQK
  - Rib(s) ØMQG
  - Shoulder
    - Left ØMQ2
    - Right ØMQ1
  - Spine
    - Lower ØMQD
    - Upper ØMQC
  - Sternum ØMQF
  - Upper Extremity
    - Left ØMQB
    - Right ØMQ9
  - Wrist
    - Left ØMQ6
    - Right ØMQ5
- Buttock
  - Left ØYQ1
  - Right ØYQØ
- Carina ØBQ2
- Carotid Bodies, Bilateral ØGQ8
- Carotid Body
  - Left ØGQ6
  - Right ØGQ7
- Carpal
  - Left ØPQN
  - Right ØPQM
- Cecum ØDQH
- Cerebellum ØØQC
- Cerebral Hemisphere ØØQ7
- Cerebral Meninges ØØQ1
- Cerebral Ventricle ØØQ6
- Cervix ØUQC
- Chest Wall ØWQ8
- Chordae Tendineae Ø2Q9
- Choroid
  - Left Ø8QB
  - Right Ø8QA
- Cisterna Chyli Ø7QL
- Clavicle
  - Left ØPQB
  - Right ØPQ9
- Clitoris ØUQJ
- Coccygeal Glomus ØGQB
- Coccyx ØQQS
- Colon
  - Ascending ØDQK
  - Descending ØDQM
  - Sigmoid ØDQN
  - Transverse ØDQL
- Conduction Mechanism Ø2Q8
- Conjunctiva
  - Left Ø8QTXZZ
  - Right Ø8QSXZZ
- Cord
  - Bilateral ØVQH
  - Left ØVQG
  - Right ØVQF
- Cornea
  - Left Ø8Q9XZZ
  - Right Ø8Q8XZZ
- Cul-de-sac ØUQF
- Diaphragm ØBQT
- Disc
  - Cervical Vertebral ØRQ3
  - Cervicothoracic Vertebral ØRQ5

Repair — continued
- Disc — continued
  - Lumbar Vertebral ØSQ2
  - Lumbosacral ØSQ4
  - Thoracic Vertebral ØRQ9
  - Thoracolumbar Vertebral ØRQB
- Duct
  - Common Bile ØFQ9
  - Cystic ØFQ8
  - Hepatic
    - Common ØFQ7
    - Left ØFQ6
    - Right ØFQ5
  - Lacrimal
    - Left Ø8QY
    - Right Ø8QX
  - Pancreatic ØFQD
    - Accessory ØFQF
  - Parotid
    - Left ØCQC
    - Right ØCQB
- Duodenum ØDQ9
- Dura Mater ØØQ2
- Ear
  - External
    - Bilateral Ø9Q2
    - Left Ø9Q1
    - Right Ø9QØ
  - External Auditory Canal
    - Left Ø9Q4
    - Right Ø9Q3
  - Inner
    - Left Ø9QE
    - Right Ø9QD
  - Middle
    - Left Ø9Q6
    - Right Ø9Q5
- Elbow Region
  - Left ØXQC
  - Right ØXQB
- Epididymis
  - Bilateral ØVQL
  - Left ØVQK
  - Right ØVQJ
- Epiglottis ØCQR
- Esophagogastric Junction ØDQ4
- Esophagus ØDQ5
  - Lower ØDQ3
  - Middle ØDQ2
  - Upper ØDQ1
- Eustachian Tube
  - Left Ø9QG
  - Right Ø9QF
- Extremity
  - Lower
    - Left ØYQB
    - Right ØYQ9
  - Upper
    - Left ØXQ7
    - Right ØXQ6
- Eye
  - Left Ø8Q1XZZ
  - Right Ø8QØXZZ
- Eyelid
  - Lower
    - Left Ø8QR
    - Right Ø8QQ
  - Upper
    - Left Ø8QP
    - Right Ø8QN
- Face ØWQ2
- Fallopian Tube
  - Left ØUQ6
  - Right ØUQ5
- Fallopian Tubes, Bilateral ØUQ7
- Femoral Region
  - Bilateral ØYQE
  - Left ØYQ8
  - Right ØYQ7
- Femoral Shaft
  - Left ØQQ9
  - Right ØQQ8
- Femur
  - Lower
    - Left ØQQC
    - Right ØQQB
  - Upper
    - Left ØQQ7
    - Right ØQQ6

Repair — continued
- Fibula
  - Left ØQQK
  - Right ØQQJ
- Finger
  - Index
    - Left ØXQP
    - Right ØXQN
  - Little
    - Left ØXQW
    - Right ØXQV
  - Middle
    - Left ØXQR
    - Right ØXQQ
  - Ring
    - Left ØXQT
    - Right ØXQS
- Finger Nail ØHQQXZZ
- Floor of mouth see Repair, Oral Cavity and Throat ØWQ3
- Foot
  - Left ØYQN
  - Right ØYQM
- Gallbladder ØFQ4
- Gingiva
  - Lower ØCQ6
  - Upper ØCQ5
- Gland
  - Adrenal
    - Bilateral ØGQ4
    - Left ØGQ2
    - Right ØGQ3
  - Lacrimal
    - Left Ø8QW
    - Right Ø8QV
  - Minor Salivary ØCQJ
  - Parotid
    - Left ØCQ9
    - Right ØCQ8
  - Pituitary ØGQØ
  - Sublingual
    - Left ØCQF
    - Right ØCQD
  - Submaxillary
    - Left ØCQH
    - Right ØCQG
  - Vestibular ØUQL
- Glenoid Cavity
  - Left ØPQ8
  - Right ØPQ7
- Glomus Jugulare ØGQC
- Hand
  - Left ØXQK
  - Right ØXQJ
- Head ØWQØ
- Heart Ø2QA
  - Left Ø2QC
  - Right Ø2QB
- Humeral Head
  - Left ØPQD
  - Right ØPQC
- Humeral Shaft
  - Left ØPQG
  - Right ØPQF
- Hymen ØUQK
- Hypothalamus ØØQA
- Ileocecal Valve ØDQC
- Ileum ØDQB
- Inguinal Region
  - Bilateral ØYQA
  - Left ØYQ6
  - Right ØYQ5
- Intestine
  - Large ØDQE
    - Left ØDQG
    - Right ØDQF
  - Small ØDQ8
- Iris
  - Left Ø8QD3ZZ
  - Right Ø8QC3ZZ
- Jaw
  - Lower ØWQ5
  - Upper ØWQ4
- Jejunum ØDQA
- Joint
  - Acromioclavicular
    - Left ØRQH
    - Right ØRQG

Repair — continued
  Joint — continued
    Ankle
      Left ØSQG
      Right ØSQF
    Carpal
      Left ØRQR
      Right ØRQQ
    Carpometacarpal
      Left ØRQT
      Right ØRQS
    Cervical Vertebral ØRQ1
    Cervicothoracic Vertebral ØRQ4
    Coccygeal ØSQ6
    Elbow
      Left ØRQM
      Right ØRQL
    Finger Phalangeal
      Left ØRQX
      Right ØRQW
    Hip
      Left ØSQB
      Right ØSQ9
    Knee
      Left ØSQD
      Right ØSQC
    Lumbar Vertebral ØSQ0
    Lumbosacral ØSQ3
    Metacarpophalangeal
      Left ØRQV
      Right ØRQU
    Metatarsal-Phalangeal
      Left ØSQN
      Right ØSQM
    Occipital-cervical ØRQ0
    Sacrococcygeal ØSQ5
    Sacroiliac
      Left ØSQ8
      Right ØSQ7
    Shoulder
      Left ØRQK
      Right ØRQJ
    Sternoclavicular
      Left ØRQF
      Right ØRQE
    Tarsal
      Left ØSQJ
      Right ØSQH
    Tarsometatarsal
      Left ØSQL
      Right ØSQK
    Temporomandibular
      Left ØRQD
      Right ØRQC
    Thoracic Vertebral ØRQ6
    Thoracolumbar Vertebral ØRQA
    Toe Phalangeal
      Left ØSQQ
      Right ØSQP
    Wrist
      Left ØRQP
      Right ØRQN
  Kidney
    Left ØTQ1
    Right ØTQ0
  Kidney Pelvis
    Left ØTQ4
    Right ØTQ3
  Knee Region
    Left ØYQG
    Right ØYQF
  Larynx ØCQS
  Leg
    Lower
      Left ØYQJ
      Right ØYQH
    Upper
      Left ØYQD
      Right ØYQC
  Lens
    Left Ø8QK3ZZ
    Right Ø8QJ3ZZ
  Lip
    Lower ØCQ1
    Upper ØCQ0
  Liver ØFQ0
    Left Lobe ØFQ2
    Right Lobe ØFQ1

Repair — continued
  Lung
    Bilateral ØBQM
    Left ØBQL
    Lower Lobe
      Left ØBQJ
      Right ØBQF
    Middle Lobe, Right ØBQD
    Right ØBQK
    Upper Lobe
      Left ØBQG
      Right ØBQC
  Lung Lingula ØBQH
  Lymphatic
    Aortic Ø7QD
    Axillary
      Left Ø7Q6
      Right Ø7Q5
    Head Ø7Q0
    Inguinal
      Left Ø7QJ
      Right Ø7QH
    Internal Mammary
      Left Ø7Q9
      Right Ø7Q8
    Lower Extremity
      Left Ø7QG
      Right Ø7QF
    Mesenteric Ø7QB
    Neck
      Left Ø7Q2
      Right Ø7Q1
    Pelvis Ø7QC
    Thoracic Duct Ø7QK
    Thorax Ø7Q7
    Upper Extremity
      Left Ø7Q4
      Right Ø7Q3
  Mandible
    Left ØNQV
    Right ØNQT
  Maxilla ØNQR
  Mediastinum ØWQC
  Medulla Oblongata ØØQD
  Mesentery ØDQV
  Metacarpal
    Left ØPQQ
    Right ØPQP
  Metatarsal
    Left ØQQP
    Right ØQQN
  Muscle
    Abdomen
      Left ØKQL
      Right ØKQK
    Extraocular
      Left Ø8QM
      Right Ø8QL
    Facial ØKQ1
    Foot
      Left ØKQW
      Right ØKQV
    Hand
      Left ØKQD
      Right ØKQC
    Head ØKQ0
    Hip
      Left ØKQP
      Right ØKQN
    Lower Arm and Wrist
      Left ØKQB
      Right ØKQ9
    Lower Leg
      Left ØKQT
      Right ØKQS
    Neck
      Left ØKQ3
      Right ØKQ2
    Papillary Ø2QD
    Perineum ØKQM
    Shoulder
      Left ØKQ6
      Right ØKQ5
    Thorax
      Left ØKQJ
      Right ØKQH
    Tongue, Palate, Pharynx ØKQ4
    Trunk
      Left ØKQG

Repair — continued
  Muscle — continued
    Trunk — continued
      Right ØKQF
    Upper Arm
      Left ØKQ8
      Right ØKQ7
    Upper Leg
      Left ØKQR
      Right ØKQQ
  Nasal Mucosa and Soft Tissue Ø9QK
  Nasopharynx Ø9QN
  Neck ØWQ6
  Nerve
    Abdominal Sympathetic Ø1QM
    Abducens ØØQL
    Accessory ØØQR
    Acoustic ØØQN
    Brachial Plexus Ø1Q3
    Cervical Ø1Q1
    Cervical Plexus Ø1Q0
    Facial ØØQM
    Femoral Ø1QD
    Glossopharyngeal ØØQP
    Head and Neck Sympathetic Ø1QK
    Hypoglossal ØØQS
    Lumbar Ø1QB
    Lumbar Plexus Ø1Q9
    Lumbar Sympathetic Ø1QN
    Lumbosacral Plexus Ø1QA
    Median Ø1Q5
    Oculomotor ØØQH
    Olfactory ØØQF
    Optic ØØQG
    Peroneal Ø1QH
    Phrenic Ø1Q2
    Pudendal Ø1QC
    Radial Ø1Q6
    Sacral Ø1QR
    Sacral Plexus Ø1QQ
    Sacral Sympathetic Ø1QP
    Sciatic Ø1QF
    Thoracic Ø1Q8
    Thoracic Sympathetic Ø1QL
    Tibial Ø1QG
    Trigeminal ØØQK
    Trochlear ØØQJ
    Ulnar Ø1Q4
    Vagus ØØQQ
  Nipple
    Left ØHQX
    Right ØHQW
  Omentum ØDQU
  Oral Cavity and Throat ØWQ3
  Orbit
    Left ØNQQ
    Right ØNQP
  Ovary
    Bilateral ØUQ2
    Left ØUQ1
    Right ØUQ0
  Palate
    Hard ØCQ2
    Soft ØCQ3
  Pancreas ØFQG
  Para-aortic Body ØGQ9
  Paraganglion Extremity ØGQF
  Parathyroid Gland ØGQR
    Inferior
      Left ØGQP
      Right ØGQN
    Multiple ØGQQ
    Superior
      Left ØGQM
      Right ØGQL
  Patella
    Left ØQQF
    Right ØQQD
  Penis ØVQS
  Pericardium Ø2QN
  Perineum
    Female ØWQN
    Male ØWQM
  Peritoneum ØDQW
  Phalanx
    Finger
      Left ØPQV
      Right ØPQT

Repair — continued
  Phalanx — continued
    Thumb
      Left ØPQS
      Right ØPQR
    Toe
      Left ØQQR
      Right ØQQQ
  Pharynx ØCQM
  Pineal Body ØGQ1
  Pleura
    Left ØBQP
    Right ØBQN
  Pons ØØQB
  Prepuce ØVQT
  Products of Conception 1ØQØ
  Prostate ØVQØ
  Radius
    Left ØPQJ
    Right ØPQH
  Rectum ØDQP
  Retina
    Left Ø8QF3ZZ
    Right Ø8QE3ZZ
  Retinal Vessel
    Left Ø8QH3ZZ
    Right Ø8QG3ZZ
  Ribs
    1 to 2 ØPQ1
    3 or More ØPQ2
  Sacrum ØQQ1
  Scapula
    Left ØPQ6
    Right ØPQ5
  Sclera
    Left Ø8Q7XZZ
    Right Ø8Q6XZZ
  Scrotum ØVQ5
  Septum
    Atrial Ø2Q5
    Nasal Ø9QM
    Ventricular Ø2QM
  Shoulder Region
    Left ØXQ3
    Right ØXQ2
  Sinus
    Accessory Ø9QP
    Ethmoid
      Left Ø9QV
      Right Ø9QU
    Frontal
      Left Ø9QT
      Right Ø9QS
    Mastoid
      Left Ø9QC
      Right Ø9QB
    Maxillary
      Left Ø9QR
      Right Ø9QQ
    Sphenoid
      Left Ø9QX
      Right Ø9QW
  Skin
    Abdomen ØHQ7XZZ
    Back ØHQ6XZZ
    Buttock ØHQ8XZZ
    Chest ØHQ5XZZ
    Ear
      Left ØHQ3XZZ
      Right ØHQ2XZZ
    Face ØHQ1XZZ
    Foot
      Left ØHQNXZZ
      Right ØHQMXZZ
    Hand
      Left ØHQGXZZ
      Right ØHQFXZZ
    Inguinal ØHQAXZZ
    Lower Arm
      Left ØHQEXZZ
      Right ØHQDXZZ
    Lower Leg
      Left ØHQLXZZ
      Right ØHQKXZZ
    Neck ØHQ4XZZ
    Perineum ØHQ9XZZ
    Scalp ØHQØXZZ
    Upper Arm
      Left ØHQCXZZ

Repair — continued
  Skin — continued
    Upper Arm — continued
      Right ØHQBXZZ
    Upper Leg
      Left ØHQJXZZ
      Right ØHQHXZZ
  Skull ØNQØ
  Spinal Cord
    Cervical ØØQW
    Lumbar ØØQY
    Thoracic ØØQX
  Spinal Meninges ØØQT
  Spleen Ø7QP
  Sternum ØPQØ
  Stomach ØDQ6
    Pylorus ØDQ7
  Subcutaneous Tissue and Fascia
    Abdomen ØJQ8
    Back ØJQ7
    Buttock ØJQ9
    Chest ØJQ6
    Face ØJQ1
    Foot
      Left ØJQR
      Right ØJQQ
    Hand
      Left ØJQK
      Right ØJQJ
    Lower Arm
      Left ØJQH
      Right ØJQG
    Lower Leg
      Left ØJQP
      Right ØJQN
    Neck
      Left ØJQ5
      Right ØJQ4
    Pelvic Region ØJQC
    Perineum ØJQB
    Scalp ØJQØ
    Upper Arm
      Left ØJQF
      Right ØJQD
    Upper Leg
      Left ØJQM
      Right ØJQL
  Tarsal
    Left ØQQM
    Right ØQQL
  Tendon
    Abdomen
      Left ØLQG
      Right ØLQF
    Ankle
      Left ØLQT
      Right ØLQS
    Foot
      Left ØLQW
      Right ØLQV
    Hand
      Left ØLQ8
      Right ØLQ7
    Head and Neck ØLQØ
    Hip
      Left ØLQK
      Right ØLQJ
    Knee
      Left ØLQR
      Right ØLQQ
    Lower Arm and Wrist
      Left ØLQ6
      Right ØLQ5
    Lower Leg
      Left ØLQP
      Right ØLQN
    Perineum ØLQH
    Shoulder
      Left ØLQ2
      Right ØLQ1
    Thorax
      Left ØLQD
      Right ØLQC
    Trunk
      Left ØLQB
      Right ØLQ9
    Upper Arm
      Left ØLQ4
      Right ØLQ3

Repair — continued
  Tendon — continued
    Upper Leg
      Left ØLQM
      Right ØLQL
  Testis
    Bilateral ØVQC
    Left ØVQB
    Right ØVQ9
  Thalamus ØØQ9
  Thumb
    Left ØXQM
    Right ØXQL
  Thymus Ø7QM
  Thyroid Gland ØGQK
    Left Lobe ØGQG
    Right Lobe ØGQH
  Thyroid Gland Isthmus ØGQJ
  Tibia
    Left ØQQH
    Right ØQQG
  Toe
    1st
      Left ØYQQ
      Right ØYQP
    2nd
      Left ØYQS
      Right ØYQR
    3rd
      Left ØYQU
      Right ØYQT
    4th
      Left ØYQW
      Right ØYQV
    5th
      Left ØYQY
      Right ØYQX
  Toe Nail ØHQRXZZ
  Tongue ØCQ7
  Tonsils ØCQP
  Tooth
    Lower ØCQX
    Upper ØCQW
  Trachea ØBQ1
  Tunica Vaginalis
    Left ØVQ7
    Right ØVQ6
  Turbinate, Nasal Ø9QL
  Tympanic Membrane
    Left Ø9Q8
    Right Ø9Q7
  Ulna
    Left ØPQL
    Right ØPQK
  Ureter
    Left ØTQ7
    Right ØTQ6
  Urethra ØTQD
  Uterine Supporting Structure ØUQ4
  Uterus ØUQ9
  Uvula ØCQN
  Vagina ØUQG
  Valve
    Aortic Ø2QF
    Mitral Ø2QG
    Pulmonary Ø2QH
    Tricuspid Ø2QJ
  Vas Deferens
    Bilateral ØVQQ
    Left ØVQP
    Right ØVQN
  Vein
    Axillary
      Left Ø5Q8
      Right Ø5Q7
    Azygos Ø5QØ
    Basilic
      Left Ø5QC
      Right Ø5QB
    Brachial
      Left Ø5QA
      Right Ø5Q9
    Cephalic
      Left Ø5QF
      Right Ø5QD
    Colic Ø6Q7
    Common Iliac
      Left Ø6QD
      Right Ø6QC

Repair — continued

Vein — continued
Coronary 02Q4
Esophageal 06Q3
External Iliac
Left 06QG
Right 06QF
External Jugular
Left 05QQ
Right 05QP
Face
Left 05QV
Right 05QT
Femoral
Left 06QN
Right 06QM
Foot
Left 06QV
Right 06QT
Gastric 06Q2
Hand
Left 05QH
Right 05QG
Hemiazygos 05Q1
Hepatic 06Q4
Hypogastric
Left 06QJ
Right 06QH
Inferior Mesenteric 06Q6
Innominate
Left 05Q4
Right 05Q3
Internal Jugular
Left 05QN
Right 05QM
Intracranial 05QL
Lower 06QY
Portal 06Q8
Pulmonary
Left 02QT
Right 02QS
Renal
Left 06QB
Right 06Q9
Saphenous
Left 06QQ
Right 06QP
Splenic 06Q1
Subclavian
Left 05Q6
Right 05Q5
Superior Mesenteric 06Q5
Upper 05QY
Vertebral
Left 05QS
Right 05QR
Vena Cava
Inferior 06Q0
Superior 02QV
Ventricle
Left 02QL
Right 02QK
Vertebra
Cervical 0PQ3
Lumbar 0QQ0
Thoracic 0PQ4
Vesicle
Bilateral 0VQ3
Left 0VQ2
Right 0VQ1
Vitreous
Left 08Q53ZZ
Right 08Q43ZZ
Vocal Cord
Left 0CQV
Right 0CQT
Vulva 0UQM
Wrist Region
Left 0XQH
Right 0XQG

Repair, obstetric laceration, periurethral 0UQMXZZ

Replacement

Acetabulum
Left 0QR5
Right 0QR4
Ampulla of Vater 0FRC
Anal Sphincter 0DRR
Aorta
Abdominal 04R0

Replacement — continued

Aorta — continued
Thoracic
Ascending/Arch 02RX
Descending 02RW
Artery
Anterior Tibial
Left 04RQ
Right 04RP
Axillary
Left 03R6
Right 03R5
Brachial
Left 03R8
Right 03R7
Celiac 04R1
Colic
Left 04R7
Middle 04R8
Right 04R6
Common Carotid
Left 03RJ
Right 03RH
Common Iliac
Left 04RD
Right 04RC
External Carotid
Left 03RN
Right 03RM
External Iliac
Left 04RJ
Right 04RH
Face 03RR
Femoral
Left 04RL
Right 04RK
Foot
Left 04RW
Right 04RV
Gastric 04R2
Hand
Left 03RF
Right 03RD
Hepatic 04R3
Inferior Mesenteric 04RB
Innominate 03R2
Internal Carotid
Left 03RL
Right 03RK
Internal Iliac
Left 04RF
Right 04RE
Internal Mammary
Left 03R1
Right 03R0
Intracranial 03RG
Lower 04RY
Peroneal
Left 04RU
Right 04RT
Popliteal
Left 04RN
Right 04RM
Posterior Tibial
Left 04RS
Right 04RR
Pulmonary
Left 02RR
Right 02RQ
Pulmonary Trunk 02RP
Radial
Left 03RC
Right 03RB
Renal
Left 04RA
Right 04R9
Splenic 04R4
Subclavian
Left 03R4
Right 03R3
Superior Mesenteric 04R5
Temporal
Left 03RT
Right 03RS
Thyroid
Left 03RV
Right 03RU
Ulnar
Left 03RA

Replacement — continued

Artery — continued
Ulnar — continued
Right 03R9
Upper 03RY
Vertebral
Left 03RQ
Right 03RP
Atrium
Left 02R7
Right 02R6
Auditory Ossicle
Left 09RA0
Right 09R90
Bladder 0TRB
Bladder Neck 0TRC
Bone
Ethmoid
Left 0NRG
Right 0NRF
Frontal 0NR1
Hyoid 0NRX
Lacrimal
Left 0NRJ
Right 0NRH
Nasal 0NRB
Occipital 0NR7
Palatine
Left 0NRL
Right 0NRK
Parietal
Left 0NR4
Right 0NR3
Pelvic
Left 0QR3
Right 0QR2
Sphenoid 0NRC
Temporal
Left 0NR6
Right 0NR5
Zygomatic
Left 0NRN
Right 0NRM
Breast
Bilateral 0HRV
Left 0HRU
Right 0HRT
Bronchus
Lingula 0BR9
Lower Lobe
Left 0BRB
Right 0BR6
Main
Left 0BR7
Right 0BR3
Middle Lobe, Right 0BR5
Upper Lobe
Left 0BR8
Right 0BR4
Buccal Mucosa 0CR4
Bursa and Ligament
Abdomen
Left 0MRJ
Right 0MRH
Ankle
Left 0MRR
Right 0MRQ
Elbow
Left 0MR4
Right 0MR3
Foot
Left 0MRT
Right 0MRS
Hand
Left 0MR8
Right 0MR7
Head and Neck 0MR0
Hip
Left 0MRM
Right 0MRL
Knee
Left 0MRP
Right 0MRN
Lower Extremity
Left 0MRW
Right 0MRV
Perineum 0MRK
Rib(s) 0MRG

Replacement — *continued*
  Bursa and Ligament — *continued*
    Shoulder
      Left ØMR2
      Right ØMR1
    Spine
      Lower ØMRD
      Upper ØMRC
    Sternum ØMRF
    Upper Extremity
      Left ØMRB
      Right ØMR9
    Wrist
      Left ØMR6
      Right ØMR5
  Carina ØBR2
  Carpal
    Left ØPRN
    Right ØPRM
  Cerebral Meninges ØØR1
  Cerebral Ventricle ØØR6
  Chordae Tendineae Ø2R9
  Choroid
    Left Ø8RB
    Right Ø8RA
  Clavicle
    Left ØPRB
    Right ØPR9
  Coccyx ØQRS
  Conjunctiva
    Left Ø8RTX
    Right Ø8RSX
  Cornea
    Left Ø8R9
    Right Ø8R8
  Diaphragm ØBRT
  Disc
    Cervical Vertebral ØRR3Ø
    Cervicothoracic Vertebral ØRR5Ø
    Lumbar Vertebral ØSR2Ø
    Lumbosacral ØSR4Ø
    Thoracic Vertebral ØRR9Ø
    Thoracolumbar Vertebral ØRRBØ
  Duct
    Common Bile ØFR9
    Cystic ØFR8
    Hepatic
      Common ØFR7
      Left ØFR6
      Right ØFR5
    Lacrimal
      Left Ø8RY
      Right Ø8RX
    Pancreatic ØFRD
      Accessory ØFRF
    Parotid
      Left ØCRC
      Right ØCRB
  Dura Mater ØØR2
  Ear
    External
      Bilateral Ø9R2
      Left Ø9R1
      Right Ø9RØ
    Inner
      Left Ø9REØ
      Right Ø9RDØ
    Middle
      Left Ø9R6Ø
      Right Ø9R5Ø
  Epiglottis ØCRR
  Esophagus ØDR5
  Eye
    Left Ø8R1
    Right Ø8RØ
  Eyelid
    Lower
      Left Ø8RR
      Right Ø8RQ
    Upper
      Left Ø8RP
      Right Ø8RN
  Femoral Shaft
    Left ØQR9
    Right ØQR8
  Femur
    Lower
      Left ØQRC
      Right ØQRB

Replacement — *continued*
  Femur — *continued*
    Upper
      Left ØQR7
      Right ØQR6
  Fibula
    Left ØQRK
    Right ØQRJ
  Finger Nail ØHRQX
  Gingiva
    Lower ØCR6
    Upper ØCR5
  Glenoid Cavity
    Left ØPR8
    Right ØPR7
  Hair ØHRSX
  Heart Ø2RAØ
  Humeral Head
    Left ØPRD
    Right ØPRC
  Humeral Shaft
    Left ØPRG
    Right ØPRF
  Iris
    Left Ø8RD3
    Right Ø8RC3
  Joint
    Acromioclavicular
      Left ØRRHØ
      Right ØRRGØ
    Ankle
      Left ØSRG
      Right ØSRF
    Carpal
      Left ØRRRØ
      Right ØRRQØ
    Carpometacarpal
      Left ØRRTØ
      Right ØRRSØ
    Cervical Vertebral ØRR1Ø
    Cervicothoracic Vertebral ØRR4Ø
    Coccygeal ØSR6Ø
    Elbow
      Left ØRRMØ
      Right ØRRLØ
    Finger Phalangeal
      Left ØRRXØ
      Right ØRRWØ
    Hip
      Left ØSRB
        Acetabular Surface ØSRE
        Femoral Surface ØSRS
      Right ØSR9
        Acetabular Surface ØSRA
        Femoral Surface ØSRR
    Knee
      Left ØSRD
        Femoral Surface ØSRU
        Tibial Surface ØSRW
      Right ØSRC
        Femoral Surface ØSRT
        Tibial Surface ØSRV
    Lumbar Vertebral ØSRØØ
    Lumbosacral ØSR3Ø
    Metacarpophalangeal
      Left ØRRVØ
      Right ØRRUØ
    Metatarsal-Phalangeal
      Left ØSRNØ
      Right ØSRMØ
    Occipital-cervical ØRRØØ
    Sacrococcygeal ØSR5Ø
    Sacroiliac
      Left ØSR8Ø
      Right ØSR7Ø
    Shoulder
      Left ØRRK
      Right ØRRJ
    Sternoclavicular
      Left ØRRFØ
      Right ØRREØ
    Tarsal
      Left ØSRJØ
      Right ØSRHØ
    Tarsometatarsal
      Left ØSRLØ
      Right ØSRKØ
    Temporomandibular
      Left ØRRDØ

Replacement — *continued*
  Joint — *continued*
    Temporomandibular — *continued*
      Right ØRRCØ
    Thoracic Vertebral ØRR6Ø
    Thoracolumbar Vertebral ØRRAØ
    Toe Phalangeal
      Left ØSRQØ
      Right ØSRPØ
    Wrist
      Left ØRRPØ
      Right ØRRNØ
  Kidney Pelvis
    Left ØTR4
    Right ØTR3
  Larynx ØCRS
  Lens
    Left Ø8RK3ØZ
    Right Ø8RJ3ØZ
  Lip
    Lower ØCR1
    Upper ØCRØ
  Mandible
    Left ØNRV
    Right ØNRT
  Maxilla ØNRR
  Mesentery ØDRV
  Metacarpal
    Left ØPRQ
    Right ØPRP
  Metatarsal
    Left ØQRP
    Right ØQRN
  Muscle
    Abdomen
      Left ØKRL
      Right ØKRK
    Facial ØKR1
    Foot
      Left ØKRW
      Right ØKRV
    Hand
      Left ØKRD
      Right ØKRC
    Head ØKRØ
    Hip
      Left ØKRP
      Right ØKRN
    Lower Arm and Wrist
      Left ØKRB
      Right ØKR9
    Lower Leg
      Left ØKRT
      Right ØKRS
    Neck
      Left ØKR3
      Right ØKR2
    Papillary Ø2RD
    Perineum ØKRM
    Shoulder
      Left ØKR6
      Right ØKR5
    Thorax
      Left ØKRJ
      Right ØKRH
    Tongue, Palate, Pharynx ØKR4
    Trunk
      Left ØKRG
      Right ØKRF
    Upper Arm
      Left ØKR8
      Right ØKR7
    Upper Leg
      Left ØKRR
      Right ØKRQ
  Nasal Mucosa and Soft Tissue Ø9RK
  Nasopharynx Ø9RN
  Nerve
    Abducens ØØRL
    Accessory ØØRR
    Acoustic ØØRN
    Cervical Ø1R1
    Facial ØØRM
    Femoral Ø1RD
    Glossopharyngeal ØØRP
    Hypoglossal ØØRS
    Lumbar Ø1RB
    Median Ø1R5
    Oculomotor ØØRH

Replacement — *continued*
  Nerve — *continued*
    Olfactory 00RF
    Optic 00RG
    Peroneal 01RH
    Phrenic 01R2
    Pudendal 01RC
    Radial 01R6
    Sacral 01RR
    Sciatic 01RF
    Thoracic 01R8
    Tibial 01RG
    Trigeminal 00RK
    Trochlear 00RJ
    Ulnar 01R4
    Vagus 00RQ
  Nipple
    Left 0HRX
    Right 0HRW
  Omentum 0DRU
  Orbit
    Left 0NRQ
    Right 0NRP
  Palate
    Hard 0CR2
    Soft 0CR3
  Patella
    Left 0QRF
    Right 0QRD
  Pericardium 02RN
  Peritoneum 0DRW
  Phalanx
    Finger
      Left 0PRV
      Right 0PRT
    Thumb
      Left 0PRS
      Right 0PRR
    Toe
      Left 0QRR
      Right 0QRQ
  Pharynx 0CRM
  Radius
    Left 0PRJ
    Right 0PRH
  Retinal Vessel
    Left 08RH3
    Right 08RG3
  Ribs
    1 to 2 0PR1
    3 or More 0PR2
  Sacrum 0QR1
  Scapula
    Left 0PR6
    Right 0PR5
  Sclera
    Left 08R7X
    Right 08R6X
  Septum
    Atrial 02R5
    Nasal 09RM
    Ventricular 02RM
  Skin
    Abdomen 0HR7
    Back 0HR6
    Buttock 0HR8
    Chest 0HR5
    Ear
      Left 0HR3
      Right 0HR2
    Face 0HR1
    Foot
      Left 0HRN
      Right 0HRM
    Hand
      Left 0HRG
      Right 0HRF
    Inguinal 0HRA
    Lower Arm
      Left 0HRE
      Right 0HRD
    Lower Leg
      Left 0HRL
      Right 0HRK
    Neck 0HR4
    Perineum 0HR9
    Scalp 0HR0
    Upper Arm
      Left 0HRC

Replacement — *continued*
  Skin — *continued*
    Upper Arm — *continued*
      Right 0HRB
    Upper Leg
      Left 0HRJ
      Right 0HRH
  Skin Substitute, Porcine Liver Derived XHRPXL2
  Skull 0NR0
  Spinal Meninges 00RT
  Sternum 0PR0
  Subcutaneous Tissue and Fascia
    Abdomen 0JR8
    Back 0JR7
    Buttock 0JR9
    Chest 0JR6
    Face 0JR1
    Foot
      Left 0JRR
      Right 0JRQ
    Hand
      Left 0JRK
      Right 0JRJ
    Lower Arm
      Left 0JRH
      Right 0JRG
    Lower Leg
      Left 0JRP
      Right 0JRN
    Neck
      Left 0JR5
      Right 0JR4
    Pelvic Region 0JRC
    Perineum 0JRB
    Scalp 0JR0
    Upper Arm
      Left 0JRF
      Right 0JRD
    Upper Leg
      Left 0JRM
      Right 0JRL
  Tarsal
    Left 0QRM
    Right 0QRL
  Tendon
    Abdomen
      Left 0LRG
      Right 0LRF
    Ankle
      Left 0LRT
      Right 0LRS
    Foot
      Left 0LRW
      Right 0LRV
    Hand
      Left 0LR8
      Right 0LR7
    Head and Neck 0LR0
    Hip
      Left 0LRK
      Right 0LRJ
    Knee
      Left 0LRR
      Right 0LRQ
    Lower Arm and Wrist
      Left 0LR6
      Right 0LR5
    Lower Leg
      Left 0LRP
      Right 0LRN
    Perineum 0LRH
    Shoulder
      Left 0LR2
      Right 0LR1
    Thorax
      Left 0LRD
      Right 0LRC
    Trunk
      Left 0LRB
      Right 0LR9
    Upper Arm
      Left 0LR4
      Right 0LR3
    Upper Leg
      Left 0LRM
      Right 0LRL
  Testis
    Bilateral 0VRC0JZ
    Left 0VRB0JZ

Replacement — *continued*
  Testis — *continued*
    Right 0VR90JZ
  Thumb
    Left 0XRM
    Right 0XRL
  Tibia
    Left 0QRH
    Right 0QRG
  Toe Nail 0HRRX
  Tongue 0CR7
  Tooth
    Lower 0CRX
    Upper 0CRW
  Trachea 0BR1
  Turbinate, Nasal 09RL
  Tympanic Membrane
    Left 09R8
    Right 09R7
  Ulna
    Left 0PRL
    Right 0PRK
  Ureter
    Left 0TR7
    Right 0TR6
  Urethra 0TRD
  Uvula 0CRN
  Valve
    Aortic 02RF
    Mitral 02RG
    Pulmonary 02RH
    Tricuspid 02RJ
  Vein
    Axillary
      Left 05R8
      Right 05R7
    Azygos 05R0
    Basilic
      Left 05RC
      Right 05RB
    Brachial
      Left 05RA
      Right 05R9
    Cephalic
      Left 05RF
      Right 05RD
    Colic 06R7
    Common Iliac
      Left 06RD
      Right 06RC
    Esophageal 06R3
    External Iliac
      Left 06RG
      Right 06RF
    External Jugular
      Left 05RQ
      Right 05RP
    Face
      Left 05RV
      Right 05RT
    Femoral
      Left 06RN
      Right 06RM
    Foot
      Left 06RV
      Right 06RT
    Gastric 06R2
    Hand
      Left 05RH
      Right 05RG
    Hemiazygos 05R1
    Hepatic 06R4
    Hypogastric
      Left 06RJ
      Right 06RH
    Inferior Mesenteric 06R6
    Innominate
      Left 05R4
      Right 05R3
    Internal Jugular
      Left 05RN
      Right 05RM
    Intracranial 05RL
    Lower 06RY
    Portal 06R8
    Pulmonary
      Left 02RT
      Right 02RS

Replacement — continued
  Vein — continued
    Renal
      Left Ø6RB
      Right Ø6R9
    Saphenous
      Left Ø6RQ
      Right Ø6RP
    Splenic Ø6R1
    Subclavian
      Left Ø5R6
      Right Ø5R5
    Superior Mesenteric Ø6R5
    Upper Ø5RY
    Vertebral
      Left Ø5RS
      Right Ø5RR
  Vena Cava
    Inferior Ø6RØ
    Superior Ø2RV
  Ventricle
    Left Ø2RL
    Right Ø2RK
  Vertebra
    Cervical ØPR3
    Lumbar ØQRØ
    Thoracic ØPR4
  Vitreous
    Left Ø8R53
    Right Ø8R43
  Vocal Cord
    Left ØCRV
    Right ØCRT
  Zooplastic Tissue, Rapid Deployment Technique
    X2RF
Replacement, hip
  Partial or total see Replacement, Lower Joints ØSR
  Resurfacing only see Supplement, Lower Joints
    ØSU
Replantation see Reposition
Replantation, scalp see Reattachment, Skin, Scalp
    ØHMØ
Reposition
  Acetabulum
    Left ØQS5
    Right ØQS4
  Ampulla of Vater ØFSC
  Anus ØDSQ
  Aorta
    Abdominal Ø4SØ
    Thoracic
      Ascending/Arch Ø2SXØZZ
      Descending Ø2SWØZZ
  Artery
    Anterior Tibial
      Left Ø4SQ
      Right Ø4SP
    Axillary
      Left Ø3S6
      Right Ø3S5
    Brachial
      Left Ø3S8
      Right Ø3S7
    Celiac Ø4S1
    Colic
      Left Ø4S7
      Middle Ø4S8
      Right Ø4S6
    Common Carotid
      Left Ø3SJ
      Right Ø3SH
    Common Iliac
      Left Ø4SD
      Right Ø4SC
    Coronary
      One Artery Ø2SØØZZ
      Two Arteries Ø2S1ØZZ
    External Carotid
      Left Ø3SN
      Right Ø3SM
    External Iliac
      Left Ø4SJ
      Right Ø4SH
    Face Ø3SR
    Femoral
      Left Ø4SL
      Right Ø4SK
    Foot
      Left Ø4SW

Reposition — continued
  Artery — continued
    Foot — continued
      Right Ø4SV
    Gastric Ø4S2
    Hand
      Left Ø3SF
      Right Ø3SD
    Hepatic Ø4S3
    Inferior Mesenteric Ø4SB
    Innominate Ø3S2
    Internal Carotid
      Left Ø3SL
      Right Ø3SK
    Internal Iliac
      Left Ø4SF
      Right Ø4SE
    Internal Mammary
      Left Ø3S1
      Right Ø3SØ
    Intracranial Ø3SG
    Lower Ø4SY
    Peroneal
      Left Ø4SU
      Right Ø4ST
    Popliteal
      Left Ø4SN
      Right Ø4SM
    Posterior Tibial
      Left Ø4SS
      Right Ø4SR
    Pulmonary
      Left Ø2SRØZZ
      Right Ø2SQØZZ
    Pulmonary Trunk Ø2SPØZZ
    Radial
      Left Ø3SC
      Right Ø3SB
    Renal
      Left Ø4SA
      Right Ø4S9
    Splenic Ø4S4
    Subclavian
      Left Ø3S4
      Right Ø3S3
    Superior Mesenteric Ø4S5
    Temporal
      Left Ø3ST
      Right Ø3SS
    Thyroid
      Left Ø3SV
      Right Ø3SU
    Ulnar
      Left Ø3SA
      Right Ø3S9
    Upper Ø3SY
    Vertebral
      Left Ø3SQ
      Right Ø3SP
  Auditory Ossicle
    Left Ø9SA
    Right Ø9S9
  Bladder ØTSB
  Bladder Neck ØTSC
  Bone
    Ethmoid
      Left ØNSG
      Right ØNSF
    Frontal ØNS1
    Hyoid ØNSX
    Lacrimal
      Left ØNSJ
      Right ØNSH
    Nasal ØNSB
    Occipital ØNS7
    Palatine
      Left ØNSL
      Right ØNSK
    Parietal
      Left ØNS4
      Right ØNS3
    Pelvic
      Left ØQS3
      Right ØQS2
    Sphenoid ØNSC
    Temporal
      Left ØNS6
      Right ØNS5

Reposition — continued
  Bone — continued
    Zygomatic
      Left ØNSN
      Right ØNSM
  Breast
    Bilateral ØHSVØZZ
    Left ØHSUØZZ
    Right ØHSTØZZ
  Bronchus
    Lingula ØBS9ØZZ
    Lower Lobe
      Left ØBSBØZZ
      Right ØBS6ØZZ
    Main
      Left ØBS7ØZZ
      Right ØBS3ØZZ
    Middle Lobe, Right ØBS5ØZZ
    Upper Lobe
      Left ØBS8ØZZ
      Right ØBS4ØZZ
  Bursa and Ligament
    Abdomen
      Left ØMSJ
      Right ØMSH
    Ankle
      Left ØMSR
      Right ØMSQ
    Elbow
      Left ØMS4
      Right ØMS3
    Foot
      Left ØMST
      Right ØMSS
    Hand
      Left ØMS8
      Right ØMS7
    Head and Neck ØMSØ
    Hip
      Left ØMSM
      Right ØMSL
    Knee
      Left ØMSP
      Right ØMSN
    Lower Extremity
      Left ØMSW
      Right ØMSV
    Perineum ØMSK
    Rib(s) ØMSG
    Shoulder
      Left ØMS2
      Right ØMS1
    Spine
      Lower ØMSD
      Upper ØMSC
    Sternum ØMSF
    Upper Extremity
      Left ØMSB
      Right ØMS9
    Wrist
      Left ØMS6
      Right ØMS5
  Carina ØBS2ØZZ
  Carpal
    Left ØPSN
    Right ØPSM
  Cecum ØDSH
  Cervix ØUSC
  Clavicle
    Left ØPSB
    Right ØPS9
  Coccyx ØQSS
  Colon
    Ascending ØDSK
    Descending ØDSM
    Sigmoid ØDSN
    Transverse ØDSL
  Cord
    Bilateral ØVSH
    Left ØVSG
    Right ØVSF
  Cul-de-sac ØUSF
  Diaphragm ØBSTØZZ
  Duct
    Common Bile ØFS9
    Cystic ØFS8
    Hepatic
      Common ØFS7
      Left ØFS6

Reposition — *continued*
  Duct — *continued*
    Hepatic — *continued*
      Right 0FS5
    Lacrimal
      Left 08SY
      Right 08SX
    Pancreatic 0FSD
      Accessory 0FSF
    Parotid
      Left 0CSC
      Right 0CSB
  Duodenum 0DS9
  Ear
    Bilateral 09S2
    Left 09S1
    Right 09S0
  Epiglottis 0CSR
  Esophagus 0DS5
  Eustachian Tube
    Left 09SG
    Right 09SF
  Eyelid
    Lower
      Left 08SR
      Right 08SQ
    Upper
      Left 08SP
      Right 08SN
  Fallopian Tube
    Left 0US6
    Right 0US5
  Fallopian Tubes, Bilateral 0US7
  Femoral Shaft
    Left 0QS9
    Right 0QS8
  Femur
    Lower
      Left 0QSC
      Right 0QSB
    Upper
      Left 0QS7
      Right 0QS6
  Fibula
    Left 0QSK
    Right 0QSJ
  Gallbladder 0FS4
  Gland
    Adrenal
      Left 0GS2
      Right 0GS3
    Lacrimal
      Left 08SW
      Right 08SV
  Glenoid Cavity
    Left 0PS8
    Right 0PS7
  Hair 0HSSXZZ
  Humeral Head
    Left 0PSD
    Right 0PSC
  Humeral Shaft
    Left 0PSG
    Right 0PSF
  Ileum 0DSB
  Intestine
    Large 0DSE
    Small 0DS8
  Iris
    Left 08SD3ZZ
    Right 08SC3ZZ
  Jejunum 0DSA
  Joint
    Acromioclavicular
      Left 0RSH
      Right 0RSG
    Ankle
      Left 0SSG
      Right 0SSF
    Carpal
      Left 0RSR
      Right 0RSQ
    Carpometacarpal
      Left 0RST
      Right 0RSS
    Cervical Vertebral 0RS1
    Cervicothoracic Vertebral 0RS4
    Coccygeal 0SS6

Reposition — *continued*
  Joint — *continued*
    Elbow
      Left 0RSM
      Right 0RSL
    Finger Phalangeal
      Left 0RSX
      Right 0RSW
    Hip
      Left 0SSB
      Right 0SS9
    Knee
      Left 0SSD
      Right 0SSC
    Lumbar Vertebral 0SS0
    Lumbosacral 0SS3
    Metacarpophalangeal
      Left 0RSV
      Right 0RSU
    Metatarsal-Phalangeal
      Left 0SSN
      Right 0SSM
    Occipital-cervical 0RS0
    Sacrococcygeal 0SS5
    Sacroiliac
      Left 0SS8
      Right 0SS7
    Shoulder
      Left 0RSK
      Right 0RSJ
    Sternoclavicular
      Left 0RSF
      Right 0RSE
    Tarsal
      Left 0SSJ
      Right 0SSH
    Tarsometatarsal
      Left 0SSL
      Right 0SSK
    Temporomandibular
      Left 0RSD
      Right 0RSC
    Thoracic Vertebral 0RS6
    Thoracolumbar Vertebral 0RSA
    Toe Phalangeal
      Left 0SSQ
      Right 0SSP
    Wrist
      Left 0RSP
      Right 0RSN
  Kidney
    Left 0TS1
    Right 0TS0
  Kidney Pelvis
    Left 0TS4
    Right 0TS3
  Kidneys, Bilateral 0TS2
  Lens
    Left 08SK3ZZ
    Right 08SJ3ZZ
  Lip
    Lower 0CS1
    Upper 0CS0
  Liver 0FS0
  Lung
    Left 0BSL0ZZ
    Lower Lobe
      Left 0BSJ0ZZ
      Right 0BSF0ZZ
    Middle Lobe, Right 0BSD0ZZ
    Right 0BSK0ZZ
    Upper Lobe
      Left 0BSG0ZZ
      Right 0BSC0ZZ
  Lung Lingula 0BSH0ZZ
  Mandible
    Left 0NSV
    Right 0NST
  Maxilla 0NSR
  Metacarpal
    Left 0PSQ
    Right 0PSP
  Metatarsal
    Left 0QSP
    Right 0QSN
  Muscle
    Abdomen
      Left 0KSL
      Right 0KSK

Reposition — *continued*
  Muscle — *continued*
    Extraocular
      Left 08SM
      Right 08SL
    Facial 0KS1
    Foot
      Left 0KSW
      Right 0KSV
    Hand
      Left 0KSD
      Right 0KSC
    Head 0KS0
    Hip
      Left 0KSP
      Right 0KSN
    Lower Arm and Wrist
      Left 0KSB
      Right 0KS9
    Lower Leg
      Left 0KST
      Right 0KSS
    Neck
      Left 0KS3
      Right 0KS2
    Perineum 0KSM
    Shoulder
      Left 0KS6
      Right 0KS5
    Thorax
      Left 0KSJ
      Right 0KSH
    Tongue, Palate, Pharynx 0KS4
    Trunk
      Left 0KSG
      Right 0KSF
    Upper Arm
      Left 0KS8
      Right 0KS7
    Upper Leg
      Left 0KSR
      Right 0KSQ
  Nasal Mucosa and Soft Tissue 09SK
  Nerve
    Abducens 00SL
    Accessory 00SR
    Acoustic 00SN
    Brachial Plexus 01S3
    Cervical 01S1
    Cervical Plexus 01S0
    Facial 00SM
    Femoral 01SD
    Glossopharyngeal 00SP
    Hypoglossal 00SS
    Lumbar 01SB
    Lumbar Plexus 01S9
    Lumbosacral Plexus 01SA
    Median 01S5
    Oculomotor 00SH
    Olfactory 00SF
    Optic 00SG
    Peroneal 01SH
    Phrenic 01S2
    Pudendal 01SC
    Radial 01S6
    Sacral 01SR
    Sacral Plexus 01SQ
    Sciatic 01SF
    Thoracic 01S8
    Tibial 01SG
    Trigeminal 00SK
    Trochlear 00SJ
    Ulnar 01S4
    Vagus 00SQ
  Nipple
    Left 0HSXXZZ
    Right 0HSWXZZ
  Orbit
    Left 0NSQ
    Right 0NSP
  Ovary
    Bilateral 0US2
    Left 0US1
    Right 0US0
  Palate
    Hard 0CS2
    Soft 0CS3
  Pancreas 0FSG
  Parathyroid Gland 0GSR

▼ **Subterms under main terms may continue to next column or page**

Resection — *continued*
  Breast — *continued*
    Left ØHTUØZZ
    Right ØHTTØZZ
    Supernumerary ØHTYØZZ
  Bronchus
    Lingula ØBT9
    Lower Lobe
      Left ØBTB
      Right ØBT6
    Main
      Left ØBT7
      Right ØBT3
    Middle Lobe, Right ØBT5
    Upper Lobe
      Left ØBT8
      Right ØBT4
  Bursa and Ligament
    Abdomen
      Left ØMTJ
      Right ØMTH
    Ankle
      Left ØMTR
      Right ØMTQ
    Elbow
      Left ØMT4
      Right ØMT3
    Foot
      Left ØMTT
      Right ØMTS
    Hand
      Left ØMT8
      Right ØMT7
    Head and Neck ØMTØ
    Hip
      Left ØMTM
      Right ØMTL
    Knee
      Left ØMTP
      Right ØMTN
    Lower Extremity
      Left ØMTW
      Right ØMTV
    Perineum ØMTK
    Rib(s) ØMTG
    Shoulder
      Left ØMT2
      Right ØMT1
    Spine
      Lower ØMTD
      Upper ØMTC
    Sternum ØMTF
    Upper Extremity
      Left ØMTB
      Right ØMT9
    Wrist
      Left ØMT6
      Right ØMT5
  Carina ØBT2
  Carotid Bodies, Bilateral ØGT8
  Carotid Body
    Left ØGT6
    Right ØGT7
  Carpal
    Left ØPTNØZZ
    Right ØPTMØZZ
  Cecum ØDTH
  Cerebral Hemisphere ØØT7
  Cervix ØUTC
  Chordae Tendineae Ø2T9
  Cisterna Chyli Ø7TL
  Clavicle
    Left ØPTBØZZ
    Right ØPT9ØZZ
  Clitoris ØUTJ
  Coccygeal Glomus ØGTB
  Coccyx ØQTSØZZ
  Colon
    Ascending ØDTK
    Descending ØDTM
    Sigmoid ØDTN
    Transverse ØDTL
  Conduction Mechanism Ø2T8
  Cord
    Bilateral ØVTH
    Left ØVTG
    Right ØVTF
  Cornea
    Left Ø8T9XZZ

Resection — *continued*
  Cornea — *continued*
    Right Ø8T8XZZ
  Cul-de-sac ØUTF
  Diaphragm ØBTT
  Disc
    Cervical Vertebral ØRT3ØZZ
    Cervicothoracic Vertebral ØRT5ØZZ
    Lumbar Vertebral ØST2ØZZ
    Lumbosacral ØST4ØZZ
    Thoracic Vertebral ØRT9ØZZ
    Thoracolumbar Vertebral ØRTBØZZ
  Duct
    Common Bile ØFT9
    Cystic ØFT8
    Hepatic
      Common ØFT7
      Left ØFT6
      Right ØFT5
    Lacrimal
      Left Ø8TY
      Right Ø8TX
    Pancreatic ØFTD
      Accessory ØFTF
    Parotid
      Left ØCTCØZZ
      Right ØCTBØZZ
  Duodenum ØDT9
  Ear
    External
      Left Ø9T1
      Right Ø9TØ
    Inner
      Left Ø9TE
      Right Ø9TD
    Middle
      Left Ø9T6
      Right Ø9T5
  Epididymis
    Bilateral ØVTL
    Left ØVTK
    Right ØVTJ
  Epiglottis ØCTR
  Esophagogastric Junction ØDT4
  Esophagus ØDT5
    Lower ØDT3
    Middle ØDT2
    Upper ØDT1
  Eustachian Tube
    Left Ø9TG
    Right Ø9TF
  Eye
    Left Ø8T1XZZ
    Right Ø8TØXZZ
  Eyelid
    Lower
      Left Ø8TR
      Right Ø8TQ
    Upper
      Left Ø8TP
      Right Ø8TN
  Fallopian Tube
    Left ØUT6
    Right ØUT5
  Fallopian Tubes, Bilateral ØUT7
  Femoral Shaft
    Left ØQT9ØZZ
    Right ØQT8ØZZ
  Femur
    Lower
      Left ØQTCØZZ
      Right ØQTBØZZ
    Upper
      Left ØQT7ØZZ
      Right ØQT6ØZZ
  Fibula
    Left ØQTKØZZ
    Right ØQTJØZZ
  Finger Nail ØHTQXZZ
  Gallbladder ØFT4
  Gland
    Adrenal
      Bilateral ØGT4
      Left ØGT2
      Right ØGT3
    Lacrimal
      Left Ø8TW
      Right Ø8TV
    Minor Salivary ØCTJØZZ

Resection — *continued*
  Gland — *continued*
    Parotid
      Left ØCT9ØZZ
      Right ØCT8ØZZ
    Pituitary ØGTØ
    Sublingual
      Left ØCTFØZZ
      Right ØCTDØZZ
    Submaxillary
      Left ØCTHØZZ
      Right ØCTGØZZ
    Vestibular ØUTL
  Glenoid Cavity
    Left ØPT8ØZZ
    Right ØPT7ØZZ
  Glomus Jugulare ØGTC
  Humeral Head
    Left ØPTDØZZ
    Right ØPTCØZZ
  Humeral Shaft
    Left ØPTGØZZ
    Right ØPTFØZZ
  Hymen ØUTK
  Ileocecal Valve ØDTC
  Ileum ØDTB
  Intestine
    Large ØDTE
      Left ØDTG
      Right ØDTF
    Small ØDT8
  Iris
    Left Ø8TD3ZZ
    Right Ø8TC3ZZ
  Jejunum ØDTA
  Joint
    Acromioclavicular
      Left ØRTHØZZ
      Right ØRTGØZZ
    Ankle
      Left ØSTGØZZ
      Right ØSTFØZZ
    Carpal
      Left ØRTRØZZ
      Right ØRTQØZZ
    Carpometacarpal
      Left ØRTTØZZ
      Right ØRTSØZZ
    Cervicothoracic Vertebral ØRT4ØZZ
    Coccygeal ØST6ØZZ
    Elbow
      Left ØRTMØZZ
      Right ØRTLØZZ
    Finger Phalangeal
      Left ØRTXØZZ
      Right ØRTWØZZ
    Hip
      Left ØSTBØZZ
      Right ØST9ØZZ
    Knee
      Left ØSTDØZZ
      Right ØSTCØZZ
    Metacarpophalangeal
      Left ØRTVØZZ
      Right ØRTUØZZ
    Metatarsal-Phalangeal
      Left ØSTNØZZ
      Right ØSTMØZZ
    Sacrococcygeal ØST5ØZZ
    Sacroiliac
      Left ØST8ØZZ
      Right ØST7ØZZ
    Shoulder
      Left ØRTKØZZ
      Right ØRTJØZZ
    Sternoclavicular
      Left ØRTFØZZ
      Right ØRTEØZZ
    Tarsal
      Left ØSTJØZZ
      Right ØSTHØZZ
    Tarsometatarsal
      Left ØSTLØZZ
      Right ØSTKØZZ
    Temporomandibular
      Left ØRTDØZZ
      Right ØRTCØZZ
    Toe Phalangeal
      Left ØSTQØZZ

Subterms under main terms may continue to next column or page

Resection — continued
Tunica Vaginalis
  Left 0VT7
  Right 0VT6
Turbinate, Nasal 09TL
Tympanic Membrane
  Left 09T8
  Right 09T7
Ulna
  Left 0PTL0ZZ
  Right 0PTK0ZZ
Ureter
  Left 0TT7
  Right 0TT6
Urethra 0TTD
Uterine Supporting Structure 0UT4
Uterus 0UT9
Uvula 0CTN
Vagina 0UTG
Valve, Pulmonary 02TH
Vas Deferens
  Bilateral 0VTQ
  Left 0VTP
  Right 0VTN
Vesicle
  Bilateral 0VT3
  Left 0VT2
  Right 0VT1
Vitreous
  Left 08T53ZZ
  Right 08T43ZZ
Vocal Cord
  Left 0CTV
  Right 0CTT
Vulva 0UTM
Resection, Left ventricular outflow tract obstruction (LVOT) see Dilation, Ventricle, Left 027L
Resection, Subaortic membrane (Left ventricular outflow tract obstruction) see Dilation, Ventricle, Left 027L
Restoration, Cardiac, Single, Rhythm 5A2204Z
RestoreAdvanced neurostimulator (SureScan) (MRI Safe) use Stimulator Generator, Multiple Array Rechargeable in 0JH
RestoreSensor neurostimulator (SureScan) (MRI Safe) use Stimulator Generator, Multiple Array Rechargeable in 0JH
RestoreUltra neurostimulator (SureScan) (MRI Safe) use Stimulator Generator, Multiple Array Rechargeable in 0JH
Restriction
Ampulla of Vater 0FVC
Anus 0DVQ
Aorta
  Abdominal 04V0
    Intraluminal Device, Branched or Fenestrated 04V0
  Thoracic
    Ascending/Arch, Intraluminal Device, Branched or Fenestrated 02VX
    Descending, Intraluminal Device, Branched or Fenestrated 02VW
Artery
  Anterior Tibial
    Left 04VQ
    Right 04VP
  Axillary
    Left 03V6
    Right 03V5
  Brachial
    Left 03V8
    Right 03V7
  Celiac 04V1
  Colic
    Left 04V7
    Middle 04V8
    Right 04V6
  Common Carotid
    Left 03VJ
    Right 03VH
  Common Iliac
    Left 04VD
    Right 04VC
  External Carotid
    Left 03VN
    Right 03VM
  External Iliac
    Left 04VJ

Restriction — continued
Artery — continued
  External Iliac — continued
    Right 04VH
  Face 03VR
  Femoral
    Left 04VL
    Right 04VK
  Foot
    Left 04VW
    Right 04VV
  Gastric 04V2
  Hand
    Left 03VF
    Right 03VD
  Hepatic 04V3
  Inferior Mesenteric 04VB
  Innominate 03V2
  Internal Carotid
    Left 03VL
    Right 03VK
  Internal Iliac
    Left 04VF
    Right 04VE
  Internal Mammary
    Left 03V1
    Right 03V0
  Intracranial 03VG
  Lower 04VY
  Peroneal
    Left 04VU
    Right 04VT
  Popliteal
    Left 04VN
    Right 04VM
  Posterior Tibial
    Left 04VS
    Right 04VR
  Pulmonary
    Left 02VR
    Right 02VQ
  Pulmonary Trunk 02VP
  Radial
    Left 03VC
    Right 03VB
  Renal
    Left 04VA
    Right 04V9
  Splenic 04V4
  Subclavian
    Left 03V4
    Right 03V3
  Superior Mesenteric 04V5
  Temporal
    Left 03VT
    Right 03VS
  Thyroid
    Left 03VV
    Right 03VU
  Ulnar
    Left 03VA
    Right 03V9
  Upper 03VY
  Vertebral
    Left 03VQ
    Right 03VP
Bladder 0TVB
Bladder Neck 0TVC
Bronchus
  Lingula 0BV9
  Lower Lobe
    Left 0BVB
    Right 0BV6
  Main
    Left 0BV7
    Right 0BV3
  Middle Lobe, Right 0BV5
  Upper Lobe
    Left 0BV8
    Right 0BV4
Carina 0BV2
Cecum 0DVH
Cervix 0UVC
Cisterna Chyli 07VL
Colon
  Ascending 0DVK
  Descending 0DVM
  Sigmoid 0DVN
  Transverse 0DVL

Restriction — continued
Duct
  Common Bile 0FV9
  Cystic 0FV8
  Hepatic
    Common 0FV7
    Left 0FV6
    Right 0FV5
  Lacrimal
    Left 08VY
    Right 08VX
  Pancreatic 0FVD
    Accessory 0FVF
  Parotid
    Left 0CVC
    Right 0CVB
Duodenum 0DV9
Esophagogastric Junction 0DV4
Esophagus 0DV5
  Lower 0DV3
  Middle 0DV2
  Upper 0DV1
Heart 02VA
Ileocecal Valve 0DVC
Ileum 0DVB
Intestine
  Large 0DVE
    Left 0DVG
    Right 0DVF
  Small 0DV8
Jejunum 0DVA
Kidney Pelvis
  Left 0TV4
  Right 0TV3
Lymphatic
  Aortic 07VD
  Axillary
    Left 07V6
    Right 07V5
  Head 07V0
  Inguinal
    Left 07VJ
    Right 07VH
  Internal Mammary
    Left 07V9
    Right 07V8
  Lower Extremity
    Left 07VG
    Right 07VF
  Mesenteric 07VB
  Neck
    Left 07V2
    Right 07V1
  Pelvis 07VC
  Thoracic Duct 07VK
  Thorax 07V7
  Upper Extremity
    Left 07V4
    Right 07V3
Rectum 0DVP
Stomach 0DV6
  Pylorus 0DV7
Trachea 0BV1
Ureter
  Left 0TV7
  Right 0TV6
Urethra 0TVD
Valve, Mitral 02VG
Vein
  Axillary
    Left 05V8
    Right 05V7
  Azygos 05V0
  Basilic
    Left 05VC
    Right 05VB
  Brachial
    Left 05VA
    Right 05V9
  Cephalic
    Left 05VF
    Right 05VD
  Colic 06V7
  Common Iliac
    Left 06VD
    Right 06VC
  Esophageal 06V3
  External Iliac
    Left 06VG

Subterms under main terms may continue to next column or page

Revision of device in — *continued*
Joint — *continued*
  Hip — *continued*
    Right — *continued*
      Femoral Surface ØSWR
    Knee
      Left ØSWD
        Femoral Surface ØSWU
        Tibial Surface ØSWW
      Right ØSWC
        Femoral Surface ØSWT
        Tibial Surface ØSWV
    Lumbar Vertebral ØSWØ
    Lumbosacral ØSW3
    Metacarpophalangeal
      Left ØRWV
      Right ØRWU
    Metatarsal-Phalangeal
      Left ØSWN
      Right ØSWM
    Occipital-cervical ØRWØ
    Sacrococcygeal ØSW5
    Sacroiliac
      Left ØSW8
      Right ØSW7
    Shoulder
      Left ØRWK
      Right ØRWJ
    Sternoclavicular
      Left ØRWF
      Right ØRWE
    Tarsal
      Left ØSWJ
      Right ØSWH
    Tarsometatarsal
      Left ØSWL
      Right ØSWK
    Temporomandibular
      Left ØRWD
      Right ØRWC
    Thoracic Vertebral ØRW6
    Thoracolumbar Vertebral ØRWA
    Toe Phalangeal
      Left ØSWQ
      Right ØSWP
    Wrist
      Left ØRWP
      Right ØRWN
  Kidney ØTW5
  Larynx ØCWS
  Lens
    Left Ø8WK
    Right Ø8WJ
  Liver ØFWØ
  Lung
    Left ØBWL
    Right ØBWK
  Lymphatic Ø7WN
    Thoracic Duct Ø7WK
  Mediastinum ØWWC
  Mesentery ØDWV
  Metacarpal
    Left ØPWQ
    Right ØPWP
  Metatarsal
    Left ØQWP
    Right ØQWN
  Mouth and Throat ØCWY
  Muscle
    Extraocular
      Left Ø8WM
      Right Ø8WL
    Lower ØKWY
    Upper ØKWX
  Nasal Mucosa and Soft Tissue Ø9WK
  Neck ØWW6
  Nerve
    Cranial ØØWE
    Peripheral Ø1WY
  Omentum ØDWU
  Ovary ØUW3
  Pancreas ØFWG
  Parathyroid Gland ØGWR
  Patella
    Left ØQWF
    Right ØQWD
  Pelvic Cavity ØWWJ
  Penis ØVWS
  Pericardial Cavity ØWWD

Revision of device in — *continued*
Perineum
  Female ØWWN
  Male ØWWM
  Peritoneal Cavity ØWWG
  Peritoneum ØDWW
  Phalanx
    Finger
      Left ØPWV
      Right ØPWT
    Thumb
      Left ØPWS
      Right ØPWR
    Toe
      Left ØQWR
      Right ØQWQ
  Pineal Body ØGW1
  Pleura ØBWQ
  Pleural Cavity
    Left ØWWB
    Right ØWW9
  Prostate and Seminal Vesicles ØVW4
  Radius
    Left ØPWJ
    Right ØPWH
  Respiratory Tract ØWWQ
  Retroperitoneum ØWWH
  Ribs
    1 to 2 ØPW1
    3 or More ØPW2
  Sacrum ØQW1
  Scapula
    Left ØPW6
    Right ØPW5
  Scrotum and Tunica Vaginalis ØVW8
  Septum
    Atrial Ø2W5
    Ventricular Ø2WM
  Sinus Ø9WY
  Skin ØHWPX
  Skull ØNWØ
  Spinal Canal ØØWU
  Spinal Cord ØØWV
  Spleen Ø7WP
  Sternum ØPWØ
  Stomach ØDW6
  Subcutaneous Tissue and Fascia
    Head and Neck ØJWS
    Lower Extremity ØJWW
    Trunk ØJWT
    Upper Extremity ØJWV
  Tarsal
    Left ØQWM
    Right ØQWL
  Tendon
    Lower ØLWY
    Upper ØLWX
  Testis ØVWD
  Thymus Ø7WM
  Thyroid Gland ØGWK
  Tibia
    Left ØQWH
    Right ØQWG
  Toe Nail ØHWRX
  Trachea ØBW1
  Tracheobronchial Tree ØBWØ
  Tympanic Membrane
    Left Ø9W8
    Right Ø9W7
  Ulna
    Left ØPWL
    Right ØPWK
  Ureter ØTW9
  Urethra ØTWD
  Uterus and Cervix ØUWD
  Vagina and Cul-de-sac ØUWH
  Valve
    Aortic Ø2WF
    Mitral Ø2WG
    Pulmonary Ø2WH
    Tricuspid Ø2WJ
  Vas Deferens ØVWR
  Vein
    Azygos Ø5WØ
    Innominate
      Left Ø5W4
      Right Ø5W3
    Lower Ø6WY
    Upper Ø5WY

Revision of device in — *continued*
Vertebra
  Cervical ØPW3
  Lumbar ØQWØ
  Thoracic ØPW4
  Vulva ØUWM
Revo MRI™ SureScan® pacemaker *use* Pacemaker, Dual Chamber in ØJH
rhBMP-2 *use* Recombinant Bone Morphogenetic Protein
Rheos® System device *use* Stimulator Generator in Subcutaneous Tissue and Fascia
Rheos® System lead *use* Stimulator Lead in Upper Arteries
Rhinopharynx *use* Nasopharynx
Rhinoplasty
  see Alteration, Nasal Mucosa and Soft Tissue Ø9ØK
  see Repair, Nasal Mucosa and Soft Tissue Ø9QK
  see Replacement, Nasal Mucosa and Soft Tissue Ø9RK
  see Supplement, Nasal Mucosa and Soft Tissue Ø9UK
Rhinorrhaphy *see* Repair, Nasal Mucosa and Soft Tissue Ø9QK
Rhinoscopy Ø9JKXZZ
Rhizotomy
  see Division, Central Nervous System and Cranial Nerves ØØ8
  see Division, Peripheral Nervous System Ø18
Rhomboid major muscle
  use Trunk Muscle, Left
  use Trunk Muscle, Right
Rhomboid minor muscle
  use Trunk Muscle, Left
  use Trunk Muscle, Right
Rhythm electrocardiogram *see* Measurement, Cardiac 4AØ2
Rhytidectomy *see* Alteration, Face ØWØ2
Right ascending lumbar vein *use* Azygos Vein
Right atrioventricular valve *use* Tricuspid Valve
Right auricular appendix *use* Atrium, Right
Right colic vein *use* Colic Vein
Right coronary sulcus *use* Heart, Right
Right gastric artery *use* Gastric Artery
Right gastroepiploic vein *use* Superior Mesenteric Vein
Right inferior phrenic vein *use* Inferior Vena Cava
Right inferior pulmonary vein *use* Pulmonary Vein, Right
Right jugular trunk *use* Lymphatic, Right Neck
Right lateral ventricle *use* Cerebral Ventricle
Right lymphatic duct *use* Lymphatic, Right Neck
Right ovarian vein *use* Inferior Vena Cava
Right second lumbar vein *use* Inferior Vena Cava
Right subclavian trunk *use* Lymphatic, Right Neck
Right subcostal vein *use* Azygos Vein
Right superior pulmonary vein *use* Pulmonary Vein, Right
Right suprarenal vein *use* Inferior Vena Cava
Right testicular vein *use* Inferior Vena Cava
Rima glottidis *use* Larynx
Risorius muscle *use* Facial Muscle
RNS System lead *use* Neurostimulator Lead in Central Nervous System and Cranial Nerves
RNS system neurostimulator generator *use* Neurostimulator Generator in Head and Facial Bones
Robotic Assisted Procedure
  Extremity
    Lower 8EØY
    Upper 8EØX
  Head and Neck Region 8EØ9
  Trunk Region 8EØW
Robotic Waterjet Ablation, Destruction, Prostate XV5Ø8A4
Rotation of fetal head
  Forceps 1ØSØ7ZZ
  Manual 1ØSØXZZ
Round ligament of uterus *use* Uterine Supporting Structure
Round window
  use Inner Ear, Left
  use Inner Ear, Right
Roux-en-Y operation
  see Bypass, Gastrointestinal System ØD1
  see Bypass, Hepatobiliary System and Pancreas ØF1

Rupture
Adhesions *see* Release
Fluid collection *see* Drainage
Ruxolitinib XW0DXT5

S

Sacral ganglion *use* Sacral Sympathetic Nerve
Sacral lymph node *use* Lymphatic, Pelvis
Sacral nerve modulation (SNM) lead *use* Stimulator Lead in Urinary System
Sacral neuromodulation lead *use* Stimulator Lead in Urinary System
Sacral splanchnic nerve *use* Sacral Sympathetic Nerve
Sacrectomy *see* Excision, Lower Bones 0QB
Sacrococcygeal ligament *use* Lower Spine Bursa and Ligament
Sacrococcygeal symphysis *use* Sacrococcygeal Joint
Sacroiliac ligament *use* Lower Spine Bursa and Ligament
Sacrospinous ligament *use* Lower Spine Bursa and Ligament
Sacrotuberous ligament *use* Lower Spine Bursa and Ligament
Salpingectomy
see Excision, Female Reproductive System 0UB
see Resection, Female Reproductive System 0UT
Salpingolysis *see* Release, Female Reproductive System 0UN
Salpingopexy
see Repair, Female Reproductive System 0UQ
see Reposition, Female Reproductive System 0US
Salpingopharyngeus muscle *use* Tongue, Palate, Pharynx Muscle
Salpingoplasty
see Repair, Female Reproductive System 0UQ
see Supplement, Female Reproductive System 0UU
Salpingorrhaphy *see* Repair, Female Reproductive System 0UQ
Salpingoscopy 0UJ88ZZ
Salpingostomy *see* Drainage, Female Reproductive System 0U9
Salpingotomy *see* Drainage, Female Reproductive System 0U9
Salpinx
use Fallopian Tube, Left
use Fallopian Tube, Right
Saphenous nerve *use* Femoral Nerve
SAPIEN transcatheter aortic valve *use* Zooplastic Tissue in Heart and Great Vessels
Sarilumab XW0
SARS-CoV-2 Antibody Detection, Serum/Plasma Nanoparticle Fluorescence XXE5XV7
SARS-CoV-2 Polymerase Chain Reaction, Nasopharyngeal Fluid XXE97U7
Sartorius muscle
use Upper Leg Muscle, Left
use Upper Leg Muscle, Right
Satralizumab-mwge XW01397
SAVAL below-the-knee (BTK) drug-eluting stent system
use Intraluminal Device, Sustained Release Drug-eluting in New Technology
use Intraluminal Device, Sustained Release Drug-eluting, Two in New Technology
use Intraluminal Device, Sustained Release Drug-eluting, Three in New Technology
use Intraluminal Device, Sustained Release Drug-eluting, Four or More in New Technology
Scalene muscle
use Neck Muscle, Left
use Neck Muscle, Right
Scan
Computerized Tomography (CT) *see* Computerized Tomography (CT Scan)
Radioisotope *see* Planar Nuclear Medicine Imaging
Scaphoid bone
use Carpal, Left
use Carpal, Right
Scapholunate ligament
use Wrist Bursa and Ligament, Left
use Wrist Bursa and Ligament, Right
Scaphotrapezium ligament
use Hand Bursa and Ligament, Left
use Hand Bursa and Ligament, Right

Scapulectomy
see Excision, Upper Bones 0PB
see Resection, Upper Bones 0PT
Scapulopexy
see Repair, Upper Bones 0PQ
see Reposition, Upper Bones 0PS
Scarpa's (vestibular) ganglion *use* Acoustic Nerve
Sclerectomy *see* Excision, Eye 08B
Sclerotherapy, mechanical *see* Destruction
Sclerotherapy, via injection of sclerosing agent
see Introduction, Destructive Agent
Sclerotomy *see* Drainage, Eye 089
Scrotectomy
see Excision, Male Reproductive System 0VB
see Resection, Male Reproductive System 0VT
Scrotoplasty
see Repair, Male Reproductive System 0VQ
see Supplement, Male Reproductive System 0VU
Scrotorrhaphy *see* Repair, Male Reproductive System 0VQ
Scrototomy *see* Drainage, Male Reproductive System 0V9
Sebaceous gland *use* Skin
Second cranial nerve *use* Optic Nerve
Section, cesarean *see* Extraction, Pregnancy 10D
Secura (DR) (VR) *use* Defibrillator Generator in 0JH
Sella turcica *use* Sphenoid Bone
Semicircular canal
use Inner Ear, Left
use Inner Ear, Right
Semimembranosus muscle
use Upper Leg Muscle, Left
use Upper Leg Muscle, Right
Semitendinosus muscle
use Upper Leg Muscle, Left
use Upper Leg Muscle, Right
Sentinel™ Cerebral Protection System (CPS) X2A5312
Seprafilm *use* Adhesion Barrier
Septal cartilage *use* Nasal Septum
Septectomy
see Excision, Ear, Nose, Sinus 09B
see Excision, Heart and Great Vessels 02B
see Resection, Ear, Nose, Sinus 09T
see Resection, Heart and Great Vessels 02T
Septoplasty
see Repair, Ear, Nose, Sinus 09Q
see Repair, Heart and Great Vessels 02Q
see Replacement, Ear, Nose, Sinus 09R
see Replacement, Heart and Great Vessels 02R
see Reposition, Ear, Nose, Sinus 09S
see Supplement, Ear, Nose, Sinus 09U
see Supplement, Heart and Great Vessels 02U
Septostomy, balloon atrial 02163Z7
Septotomy *see* Drainage, Ear, Nose, Sinus 099
Sequestrectomy, bone *see* Extirpation
Serratus anterior muscle
use Thorax Muscle, Left
use Thorax Muscle, Right
Serratus posterior muscle
use Trunk Muscle, Left
use Trunk Muscle, Right
Seventh cranial nerve *use* Facial Nerve
Shapshot_NIR 8E02XDZ
Sheffield hybrid external fixator
use External Fixation Device, Hybrid in 0PH
use External Fixation Device, Hybrid in 0PS
use External Fixation Device, Hybrid in 0QH
use External Fixation Device, Hybrid in 0QS
Sheffield ring external fixator
use External Fixation Device, Ring in 0PH
use External Fixation Device, Ring in 0PS
use External Fixation Device, Ring in 0QH
use External Fixation Device, Ring in 0QS
Shirodkar cervical cerclage 0UVC7ZZ
Shock Wave Therapy, Musculoskeletal 6A93
Shockwave Intravascular Lithotripsy (Shockwave IVL) *see* Fragmentation
Short gastric artery *use* Splenic Artery
Shortening
see Excision
see Repair
see Reposition
Shunt creation *see* Bypass
Sialoadenectomy
Complete *see* Resection, Mouth and Throat 0CT

Sialoadenectomy — *continued*
Partial *see* Excision, Mouth and Throat 0CB
Sialodochoplasty
see Repair, Mouth and Throat 0CQ
see Replacement, Mouth and Throat 0CR
see Supplement, Mouth and Throat 0CU
Sialoectomy
see Excision, Mouth and Throat 0CB
see Resection, Mouth and Throat 0CT
Sialography *see* Plain Radiography, Ear, Nose, Mouth and Throat B90
Sialolithotomy *see* Extirpation, Mouth and Throat 0CC
S-ICD™ lead *use* Subcutaneous Defibrillator Lead in Subcutaneous Tissue and Fascia
Sigmoid artery *use* Inferior Mesenteric Artery
Sigmoid flexure *use* Sigmoid Colon
Sigmoid vein *use* Inferior Mesenteric Vein
Sigmoidectomy
see Excision, Gastrointestinal System 0DB
see Resection, Gastrointestinal System 0DT
Sigmoidorrhaphy *see* Repair, Gastrointestinal System 0DQ
Sigmoidoscopy 0DJD8ZZ
Sigmoidotomy *see* Drainage, Gastrointestinal System 0D9
Single lead pacemaker (atrium) (ventricle) *use* Pacemaker, Single Chamber in 0JH
Single lead rate responsive pacemaker (atrium) (ventricle) *use* Pacemaker, Single Chamber Rate Responsive in 0JH
Single-use Duodenoscope XFJ
Single-use Oversleeve with Intraoperative Colonic Irrigation XDPH8K7
Sinoatrial node *use* Conduction Mechanism
Sinogram
Abdominal Wall *see* Fluoroscopy, Abdomen and Pelvis BW11
Chest Wall *see* Plain Radiography, Chest BW03
Retroperitoneum *see* Fluoroscopy, Abdomen and Pelvis BW11
Sinus venosus *use* Atrium, Right
Sinusectomy
see Excision, Ear, Nose, Sinus 09B
see Resection, Ear, Nose, Sinus 09T
Sinusoscopy 09JY4ZZ
Sinusotomy *see* Drainage, Ear, Nose, Sinus 099
Sirolimus-eluting coronary stent *use* Intraluminal Device, Drug-eluting in Heart and Great Vessels
Sixth cranial nerve *use* Abducens Nerve
Size reduction, breast *see* Excision, Skin and Breast 0HB
SJM Biocor® Stented Valve System *use* Zooplastic Tissue in Heart and Great Vessels
Skene's (paraurethral) gland *use* Vestibular Gland
Skin Substitute, Porcine Liver Derived, Replacement XHRPXL2
Sling
Fascial, orbicularis muscle (mouth) *see* Supplement, Muscle, Facial 0KU1
Levator muscle, for urethral suspension *see* Reposition, Bladder Neck 0TSC
Pubococcygeal, for urethral suspension *see* Reposition, Bladder Neck 0TSC
Rectum *see* Reposition, Rectum 0DSP
Small bowel series *see* Fluoroscopy, Bowel, Small BD13
Small saphenous vein
use Saphenous Vein, Left
use Saphenous Vein, Right
Snapshot_NIR 8E02XDZ
Snaring, polyp, colon *see* Excision, Gastrointestinal System 0DB
Solar (celiac) plexus *use* Abdominal Sympathetic Nerve
Soleus muscle
use Lower Leg Muscle, Left
use Lower Leg Muscle, Right
Soliris® *use* Eculizumab
Spacer
Insertion of device in
Disc
Lumbar Vertebral 0SH2
Lumbosacral 0SH4
Joint
Acromioclavicular
Left 0RHH
Right 0RHG

Spacer — *continued*
  Insertion of device in — *continued*
    Joint — *continued*
      Ankle
        Left ØSHG
        Right ØSHF
      Carpal
        Left ØRHR
        Right ØRHQ
      Carpometacarpal
        Left ØRHT
        Right ØRHS
      Cervical Vertebral ØRH1
      Cervicothoracic Vertebral ØRH4
      Coccygeal ØSH6
      Elbow
        Left ØRHM
        Right ØRHL
      Finger Phalangeal
        Left ØRHX
        Right ØRHW
      Hip
        Left ØSHB
        Right ØSH9
      Knee
        Left ØSHD
        Right ØSHC
      Lumbar Vertebral ØSHØ
      Lumbosacral ØSH3
      Metacarpophalangeal
        Left ØRHV
        Right ØRHU
      Metatarsal-Phalangeal
        Left ØSHN
        Right ØSHM
      Occipital-cervical ØRHØ
      Sacrococcygeal ØSH5
      Sacroiliac
        Left ØSH8
        Right ØSH7
      Shoulder
        Left ØRHK
        Right ØRHJ
      Sternoclavicular
        Left ØRHF
        Right ØRHE
      Tarsal
        Left ØSHJ
        Right ØSHH
      Tarsometatarsal
        Left ØSHL
        Right ØSHK
      Temporomandibular
        Left ØRHD
        Right ØRHC
      Thoracic Vertebral ØRH6
      Thoracolumbar Vertebral ØRHA
      Toe Phalangeal
        Left ØSHQ
        Right ØSHP
      Wrist
        Left ØRHP
        Right ØRHN
  Removal of device from
    Acromioclavicular
      Left ØRPH
      Right ØRPG
    Ankle
      Left ØSPG
      Right ØSPF
    Carpal
      Left ØRPR
      Right ØRPQ
    Carpometacarpal
      Left ØRPT
      Right ØRPS
    Cervical Vertebral ØRP1
    Cervicothoracic Vertebral ØRP4
    Coccygeal ØSP6
    Elbow
      Left ØRPM
      Right ØRPL
    Finger Phalangeal
      Left ØRPX
      Right ØRPW
    Hip
      Left ØSPB
      Right ØSP9

Spacer — *continued*
  Removal of device from — *continued*
    Knee
      Left ØSPD
      Right ØSPC
    Lumbar Vertebral ØSPØ
    Lumbosacral ØSP3
    Metacarpophalangeal
      Left ØRPV
      Right ØRPU
    Metatarsal-Phalangeal
      Left ØSPN
      Right ØSPM
    Occipital-cervical ØRPØ
    Sacrococcygeal ØSP5
    Sacroiliac
      Left ØSP8
      Right ØSP7
    Shoulder
      Left ØRPK
      Right ØRPJ
    Sternoclavicular
      Left ØRPF
      Right ØRPE
    Tarsal
      Left ØSPJ
      Right ØSPH
    Tarsometatarsal
      Left ØSPL
      Right ØSPK
    Temporomandibular
      Left ØRPD
      Right ØRPC
    Thoracic Vertebral ØRP6
    Thoracolumbar Vertebral ØRPA
    Toe Phalangeal
      Left ØSPQ
      Right ØSPP
    Wrist
      Left ØRPP
      Right ØRPN
  Revision of device in
    Acromioclavicular
      Left ØRWH
      Right ØRWG
    Ankle
      Left ØSWG
      Right ØSWF
    Carpal
      Left ØRWR
      Right ØRWQ
    Carpometacarpal
      Left ØRWT
      Right ØRWS
    Cervical Vertebral ØRW1
    Cervicothoracic Vertebral ØRW4
    Coccygeal ØSW6
    Elbow
      Left ØRWM
      Right ØRWL
    Finger Phalangeal
      Left ØRWX
      Right ØRWW
    Hip
      Left ØSWB
      Right ØSW9
    Knee
      Left ØSWD
      Right ØSWC
    Lumbar Vertebral ØSWØ
    Lumbosacral ØSW3
    Metacarpophalangeal
      Left ØRWV
      Right ØRWU
    Metatarsal-Phalangeal
      Left ØSWN
      Right ØSWM
    Occipital-cervical ØRWØ
    Sacrococcygeal ØSW5
    Sacroiliac
      Left ØSW8
      Right ØSW7
    Shoulder
      Left ØRWK
      Right ØRWJ
    Sternoclavicular
      Left ØRWF
      Right ØRWE

Spacer — *continued*
  Revision of device in — *continued*
    Tarsal
      Left ØSWJ
      Right ØSWH
    Tarsometatarsal
      Left ØSWL
      Right ØSWK
    Temporomandibular
      Left ØRWD
      Right ØRWC
    Thoracic Vertebral ØRW6
    Thoracolumbar Vertebral ØRWA
    Toe Phalangeal
      Left ØSWQ
      Right ØSWP
    Wrist
      Left ØRWP
      Right ØRWN
Spacer, Articulating (Antibiotic) *use* Articulating Spacer in Lower Joints
Spacer, Static (Antibiotic) *use* Spacer in Lower Joints
Spectroscopy
  Intravascular Near Infrared 8E023DZ
  Near Infrared *see* Physiological Systems and Anatomical Regions 8E0
Speech Assessment F00
Speech therapy *see* Speech Treatment, Rehabilitation F06
Speech Treatment F06
Sphenoidectomy
  see Excision, Ear, Nose, Sinus 09B
  see Excision, Head and Facial Bones ØNB
  see Resection, Ear, Nose, Sinus 09T
  see Resection, Head and Facial Bones ØNT
Sphenoidotomy *see* Drainage, Ear, Nose, Sinus 099
Sphenomandibular ligament *use* Head and Neck Bursa and Ligament
Sphenopalatine (pterygopalatine) ganglion *use* Head and Neck Sympathetic Nerve
Sphincterorrhaphy, anal *see* Repair, Anal Sphincter ØDQR
Sphincterotomy, anal
  see Division, Anal Sphincter ØD8R
  see Drainage, Anal Sphincter ØD9R
Spinal cord neurostimulator lead *use* Neurostimulator Lead in Central Nervous System and Cranial Nerves
Spinal growth rods, magnetically controlled *use* Magnetically Controlled Growth Rod(s) in New Technology
Spinal nerve, cervical *use* Cervical Nerve
Spinal nerve, lumbar *use* Lumbar Nerve
Spinal nerve, sacral *use* Sacral Nerve
Spinal nerve, thoracic *use* Thoracic Nerve
Spinal Stabilization Device
  Facet Replacement
    Cervical Vertebral ØRH1
    Cervicothoracic Vertebral ØRH4
    Lumbar Vertebral ØSHØ
    Lumbosacral ØSH3
    Occipital-cervical ØRHØ
    Thoracic Vertebral ØRH6
    Thoracolumbar Vertebral ØRHA
  Interspinous Process
    Cervical Vertebral ØRH1
    Cervicothoracic Vertebral ØRH4
    Lumbar Vertebral ØSHØ
    Lumbosacral ØSH3
    Occipital-cervical ØRHØ
    Thoracic Vertebral ØRH6
    Thoracolumbar Vertebral ØRHA
  Pedicle-Based
    Cervical Vertebral ØRH1
    Cervicothoracic Vertebral ØRH4
    Lumbar Vertebral ØSHØ
    Lumbosacral ØSH3
    Occipital-cervical ØRHØ
    Thoracic Vertebral ØRH6
    Thoracolumbar Vertebral ØRHA
SpineJack® system *use* Synthetic Substitute, Mechanically Expandable (Paired) in New Technology
Spinous process
  use Cervical Vertebra
  use Lumbar Vertebra
  use Thoracic Vertebra
Spiral ganglion *use* Acoustic Nerve

Spiration IBV™ Valve System *use* Intraluminal Device, Endobronchial Valve in Respiratory System

Splenectomy
  see Excision, Lymphatic and Hemic Systems 07B
  see Resection, Lymphatic and Hemic Systems 07T

Splenic flexure *use* Transverse Colon

Splenic plexus *use* Abdominal Sympathetic Nerve

Splenius capitis muscle *use* Head Muscle

Splenius cervicis muscle
  use Neck Muscle, Left
  use Neck Muscle, Right

Splenolysis *see* Release, Lymphatic and Hemic Systems 07N

Splenopexy
  see Repair, Lymphatic and Hemic Systems 07Q
  see Reposition, Lymphatic and Hemic Systems 07S

Splenoplasty *see* Repair, Lymphatic and Hemic Systems 07Q

Splenorrhaphy *see* Repair, Lymphatic and Hemic Systems 07Q

Splenotomy *see* Drainage, Lymphatic and Hemic Systems 079

Splinting, musculoskeletal *see* Immobilization, Anatomical Regions 2W3

SPRAVATO™ *use* Esketamine Hydrochloride

SPY PINPOINT fluorescence imaging system
  see Monitoring, Physiological Systems 4A1
  see Other Imaging, Hepatobiliary System and Pancreas BF5

SPY system intraoperative fluorescence cholangiography *see* Other Imaging, Hepatobiliary System and Pancreas BF5

SPY system intravascular fluorescence angiography *see* Monitoring, Physiological Systems 4A1

Staged hepatectomy
  see Division, Hepatobiliary System and Pancreas 0F8
  see Resection, Hepatobiliary System and Pancreas 0FT

Stapedectomy
  see Excision, Ear, Nose, Sinus 09B
  see Resection, Ear, Nose, Sinus 09T

Stapediolysis *see* Release, Ear, Nose, Sinus 09N

Stapedioplasty
  see Repair, Ear, Nose, Sinus 09Q
  see Replacement, Ear, Nose, Sinus 09R
  see Supplement, Ear, Nose, Sinus 09U

Stapedotomy *see* Drainage, Ear, Nose, Sinus 099

Stapes
  use Auditory Ossicle, Left
  use Auditory Ossicle, Right

Static Spacer (Antibiotic) *use* Spacer in Lower Joints

STELARA® *use* Other New Technology Therapeutic Substance

Stellate ganglion *use* Head and Neck Sympathetic Nerve

Stem cell transplant *see* Transfusion, Circulatory 302

Stensen's duct
  use Parotid Duct, Left
  use Parotid Duct, Right

Stent, intraluminal (cardiovascular) (gastrointestinal) (hepatobiliary) (urinary) *use* Intraluminal Device

Stent retriever thrombectomy *see* Extirpation, Upper Arteries 03C

Stented tissue valve *use* Zooplastic Tissue in Heart and Great Vessels

Stereotactic Radiosurgery
  Abdomen DW23
  Adrenal Gland DG22
  Bile Ducts DF22
  Bladder DT22
  Bone Marrow D720
  Brain D020
  Brain Stem D021
  Breast
    Left DM20
    Right DM21
  Bronchus DB21
  Cervix DU21
  Chest DW22
  Chest Wall DB27
  Colon DD25
  Diaphragm DB28
  Duodenum DD22
  Ear D920
  Esophagus DD20

Stereotactic Radiosurgery — *continued*
  Eye D820
  Gallbladder DF21
  Gamma Beam
    Abdomen DW23JZZ
    Adrenal Gland DG22JZZ
    Bile Ducts DF22JZZ
    Bladder DT22JZZ
    Bone Marrow D720JZZ
    Brain D020JZZ
    Brain Stem D021JZZ
    Breast
      Left DM20JZZ
      Right DM21JZZ
    Bronchus DB21JZZ
    Cervix DU21JZZ
    Chest DW22JZZ
    Chest Wall DB27JZZ
    Colon DD25JZZ
    Diaphragm DB28JZZ
    Duodenum DD22JZZ
    Ear D920JZZ
    Esophagus DD20JZZ
    Eye D820JZZ
    Gallbladder DF21JZZ
    Gland
      Adrenal DG22JZZ
      Parathyroid DG24JZZ
      Pituitary DG20JZZ
      Thyroid DG25JZZ
    Glands, Salivary D926JZZ
    Head and Neck DW21JZZ
    Ileum DD24JZZ
    Jejunum DD23JZZ
    Kidney DT20JZZ
    Larynx D92BJZZ
    Liver DF20JZZ
    Lung DB22JZZ
    Lymphatics
      Abdomen D726JZZ
      Axillary D724JZZ
      Inguinal D728JZZ
      Neck D723JZZ
      Pelvis D727JZZ
      Thorax D725JZZ
    Mediastinum DB26JZZ
    Mouth D924JZZ
    Nasopharynx D92DJZZ
    Neck and Head DW21JZZ
    Nerve, Peripheral D027JZZ
    Nose D921JZZ
    Ovary DU20JZZ
    Palate
      Hard D928JZZ
      Soft D929JZZ
    Pancreas DF23JZZ
    Parathyroid Gland DG24JZZ
    Pelvic Region DW26JZZ
    Pharynx D92CJZZ
    Pineal Body DG21JZZ
    Pituitary Gland DG20JZZ
    Pleura DB25JZZ
    Prostate DV20JZZ
    Rectum DD27JZZ
    Sinuses D927JZZ
    Spinal Cord D026JZZ
    Spleen D722JZZ
    Stomach DD21JZZ
    Testis DV21JZZ
    Thymus D721JZZ
    Thyroid Gland DG25JZZ
    Tongue D925JZZ
    Trachea DB20JZZ
    Ureter DT21JZZ
    Urethra DT23JZZ
    Uterus DU22JZZ
  Gland
    Adrenal DG22
    Parathyroid DG24
    Pituitary DG20
    Thyroid DG25
  Glands, Salivary D926
  Head and Neck DW21
  Ileum DD24
  Jejunum DD23
  Kidney DT20
  Larynx D92B
  Liver DF20
  Lung DB22

Stereotactic Radiosurgery — *continued*
  Lymphatics
    Abdomen D726
    Axillary D724
    Inguinal D728
    Neck D723
    Pelvis D727
    Thorax D725
  Mediastinum DB26
  Mouth D924
  Nasopharynx D92D
  Neck and Head DW21
  Nerve, Peripheral D027
  Nose D921
  Other Photon
    Abdomen DW23DZZ
    Adrenal Gland DG22DZZ
    Bile Ducts DF22DZZ
    Bladder DT22DZZ
    Bone Marrow D720DZZ
    Brain D020DZZ
    Brain Stem D021DZZ
    Breast
      Left DM20DZZ
      Right DM21DZZ
    Bronchus DB21DZZ
    Cervix DU21DZZ
    Chest DW22DZZ
    Chest Wall DB27DZZ
    Colon DD25DZZ
    Diaphragm DB28DZZ
    Duodenum DD22DZZ
    Ear D920DZZ
    Esophagus DD20DZZ
    Eye D820DZZ
    Gallbladder DF21DZZ
    Gland
      Adrenal DG22DZZ
      Parathyroid DG24DZZ
      Pituitary DG20DZZ
      Thyroid DG25DZZ
    Glands, Salivary D926DZZ
    Head and Neck DW21DZZ
    Ileum DD24DZZ
    Jejunum DD23DZZ
    Kidney DT20DZZ
    Larynx D92BDZZ
    Liver DF20DZZ
    Lung DB22DZZ
    Lymphatics
      Abdomen D726DZZ
      Axillary D724DZZ
      Inguinal D728DZZ
      Neck D723DZZ
      Pelvis D727DZZ
      Thorax D725DZZ
    Mediastinum DB26DZZ
    Mouth D924DZZ
    Nasopharynx D92DDZZ
    Neck and Head DW21DZZ
    Nerve, Peripheral D027DZZ
    Nose D921DZZ
    Ovary DU20DZZ
    Palate
      Hard D928DZZ
      Soft D929DZZ
    Pancreas DF23DZZ
    Parathyroid Gland DG24DZZ
    Pelvic Region DW26DZZ
    Pharynx D92CDZZ
    Pineal Body DG21DZZ
    Pituitary Gland DG20DZZ
    Pleura DB25DZZ
    Prostate DV20DZZ
    Rectum DD27DZZ
    Sinuses D927DZZ
    Spinal Cord D026DZZ
    Spleen D722DZZ
    Stomach DD21DZZ
    Testis DV21DZZ
    Thymus D721DZZ
    Thyroid Gland DG25DZZ
    Tongue D925DZZ
    Trachea DB20DZZ
    Ureter DT21DZZ
    Urethra DT23DZZ
    Uterus DU22DZZ
  Ovary DU20

▽ **Subterms under main terms may continue to next column or page**

Stereotactic Radiosurgery — *continued*
  Palate
    Hard D928
    Soft D929
  Pancreas DF23
  Parathyroid Gland DG24
  Particulate
    Abdomen DW23HZZ
    Adrenal Gland DG22HZZ
    Bile Ducts DF22HZZ
    Bladder DT22HZZ
    Bone Marrow D720HZZ
    Brain D020HZZ
    Brain Stem D021HZZ
    Breast
      Left DM20HZZ
      Right DM21HZZ
    Bronchus DB21HZZ
    Cervix DU21HZZ
    Chest DW22HZZ
    Chest Wall DB27HZZ
    Colon DD25HZZ
    Diaphragm DB28HZZ
    Duodenum DD22HZZ
    Ear D920HZZ
    Esophagus DD20HZZ
    Eye D820HZZ
    Gallbladder DF21HZZ
    Gland
      Adrenal DG22HZZ
      Parathyroid DG24HZZ
      Pituitary DG20HZZ
      Thyroid DG25HZZ
    Glands, Salivary D926HZZ
    Head and Neck DW21HZZ
    Ileum DD24HZZ
    Jejunum DD23HZZ
    Kidney DT20HZZ
    Larynx D92BHZZ
    Liver DF20HZZ
    Lung DB22HZZ
    Lymphatics
      Abdomen D726HZZ
      Axillary D724HZZ
      Inguinal D728HZZ
      Neck D723HZZ
      Pelvis D727HZZ
      Thorax D725HZZ
    Mediastinum DB26HZZ
    Mouth D924HZZ
    Nasopharynx D92DHZZ
    Neck and Head DW21HZZ
    Nerve, Peripheral D027HZZ
    Nose D921HZZ
    Ovary DU20HZZ
    Palate
      Hard D928HZZ
      Soft D929HZZ
    Pancreas DF23HZZ
    Parathyroid Gland DG24HZZ
    Pelvic Region DW26HZZ
    Pharynx D92CHZZ
    Pineal Body DG21HZZ
    Pituitary Gland DG20HZZ
    Pleura DB25HZZ
    Prostate DV20HZZ
    Rectum DD27HZZ
    Sinuses D927HZZ
    Spinal Cord D026HZZ
    Spleen D722HZZ
    Stomach DD21HZZ
    Testis DV21HZZ
    Thymus D721HZZ
    Thyroid Gland DG25HZZ
    Tongue D925HZZ
    Trachea DB20HZZ
    Ureter DT21HZZ
    Urethra DT23HZZ
    Uterus DU22HZZ
  Pelvic Region DW26
  Pharynx D92C
  Pineal Body DG21
  Pituitary Gland DG20
  Pleura DB25
  Prostate DV20
  Rectum DD27
  Sinuses D927
  Spinal Cord D026
  Spleen D722

Stereotactic Radiosurgery — *continued*
  Stomach DD21
  Testis DV21
  Thymus D721
  Thyroid Gland DG25
  Tongue D925
  Trachea DB20
  Ureter DT21
  Urethra DT23
  Uterus DU22
Steripath® Micro™ Blood Collection System
  XXE5XR7
Sternoclavicular ligament
  use Shoulder Bursa and Ligament, Left
  use Shoulder Bursa and Ligament, Right
Sternocleidomastoid artery
  use Thyroid Artery, Left
  use Thyroid Artery, Right
Sternocleidomastoid muscle
  use Neck Muscle, Left
  use Neck Muscle, Right
Sternocostal ligament *use* Sternum Bursa and Ligament
Sternotomy
  see Division, Sternum 0P80
  see Drainage, Sternum 0P90
Stimulation, cardiac
  Cardioversion 5A2204Z
  Electrophysiologic testing *see* Measurement, Cardiac 4A02
Stimulator Generator
  Insertion of device in
    Abdomen 0JH8
    Back 0JH7
    Chest 0JH6
  Multiple Array
    Abdomen 0JH8
    Back 0JH7
    Chest 0JH6
  Multiple Array Rechargeable
    Abdomen 0JH8
    Back 0JH7
    Chest 0JH6
  Removal of device from, Subcutaneous Tissue and Fascia, Trunk 0JPT
  Revision of device in, Subcutaneous Tissue and Fascia, Trunk 0JWT
  Single Array
    Abdomen 0JH8
    Back 0JH7
    Chest 0JH6
  Single Array Rechargeable
    Abdomen 0JH8
    Back 0JH7
    Chest 0JH6
Stimulator Lead
  Insertion of device in
    Anal Sphincter 0DHR
    Artery
      Left 03HL
      Right 03HK
    Bladder 0THB
    Muscle
      Lower 0KHY
      Upper 0KHX
    Stomach 0DH6
    Ureter 0TH9
  Removal of device from
    Anal Sphincter 0DPR
    Artery, Upper 03PY
    Bladder 0TPB
    Muscle
      Lower 0KPY
      Upper 0KPX
    Stomach 0DP6
    Ureter 0TP9
  Revision of device in
    Anal Sphincter 0DWR
    Artery, Upper 03WY
    Bladder 0TWB
    Muscle
      Lower 0KWY
      Upper 0KWX
    Stomach 0DW6
    Ureter 0TW9
Stoma
  Excision
    Abdominal Wall 0WBFXZ2

Stoma — *continued*
  Excision — *continued*
    Neck 0WB6XZ2
  Repair
    Abdominal Wall 0WQFXZ2
    Neck 0WQ6XZ2
Stomatoplasty
  see Repair, Mouth and Throat 0CQ
  see Replacement, Mouth and Throat 0CR
  see Supplement, Mouth and Throat 0CU
Stomatorrhaphy *see* Repair, Mouth and Throat 0CQ
StrataGraft® *use* Bioengineered Allogeneic Construct
Stratos LV *use* Cardiac Resynchronization Pacemaker Pulse Generator in 0JH
Stress test 4A02XM4, 4A12XM4
Stripping *see* Extraction
Study
  Electrophysiologic stimulation, cardiac *see* Measurement, Cardiac 4A02
  Ocular motility 4A07X7Z
  Pulmonary airway flow measurement *see* Measurement, Respiratory 4A09
  Visual acuity 4A07X0Z
Styloglossus muscle *use* Tongue, Palate, Pharynx Muscle
Stylomandibular ligament *use* Head and Neck Bursa and Ligament
Stylopharyngeus muscle *use* Tongue, Palate, Pharynx Muscle
Subacromial bursa
  use Shoulder Bursa and Ligament, Left
  use Shoulder Bursa and Ligament, Right
Subaortic (common iliac) lymph node *use* Lymphatic, Pelvis
Subarachnoid space, spinal *use* Spinal Canal
Subclavicular (apical) lymph node
  use Lymphatic, Left Axillary
  use Lymphatic, Right Axillary
Subclavius muscle
  use Thorax Muscle, Left
  use Thorax Muscle, Right
Subclavius nerve *use* Brachial Plexus
Subcostal artery *use* Upper Artery
Subcostal muscle
  use Thorax Muscle, Left
  use Thorax Muscle, Right
Subcostal nerve *use* Thoracic Nerve
Subcutaneous Defibrillator Lead
  Insertion of device in, Subcutaneous Tissue and Fascia, Chest 0JH6
  Removal of device from, Subcutaneous Tissue and Fascia, Trunk 0JPT
  Revision of device in, Subcutaneous Tissue and Fascia, Trunk 0JWT
Subcutaneous injection reservoir, port *use* Vascular Access Device, Totally Implantable in Subcutaneous Tissue and Fascia
Subcutaneous injection reservoir, pump *use* Infusion Device, Pump in Subcutaneous Tissue and Fascia
Subdermal progesterone implant *use* Contraceptive Device in Subcutaneous Tissue and Fascia
Subdural space, spinal *use* Spinal Canal
Submandibular ganglion
  use Facial Nerve
  use Head and Neck Sympathetic Nerve
Submandibular gland
  use Submaxillary Gland, Left
  use Submaxillary Gland, Right
Submandibular lymph node *use* Lymphatic, Head
Submandibular space *use* Subcutaneous Tissue and Fascia, Face
Submaxillary ganglion *use* Head and Neck Sympathetic Nerve
Submaxillary lymph node *use* Lymphatic, Head
Submental artery *use* Face Artery
Submental lymph node *use* Lymphatic, Head
Submucous (Meissner's) plexus *use* Abdominal Sympathetic Nerve
Suboccipital nerve *use* Cervical Nerve
Suboccipital venous plexus
  use Vertebral Vein, Left
  use Vertebral Vein, Right
Subparotid lymph node *use* Lymphatic, Head
Subscapular aponeurosis
  use Subcutaneous Tissue and Fascia, Left Upper Arm

Subscapular aponeurosis — *continued*
use Subcutaneous Tissue and Fascia, Right Upper Arm
Subscapular artery
use Axillary Artery, Left
use Axillary Artery, Right
Subscapular (posterior) lymph node
use Lymphatic, Axillary, Left
use Lymphatic, Axillary, Right
Subscapularis muscle
use Shoulder Muscle, Left
use Shoulder Muscle, Right
Substance Abuse Treatment
Counseling
Family, for substance abuse, Other Family Counseling HZ63ZZZ
Group
12-Step HZ43ZZZ
Behavioral HZ41ZZZ
Cognitive HZ40ZZZ
Cognitive-Behavioral HZ42ZZZ
Confrontational HZ48ZZZ
Continuing Care HZ49ZZZ
Infectious Disease
Post-Test HZ4CZZZ
Pre-Test HZ4CZZZ
Interpersonal HZ44ZZZ
Motivational Enhancement HZ47ZZZ
Psychoeducation HZ46ZZZ
Spiritual HZ4BZZZ
Vocational HZ45ZZZ
Individual
12-Step HZ33ZZZ
Behavioral HZ31ZZZ
Cognitive HZ30ZZZ
Cognitive-Behavioral HZ32ZZZ
Confrontational HZ38ZZZ
Continuing Care HZ39ZZZ
Infectious Disease
Post-Test HZ3CZZZ
Pre-Test HZ3CZZZ
Interpersonal HZ34ZZZ
Motivational Enhancement HZ37ZZZ
Psychoeducation HZ36ZZZ
Spiritual HZ3BZZZ
Vocational HZ35ZZZ
Detoxification Services, for substance abuse HZ2ZZZZ
Medication Management
Antabuse HZ83ZZZ
Bupropion HZ87ZZZ
Clonidine HZ86ZZZ
Levo-alpha-acetyl-methadol (LAAM) HZ82ZZZ
Methadone Maintenance HZ81ZZZ
Naloxone HZ85ZZZ
Naltrexone HZ84ZZZ
Nicotine Replacement HZ80ZZZ
Other Replacement Medication HZ89ZZZ
Psychiatric Medication HZ88ZZZ
Pharmacotherapy
Antabuse HZ93ZZZ
Bupropion HZ97ZZZ
Clonidine HZ96ZZZ
Levo-alpha-acetyl-methadol (LAAM) HZ92ZZZ
Methadone Maintenance HZ91ZZZ
Naloxone HZ95ZZZ
Naltrexone HZ94ZZZ
Nicotine Replacement HZ90ZZZ
Psychiatric Medication HZ98ZZZ
Replacement Medication, Other HZ99ZZZ
Psychotherapy
12-Step HZ53ZZZ
Behavioral HZ51ZZZ
Cognitive HZ50ZZZ
Cognitive-Behavioral HZ52ZZZ
Confrontational HZ58ZZZ
Interactive HZ55ZZZ
Interpersonal HZ54ZZZ
Motivational Enhancement HZ57ZZZ
Psychoanalysis HZ5BZZZ
Psychodynamic HZ5CZZZ
Psychoeducation HZ56ZZZ
Psychophysiological HZ5DZZZ
Supportive HZ59ZZZ
Substantia nigra *use* Basal Ganglia

Subtalar (talocalcaneal) joint
use Tarsal Joint, Left
use Tarsal Joint, Right
Subtalar ligament
use Foot Bursa and Ligament, Left
use Foot Bursa and Ligament, Right
Subthalamic nucleus *use* Basal Ganglia
Suction curettage (D&C), nonobstetric *see* Extraction, Endometrium 0UDB
Suction curettage, obstetric post-delivery *see* Extraction, Products of Conception, Retained 10D1
Superficial circumflex iliac vein
use Saphenous Vein, Left
use Saphenous Vein, Right
Superficial epigastric artery
use Femoral Artery, Left
use Femoral Artery, Right
Superficial epigastric vein
use Saphenous Vein, Left
use Saphenous Vein, Right
Superficial Inferior Epigastric Artery Flap
Replacement
Bilateral 0HRV078
Left 0HRU078
Right 0HRT078
Transfer
Left 0KXG
Right 0KXF
Superficial palmar arch
use Hand Artery, Left
use Hand Artery, Right
Superficial palmar venous arch
use Hand Vein, Left
use Hand Vein, Right
Superficial temporal artery
use Temporal Artery, Left
use Temporal Artery, Right
Superficial transverse perineal muscle *use* Perineum Muscle
Superior cardiac nerve *use* Thoracic Sympathetic Nerve
Superior cerebellar vein *use* Intracranial Vein
Superior cerebral vein *use* Intracranial Vein
Superior clunic (cluneal) nerve *use* Lumbar Nerve
Superior epigastric artery
use Internal Mammary Artery, Left
use Internal Mammary Artery, Right
Superior genicular artery
use Popliteal Artery, Left
use Popliteal Artery, Right
Superior gluteal artery
use Internal Iliac Artery, Left
use Internal Iliac Artery, Right
Superior gluteal nerve *use* Lumbar Plexus
Superior hypogastric plexus *use* Abdominal Sympathetic Nerve
Superior labial artery *use* Face Artery
Superior laryngeal artery
use Thyroid Artery, Left
use Thyroid Artery, Right
Superior laryngeal nerve *use* Vagus Nerve
Superior longitudinal muscle *use* Tongue, Palate, Pharynx Muscle
Superior mesenteric ganglion *use* Abdominal Sympathetic Nerve
Superior mesenteric lymph node *use* Lymphatic, Mesenteric
Superior mesenteric plexus *use* Abdominal Sympathetic Nerve
Superior oblique muscle
use Extraocular Muscle, Left
use Extraocular Muscle, Right
Superior olivary nucleus *use* Pons
Superior rectal artery *use* Inferior Mesenteric Artery
Superior rectal vein *use* Inferior Mesenteric Vein
Superior rectus muscle
use Extraocular Muscle, Left
use Extraocular Muscle, Right
Superior tarsal plate
use Upper Eyelid, Left
use Upper Eyelid, Right
Superior thoracic artery
use Axillary Artery, Left
use Axillary Artery, Right
Superior thyroid artery
use External Carotid Artery, Left
use External Carotid Artery, Right

Superior thyroid artery — *continued*
use Thyroid Artery, Left
use Thyroid Artery, Right
Superior turbinate *use* Nasal Turbinate
Superior ulnar collateral artery
use Brachial Artery, Left
use Brachial Artery, Right
Supersaturated Oxygen therapy 5A0512C, 5A0522C
Supplement
Abdominal Wall 0WUF
Acetabulum
Left 0QU5
Right 0QU4
Ampulla of Vater 0FUC
Anal Sphincter 0DUR
Ankle Region
Left 0YUL
Right 0YUK
Anus 0DUQ
Aorta
Abdominal 04U0
Thoracic
Ascending/Arch 02UX
Descending 02UW
Arm
Lower
Left 0XUF
Right 0XUD
Upper
Left 0XU9
Right 0XU8
Artery
Anterior Tibial
Left 04UQ
Right 04UP
Axillary
Left 03U6
Right 03U5
Brachial
Left 03U8
Right 03U7
Celiac 04U1
Colic
Left 04U7
Middle 04U8
Right 04U6
Common Carotid
Left 03UJ
Right 03UH
Common Iliac
Left 04UD
Right 04UC
Coronary
Four or More Arteries 02U3
One Artery 02U0
Three Arteries 02U2
Two Arteries 02U1
External Carotid
Left 03UN
Right 03UM
External Iliac
Left 04UJ
Right 04UH
Face 03UR
Femoral
Left 04UL
Right 04UK
Foot
Left 04UW
Right 04UV
Gastric 04U2
Hand
Left 03UF
Right 03UD
Hepatic 04U3
Inferior Mesenteric 04UB
Innominate 03U2
Internal Carotid
Left 03UL
Right 03UK
Internal Iliac
Left 04UF
Right 04UE
Internal Mammary
Left 03U1
Right 03U0
Intracranial 03UG
Lower 04UY

Supplement — *continued*
  Finger — *continued*
    Middle — *continued*
      Right ØXUQ
    Ring
      Left ØXUT
      Right ØXUS
  Foot
    Left ØYUN
    Right ØYUM
  Gingiva
    Lower ØCU6
    Upper ØCU5
  Glenoid Cavity
    Left ØPU8
    Right ØPU7
  Hand
    Left ØXUK
    Right ØXUJ
  Head ØWUØ
  Heart Ø2UA
  Humeral Head
    Left ØPUD
    Right ØPUC
  Humeral Shaft
    Left ØPUG
    Right ØPUF
  Hymen ØUUK
  Ileocecal Valve ØDUC
  Ileum ØDUB
  Inguinal Region
    Bilateral ØYUA
    Left ØYU6
    Right ØYU5
  Intestine
    Large ØDUE
      Left ØDUG
      Right ØDUF
    Small ØDU8
  Iris
    Left Ø8UD
    Right Ø8UC
  Jaw
    Lower ØWU5
    Upper ØWU4
  Jejunum ØDUA
  Joint
    Acromioclavicular
      Left ØRUH
      Right ØRUG
    Ankle
      Left ØSUG
      Right ØSUF
    Carpal
      Left ØRUR
      Right ØRUQ
    Carpometacarpal
      Left ØRUT
      Right ØRUS
    Cervical Vertebral ØRU1
    Cervicothoracic Vertebral ØRU4
    Coccygeal ØSU6
    Elbow
      Left ØRUM
      Right ØRUL
    Finger Phalangeal
      Left ØRUX
      Right ØRUW
    Hip
      Left ØSUB
        Acetabular Surface ØSUE
        Femoral Surface ØSUS
      Right ØSU9
        Acetabular Surface ØSUA
        Femoral Surface ØSUR
    Knee
      Left ØSUD
        Femoral Surface ØSUUØ9Z
        Tibial Surface ØSUWØ9Z
      Right ØSUC
        Femoral Surface ØSUTØ9Z
        Tibial Surface ØSUVØ9Z
    Lumbar Vertebral ØSUØ
    Lumbosacral ØSU3
    Metacarpophalangeal
      Left ØRUV
      Right ØRUU
    Metatarsal-Phalangeal
      Left ØSUN

Supplement — *continued*
  Joint — *continued*
    Metatarsal-Phalangeal — *continued*
      Right ØSUM
    Occipital-cervical ØRUØ
    Sacrococcygeal ØSU5
    Sacroiliac
      Left ØSU8
      Right ØSU7
    Shoulder
      Left ØRUK
      Right ØRUJ
    Sternoclavicular
      Left ØRUF
      Right ØRUE
    Tarsal
      Left ØSUJ
      Right ØSUH
    Tarsometatarsal
      Left ØSUL
      Right ØSUK
    Temporomandibular
      Left ØRUD
      Right ØRUC
    Thoracic Vertebral ØRU6
    Thoracolumbar Vertebral ØRUA
    Toe Phalangeal
      Left ØSUQ
      Right ØSUP
    Wrist
      Left ØRUP
      Right ØRUN
  Kidney Pelvis
    Left ØTU4
    Right ØTU3
  Knee Region
    Left ØYUG
    Right ØYUF
  Larynx ØCUS
  Leg
    Lower
      Left ØYUJ
      Right ØYUH
    Upper
      Left ØYUD
      Right ØYUC
  Lip
    Lower ØCU1
    Upper ØCUØ
  Lymphatic
    Aortic Ø7UD
    Axillary
      Left Ø7U6
      Right Ø7U5
    Head Ø7UØ
    Inguinal
      Left Ø7UJ
      Right Ø7UH
    Internal Mammary
      Left Ø7U9
      Right Ø7U8
    Lower Extremity
      Left Ø7UG
      Right Ø7UF
    Mesenteric Ø7UB
    Neck
      Left Ø7U2
      Right Ø7U1
    Pelvis Ø7UC
    Thoracic Duct Ø7UK
    Thorax Ø7U7
    Upper Extremity
      Left Ø7U4
      Right Ø7U3
  Mandible
    Left ØNUV
    Right ØNUT
  Maxilla ØNUR
  Mediastinum ØWUC
  Mesentery ØDUV
  Metacarpal
    Left ØPUQ
    Right ØPUP
  Metatarsal
    Left ØQUP
    Right ØQUN
  Muscle
    Abdomen
      Left ØKUL

Supplement — *continued*
  Muscle — *continued*
    Abdomen — *continued*
      Right ØKUK
    Extraocular
      Left Ø8UM
      Right Ø8UL
    Facial ØKU1
    Foot
      Left ØKUW
      Right ØKUV
    Hand
      Left ØKUD
      Right ØKUC
    Head ØKUØ
    Hip
      Left ØKUP
      Right ØKUN
    Lower Arm and Wrist
      Left ØKUB
      Right ØKU9
    Lower Leg
      Left ØKUT
      Right ØKUS
    Neck
      Left ØKU3
      Right ØKU2
    Papillary Ø2UD
    Perineum ØKUM
    Shoulder
      Left ØKU6
      Right ØKU5
    Thorax
      Left ØKUJ
      Right ØKUH
    Tongue, Palate, Pharynx ØKU4
    Trunk
      Left ØKUG
      Right ØKUF
    Upper Arm
      Left ØKU8
      Right ØKU7
    Upper Leg
      Left ØKUR
      Right ØKUQ
  Nasal Mucosa and Soft Tissue Ø9UK
  Nasopharynx Ø9UN
  Neck ØWU6
  Nerve
    Abducens ØØUL
    Accessory ØØUR
    Acoustic ØØUN
    Cervical Ø1U1
    Facial ØØUM
    Femoral Ø1UD
    Glossopharyngeal ØØUP
    Hypoglossal ØØUS
    Lumbar Ø1UB
    Median Ø1U5
    Oculomotor ØØUH
    Olfactory ØØUF
    Optic ØØUG
    Peroneal Ø1UH
    Phrenic Ø1U2
    Pudendal Ø1UC
    Radial Ø1U6
    Sacral Ø1UR
    Sciatic Ø1UF
    Thoracic Ø1U8
    Tibial Ø1UG
    Trigeminal ØØUK
    Trochlear ØØUJ
    Ulnar Ø1U4
    Vagus ØØUQ
  Nipple
    Left ØHUX
    Right ØHUW
  Omentum ØDUU
  Orbit
    Left ØNUQ
    Right ØNUP
  Palate
    Hard ØCU2
    Soft ØCU3
  Patella
    Left ØQUF
    Right ØQUD
  Penis ØVUS
  Pericardium Ø2UN

Supplement — *continued*
　Vein — *continued*
　　Vertebral
　　　Left Ø5US
　　　Right Ø5UR
　Vena Cava
　　Inferior Ø6UØ
　　Superior Ø2UV
　Ventricle
　　Left Ø2UL
　　Right Ø2UK
　Vertebra
　　Cervical ØPU3
　　Lumbar ØQUØ
　　　Mechanically Expandable (Paired) Synthetic Substitute XNUØ356
　　Thoracic ØPU4
　　　Mechanically Expandable (Paired) Synthetic Substitute XNU4356
　Vesicle
　　Bilateral ØVU3
　　Left ØVU2
　　Right ØVU1
　Vocal Cord
　　Left ØCUV
　　Right ØCUT
　Vulva ØUUM
　Wrist Region
　　Left ØXUH
　　Right ØXUG
Supraclavicular (Virchow's) lymph node
　use Lymphatic, Left Neck
　use Lymphatic, Right Neck
Supraclavicular nerve *use* Cervical Plexus
Suprahyoid lymph node *use* Lymphatic, Head
Suprahyoid muscle
　use Neck Muscle, Left
　use Neck Muscle, Right
Suprainguinal lymph node *use* Lymphatic, Pelvis
Supraorbital vein
　use Face Vein, Left
　use Face Vein, Right
Suprarenal gland
　use Adrenal Gland
　use Adrenal Gland, Bilateral
　use Adrenal Gland, Left
　use Adrenal Gland, Right
Suprarenal plexus *use* Abdominal Sympathetic Nerve
Suprascapular nerve *use* Brachial Plexus
Supraspinatus fascia
　use Subcutaneous Tissue and Fascia, Left Upper Arm
　use Subcutaneous Tissue and Fascia, Right Upper Arm
Supraspinatus muscle
　use Shoulder Muscle, Left
　use Shoulder Muscle, Right
Supraspinous ligament
　use Lower Spine Bursa and Ligament
　use Upper Spine Bursa and Ligament
Suprasternal notch *use* Sternum
Supratrochlear lymph node
　use Lymphatic, Left Upper Extremity
　use Lymphatic, Right Upper Extremity
Sural artery
　use Popliteal Artery, Left
　use Popliteal Artery, Right
Surpass Streamline™ Flow Diverter *use* Intraluminal Device, Flow Diverter in Ø3V
Suspension
　Bladder Neck *see* Reposition, Bladder Neck ØTSC
　Kidney *see* Reposition, Urinary System ØTS
　Urethra *see* Reposition, Urinary System ØTS
　Urethrovesical *see* Reposition, Bladder Neck ØTSC
　Uterus *see* Reposition, Uterus ØUS9
　Vagina *see* Reposition, Vagina ØUSG
Sustained Release Drug-eluting Intraluminal Device
　Dilation
　　Anterior Tibial
　　　Left X27Q385
　　　Right X27P385
　　Femoral
　　　Left X27J385
　　　Right X27H385
　　Peroneal
　　　Left X27U385

Sustained Release Drug-eluting Intraluminal Device — *continued*
　Dilation — *continued*
　　Peroneal — *continued*
　　　Right X27T385
　　Popliteal
　　　Left Distal X27N385
　　　Left Proximal X27L385
　　　Right Distal X27M385
　　　Right Proximal X27K385
　　Posterior Tibial
　　　Left X27S385
　　　Right X27R385
　Four or More
　　Anterior Tibial
　　　Left X27Q3C5
　　　Right X27P3C5
　　Femoral
　　　Left X27J3C5
　　　Right X27H3C5
　　Peroneal
　　　Left X27U3C5
　　　Right X27T3C5
　　Popliteal
　　　Left Distal X27N3C5
　　　Left Proximal X27L3C5
　　　Right Distal X27M3C5
　　　Right Proximal X27K3C5
　　Posterior Tibial
　　　Left X27S3C5
　　　Right X27R3C5
　Three
　　Anterior Tibial
　　　Left X27Q3B5
　　　Right X27P3B5
　　Femoral
　　　Left X27J3B5
　　　Right X27H3B5
　　Peroneal
　　　Left X27U3B5
　　　Right X27T3B5
　　Popliteal
　　　Left Distal X27N3B5
　　　Left Proximal X27L3B5
　　　Right Distal X27M3B5
　　　Right Proximal X27K3B5
　　Posterior Tibial
　　　Left X27S3B5
　　　Right X27R3B5
　Two
　　Anterior Tibial
　　　Left X27Q395
　　　Right X27P395
　　Femoral
　　　Left X27J395
　　　Right X27H395
　　Peroneal
　　　Left X27U395
　　　Right X27T395
　　Popliteal
　　　Left Distal X27N395
　　　Left Proximal X27L395
　　　Right Distal X27M395
　　　Right Proximal X27K395
　　Posterior Tibial
　　　Left X27S395
　　　Right X27R395
Suture
　Laceration repair *see* Repair
　Ligation *see* Occlusion
Suture Removal
　Extremity
　　Lower 8EØYXY8
　　Upper 8EØXXY8
　Head and Neck Region 8EØ9XY8
　Trunk Region 8EØWXY8
Sutureless valve, Perceval *use* Zooplastic Tissue, Rapid Deployment Technique in New Technology
Sweat gland *use* Skin
Sympathectomy *see* Excision, Peripheral Nervous System Ø1B
SynCardia (temporary) total artificial heart (TAH) *use* Synthetic Substitute, Pneumatic in Ø2R
SynCardia Total Artificial Heart *use* Synthetic Substitute
Synchra CRT-P *use* Cardiac Resynchronization Pacemaker Pulse Generator in ØJH

SynchroMed pump *use* Infusion Device, Pump in Subcutaneous Tissue and Fascia
Synechiotomy, iris *see* Release, Eye Ø8N
Synovectomy
　Lower joint *see* Excision, Lower Joints ØSB
　Upper joint *see* Excision, Upper Joints ØRB
Synthetic Human Angiotensin II XWØ
Systemic Nuclear Medicine Therapy
　Abdomen CW7Ø
　Anatomical Regions, Multiple CW7YYZZ
　Chest CW73
　Thyroid CW7G
　Whole Body CW7N

T

Tagraxofusp-erzs Antineoplastic XWØ
Takedown
　Arteriovenous shunt *see* Removal of device from, Upper Arteries Ø3P
　Arteriovenous shunt, with creation of new shunt *see* Bypass, Upper Arteries Ø31
　Stoma
　　see Excision
　　see Reposition
Talent® Converter *use* Intraluminal Device
Talent® Occluder *use* Intraluminal Device
Talent® Stent Graft (abdominal) (thoracic) *use* Intraluminal Device
Talocalcaneal (subtalar) joint
　use Tarsal Joint, Left
　use Tarsal Joint, Right
Talocalcaneal ligament
　use Foot Bursa and Ligament, Left
　use Foot Bursa and Ligament, Right
Talocalcaneonavicular joint
　use Tarsal Joint, Left
　use Tarsal Joint, Right
Talocalcaneonavicular ligament
　use Foot Bursa and Ligament, Left
　use Foot Bursa and Ligament, Right
Talocrural joint
　use Ankle Joint, Left
　use Joint, Ankle, Right
Talofibular ligament
　use Ankle Bursa and Ligament, Left
　use Ankle Bursa and Ligament, Right
Talus bone
　use Tarsal, Left
　use Tarsal, Right
TandemHeart® System *use* Short-term External Heart Assist System in Heart and Great Vessels
Tarsectomy
　see Excision, Lower Bones ØQB
　see Resection, Lower Bones ØQT
Tarsometatarsal ligament
　use Foot Bursa and Ligament, Left
　use Foot Bursa and Ligament, Right
Tarsorrhaphy *see* Repair, Eye Ø8Q
Tattooing
　Cornea 3EØCXMZ
　Skin *see* Introduction of substance in or on, Skin 3EØØ
TAXUS® Liberté® Paclitaxel-eluting Coronary Stent System *use* Intraluminal Device, Drug-eluting in Heart and Great Vessels
TBNA (transbronchial needle aspiration)
　Fluid or gas *see* Drainage, Respiratory System ØB9
　Tissue biopsy *see* Extraction, Respiratory System ØBD
Tecartus™ *use* Brexucabtagene Autoleucel Immunotherapy
TECENTRIQ® *use* Atezolizumab Antineoplastic
Telemetry 4A12X4Z
　Ambulatory 4A12X45
Temperature gradient study 4AØZXKZ
Temporal lobe *use* Cerebral Hemisphere
Temporalis muscle *use* Head Muscle
Temporoparietalis muscle *use* Head Muscle
Tendolysis *see* Release, Tendons ØLN
Tendonectomy
　see Excision, Tendons ØLB
　see Resection, Tendons ØLT
Tendonoplasty, tenoplasty
　see Repair, Tendons ØLQ
　see Replacement, Tendons ØLR

Transverse Rectus Abdominis Myocutaneous Flap — *continued*
  Replacement — *continued*
    Left ØHRUØ76
    Right ØHRTØ76
  Transfer
    Left ØKXL
    Right ØKXK
Transverse scapular ligament
  use Shoulder Bursa and Ligament, Left
  use Shoulder Bursa and Ligament, Right
Transverse thoracis muscle
  use Thorax Muscle, Left
  use Thorax Muscle, Right
Transversospinalis muscle
  use Trunk Muscle, Left
  use Trunk Muscle, Right
Transversus abdominis muscle
  use Abdomen Muscle, Left
  use Abdomen Muscle, Right
Trapezium bone
  use Carpal, Left
  use Carpal, Right
Trapezius muscle
  use Trunk Muscle, Left
  use Trunk Muscle, Right
Trapezoid bone
  use Carpal, Left
  use Carpal, Right
Triceps brachii muscle
  use Upper Arm Muscle, Left
  use Upper Arm Muscle, Right
Tricuspid annulus *use* Tricuspid Valve
Trifacial nerve *use* Trigeminal Nerve
Trifecta™ Valve (aortic) *use* Zooplastic Tissue in Heart and Great Vessels
Trigone of bladder *use* Bladder
TriGuard 3™ CEPD (cerebral embolic protection device) X2A6325
Trilaciclib XWØ
Trimming, excisional *see* Excision
Triquetral bone
  use Carpal, Left
  use Carpal, Right
Trochanteric bursa
  use Hip Bursa and Ligament, Left
  use Hip Bursa and Ligament, Right
TUMT (transurethral microwave thermotherapy of prostate) ØV5Ø7ZZ
TUNA (transurethral needle ablation of prostate) ØV5Ø7ZZ
Tunneled central venous catheter *use* Vascular Access Device, Tunneled in Subcutaneous Tissue and Fascia
Tunneled spinal (intrathecal) catheter *use* Infusion Device
Turbinectomy
  see Excision, Ear, Nose, Sinus 09B
  see Resection, Ear, Nose, Sinus 09T
Turbinoplasty
  see Repair, Ear, Nose, Sinus 09Q
  see Replacement, Ear, Nose, Sinus 09R
  see Supplement, Ear, Nose, Sinus 09U
Turbinotomy
  see Division, Ear, Nose, Sinus 098
  see Drainage, Ear, Nose, Sinus 099
TURP (transurethral resection of prostate) ØVBØ7ZZ
  see Excision, Prostate ØVB9
  see Resection, Prostate ØVT9
Twelfth cranial nerve *use* Hypoglossal Nerve
Two lead pacemaker *use* Pacemaker, Dual Chamber in ØJH
Tympanic cavity
  use Middle Ear, Left
  use Middle Ear, Right
Tympanic nerve *use* Glossopharyngeal Nerve
Tympanic part of temoporal bone
  use Temporal Bone, Left
  use Temporal Bone, Right
Tympanogram *see* Hearing Assessment, Diagnostic Audiology F13
Tympanoplasty
  see Repair, Ear, Nose, Sinus 09Q
  see Replacement, Ear, Nose, Sinus 09R
  see Supplement, Ear, Nose, Sinus 09U

Tympanosympathectomy *see* Excision, Nerve, Head and Neck Sympathetic 01BK
Tympanotomy *see* Drainage, Ear, Nose, Sinus 099
TYRX Antibacterial Envelope *use* Anti-Infective Envelope

U

Ulnar collateral carpal ligament
  use Wrist Bursa and Ligament, Left
  use Wrist Bursa and Ligament, Right
Ulnar collateral ligament
  use Elbow Bursa and Ligament, Left
  use Elbow Bursa and Ligament, Right
Ulnar notch
  use Radius, Left
  use Radius, Right
Ulnar vein
  use Brachial Vein, Left
  use Brachial Vein, Right
Ultrafiltration
  Hemodialysis *see* Performance, Urinary 5A1D
  Therapeutic plasmapheresis *see* Pheresis, Circulatory 6A55
Ultraflex™ Precision Colonic Stent System *use* Intraluminal Device
ULTRAPRO Hernia System (UHS) *use* Synthetic Substitute
ULTRAPRO Partially Absorbable Lightweight Mesh *use* Synthetic Substitute
ULTRAPRO Plug *use* Synthetic Substitute
Ultrasonic osteogenic stimulator
  use Bone Growth Stimulator in Head and Facial Bones
  use Bone Growth Stimulator in Lower Bones
  use Bone Growth Stimulator in Upper Bones
Ultrasonography
  Abdomen BW40ZZZ
  Abdomen and Pelvis BW41ZZZ
  Abdominal Wall BH49ZZZ
  Aorta
    Abdominal, Intravascular B440ZZ3
    Thoracic, Intravascular B340ZZ3
  Appendix BD48ZZZ
  Artery
    Brachiocephalic-Subclavian, Right, Intravascular B341ZZ3
    Celiac and Mesenteric, Intravascular B44KZZ3
    Common Carotid
      Bilateral, Intravascular B345ZZ3
      Left, Intravascular B344ZZ3
      Right, Intravascular B343ZZ3
    Coronary
      Multiple B241YZZ
        Intravascular B241ZZ3
        Transesophageal B241ZZ4
      Single B240YZZ
        Intravascular B240ZZ3
        Transesophageal B240ZZ4
    Femoral, Intravascular B44LZZ3
    Inferior Mesenteric, Intravascular B445ZZ3
    Internal Carotid
      Bilateral, Intravascular B348ZZ3
      Left, Intravascular B347ZZ3
      Right, Intravascular B346ZZ3
    Intra-Abdominal, Other, Intravascular B44BZZ3
    Intracranial, Intravascular B34RZZ3
    Lower Extremity
      Bilateral, Intravascular B44HZZ3
      Left, Intravascular B44GZZ3
      Right, Intravascular B44FZZ3
    Mesenteric and Celiac, Intravascular B44KZZ3
    Ophthalmic, Intravascular B34VZZ3
    Penile, Intravascular B44NZZ3
    Pulmonary
      Left, Intravascular B34TZZ3
      Right, Intravascular B34SZZ3
    Renal
      Bilateral, Intravascular B448ZZ3
      Left, Intravascular B447ZZ3
      Right, Intravascular B446ZZ3
    Subclavian, Left, Intravascular B342ZZ3
    Superior Mesenteric, Intravascular B444ZZ3
    Upper Extremity
      Bilateral, Intravascular B34KZZ3
      Left, Intravascular B34JZZ3

Ultrasonography — *continued*
  Artery — *continued*
    Upper Extremity — *continued*
      Right, Intravascular B34HZZ3
  Bile Duct BF40ZZZ
  Bile Duct and Gallbladder BF43ZZZ
  Bladder BT40ZZZ
    and Kidney BT4JZZZ
  Brain B040ZZZ
  Breast
    Bilateral BH42ZZZ
    Left BH41ZZZ
    Right BH40ZZZ
  Chest Wall BH4BZZZ
  Coccyx BR4FZZZ
  Connective Tissue
    Lower Extremity BL41ZZZ
    Upper Extremity BL40ZZZ
  Duodenum BD49ZZZ
  Elbow
    Left, Densitometry BP4HZZ1
    Right, Densitometry BP4GZZ1
  Esophagus BD41ZZZ
  Extremity
    Lower BH48ZZZ
    Upper BH47ZZZ
  Eye
    Bilateral B847ZZZ
    Left B846ZZZ
    Right B845ZZZ
  Fallopian Tube
    Bilateral BU42
    Left BU41
    Right BU40
  Fetal Umbilical Cord BY47ZZZ
  Fetus
    First Trimester, Multiple Gestation BY4BZZZ
    Second Trimester, Multiple Gestation BY4DZZZ
    Single
      First Trimester BY49ZZZ
      Second Trimester BY4CZZZ
      Third Trimester BY4FZZZ
    Third Trimester, Multiple Gestation BY4GZZZ
  Gallbladder BF42ZZZ
  Gallbladder and Bile Duct BF43ZZZ
  Gastrointestinal Tract BD47ZZZ
  Gland
    Adrenal
      Bilateral BG42ZZZ
      Left BG41ZZZ
      Right BG40ZZZ
    Parathyroid BG43ZZZ
    Thyroid BG44ZZZ
  Hand
    Left, Densitometry BP4PZZ1
    Right, Densitometry BP4NZZ1
  Head and Neck BH4CZZZ
  Heart
    Left B245YZZ
      Intravascular B245ZZ3
      Transesophageal B245ZZ4
    Pediatric B24DYZZ
      Intravascular B24DZZ3
      Transesophageal B24DZZ4
    Right B244YZZ
      Intravascular B244ZZ3
      Transesophageal B244ZZ4
    Right and Left B246YZZ
      Intravascular B246ZZ3
      Transesophageal B246ZZ4
  Heart with Aorta B24BYZZ
    Intravascular B24BZZ3
    Transesophageal B24BZZ4
  Hepatobiliary System, All BF4CZZZ
  Hip
    Bilateral BQ42ZZZ
    Left BQ41ZZZ
    Right BQ40ZZZ
  Kidney
    and Bladder BT4JZZZ
    Bilateral BT43ZZZ
    Left BT42ZZZ
    Right BT41ZZZ
    Transplant BT49ZZZ
  Knee
    Bilateral BQ49ZZZ
    Left BQ48ZZZ
    Right BQ47ZZZ

Ultrasonography — continued
Liver BF45ZZZ
Liver and Spleen BF46ZZZ
Mediastinum BB4CZZZ
Neck BW4FZZZ
Ovary
    Bilateral BU45
    Left BU44
    Right BU43
Ovary and Uterus BU4C
Pancreas BF47ZZZ
Pelvic Region BW4GZZZ
Pelvis and Abdomen BW41ZZZ
Penis BV4BZZZ
Pericardium B24CYZZ
    Intravascular B24CZZ3
    Transesophageal B24CZZ4
Placenta BY48ZZZ
Pleura BB4BZZZ
Prostate and Seminal Vesicle BV49ZZZ
Rectum BD4CZZZ
Sacrum BR4FZZZ
Scrotum BV44ZZZ
Seminal Vesicle and Prostate BV49ZZZ
Shoulder
    Left, Densitometry BP49ZZ1
    Right, Densitometry BP48ZZ1
Spinal Cord B04BZZZ
Spine
    Cervical BR40ZZZ
    Lumbar BR49ZZZ
    Thoracic BR47ZZZ
Spleen and Liver BF46ZZZ
Stomach BD42ZZZ
Tendon
    Lower Extremity BL43ZZZ
    Upper Extremity BL42ZZZ
Ureter
    Bilateral BT48ZZZ
    Left BT47ZZZ
    Right BT46ZZZ
Urethra BT45ZZZ
Uterus BU46
Uterus and Ovary BU4C
Vein
    Jugular
        Left, Intravascular B544ZZ3
        Right, Intravascular B543ZZ3
    Lower Extremity
        Bilateral, Intravascular B54DZZ3
        Left, Intravascular B54CZZ3
        Right, Intravascular B54BZZ3
    Portal, Intravascular B54TZZ3
    Renal
        Bilateral, Intravascular B54LZZ3
        Left, Intravascular B54KZZ3
        Right, Intravascular B54JZZ3
    Spanchnic, Intravascular B54TZZ3
    Subclavian
        Left, Intravascular B547ZZ3
        Right, Intravascular B546ZZ3
    Upper Extremity
        Bilateral, Intravascular B54PZZ3
        Left, Intravascular B54NZZ3
        Right, Intravascular B54MZZ3
    Vena Cava
        Inferior, Intravascular B549ZZ3
        Superior, Intravascular B548ZZ3
    Wrist
        Left, Densitometry BP4MZZ1
        Right, Densitometry BP4LZZ1
Ultrasound bone healing system
use Bone Growth Stimulator in Head and Facial
      Bones
use Bone Growth Stimulator in Lower Bones
use Bone Growth Stimulator in Upper Bones
Ultrasound Therapy
Heart 6A75
No Qualifier 6A75
Vessels
    Head and Neck 6A75
    Other 6A75
    Peripheral 6A75
Ultraviolet Light Therapy, Skin 6A80
Umbilical artery
use Internal Iliac Artery, Left
use Internal Iliac Artery, Right
use Lower Artery

Uniplanar external fixator
use External Fixation Device, Monoplanar in ØPH
use External Fixation Device, Monoplanar in ØPS
use External Fixation Device, Monoplanar in ØQH
use External Fixation Device, Monoplanar in ØQS
Upper GI series see Fluoroscopy, Gastrointestinal, Upper BD15
Ureteral orifice
use Ureter
use Ureter, Left
use Ureter, Right
use Ureters, Bilateral
Ureterectomy
see Excision, Urinary System ØTB
see Resection, Urinary System ØTT
Ureterocolostomy see Bypass, Urinary System ØT1
Ureterocystostomy see Bypass, Urinary System ØT1
Ureteroenterostomy see Bypass, Urinary System ØT1
Ureteroileostomy see Bypass, Urinary System ØT1
Ureterolithotomy see Extirpation, Urinary System ØTC
Ureterolysis see Release, Urinary System ØTN
Ureteroneocystostomy
see Bypass, Urinary System ØT1
see Reposition, Urinary System ØTS
Ureteropelvic junction (UPJ)
use Kidney Pelvis, Left
use Kidney Pelvis, Right
Ureteropexy
see Repair, Urinary System ØTQ
see Reposition, Urinary System ØTS
Ureteroplasty
see Repair, Urinary System ØTQ
see Replacement, Urinary System ØTR
see Supplement, Urinary System ØTU
Ureteroplication see Restriction, Urinary System ØTV
Ureteropyelography see Fluoroscopy, Urinary System BT1
Ureterorrhaphy see Repair, Urinary System ØTQ
Ureteroscopy ØTJ98ZZ
Ureterostomy
see Bypass, Urinary System ØT1
see Drainage, Urinary System ØT9
Ureterotomy see Drainage, Urinary System ØT9
Ureteroureterostomy see Bypass, Urinary System ØT1
Ureterovesical orifice
use Ureter
use Ureter, Left
use Ureter, Right
use Ureters, Bilateral
Urethral catheterization, indwelling ØT9B70Z
Urethrectomy
see Excision, Urethra ØTBD
see Resection, Urethra ØTTD
Urethrolithotomy see Extirpation, Urethra ØTCD
Urethrolysis see Release, Urethra ØTND
Urethropexy
see Repair, Urethra ØTQD
see Reposition, Urethra ØTSD
Urethroplasty
see Repair, Urethra ØTQD
see Replacement, Urethra ØTRD
see Supplement, Urethra ØTUD
Urethrorrhaphy see Repair, Urethra ØTQD
Urethroscopy ØTJD8ZZ
Urethrotomy see Drainage, Urethra ØT9D
Uridine Triacetate XWØDX82
Urinary incontinence stimulator lead use Stimulator Lead in Urinary System
Urography see Fluoroscopy, Urinary System BT1
Ustekinumab use Other New Technology Therapeutic Substance
Uterine Artery
use Internal Iliac Artery, Left
use Internal Iliac Artery, Right
Uterine artery embolization (UAE) see Occlusion, Lower Arteries Ø4L
Uterine cornu use Uterus
Uterine tube
use Fallopian Tube, Left
use Fallopian Tube, Right
Uterine vein
use Hypogastric Vein, Left
use Hypogastric Vein, Right
Uvulectomy
see Excision, Uvula ØCBN
see Resection, Uvula ØCTN

Uvulorrhaphy see Repair, Uvula ØCQN
Uvulotomy see Drainage, Uvula ØC9N

V

Vabomere™ use Meropenem-vaborbactam Anti-infective
Vaccination see Introduction of Serum, Toxoid, and Vaccine
Vacuum extraction, obstetric 10D07Z6
Vaginal artery
use Internal Iliac Artery, Left
use Internal Iliac Artery, Right
Vaginal pessary use Intraluminal Device, Pessary in Female Reproductive System
Vaginal vein
use Hypogastric Vein, Left
use Hypogastric Vein, Right
Vaginectomy
see Excision, Vagina ØUBG
see Resection, Vagina ØUTG
Vaginofixation
see Repair, Vagina ØUQG
see Reposition, Vagina ØUSG
Vaginoplasty
see Repair, Vagina ØUQG
see Supplement, Vagina ØUUG
Vaginorrhaphy see Repair, Vagina ØUQG
Vaginoscopy ØUJH8ZZ
Vaginotomy see Drainage, Female Reproductive System ØU9
Vagotomy see Division, Nerve, Vagus ØØ8Q
Valiant Thoracic Stent Graft use Intraluminal Device
Valvotomy, valvulotomy
see Division, Heart and Great Vessels Ø28
see Release, Heart and Great Vessels Ø2N
Valvuloplasty
see Repair, Heart and Great Vessels Ø2Q
see Replacement, Heart and Great Vessels Ø2R
see Supplement, Heart and Great Vessels Ø2U
Valvuloplasty, Alfieri Stitch see Restriction, Valve, Mitral Ø2VG
Vascular Access Device
Totally Implantable
    Insertion of device in
        Abdomen ØJH8
        Chest ØJH6
        Lower Arm
            Left ØJHH
            Right ØJHG
        Lower Leg
            Left ØJHP
            Right ØJHN
        Upper Arm
            Left ØJHF
            Right ØJHD
        Upper Leg
            Left ØJHM
            Right ØJHL
    Removal of device from
        Lower Extremity ØJPW
        Trunk ØJPT
        Upper Extremity ØJPV
    Revision of device in
        Lower Extremity ØJWW
        Trunk ØJWT
        Upper Extremity ØJWV
Tunneled
    Insertion of device in
        Abdomen ØJH8
        Chest ØJH6
        Lower Arm
            Left ØJHH
            Right ØJHG
        Lower Leg
            Left ØJHP
            Right ØJHN
        Upper Arm
            Left ØJHF
            Right ØJHD
        Upper Leg
            Left ØJHM
            Right ØJHL
    Removal of device from
        Lower Extremity ØJPW
        Trunk ØJPT
        Upper Extremity ØJPV

Vascular Access Device — *continued*
    Tunneled — *continued*
        Revision of device in
            Lower Extremity ØJWW
            Trunk ØJWT
            Upper Extremity ØJWV
Vasectomy *see* Excision, Male Reproductive System ØVB
Vasography
    see Fluoroscopy, Male Reproductive System BV1
    see Plain Radiography, Male Reproductive System BVØ
Vasoligation *see* Occlusion, Male Reproductive System ØVL
Vasorrhaphy *see* Repair, Male Reproductive System ØVQ
Vasostomy *see* Bypass, Male Reproductive System ØV1
Vasotomy
    Drainage *see* Drainage, Male Reproductive System ØV9
    With ligation *see* Occlusion, Male Reproductive System ØVL
Vasovasostomy *see* Repair, Male Reproductive System ØVQ
Vastus intermedius muscle
    use Upper Leg Muscle, Left
    use Upper Leg Muscle, Right
Vastus lateralis muscle
    use Upper Leg Muscle, Left
    use Upper Leg Muscle, Right
Vastus medialis muscle
    use Upper Leg Muscle, Left
    use Upper Leg Muscle, Right
VCG (vectorcardiogram) *see* Measurement, Cardiac 4A02
Vectra® Vascular Access Graft *use* Vascular Access Device, Tunneled in Subcutaneous Tissue and Fascia
Veklury *use* Remdesivir Anti-infective
Venclexta® *use* Venetoclax Antineoplastic
Venectomy
    see Excision, Lower Veins Ø6B
    see Excision, Upper Veins Ø5B
Venetoclax Antineoplastic XW0DXR5
Venography
    see Fluoroscopy, Veins B51
    see Plain Radiography, Veins B50
Venorrhaphy
    see Repair, Lower Veins Ø6Q
    see Repair, Upper Veins Ø5Q
Venotripsy
    see Occlusion, Lower Veins Ø6L
    see Occlusion, Upper Veins Ø5L
Ventricular fold *use* Larynx
Ventriculoatriostomy *see* Bypass, Central Nervous System and Cranial Nerves 001
Ventriculocisternostomy *see* Bypass, Central Nervous System and Cranial Nerves 001
Ventriculogram, cardiac
    Combined left and right heart *see* Fluoroscopy, Heart, Right and Left B216
    Left ventricle *see* Fluoroscopy, Heart, Left B215
    Right ventricle *see* Fluoroscopy, Heart, Right B214
Ventriculopuncture, through previously implanted catheter 8C01X6J
Ventriculoscopy 00J04ZZ
Ventriculostomy
    External drainage *see* Drainage, Cerebral Ventricle 0096
    Internal shunt *see* Bypass, Cerebral Ventricle 0016
Ventriculovenostomy *see* Bypass, Cerebral Ventricle 0016
Ventrio™ Hernia Patch *use* Synthetic Substitute
VEP (visual evoked potential) 4A07X0Z
Vermiform appendix *use* Appendix
Vermilion border
    use Lower Lip
    use Upper Lip
Versa *use* Pacemaker, Dual Chamber in ØJH
Version, obstetric
    External 10S0XZZ
    Internal 10S07ZZ

Vertebral arch
    use Cervical Vertebra
    use Lumbar Vertebra
    use Thoracic Vertebra
Vertebral body
    use Cervical Vertebra
    use Lumbar Vertebra
    use Thoracic Vertebra
Vertebral canal *use* Spinal Canal
Vertebral foramen
    use Cervical Vertebra
    use Lumbar Vertebra
    use Thoracic Vertebra
Vertebral lamina
    use Cervical Vertebra
    use Lumbar Vertebra
    use Thoracic Vertebra
Vertebral pedicle
    use Cervical Vertebra
    use Lumbar Vertebra
    use Thoracic Vertebra
Vesical vein
    use Hypogastric Vein, Left
    use Hypogastric Vein, Right
Vesicotomy *see* Drainage, Urinary System ØT9
Vesiculectomy
    see Excision, Male Reproductive System ØVB
    see Resection, Male Reproductive System ØVT
Vesiculogram, seminal *see* Plain Radiography, Male Reproductive System BVØ
Vesiculotomy *see* Drainage, Male Reproductive System ØV9
Vestibular Assessment F15Z
Vestibular (Scarpa's) ganglion *use* Acoustic Nerve
Vestibular nerve *use* Acoustic Nerve
Vestibular Treatment F0C
Vestibulocochlear nerve *use* Acoustic Nerve
VH-IVUS (virtual histology intravascular ultrasound) *see* Ultrasonography, Heart B24
Virchow's (supraclavicular) lymph node
    use Lymphatic, Left Neck
    use Lymphatic, Right Neck
Virtuoso (II) (DR) (VR) *use* Defibrillator Generator in ØJH
Vistogard(R) *use* Uridine Triacetate
Vitrectomy
    see Excision, Eye Ø8B
    see Resection, Eye Ø8T
Vitreous body
    use Vitreous, Left
    use Vitreous, Right
Viva (XT) (S) *use* Cardiac Resynchronization Defibrillator Pulse Generator in ØJH
Vocal fold
    use Vocal Cord, Left
    use Vocal Cord, Right
Vocational
    Assessment *see* Activities of Daily Living Assessment, Rehabilitation F02
    Retraining *see* Activities of Daily Living Treatment, Rehabilitation F08
Volar (palmar) digital vein
    use Hand Vein, Left
    use Hand Vein, Right
Volar (palmar) metacarpal vein
    use Hand Vein, Left
    use Hand Vein, Right
Vomer bone *use* Nasal Septum
Vomer of nasal septum *use* Nasal Bone
Voraxaze *use* Glucarpidase
Vulvectomy
    see Excision, Female Reproductive System ØUB
    see Resection, Female Reproductive System ØUT
V-Wave Interatrial Shunt System *use* Synthetic Substitute
VYXEOS™ *use* Cytarabine and Daunorubicin Liposome Antineoplastic

W

WALLSTENT® Endoprosthesis *use* Intraluminal Device
Washing *see* Irrigation

WavelinQ EndoAVF system
    Radial Artery, Left 031C3ZF
    Radial Artery, Right 031B3ZF
    Ulnar Artery, Left 031A3ZF
    Ulnar Artery, Right 03193ZF
Wedge resection, pulmonary *see* Excision, Respiratory System ØBB
Whole Blood Nucleic Acid-base Microbial Detection XXE5XM5
Window *see* Drainage
Wiring, dental 2W31X9Z

X

Xact Carotid Stent System *use* Intraluminal Device
XENLETA™ *use* Lefamulin Anti-infective
Xenograft *use* Zooplastic Tissue in Heart and Great Vessels
XIENCE Everolimus Eluting Coronary Stent System *use* Intraluminal Device, Drug-eluting in Heart and Great Vessels
Xiphoid process *use* Sternum
XLIF® System *use* Interbody Fusion Device in Lower Joints
XOSPATA® *use* Gilteritinib Antineoplastic
X-ray *see* Plain Radiography
X-STOP® Spacer
    use Spinal Stabilization Device, Interspinous Process in ØRH
    use Spinal Stabilization Device, Interspinous Process in ØSH

Y

Yescarta® *use* Axicabtagene Ciloleucel Immunotherapy
Yoga Therapy 8E0ZXY4

Z

Zenith AAA Endovascular Graft *use* Intraluminal Device
Zenith Flex® AAA Endovascular Graft *use* Intraluminal Device
Zenith TX2® TAA Endovascular Graft *use* Intraluminal Device
Zenith® Fenestrated AAA Endovascular Graft
    use Intraluminal Device, Branched or Fenestrated, One or Two Arteries in 04V
    use Intraluminal Device, Branched or Fenestrated, Three or More Arteries in 04V
Zenith® Renu™ AAA Ancillary Graft *use* Intraluminal Device
ZEPZELCA™ *use* Lurbinectedin
ZERBAXA® *use* Ceftolozane/Tazobactam Anti-infective
Zilver® PTX® (paclitaxel) Drug-Eluting Peripheral Stent
    use Intraluminal Device, Drug-eluting in Lower Arteries
    use Intraluminal Device, Drug-eluting in Upper Arteries
Zimmer® NexGen® LPS Mobile Bearing Knee *use* Synthetic Substitute
Zimmer® NexGen® LPS-Flex Mobile Knee *use* Synthetic Substitute
ZINPLAVA™ *use* Bezlotoxumab Monoclonal Antibody
Zonule of Zinn
    use Lens, Left
    use Lens, Right
Zooplastic Tissue, Rapid Deployment Technique, Replacement X2RF
Zotarolimus-eluting Coronary Stent *use* Intraluminal Device, Drug-eluting in Heart and Great Vessels
Z-plasty, skin for scar contracture *see* Release, Skin and Breast ØHN
ZULRESSO™ *use* Brexanolone
Zygomatic process of frontal bone *use* Frontal Bone
Zygomatic process of temporal bone
    use Temporal Bone, Left
    use Temporal Bone, Right
Zygomaticus muscle *use* Facial Muscle
Zyvox *use* Oxazolidinones

ICD-10-PCS Tables

Central Nervous System and Cranial Nerves 001–00X

Character Meanings

This Character Meaning table is provided as a guide to assist the user in the identification of character members that may be found in this section of code tables. It **SHOULD NOT** be used to build a PCS code.

Operation–Character 3		Body Part–Character 4		Approach–Character 5		Device–Character 6		Qualifier–Character 7	
1	Bypass	0	Brain	0	Open	0	Drainage Device	0	Nasopharynx
2	Change	1	Cerebral Meninges	3	Percutaneous	1	Radioactive Element	1	Mastoid Sinus
5	Destruction	2	Dura Mater	4	Percutaneous Endoscopic	2	Monitoring Device	2	Atrium
7	Dilation	3	Epidural Space, Intracranial	X	External	3	Infusion Device	3	Blood Vessel
8	Division	4	Subdural Space, Intracranial			4	Radioactive Element, Cesium-131 Collagen Implant	4	Pleural Cavity
9	Drainage	5	Subarachnoid Space, Intracranial			7	Autologous Tissue Substitute	5	Intestine
B	Excision	6	Cerebral Ventricle			J	Synthetic Substitute	6	Peritoneal Cavity
C	Extirpation	7	Cerebral Hemisphere			K	Nonautologous Tissue Substitute	7	Urinary Tract
D	Extraction	8	Basal Ganglia			M	Neurostimulator Lead	8	Bone Marrow
F	Fragmentation	9	Thalamus			Y	Other Device	9	Fallopian Tube
H	Insertion	A	Hypothalamus			Z	No Device	A	Subgaleal Space
J	Inspection	B	Pons					B	Cerebral Cisterns
K	Map	C	Cerebellum					F	Olfactory Nerve
N	Release	D	Medulla Oblongata					G	Optic Nerve
P	Removal	E	Cranial Nerve					H	Oculomotor Nerve
Q	Repair	F	Olfactory Nerve					J	Trochlear Nerve
R	Replacement	G	Optic Nerve					K	Trigeminal Nerve
S	Reposition	H	Oculomotor Nerve					L	Abducens Nerve
T	Resection	J	Trochlear Nerve					M	Facial Nerve
U	Supplement	K	Trigeminal Nerve					N	Acoustic Nerve
W	Revision	L	Abducens Nerve					P	Glossopharyngeal Nerve
X	Transfer	M	Facial Nerve					Q	Vagus Nerve
		N	Acoustic Nerve					R	Accessory Nerve
		P	Glossopharyngeal Nerve					S	Hypoglossal Nerve
		Q	Vagus Nerve					X	Diagnostic
		R	Accessory Nerve					Z	No Qualifier
		S	Hypoglossal Nerve						
		T	Spinal Meninges						
		U	Spinal Canal						
		V	Spinal Cord						
		W	Cervical Spinal Cord						
		X	Thoracic Spinal Cord						
		Y	Lumbar Spinal Cord						

AHA Coding Clinic for table 001

2021, 2Q, 19	Electromagnetic stealth guided ventriculoperitoneal shunt insertion with endoscopy
2019, 4Q, 21-22	Cerebral ventricle bypass Qualifier
2018, 4Q, 86	Placement of lumboatrial shunt
2017, 4Q, 39-41	Dilation and bypass of cerebral ventricle
2015, 2Q, 9	Revision of ventriculoperitoneal (VP) shunt
2013, 2Q, 36	Insertion of ventriculoperitoneal shunt with laparoscopic assistance

AHA Coding Clinic for table 005

2021, 2Q, 17	Dorsal root entry zone procedure

AHA Coding Clinic for table 007

2017, 4Q, 39-41	Dilation and bypass of cerebral ventricle

AHA Coding Clinic for table 009

2018, 4Q, 85	Externalization of lumboatrial shunt
2017, 1Q, 50	Failed lumbar puncture
2015, 3Q, 10	Open evacuation of subdural hematoma
2015, 3Q, 11	Percutaneous drainage of subdural hematoma
2015, 3Q, 12	Subdural evacuation portal system (SEPS) placement
2015, 3Q, 12	Placement of ventriculostomy catheter via burr hole
2015, 2Q, 30	Drainage of syrinx
2015, 1Q, 31	Intrathecal chemotherapy
2014, 1Q, 8	Diagnostic lumbar tap
2014, 1Q, 8	Lumbar drainage port aspiration

AHA Coding Clinic for table 00B

2017, 3Q, 17	Resection of schwannoma and placement of DuraGen and Lorenz cranial plating system
2016, 2Q, 12	Resection of malignant neoplasm of infratemporal fossa
2016, 2Q, 18	Amygdalohippocampectomy
2014, 4Q, 34	Resection of brain malignancy with implantation of chemotherapeutic wafer
2014, 3Q, 24	Repair of lipomyelomeningocele and tethered cord

AHA Coding Clinic for table 00C

2019, 3Q, 4	Evacuation of subdural hematoma and control of bleeding artery
2019, 2Q, 36	Evacuation of hematoma using NICO Brainpath® technology
2017, 4Q, 48	New and revised body part values - Extirpation spinal canal
2016, 2Q, 29	Decompressive craniectomy with cryopreservation and storage of bone flap
2015, 3Q, 10	Open evacuation of subdural hematoma
2015, 3Q, 11	Percutaneous drainage of subdural hematoma
2015, 3Q, 13	Evacuation of intracerebral hematoma

AHA Coding Clinic for table 00D

2015, 3Q, 13	Nonexcisional debridement of cranial wound with removal and replacement of hardware

AHA Coding Clinic for table 00H

2020, 4Q, 43-44	Insertion of radioactive element
2020, 2Q, 15	Ommaya Reservoir with Ventricular Catheter Placement
2020, 2Q, 16	Ommaya Reservoir Placement for Cerebrospinal Fluid Infusion Therapy
2017, 4Q, 30-31	Radiotherapeutic brain implant
2017, 3Q, 13	Implantation of bilateral neurostimulator electrodes
2014, 3Q, 19	End of life replacement of Baclofen pump

AHA Coding Clinic for table 00J

2021, 2Q, 19	Electromagnetic stealth guided ventriculoperitoneal shunt insertion with endoscopy
2019, 2Q, 36	Evacuation of hematoma using NICO Brainpath® technology
2017, 1Q, 50	Failed lumbar puncture

AHA Coding Clinic for table 00N

2019, 2Q, 19	Cervical spinal fusion, decompression and placement of interfacet stabilization device
2019, 1Q, 28	Decompressive laminectomy of both spinal cord and nerve roots
2018, 3Q, 30	Decompressive laminectomy (release of spinal cord versus release of spinal meninges)
2017, 3Q, 10	Repair of Chiari malformation
2017, 2Q, 23	Decompression of spinal cord and placement of instrumentation
2016, 2Q, 29	Decompressive craniectomy with cryopreservation and storage of bone flap
2015, 2Q, 20	Cervical laminoplasty
2015, 2Q, 21	Multiple decompressive cervical laminectomies
2015, 2Q, 34	Decompressive laminectomy
2014, 3Q, 24	Repair of lipomyelomeningocele and tethered cord

AHA Coding Clinic for table 00P

2014, 3Q, 19	End of life replacement of Baclofen pump

AHA Coding Clinic for table 00Q

2014, 3Q, 7	Hemi-cranioplasty for repair of cranial defect
2013, 3Q, 25	Fracture of frontal bone with repair and coagulation for hemostasis

AHA Coding Clinic for table 00S

2014, 4Q, 35	Reimplantation of buccal nerve

AHA Coding Clinic for table 00U

2018, 1Q, 9	Craniectomy with DuraGaurd placement
2017, 4Q, 62	Added and revised device values - Nerve substitutes
2017, 3Q, 10	Repair of Chiari malformation
2017, 3Q, 17	Resection of schwannoma and placement of DuraGen and Lorenz cranial plating system
2015, 4Q, 39	Dural patch graft
2014, 3Q, 24	Repair of lipomyelomeningocele and tethered cord

AHA Coding Clinic for table 00W

2018, 4Q, 86	Placement of lumboatrial shunt

Brain

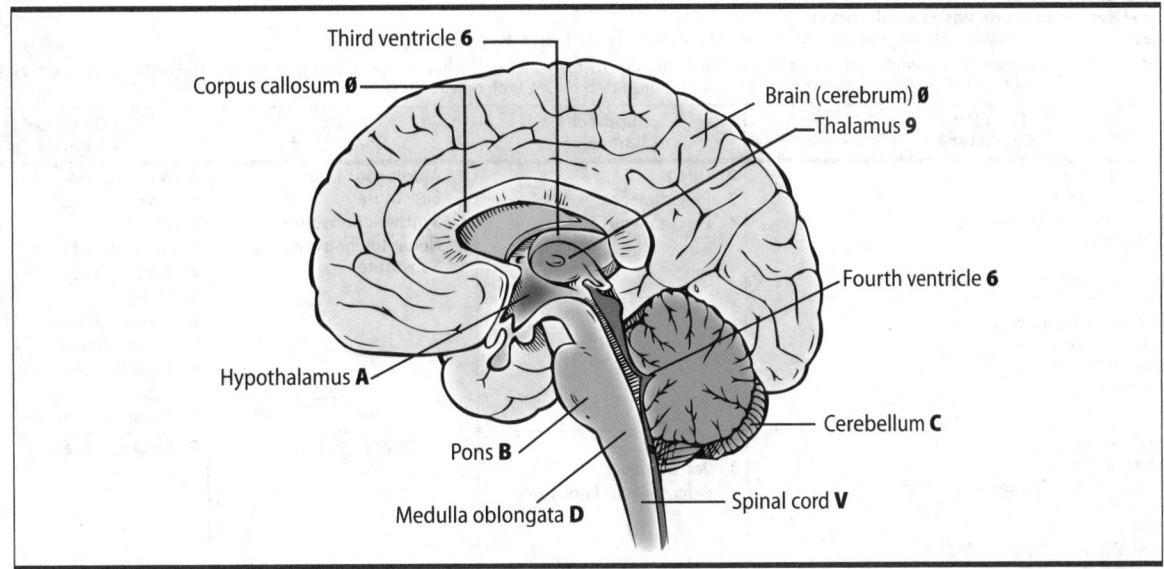

Third ventricle **6**
Corpus callosum **Ø**
Brain (cerebrum) **Ø**
Thalamus **9**
Fourth ventricle **6**
Hypothalamus **A**
Cerebellum **C**
Pons **B**
Spinal cord **V**
Medulla oblongata **D**

Cranial Nerves

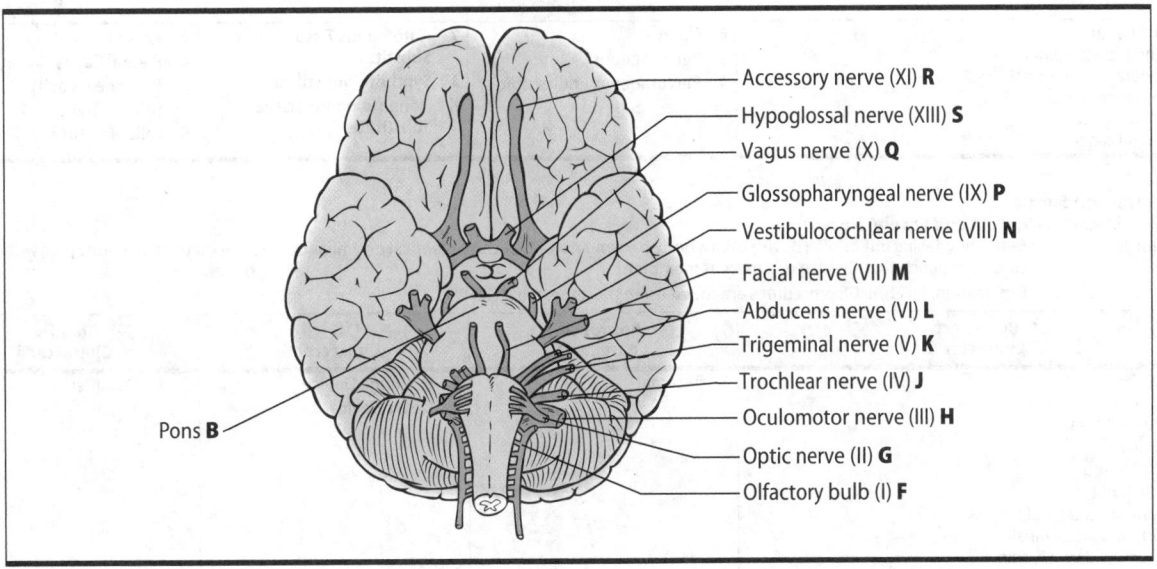

Accessory nerve (XI) **R**
Hypoglossal nerve (XIII) **S**
Vagus nerve (X) **Q**
Glossopharyngeal nerve (IX) **P**
Vestibulocochlear nerve (VIII) **N**
Facial nerve (VII) **M**
Abducens nerve (VI) **L**
Trigeminal nerve (V) **K**
Trochlear nerve (IV) **J**
Oculomotor nerve (III) **H**
Optic nerve (II) **G**
Olfactory bulb (I) **F**
Pons **B**

Central Nervous System and Cranial Nerves

Ø   **Medical and Surgical**
Ø   **Central Nervous System and Cranial Nerves**
1   **Bypass**   Definition: Altering the route of passage of the contents of a tubular body part

                         Explanation: Rerouting contents of a body part to a downstream area of the normal route, to a similar route and body part, or to an abnormal route and dissimilar body part. Includes one or more anastomoses, with or without the use of a device.

Body Part Character 4	Approach Character 5	Device Character 6	Qualifier Character 7
6 Cerebral Ventricle Aqueduct of Sylvius Cerebral aqueduct (Sylvius) Choroid plexus Ependyma Foramen of Monro (intraventricular) Fourth ventricle Interventricular foramen (Monro) Left lateral ventricle Right lateral ventricle Third ventricle	Ø Open 3 Percutaneous 4 Percutaneous Endoscopic	7 Autologous Tissue Substitute J Synthetic Substitute K Nonautologous Tissue Substitute	Ø Nasopharynx 1 Mastoid Sinus 2 Atrium 3 Blood Vessel 4 Pleural Cavity 5 Intestine 6 Peritoneal Cavity 7 Urinary Tract 8 Bone Marrow A Subgaleal Space B Cerebral Cisterns
6 Cerebral Ventricle Aqueduct of Sylvius Cerebral aqueduct (Sylvius) Choroid plexus Ependyma Foramen of Monro (intraventricular) Fourth ventricle Interventricular foramen (Monro) Left lateral ventricle Right lateral ventricle Third ventricle	Ø Open 3 Percutaneous 4 Percutaneous Endoscopic	Z No Device	B Cerebral Cisterns
U Spinal Canal Epidural space, spinal Extradural space, spinal Subarachnoid space, spinal Subdural space, spinal Vertebral canal	Ø Open 3 Percutaneous 4 Percutaneous Endoscopic	7 Autologous Tissue Substitute J Synthetic Substitute K Nonautologous Tissue Substitute	2 Atrium 4 Pleural Cavity 6 Peritoneal Cavity 7 Urinary Tract 9 Fallopian Tube

Ø   **Medical and Surgical**
Ø   **Central Nervous System and Cranial Nerves**
2   **Change**   Definition: Taking out or off a device from a body part and putting back an identical or similar device in or on the same body part without cutting or puncturing the skin or a mucous membrane

                         Explanation: All CHANGE procedures are coded using the approach EXTERNAL

Body Part Character 4	Approach Character 5	Device Character 6	Qualifier Character 7
Ø Brain Cerebrum Corpus callosum Encephalon **E Cranial Nerve** **U Spinal Canal** Epidural space, spinal Extradural space, spinal Subarachnoid space, spinal Subdural space, spinal Vertebral canal	X External	Ø Drainage Device Y Other Device	Z No Qualifier

Non-OR   All body part, approach, device, and qualifier values

Ø   Medical and Surgical
Ø   Central Nervous System and Cranial Nerves
5   Destruction   Definition: Physical eradication of all or a portion of a body part by the direct use of energy, force, or a destructive agent
                     Explanation: None of the body part is physically taken out

Body Part Character 4		Approach Character 5	Device Character 6	Qualifier Character 7

Ø Brain
Cerebrum
Corpus callosum
Encephalon
1 Cerebral Meninges
Arachnoid mater,
   intracranial
Leptomeninges,
   intracranial
Pia mater, intracranial
2 Dura Mater
Diaphragma sellae
Dura mater, intracranial
Falx cerebri
Tentorium cerebelli
6 Cerebral Ventricle
Aqueduct of Sylvius
Cerebral aqueduct
   (Sylvius)
Choroid plexus
Ependyma
Foramen of Monro
   (intraventricular)
Fourth ventricle
Interventricular foramen
   (Monro)
Left lateral ventricle
Right lateral ventricle
Third ventricle
7 Cerebral Hemisphere
Frontal lobe
Occipital lobe
Parietal lobe
Temporal lobe
8 Basal Ganglia
Basal nuclei
Claustrum
Corpus striatum
Globus pallidus
Substantia nigra
Subthalamic nucleus
9 Thalamus
Epithalamus
Geniculate nucleus
Metathalamus
Pulvinar
A Hypothalamus
Mammillary body
B Pons
Apneustic center
Basis pontis
Locus ceruleus
Pneumotaxic center
Pontine tegmentum
Superior olivary nucleus
C Cerebellum
Culmen
D Medulla Oblongata
Myelencephalon
F Olfactory Nerve
First cranial nerve
Olfactory bulb
G Optic Nerve
Optic chiasma
Second cranial nerve
	H Oculomotor Nerve
	Third cranial nerve
	J Trochlear Nerve
	Fourth cranial nerve
	K Trigeminal Nerve
	Fifth cranial nerve
	Gasserian ganglion
	Mandibular nerve
	Maxillary nerve
	Ophthalmic nerve
	Trifacial nerve
	L Abducens Nerve
	Sixth cranial nerve
	M Facial Nerve
	Chorda tympani
	Geniculate ganglion
	Greater superficial petrosal
	   nerve
	Nerve to the stapedius
	Parotid plexus
	Posterior auricular nerve
	Seventh cranial nerve
	Submandibular ganglion
	N Acoustic Nerve
	Cochlear nerve
	Eighth cranial nerve
	Scarpa's (vestibular)
	   ganglion
	Spiral ganglion
	Vestibular (Scarpa's)
	   ganglion
	Vestibular nerve
	Vestibulocochlear nerve
	P Glossopharyngeal Nerve
	Carotid sinus nerve
	Ninth cranial nerve
	Tympanic nerve
	Q Vagus Nerve
	Anterior vagal trunk
	Pharyngeal plexus
	Pneumogastric nerve
	Posterior vagal trunk
	Pulmonary plexus
	Recurrent laryngeal nerve
	Superior laryngeal nerve
	Tenth cranial nerve
	R Accessory Nerve
	Eleventh cranial nerve
	S Hypoglossal Nerve
	Twelfth cranial nerve
	T Spinal Meninges
	Arachnoid mater, spinal
	Denticulate (dentate)
	   ligament
	Dura mater, spinal
	Filum terminale
	Leptomeninges, spinal
	Pia mater, spinal
	W Cervical Spinal Cord
	Dorsal root ganglion
	X Thoracic Spinal Cord
	Dorsal root ganglion
	Y Lumbar Spinal Cord
	Cauda equina
	Conus medullaris
	Dorsal root ganglion
		Ø Open
		3 Percutaneous
		4 Percutaneous Endoscopic
			Z No Device	**Z No Qualifier**

Non-OR   ØØ5[F,G,H,J,K,L,M,N,P,Q,R,S][Ø,3,4]ZZ

NC Noncovered Procedure   LC Limited Coverage   QA Questionable OB Admit   NT New Tech Add-on   ⊞ Combination Member   ♂ Male   ♀ Female

ICD-10-PCS 2022   135

Ø   Medical and Surgical
Ø   Central Nervous System and Cranial Nerves
7   Dilation   Definition: Expanding an orifice or the lumen of a tubular body part

Explanation: The orifice can be a natural orifice or an artificially created orifice. Accomplished by stretching a tubular body part using intraluminal pressure or by cutting part of the orifice or wall of the tubular body part.

Body Part Character 4	Approach Character 5	Device Character 6	Qualifier Character 7

6   Cerebral Ventricle
     Aqueduct of Sylvius
     Cerebral aqueduct (Sylvius)
     Choroid plexus
     Ependyma
     Foramen of Monro (intraventricular)
     Fourth ventricle
     Interventricular foramen (Monro)
     Left lateral ventricle
     Right lateral ventricle
     Third ventricle
	Ø Open
	3 Percutaneous
	4 Percutaneous Endoscopic
		Z No Device	**Z** No Qualifier

Ø   Medical and Surgical
Ø   Central Nervous System and Cranial Nerves
8   Division   Definition: Cutting into a body part, without draining fluids and/or gases from the body part, in order to separate or transect a body part

Explanation: All or a portion of the body part is separated into two or more portions

Body Part Character 4		Approach Character 5	Device Character 6	Qualifier Character 7

Ø   Brain
    Cerebrum
    Corpus callosum
    Encephalon
7   Cerebral Hemisphere
    Frontal lobe
    Occipital lobe
    Parietal lobe
    Temporal lobe
8   Basal Ganglia
    Basal nuclei
    Claustrum
    Corpus striatum
    Globus pallidus
    Substantia nigra
    Subthalamic nucleus
F   Olfactory Nerve
    First cranial nerve
    Olfactory bulb
G   Optic Nerve
    Optic chiasma
    Second cranial nerve
H   Oculomotor Nerve
    Third cranial nerve
J   Trochlear Nerve
    Fourth cranial nerve
K   Trigeminal Nerve
    Fifth cranial nerve
    Gasserian ganglion
    Mandibular nerve
    Maxillary nerve
    Ophthalmic nerve
    Trifacial nerve
L   Abducens Nerve
    Sixth cranial nerve
M   Facial Nerve
    Chorda tympani
    Geniculate ganglion
    Greater superficial petrosal
      nerve
    Nerve to the stapedius
    Parotid plexus
    Posterior auricular nerve
    Seventh cranial nerve
    Submandibular ganglion
	N Acoustic Nerve
	    Cochlear nerve
	    Eighth cranial nerve
	    Scarpa's (vestibular)
	      ganglion
	    Spiral ganglion
	    Vestibular (Scarpa's)
	      ganglion
	    Vestibular nerve
	    Vestibulocochlear nerve
	P Glossopharyngeal Nerve
	    Carotid sinus nerve
	    Ninth cranial nerve
	    Tympanic nerve
	Q Vagus Nerve
	    Anterior vagal trunk
	    Pharyngeal plexus
	    Pneumogastric nerve
	    Posterior vagal trunk
	    Pulmonary plexus
	    Recurrent laryngeal nerve
	    Superior laryngeal nerve
	    Tenth cranial nerve
	R Accessory Nerve
	    Eleventh cranial nerve
	S Hypoglossal Nerve
	    Twelfth cranial nerve
	W Cervical Spinal Cord
	    Dorsal root ganglion
	X Thoracic Spinal Cord
	    Dorsal root ganglion
	Y Lumbar Spinal Cord
	    Cauda equina
	    Conus medullaris
	    Dorsal root ganglion
		Ø Open
		3 Percutaneous
		4 Percutaneous Endoscopic
			Z No Device	**Z** No Qualifier

Ø   **Medical and Surgical**
Ø   **Central Nervous System and Cranial Nerves**
9   **Drainage**   Definition: Taking or letting out fluids and/or gases from a body part

               Explanation: The qualifier DIAGNOSTIC is used to identify drainage procedures that are biopsies

Body Part Character 4		Approach Character 5	Device Character 6	Qualifier Character 7

Ø Brain
  Cerebrum
  Corpus callosum
  Encephalon
1 Cerebral Meninges
  Arachnoid mater,
    intracranial
  Leptomeninges,
    intracranial
  Pia mater, intracranial
2 Dura Mater
  Diaphragma sellae
  Dura mater, intracranial
  Falx cerebri
  Tentorium cerebelli
3 Epidural Space,
Intracranial
  Extradural space,
    intracranial
4 Subdural Space,
Intracranial
5 Subarachnoid Space,
Intracranial
6 Cerebral Ventricle
  Aqueduct of Sylvius
  Cerebral aqueduct
    (Sylvius)
  Choroid plexus
  Ependyma
  Foramen of Monro
    (intraventricular)
  Fourth ventricle
  Interventricular foramen
    (Monro)
  Left lateral ventricle
  Right lateral ventricle
  Third ventricle
7 Cerebral Hemisphere
  Frontal lobe
  Occipital lobe
  Parietal lobe
  Temporal lobe
8 Basal Ganglia
  Basal nuclei
  Claustrum
  Corpus striatum
  Globus pallidus
  Substantia nigra
  Subthalamic nucleus
9 Thalamus
  Epithalamus
  Geniculate nucleus
  Metathalamus
  Pulvinar
A Hypothalamus
  Mammillary body
B Pons
  Apneustic center
  Basis pontis
  Locus ceruleus
  Pneumotaxic center
  Pontine tegmentum
  Superior olivary nucleus
C Cerebellum
  Culmen
D Medulla Oblongata
  Myelencephalon
F Olfactory Nerve
  First cranial nerve
  Olfactory bulb
	G Optic Nerve
	  Optic chiasma
	  Second cranial nerve
	H Oculomotor Nerve
	  Third cranial nerve
	J Trochlear Nerve
	  Fourth cranial nerve
	K Trigeminal Nerve
	  Fifth cranial nerve
	  Gasserian ganglion
	  Mandibular nerve
	  Maxillary nerve
	  Ophthalmic nerve
	  Trifacial nerve
	L Abducens Nerve
	  Sixth cranial nerve
	M Facial Nerve
	  Chorda tympani
	  Geniculate ganglion
	  Greater superficial petrosal
	    nerve
	  Nerve to the stapedius
	  Parotid plexus
	  Posterior auricular nerve
	  Seventh cranial nerve
	  Submandibular ganglion
	N Acoustic Nerve
	  Cochlear nerve
	  Eighth cranial nerve
	  Scarpa's (vestibular) ganglion
	  Spiral ganglion
	  Vestibular (Scarpa's) ganglion
	  Vestibular nerve
	  Vestibulocochlear nerve
	P Glossopharyngeal Nerve
	  Carotid sinus nerve
	  Ninth cranial nerve
	  Tympanic nerve
	Q Vagus Nerve
	  Anterior vagal trunk
	  Pharyngeal plexus
	  Pneumogastric nerve
	  Posterior vagal trunk
	  Pulmonary plexus
	  Recurrent laryngeal nerve
	  Superior laryngeal nerve
	  Tenth cranial nerve
	R Accessory Nerve
	  Eleventh cranial nerve
	S Hypoglossal Nerve
	  Twelfth cranial nerve
	T Spinal Meninges
	  Arachnoid mater, spinal
	  Denticulate (dentate)
	    ligament
	  Dura mater, spinal
	  Filum terminale
	  Leptomeninges, spinal
	  Pia mater, spinal
	U Spinal Canal
	  Epidural space, spinal
	  Extradural space, spinal
	  Subarachnoid space, spinal
	  Subdural space, spinal
	  Vertebral canal
	W Cervical Spinal Cord
	  Dorsal root ganglion
	X Thoracic Spinal Cord
	  Dorsal root ganglion
	Y Lumbar Spinal Cord
	  Cauda equina
	  Conus medullaris
	  Dorsal root ganglion
		Ø Open
		3 Percutaneous
		4 Percutaneous Endoscopic
			Ø Drainage Device	**Z No Qualifier**

Non-OR	ØØ9[T,W,X,Y]3ØZ
Non-OR	ØØ9U[3,4]ØZ

ØØ9 Continued on next page

NC Noncovered Procedure   LC Limited Coverage   QA Questionable OB Admit   NT New Tech Add-on   ⊞ Combination Member   ♂ Male   ♀ Female

Ø   **Medical and Surgical**   *009 Continued*

Ø   **Central Nervous System and Cranial Nerves**

9   **Drainage**   Definition: Taking or letting out fluids and/or gases from a body part

                      Explanation: The qualifier DIAGNOSTIC is used to identify drainage procedures that are biopsies

Body Part Character 4		Approach Character 5	Device Character 6	Qualifier Character 7

Ø Brain
Cerebrum
Corpus callosum
Encephalon
1 Cerebral Meninges
Arachnoid mater,
   intracranial
Leptomeninges,
   intracranial
Pia mater, intracranial
2 Dura Mater
Diaphragma sellae
Dura mater, intracranial
Falx cerebri
Tentorium cerebelli
**3 Epidural Space,
Intracranial**
Extradural space,
   intracranial
**4 Subdural Space,
Intracranial**
**5 Subarachnoid Space,
Intracranial**
6 Cerebral Ventricle
Aqueduct of Sylvius
Cerebral aqueduct
   (Sylvius)
Choroid plexus
Ependyma
Foramen of Monro
   (intraventricular)
Fourth ventricle
Interventricular foramen
   (Monro)
Left lateral ventricle
Right lateral ventricle
Third ventricle
7 Cerebral Hemisphere
Frontal lobe
Occipital lobe
Parietal lobe
Temporal lobe
8 Basal Ganglia
Basal nuclei
Claustrum
Corpus striatum
Globus pallidus
Substantia nigra
Subthalamic nucleus
9 Thalamus
Epithalamus
Geniculate nucleus
Metathalamus
Pulvinar
A Hypothalamus
Mammillary body
B Pons
Apneustic center
Basis pontis
Locus ceruleus
Pneumotaxic center
Pontine tegmentum
Superior olivary nucleus
C Cerebellum
Culmen
D Medulla Oblongata
Myelencephalon
F Olfactory Nerve
First cranial nerve
Olfactory bulb
	G Optic Nerve
	Optic chiasma
	Second cranial nerve
	H Oculomotor Nerve
	Third cranial nerve
	J Trochlear Nerve
	Fourth cranial nerve
	K Trigeminal Nerve
	Fifth cranial nerve
	Gasserian ganglion
	Mandibular nerve
	Maxillary nerve
	Ophthalmic nerve
	Trifacial nerve
	L Abducens Nerve
	Sixth cranial nerve
	M Facial Nerve
	Chorda tympani
	Geniculate ganglion
	Greater superficial petrosal
	   nerve
	Nerve to the stapedius
	Parotid plexus
	Posterior auricular nerve
	Seventh cranial nerve
	Submandibular ganglion
	N Acoustic Nerve
	Cochlear nerve
	Eighth cranial nerve
	Scarpa's (vestibular) ganglion
	Spiral ganglion
	Vestibular (Scarpa's) ganglion
	Vestibular nerve
	Vestibulocochlear nerve
	P Glossopharyngeal Nerve
	Carotid sinus nerve
	Ninth cranial nerve
	Tympanic nerve
	Q Vagus Nerve
	Anterior vagal trunk
	Pharyngeal plexus
	Pneumogastric nerve
	Posterior vagal trunk
	Pulmonary plexus
	Recurrent laryngeal nerve
	Superior laryngeal nerve
	Tenth cranial nerve
	R Accessory Nerve
	Eleventh cranial nerve
	S Hypoglossal Nerve
	Twelfth cranial nerve
	T Spinal Meninges
	Arachnoid mater, spinal
	Denticulate (dentate)
	   ligament
	Dura mater, spinal
	Filum terminale
	Leptomeninges, spinal
	Pia mater, spinal
	U Spinal Canal
	Epidural space, spinal
	Extradural space, spinal
	Subarachnoid space, spinal
	Subdural space, spinal
	Vertebral canal
	W Cervical Spinal Cord
	Dorsal root ganglion
	X Thoracic Spinal Cord
	Dorsal root ganglion
	Y Lumbar Spinal Cord
	Cauda equina
	Conus medullaris
	Dorsal root ganglion
		Ø Open
		3 Percutaneous
		4 Percutaneous Endoscopic
			Z No Device	**X Diagnostic**
				Z No Qualifier

Non-OR	009[Ø,1,2,3,4,5,6,7,8,9,A,B,C,D,F,G,H,J,K,L,M,N,P,Q,R,S][3,4]ZX
Non-OR	009[T,W,X,Y]3Z[X,Z]
Non-OR	009U[3,4]Z[X,Z]

Ø   **Medical and Surgical**
Ø   **Central Nervous System and Cranial Nerves**
B   **Excision**   Definition: Cutting out or off, without replacement, a portion of a body part
                 Explanation: The qualifier DIAGNOSTIC is used to identify excision procedures that are biopsies

Body Part Character 4		Approach Character 5	Device Character 6	Qualifier Character 7
Ø Brain Cerebrum Corpus callosum Encephalon **1 Cerebral Meninges** Arachnoid mater, intracranial Leptomeninges, intracranial Pia mater, intracranial **2 Dura Mater** Diaphragma sellae Dura mater, intracranial Falx cerebri Tentorium cerebelli **6 Cerebral Ventricle** Aqueduct of Sylvius Cerebral aqueduct (Sylvius) Choroid plexus Ependyma Foramen of Monro (intraventricular) Fourth ventricle Interventricular foramen (Monro) Left lateral ventricle Right lateral ventricle Third ventricle **7 Cerebral Hemisphere** Frontal lobe Occipital lobe Parietal lobe Temporal lobe **8 Basal Ganglia** Basal nuclei Claustrum Corpus striatum Globus pallidus Substantia nigra Subthalamic nucleus **9 Thalamus** Epithalamus Geniculate nucleus Metathalamus Pulvinar **A Hypothalamus** Mammillary body **B Pons** Apneustic center Basis pontis Locus ceruleus Pneumotaxic center Pontine tegmentum Superior olivary nucleus **C Cerebellum** Culmen **D Medulla Oblongata** Myelencephalon **F Olfactory Nerve** First cranial nerve Olfactory bulb **G Optic Nerve** Optic chiasma Second cranial nerve	**H Oculomotor Nerve** Third cranial nerve **J Trochlear Nerve** Fourth cranial nerve **K Trigeminal Nerve** Fifth cranial nerve Gasserian ganglion Mandibular nerve Maxillary nerve Ophthalmic nerve Trifacial nerve **L Abducens Nerve** Sixth cranial nerve **M Facial Nerve** Chorda tympani Geniculate ganglion Greater superficial petrosal nerve Nerve to the stapedius Parotid plexus Posterior auricular nerve Seventh cranial nerve Submandibular ganglion **N Acoustic Nerve** Cochlear nerve Eighth cranial nerve Scarpa's (vestibular) ganglion Spiral ganglion Vestibular (Scarpa's) ganglion Vestibular nerve Vestibulocochlear nerve **P Glossopharyngeal Nerve** Carotid sinus nerve Ninth cranial nerve Tympanic nerve **Q Vagus Nerve** Anterior vagal trunk Pharyngeal plexus Pneumogastric nerve Posterior vagal trunk Pulmonary plexus Recurrent laryngeal nerve Superior laryngeal nerve Tenth cranial nerve **R Accessory Nerve** Eleventh cranial nerve **S Hypoglossal Nerve** Twelfth cranial nerve **T Spinal Meninges** Arachnoid mater, spinal Denticulate (dentate) ligament Dura mater, spinal Filum terminale Leptomeninges, spinal Pia mater, spinal **W Cervical Spinal Cord** Dorsal root ganglion **X Thoracic Spinal Cord** Dorsal root ganglion **Y Lumbar Spinal Cord** Cauda equina Conus medullaris Dorsal root ganglion	**Ø Open** **3 Percutaneous** **4 Percutaneous Endoscopic**	**Z No Device**	**X Diagnostic** **Z No Qualifier**

Non-OR   ØØB[F,G,H,J,K,L,M,N,P,Q,R,S][3,4]ZX

0   **Medical and Surgical**
0   **Central Nervous System and Cranial Nerves**
C   **Extirpation**   Definition: Taking or cutting out solid matter from a body part

Explanation: The solid matter may be an abnormal byproduct of a biological function or a foreign body; it may be imbedded in a body part or in the lumen of a tubular body part. The solid matter may or may not have been previously broken into pieces.

Body Part Character 4		Approach Character 5	Device Character 6	Qualifier Character 7

0 **Brain**
  Cerebrum
  Corpus callosum
  Encephalon
1 **Cerebral Meninges**
  Arachnoid mater,
    intracranial
  Leptomeninges,
    intracranial
  Pia mater, intracranial
2 **Dura Mater**
  Diaphragma sellae
  Dura mater, intracranial
  Falx cerebri
  Tentorium cerebelli
3 **Epidural Space,**
  Intracranial
  Extradural space,
    intracranial
4 **Subdural Space,**
  Intracranial
5 **Subarachnoid Space,**
  Intracranial
6 **Cerebral Ventricle**
  Aqueduct of Sylvius
  Cerebral aqueduct
    (Sylvius)
  Choroid plexus
  Ependyma
  Foramen of Monro
    (intraventricular)
  Fourth ventricle
  Interventricular foramen
    (Monro)
  Left lateral ventricle
  Right lateral ventricle
  Third ventricle
7 **Cerebral Hemisphere**
  Frontal lobe
  Occipital lobe
  Parietal lobe
  Temporal lobe
8 **Basal Ganglia**
  Basal nuclei
  Claustrum
  Corpus striatum
  Globus pallidus
  Substantia nigra
  Subthalamic nucleus
9 **Thalamus**
  Epithalamus
  Geniculate nucleus
  Metathalamus
  Pulvinar
A **Hypothalamus**
  Mammillary body
B **Pons**
  Apneustic center
  Basis pontis
  Locus ceruleus
  Pneumotaxic center
  Pontine tegmentum
  Superior olivary nucleus
C **Cerebellum**
  Culmen
D **Medulla Oblongata**
  Myelencephalon
F **Olfactory Nerve**
  First cranial nerve
  Olfactory bulb
	G **Optic Nerve**
	  Optic chiasma
	  Second cranial nerve
	H **Oculomotor Nerve**
	  Third cranial nerve
	J **Trochlear Nerve**
	  Fourth cranial nerve
	K **Trigeminal Nerve**
	  Fifth cranial nerve
	  Gasserian ganglion
	  Mandibular nerve
	  Maxillary nerve
	  Ophthalmic nerve
	  Trifacial nerve
	L **Abducens Nerve**
	  Sixth cranial nerve
	M **Facial Nerve**
	  Chorda tympani
	  Geniculate ganglion
	  Greater superficial petrosal
	    nerve
	  Nerve to the stapedius
	  Parotid plexus
	  Posterior auricular nerve
	  Seventh cranial nerve
	  Submandibular ganglion
	N **Acoustic Nerve**
	  Cochlear nerve
	  Eighth cranial nerve
	  Scarpa's (vestibular)
	    ganglion
	  Spiral ganglion
	  Vestibular (Scarpa's)
	    ganglion
	  Vestibular nerve
	  Vestibulocochlear nerve
	P **Glossopharyngeal Nerve**
	  Carotid sinus nerve
	  Ninth cranial nerve
	  Tympanic nerve
	Q **Vagus Nerve**
	  Anterior vagal trunk
	  Pharyngeal plexus
	  Pneumogastric nerve
	  Posterior vagal trunk
	  Pulmonary plexus
	  Recurrent laryngeal nerve
	  Superior laryngeal nerve
	  Tenth cranial nerve
	R **Accessory Nerve**
	  Eleventh cranial nerve
	S **Hypoglossal Nerve**
	  Twelfth cranial nerve
	T **Spinal Meninges**
	  Arachnoid mater, spinal
	  Denticulate (dentate)
	    ligament
	  Dura mater, spinal
	  Filum terminale
	  Leptomeninges, spinal
	  Pia mater, spinal
	U **Spinal Canal**
	W **Cervical Spinal Cord**
	  Dorsal root ganglion
	X **Thoracic Spinal Cord**
	  Dorsal root ganglion
	Y **Lumbar Spinal Cord**
	  Cauda equina
	  Conus medullaris
	  Dorsal root ganglion
		0 Open
		3 Percutaneous
		4 Percutaneous Endoscopic
			Z No Device	**Z** No Qualifier

Ø   Medical and Surgical
Ø   Central Nervous System and Cranial Nerves
D   Extraction   Definition: Pulling or stripping out or off all or a portion of a body part by the use of force

Explanation: The qualifier DIAGNOSTIC is used to identify extraction procedures that are biopsies

Body Part Character 4		Approach Character 5	Device Character 6	Qualifier Character 7
Ø Brain Cerebrum Corpus callosum Encephalon	**M Facial Nerve** Chorda tympani Geniculate ganglion Greater superficial petrosal nerve Nerve to the stapedius Parotid plexus Posterior auricular nerve Seventh cranial nerve Submandibular ganglion	**Ø Open** **3 Percutaneous** **4 Percutaneous Endoscopic**	**Z No Device**	**Z No Qualifier**
1 Cerebral Meninges Arachnoid mater, intracranial Leptomeninges, intracranial Pia mater, intracranial				
2 Dura Mater Diaphragma sellae Dura mater, intracranial Falx cerebri Tentorium cerebelli	**N Acoustic Nerve** Cochlear nerve Eighth cranial nerve Scarpa's (vestibular) ganglion Spiral ganglion Vestibular (Scarpa's) ganglion Vestibular nerve Vestibulocochlear nerve			
7 Cerebral Hemisphere Frontal lobe Occipital lobe Parietal lobe Temporal lobe				
F Olfactory Nerve First cranial nerve Olfactory bulb	**P Glossopharyngeal Nerve** Carotid sinus nerve Ninth cranial nerve Tympanic nerve			
G Optic Nerve Optic chiasma Second cranial nerve	**Q Vagus Nerve** Anterior vagal trunk Pharyngeal plexus Pneumogastric nerve Posterior vagal trunk Pulmonary plexus Recurrent laryngeal nerve Superior laryngeal nerve Tenth cranial nerve			
H Oculomotor Nerve Third cranial nerve				
J Trochlear Nerve Fourth cranial nerve	**R Accessory Nerve** Eleventh cranial nerve			
K Trigeminal Nerve Fifth cranial nerve Gasserian ganglion Mandibular nerve Maxillary nerve Ophthalmic nerve Trifacial nerve	**S Hypoglossal Nerve** Twelfth cranial nerve			
	T Spinal Meninges Arachnoid mater, spinal Denticulate (dentate) ligament Dura mater, spinal Filum terminale Leptomeninges, spinal Pia mater, spinal			
L Abducens Nerve Sixth cranial nerve				

NC Noncovered Procedure   **LC** Limited Coverage   **QA** Questionable OB Admit   **NT** New Tech Add-on   ⊞ Combination Member   ♂ Male   ♀ Female

ICD-10-PCS 2022   **141**

Ø   **Medical and Surgical**
Ø   **Central Nervous System and Cranial Nerves**
F   **Fragmentation**   Definition: Breaking solid matter in a body part into pieces

       Explanation: Physical force (e.g., manual, ultrasonic) applied directly or indirectly is used to break the solid matter into pieces. The solid matter may be an abnormal byproduct of a biological function or a foreign body. The pieces of solid matter are not taken out.

Body Part Character 4	Approach Character 5	Device Character 6	Qualifier Character 7

3 Epidural Space, Intracranial `NC`
    Extradural space, intracranial
4 Subdural Space, Intracranial `NC`
5 Subarachnoid Space, Intracranial `NC`
6 Cerebral Ventricle `NC`
    Aqueduct of Sylvius
    Cerebral aqueduct (Sylvius)
    Choroid plexus
    Ependyma
    Foramen of Monro (intraventricular)
    Fourth ventricle
    Interventricular foramen (Monro)
    Left lateral ventricle
    Right lateral ventricle
    Third ventricle
U Spinal Canal
    Epidural space, spinal
    Extradural space, spinal
    Subarachnoid space, spinal
    Subdural space, spinal
    Vertebral canal
	Ø Open
	3 Percutaneous
	4 Percutaneous Endoscopic
	X External
		Z No Device	**Z** No Qualifier

Non-OR   ØØF[3,4,5,6]XZZ
`NC`   ØØF[3,4,5,6]XZZ

Ø   **Medical and Surgical**
Ø   **Central Nervous System and Cranial Nerves**
H   **Insertion**   Definition: Putting in a nonbiological appliance that monitors, assists, performs, or prevents a physiological function but does not physically take the place of a body part

       Explanation: None

Body Part Character 4	Approach Character 5	Device Character 6	Qualifier Character 7

Ø Brain ⊞
    Cerebrum
    Corpus callosum
    Encephalon
	Ø Open	**1** Radioactive Element
		2 Monitoring Device
		3 Infusion Device
		4 Radioactive Element, Cesium-131
		    Collagen Implant
		M Neurostimulator Lead
		Y Other Device
			Z No Qualifier

Ø Brain ⊞
    Cerebrum
    Corpus callosum
    Encephalon
	3 Percutaneous
	4 Percutaneous Endoscopic
		1 Radioactive Element
		2 Monitoring Device
		3 Infusion Device
		M Neurostimulator Lead
		Y Other Device
			Z No Qualifier

6 Cerebral Ventricle ⊞
    Aqueduct of Sylvius
    Cerebral aqueduct (Sylvius)
    Choroid plexus
    Ependyma
    Foramen of Monro (intraventricular)
    Fourth ventricle Interventricular foramen
      (Monro)
    Left lateral ventricle
    Right lateral ventricle
    Third ventricle
E Cranial Nerve ⊞
U Spinal Canal ⊞
    Epidural space, spinal
    Extradural space, spinal
    Subarachnoid space, spinal
    Subdural space, spinal
    Vertebral canal
V Spinal Cord ⊞
    Dorsal root ganglion
	Ø Open
	3 Percutaneous
	4 Percutaneous Endoscopic
		1 Radioactive Element
		2 Monitoring Device
		3 Infusion Device
		M Neurostimulator Lead
		Y Other Device
			Z No Qualifier

DRG Non-OR	ØØHØØ4Z	**See Appendix L for Procedure Combinations**	
Non-OR	ØØH[E,U,V]32Z	⊞ ØØHØØMZ	
Non-OR	ØØH[E,U][3,4]YZ	⊞ ØØHØ[3,4]MZ	
Non-OR	ØØH[U,V][Ø,3,4]3Z	⊞ ØØH[6,E,U,V][Ø,3,4]MZ	

---

0   Medical and Surgical
0   Central Nervous System and Cranial Nerves
J   Inspection   Definition: Visually and/or manually exploring a body part

Explanation: Visual exploration may be performed with or without optical instrumentation. Manual exploration may be performed directly or through intervening body layers.

Body Part Character 4	Approach Character 5	Device Character 6	Qualifier Character 7
0 Brain Cerebrum Corpus callosum Encephalon **E Cranial Nerve** **U Spinal Canal** Epidural space, spinal Extradural space, spinal Subarachnoid space, spinal Subdural space, spinal Vertebral canal **V Spinal Cord** Dorsal root ganglion	**0** Open **3** Percutaneous **4** Percutaneous Endoscopic	**Z** No Device	**Z** No Qualifier

Non-OR	00J[0,E,U,V]3ZZ

0   Medical and Surgical
0   Central Nervous System and Cranial Nerves
K   Map   Definition: Locating the route of passage of electrical impulses and/or locating functional areas in a body part

Explanation: Applicable only to the cardiac conduction mechanism and the central nervous system

Body Part Character 4	Approach Character 5	Device Character 6	Qualifier Character 7
0 Brain Cerebrum Corpus callosum Encephalon **7 Cerebral Hemisphere** Frontal lobe Occipital lobe Parietal lobe Temporal lobe **8 Basal Ganglia** Basal nuclei Claustrum Corpus striatum Globus pallidus Substantia nigra Subthalamic nucleus **9 Thalamus** Epithalamus Geniculate nucleus Metathalamus Pulvinar **A Hypothalamus** Mammillary body **B Pons** Apneustic center Basis pontis Locus ceruleus Pneumotaxic center Pontine tegmentum Superior olivary nucleus **C Cerebellum** Culmen **D Medulla Oblongata** Myelencephalon	**0** Open **3** Percutaneous **4** Percutaneous Endoscopic	**Z** No Device	**Z** No Qualifier

NC Noncovered Procedure   LC Limited Coverage   QA Questionable OB Admit   NT New Tech Add-on   ⊞ Combination Member   ♂ Male   ♀ Female

ICD-10-PCS 2022   **143**

Ø   **Medical and Surgical**
Ø   **Central Nervous System and Cranial Nerves**
N   **Release**   Definition: Freeing a body part from an abnormal physical constraint by cutting or by the use of force
                          Explanation: Some of the restraining tissue may be taken out but none of the body part is taken out

Body Part Character 4		Approach Character 5	Device Character 6	Qualifier Character 7

Ø Brain
Cerebrum
Corpus callosum
Encephalon
1 Cerebral Meninges
Arachnoid mater,
   intracranial
Leptomeninges,
   intracranial
Pia mater, intracranial
2 Dura Mater
Diaphragma sellae
Dura mater, intracranial
Falx cerebri
Tentorium cerebelli
6 Cerebral Ventricle
Aqueduct of Sylvius
Cerebral aqueduct
   (Sylvius)
Choroid plexus
Ependyma
Foramen of Monro
   (intraventricular)
Fourth ventricle
Interventricular foramen
   (Monro)
Left lateral ventricle
Right lateral ventricle
Third ventricle
7 Cerebral Hemisphere
Frontal lobe
Occipital lobe
Parietal lobe
Temporal lobe
8 Basal Ganglia
Basal nuclei
Claustrum
Corpus striatum
Globus pallidus
Substantia nigra
Subthalamic nucleus
9 Thalamus
Epithalamus
Geniculate nucleus
Metathalamus
Pulvinar
A Hypothalamus
Mammillary body
B Pons
Apneustic center
Basis pontis
Locus ceruleus
Pneumotaxic center
Pontine tegmentum
Superior olivary nucleus
C Cerebellum
Culmen
D Medulla Oblongata
Myelencephalon
F Olfactory Nerve
First cranial nerve
Olfactory bulb
G Optic Nerve
Optic chiasma
Second cranial nerve
	H Oculomotor Nerve
	Third cranial nerve
	J Trochlear Nerve
	Fourth cranial nerve
	K Trigeminal Nerve
	Fifth cranial nerve
	Gasserian ganglion
	Mandibular nerve
	Maxillary nerve
	Ophthalmic nerve
	Trifacial nerve
	L Abducens Nerve
	Sixth cranial nerve
	M Facial Nerve
	Chorda tympani
	Geniculate ganglion
	Greater superficial petrosal
	   nerve
	Nerve to the stapedius
	Parotid plexus
	Posterior auricular nerve
	Seventh cranial nerve
	Submandibular ganglion
	N Acoustic Nerve
	Cochlear nerve
	Eighth cranial nerve
	Scarpa's (vestibular)
	   ganglion
	Spiral ganglion
	Vestibular (Scarpa's)
	   ganglion
	Vestibular nerve
	Vestibulocochlear nerve
	P Glossopharyngeal Nerve
	Carotid sinus nerve
	Ninth cranial nerve
	Tympanic nerve
	Q Vagus Nerve
	Anterior vagal trunk
	Pharyngeal plexus
	Pneumogastric nerve
	Posterior vagal trunk
	Pulmonary plexus
	Recurrent laryngeal nerve
	Superior laryngeal nerve
	Tenth cranial nerve
	R Accessory Nerve
	Eleventh cranial nerve
	S Hypoglossal Nerve
	Twelfth cranial nerve
	T Spinal Meninges
	Arachnoid mater, spinal
	Denticulate (dentate)
	   ligament
	Dura mater, spinal
	Filum terminale
	Leptomeninges, spinal
	Pia mater, spinal
	W Cervical Spinal Cord
	Dorsal root ganglion
	X Thoracic Spinal Cord
	Dorsal root ganglion
	Y Lumbar Spinal Cord
	Cauda equina
	Conus medullaris
	Dorsal root ganglion
		Ø Open
		3 Percutaneous
		4 Percutaneous Endoscopic
			Z No Device	**Z No Qualifier**

Ø   **Medical and Surgical**
Ø   **Central Nervous System and Cranial Nerves**
P   **Removal**   Definition: Taking out or off a device from a body part

                    Explanation: If a device is taken out and a similar device put in without cutting or puncturing the skin or mucous membrane, the procedure is coded to the root operation CHANGE. Otherwise, the procedure for taking out a device is coded to the root operation REMOVAL.

Body Part Character 4	Approach Character 5	Device Character 6	Qualifier Character 7
Ø Brain Cerebrum Corpus callosum Encephalon **V Spinal Cord** Dorsal root ganglion	**Ø** Open **3** Percutaneous **4** Percutaneous Endoscopic	**Ø** Drainage Device **2** Monitoring Device **3** Infusion Device **7** Autologous Tissue Substitute **J** Synthetic Substitute **K** Nonautologous Tissue Substitute **M** Neurostimulator Lead **Y** Other Device	**Z** No Qualifier
Ø Brain Cerebrum Corpus callosum Encephalon **V Spinal Cord** Dorsal root ganglion	**X** External	**Ø** Drainage Device **2** Monitoring Device **3** Infusion Device **M** Neurostimulator Lead	**Z** No Qualifier
6 Cerebral Ventricle Aqueduct of Sylvius Cerebral aqueduct (Sylvius) Choroid plexus Ependyma Foramen of Monro (intraventricular) Fourth ventricle Interventricular foramen (Monro) Left lateral ventricle Right lateral ventricle Third ventricle **U Spinal Canal** Epidural space, spinal Extradural space, spinal Subarachnoid space, spinal Subdural space, spinal Vertebral canal	**Ø** Open **3** Percutaneous **4** Percutaneous Endoscopic	**Ø** Drainage Device **2** Monitoring Device **3** Infusion Device **J** Synthetic Substitute **M** Neurostimulator Lead **Y** Other Device	**Z** No Qualifier
6 Cerebral Ventricle Aqueduct of Sylvius Cerebral aqueduct (Sylvius) Choroid plexus Ependyma Foramen of Monro (intraventricular) Fourth ventricle Interventricular foramen (Monro) Left lateral ventricle Right lateral ventricle Third ventricle **U Spinal Canal** Epidural space, spinal Extradural space, spinal Subarachnoid space, spinal Subdural space, spinal Vertebral canal	**X** External	**Ø** Drainage Device **2** Monitoring Device **3** Infusion Device **M** Neurostimulator Lead	**Z** No Qualifier
E Cranial Nerve	**Ø** Open **3** Percutaneous **4** Percutaneous Endoscopic	**Ø** Drainage Device **2** Monitoring Device **3** Infusion Device **7** Autologous Tissue Substitute **M** Neurostimulator Lead **Y** Other Device	**Z** No Qualifier
E Cranial Nerve	**X** External	**Ø** Drainage Device **2** Monitoring Device **3** Infusion Device **M** Neurostimulator Lead	**Z** No Qualifier

Non-OR   00P[0,V]3[0,2,3]Z
Non-OR   00P[0,V][3,4]YZ
Non-OR   00P[0,V]X[0,2,3,M]Z
Non-OR   00P[6,U]3[0,2,3]Z
Non-OR   00P[6,U][3,4]YZ
Non-OR   00P[6,U]X[0,2,3,M]Z
Non-OR   00PE3[0,2,3]Z
Non-OR   00PE[3,4]YZ
Non-OR   00PEX[0,2,3,M]Z

NC Noncovered Procedure   **LC** Limited Coverage   **QA** Questionable OB Admit   **NT** New Tech Add-on   ✚ Combination Member   ♂ Male   ♀ Female

Ø   Medical and Surgical
Ø   Central Nervous System and Cranial Nerves
Q   Repair   Definition: Restoring, to the extent possible, a body part to its normal anatomic structure and function

Explanation: Used only when the method to accomplish the repair is not one of the other root operations

Body Part Character 4		Approach Character 5	Device Character 6	Qualifier Character 7

Ø   Brain
Cerebrum
Corpus callosum
Encephalon
1   Cerebral Meninges
Arachnoid mater,
    intracranial
Leptomeninges,
    intracranial
Pia mater, intracranial
2   Dura Mater
Diaphragma sellae
Dura mater, intracranial
Falx cerebri
Tentorium cerebelli
6   Cerebral Ventricle
Aqueduct of Sylvius
Cerebral aqueduct
    (Sylvius)
Choroid plexus
Ependyma
Foramen of Monro
    (intraventricular)
Fourth ventricle
Interventricular foramen
    (Monro)
Left lateral ventricle
Right lateral ventricle
Third ventricle
7   Cerebral Hemisphere
Frontal lobe
Occipital lobe
Parietal lobe
Temporal lobe
8   Basal Ganglia
Basal nuclei
Claustrum
Corpus striatum
Globus pallidus
Substantia nigra
Subthalamic nucleus
9   Thalamus
Epithalamus
Geniculate nucleus
Metathalamus
Pulvinar
A   Hypothalamus
Mammillary body
B   Pons
Apneustic center
Basis pontis
Locus ceruleus
Pneumotaxic center
Pontine tegmentum
Superior olivary nucleus
C   Cerebellum
Culmen
D   Medulla Oblongata
Myelencephalon
F   Olfactory Nerve
First cranial nerve
Olfactory bulb
G   Optic Nerve
Optic chiasma
Second cranial nerve
	H Oculomotor Nerve
	Third cranial nerve
	J Trochlear Nerve
	Fourth cranial nerve
	K Trigeminal Nerve
	Fifth cranial nerve
	Gasserian ganglion
	Mandibular nerve
	Maxillary nerve
	Ophthalmic nerve
	Trifacial nerve
	L Abducens Nerve
	Sixth cranial nerve
	M Facial Nerve
	Chorda tympani
	Geniculate ganglion
	Greater superficial petrosal
	    nerve
	Nerve to the stapedius
	Parotid plexus
	Posterior auricular nerve
	Seventh cranial nerve
	Submandibular ganglion
	N Acoustic Nerve
	Cochlear nerve
	Eighth cranial nerve
	Scarpa's (vestibular)
	    ganglion
	Spiral ganglion
	Vestibular (Scarpa's)
	    ganglion
	Vestibular nerve
	Vestibulocochlear nerve
	P Glossopharyngeal Nerve
	Carotid sinus nerve
	Ninth cranial nerve
	Tympanic nerve
	Q Vagus Nerve
	Anterior vagal trunk
	Pharyngeal plexus
	Pneumogastric nerve
	Posterior vagal trunk
	Pulmonary plexus
	Recurrent laryngeal nerve
	Superior laryngeal nerve
	Tenth cranial nerve
	R Accessory Nerve
	Eleventh cranial nerve
	S Hypoglossal Nerve
	Twelfth cranial nerve
	T Spinal Meninges
	Arachnoid mater, spinal
	Denticulate (dentate)
	    ligament
	Dura mater, spinal
	Filum terminale
	Leptomeninges, spinal
	Pia mater, spinal
	W Cervical Spinal Cord
	Dorsal root ganglion
	X Thoracic Spinal Cord
	Dorsal root ganglion
	Y Lumbar Spinal Cord
	Cauda equina
	Conus medullaris
	Dorsal root ganglion
		Ø Open
		3 Percutaneous
		4 Percutaneous Endoscopic
			Z No Device	**Z No Qualifier**

| Non-OR Procedure | DRG Non-OR Procedure | Valid OR Procedure | HAC Associated Procedure | Combination Only | New/Revised GREEN |

146   ICD-10-PCS 2022

ØØQ–ØØQ

Ø   **Medical and Surgical**
Ø   **Central Nervous System and Cranial Nerves**
R   **Replacement**   Definition: Putting in or on biological or synthetic material that physically takes the place and/or function of all or a portion of a body part

                 Explanation: The body part may have been taken out or replaced, or may be taken out, physically eradicated, or rendered nonfunctional during the REPLACEMENT procedure. A REMOVAL procedure is coded for taking out the device used in a previous replacement procedure.

Body Part Character 4		Approach Character 5	Device Character 6	Qualifier Character 7

1 Cerebral Meninges
  Arachnoid mater,
    intracranial
  Leptomeninges,
    intracranial
  Pia mater, intracranial
2 Dura Mater
  Diaphragma sellae
  Dura mater, intracranial
  Falx cerebri
  Tentorium cerebelli
6 Cerebral Ventricle
  Aqueduct of Sylvius
  Cerebral aqueduct
    (Sylvius)
  Choroid plexus
  Ependyma
  Foramen of Monro
    (intraventricular)
  Fourth ventricle
  Interventricular foramen·
    (Monro)
  Left lateral ventricle
  Right lateral ventricle
  Third ventricle
F Olfactory Nerve
  First cranial nerve
  Olfactory bulb
G Optic Nerve
  Optic chiasma
  Second cranial nerve
H Oculomotor Nerve
  Third cranial nerve
J Trochlear Nerve
  Fourth cranial nerve
K Trigeminal Nerve
  Fifth cranial nerve
  Gasserian ganglion
  Mandibular nerve
  Maxillary nerve
  Ophthalmic nerve
  Trifacial nerve
L Abducens Nerve
  Sixth cranial nerve
	M Facial Nerve
	  Chorda tympani
	  Geniculate ganglion
	  Greater superficial petrosal
	    nerve
	  Nerve to the stapedius
	  Parotid plexus
	  Posterior auricular nerve
	  Seventh cranial nerve
	  Submandibular ganglion
	N Acoustic Nerve
	  Cochlear nerve
	  Eighth cranial nerve
	  Scarpa's (vestibular)
	    ganglion
	  Spiral ganglion
	  Vestibular (Scarpa's)
	    ganglion
	  Vestibular nerve
	  Vestibulocochlear nerve
	P Glossopharyngeal Nerve
	  Carotid sinus nerve
	  Ninth cranial nerve
	  Tympanic nerve
	Q Vagus Nerve
	  Anterior vagal trunk
	  Pharyngeal plexus
	  Pneumogastric nerve
	  Posterior vagal trunk
	  Pulmonary plexus
	  Recurrent laryngeal nerve
	  Superior laryngeal nerve
	  Tenth cranial nerve
	R Accessory Nerve
	  Eleventh cranial nerve
	S Hypoglossal Nerve
	  Twelfth cranial nerve
	T Spinal Meninges
	  Arachnoid mater, spinal
	  Denticulate (dentate)
	    ligament
	  Dura mater, spinal
	  Filum terminale
	  Leptomeninges, spinal
	  Pia mater, spinal
		Ø Open
		4 Percutaneous Endoscopic
			7 Autologous Tissue
			  Substitute
			J Synthetic Substitute
			K Nonautologous Tissue
			  Substitute
				Z No Qualifier

NC Noncovered Procedure   **LC** Limited Coverage   **QA** Questionable OB Admit   **NT** New Tech Add-on   ⊞ Combination Member   ♂ Male   ♀ Female

ICD-10-PCS 2022   **147**

0   Medical and Surgical
0   Central Nervous System and Cranial Nerves
S   Reposition   Definition: Moving to its normal location, or other suitable location, all or a portion of a body part

Explanation: The body part is moved to a new location from an abnormal location, or from a normal location where it is not functioning correctly. The body part may or may not be cut out or off to be moved to the new location.

Body Part Character 4		Approach Character 5	Device Character 6	Qualifier Character 7

F   **Olfactory Nerve**
    First cranial nerve
    Olfactory bulb
G   **Optic Nerve**
    Optic chiasma
    Second cranial nerve
H   **Oculomotor Nerve**
    Third cranial nerve
J   **Trochlear Nerve**
    Fourth cranial nerve
K   **Trigeminal Nerve**
    Fifth cranial nerve
    Gasserian ganglion
    Mandibular nerve
    Maxillary nerve
    Ophthalmic nerve
    Trifacial nerve
L   **Abducens Nerve**
    Sixth cranial nerve
M   **Facial Nerve**
    Chorda tympani
    Geniculate ganglion
    Greater superficial petrosal
      nerve
    Nerve to the stapedius
    Parotid plexus
    Posterior auricular nerve
    Seventh cranial nerve
    Submandibular ganglion
	N **Acoustic Nerve**
	    Cochlear nerve
	    Eighth cranial nerve
	    Scarpa's (vestibular)
	      ganglion
	    Spiral ganglion
	    Vestibular (Scarpa's)
	      ganglion
	    Vestibular nerve
	    Vestibulocochlear nerve
	P **Glossopharyngeal Nerve**
	    Carotid sinus nerve
	    Ninth cranial nerve
	    Tympanic nerve
	Q **Vagus Nerve**
	    Anterior vagal trunk
	    Pharyngeal plexus
	    Pneumogastric nerve
	    Posterior vagal trunk
	    Pulmonary plexus
	    Recurrent laryngeal nerve
	    Superior laryngeal nerve
	    Tenth cranial nerve
	R **Accessory Nerve**
	    Eleventh cranial nerve
	S **Hypoglossal Nerve**
	    Twelfth cranial nerve
	W **Cervical Spinal Cord**
	    Dorsal root ganglion
	X **Thoracic Spinal Cord**
	    Dorsal root ganglion
	Y **Lumbar Spinal Cord**
	    Cauda equina
	    Conus medullaris
	    Dorsal root ganglion
		0 Open
		3 Percutaneous
		4 Percutaneous Endoscopic
			Z No Device	**Z** No Qualifier

0   Medical and Surgical
0   Central Nervous System and Cranial Nerves
T   Resection   Definition: Cutting out or off, without replacement, all of a body part

Explanation: None

Body Part Character 4	Approach Character 5	Device Character 6	Qualifier Character 7

7   **Cerebral Hemisphere**
    Frontal lobe
    Occipital lobe
    Parietal lobe
    Temporal lobe
	0 Open
	3 Percutaneous
	4 Percutaneous Endoscopic
		Z No Device	**Z** No Qualifier

Ø   **Medical and Surgical**
Ø   **Central Nervous System and Cranial Nerves**
U   **Supplement**   Definition: Putting in or on biological or synthetic material that physically reinforces and/or augments the function of a portion of a body part

Explanation: The biological material is non-living, or is living and from the same individual. The body part may have been previously replaced, and the SUPPLEMENT procedure is performed to physically reinforce and/or augment the function of the replaced body part.

Body Part Character 4		Approach Character 5	Device Character 6	Qualifier Character 7

1 Cerebral Meninges
  Arachnoid mater,
    intracranial
  Leptomeninges,
    intracranial
  Pia mater, intracranial
2 Dura Mater
  Diaphragma sellae
  Dura mater, intracranial
  Falx cerebri
  Tentorium cerebelli
6 Cerebral Ventricle
  Aqueduct of Sylvius
  Cerebral aqueduct
    (Sylvius)
  Choroid plexus
  Ependyma
  Foramen of Monro
    (intraventricular)
  Fourth ventricle
  Interventricular foramen
    (Monro)
  Left lateral ventricle
  Right lateral ventricle
  Third ventricle
F Olfactory Nerve
  First cranial nerve
  Olfactory bulb
G Optic Nerve
  Optic chiasma
  Second cranial nerve
H Oculomotor Nerve
  Third cranial nerve
J Trochlear Nerve
  Fourth cranial nerve
K Trigeminal Nerve
  Fifth cranial nerve
  Gasserian ganglion
  Mandibular nerve
  Maxillary nerve
  Ophthalmic nerve
  Trifacial nerve
L Abducens Nerve
  Sixth cranial nerve
	M Facial Nerve
	  Chorda tympani
	  Geniculate ganglion
	  Greater superficial petrosal
	    nerve
	  Nerve to the stapedius
	  Parotid plexus
	  Posterior auricular nerve
	  Seventh cranial nerve
	  Submandibular ganglion
	N Acoustic Nerve
	  Cochlear nerve
	  Eighth cranial nerve
	  Scarpa's (vestibular)
	    ganglion
	  Spiral ganglion
	  Vestibular (Scarpa's)
	    ganglion
	  Vestibular nerve
	  Vestibulocochlear nerve
	P Glossopharyngeal Nerve
	  Carotid sinus nerve
	  Ninth cranial nerve
	  Tympanic nerve
	Q Vagus Nerve
	  Anterior vagal trunk
	  Pharyngeal plexus
	  Pneumogastric nerve
	  Posterior vagal trunk
	  Pulmonary plexus
	  Recurrent laryngeal nerve
	  Superior laryngeal nerve
	  Tenth cranial nerve
	R Accessory Nerve
	  Eleventh cranial nerve
	S Hypoglossal Nerve
	  Twelfth cranial nerve
	T Spinal Meninges
	  Arachnoid mater, spinal
	  Denticulate (dentate)
	    ligament
	  Dura mater, spinal
	  Filum terminale
	  Leptomeninges, spinal
	  Pia mater, spinal
		Ø Open
		3 Percutaneous
		4 Percutaneous Endoscopic
			7 Autologous Tissue
			    Substitute
			J Synthetic Substitute
			K Nonautologous Tissue
			    Substitute
				Z No Qualifier

0   Medical and Surgical
0   Central Nervous System and Cranial Nerves
W   Revision   Definition: Correcting, to the extent possible, a portion of a malfunctioning device or the position of a displaced device

              Explanation: Revision can include correcting a malfunctioning or displaced device by taking out or putting in components of the device such as a screw or pin

Body Part Character 4	Approach Character 5	Device Character 6	Qualifier Character 7
0 Brain Cerebrum Corpus callosum Encephalon **V Spinal Cord** Dorsal root ganglion	**0** Open **3** Percutaneous **4** Percutaneous Endoscopic	**0** Drainage Device **2** Monitoring Device **3** Infusion Device **7** Autologous Tissue Substitute **J** Synthetic Substitute **K** Nonautologous Tissue Substitute **M** Neurostimulator Lead **Y** Other Device	**Z** No Qualifier
0 Brain Cerebrum Corpus callosum Encephalon **V Spinal Cord** Dorsal root ganglion	**X** External	**0** Drainage Device **2** Monitoring Device **3** Infusion Device **7** Autologous Tissue Substitute **J** Synthetic Substitute **K** Nonautologous Tissue Substitute **M** Neurostimulator Lead	**Z** No Qualifier
6 Cerebral Ventricle Aqueduct of Sylvius Cerebral aqueduct (Sylvius) Choroid plexus Ependyma Foramen of Monro (intraventricular) Fourth ventricle Interventricular foramen (Monro) Left lateral ventricle Right lateral ventricle Third ventricle **U Spinal Canal** Epidural space, spinal Extradural space, spinal Subarachnoid space, spinal Subdural space, spinal Vertebral canal	**0** Open **3** Percutaneous **4** Percutaneous Endoscopic	**0** Drainage Device **2** Monitoring Device **3** Infusion Device **J** Synthetic Substitute **M** Neurostimulator Lead **Y** Other Device	**Z** No Qualifier
6 Cerebral Ventricle Aqueduct of Sylvius Cerebral aqueduct (Sylvius) Choroid plexus Ependyma Foramen of Monro (intraventricular) Fourth ventricle Interventricular foramen (Monro) Left lateral ventricle Right lateral ventricle Third ventricle **U Spinal Canal** Epidural space, spinal Extradural space, spinal Subarachnoid space, spinal Subdural space, spinal Vertebral canal	**X** External	**0** Drainage Device **2** Monitoring Device **3** Infusion Device **J** Synthetic Substitute **M** Neurostimulator Lead	**Z** No Qualifier
E Cranial Nerve	**0** Open **3** Percutaneous **4** Percutaneous Endoscopic	**0** Drainage Device **2** Monitoring Device **3** Infusion Device **7** Autologous Tissue Substitute **M** Neurostimulator Lead **Y** Other Device	**Z** No Qualifier
E Cranial Nerve	**X** External	**0** Drainage Device **2** Monitoring Device **3** Infusion Device **7** Autologous Tissue Substitute **M** Neurostimulator Lead	**Z** No Qualifier

Non-OR	00W[0,V][3,4]YZ
Non-OR	00W[0,V]X[0,2,3,7,J,K,M]Z
Non-OR	00W[6,U][3,4]YZ
Non-OR	00W[6,U]X[0,2,3,J,M]Z
Non-OR	00WE[3,4]YZ
Non-OR	00WEX[0,2,3,7,M]Z

Ø   **Medical and Surgical**
Ø   **Central Nervous System and Cranial Nerves**
X   **Transfer**   Definition: Moving, without taking out, all or a portion of a body part to another location to take over the function of all or a portion of a body part
                          Explanation: The body part transferred remains connected to its vascular and nervous supply

Body Part Character 4	Approach Character 5	Device Character 6	Qualifier Character 7
F Olfactory Nerve First cranial nerve Olfactory bulb **G Optic Nerve** Optic chiasma Second cranial nerve **H Oculomotor Nerve** Third cranial nerve **J Trochlear Nerve** Fourth cranial nerve **K Trigeminal Nerve** Fifth cranial nerve Gasserian ganglion Mandibular nerve Maxillary nerve Ophthalmic nerve Trifacial nerve **L Abducens Nerve** Sixth cranial nerve **M Facial Nerve** Chorda tympani Geniculate ganglion Greater superficial petrosal nerve Nerve to the stapedius Parotid plexus Posterior auricular nerve Seventh cranial nerve Submandibular ganglion **N Acoustic Nerve** Cochlear nerve Eighth cranial nerve Scarpa's (vestibular) ganglion Spiral ganglion Vestibular (Scarpa's) ganglion Vestibular nerve Vestibulocochlear nerve **P Glossopharyngeal Nerve** Carotid sinus nerve Ninth cranial nerve Tympanic nerve **Q Vagus Nerve** Anterior vagal trunk Pharyngeal plexus Pneumogastric nerve Posterior vagal trunk Pulmonary plexus Recurrent laryngeal nerve Superior laryngeal nerve Tenth cranial nerve **R Accessory Nerve** Eleventh cranial nerve **S Hypoglossal Nerve** Twelfth cranial nerve	**Ø Open** **4 Percutaneous Endoscopic**	**Z No Device**	**F Olfactory Nerve** **G Optic Nerve** **H Oculomotor Nerve** **J Trochlear Nerve** **K Trigeminal Nerve** **L Abducens Nerve** **M Facial Nerve** **N Acoustic Nerve** **P Glossopharyngeal Nerve** **Q Vagus Nerve** **R Accessory Nerve** **S Hypoglossal Nerve**

Peripheral Nervous System Ø12–Ø1X

Character Meanings

This Character Meaning table is provided as a guide to assist the user in the identification of character members that may be found in this section of code tables. It **SHOULD NOT** be used to build a PCS code.

Operation–Character 3	Body Part–Character 4	Approach–Character 5	Device–Character 6	Qualifier–Character 7
2 Change	Ø Cervical Plexus	Ø Open	Ø Drainage Device	1 Cervical Nerve
5 Destruction	1 Cervical Nerve	3 Percutaneous	1 Radioactive Element	2 Phrenic Nerve
8 Division	2 Phrenic Nerve	4 Percutaneous Endoscopic	2 Monitoring Device	4 Ulnar Nerve
9 Drainage	3 Brachial Plexus	X External	7 Autologous Tissue Substitute	5 Median Nerve
B Excision	4 Ulnar Nerve		J Synthetic Substitute	6 Radial Nerve
C Extirpation	5 Median Nerve		K Nonautologous Tissue Substitute	8 Thoracic Nerve
D Extraction	6 Radial Nerve		M Neurostimulator Lead	B Lumbar Nerve
H Insertion	8 Thoracic Nerve		Y Other Device	C Perineal Nerve
J Inspection	9 Lumbar Plexus		Z No Device	D Femoral Nerve
N Release	A Lumbosacral Plexus			F Sciatic Nerve
P Removal	B Lumbar Nerve			G Tibial Nerve
Q Repair	C Pudendal Nerve			H Peroneal Nerve
R Replacement	D Femoral Nerve			X Diagnostic
S Reposition	F Sciatic Nerve			Z No Qualifier
U Supplement	G Tibial Nerve			
W Revision	H Peroneal Nerve			
X Transfer	K Head and Neck Sympathetic Nerve			
	L Thoracic Sympathetic Nerve			
	M Abdominal Sympathetic Nerve			
	N Lumbar Sympathetic Nerve			
	P Sacral Sympathetic Nerve			
	Q Sacral Plexus			
	R Sacral Nerve			
	Y Peripheral Nerve			

AHA Coding Clinic for table Ø1B
2018, 2Q, 22   Excision of synovial cyst
2017, 2Q, 19   Thoracic outlet decompression with sympathectomy

AHA Coding Clinic for table Ø1H
2020, 4Q, 43-44   Insertion of radioactive element

AHA Coding Clinic for table Ø1N
2019, 1Q, 28   Decompressive laminectomy of both spinal cord and nerve roots
2018, 2Q, 22   Excision of synovial cyst
2017, 2Q, 19   Thoracic outlet decompression with sympathectomy
2016, 2Q, 16   Decompressive laminectomy/foraminotomy and lumbar discectomy
2016, 2Q, 17   Removal of longitudinal ligament to decompress cervical nerve root
2016, 2Q, 23   Thoracic outlet syndrome and release of brachial plexus
2015, 2Q, 34   Decompressive laminectomy
2014, 3Q, 33   Radial fracture treatment with open reduction internal fixation, and release of carpal ligament

AHA Coding Clinic for table Ø1Q
2019, 3Q, 32   Breast reconstruction with neurotization

AHA Coding Clinic for table Ø1U
2019, 3Q, 32   Breast reconstruction with neurotization
2017, 4Q, 62   Added and revised device values - Nerve substitutes

Median and Ulnar Nerves

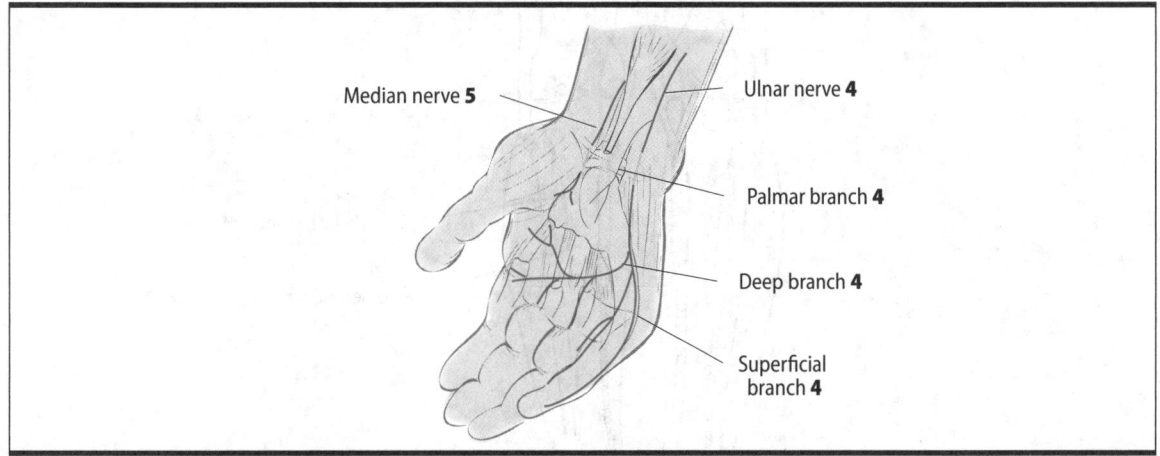

Median nerve **5**   Ulnar nerve **4**
Palmar branch **4**
Deep branch **4**
Superficial branch **4**

Peripheral Nervous System

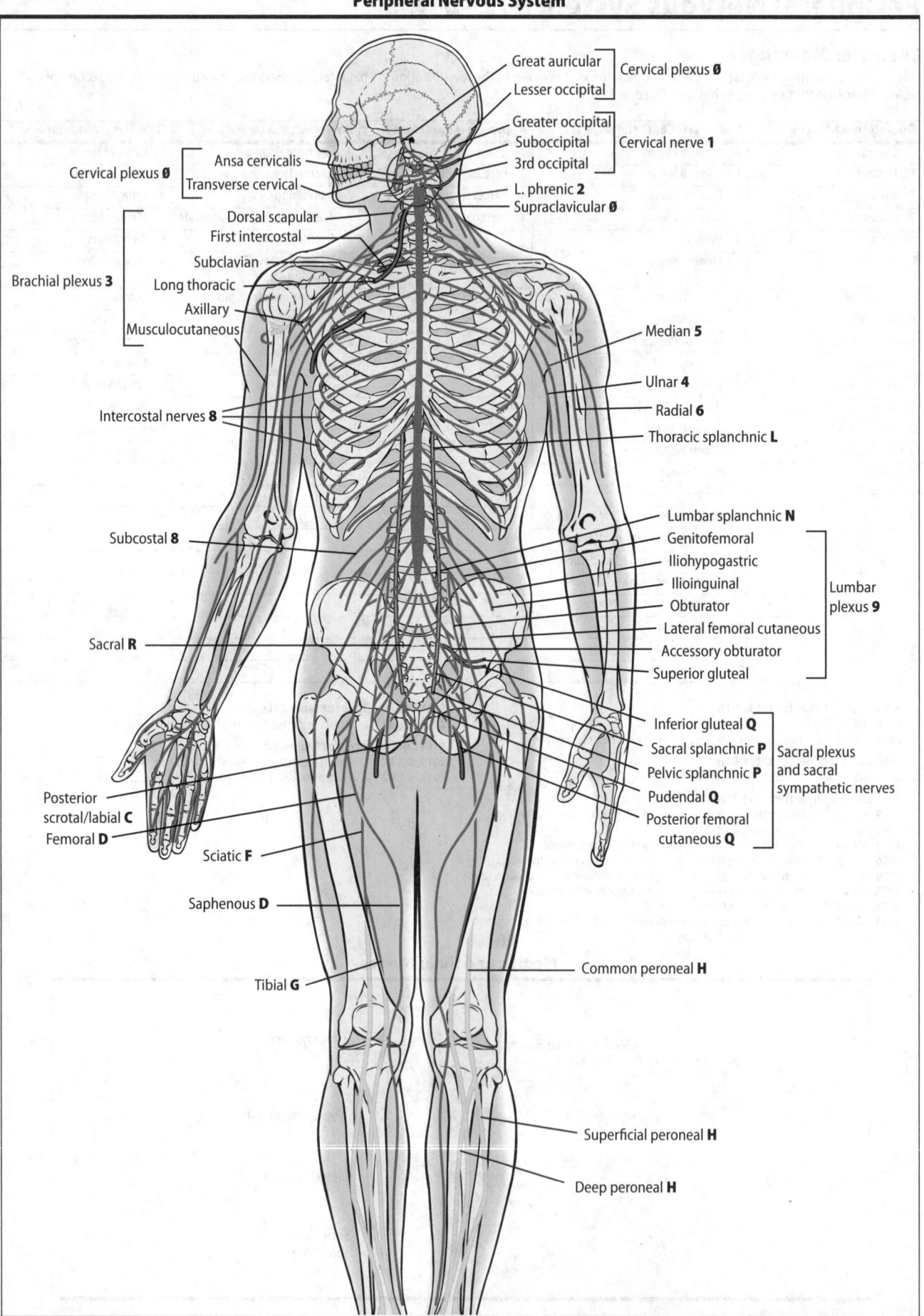

Great auricular
Lesser occipital
} Cervical plexus **Ø**

Greater occipital
Suboccipital
3rd occipital
} Cervical nerve **1**

Cervical plexus **Ø**

Ansa cervicalis
Transverse cervical

L. phrenic **2**
Supraclavicular **Ø**

Dorsal scapular
First intercostal
Subclavian
Long thoracic
Axillary
Musculocutaneous
} Brachial plexus **3**

Median **5**
Ulnar **4**
Radial **6**
Thoracic splanchnic **L**

Intercostal nerves **8**

Subcostal **8**

Lumbar splanchnic **N**
Genitofemoral
Iliohypogastric
Ilioinguinal
Obturator
Lateral femoral cutaneous
Accessory obturator
Superior gluteal
} Lumbar plexus **9**

Sacral **R**

Inferior gluteal **Q**
Sacral splanchnic **P**
Pelvic splanchnic **P**
Pudendal **Q**
Posterior femoral cutaneous **Q**
} Sacral plexus and sacral sympathetic nerves

Posterior scrotal/labial **C**
Femoral **D**
Sciatic **F**

Saphenous **D**

Common peroneal **H**

Tibial **G**

Superficial peroneal **H**

Deep peroneal **H**

Ø   **Medical and Surgical**
1   **Peripheral Nervous System**
2   **Change**   Definition: Taking out or off a device from a body part and putting back an identical or similar device in or on the same body part without cutting or puncturing the skin or a mucous membrane
           Explanation: All CHANGE procedures are coded using the approach EXTERNAL

Body Part Character 4	Approach Character 5	Device Character 6	Qualifier Character 7
Y Peripheral Nerve	X External	Ø Drainage Device Y Other Device	Z No Qualifier

Non-OR   All body part, approach, device, and qualifier values

---

Ø   **Medical and Surgical**
1   **Peripheral Nervous System**   Definition: Physical eradication of all or a portion of a body part by the direct use of energy, force, or a destructive agent
5   **Destruction**   Explanation: None of the body part is physically taken out

Body Part Character 4		Approach Character 5	Device Character 6	Qualifier Character 7

Ø   **Cervical Plexus**
    Ansa cervicalis
    Cutaneous (transverse) cervical nerve
    Great auricular nerve
    Lesser occipital nerve
    Supraclavicular nerve
    Transverse (cutaneous) cervical nerve
1   **Cervical Nerve**
    Greater occipital nerve
    Spinal nerve, cervical
    Suboccipital nerve
    Third occipital nerve
2   **Phrenic Nerve**
    Accessory phrenic nerve
3   **Brachial Plexus**
    Axillary nerve
    Dorsal scapular nerve
    First intercostal nerve
    Long thoracic nerve
    Musculocutaneous nerve
    Subclavius nerve
    Suprascapular nerve
4   **Ulnar Nerve**
    Cubital nerve
5   **Median Nerve**
    Anterior interosseous nerve
    Palmar cutaneous nerve
6   **Radial Nerve**
    Dorsal digital nerve
    Musculospiral nerve
    Palmar cutaneous nerve
    Posterior interosseous nerve
8   **Thoracic Nerve**
    Intercostal nerve
    Intercostobrachial nerve
    Spinal nerve, thoracic
    Subcostal nerve
9   **Lumbar Plexus**
    Accessory obturator nerve
    Genitofemoral nerve
    Iliohypogastric nerve
    Ilioinguinal nerve
    Lateral femoral cutaneous nerve
    Obturator nerve
    Superior gluteal nerve
A   **Lumbosacral Plexus**
B   **Lumbar Nerve**
    Lumbosacral trunk
    Spinal nerve, lumbar
    Superior clunic (cluneal) nerve
C   **Pudendal Nerve**
    Posterior labial nerve
    Posterior scrotal nerve
D   **Femoral Nerve**
    Anterior crural nerve
    Saphenous nerve
F   **Sciatic Nerve**
    Ischiatic nerve
G   **Tibial Nerve**
    Lateral plantar nerve
    Medial plantar nerve
    Medial popliteal nerve
    Medial sural cutaneous nerve
	H **Peroneal Nerve**
	    Common fibular nerve
	    Common peroneal nerve
	    External popliteal nerve
	    Lateral sural cutaneous nerve
	K **Head and Neck Sympathetic Nerve**
	    Cavernous plexus
	    Cervical ganglion
	    Ciliary ganglion
	    Internal carotid plexus
	    Otic ganglion
	    Pterygopalatine (sphenopalatine)
	      ganglion
	    Sphenopalatine (pterygopalatine)
	      ganglion
	    Stellate ganglion
	    Submandibular ganglion
	    Submaxillary ganglion
	L **Thoracic Sympathetic Nerve**
	    Cardiac plexus
	    Esophageal plexus
	    Greater splanchnic nerve
	    Inferior cardiac nerve
	    Least splanchnic nerve
	    Lesser splanchnic nerve
	    Middle cardiac nerve
	    Pulmonary plexus
	    Superior cardiac nerve
	    Thoracic aortic plexus
	    Thoracic ganglion
	M **Abdominal Sympathetic Nerve**
	    Abdominal aortic plexus
	    Auerbach's (myenteric) plexus
	    Celiac (solar) plexus
	    Celiac ganglion
	    Gastric plexus
	    Hepatic plexus
	    Inferior hypogastric plexus
	    Inferior mesenteric ganglion
	    Inferior mesenteric plexus
	    Meissner's (submucous) plexus
	    Myenteric (Auerbach's) plexus
	    Pancreatic plexus
	    Pelvic splanchnic nerve
	    Renal nerve
	    Renal plexus
	    Solar (celiac) plexus
	    Splenic plexus
	    Submucous (Meissner's) plexus
	    Superior hypogastric plexus
	    Superior mesenteric ganglion
	    Superior mesenteric plexus
	    Suprarenal plexus
	N **Lumbar Sympathetic Nerve**
	    Lumbar ganglion
	    Lumbar splanchnic nerve
	P **Sacral Sympathetic Nerve**
	    Ganglion impar (ganglion of
	      Walther)
	    Pelvic splanchnic nerve
	    Sacral ganglion
	    Sacral splanchnic nerve
	Q **Sacral Plexus**
	    Inferior gluteal nerve
	    Posterior femoral cutaneous nerve
	    Pudendal nerve
	R **Sacral Nerve**
	    Spinal nerve, sacral
		Ø Open
		3 Percutaneous
		4 Percutaneous
		     Endoscopic
			Z No Device	Z No Qualifier

Non-OR   Ø15[Ø,2,3,4,5,6,9,A,C,D,F,G,H,Q][Ø,3,4]ZZ   **Non-OR**   Ø15[1,8,B,R]3ZZ

NC Noncovered Procedure   **LC** Limited Coverage   **QA** Questionable OB Admit   **NT** New Tech Add-on   ⊞ Combination Member   ♂ Male   ♀ Female

ICD-10-PCS 2022   155

Ø12–Ø15

Peripheral Nervous System

Ø Medical and Surgical
1 Peripheral Nervous System
8 Division   Definition: Cutting into a body part, without draining fluids and/or gases from the body part, in order to separate or transect a body part
                 Explanation: All or a portion of the body part is separated into two or more portions

Body Part Character 4	Approach Character 5	Device Character 6	Qualifier Character 7
Ø Cervical Plexus Ansa cervicalis Cutaneous (transverse) cervical nerve Great auricular nerve Lesser occipital nerve Supraclavicular nerve Transverse (cutaneous) cervical nerve **1 Cervical Nerve** Greater occipital nerve Spinal nerve, cervical Suboccipital nerve Third occipital nerve **2 Phrenic Nerve** Accessory phrenic nerve **3 Brachial Plexus** Axillary nerve Dorsal scapular nerve First intercostal nerve Long thoracic nerve Musculocutaneous nerve Subclavius nerve Suprascapular nerve **4 Ulnar Nerve** Cubital nerve **5 Median Nerve** Anterior interosseous nerve Palmar cutaneous nerve **6 Radial Nerve** Dorsal digital nerve Musculospiral nerve Palmar cutaneous nerve Posterior interosseous nerve **8 Thoracic Nerve** Intercostal nerve Intercostobrachial nerve Spinal nerve, thoracic Subcostal nerve **9 Lumbar Plexus** Accessory obturator nerve Genitofemoral nerve Iliohypogastric nerve Ilioinguinal nerve Lateral femoral cutaneous nerve Obturator nerve Superior gluteal nerve **A Lumbosacral Plexus** **B Lumbar Nerve** Lumbosacral trunk Spinal nerve, lumbar Superior clunic (cluneal) nerve **C Pudendal Nerve** Posterior labial nerve Posterior scrotal nerve **D Femoral Nerve** Anterior crural nerve Saphenous nerve **F Sciatic Nerve** Ischiatic nerve **G Tibial Nerve** Lateral plantar nerve Medial plantar nerve Medial popliteal nerve Medial sural cutaneous nerve	**H Peroneal Nerve** Common fibular nerve Common peroneal nerve External popliteal nerve Lateral sural cutaneous nerve **K Head and Neck Sympathetic Nerve** Cavernous plexus Cervical ganglion Ciliary ganglion Internal carotid plexus Otic ganglion Pterygopalatine (sphenopalatine) ganglion Sphenopalatine (pterygopalatine) ganglion Stellate ganglion Submandibular ganglion Submaxillary ganglion **L Thoracic Sympathetic Nerve** Cardiac plexus Esophageal plexus Greater splanchnic nerve Inferior cardiac nerve Least splanchnic nerve Lesser splanchnic nerve Middle cardiac nerve Pulmonary plexus Superior cardiac nerve Thoracic aortic plexus Thoracic ganglion **M Abdominal Sympathetic Nerve** Abdominal aortic plexus Auerbach's (myenteric) plexus Celiac (solar) plexus Celiac ganglion Gastric plexus Hepatic plexus Inferior hypogastric plexus Inferior mesenteric ganglion Inferior mesenteric plexus Meissner's (submucous) plexus Myenteric (Auerbach's) plexus Pancreatic plexus Pelvic splanchnic nerve Renal nerve Renal plexus Solar (celiac) plexus Splenic plexus Submucous (Meissner's) plexus Superior hypogastric plexus Superior mesenteric ganglion Superior mesenteric plexus Suprarenal plexus **N Lumbar Sympathetic Nerve** Lumbar ganglion Lumbar splanchnic nerve **P Sacral Sympathetic Nerve** Ganglion impar (ganglion of Walther) Pelvic splanchnic nerve Sacral ganglion Sacral splanchnic nerve **Q Sacral Plexus** Inferior gluteal nerve Posterior femoral cutaneous nerve Pudendal nerve **R Sacral Nerve** Spinal nerve, sacral	**Ø Open** **3 Percutaneous** **4 Percutaneous Endoscopic**	**Z No Device**	**Z No Qualifier**

Ø   **Medical and Surgical**
1   **Peripheral Nervous System**
9   **Drainage**   Definition: Taking or letting out fluids and/or gases from a body part
                   Explanation: The qualifier DIAGNOSTIC is used to identify drainage procedures that are biopsies

Body Part Character 4		Approach Character 5	Device Character 6	Qualifier Character 7

Ø **Cervical Plexus**
  Ansa cervicalis
  Cutaneous (transverse) cervical
    nerve
  Great auricular nerve
  Lesser occipital nerve
  Supraclavicular nerve
  Transverse (cutaneous) cervical
    nerve
1 **Cervical Nerve**
  Greater occipital nerve
  Spinal nerve, cervical
  Suboccipital nerve
  Third occipital nerve
2 **Phrenic Nerve**
  Accessory phrenic nerve
3 **Brachial Plexus**
  Axillary nerve
  Dorsal scapular nerve
  First intercostal nerve
  Long thoracic nerve
  Musculocutaneous nerve
  Subclavius nerve
  Suprascapular nerve
4 **Ulnar Nerve**
  Cubital nerve
5 **Median Nerve**
  Anterior interosseous nerve
  Palmar cutaneous nerve
6 **Radial Nerve**
  Dorsal digital nerve
  Musculospiral nerve
  Palmar cutaneous nerve
  Posterior interosseous nerve
8 **Thoracic Nerve**
  Intercostal nerve
  Intercostobrachial nerve
  Spinal nerve, thoracic
  Subcostal nerve
9 **Lumbar Plexus**
  Accessory obturator nerve
  Genitofemoral nerve
  Iliohypogastric nerve
  Ilioinguinal nerve
  Lateral femoral cutaneous
    nerve
  Obturator nerve
  Superior gluteal nerve
A **Lumbosacral Plexus**
B **Lumbar Nerve**
  Lumbosacral trunk
  Spinal nerve, lumbar
  Superior clunic (cluneal) nerve
C **Pudendal Nerve**
  Posterior labial nerve
  Posterior scrotal nerve
D **Femoral Nerve**
  Anterior crural nerve
  Saphenous nerve
F **Sciatic Nerve**
  Ischiatic nerve
G **Tibial Nerve**
  Lateral plantar nerve
  Medial plantar nerve
  Medial popliteal nerve
  Medial sural cutaneous nerve
	H **Peroneal Nerve**
	  Common fibular nerve
	  Common peroneal nerve
	  External popliteal nerve
	  Lateral sural cutaneous nerve
	K **Head and Neck Sympathetic**
	  Nerve
	  Cavernous plexus
	  Cervical ganglion
	  Ciliary ganglion
	  Internal carotid plexus
	  Otic ganglion
	  Pterygopalatine
	    (sphenopalatine) ganglion
	  Sphenopalatine
	    (pterygopalatine) ganglion
	  Stellate ganglion
	  Submandibular ganglion
	  Submaxillary ganglion
	L **Thoracic Sympathetic Nerve**
	  Cardiac plexus
	  Esophageal plexus
	  Greater splanchnic nerve
	  Inferior cardiac nerve
	  Least splanchnic nerve
	  Lesser splanchnic nerve
	  Middle cardiac nerve
	  Pulmonary plexus
	  Superior cardiac nerve
	  Thoracic aortic plexus
	  Thoracic ganglion
	M **Abdominal Sympathetic**
	  Nerve
	  Abdominal aortic plexus
	  Auerbach's (myenteric) plexus
	  Celiac (solar) plexus
	  Celiac ganglion
	  Gastric plexus
	  Hepatic plexus
	  Inferior hypogastric plexus
	  Inferior mesenteric ganglion
	  Inferior mesenteric plexus
	  Meissner's (submucous) plexus
	  Myenteric (Auerbach's) plexus
	  Pancreatic plexus
	  Pelvic splanchnic nerve
	  Renal nerve
	  Renal plexus
	  Solar (celiac) plexus
	  Splenic plexus
	  Submucous (Meissner's) plexus
	  Superior hypogastric plexus
	  Superior mesenteric ganglion
	  Superior mesenteric plexus
	  Suprarenal plexus
	N **Lumbar Sympathetic Nerve**
	  Lumbar ganglion
	  Lumbar splanchnic nerve
	P **Sacral Sympathetic Nerve**
	  Ganglion impar (ganglion of
	    Walther)
	  Pelvic splanchnic nerve
	  Sacral ganglion
	  Sacral splanchnic nerve
	Q **Sacral Plexus**
	  Inferior gluteal nerve
	  Posterior femoral cutaneous
	    nerve
	  Pudendal nerve
	R **Sacral Nerve**
	  Spinal nerve, sacral
		Ø Open
		3 Percutaneous
		4 Percutaneous Endoscopic
			Ø Drainage Device	Z No Qualifier

Non-OR   019[Ø,1,2,3,4,5,6,8,9,A,B,C,D,F,G,H,K,L,M,N,P,Q,R]3ØZ

019 Continued on next page

NC Noncovered Procedure   LC Limited Coverage   QA Questionable OB Admit   NT New Tech Add-on   ⊞ Combination Member   ♂ Male   ♀ Female

Peripheral Nervous System

Ø	**Medical and Surgical**
1	**Peripheral Nervous System**
9	**Drainage** Definition: Taking or letting out fluids and/or gases from a body part

Ø19 Continued

Explanation: The qualifier DIAGNOSTIC is used to identify drainage procedures that are biopsies

Body Part Character 4		Approach Character 5	Device Character 6	Qualifier Character 7

Ø Cervical Plexus
Ansa cervicalis
Cutaneous (transverse) cervical
  nerve
Great auricular nerve
Lesser occipital nerve
Supraclavicular nerve
Transverse (cutaneous) cervical
  nerve
1 Cervical Nerve
Greater occipital nerve
Spinal nerve, cervical
Suboccipital nerve
Third occipital nerve
2 Phrenic Nerve
Accessory phrenic nerve
3 Brachial Plexus
Axillary nerve
Dorsal scapular nerve
First intercostal nerve
Long thoracic nerve
Musculocutaneous nerve
Subclavius nerve
Suprascapular nerve
4 Ulnar Nerve
Cubital nerve
5 Median Nerve
Anterior interosseous nerve
Palmar cutaneous nerve
6 Radial Nerve
Dorsal digital nerve
Musculospiral nerve
Palmar cutaneous nerve
Posterior interosseous nerve
8 Thoracic Nerve
Intercostal nerve
Intercostobrachial nerve
Spinal nerve, thoracic
Subcostal nerve
9 Lumbar Plexus
Accessory obturator nerve
Genitofemoral nerve
Iliohypogastric nerve
Ilioinguinal nerve
Lateral femoral cutaneous
  nerve
Obturator nerve
Superior gluteal nerve
A Lumbosacral Plexus
B Lumbar Nerve
Lumbosacral trunk
Spinal nerve, lumbar
Superior clunic (cluneal) nerve
C Pudendal Nerve
Posterior labial nerve
Posterior scrotal nerve
D Femoral Nerve
Anterior crural nerve
Saphenous nerve
F Sciatic Nerve
Ischiatic nerve
G Tibial Nerve
Lateral plantar nerve
Medial plantar nerve
Medial popliteal nerve
Medial sural cutaneous nerve
	H Peroneal Nerve
	Common fibular nerve
	Common peroneal nerve
	External popliteal nerve
	Lateral sural cutaneous nerve
	**K Head and Neck Sympathetic
	Nerve**
	Cavernous plexus
	Cervical ganglion
	Ciliary ganglion
	Internal carotid plexus
	Otic ganglion
	Pterygopalatine
	  (sphenopalatine) ganglion
	Sphenopalatine
	  (pterygopalatine) ganglion
	Stellate ganglion
	Submandibular ganglion
	Submaxillary ganglion
	L Thoracic Sympathetic Nerve
	Cardiac plexus
	Esophageal plexus
	Greater splanchnic nerve
	Inferior cardiac nerve
	Least splanchnic nerve
	Lesser splanchnic nerve
	Middle cardiac nerve
	Pulmonary plexus
	Superior cardiac nerve
	Thoracic aortic plexus
	Thoracic ganglion
	**M Abdominal Sympathetic
	Nerve**
	Abdominal aortic plexus
	Auerbach's (myenteric) plexus
	Celiac (solar) plexus
	Celiac ganglion
	Gastric plexus
	Hepatic plexus
	Inferior hypogastric plexus
	Inferior mesenteric ganglion
	Inferior mesenteric plexus
	Meissner's (submucous) plexus
	Myenteric (Auerbach's) plexus
	Pancreatic plexus
	Pelvic splanchnic nerve
	Renal nerve
	Renal plexus
	Solar (celiac) plexus
	Splenic plexus
	Submucous (Meissner's) plexus
	Superior hypogastric plexus
	Superior mesenteric ganglion
	Superior mesenteric plexus
	Suprarenal plexus
	N Lumbar Sympathetic Nerve
	Lumbar ganglion
	Lumbar splanchnic nerve
	P Sacral Sympathetic Nerve
	Ganglion impar (ganglion of
	  Walther)
	Pelvic splanchnic nerve
	Sacral ganglion
	Sacral splanchnic nerve
	Q Sacral Plexus
	Inferior gluteal nerve
	Posterior femoral cutaneous
	  nerve
	Pudendal nerve
	R Sacral Nerve
	Spinal nerve, sacral
		Ø Open
		3 Percutaneous
		4 Percutaneous Endoscopic
			Z No Device	**X Diagnostic**
				Z No Qualifier

Non-OR	Ø19[Ø,1,2,3,4,5,6,8,9,A,B,C,D,F,G,H,Q,R][3,4]ZX
Non-OR	Ø19[Ø,1,2,3,4,5,6,8,9,A,B,C,D,F,G,H,K,L,M,N,P,Q,R]3ZZ

Ø   **Medical and Surgical**
1   **Peripheral Nervous System**
B   **Excision**   Definition: Cutting out or off, without replacement, a portion of a body part

                Explanation: The qualifier DIAGNOSTIC is used to identify excision procedures that are biopsies

Body Part Character 4		Approach Character 5	Device Character 6	Qualifier Character 7

Ø   **Cervical Plexus**
    Ansa cervicalis
    Cutaneous (transverse) cervical
      nerve
    Great auricular nerve
    Lesser occipital nerve
    Supraclavicular nerve
    Transverse (cutaneous) cervical
      nerve
1   **Cervical Nerve**
    Greater occipital nerve
    Spinal nerve, cervical
    Suboccipital nerve
    Third occipital nerve
2   **Phrenic Nerve**
    Accessory phrenic nerve
3   **Brachial Plexus**
    Axillary nerve
    Dorsal scapular nerve
    First intercostal nerve
    Long thoracic nerve
    Musculocutaneous nerve
    Subclavius nerve
    Suprascapular nerve
4   **Ulnar Nerve**
    Cubital nerve
5   **Median Nerve**
    Anterior interosseous nerve
    Palmar cutaneous nerve
6   **Radial Nerve**
    Dorsal digital nerve
    Musculospiral nerve
    Palmar cutaneous nerve
    Posterior interosseous nerve
8   **Thoracic Nerve**
    Intercostal nerve
    Intercostobrachial nerve
    Spinal nerve, thoracic
    Subcostal nerve
9   **Lumbar Plexus**
    Accessory obturator nerve
    Genitofemoral nerve
    Iliohypogastric nerve
    Ilioinguinal nerve
    Lateral femoral cutaneous
      nerve
    Obturator nerve
    Superior gluteal nerve
A   **Lumbosacral Plexus**
B   **Lumbar Nerve**
    Lumbosacral trunk
    Spinal nerve, lumbar
    Superior clunic (cluneal) nerve
C   **Pudendal Nerve**
    Posterior labial nerve
    Posterior scrotal nerve
D   **Femoral Nerve**
    Anterior crural nerve
    Saphenous nerve
F   **Sciatic Nerve**
    Ischiatic nerve
G   **Tibial Nerve**
    Lateral plantar nerve
    Medial plantar nerve
    Medial popliteal nerve
    Medial sural cutaneous nerve
	H **Peroneal Nerve**
	    Common fibular nerve
	    Common peroneal nerve
	    External popliteal nerve
	    Lateral sural cutaneous nerve
	K **Head and Neck Sympathetic**
	    Nerve
	    Cavernous plexus
	    Cervical ganglion
	    Ciliary ganglion
	    Internal carotid plexus
	    Otic ganglion
	    Pterygopalatine
	      (sphenopalatine) ganglion
	    Sphenopalatine
	      (pterygopalatine) ganglion
	    Stellate ganglion
	    Submandibular ganglion
	    Submaxillary ganglion
	L **Thoracic Sympathetic**
	    Nerve
	    Cardiac plexus
	    Esophageal plexus
	    Greater splanchnic nerve
	    Inferior cardiac nerve
	    Least splanchnic nerve
	    Lesser splanchnic nerve
	    Middle cardiac nerve
	    Pulmonary plexus
	    Superior cardiac nerve
	    Thoracic aortic plexus
	    Thoracic ganglion
	M **Abdominal Sympathetic**
	    Nerve
	    Abdominal aortic plexus
	    Auerbach's (myenteric) plexus
	    Celiac (solar) plexus
	    Celiac ganglion
	    Gastric plexus
	    Hepatic plexus
	    Inferior hypogastric plexus
	    Inferior mesenteric ganglion
	    Inferior mesenteric plexus
	    Meissner's (submucous) plexus
	    Myenteric (Auerbach's) plexus
	    Pancreatic plexus
	    Pelvic splanchnic nerve
	    Renal nerve
	    Renal plexus
	    Solar (celiac) plexus
	    Splenic plexus
	    Submucous (Meissner's) plexus
	    Superior hypogastric plexus
	    Superior mesenteric ganglion
	    Superior mesenteric plexus
	    Suprarenal plexus
	N **Lumbar Sympathetic Nerve**
	    Lumbar ganglion
	    Lumbar splanchnic nerve
	P **Sacral Sympathetic Nerve**
	    Ganglion impar (ganglion of
	      Walther)
	    Pelvic splanchnic nerve
	    Sacral ganglion
	    Sacral splanchnic nerve
	Q **Sacral Plexus**
	    Inferior gluteal nerve
	    Posterior femoral cutaneous
	      nerve
	    Pudendal nerve
	R **Sacral Nerve**
	    Spinal nerve, sacral
		Ø Open
		3 Percutaneous
		4 Percutaneous Endoscopic
			Z No Device	**X** Diagnostic
				Z No Qualifier

Non-OR   Ø1B[Ø,1,2,3,4,5,6,8,9,A,B,C,D,F,G,H,Q,R][3,4]ZX

NC Noncovered Procedure   LC Limited Coverage   QA Questionable OB Admit   NT New Tech Add-on   ⊞ Combination Member   ♂ Male   ♀ Female

ICD-10-PCS 2022   **159**

Ø1B–Ø1B

Peripheral Nervous System

0   **Medical and Surgical**
1   **Peripheral Nervous System**
C   **Extirpation**   Definition: Taking or cutting out solid matter from a body part
                 Explanation: The solid matter may be an abnormal byproduct of a biological function or a foreign body; it may be imbedded in a body part or in the lumen of a tubular body part. The solid matter may or may not have been previously broken into pieces.

Body Part Character 4	Approach Character 5	Device Character 6	Qualifier Character 7

0 Cervical Plexus
  Ansa cervicalis
  Cutaneous (transverse) cervical
    nerve
  Great auricular nerve
  Lesser occipital nerve
  Supraclavicular nerve
  Transverse (cutaneous) cervical
    nerve
1 Cervical Nerve
  Greater occipital nerve
  Spinal nerve, cervical
  Suboccipital nerve
  Third occipital nerve
2 Phrenic Nerve
  Accessory phrenic nerve
3 Brachial Plexus
  Axillary nerve
  Dorsal scapular nerve
  First intercostal nerve
  Long thoracic nerve
  Musculocutaneous nerve
  Subclavius nerve
  Suprascapular nerve
4 Ulnar Nerve
  Cubital nerve
5 Median Nerve
  Anterior interosseous nerve
  Palmar cutaneous nerve
6 Radial Nerve
  Dorsal digital nerve
  Musculospiral nerve
  Palmar cutaneous nerve
  Posterior interosseous nerve
8 Thoracic Nerve
  Intercostal nerve
  Intercostobrachial nerve
  Spinal nerve, thoracic
  Subcostal nerve
9 Lumbar Plexus
  Accessory obturator nerve
  Genitofemoral nerve
  Iliohypogastric nerve
  Ilioinguinal nerve
  Lateral femoral cutaneous
    nerve
  Obturator nerve
  Superior gluteal nerve
A Lumbosacral Plexus
B Lumbar Nerve
  Lumbosacral trunk
  Spinal nerve, lumbar
  Superior clunic (cluneal) nerve
C Pudendal Nerve
  Posterior labial nerve
  Posterior scrotal nerve
D Femoral Nerve
  Anterior crural nerve
  Saphenous nerve
F Sciatic Nerve
  Ischiatic nerve
G Tibial Nerve
  Lateral plantar nerve
  Medial plantar nerve
  Medial popliteal nerve
  Medial sural cutaneous nerve
	0 Open
	3 Percutaneous
	4 Percutaneous Endoscopic
		Z No Device	**Z No Qualifier**

H Peroneal Nerve
  Common fibular nerve
  Common peroneal nerve
  External popliteal nerve
  Lateral sural cutaneous nerve
K Head and Neck Sympathetic
  Nerve
  Cavernous plexus
  Cervical ganglion
  Ciliary ganglion
  Internal carotid plexus
  Otic ganglion
  Pterygopalatine
    (sphenopalatine) ganglion
  Sphenopalatine
    (pterygopalatine) ganglion
  Stellate ganglion
  Submandibular ganglion
  Submaxillary ganglion
L Thoracic Sympathetic Nerve
  Cardiac plexus
  Esophageal plexus
  Greater splanchnic nerve
  Inferior cardiac nerve
  Least splanchnic nerve
  Lesser splanchnic nerve
  Middle cardiac nerve
  Pulmonary plexus
  Superior cardiac nerve
  Thoracic aortic plexus
  Thoracic ganglion
M Abdominal Sympathetic
  Nerve
  Abdominal aortic plexus
  Auerbach's (myenteric) plexus
  Celiac (solar) plexus
  Celiac ganglion
  Gastric plexus
  Hepatic plexus
  Inferior hypogastric plexus
  Inferior mesenteric ganglion
  Inferior mesenteric plexus
  Meissner's (submucous) plexus
  Myenteric (Auerbach's) plexus
  Pancreatic plexus
  Pelvic splanchnic nerve
  Renal nerve
  Renal plexus
  Solar (celiac) plexus
  Splenic plexus
  Submucous (Meissner's) plexus
  Superior hypogastric plexus
  Superior mesenteric ganglion
  Superior mesenteric plexus
  Suprarenal plexus
N Lumbar Sympathetic Nerve
  Lumbar ganglion
  Lumbar splanchnic nerve
P Sacral Sympathetic Nerve
  Ganglion impar (ganglion of
    Walther)
  Pelvic splanchnic nerve
  Sacral ganglion
  Sacral splanchnic nerve
Q Sacral Plexus
  Inferior gluteal nerve
  Posterior femoral cutaneous
    nerve
  Pudendal nerve
R Sacral Nerve
  Spinal nerve, sacral			

0　Medical and Surgical
1　Peripheral Nervous System
D　Extraction　　Definition: Pulling or stripping out or off all or a portion of a body part by the use of force
　　　　　　　　　　Explanation: The qualifier DIAGNOSTIC is used to identify extraction procedures that are biopsies

Body Part Character 4		Approach Character 5	Device Character 6	Qualifier Character 7
0　Cervical Plexus 　　Ansa cervicalis 　　Cutaneous (transverse) cervical 　　　nerve 　　Great auricular nerve 　　Lesser occipital nerve 　　Supraclavicular nerve 　　Transverse (cutaneous) cervical 　　　nerve **1　Cervical Nerve** 　　Greater occipital nerve 　　Spinal nerve, cervical 　　Suboccipital nerve 　　Third occipital nerve **2　Phrenic Nerve** 　　Accessory phrenic nerve **3　Brachial Plexus** 　　Axillary nerve 　　Dorsal scapular nerve 　　First intercostal nerve 　　Long thoracic nerve 　　Musculocutaneous nerve 　　Subclavius nerve 　　Suprascapular nerve **4　Ulnar Nerve** 　　Cubital nerve **5　Median Nerve** 　　Anterior interosseous nerve 　　Palmar cutaneous nerve **6　Radial Nerve** 　　Dorsal digital nerve 　　Musculospiral nerve 　　Palmar cutaneous nerve 　　Posterior interosseous nerve **8　Thoracic Nerve** 　　Intercostal nerve 　　Intercostobrachial nerve 　　Spinal nerve, thoracic 　　Subcostal nerve **9　Lumbar Plexus** 　　Accessory obturator nerve 　　Genitofemoral nerve 　　Iliohypogastric nerve 　　Ilioinguinal nerve 　　Lateral femoral cutaneous nerve 　　Obturator nerve 　　Superior gluteal nerve **A　Lumbosacral Plexus** **B　Lumbar Nerve** 　　Lumbosacral trunk 　　Spinal nerve, lumbar 　　Superior clunic (cluneal) nerve **C　Pudendal Nerve]** 　　Posterior labial nerve 　　Posterior scrotal nerve **D　Femoral Nerve** 　　Anterior crural nerve 　　Saphenous nerve **F　Sciatic Nerve** 　　Ischiatic nerve **G　Tibial Nerve** 　　Lateral plantar nerve 　　Medial plantar nerve 　　Medial popliteal nerve 　　Medial sural cutaneous nerve	**H　Peroneal Nerve** 　　Common fibular nerve 　　Common peroneal nerve 　　External popliteal nerve 　　Lateral sural cutaneous nerve **K　Head and Neck Sympathetic 　　Nerve** 　　Cavernous plexus 　　Cervical ganglion 　　Ciliary ganglion 　　Internal carotid plexus 　　Otic ganglion 　　Pterygopalatine 　　　(sphenopalatine) ganglion 　　Sphenopalatine 　　　(pterygopalatine) ganglion 　　Stellate ganglion 　　Submandibular ganglion 　　Submaxillary ganglion **L　Thoracic Sympathetic Nerve** 　　Cardiac plexus 　　Esophageal plexus 　　Greater splanchnic nerve 　　Inferior cardiac nerve 　　Least splanchnic nerve 　　Lesser splanchnic nerve 　　Middle cardiac nerve 　　Pulmonary plexus 　　Superior cardiac nerve 　　Thoracic aortic plexus 　　Thoracic ganglion **M　Abdominal Sympathetic Nerve** 　　Abdominal aortic plexus 　　Auerbach's (myenteric) plexus 　　Celiac (solar) plexus 　　Celiac ganglion 　　Gastric plexus 　　Hepatic plexus 　　Inferior hypogastric plexus 　　Inferior mesenteric ganglion 　　Inferior mesenteric plexus 　　Meissner's (submucous) plexus 　　Myenteric (Auerbach's) plexus 　　Pancreatic plexus 　　Pelvic splanchnic nerve 　　Renal nerve 　　Renal plexus 　　Solar (celiac) plexus 　　Splenic plexus 　　Submucous (Meissner's) plexus 　　Superior hypogastric plexus 　　Superior mesenteric ganglion 　　Superior mesenteric plexus 　　Suprarenal plexus **N　Lumbar Sympathetic Nerve** 　　Lumbar ganglion 　　Lumbar splanchnic nerve **P　Sacral Sympathetic Nerve** 　　Ganglion impar (ganglion of 　　　Walther) 　　Pelvic splanchnic nerve 　　Sacral ganglion 　　Sacral splanchnic nerve **Q　Sacral Plexus** 　　Inferior gluteal nerve 　　Posterior femoral cutaneous 　　　nerve 　　Pudendal nerve **R　Sacral Nerve** 　　Spinal nerve, sacral	**0　Open** **3　Percutaneous** **4　Percutaneous Endoscopic**	**Z　No Device**	**Z　No Qualifier**

NC Noncovered Procedure　　LC Limited Coverage　　OA Questionable OB Admit　　NT New Tech Add-on　　⊞ Combination Member　　♂ Male　　♀ Female
ICD-10-PCS 2022　　161

01D–01D

Peripheral Nervous System

Ø   **Medical and Surgical**
1   **Peripheral Nervous System**
H   **Insertion**   Definition: Putting in a nonbiological appliance that monitors, assists, performs, or prevents a physiological function but does not physically take the place of a body part

Explanation: None

Body Part Character 4		Approach Character 5	Device Character 6	Qualifier Character 7
Y Peripheral Nerve	⊞	Ø Open 3 Percutaneous 4 Percutaneous Endoscopic	1 Radioactive Element 2 Monitoring Device M Neurostimulator Lead Y Other Device	Z No Qualifier

Non-OR	01HY31Z	
Non-OR	01HY[3,4]YZ	**See Appendix L for Procedure Combinations** ⊞ 01HY[0,3,4]MZ

Ø   **Medical and Surgical**
1   **Peripheral Nervous System**
J   **Inspection**   Definition: Visually and/or manually exploring a body part

Explanation: Visual exploration may be performed with or without optical instrumentation. Manual exploration may be performed directly or through intervening body layers.

Body Part Character 4	Approach Character 5	Device Character 6	Qualifier Character 7
Y Peripheral Nerve	Ø Open 3 Percutaneous 4 Percutaneous Endoscopic	Z No Device	Z No Qualifier

Non-OR	01JY3ZZ

Ø   **Medical and Surgical**
1   **Peripheral Nervous System**
N   **Release**   Definition: Freeing a body part from an abnormal physical constraint by cutting or by the use of force
            Explanation: Some of the restraining tissue may be taken out but none of the body part is taken out

Body Part Character 4		Approach Character 5	Device Character 6	Qualifier Character 7

Ø Cervical Plexus
Ansa cervicalis
Cutaneous (transverse) cervical
  nerve
Great auricular nerve
Lesser occipital nerve
Supraclavicular nerve
Transverse (cutaneous) cervical
  nerve
1 Cervical Nerve
Greater occipital nerve
Spinal nerve, cervical
Suboccipital nerve
Third occipital nerve
2 Phrenic Nerve
Accessory phrenic nerve
3 Brachial Plexus
Axillary nerve
Dorsal scapular nerve
First intercostal nerve
Long thoracic nerve
Musculocutaneous nerve
Subclavius nerve
Suprascapular nerve
4 Ulnar Nerve
Cubital nerve
5 Median Nerve
Anterior interosseous nerve
Palmar cutaneous nerve
6 Radial Nerve
Dorsal digital nerve
Musculospiral nerve
Palmar cutaneous nerve
Posterior interosseous nerve
8 Thoracic Nerve
Intercostal nerve
Intercostobrachial nerve
Spinal nerve, thoracic
Subcostal nerve
9 Lumbar Plexus
Accessory obturator nerve
Genitofemoral nerve
Iliohypogastric nerve
Ilioinguinal nerve
Lateral femoral cutaneous nerve
Obturator nerve
Superior gluteal nerve
A Lumbosacral Plexus
B Lumbar Nerve
Lumbosacral trunk
Spinal nerve, lumbar
Superior clunic (cluneal) nerve
C Pudendal Nerve
Posterior labial nerve
Posterior scrotal nerve
D Femoral Nerve
Anterior crural nerve
Saphenous nerve
F Sciatic Nerve
Ischiatic nerve
G Tibial Nerve
Lateral plantar nerve
Medial plantar nerve
Medial popliteal nerve
Medial sural cutaneous nerve
	H Peroneal Nerve
	Common fibular nerve
	Common peroneal nerve
	External popliteal nerve
	Lateral sural cutaneous nerve
	K Head and Neck Sympathetic Nerve
	Cavernous plexus
	Cervical ganglion
	Ciliary ganglion
	Internal carotid plexus
	Otic ganglion
	Pterygopalatine
	  (sphenopalatine) ganglion
	Sphenopalatine
	  (pterygopalatine) ganglion
	Stellate ganglion
	Submandibular ganglion
	Submaxillary ganglion
	L Thoracic Sympathetic Nerve
	Cardiac plexus
	Esophageal plexus
	Greater splanchnic nerve
	Inferior cardiac nerve
	Least splanchnic nerve
	Lesser splanchnic nerve
	Middle cardiac nerve
	Pulmonary plexus
	Superior cardiac nerve
	Thoracic aortic plexus
	Thoracic ganglion
	M Abdominal Sympathetic Nerve
	Abdominal aortic plexus
	Auerbach's (myenteric) plexus
	Celiac (solar) plexus
	Celiac ganglion
	Gastric plexus
	Hepatic plexus
	Inferior hypogastric plexus
	Inferior mesenteric ganglion
	Inferior mesenteric plexus
	Meissner's (submucous) plexus
	Myenteric (Auerbach's) plexus
	Pancreatic plexus
	Pelvic splanchnic nerve
	Renal nerve
	Renal plexus
	Solar (celiac) plexus
	Splenic plexus
	Submucous (Meissner's) plexus
	Superior hypogastric plexus
	Superior mesenteric ganglion
	Superior mesenteric plexus
	Suprarenal plexus
	N Lumbar Sympathetic Nerve
	Lumbar ganglion
	Lumbar splanchnic nerve
	P Sacral Sympathetic Nerve
	Ganglion impar (ganglion of
	  Walther)
	Pelvic splanchnic nerve
	Sacral ganglion
	Sacral splanchnic nerve
	Q Sacral Plexus
	Inferior gluteal nerve
	Posterior femoral cutaneous
	  nerve
	Pudendal nerve
	R Sacral Nerve
	Spinal nerve, sacral
		Ø Open
		3 Percutaneous
		4 Percutaneous Endoscopic
			Z No Device	**Z No Qualifier**

NC Noncovered Procedure   **LC** Limited Coverage   **QA** Questionable OB Admit   **NT** New Tech Add-on   ⊞ Combination Member   ♂ Male   ♀ Female

ICD-10-PCS 2022   163

Ø1N–Ø1N

0 **Medical and Surgical**
1 **Peripheral Nervous System**
P **Removal**   Definition: Taking out or off a device from a body part

Explanation: If a device is taken out and a similar device put in without cutting or puncturing the skin or mucous membrane, the procedure is coded to the root operation CHANGE. Otherwise, the procedure for taking out a device is coded to the root operation REMOVAL.

Body Part Character 4	Approach Character 5	Device Character 6	Qualifier Character 7
Y Peripheral Nerve	**0** Open **3** Percutaneous **4** Percutaneous Endoscopic	**0** Drainage Device **2** Monitoring Device **7** Autologous Tissue Substitute **M** Neurostimulator Lead **Y** Other Device	**Z** No Qualifier
Y Peripheral Nerve	**X** External	**0** Drainage Device **2** Monitoring Device **M** Neurostimulator Lead	**Z** No Qualifier

Non-OR 01PY3[0,2]Z
Non-OR 01PY[3,4]YZ
Non-OR 01PYX[0,2,M]Z

Peripheral Nervous System

0   **Medical and Surgical**
1   **Peripheral Nervous System**
Q   **Repair**   Definition: Restoring, to the extent possible, a body part to its normal anatomic structure and function
                          Explanation: Used only when the method to accomplish the repair is not one of the other root operations

Body Part Character 4		Approach Character 5	Device Character 6	Qualifier Character 7

0 **Cervical Plexus**
    Ansa cervicalis
    Cutaneous (transverse) cervical
        nerve
    Great auricular nerve
    Lesser occipital nerve
    Supraclavicular nerve
    Transverse (cutaneous) cervical
        nerve
1 **Cervical Nerve**
    Greater occipital nerve
    Spinal nerve, cervical
    Suboccipital nerve
    Third occipital nerve
2 **Phrenic Nerve**
    Accessory phrenic nerve
3 **Brachial Plexus**
    Axillary nerve
    Dorsal scapular nerve
    First intercostal nerve
    Long thoracic nerve
    Musculocutaneous nerve
    Subclavius nerve
    Suprascapular nerve
4 **Ulnar Nerve**
    Cubital nerve
5 **Median Nerve**
    Anterior interosseous nerve
    Palmar cutaneous nerve
6 **Radial Nerve**
    Dorsal digital nerve
    Musculospiral nerve
    Palmar cutaneous nerve
    Posterior interosseous nerve
8 **Thoracic Nerve**
    Intercostal nerve
    Intercostobrachial nerve
    Spinal nerve, thoracic
    Subcostal nerve
9 **Lumbar Plexus**
    Accessory obturator nerve
    Genitofemoral nerve
    Iliohypogastric nerve
    Ilioinguinal nerve
    Lateral femoral cutaneous
        nerve
    Obturator nerve
    Superior gluteal nerve
A **Lumbosacral Plexus**
B **Lumbar Nerve**
    Lumbosacral trunk
    Spinal nerve, lumbar
    Superior clunic (cluneal) nerve
C **Pudendal Nerve**
    Posterior labial nerve
    Posterior scrotal nerve
D **Femoral Nerve**
    Anterior crural nerve
    Saphenous nerve
F **Sciatic Nerve**
    Ischiatic nerve
G **Tibial Nerve**
    Lateral plantar nerve
    Medial plantar nerve
    Medial popliteal nerve
    Medial sural cutaneous nerve
	H **Peroneal Nerve**
	    Common fibular nerve
	    Common peroneal nerve
	    External popliteal nerve
	    Lateral sural cutaneous nerve
	K **Head and Neck Sympathetic**
	    Nerve
	    Cavernous plexus
	    Cervical ganglion
	    Ciliary ganglion
	    Internal carotid plexus
	    Otic ganglion
	    Pterygopalatine
	        (sphenopalatine) ganglion
	    Sphenopalatine
	        (pterygopalatine) ganglion
	    Stellate ganglion
	    Submandibular ganglion
	    Submaxillary ganglion
	L **Thoracic Sympathetic Nerve**
	    Cardiac plexus
	    Esophageal plexus
	    Greater splanchnic nerve
	    Inferior cardiac nerve
	    Least splanchnic nerve
	    Lesser splanchnic nerve
	    Middle cardiac nerve
	    Pulmonary plexus
	    Superior cardiac nerve
	    Thoracic aortic plexus
	    Thoracic ganglion
	M **Abdominal Sympathetic**
	    Nerve
	    Abdominal aortic plexus
	    Auerbach's (myenteric) plexus
	    Celiac (solar) plexus
	    Celiac ganglion
	    Gastric plexus
	    Hepatic plexus
	    Inferior hypogastric plexus
	    Inferior mesenteric ganglion
	    Inferior mesenteric plexus
	    Meissner's (submucous) plexus
	    Myenteric (Auerbach's) plexus
	    Pancreatic plexus
	    Pelvic splanchnic nerve
	    Renal nerve
	    Renal plexus
	    Solar (celiac) plexus
	    Splenic plexus
	    Submucous (Meissner's) plexus
	    Superior hypogastric plexus
	    Superior mesenteric ganglion
	    Superior mesenteric plexus
	    Suprarenal plexus
	N **Lumbar Sympathetic Nerve**
	    Lumbar ganglion
	    Lumbar splanchnic nerve
	P **Sacral Sympathetic Nerve**
	    Ganglion impar (ganglion of
	        Walther)
	    Pelvic splanchnic nerve
	    Sacral ganglion
	    Sacral splanchnic nerve
	Q **Sacral Plexus**
	    Inferior gluteal nerve
	    Posterior femoral cutaneous
	        nerve
	    Pudendal nerve
	R **Sacral Nerve**
	    Spinal nerve, sacral
		0 Open
		3 Percutaneous
		4 Percutaneous Endoscopic
			Z No Device	**Z** No Qualifier

NC Noncovered Procedure   **LC** Limited Coverage   **QA** Questionable OB Admit   **NT** New Tech Add-on   **⊞** Combination Member   ♂ Male   ♀ Female

ICD-10-PCS 2022   **165**

Peripheral Nervous System

01Q–01Q

Peripheral Nervous System

Ø   Medical and Surgical
1   Peripheral Nervous System
R   Replacement   Definition: Putting in or on biological or synthetic material that physically takes the place and/or function of all or a portion of a body part

Explanation: The body part may have been taken out or replaced, or may be taken out, physically eradicated, or rendered nonfunctional during the REPLACEMENT procedure. A REMOVAL procedure is coded for taking out the device used in a previous replacement procedure.

Body Part Character 4	Approach Character 5	Device Character 6	Qualifier Character 7
1 Cervical Nerve Greater occipital nerve Spinal nerve, cervical Suboccipital nerve Third occipital nerve **2 Phrenic Nerve** Accessory phrenic nerve **4 Ulnar Nerve** Cubital nerve **5 Median Nerve** Anterior interosseous nerve Palmar cutaneous nerve **6 Radial Nerve** Dorsal digital nerve Musculospiral nerve Palmar cutaneous nerve Posterior interosseous nerve **8 Thoracic Nerve** Intercostal nerve Intercostobrachial nerve Spinal nerve, thoracic Subcostal nerve **B Lumbar Nerve** Lumbosacral trunk Spinal nerve, lumbar Superior clunic (cluneal) nerve **C Pudendal Nerve** Posterior labial nerve Posterior scrotal nerve **D Femoral Nerve** Anterior crural nerve Saphenous nerve **F Sciatic Nerve** Ischiatic nerve **G Tibial Nerve** Lateral plantar nerve Medial plantar nerve Medial popliteal nerve Medial sural cutaneous nerve **H Peroneal Nerve** Common fibular nerve Common peroneal nerve External popliteal nerve Lateral sural cutaneous nerve **R Sacral Nerve** Spinal nerve, sacral	**Ø** Open **4** Percutaneous Endoscopic	**7** Autologous Tissue Substitute **J** Synthetic Substitute **K** Nonautologous Tissue Substitute	**Z** No Qualifier

0 Medical and Surgical
1 Peripheral Nervous System
S Reposition   Definition: Moving to its normal location, or other suitable location, all or a portion of a body part

                 Explanation: The body part is moved to a new location from an abnormal location, or from a normal location where it is not functioning correctly. The body part may or may not be cut out or off to be moved to the new location.

Body Part Character 4	Approach Character 5	Device Character 6	Qualifier Character 7
0 Cervical Plexus Ansa cervicalis Cutaneous (transverse) cervical nerve Great auricular nerve Lesser occipital nerve Supraclavicular nerve Transverse (cutaneous) cervical nerve **1 Cervical Nerve** Greater occipital nerve Spinal nerve, cervical Suboccipital nerve Third occipital nerve **2 Phrenic Nerve** Accessory phrenic nerve **3 Brachial Plexus** Axillary nerve Dorsal scapular nerve First intercostal nerve Long thoracic nerve Musculocutaneous nerve Subclavius nerve Suprascapular nerve **4 Ulnar Nerve** Cubital nerve **5 Median Nerve** Anterior interosseous nerve Palmar cutaneous nerve **6 Radial Nerve** Dorsal digital nerve Musculospiral nerve Palmar cutaneous nerve Posterior interosseous nerve **8 Thoracic Nerve** Intercostal nerve Intercostobrachial nerve Spinal nerve, thoracic Subcostal nerve **9 Lumbar Plexus** Accessory obturator nerve Genitofemoral nerve Iliohypogastric nerve Ilioinguinal nerve Lateral femoral cutaneous nerve Obturator nerve Superior gluteal nerve **A Lumbosacral Plexus** **B Lumbar Nerve** Lumbosacral trunk Spinal nerve, lumbar Superior clunic (cluneal) nerve **C Pudendal Nerve** Posterior labial nerve Posterior scrotal nerve **D Femoral Nerve** Anterior crural nerve Saphenous nerve **F Sciatic Nerve** Ischiatic nerve **G Tibial Nerve** Lateral plantar nerve Medial plantar nerve Medial popliteal nerve Medial sural cutaneous nerve **H Peroneal Nerve** Common fibular nerve Common peroneal nerve External popliteal nerve Lateral sural cutaneous nerve **Q Sacral Plexus** Inferior gluteal nerve Posterior femoral cutaneous nerve Pudendal nerve **R Sacral Nerve** Spinal nerve, sacral	**0 Open** **3 Percutaneous** **4 Percutaneous Endoscopic**	**Z No Device**	**Z No Qualifier**

Peripheral Nervous System (side tab)

Ø   **Medical and Surgical**
1   **Peripheral Nervous System**
U   **Supplement**   Definition: Putting in or on biological or synthetic material that physically reinforces and/or augments the function of a portion of a body part
          Explanation: The biological material is non-living, or is living and from the same individual. The body part may have been previously replaced, and the SUPPLEMENT procedure is performed to physically reinforce and/or augment the function of the replaced body part.

Body Part Character 4	Approach Character 5	Device Character 6	Qualifier Character 7

1 Cervical Nerve
  Greater occipital nerve
  Spinal nerve, cervical
  Suboccipital nerve
  Third occipital nerve
2 Phrenic Nerve
  Accessory phrenic nerve
4 Ulnar Nerve
  Cubital nerve
5 Median Nerve
  Anterior interosseous nerve
  Palmar cutaneous nerve
6 Radial Nerve
  Dorsal digital nerve
  Musculospiral nerve
  Palmar cutaneous nerve
  Posterior interosseous nerve
8 Thoracic Nerve
  Intercostal nerve
  Intercostobrachial nerve
  Spinal nerve, thoracic
  Subcostal nerve
B Lumbar Nerve
  Lumbosacral trunk
  Spinal nerve, lumbar
  Superior clunic (cluneal) nerve
C Pudendal Nerve
  Posterior labial nerve
  Posterior scrotal nerve
D Femoral Nerve
  Anterior crural nerve
  Saphenous nerve
F Sciatic Nerve
  Ischiatic nerve
G Tibial Nerve
  Lateral plantar nerve
  Medial plantar nerve
  Medial popliteal nerve
  Medial sural cutaneous nerve
H Peroneal Nerve
  Common fibular nerve
  Common peroneal nerve
  External popliteal nerve
  Lateral sural cutaneous nerve
R Sacral Nerve
  Spinal nerve, sacral
	Ø Open
	3 Percutaneous
	4 Percutaneous Endoscopic
		7 Autologous Tissue Substitute
		J Synthetic Substitute
		K Nonautologous Tissue Substitute
			Z No Qualifier

Ø   **Medical and Surgical**
1   **Peripheral Nervous System**
W   **Revision**   Definition: Correcting, to the extent possible, a portion of a malfunctioning device or the position of a displaced device
          Explanation: Revision can include correcting a malfunctioning or displaced device by taking out or putting in components of the device such as a screw or pin

Body Part Character 4	Approach Character 5	Device Character 6	Qualifier Character 7
Y Peripheral Nerve	**Ø** Open **3** Percutaneous **4** Percutaneous Endoscopic	**Ø** Drainage Device **2** Monitoring Device **7** Autologous Tissue Substitute **M** Neurostimulator Lead **Y** Other Device	**Z** No Qualifier
Y Peripheral Nerve	**X** External	**Ø** Drainage Device **2** Monitoring Device **7** Autologous Tissue Substitute **M** Neurostimulator Lead	**Z** No Qualifier

Non-OR   Ø1WY[3,4]YZ
Non-OR   Ø1WYX[Ø,2,7,M]Z

Ø   Medical and Surgical
1   Peripheral Nervous System
X   Transfer   Definition: Moving, without taking out, all or a portion of a body part to another location to take over the function of all or a portion of a body part
         Explanation: The body part transferred remains connected to its vascular and nervous supply

Body Part Character 4	Approach Character 5	Device Character 6	Qualifier Character 7

1   Cervical Nerve
    Greater occipital nerve
    Spinal nerve, cervical
    Suboccipital nerve
    Third occipital nerve
2   Phrenic Nerve
    Accessory phrenic nerve
	Ø Open
	4 Percutaneous Endoscopic
		Z No Device	**1 Cervical Nerve**
			2 Phrenic Nerve

4   Ulnar Nerve
    Cubital nerve
5   Median Nerve
    Anterior interosseous nerve
    Palmar cutaneous nerve
6   Radial Nerve
    Dorsal digital nerve
    Musculospiral nerve
    Palmar cutaneous nerve
    Posterior interosseous nerve
	Ø Open
	4 Percutaneous Endoscopic
		Z No Device	**4 Ulnar Nerve**
			5 Median Nerve
			6 Radial Nerve

8   Thoracic Nerve
    Intercostal nerve
    Intercostobrachial nerve
    Spinal nerve, thoracic
    Subcostal nerve
	Ø Open
	4 Percutaneous Endoscopic
		Z No Device	**8 Thoracic Nerve**

B   Lumbar Nerve
    Lumbosacral trunk
    Spinal nerve, lumbar
    Superior clunic (cluneal) nerve
C   Pudendal Nerve
    Posterior labial nerve
    Posterior scrotal nerve
	Ø Open
	4 Percutaneous Endoscopic
		Z No Device	**B Lumbar Nerve**
			C Perineal Nerve

D   Femoral Nerve
    Anterior crural nerve
    Saphenous nerve
F   Sciatic Nerve
    Ischiatic nerve
G   Tibial Nerve
    Lateral plantar nerve
    Medial plantar nerve
    Medial popliteal nerve
    Medial sural cutaneous nerve
H   Peroneal Nerve
    Common fibular nerve
    Common peroneal nerve
    External popliteal nerve
    Lateral sural cutaneous nerve
	Ø Open
	4 Percutaneous Endoscopic
		Z No Device	**D Femoral Nerve**
			F Sciatic Nerve
			G Tibial Nerve
			H Peroneal Nerve

NC Noncovered Procedure   **LC** Limited Coverage   **QA** Questionable OB Admit   **NT** New Tech Add-on   ⊞ Combination Member   ♂ Male   ♀ Female

ICD-10-PCS 2022   **169**

01X–01X

Heart and Great Vessels Ø21–Ø2Y

Character Meanings

This Character Meaning table is provided as a guide to assist the user in the identification of character members that may be found in this section of code tables. It **SHOULD NOT** be used to build a PCS code.

Operation–Character 3	Body Part–Character 4	Approach–Character 5	Device–Character 6	Qualifier–Character 7
1 Bypass	Ø Coronary Artery, One Artery	Ø Open	Ø Monitoring Device, Pressure Sensor	Ø Allogeneic OR Ultrasonic
4 Creation	1 Coronary Artery, Two Arteries	3 Percutaneous	2 Monitoring Device	1 Syngeneic
5 Destruction	2 Coronary Artery, Three Arteries	4 Percutaneous Endoscopic	3 Infusion Device	2 Zooplastic OR Common Atrioventricular Valve
7 Dilation	3 Coronary Artery, Four or More Arteries	X External	4 Intraluminal Device, Drug-eluting	3 Coronary Artery
8 Division	4 Coronary Vein		5 Intraluminal Device, Drug-eluting, Two	4 Coronary Vein
B Excision	5 Atrial Septum		6 Intraluminal Device, Drug-eluting, Three	5 Coronary Circulation
C Extirpation	6 Atrium, Right		7 Intraluminal Device, Drug-eluting, Four or More OR Autologous Tissue Substitute	6 Bifurcation OR Atrium, Right
F Fragmentation	7 Atrium, Left		8 Zooplastic Tissue	7 Atrium, Left OR Orbital Atherectomy Technique
H Insertion	8 Conduction Mechanism		9 Autologous Venous Tissue	8 Internal Mammary, Right
J Inspection	9 Chordae Tendineae		A Autologous Arterial Tissue	9 Internal Mammary, Left
K Map	A Heart		C Extraluminal Device	A Innominate Artery
L Occlusion	B Heart, Right		D Intraluminal Device	B Subclavian
N Release	C Heart, Left		E Intraluminal Device, Two OR Intraluminal Device, Branched or Fenestrated, One or Two Arteries	C Thoracic Artery
P Removal	D Papillary Muscle		F Intraluminal Device, Three OR Intraluminal Device, Branched or Fenestrated, Three or More Arteries	D Carotid
Q Repair	F Aortic Valve		G Intraluminal Device, Four or More	E Atrioventricular Valve, Left
R Replacement	G Mitral Valve		J Synthetic Substitute OR Cardiac Lead, Pacemaker	F Abdominal Artery
S Reposition	H Pulmonary Valve		K Nonautologous Tissue Substitute OR Cardiac Lead, Defibrillator	G Atrioventricular Valve, Right OR Axillary Artery
T Resection	J Tricuspid Valve		L Biologic with Synthetic Substitute, Autoregulated Electrohydraulic	H Transapical OR Brachial Artery
U Supplement	K Ventricle, Right		M Cardiac Lead OR Synthetic Substitute, Pneumatic	J Truncal Valve OR Temporary OR Intraoperative
V Restriction	L Ventricle, Left		N Intracardiac Pacemaker	K Left Atrial Appendage
			Q Implantable Heart Assist System	L In Existing Conduit
			R Short-term External Heart Assist System	M Native Site
W Revision	M Ventricular Septum		T Intraluminal Device, Radioactive	P Pulmonary Trunk
Y Transplantation	N Pericardium		Y Other Device	Q Pulmonary Artery, Right
	P Pulmonary Trunk		Z No Device	R Pulmonary Artery, Left
	Q Pulmonary Artery, Right			S Pulmonary Vein, Right OR Biventricular
	R Pulmonary Artery, Left			T Pulmonary Vein, Left OR Ductus Arteriosus
	S Pulmonary Vein, Right			U Pulmonary Vein, Confluence
	T Pulmonary Vein, Left			V Lower Extremity Artery
	V Superior Vena Cava			W Aorta
	W Thoracic Aorta, Descending			X Diagnostic
	X Thoracic Aorta, Ascending/Arch			Z No Qualifier
	Y Great Vessel			

AHA Coding Clinic for table Ø21

2020, 4Q, 44-45	Atrium bypass qualifier
2020, 1Q, 24	Pulmonary artery unifocalization
2020, 1Q, 37	Bypass of ascending aorta to brachiocephalic artery
2019, 4Q, 23	Bypass thoracic aorta to innominate artery
2019, 3Q, 30	Aortic aneurysm repair with debranching of common carotid and brachiocephalic arteries
2018, 4Q, 45-46	Descending thoracic aorta bypass
2018, 3Q, 8	Coronary artery bypass graft surgery (revision versus total redo)
2018, 3Q, 26	Coronary artery bypass graft surgery with endarterectomy
2017, 4Q, 56	Added approach values - Percutaneous heart valve procedures
2017, 1Q, 19	Norwood Sano procedure
2016, 4Q, 80-81	Thoracic aorta, ascending/arch and descending
2016, 4Q, 82-83	Coronary artery, number of arteries
2016, 4Q, 102-109	Correction of congenital heart defects
2016, 4Q, 144	Repair of atrial septal defect and anomalous pulmonary venous return
2016, 4Q, 145	Modified Warden procedure for repair of septal defect and right partial anomalous pulmonary venous return
2016, 1Q, 27	Aortocoronary bypass graft utilizing Y-graft
2015, 4Q, 22, 24	Congenital heart corrective procedures
2015, 3Q, 16	Revision of previous truncus arteriosus surgery with ventricle to pulmonary artery conduit
2014, 3Q, 3	Blalock-Taussig shunt procedure
2014, 3Q, 8	Coronary artery bypass graft utilizing internal mammary as pedicle graft
2014, 3Q, 20	MAZE procedure performed with coronary artery bypass graft
2014, 3Q, 29	Fontan completion procedure stage II
2014, 3Q, 30	Creation of conduit from right ventricle to pulmonary artery
2014, 1Q, 10	Repair of thoracic aortic aneurysm & coronary artery bypass graft
2013, 2Q, 37	Coronary artery release performed during coronary artery bypass graft

AHA Coding Clinic for table Ø24

2016, 4Q, 101	Root operation Creation
2016, 4Q, 102-109	Correction of congenital heart defects

AHA Coding Clinic for table Ø25

2020, 1Q, 32	Ablation convergent procedure (catheter-based and thoracoscopic ablations)
2018, 3Q, 27	Alcohol septal ablation
2016, 4Q, 80-81	Thoracic aorta, ascending/arch and descending
2016, 3Q, 43-44	Peri-pulmonary catheter ablation
2016, 3Q, 44-45	Maze procedure
2016, 2Q, 17	Photodynamic therapy for treatment of malignant mesothelioma
2014, 4Q, 47	Catheter ablation of peripulmonary veins
2014, 3Q, 19	Ablation of ventricular tachycardia with Impella® support
2014, 3Q, 20	MAZE procedure performed with coronary artery bypass graft
2013, 2Q, 38	Catheter ablation to treat atrial fibrillation

AHA Coding Clinic for table Ø27

2018, 3Q, 7	Coronary brachytherapy with angioplasty
2018, 3Q, 10	Disruption of perma-catheter fibrin sheath via angioplasty of superior vena cava
2018, 2Q, 24	Coronary artery bifurcation
2017, 4Q, 32-33	Corrective surgery of left ventricular outflow tract obstruction
2016, 4Q, 80-81	Thoracic aorta, ascending/arch and descending
2016, 4Q, 82-83	Coronary artery, number of arteries
2016, 4Q, 84-85	Coronary Artery, number of stents
2016, 4Q, 86-88	Coronary and peripheral artery bifurcation
2016, 1Q, 16	Pulmonary valvotomy and dilation of annulus
2015, 4Q, 13	New Section X codes—New Technology procedures
2015, 3Q, 9	Failed attempt to treat coronary artery occlusion
2015, 3Q, 10	Coronary angioplasty with unsuccessful stent insertion
2015, 3Q, 16	Revision of previous truncus arteriosus surgery with ventricle to pulmonary artery conduit
2015, 2Q, 3-5	Coronary artery intervention site
2014, 2Q, 4	Coronary angioplasty of bypassed vessel

AHA Coding Clinic for table Ø2B

2019, 3Q, 32	Endomyocardial biopsy and right heart catheterization
2019, 2Q, 20	Pericardiectomy for constrictive pericarditis
2017, 1Q, 38	Mitral valve repair and chordae tendineae transfer
2016, 4Q, 80-81	Thoracic aorta, ascending/arch and descending
2015, 2Q, 23	Annuloplasty ring

AHA Coding Clinic for table Ø2C

2019, 4Q, 25	Coronary artery to root operation Supplement
2018, 3Q, 26	Coronary artery bypass graft surgery with endarterectomy
2018, 2Q, 24	Coronary artery bifurcation
2017, 2Q, 23	Thrombectomy via Fogarty catheter
2016, 4Q, 80-81	Thoracic aorta, ascending/arch and descending
2016, 4Q, 82-83	Coronary artery, number of arteries
2016, 4Q, 86-87	Coronary and peripheral artery bifurcation
2016, 2Q, 24	Repair/decalcification of mitral valve
2016, 2Q, 25	Aortic valve surgery with excision of calcium deposits

AHA Coding Clinic for table Ø2F

2020, 4Q, 45-49	New fragmentation tables
2020, 4Q, 49-50	Intravascular ultrasound assisted thrombolysis
2020, 4Q, 50	Intravascular lithotripsy

AHA Coding Clinic for table Ø2H

2021, 2Q, 23	Clarification of lead placement in bundle of HIS
2019, 4Q, 23-24	Coronary artery Body Part to root operation Insertion
2019, 3Q, 19	Insertion of left ventricular catheter
2019, 3Q, 23	Placement of pacemaker lead in Bundle of HIS
2019, 1Q, 24	Replacement of left ventricular assist device with retention of outflow graft
2018, 4Q, 94	Insertion and removal of failed Watchman™ device
2018, 2Q, 3-5	Intra-aortic balloon pump
2018, 2Q, 19	Pacing lead attached to automatic implantable cardioverter defibrillator
2017, 4Q, 42-45	Insertion of external heart assist devices
2017, 4Q, 63-64	Added and revised device values - Vascular access reservoir
2017, 4Q, 104	Placement of Watchman™ left atrial appendage device
2017, 3Q, 11	Placement of peripherally inserted central catheter using 3CG ECG technology
2017, 2Q, 24	Tunneled catheter versus totally implantable catheter
2017, 2Q, 26	Exchange of tunneled catheter
2017, 1Q, 10-11	External heart assist device
2016, 4Q, 80-81	Thoracic aorta, ascending/arch and descending
2016, 4Q, 95	Intracardiac pacemaker
2016, 4Q, 137-138	Heart assist device systems
2016, 2Q, 15	Removal and replacement of tunneled internal jugular catheter
2015, 4Q, 14	New Section X codes—New Technology procedures
2015, 4Q, 26-31	Vascular access devices
2015, 3Q, 35	Swan Ganz catheterization
2015, 2Q, 31	Leadless pacemaker insertion
2015, 2Q, 33	Totally implantable central venous access device (Port-a-Cath)
2013, 3Q, 18	Placement of peripherally inserted central catheter (PICC)

AHA Coding Clinic for table Ø2J

2015, 3Q, 9	Failed attempt to treat coronary artery occlusion

AHA Coding Clinic for table Ø2K

2020, 1Q, 32	Ablation convergent procedure (catheter-based and thoracoscopic ablations)

AHA Coding Clinic for table Ø2L

2018, 4Q, 94	Insertion and removal of failed Watchman™ device
2017, 4Q, 31	Resuscitative endovascular balloon occlusion of the aorta
2017, 4Q, 33-34	Occlusion/ligation of pulmonary trunk & right pulmonary artery
2016, 4Q, 102-109	Correction of congenital heart defects
2016, 2Q, 26	Embolization of pulmonary arteriovenous fistula
2015, 4Q, 23	Congenital heart corrective procedures
2014, 3Q, 20	MAZE procedure performed with coronary artery bypass graft

AHA Coding Clinic for table Ø2N

2019, 2Q, 13	Unroofing of anomalous coronary artery
2019, 2Q, 20	Pericardiectomy for constrictive pericarditis
2017, 4Q, 35	Release of myocardial bridge
2016, 4Q, 80-81	Thoracic aorta, ascending/arch and descending
2014, 3Q, 16	Repair of Tetralogy of Fallot

AHA Coding Clinic for table Ø2P

2019, 1Q, 24	Replacement of left ventricular assist device with retention of outflow graft
2018, 4Q, 52-54	Percutaneous extracorporeal membrane oxygenation
2018, 4Q, 85	Externalization of lumboatrial shunt
2018, 4Q, 94	Insertion and removal of failed Watchman™ device
2018, 2Q, 3-5	Intra-aortic balloon pump
2017, 4Q, 42-45	Insertion of external heart assist devices
2017, 4Q, 104	Placement of Watchman™ left atrial appendage device
2017, 3Q, 18	Intra-aortic balloon pump removal
2017, 2Q, 24	Tunneled catheter versus totally implantable catheter
2017, 2Q, 26	Exchange of tunneled catheter
2017, 1Q, 11	External heart assist device
2017, 1Q, 13	SynCardia total artificial heart
2016, 4Q, 95-96	Intracardiac pacemaker
2016, 4Q, 137-139	Heart assist device systems
2016, 3Q, 19	Nonoperative removal of peripherally inserted central catheter
2016, 2Q, 15	Removal and replacement of tunneled internal jugular catheter
2015, 4Q, 31	Vascular access devices
2015, 3Q, 33	Approach values for repositioning and removal of cardiac lead

AHA Coding Clinic for table Ø2Q

2018, 1Q, 12	Percutaneous balloon valvuloplasty & cardiac catheterization with ventriculogram
2017, 1Q, 18	Sutureless repair of pulmonary vein stenosis
2016, 4Q, 80-81	Thoracic aorta, ascending/arch and descending
2016, 4Q, 82-83	Coronary artery, number of arteries
2016, 4Q, 101	Root operation Creation
2016, 4Q, 102-109	Correction of congenital heart defects
2015, 4Q, 23	Congenital heart corrective procedures
2015, 3Q, 16	Vascular ring surgery and double aortic arch
2015, 2Q, 23	Annuloplasty ring
2013, 3Q, 26	Transcatheter replacement of heart valve (TAVR) with measurements

AHA Coding Clinic for table Ø2R

2020, 1Q, 25	Elephant trunk repair of aortic dissection
2019, 4Q, 24	Coronary artery Body Part to root operation Insertion
2019, 4Q, 46	Cerebral embolic filtration
2019, 3Q, 23	Replacement of atrioventricular valve
2019, 3Q, 24	Valve sparing aortic root replacement with modified Gleason Vascutek® graft to ascending aorta
2019, 1Q, 31	Transcatheter aortic valve in valve replacement
2018, 3Q, 11	Transcatheter aortic valve replacement via transaortic approach
2018, 1Q, 12	Percutaneous balloon valvuloplasty & cardiac catheterization with ventriculogram
2017, 4Q, 55-56	Added approach values - Percutaneous heart valve procedures
2017, 1Q, 13	SynCardia total artificial heart
2016, 4Q, 80-81	Thoracic aorta, ascending/arch and descending
2016, 3Q, 32	Transcatheter tricuspid valve replacement
2014, 1Q, 10	Repair of thoracic aortic aneurysm & coronary artery bypass graft

AHA Coding Clinic for table Ø2S

2016, 4Q, 80-81	Thoracic aorta, ascending/arch and descending
2016, 4Q, 82-83	Coronary artery, number of arteries
2016, 4Q, 102-109	Correction of congenital heart defects
2015, 4Q, 23	Congenital heart corrective procedures

AHA Coding Clinic for table Ø2U

2020, 4Q, 52	Transapical mitral valve repair with device
2020, 1Q, 24	Pulmonary artery unifocalization
2019, 4Q, 25	Coronary artery to root operation Supplement
2018, 1Q, 12	Percutaneous balloon valvuloplasty & cardiac catheterization with ventriculogram
2017, 4Q, 36	Alfieri stitch procedure
2017, 3Q, 7	Senning procedure (arterial switch)
2017, 1Q, 19	Norwood Sano procedure
2016, 4Q, 80-81	Thoracic aorta, ascending/arch and descending
2016, 4Q, 101	Root operation Creation
2016, 4Q, 102-109	Correction of congenital heart defects
2016, 2Q, 23	Repair of tetralogy of Fallot with autologous pericardial patch graft
2016, 2Q, 26	Aortic valve replacement with aortic root enlargement
2015, 4Q, 22-24	Congenital heart corrective procedures
2015, 3Q, 16	Revision of previous truncus arteriosus surgery with ventricle to pulmonary artery conduit
2015, 2Q, 23	Annuloplasty ring
2014, 3Q, 16	Repair of Tetralogy of Fallot

AHA Coding Clinic for table Ø2V

2020, 1Q, 25	Elephant trunk repair of aortic dissection
2017, 4Q, 35-36	Alfieri stitch procedure
2016, 4Q, 80-81	Thoracic aorta, ascending/arch and descending
2016, 4Q, 89-92	Branched and fenestrated endograft repair of aneurysms

AHA Coding Clinic for table Ø2W

2019, 1Q, 24	Replacement of left ventricular assist device with retention of outflow graft
2018, 3Q, 8	Coronary artery bypass graft surgery (revision versus total redo)
2018, 3Q, 9	Fibrin sheath stripping of malfunctioning port-a-cath
2018, 1Q, 17	Repositioning of Impella short-term external heart assist device
2017, 4Q, 42-45	Insertion of external heart assist devices
2017, 4Q, 55-56	Added approach values - Percutaneous heart valve procedures
2016, 4Q, 85	Coronary Artery, number of stents
2016, 4Q, 95-96	Intracardiac pacemaker
2015, 3Q, 32	Approach values for repositioning and removal of cardiac lead
2014, 3Q, 31	Closure of paravalvular leak using Amplatzer® vascular plug

AHA Coding Clinic for table Ø2Y

| 2013, 3Q, 18 | Heart transplant surgery |

Coronary Arteries

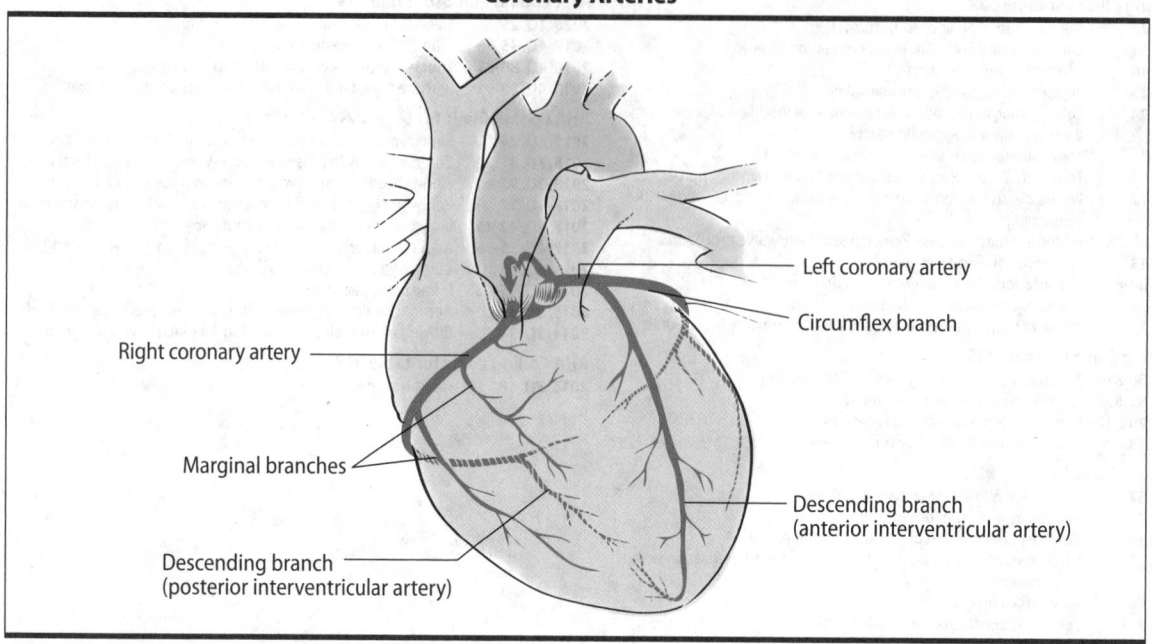

Left coronary artery

Circumflex branch

Right coronary artery

Marginal branches

Descending branch
(anterior interventricular artery)

Descending branch
(posterior interventricular artery)

Heart Anatomy

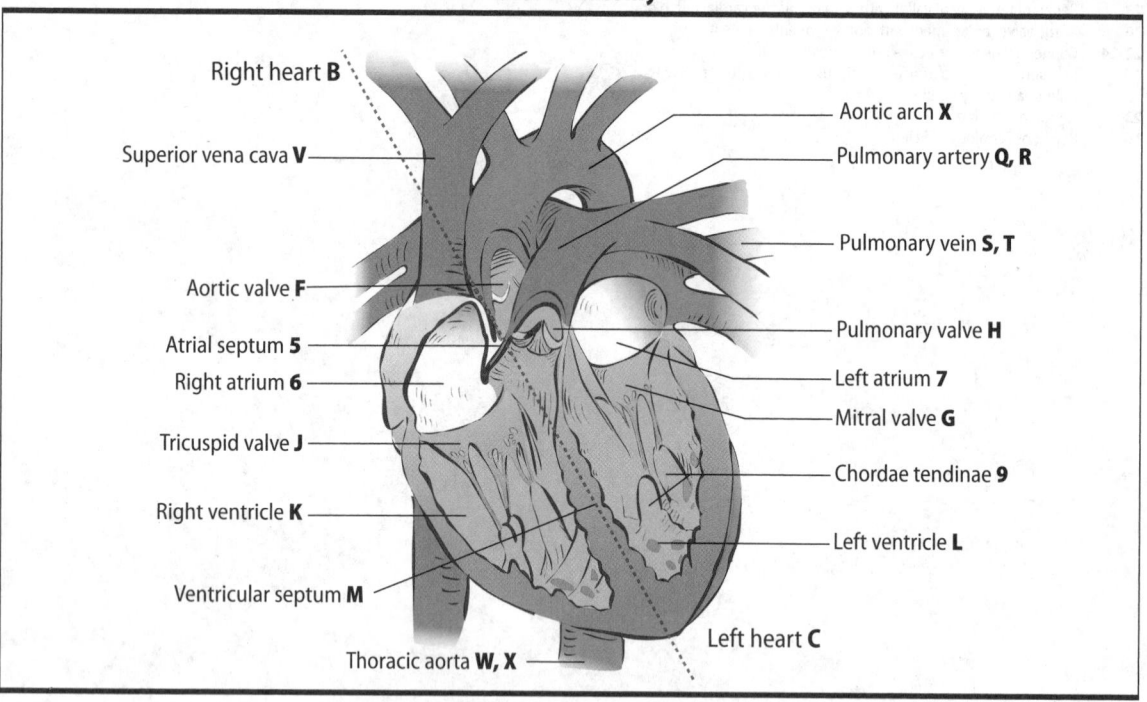

Right heart **B**

Superior vena cava **V**

Aortic valve **F**

Atrial septum **5**

Right atrium **6**

Tricuspid valve **J**

Right ventricle **K**

Ventricular septum **M**

Thoracic aorta **W, X**

Aortic arch **X**

Pulmonary artery **Q, R**

Pulmonary vein **S, T**

Pulmonary valve **H**

Left atrium **7**

Mitral valve **G**

Chordae tendinae **9**

Left ventricle **L**

Left heart **C**

Ø Medical and Surgical
2 Heart and Great Vessels
1 Bypass   Definition: Altering the route of passage of the contents of a tubular body part

Explanation: Rerouting contents of a body part to a downstream area of the normal route, to a similar route and body part, or to an abnormal route and dissimilar body part. Includes one or more anastomoses, with or without the use of a device.

Body Part Character 4	Approach Character 5	Device Character 6	Qualifier Character 7
Ø Coronary Artery, One Artery **1** Coronary Artery, Two Arteries **2** Coronary Artery, Three Arteries **3** Coronary Artery, Four or More Arteries	**Ø** Open	**8** Zooplastic Tissue **9** Autologous Venous Tissue **A** Autologous Arterial Tissue **J** Synthetic Substitute **K** Nonautologous Tissue Substitute	**3** Coronary Artery **8** Internal Mammary, Right **9** Internal Mammary, Left **C** Thoracic Artery **F** Abdominal Artery **W** Aorta
Ø Coronary Artery, One Artery **1** Coronary Artery, Two Arteries **2** Coronary Artery, Three Arteries **3** Coronary Artery, Four or More Arteries	**Ø** Open	**Z** No Device	**3** Coronary Artery **8** Internal Mammary, Right **9** Internal Mammary, Left **C** Thoracic Artery **F** Abdominal Artery
Ø Coronary Artery, One Artery **1** Coronary Artery, Two Arteries **2** Coronary Artery, Three Arteries **3** Coronary Artery, Four or More Arteries	**3** Percutaneous	**4** Intraluminal Device, Drug-eluting **D** Intraluminal Device	**4** Coronary Vein
Ø Coronary Artery, One Artery **1** Coronary Artery, Two Arteries **2** Coronary Artery, Three Arteries **3** Coronary Artery, Four or More Arteries	**4** Percutaneous Endoscopic	**4** Intraluminal Device, Drug-eluting **D** Intraluminal Device	**4** Coronary Vein
Ø Coronary Artery, One Artery **1** Coronary Artery, Two Arteries **2** Coronary Artery, Three Arteries **3** Coronary Artery, Four or More Arteries	**4** Percutaneous Endoscopic	**8** Zooplastic Tissue **9** Autologous Venous Tissue **A** Autologous Arterial Tissue **J** Synthetic Substitute **K** Nonautologous Tissue Substitute	**3** Coronary Artery **8** Internal Mammary, Right **9** Internal Mammary, Left **C** Thoracic Artery **F** Abdominal Artery **W** Aorta
Ø Coronary Artery, One Artery **1** Coronary Artery, Two Arteries **2** Coronary Artery, Three Arteries **3** Coronary Artery, Four or More Arteries	**4** Percutaneous Endoscopic	**Z** No Device	**3** Coronary Artery **8** Internal Mammary, Right **9** Internal Mammary, Left **C** Thoracic Artery **F** Abdominal Artery
6 Atrium, Right Atrium dextrum cordis Right auricular appendix Sinus venosus	**Ø** Open **4** Percutaneous Endoscopic	**8** Zooplastic Tissue **9** Autologous Venous Tissue **A** Autologous Arterial Tissue **J** Synthetic Substitute **K** Nonautologous Tissue Substitute	**P** Pulmonary Trunk **Q** Pulmonary Artery, Right **R** Pulmonary Artery, Left
6 Atrium, Right Atrium dextrum cordis Right auricular appendix Sinus venosus	**Ø** Open **4** Percutaneous Endoscopic	**Z** No Device	**7** Atrium, Left **P** Pulmonary Trunk **Q** Pulmonary Artery, Right **R** Pulmonary Artery, Left
6 Atrium, Right Atrium dextrum cordis Right auricular appendix Sinus venosus	**3** Percutaneous	**Z** No Device	**7** Atrium, Left
7 Atrium, Left Atrium pulmonale Left auricular appendix	**Ø** Open **4** Percutaneous Endoscopic	**8** Zooplastic Tissue **9** Autologous Venous Tissue **A** Autologous Arterial Tissue **J** Synthetic Substitute **K** Nonautologous Tissue Substitute **Z** No Device	**P** Pulmonary Trunk **Q** Pulmonary Artery, Right **R** Pulmonary Artery, Left **S** Pulmonary Vein, Right **T** Pulmonary Vein, Left **U** Pulmonary Vein, Confluence
7 Atrium, Left Atrium pulmonale Left auricular appendix	**3** Percutaneous	**J** Synthetic Substitute	**6** Atrium, Right
K Ventricle, Right Conus arteriosus **L** Ventricle, Left	**Ø** Open **4** Percutaneous Endoscopic	**8** Zooplastic Tissue **9** Autologous Venous Tissue **A** Autologous Arterial Tissue **J** Synthetic Substitute **K** Nonautologous Tissue Substitute	**P** Pulmonary Trunk **Q** Pulmonary Artery, Right **R** Pulmonary Artery, Left

HAC Ø21[Ø,1,2,3]Ø[8,9,A,J,K][3,8,9,C,F,W] when reported with SDx J98.51 or J98.59
HAC Ø21[Ø,1,2,3]ØZ[3,8,9,C,F] when reported with SDx J98.51 or J98.59
HAC Ø21[Ø,1,2,3]4[8,9,A,J,K][3,8,9,C,F,W] when reported with SDx J98.51 or J98.59
HAC Ø21[Ø,1,2,3]4Z[3,8,9,C,F] when reported with SDx J98.51 or J98.59

Ø21 Continued on next page

NC Noncovered Procedure   **LC** Limited Coverage   **QA** Questionable OB Admit   **NT** New Tech Add-on   ⊞ Combination Member   ♂ Male   ♀ Female

Ø	**Medical and Surgical**		
2	**Heart and Great Vessels**		
1	**Bypass**	Definition: Altering the route of passage of the contents of a tubular body part	

Ø21 Continued

Explanation: Rerouting contents of a body part to a downstream area of the normal route, to a similar route and body part, or to an abnormal route and dissimilar body part. Includes one or more anastomoses, with or without the use of a device.

Body Part Character 4	Approach Character 5	Device Character 6	Qualifier Character 7
K Ventricle, Right Conus arteriosus L Ventricle, Left	Ø Open 4 Percutaneous Endoscopic	Z No Device	5 Coronary Circulation 8 Internal Mammary, Right 9 Internal Mammary, Left C Thoracic Artery F Abdominal Artery P Pulmonary Trunk Q Pulmonary Artery, Right R Pulmonary Artery, Left W Aorta

P Pulmonary Trunk
Q Pulmonary Artery, Right
R Pulmonary Artery, Left
   Arterial canal (duct)
   Botallo's duct
   Pulmoaortic canal
	Ø Open
	4 Percutaneous Endoscopic
		8 Zooplastic Tissue
		9 Autologous Venous Tissue
		A Autologous Arterial Tissue
		J Synthetic Substitute
		K Nonautologous Tissue Substitute
		Z No Device
			A Innominate Artery
			B Subclavian
			D Carotid

V Superior Vena Cava Precava	Ø Open 4 Percutaneous Endoscopic	8 Zooplastic Tissue 9 Autologous Venous Tissue A Autologous Arterial Tissue J Synthetic Substitute K Nonautologous Tissue Substitute Z No Device	P Pulmonary Trunk Q Pulmonary Artery, Right R Pulmonary Artery, Left S Pulmonary Vein, Right T Pulmonary Vein, Left U Pulmonary Vein, Confluence
W Thoracic Aorta, Descending	Ø Open	8 Zooplastic Tissue 9 Autologous Venous Tissue A Autologous Arterial Tissue J Synthetic Substitute K Nonautologous Tissue Substitute	A Innominate Artery B Subclavian D Carotid F Abdominal Artery G Axillary Artery H Brachial Artery P Pulmonary Trunk Q Pulmonary Artery, Right R Pulmonary Artery, Left V Lower Extremity Artery
W Thoracic Aorta, Descending	Ø Open	Z No Device	A Innominate Artery B Subclavian D Carotid P Pulmonary Trunk Q Pulmonary Artery, Right R Pulmonary Artery, Left
W Thoracic Aorta, Descending	4 Percutaneous Endoscopic	8 Zooplastic Tissue 9 Autologous Venous Tissue A Autologous Arterial Tissue J Synthetic Substitute K Nonautologous Tissue Substitute Z No Device	A Innominate Artery B Subclavian D Carotid P Pulmonary Trunk Q Pulmonary Artery, Right R Pulmonary Artery, Left

X Thoracic Aorta, Ascending/Arch
   Aortic arch
   Ascending aorta
	Ø Open
	4 Percutaneous Endoscopic
		8 Zooplastic Tissue
		9 Autologous Venous Tissue
		A Autologous Arterial Tissue
		J Synthetic Substitute
		K Nonautologous Tissue Substitute
		Z No Device
			A Innominate Artery
			B Subclavian
			D Carotid
			P Pulmonary Trunk
			Q Pulmonary Artery, Right
			R Pulmonary Artery, Left

Ø	**Medical and Surgical**		
2	**Heart and Great Vessels**		
4	**Creation**	Definition: Putting in or on biological or synthetic material to form a new body part that to the extent possible replicates the anatomic structure or function of an absent body part	

Explanation: Used for gender reassignment surgery and corrective procedures in individuals with congenital anomalies

Body Part Character 4	Approach Character 5	Device Character 6	Qualifier Character 7
F Aortic Valve Aortic annulus	Ø Open	7 Autologous Tissue 8 Zooplastic Tissue J Synthetic Substitute K Nonautologous Tissue Substitute	J Truncal Valve

G Mitral Valve
   Bicuspid valve
   Left atrioventricular valve
   Mitral annulus
J Tricuspid Valve
   Right atrioventricular valve
   Tricuspid annulus
	Ø Open	7 Autologous Tissue
		8 Zooplastic Tissue
		J Synthetic Substitute
		K Nonautologous Tissue Substitute
			2 Common Atrioventricular Valve

Non-OR Procedure   DRG Non-OR Procedure   Valid OR Procedure   HAC Associated Procedure   Combination Only   New/Revised GREEN

Ø   Medical and Surgical
2   Heart and Great Vessels
5   Destruction   Definition: Physical eradication of all or a portion of a body part by the direct use of energy, force, or a destructive agent
                       Explanation: None of the body part is physically taken out

Body Part Character 4	Approach Character 5	Device Character 6	Qualifier Character 7
4 Coronary Vein	Ø Open	Z No Device	Z No Qualifier
5 Atrial Septum Interatrial septum	3 Percutaneous 4 Percutaneous Endoscopic		

6   Atrium, Right
     Atrium dextrum cordis
     Right auricular appendix
     Sinus venosus			

8   Conduction Mechanism
     Atrioventricular node
     Bundle of His
     Bundle of Kent
     Sinoatrial node			

9 Chordae Tendineae			
D Papillary Muscle			
F Aortic Valve Aortic annulus			

G   Mitral Valve
     Bicuspid valve
     Left atrioventricular valve
     Mitral annulus			

H   Pulmonary Valve
     Pulmonary annulus
     Pulmonic valve			

J   Tricuspid Valve
     Right atrioventricular valve
     Tricuspid annulus			

K Ventricle, Right Conus arteriosus			
L Ventricle, Left			
M Ventricular Septum Interventricular septum			
N Pericardium			
P Pulmonary Trunk			
Q Pulmonary Artery, Right			

R   Pulmonary Artery, Left
     Arterial canal (duct)
     Botallo's duct
     Pulmoaortic canal			

S   Pulmonary Vein, Right
     Right inferior pulmonary vein
     Right superior pulmonary vein			

T   Pulmonary Vein, Left
     Left inferior pulmonary vein
     Left superior pulmonary vein			

V Superior Vena Cava Precava			
W Thoracic Aorta, Descending			

X   Thoracic Aorta, Ascending/Arch
     Aortic arch
     Ascending aorta			

7   Atrium, Left
     Atrium pulmonale
     Left auricular appendix
	Ø Open
	3 Percutaneous
	4 Percutaneous Endoscopic
		Z No Device	K Left Atrial Appendage
			Z No Qualifier

DRG Non-OR   Ø257[Ø,3,4]ZK

NC Noncovered Procedure   LC Limited Coverage   QA Questionable OB Admit   NT New Tech Add-on   ⊞ Combination Member   ♂ Male   ♀ Female

ICD-10-PCS 2022   177

Ø   Medical and Surgical
2   Heart and Great Vessels
7   Dilation   Definition: Expanding an orifice or the lumen of a tubular body part

Explanation: The orifice can be a natural orifice or an artificially created orifice. Accomplished by stretching a tubular body part using intraluminal pressure or by cutting part of the orifice or wall of the tubular body part.

Body Part Character 4	Approach Character 5	Device Character 6	Qualifier Character 7

Ø   Coronary Artery, One Artery
1   Coronary Artery, Two Arteries
2   Coronary Artery, Three Arteries
3   Coronary Artery, Four or More Arteries
	Ø Open
	3 Percutaneous
	4 Percutaneous Endoscopic
		4 Intraluminal Device,
		    Drug-eluting
		5 Intraluminal Device, Drug-eluting,
		    Two
		6 Intraluminal Device, Drug-eluting,
		    Three
		7 Intraluminal Device, Drug-eluting,
		    Four or More
		D Intraluminal Device
		E Intraluminal Device, Two
		F Intraluminal Device, Three
		G Intraluminal Device, Four or More
		T Intraluminal Device, Radioactive
		Z No Device
			6 Bifurcation
			Z No Qualifier

F   Aortic Valve
    Aortic annulus
G   Mitral Valve
    Bicuspid valve
    Left atrioventricular valve
    Mitral annulus
H   Pulmonary Valve
    Pulmonary annulus
    Pulmonic valve
J   Tricuspid Valve
    Right atrioventricular valve
    Tricuspid annulus
K   Ventricle, Right
    Conus arteriosus
L   Ventricle, Left
P   Pulmonary Trunk
Q   Pulmonary Artery, Right
S   Pulmonary Vein, Right
    Right inferior pulmonary vein
    Right superior pulmonary vein
T   Pulmonary Vein, Left
    Left inferior pulmonary vein
    Left superior pulmonary vein
V   Superior Vena Cava
    Precava
W   Thoracic Aorta, Descending
X   Thoracic Aorta, Ascending/Arch
    Aortic arch
    Ascending aorta
	Ø Open
	3 Percutaneous
	4 Percutaneous Endoscopic
		4 Intraluminal Device,
		    Drug-eluting
		D Intraluminal Device
		Z No Device
			Z No Qualifier

R   Pulmonary Artery, Left
    Arterial canal (duct)
    Botallo's duct
    Pulmoaortic canal
	Ø Open
	3 Percutaneous
	4 Percutaneous Endoscopic
		4 Intraluminal Device,
		    Drug-eluting
		D Intraluminal Device
		Z No Device
			T Ductus Arteriosus
			Z No Qualifier

Ø   Medical and Surgical
2   Heart and Great Vessels
8   Division   Definition: Cutting into a body part, without draining fluids and/or gases from the body part, in order to separate or transect a body part

Explanation: All or a portion of the body part is separated into two or more portions

Body Part Character 4	Approach Character 5	Device Character 6	Qualifier Character 7

8   Conduction Mechanism
    Atrioventricular node
    Bundle of His
    Bundle of Kent
    Sinoatrial node
9   Chordae Tendineae
D   Papillary Muscle
	Ø Open
	3 Percutaneous
	4 Percutaneous Endoscopic
		Z No Device	Z No Qualifier

Ø   **Medical and Surgical**
2   **Heart and Great Vessels**
B   **Excision**   Definition: Cutting out or off, without replacement, a portion of a body part

                 Explanation: The qualifier DIAGNOSTIC is used to identify excision procedures that are biopsies

Body Part Character 4	Approach Character 5	Device Character 6	Qualifier Character 7

4   Coronary Vein
5   Atrial Septum
     Interatrial septum
6   Atrium, Right
     Atrium dextrum cordis
     Right auricular appendix
     Sinus venosus
8   Conduction Mechanism
     Atrioventricular node
     Bundle of His
     Bundle of Kent
     Sinoatrial node
9   Chordae Tendineae
D   Papillary Muscle
F   Aortic Valve
     Aortic annulus
G   Mitral Valve
     Bicuspid valve
     Left atrioventricular valve
     Mitral annulus
H   Pulmonary Valve
     Pulmonary annulus
     Pulmonic valve
J   Tricuspid Valve
     Right atrioventricular valve
     Tricuspid annulus
K   Ventricle, Right   NC
     Conus arteriosus
L   Ventricle, Left   NC
M   Ventricular Septum
     Interventricular septum
N   Pericardium
P   Pulmonary Trunk
Q   Pulmonary Artery, Right
R   Pulmonary Artery, Left
     Arterial canal (duct)
     Botallo's duct
     Pulmoaortic canal
S   Pulmonary Vein, Right
     Right inferior pulmonary vein
     Right superior pulmonary vein
T   Pulmonary Vein, Left
     Left inferior pulmonary vein
     Left superior pulmonary vein
V   Superior Vena Cava
     Precava
W   Thoracic Aorta, Descending
X   Thoracic Aorta, Ascending/Arch
     Aortic arch
     Ascending aorta
	Ø Open
	3 Percutaneous
	4 Percutaneous Endoscopic
		Z No Device	**X** Diagnostic
			Z No Qualifier

7   Atrium, Left
     Atrium pulmonale
     Left auricular appendix
	Ø Open
	3 Percutaneous
	4 Percutaneous Endoscopic
		Z No Device	**K** Left Atrial Appendage
			X Diagnostic
			Z No Qualifier

DRG Non-OR   Ø2B7[Ø,3,4]ZK
Non-OR   Ø2B[4,5,6,8,9,D,F,G,H,J,K,L,M][Ø,3,4]ZX
NC   Ø2B[K,L][Ø,3,4]ZZ

NC Noncovered Procedure   **LC** Limited Coverage   **QA** Questionable OB Admit   **NT** New Tech Add-on   ⊞ Combination Member   ♂ Male   ♀ Female

ICD-10-PCS 2022   **179**

Ø2B–Ø2B

Ø **Medical and Surgical**
2 **Heart and Great Vessels**
C **Extirpation**   Definition: Taking or cutting out solid matter from a body part

Explanation: The solid matter may be an abnormal byproduct of a biological function or a foreign body; it may be imbedded in a body part or in the lumen of a tubular body part. The solid matter may or may not have been previously broken into pieces.

Body Part Character 4	Approach Character 5	Device Character 6	Qualifier Character 7
Ø Coronary Artery, One Artery **1** Coronary Artery, Two Arteries **2** Coronary Artery, Three Arteries **3** Coronary Artery, Four or More Arteries	**Ø** Open **4** Percutaneous Endoscopic	**Z** No Device	**6** Bifurcation **Z** No Qualifier
Ø Coronary Artery, One Artery **1** Coronary Artery, Two Arteries **2** Coronary Artery, Three Arteries **3** Coronary Artery, Four or More Arteries	**3** Percutaneous	**Z** No Device	**6** Bifurcation **7** Orbital Atherectomy Technique **Z** No Qualifier
4 Coronary Vein **5** Atrial Septum Interatrial septum **6** Atrium, Right Atrium dextrum cordis Right auricular appendix Sinus venosus **7** Atrium, Left Atrium pulmonale Left auricular appendix **8** Conduction Mechanism Atrioventricular node Bundle of His Bundle of Kent Sinoatrial node **9** Chordae Tendineae **D** Papillary Muscle **F** Aortic Valve Aortic annulus **G** Mitral Valve Bicuspid valve Left atrioventricular valve Mitral annulus **H** Pulmonary Valve Pulmonary annulus Pulmonic valve **J** Tricuspid Valve Right atrioventricular valve Tricuspid annulus **K** Ventricle, Right Conus arteriosus **L** Ventricle, Left **M** Ventricular Septum Interventricular septum **N** Pericardium **P** Pulmonary Trunk **Q** Pulmonary Artery, Right **R** Pulmonary Artery, Left Arterial canal (duct) Botallo's duct Pulmoaortic canal **S** Pulmonary Vein, Right Right inferior pulmonary vein Right superior pulmonary vein **T** Pulmonary Vein, Left Left inferior pulmonary vein Left superior pulmonary vein **V** Superior Vena Cava Precava **W** Thoracic Aorta, Descending **X** Thoracic Aorta, Ascending/Arch Aortic arch Ascending aorta	**Ø** Open **3** Percutaneous **4** Percutaneous Endoscopic	**Z** No Device	**Z** No Qualifier

02C–02C

Non-OR Procedure   DRG Non-OR Procedure   Valid OR Procedure   HAC Associated Procedure   Combination Only   New/Revised GREEN
180   ICD-10-PCS 2022

Ø	**Medical and Surgical**	
2	**Heart and Great Vessels**	
F	**Fragmentation**	Definition: Breaking solid matter in a body part into pieces
		Explanation: Physical force (e.g., manual, ultrasonic) applied directly or indirectly is used to break the solid matter into pieces. The solid matter may be an abnormal byproduct of a biological function or a foreign body. The pieces of solid matter are not taken out.

Body Part Character 4	Approach Character 5	Device Character 6	Qualifier Character 7
Ø Coronary Artery, One Artery **1** Coronary Artery, Two Arteries **2** Coronary Artery, Three Arteries **3** Coronary Artery, Four or More Arteries	**3** Percutaneous	**Z** No Device	**Z** No Qualifier
N Pericardium NC	**Ø** Open **3** Percutaneous **4** Percutaneous Endoscopic **X** External	**Z** No Device	**Z** No Qualifier

P Pulmonary Trunk
Q Pulmonary Artery, Right
R Pulmonary Artery, Left
    Arterial canal (duct)
    Botallo's duct
    Pulmoaortic canal
S Pulmonary Vein, Right
    Right inferior pulmonary vein
    Right superior pulmonary vein
T Pulmonary Vein, Left
    Left inferior pulmonary vein
    Left superior pulmonary vein
	3 Percutaneous	**Z** No Device	**Ø** Ultrasonic
			Z No Qualifier

Non-OR   Ø2FNXZZ
NC   Ø2FNXZZ

NC Noncovered Procedure   LC Limited Coverage   QA Questionable OB Admit   NT New Tech Add-on   ⊞ Combination Member   ♂ Male   ♀ Female

ICD-10-PCS 2022   181

Heart and Great Vessels

Ø   **Medical and Surgical**
2   **Heart and Great Vessels**
H   **Insertion**   Definition: Putting in a nonbiological appliance that monitors, assists, performs, or prevents a physiological function but does not physically take the place of a body part
                   Explanation: None

Body Part Character 4	Approach Character 5	Device Character 6	Qualifier Character 7
Ø Coronary Artery, One Artery **1** Coronary Artery, Two Arteries **2** Coronary Artery, Three Arteries **3** Coronary Artery, Four or More Arteries	**Ø** Open **3** Percutaneous **4** Percutaneous Endoscopic	**D** Intraluminal Device **Y** Other Device	**Z** No Qualifier

4   Coronary Vein ⊞
6   Atrium, Right ⊞
     Atrium dextrum cordis
     Right auricular appendix
     Sinus venosus
7   Atrium, Left ⊞
     Atrium pulmonale
     Left auricular appendix
K   Ventricle, Right ⊞
     Conus arteriosus
L   Ventricle, Left ⊞
	Ø Open
	3 Percutaneous
	4 Percutaneous Endoscopic
		Ø Monitoring Device, Pressure Sensor
		2 Monitoring Device
		3 Infusion Device
		D Intraluminal Device
		J Cardiac Lead, Pacemaker
		K Cardiac Lead, Defibrillator
		M Cardiac Lead
		N Intracardiac Pacemaker
		Y Other Device
			Z No Qualifier

A Heart `LC` `NC`	**Ø** Open **3** Percutaneous **4** Percutaneous Endoscopic	**Q** Implantable Heart Assist System **Y** Other Device	**Z** No Qualifier
A Heart ⊞	**Ø** Open **3** Percutaneous **4** Percutaneous Endoscopic	**R** Short-term External Heart Assist System	**J** Intraoperative **S** Biventricular **Z** No Qualifier
N Pericardium ⊞	**Ø** Open **3** Percutaneous **4** Percutaneous Endoscopic	**Ø** Monitoring Device, Pressure Sensor **2** Monitoring Device **J** Cardiac Lead, Pacemaker **K** Cardiac Lead, Defibrillator **M** Cardiac Lead **Y** Other Device	**Z** No Qualifier

P   Pulmonary Trunk
Q   Pulmonary Artery, Right
R   Pulmonary Artery, Left
     Arterial canal (duct)
     Botallo's duct
     Pulmoaortic canal
S   Pulmonary Vein, Right
     Right inferior pulmonary vein
     Right superior pulmonary vein
T   Pulmonary Vein, Left
     Left inferior pulmonary vein
     Left superior pulmonary vein
V   Superior Vena Cava
     Precava
W   Thoracic Aorta, Descending
	Ø Open
	3 Percutaneous
	4 Percutaneous Endoscopic
		Ø Monitoring Device, Pressure Sensor
		2 Monitoring Device
		3 Infusion Device
		D Intraluminal Device
		Y Other Device
			Z No Qualifier

X   Thoracic Aorta, Ascending/Arch ⊞
     Aortic arch
     Ascending aorta
	Ø Open
	3 Percutaneous
	4 Percutaneous Endoscopic
		Ø Monitoring Device, Pressure Sensor
		2 Monitoring Device
		3 Infusion Device
		D Intraluminal Device
			Z No Qualifier

DRG Non-OR	Ø2H[4,6,7,K,L][Ø,3,4][J,M]Z	**HAC**	Ø2H43[J,K,M]Z when reported with SDx K68.11 or T81.4Ø-T81.49, T82.6-T82.7 with 7th character A
DRG Non-OR	Ø2HK32Z		
DRG Non-OR	Ø2HN[Ø,3,4][J,M]Z	**HAC**	Ø2H[6,K]33Z when reported with SDx J95.811
Non-OR	Ø2H[4,6,7,L]3[2,3]Z	**HAC**	Ø2H[6,7]3[J,M]Z when reported with SDx K68.11 or T81.4Ø-T81.49, T82.6-T82.7 with 7th character A
Non-OR	Ø2H[6,7]3MZ		
Non-OR	Ø2HK3[Ø,3]Z	**HAC**	Ø2H[K,L]3JZ when reported with SDx K68.11 or T81.4Ø-T81.49, T82.6-T82.7 with 7th character A
Non-OR	Ø2HN32Z		
Non-OR	Ø2HP[Ø,3,4][Ø,2,3]Z	**HAC**	Ø2HN[Ø,3,4][J,M]Z when reported with SDx K68.11 or T81.4Ø-T81.49, T82.6-T82.7 with 7th character A
Non-OR	Ø2H[Q,R][Ø,3,4][2,3]Z		
Non-OR	Ø2H[S,T,V,W][Ø,3,4]3Z	**HAC**	Ø2H[S,T,V][3,4]3Z when reported with SDx J95.811
Non-OR	Ø2H[S,T,V,W]32Z	`LC`	Ø2HAØQZ
Non-OR	Ø2HW[Ø,3]ØZ	`NC`	Ø2HA[3,4]QZ
Non-OR	Ø2HX[Ø,3,4][Ø,3]Z		

See Appendix L for Procedure Combinations
   ⊞   Ø2H[4,6,7,K,L][Ø,3,4][J,K,M]Z
   ⊞   Ø2HA[Ø,4]R[S,Z]
   ⊞   Ø2HA3RS
   ⊞   Ø2HN[Ø,3,4][J,K,M]Z

Ø Medical and Surgical
2 Heart and Great Vessels
J Inspection   Definition: Visually and/or manually exploring a body part

Explanation: Visual exploration may be performed with or without optical instrumentation. Manual exploration may be performed directly or through intervening body layers.

Body Part Character 4	Approach Character 5	Device Character 6	Qualifier Character 7
A Heart **Y** Great Vessel	**Ø** Open **3** Percutaneous **4** Percutaneous Endoscopic	**Z** No Device	**Z** No Qualifier

Non-OR   02J[A,Y]3ZZ

Ø Medical and Surgical
2 Heart and Great Vessels
K Map   Definition: Locating the route of passage of electrical impulses and/or locating functional areas in a body part

Explanation: Applicable only to the cardiac conduction mechanism and the central nervous system

Body Part Character 4	Approach Character 5	Device Character 6	Qualifier Character 7

8 Conduction Mechanism
   Atrioventricular node
   Bundle of His
   Bundle of Kent
   Sinoatrial node
	Ø Open
	3 Percutaneous
	4 Percutaneous Endoscopic
		Z No Device	**Z** No Qualifier

DRG Non-OR   02K8[0,3,4]ZZ

Ø Medical and Surgical
2 Heart and Great Vessels
L Occlusion   Definition: Completely closing an orifice or the lumen of a tubular body part

Explanation: The orifice can be a natural orifice or an artificially created orifice

Body Part Character 4	Approach Character 5	Device Character 6	Qualifier Character 7

7 Atrium, Left
   Atrium pulmonale
   Left auricular appendix
	Ø Open
	3 Percutaneous
	4 Percutaneous Endoscopic
		C Extraluminal Device
		D Intraluminal Device
		Z No Device
			K Left Atrial Appendage

H Pulmonary Valve
   Pulmonary annulus
   Pulmonic valve
P Pulmonary Trunk
Q Pulmonary Artery, Right
S Pulmonary Vein, Right
   Right inferior pulmonary vein
   Right superior pulmonary vein
T Pulmonary Vein, Left
   Left inferior pulmonary vein
   Left superior pulmonary vein
V Superior Vena Cava
   Precava
	Ø Open
	3 Percutaneous
	4 Percutaneous Endoscopic
		C Extraluminal Device
		D Intraluminal Device
		Z No Device
			Z No Qualifier

R Pulmonary Artery, Left
   Arterial canal (duct)
   Botallo's duct
   Pulmoaortic canal
	Ø Open
	3 Percutaneous
	4 Percutaneous Endoscopic
		C Extraluminal Device
		D Intraluminal Device
		Z No Device
			T Ductus Arteriosus
			Z No Qualifier

W Thoracic Aorta, Descending	**3** Percutaneous	**D** Intraluminal Device	**J** Temporary

DRG Non-OR   02L7[0,3,4][C,D,Z]K

Heart and Great Vessels

Ø   **Medical and Surgical**
2   **Heart and Great Vessels**
N   **Release**   Definition: Freeing a body part from an abnormal physical constraint by cutting or by the use of force
                               Explanation: Some of the restraining tissue may be taken out but none of the body part is taken out

Body Part Character 4	Approach Character 5	Device Character 6	Qualifier Character 7

Ø Coronary Artery, One Artery
1 Coronary Artery, Two Arteries
2 Coronary Artery, Three Arteries
3 Coronary Artery, Four or More Arteries
4 Coronary Vein
5 Atrial Septum
   Interatrial septum
6 Atrium, Right
   Atrium dextrum cordis
   Right auricular appendix
   Sinus venosus
7 Atrium, Left
   Atrium pulmonale
   Left auricular appendix
8 Conduction Mechanism
   Atrioventricular node
   Bundle of His
   Bundle of Kent
   Sinoatrial node
9 Chordae Tendineae
D Papillary Muscle
F Aortic Valve
   Aortic annulus
G Mitral Valve
   Bicuspid valve
   Left atrioventricular valve
   Mitral annulus
H Pulmonary Valve
   Pulmonary annulus
   Pulmonic valve
J Tricuspid Valve
   Right atrioventricular valve
   Tricuspid annulus
K Ventricle, Right
   Conus arteriosus
L Ventricle, Left
M Ventricular Septum
   Interventricular septum
N Pericardium
P Pulmonary Trunk
Q Pulmonary Artery, Right
R Pulmonary Artery, Left
   Arterial canal (duct)
   Botallo's duct
   Pulmoaortic canal
S Pulmonary Vein, Right
   Right inferior pulmonary vein
   Right superior pulmonary vein
T Pulmonary Vein, Left
   Left inferior pulmonary vein
   Left superior pulmonary vein
V Superior Vena Cava
   Precava
W Thoracic Aorta, Descending
X Thoracic Aorta, Ascending/Arch
   Aortic arch
   Ascending aorta
	Ø Open
	3 Percutaneous
	4 Percutaneous Endoscopic
		Z No Device	Z No Qualifier

Ø   Medical and Surgical
2   Heart and Great Vessels
P   Removal   Definition: Taking out or off a device from a body part

Explanation: If a device is taken out and a similar device put in without cutting or puncturing the skin or mucous membrane, the procedure is coded to the root operation CHANGE. Otherwise, the procedure for taking out a device is coded to the root operation REMOVAL.

Body Part Character 4	Approach Character 5	Device Character 6	Qualifier Character 7
A Heart	Ø Open 3 Percutaneous 4 Percutaneous Endoscopic	2 Monitoring Device 3 Infusion Device 7 Autologous Tissue Substitute 8 Zooplastic Tissue C Extraluminal Device D Intraluminal Device J Synthetic Substitute K Nonautologous Tissue Substitute M Cardiac Lead N Intracardiac Pacemaker Q Implantable Heart Assist System Y Other Device	Z No Qualifier
A Heart ⊞	Ø Open 3 Percutaneous 4 Percutaneous Endoscopic	R Short-term External Heart Assist System	S Biventricular Z No Qualifier
A Heart	X External	2 Monitoring Device 3 Infusion Device D Intraluminal Device M Cardiac Lead	Z No Qualifier
Y Great Vessel	Ø Open 3 Percutaneous 4 Percutaneous Endoscopic	2 Monitoring Device 3 Infusion Device 7 Autologous Tissue Substitute 8 Zooplastic Tissue C Extraluminal Device D Intraluminal Device J Synthetic Substitute K Nonautologous Tissue Substitute Y Other Device	Z No Qualifier
Y Great Vessel	X External	2 Monitoring Device 3 Infusion Device D Intraluminal Device	Z No Qualifier

Non-OR   Ø2PA3[2,3,D]Z
Non-OR   Ø2PA[3,4]YZ
Non-OR   Ø2PAX[2,3,D,M]Z
Non-OR   Ø2PY3[2,3,D]Z
Non-OR   Ø2PY[3,4]YZ
Non-OR   Ø2PYX[2,3,D]Z
HAC   Ø2PA[Ø,3,4]MZ when reported with SDx K68.11 or T81.4Ø-T81.49, T82.6-T82.7 with 7th character A
HAC   Ø2PAXMZ when reported with SDx K68.11 or T81.4Ø-T81.49, T82.6-T82.7 with 7th character A

See Appendix L for Procedure Combinations
⊞   Ø2PA[Ø,3,4]RZ

NC Noncovered Procedure   LC Limited Coverage   QA Questionable OB Admit   NT New Tech Add-on

Heart and Great Vessels

Ø **Medical and Surgical**
2 **Heart and Great Vessels**
Q **Repair**   Definition: Restoring, to the extent possible, a body part to its normal anatomic structure and function
                     Explanation: Used only when the method to accomplish the repair is not one of the other root operations

Body Part Character 4	Approach Character 5	Device Character 6	Qualifier Character 7

Ø Coronary Artery, One Artery
1 Coronary Artery, Two Arteries
2 Coronary Artery, Three Arteries
3 Coronary Artery, Four or More
   Arteries
4 Coronary Vein
5 Atrial Septum
   Interatrial septum
6 Atrium, Right
   Atrium dextrum cordis
   Right auricular appendix
   Sinus venosus
7 Atrium, Left
   Atrium pulmonale
   Left auricular appendix
8 Conduction Mechanism
   Atrioventricular node
   Bundle of His
   Bundle of Kent
   Sinoatrial node
9 Chordae Tendineae
A Heart
B Heart, Right
   Right coronary sulcus
C Heart, Left
   Left coronary sulcus
   Obtuse margin
D Papillary Muscle
H Pulmonary Valve
   Pulmonary annulus
   Pulmonic valve
K Ventricle, Right
   Conus arteriosus
L Ventricle, Left
M Ventricular Septum
   Interventricular septum
N Pericardium
P Pulmonary Trunk
Q Pulmonary Artery, Right
R Pulmonary Artery, Left
   Arterial canal (duct)
   Botallo's duct
   Pulmoaortic canal
S Pulmonary Vein, Right
   Right inferior pulmonary vein
   Right superior pulmonary vein
T Pulmonary Vein, Left
   Left inferior pulmonary vein
   Left superior pulmonary vein
V Superior Vena Cava
   Precava
W Thoracic Aorta, Descending
X Thoracic Aorta, Ascending/Arch
   Aortic arch
   Ascending aorta
	Ø Open
	3 Percutaneous
	4 Percutaneous Endoscopic
		Z No Device	Z No Qualifier

F Aortic Valve Aortic annulus	Ø Open 3 Percutaneous 4 Percutaneous Endoscopic	Z No Device	J Truncal Valve Z No Qualifier

G Mitral Valve
   Bicuspid valve
   Left atrioventricular valve
   Mitral annulus
	Ø Open
	3 Percutaneous
	4 Percutaneous Endoscopic
		Z No Device	E Atrioventricular Valve, Left
			Z No Qualifier

J Tricuspid Valve
   Right atrioventricular valve
   Tricuspid annulus
	Ø Open
	3 Percutaneous
	4 Percutaneous Endoscopic
		Z No Device	G Atrioventricular Valve, Right
			Z No Qualifier

Ø   Medical and Surgical
2   Heart and Great Vessels
R   Replacement   Definition: Putting in or on biological or synthetic material that physically takes the place and/or function of all or a portion of a body part

Explanation: The body part may have been taken out or replaced, or may be taken out, physically eradicated, or rendered nonfunctional during the REPLACEMENT procedure. A REMOVAL procedure is coded for taking out the device used in a previous replacement procedure.

Body Part Character 4	Approach Character 5	Device Character 6	Qualifier Character 7
5 Atrial Septum Interatrial septum **6 Atrium, Right** Atrium dextrum cordis Right auricular appendix Sinus venosus **7 Atrium, Left** Atrium pulmonale Left auricular appendix **9 Chordae Tendineae** **D Papillary Muscle** **K Ventricle, Right** `LC` `NC` ⊞ Conus arteriosus **L Ventricle, Left** `LC` `NC` ⊞ **M Ventricular Septum** Interventricular septum **N Pericardium** **P Pulmonary Trunk** **Q Pulmonary Artery, Right** **R Pulmonary Artery, Left** Arterial canal (duct) Botallo's duct Pulmoaortic canal **S Pulmonary Vein, Right** Right inferior pulmonary vein Right superior pulmonary vein **T Pulmonary Vein, Left** Left inferior pulmonary vein Left superior pulmonary vein **V Superior Vena Cava** Precava **W Thoracic Aorta, Descending** **X Thoracic Aorta, Ascending/Arch** Aortic arch Ascending aorta	**Ø Open** **4 Percutaneous Endoscopic**	**7 Autologous Tissue Substitute** **8 Zooplastic Tissue** **J Synthetic Substitute** **K Nonautologous Tissue Substitute**	**Z No Qualifier**
A Heart	Ø Open	L Biologic with Synthetic Substitute, Autoregulated Electrohydraulic M Synthetic Substitute, Pneumatic	Z No Qualifier
F Aortic Valve Aortic annulus **G Mitral Valve** Bicuspid valve Left atrioventricular valve Mitral annulus **J Tricuspid Valve** Right atrioventricular valve Tricuspid annulus	**Ø Open** **4 Percutaneous Endoscopic**	**7 Autologous Tissue Substitute** **8 Zooplastic Tissue** **J Synthetic Substitute** **K Nonautologous Tissue Substitute**	**Z No Qualifier**
F Aortic Valve Aortic annulus **G Mitral Valve** Bicuspid valve Left atrioventricular valve Mitral annulus **J Tricuspid Valve** Right atrioventricular valve Tricuspid annulus	**3 Percutaneous**	**7 Autologous Tissue Substitute** **8 Zooplastic Tissue** **J Synthetic Substitute** **K Nonautologous Tissue Substitute**	**H Transapical** **Z No Qualifier**
H Pulmonary Valve Pulmonary annulus Pulmonic valve	**Ø Open** **4 Percutaneous Endoscopic**	**7 Autologous Tissue Substitute** **8 Zooplastic Tissue** **J Synthetic Substitute** **K Nonautologous Tissue Substitute**	**Z No Qualifier**
H Pulmonary Valve Pulmonary annulus Pulmonic valve	**3 Percutaneous**	**7 Autologous Tissue Substitute** **J Synthetic Substitute** **K Nonautologous Tissue Substitute**	**H Transapical** **Z No Qualifier**
H Pulmonary Valve Pulmonary annulus Pulmonic valve	**3 Percutaneous**	**8 Zooplastic Tissue**	**H Transapical** **L In Existing Conduit** **M Native Site** **Z No Qualifier**

`LC`   02RKØJZ with 02RLØJZ with diagnosis code Z00.6
`NC`   02RKØJZ with 02RLØJZ without diagnosis code Z00.6

See Appendix L for Procedure Combinations
   ⊞   02R[K,L]ØJZ

`NC` Noncovered Procedure   `LC` Limited Coverage   `QA` Questionable OB Admit   `NT` New Tech Add-on   ⊞ Combination Member   ♂ Male   ♀ Female

Ø   Medical and Surgical
2   Heart and Great Vessels
S   Reposition   Definition: Moving to its normal location, or other suitable location, all or a portion of a body part

Explanation: The body part is moved to a new location from an abnormal location, or from a normal location where it is not functioning correctly. The body part may or may not be cut out or off to be moved to the new location.

Body Part Character 4	Approach Character 5	Device Character 6	Qualifier Character 7

Ø   Coronary Artery, One Artery
1   Coronary Artery, Two Arteries
P   Pulmonary Trunk
Q   Pulmonary Artery, Right
R   Pulmonary Artery, Left
    Arterial canal (duct)
    Botallo's duct
    Pulmoaortic canal
S   Pulmonary Vein, Right
    Right inferior pulmonary vein
    Right superior pulmonary vein
T   Pulmonary Vein, Left
    Left inferior pulmonary vein
    Left superior pulmonary vein
V   Superior Vena Cava
    Precava
W   Thoracic Aorta, Descending
X   Thoracic Aorta, Ascending/Arch
    Aortic arch
    Ascending aorta
	Ø Open	**Z** No Device	**Z** No Qualifier

Ø   Medical and Surgical
2   Heart and Great Vessels
T   Resection   Definition: Cutting out or off, without replacement, all of a body part

Explanation: None

Body Part Character 4	Approach Character 5	Device Character 6	Qualifier Character 7

5   Atrial Septum
    Interatrial septum
8   Conduction Mechanism
    Atrioventricular node
    Bundle of His
    Bundle of Kent
    Sinoatrial node
9   Chordae Tendineae
D   Papillary Muscle
H   Pulmonary Valve
    Pulmonary annulus
    Pulmonic valve
M   Ventricular Septum
    Interventricular septum
N   Pericardium
	Ø Open
	3 Percutaneous
	4 Percutaneous Endoscopic
		Z No Device	**Z** No Qualifier

Ø   Medical and Surgical
2   Heart and Great Vessels
U   Supplement   Definition: Putting in or on biological or synthetic material that physically reinforces and/or augments the function of a portion of a body part

Explanation: The biological material is non-living, or is living and from the same individual. The body part may have been previously replaced, and the SUPPLEMENT procedure is performed to physically reinforce and/or augment the function of the replaced body part.

Body Part Character 4	Approach Character 5	Device Character 6	Qualifier Character 7

Ø Coronary Artery, One Artery
1 Coronary Artery, Two Arteries
2 Coronary Artery, Three Arteries
3 Coronary Artery, Four or More
   Arteries
5 Atrial Septum
   Interatrial septum
6 Atrium, Right
   Atrium dextrum cordis
   Right auricular appendix
   Sinus venosus
7 Atrium, Left
   Atrium pulmonale
   Left auricular appendix
9 Chordae Tendineae
A Heart
D Papillary Muscle
H Pulmonary Valve
   Pulmonary annulus
   Pulmonic valve
K Ventricle, Right
   Conus arteriosus
L Ventricle, Left
M Ventricular Septum
   Interventricular septum
N Pericardium
P Pulmonary Trunk
Q Pulmonary Artery, Right
R Pulmonary Artery, Left
   Arterial canal (duct)
   Botallo's duct
   Pulmoaortic canal
S Pulmonary Vein, Right
   Right inferior pulmonary vein
   Right superior pulmonary vein
T Pulmonary Vein, Left
   Left inferior pulmonary vein
   Left superior pulmonary vein
V Superior Vena Cava
   Precava
W Thoracic Aorta, Descending
X Thoracic Aorta, Ascending/Arch
   Aortic arch
   Ascending aorta
	Ø Open
	3 Percutaneous
	4 Percutaneous Endoscopic
		7 Autologous Tissue Substitute
		8 Zooplastic Tissue
		J Synthetic Substitute
		K Nonautologous Tissue Substitute
			Z No Qualifier

F Aortic Valve Aortic annulus	**Ø** Open **3** Percutaneous **4** Percutaneous Endoscopic	**7** Autologous Tissue Substitute **8** Zooplastic Tissue **J** Synthetic Substitute **K** Nonautologous Tissue Substitute	**J** Truncal Valve **Z** No Qualifier

G Mitral Valve
   Bicuspid valve
   Left atrioventricular valve
   Mitral annulus
	Ø Open
	4 Percutaneous Endoscopic
		7 Autologous Tissue Substitute
		8 Zooplastic Tissue
		J Synthetic Substitute
		K Nonautologous Tissue Substitute
			E Atrioventricular Valve, Left
			Z No Qualifier

G Mitral Valve
   Bicuspid valve
   Left atrioventricular valve
   Mitral annulus
	3 Percutaneous	**7** Autologous Tissue Substitute
		8 Zooplastic Tissue
		K Nonautologous Tissue Substitute
			E Atrioventricular Valve, Left
			Z No Qualifier

G Mitral Valve
   Bicuspid valve
   Left atrioventricular valve
   Mitral annulus
	3 Percutaneous	**J** Synthetic Substitute	**E** Atrioventricular Valve, Left
			H Transapical
			Z No Qualifier

J Tricuspid Valve
   Right atrioventricular valve
   Tricuspid annulus
	Ø Open
	3 Percutaneous
	4 Percutaneous Endoscopic
		7 Autologous Tissue Substitute
		8 Zooplastic Tissue
		J Synthetic Substitute
		K Nonautologous Tissue Substitute
			G Atrioventricular Valve, Right
			Z No Qualifier

DRG Non-OR   Ø2U7[3,4]JZ

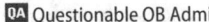

NC Noncovered Procedure   **LC** Limited Coverage   **QA** Questionable OB Admit   **NT** New Tech Add-on   ⊞ Combination Member   ♂ Male   ♀ Female

ICD-10-PCS 2022   189

Ø2U–Ø2U

Ø   **Medical and Surgical**
2   **Heart and Great Vessels**
V   **Restriction**   Definition: Partially closing an orifice or the lumen of a tubular body part
                        Explanation: The orifice can be a natural orifice or an artificially created orifice

Body Part Character 4	Approach Character 5	Device Character 6	Qualifier Character 7
A Heart	**Ø** Open **3** Percutaneous **4** Percutaneous Endoscopic	**C** Extraluminal Device **Z** No Device	**Z** No Qualifier

G Mitral Valve
     Bicuspid valve
     Left atrioventricular valve
     Mitral annulus
	Ø Open
	3 Percutaneous
	4 Percutaneous Endoscopic
		Z No Device	**Z** No Qualifier

L Ventricle, Left
P Pulmonary Trunk
Q Pulmonary Artery, Right
S Pulmonary Vein, Right
     Right inferior pulmonary vein
     Right superior pulmonary vein
T Pulmonary Vein, Left
     Left inferior pulmonary vein
     Left superior pulmonary vein
V Superior Vena Cava
     Precava
	Ø Open
	3 Percutaneous
	4 Percutaneous Endoscopic
		C Extraluminal Device
		D Intraluminal Device
		Z No Device
			Z No Qualifier

R Pulmonary Artery, Left
     Arterial canal (duct)
     Botallo's duct
     Pulmoaortic canal
	Ø Open
	3 Percutaneous
	4 Percutaneous Endoscopic
		C Extraluminal Device
		D Intraluminal Device
		Z No Device
			T Ductus Arteriosus
			Z No Qualifier

W Thoracic Aorta, Descending
X Thoracic Aorta, Ascending/Arch
     Aortic arch
     Ascending aorta
	Ø Open
	3 Percutaneous
	4 Percutaneous Endoscopic
		C Extraluminal Device
		D Intraluminal Device
		E Intraluminal Device, Branched or
		     Fenestrated, One or Two Arteries
		F Intraluminal Device, Branched or
		     Fenestrated, Three or More Arteries
		Z No Device
			Z No Qualifier

0 Medical and Surgical
2 Heart and Great Vessels
W Revision   Definition: Correcting, to the extent possible, a portion of a malfunctioning device or the position of a displaced device
       Explanation: Revision can include correcting a malfunctioning or displaced device by taking out or putting in components of the device such as a screw or pin

Body Part Character 4	Approach Character 5	Device Character 6	Qualifier Character 7
5 Atrial Septum Interatrial septum **M Ventricular Septum** Interventricular septum	**0** Open **4** Percutaneous Endoscopic	**J** Synthetic Substitute	**Z** No Qualifier
A Heart `LC` `NC` ⊞	**0** Open **3** Percutaneous **4** Percutaneous Endoscopic	**2** Monitoring Device **3** Infusion Device **7** Autologous Tissue Substitute **8** Zooplastic Tissue **C** Extraluminal Device **D** Intraluminal Device **J** Synthetic Substitute **K** Nonautologous Tissue Substitute **M** Cardiac Lead **N** Intracardiac Pacemaker **Q** Implantable Heart Assist System **Y** Other Device	**Z** No Qualifier
A Heart ⊞	**0** Open **3** Percutaneous **4** Percutaneous Endoscopic	**R** Short-term External Heart Assist System	**S** Biventricular **Z** No Qualifier
A Heart	**X** External	**2** Monitoring Device **3** Infusion Device **7** Autologous Tissue Substitute **8** Zooplastic Tissue **C** Extraluminal Device **D** Intraluminal Device **J** Synthetic Substitute **K** Nonautologous Tissue Substitute **M** Cardiac Lead **N** Intracardiac Pacemaker **Q** Implantable Heart Assist System	**Z** No Qualifier
A Heart	**X** External	**R** Short-term External Heart Assist System	**S** Biventricular **Z** No Qualifier
F Aortic Valve Aortic annulus **G Mitral Valve** Bicuspid valve Left atrioventricular valve Mitral annulus **H Pulmonary Valve** Pulmonary annulus Pulmonic valve **J Tricuspid Valve** Right atrioventricular valve Tricuspid annulus	**0** Open **3** Percutaneous **4** Percutaneous Endoscopic	**7** Autologous Tissue Substitute **8** Zooplastic Tissue **J** Synthetic Substitute **K** Nonautologous Tissue Substitute	**Z** No Qualifier
Y Great Vessel	**0** Open **3** Percutaneous **4** Percutaneous Endoscopic	**2** Monitoring Device **3** Infusion Device **7** Autologous Tissue Substitute **8** Zooplastic Tissue **C** Extraluminal Device **D** Intraluminal Device **J** Synthetic Substitute **K** Nonautologous Tissue Substitute **Y** Other Device	**Z** No Qualifier
Y Great Vessel	**X** External	**2** Monitoring Device **3** Infusion Device **7** Autologous Tissue Substitute **8** Zooplastic Tissue **C** Extraluminal Device **D** Intraluminal Device **J** Synthetic Substitute **K** Nonautologous Tissue Substitute	**Z** No Qualifier

Non-OR 02WA3[2,3,D]Z	**HAC**	02WA[0,3,4]MZ when reported with T81.40–T81.49, T82.6–T82.7 with 7th character A
Non-OR 02WA[3,4]YZ	`LC`	02WA0[J,Q]Z
Non-OR 02WAX[2,3,7,8,C,D,J,K,M,N,Q]Z	`NC`	02WA[3,4]QZ
Non-OR 02WAXRZ		
Non-OR 02WY3[2,3,D]Z	**See Appendix L for Procedure Combinations**	
Non-OR 02WY[3,4]YZ	⊞	02WA[0,3,4]QZ
Non-OR 02WYX[2,3,7,8,C,D,J,K]Z	⊞	02WA[0,3,4]RZ

`NC` Noncovered Procedure   `LC` Limited Coverage   `QA` Questionable OB Admit   `NT` New Tech Add-on   ⊞ Combination Member   ♂ Male   ♀ Female

Heart and Great Vessels

Ø **Medical and Surgical**
2 **Heart and Great Vessels**
Y **Transplantation** Definition: Putting in or on all or a portion of a living body part taken from another individual or animal to physically take the place and/or function of all or a portion of a similar body part

          Explanation: The native body part may or may not be taken out, and the transplanted body part may take over all or a portion of its function

Body Part Character 4	Approach Character 5	Device Character 6	Qualifier Character 7
A Heart **LC**	Ø Open	Z No Device	Ø Allogeneic 1 Syngeneic 2 Zooplastic

LC   Ø2YAØZ[Ø,1,2]

Upper Arteries Ø31–Ø3W

Character Meanings

This Character Meaning table is provided as a guide to assist the user in the identification of character members that may be found in this section of code tables. It **SHOULD NOT** be used to build a PCS code.

Operation–Character 3	Body Part–Character 4	Approach–Character 5	Device–Character 6	Qualifier–Character 7
1 Bypass	Ø Internal Mammary Artery, Right	Ø Open	Ø Drainage Device	Ø Upper Arm Artery, Right OR Ultrasonic
5 Destruction	1 Internal Mammary Artery, Left	3 Percutaneous	2 Monitoring Device	1 Upper Arm Artery, Left OR Drug-Coated Balloon
7 Dilation	2 Innominate Artery	4 Percutaneous Endoscopic	3 Infusion Device	2 Upper Arm Artery, Bilateral
9 Drainage	3 Subclavian Artery, Right	X External	4 Intraluminal Device, Drug-eluting	3 Lower Arm Artery, Right
B Excision	4 Subclavian Artery, Left		5 Intraluminal Device, Drug-eluting, Two	4 Lower Arm Artery, Left
C Extirpation	5 Axillary Artery, Right		6 Intraluminal Device, Drug-eluting, Three	5 Lower Arm Artery, Bilateral
F Fragmentation	6 Axillary Artery, Left		7 Intraluminal Device, Drug-eluting, Four or More OR Autologous Tissue Substitute	6 Upper Leg Artery, Right
H Insertion	7 Brachial Artery, Right		9 Autologous Venous Tissue	7 Upper Leg Artery, Left OR Stent Retriever
J Inspection	8 Brachial Artery, Left		A Autologous Arterial Tissue	8 Upper Leg Artery, Bilateral
L Occlusion	9 Ulnar Artery, Right		B Intraluminal Device, Bioactive	9 Lower Leg Artery, Right
N Release	A Ulnar Artery, Left		C Extraluminal Device	B Lower Leg Artery, Left
P Removal	B Radial Artery, Right		D Intraluminal Device	C Lower Leg Artery, Bilateral
Q Repair	C Radial Artery, Left		E Intraluminal Device, Two	D Upper Arm Vein
R Replacement	D Hand Artery, Right		F Intraluminal Device, Three	F Lower Arm Vein
S Reposition	F Hand Artery, Left		G Intraluminal Device, Four or More	G Intracranial Artery
U Supplement	G Intracranial Artery		H Intraluminal Device, Flow Diverter	J Extracranial Artery, Right
V Restriction	H Common Carotid Artery, Right		J Synthetic Substitute	K Extracranial Artery, Left
W Revision	J Common Carotid Artery, Left		K Nonautologous Tissue Substitute	M Pulmonary Artery, Right
	K Internal Carotid Artery, Right		M Stimulator Lead	N Pulmonary Artery, Left
	L Internal Carotid Artery, Left		Y Other Device	T Abdominal Artery
	M External Carotid Artery, Right		Z No Device	V Superior Vena Cava
	N External Carotid Artery, Left			W Lower Extremity Vein
	P Vertebral Artery, Right			X Diagnostic
	Q Vertebral Artery, Left			Y Upper Artery
	R Face Artery			Z No Qualifier
	S Temporal Artery, Right			
	T Temporal Artery, Left			
	U Thyroid Artery, Right			
	V Thyroid Artery, Left			
	Y Upper Artery			

Upper Arteries

AHA Coding Clinic for table Ø31

2019, 4Q, 26	Upper artery bypass Qualifier
2019, 4Q, 26	Percutaneous approach upper artery bypass
2017, 4Q, 64-65	New qualifier values - Left to right carotid bypass
2017, 2Q, 22	Carotid artery to subclavian artery transposition
2017, 1Q, 31	Left to right common carotid artery bypass
2016, 3Q, 37	Insertion of arteriovenous graft using HeRO device
2016, 3Q, 39	Revision of arteriovenous graft
2013, 4Q, 125	Stage II cephalic vein transposition (superficialization) of arteriovenous fistula
2013, 1Q, 27	Creation of radial artery fistula

AHA Coding Clinic for table Ø37

2020, 4Q, 70-71	Cerebral embolic filtration extracorporeal flow reversal circuit
2019, 4Q, 27	Bifurcation Qualifier
2019, 3Q, 29	Transcarotid arterial catheterization
2018, 2Q, 24	Coronary artery bifurcation
2016, 4Q, 86	Peripheral artery, number of stents
2016, 4Q, 86-87	Coronary and peripheral artery bifurcation
2015, 1Q, 32	Deployment of stent for herniated/migrated coil in basilar artery

AHA Coding Clinic for table Ø3B

| 2016, 2Q, 12 | Resection of malignant neoplasm of infratemporal fossa |

AHA Coding Clinic for table Ø3C

2021, 2Q, 13	Thromboendarterectomy with deconstruction of internal carotid artery
2020, 3Q, 38	Thrombectomy of arteriovenous fistula with angioplasty and stent placement
2019, 4Q, 27	Bifurcation Qualifier
2018, 4Q, 47-48	Endovascular thrombectomy with stent retriever
2018, 2Q, 24	Coronary artery bifurcation
2017, 4Q, 64-65	New qualifier values - Left to right carotid bypass
2017, 2Q, 23	Thrombectomy via Fogarty catheter
2016, 4Q, 86-87	Coronary and peripheral artery bifurcation
2016, 2Q, 11	Carotid endarterectomy with patch angioplasty
2015, 1Q, 29	Discontinued carotid endarterectomy

AHA Coding Clinic for table Ø3F

2020, 4Q, 45-49	New fragmentation tables
2020, 4Q, 49-50	Intravascular ultrasound assisted thrombolysis
2020, 4Q, 50	Intravascular lithotripsy

AHA Coding Clinic for table Ø3H

| 2020, 1Q, 25 | Elephant trunk repair of aortic dissection |
| 2016, 2Q, 32 | Arterial catheter placement |

AHA Coding Clinic for table Ø3J

| 2021, 1Q, 16 | Placement of Sentinel™ embolic protection device with deployment of single filter |
| 2015, 1Q, 29 | Discontinued carotid endarterectomy |

AHA Coding Clinic for table Ø3L

2021, 2Q, 13	Thromboendarterectomy with deconstruction of internal carotid artery
2016, 2Q, 30	Clipping (occlusion) of cerebral artery, decompressive craniectomy and storage of bone flap in abdominal wall
2014, 4Q, 20	Control of epistaxis
2014, 4Q, 37	Endovascular embolization of arteriovenous malformation using Onyx-18 liquid

AHA Coding Clinic for table Ø3Q

| 2017, 1Q, 31 | Left to right common carotid artery bypass |

AHA Coding Clinic for table Ø3S

| 2017, 2Q, 22 | Carotid artery to subclavian artery transposition |
| 2015, 3Q, 27 | Moyamoya disease and hemispheric pial synagiosis with craniotomy |

AHA Coding Clinic for table Ø3U

| 2019, 1Q, 22 | Cerebral artery fusiform aneurysm repair via wrapping |
| 2016, 2Q, 11 | Carotid endarterectomy with patch angioplasty |

AHA Coding Clinic for table Ø3V

2019, 4Q, 27-28	Aneurysm treatment using flow diverter stent
2019, 1Q, 22	Cerebral artery fusiform aneurysm repair via wrapping
2016, 1Q, 19	Embolization of superior hypophyseal aneurysm using stent-assisted coil

AHA Coding Clinic for table Ø3W

| 2016, 3Q, 39 | Revision of arteriovenous graft |
| 2015, 1Q, 32 | Deployment of stent for herniated/migrated coil in basilar artery |

Upper Arteries

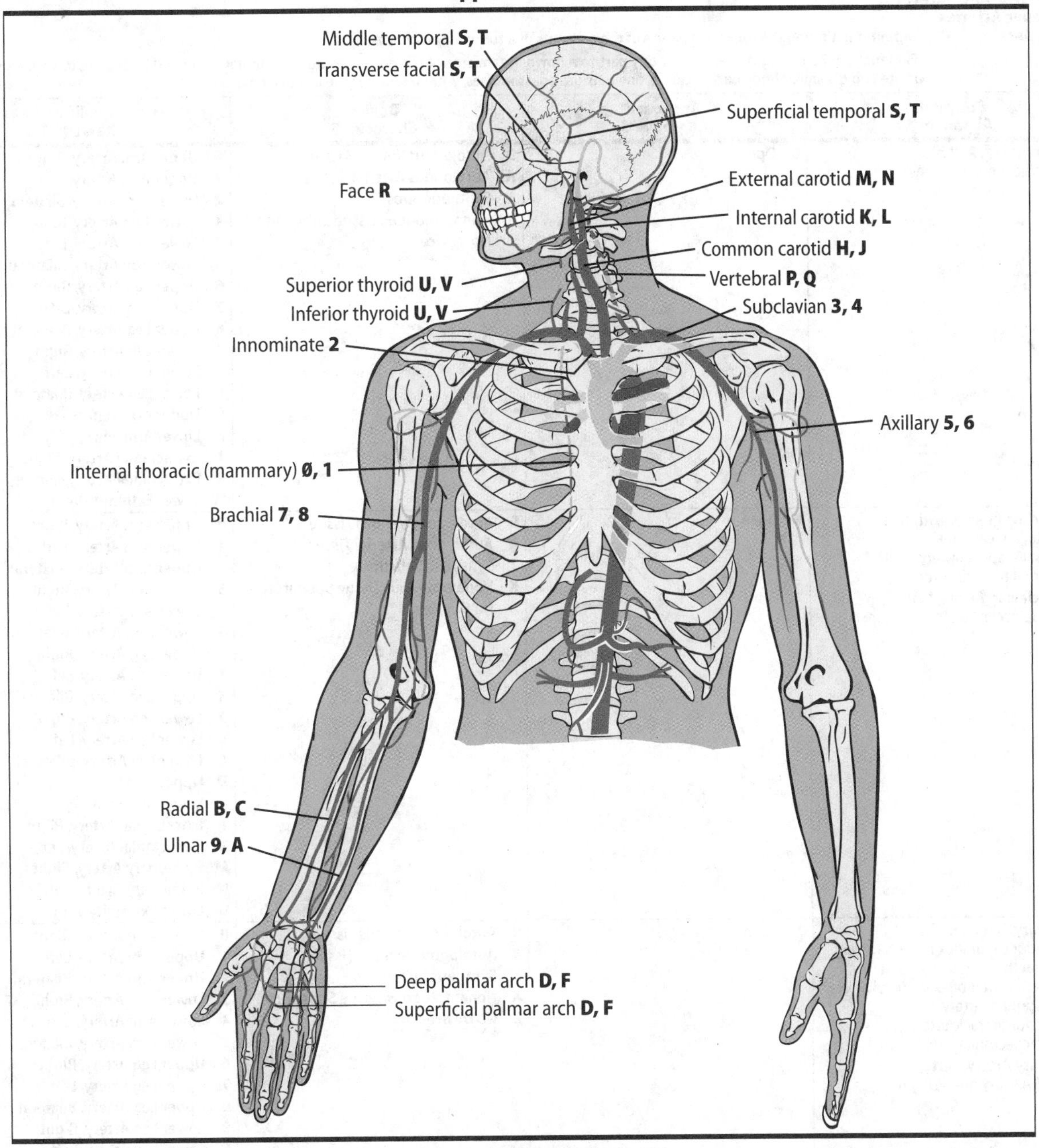

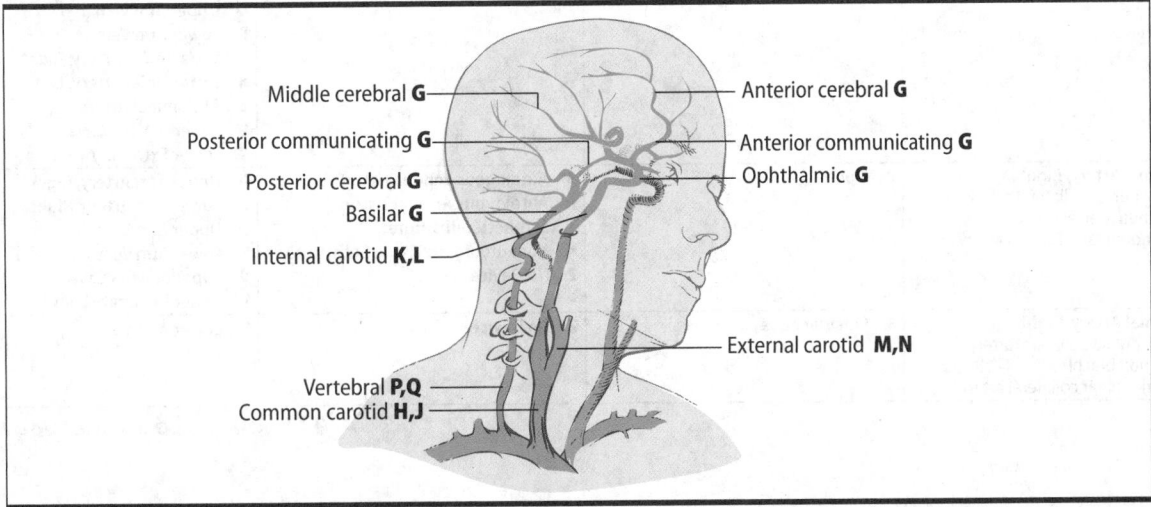

Middle temporal **S, T**
Transverse facial **S, T**
Superficial temporal **S, T**
Face **R**
External carotid **M, N**
Internal carotid **K, L**
Common carotid **H, J**
Vertebral **P, Q**
Superior thyroid **U, V**
Inferior thyroid **U, V**
Subclavian **3, 4**
Innominate **2**
Axillary **5, 6**
Internal thoracic (mammary) **Ø, 1**
Brachial **7, 8**
Radial **B, C**
Ulnar **9, A**
Deep palmar arch **D, F**
Superficial palmar arch **D, F**

Head and Neck Arteries

Middle cerebral **G**
Anterior cerebral **G**
Posterior communicating **G**
Anterior communicating **G**
Posterior cerebral **G**
Ophthalmic **G**
Basilar **G**
Internal carotid **K,L**
External carotid **M,N**
Vertebral **P,Q**
Common carotid **H,J**

Ø   Medical and Surgical
3   Upper Arteries
1   Bypass   Definition: Altering the route of passage of the contents of a tubular body part

Explanation: Rerouting contents of a body part to a downstream area of the normal route, to a similar route and body part, or to an abnormal route and dissimilar body part. Includes one or more anastomoses, with or without the use of a device.

Body Part Character 4	Approach Character 5	Device Character 6	Qualifier Character 7
2 Innominate Artery Brachiocephalic artery Brachiocephalic trunk	Ø Open	9 Autologous Venous Tissue A Autologous Arterial Tissue J Synthetic Substitute K Nonautologous Tissue Substitute Z No Device	Ø Upper Arm Artery, Right 1 Upper Arm Artery, Left 2 Upper Arm Artery, Bilateral 3 Lower Arm Artery, Right 4 Lower Arm Artery, Left 5 Lower Arm Artery, Bilateral 6 Upper Leg Artery, Right 7 Upper Leg Artery, Left 8 Upper Leg Artery, Bilateral 9 Lower Leg Artery, Right B Lower Leg Artery, Left C Lower Leg Artery, Bilateral D Upper Arm Vein F Lower Arm Vein J Extracranial Artery, Right K Extracranial Artery, Left W Lower Extremity Vein
3 Subclavian Artery, Right Costocervical trunk Dorsal scapular artery Internal thoracic artery 4 Subclavian Artery, Left *See 3 Subclavian Artery, Right*	Ø Open	9 Autologous Venous Tissue A Autologous Arterial Tissue J Synthetic Substitute K Nonautologous Tissue Substitute Z No Device	Ø Upper Arm Artery, Right 1 Upper Arm Artery, Left 2 Upper Arm Artery, Bilateral 3 Lower Arm Artery, Right 4 Lower Arm Artery, Left 5 Lower Arm Artery, Bilateral 6 Upper Leg Artery, Right 7 Upper Leg Artery, Left 8 Upper Leg Artery, Bilateral 9 Lower Leg Artery, Right B Lower Leg Artery, Left C Lower Leg Artery, Bilateral D Upper Arm Vein F Lower Arm Vein J Extracranial Artery, Right K Extracranial Artery, Left M Pulmonary Artery, Right N Pulmonary Artery, Left W Lower Extremity Vein
5 Axillary Artery, Right Anterior circumflex humeral artery Lateral thoracic artery Posterior circumflex humeral artery Subscapular artery Superior thoracic artery Thoracoacromial artery 6 Axillary Artery, Left *See 5 Axillary Artery, Right*	Ø Open	9 Autologous Venous Tissue A Autologous Arterial Tissue J Synthetic Substitute K Nonautologous Tissue Substitute Z No Device	Ø Upper Arm Artery, Right 1 Upper Arm Artery, Left 2 Upper Arm Artery, Bilateral 3 Lower Arm Artery, Right 4 Lower Arm Artery, Left 5 Lower Arm Artery, Bilateral 6 Upper Leg Artery, Right 7 Upper Leg Artery, Left 8 Upper Leg Artery, Bilateral 9 Lower Leg Artery, Right B Lower Leg Artery, Left C Lower Leg Artery, Bilateral D Upper Arm Vein F Lower Arm Vein J Extracranial Artery, Right K Extracranial Artery, Left T Abdominal Artery V Superior Vena Cava W Lower Extremity Vein
7 Brachial Artery, Right Inferior ulnar collateral artery Profunda brachii Superior ulnar collateral artery	Ø Open	9 Autologous Venous Tissue A Autologous Arterial Tissue J Synthetic Substitute K Nonautologous Tissue Substitute Z No Device	Ø Upper Arm Artery, Right 3 Lower Arm Artery, Right D Upper Arm Vein F Lower Arm Vein V Superior Vena Cava W Lower Extremity Vein
7 Brachial Artery, Right Inferior ulnar collateral artery Profunda brachii Superior ulnar collateral artery	3 Percutaneous	Z No Device	F Lower Arm Vein

Ø31 Continued on next page

Ø   **Medical and Surgical**
3   **Upper Arteries**
1   **Bypass**   Definition: Altering the route of passage of the contents of a tubular body part

Ø31 Continued

Explanation: Rerouting contents of a body part to a downstream area of the normal route, to a similar route and body part, or to an abnormal route and dissimilar body part. Includes one or more anastomoses, with or without the use of a device.

Body Part Character 4	Approach Character 5	Device Character 6	Qualifier Character 7
8 **Brachial Artery, Left** Inferior ulnar collateral artery Profunda brachii Superior ulnar collateral artery	Ø Open	9 Autologous Venous Tissue A Autologous Arterial Tissue J Synthetic Substitute K Nonautologous Tissue Substitute Z No Device	1 Upper Arm Artery, Left 4 Lower Arm Artery, Left D Upper Arm Vein F Lower Arm Vein V Superior Vena Cava W Lower Extremity Vein
8 **Brachial Artery, Left** Inferior ulnar collateral artery Profunda brachii Superior ulnar collateral artery	3 Percutaneous	Z No Device	F Lower Arm Vein
9 **Ulnar Artery, Right** Anterior ulnar recurrent artery Common interosseous artery Posterior ulnar recurrent artery B **Radial Artery, Right** Radial recurrent artery	Ø Open	9 Autologous Venous Tissue A Autologous Arterial Tissue J Synthetic Substitute K Nonautologous Tissue Substitute Z No Device	3 Lower Arm Artery, Right F Lower Arm Vein
9 **Ulnar Artery, Right** Anterior ulnar recurrent artery Common interosseous artery Posterior ulnar recurrent artery B **Radial Artery, Right** Radial recurrent artery	3 Percutaneous	Z No Device	F Lower Arm Vein
A **Ulnar Artery, Left** Anterior ulnar recurrent artery Common interosseous artery Posterior ulnar recurrent artery C **Radial Artery, Left** Radial recurrent artery	Ø Open	9 Autologous Venous Tissue A Autologous Arterial Tissue J Synthetic Substitute K Nonautologous Tissue Substitute Z No Device	4 Lower Arm Artery, Left F Lower Arm Vein
A **Ulnar Artery, Left** Anterior ulnar recurrent artery Common interosseous artery Posterior ulnar recurrent artery C **Radial Artery, Left** Radial recurrent artery	3 Percutaneous	Z No Device	F Lower Arm Vein

G   **Intracranial Artery**
Anterior cerebral artery
Anterior choroidal artery
Anterior communicating artery
Basilar artery
Circle of Willis
Internal carotid artery, intracranial
   portion
Middle cerebral artery
Ophthalmic artery
Posterior cerebral artery
Posterior communicating artery
Posterior inferior cerebellar artery
   (PICA)
S   **Temporal Artery, Right**
Middle temporal artery
Superficial temporal artery
Transverse facial artery
T   **Temporal Artery, Left**
See S Temporal Artery, Right
	Ø Open	9 Autologous Venous Tissue
		A Autologous Arterial Tissue
		J Synthetic Substitute
		K Nonautologous Tissue Substitute
		Z No Device
			G Intracranial Artery

H **Common Carotid Artery, Right** J **Common Carotid Artery, Left**	Ø Open	9 Autologous Venous Tissue A Autologous Arterial Tissue J Synthetic Substitute K Nonautologous Tissue Substitute Z No Device	G Intracranial Artery J Extracranial Artery, Right K Extracranial Artery, Left Y Upper Artery

Ø31 Continued on next page

NC Noncovered Procedure   **LC** Limited Coverage   **QA** Questionable OB Admit   **NT** New Tech Add-on   ⊞ Combination Member   ♂Male   ♀Female

ICD-10-PCS 2022   **197**

Ø31–Ø31

0   **Medical and Surgical**
3   **Upper Arteries**   *031 Continued*
1   **Bypass**   Definition: Altering the route of passage of the contents of a tubular body part

                              Explanation: Rerouting contents of a body part to a downstream area of the normal route, to a similar route and body part, or to an abnormal route and dissimilar body part. Includes one or more anastomoses, with or without the use of a device.

Body Part Character 4	Approach Character 5	Device Character 6	Qualifier Character 7

K   **Internal Carotid Artery, Right**
     Caroticotympanic artery
     Carotid sinus
L   **Internal Carotid Artery, Left**
     Caroticotympanic artery
     Carotid sinus
M   **External Carotid Artery, Right**
     Ascending pharyngeal artery
     Internal maxillary artery
     Lingual artery
     Maxillary artery
     Occipital artery
     Posterior auricular artery
     Superior thyroid artery
N   **External Carotid Artery, Left**
     Ascending pharyngeal artery
     Internal maxillary artery
     Lingual artery
     Maxillary artery
     Occipital artery
     Posterior auricular artery
     Superior thyroid artery
	0 Open	**9** Autologous Venous Tissue
		A Autologous Arterial Tissue
		J Synthetic Substitute
		K Nonautologous Tissue Substitute
		Z No Device
			J Extracranial Artery, Right
			K Extracranial Artery, Left

Ø   **Medical and Surgical**
3   **Upper Arteries**
5   **Destruction**   Definition: Physical eradication of all or a portion of a body part by the direct use of energy, force, or a destructive agent
                       Explanation: None of the body part is physically taken out

Body Part Character 4		Approach Character 5	Device Character 6	Qualifier Character 7

Ø **Internal Mammary Artery, Right**
  Anterior intercostal artery
  Internal thoracic artery
  Musculophrenic artery
  Pericardiophrenic artery
  Superior epigastric artery
1 **Internal Mammary Artery, Left**
  See Ø *Internal Mammary Artery, Right*
2 **Innominate Artery**
  Brachiocephalic artery
  Brachiocephalic trunk
3 **Subclavian Artery, Right**
  Costocervical trunk
  Dorsal scapular artery
  Internal thoracic artery
4 **Subclavian Artery, Left**
  See 3 *Subclavian Artery, Right*
5 **Axillary Artery, Right**
  Anterior circumflex humeral
    artery
  Lateral thoracic artery
  Posterior circumflex humeral
    artery
  Subscapular artery
  Superior thoracic artery
  Thoracoacromial artery
6 **Axillary Artery, Left**
  See 5 *Axillary Artery, Right*
7 **Brachial Artery, Right**
  Inferior ulnar collateral artery
  Profunda brachii
  Superior ulnar collateral artery
8 **Brachial Artery, Left**
  See 7 *Brachial Artery, Right*
9 **Ulnar Artery, Right**
  Anterior ulnar recurrent artery
  Common interosseous artery
  Posterior ulnar recurrent artery
A **Ulnar Artery, Left**
  See 9 *Ulnar Artery, Right*
B **Radial Artery, Right**
  Radial recurrent artery
C **Radial Artery, Left**
  See B *Radial Artery, Right*
D **Hand Artery, Right**
  Deep palmar arch
  Princeps pollicis artery
  Radialis indicis
  Superficial palmar arch
F **Hand Artery, Left**
  See D *Hand Artery, Right*
G **Intracranial Artery**
  Anterior cerebral artery
  Anterior choroidal artery
  Anterior communicating artery
  Basilar artery
  Circle of Willis
  Internal carotid artery,
    intracranial portion
  Middle cerebral artery
  Ophthalmic artery
  Posterior cerebral artery
  Posterior communicating artery
  Posterior inferior cerebellar
    artery (PICA)
	H **Common Carotid Artery, Right**
	J **Common Carotid Artery, Left**
	K **Internal Carotid Artery, Right**
	  Caroticotympanic artery
	  Carotid sinus
	L **Internal Carotid Artery, Left**
	  See K *Internal Carotid Artery, Right*
	M **External Carotid Artery, Right**
	  Ascending pharyngeal artery
	  Internal maxillary artery
	  Lingual artery
	  Maxillary artery
	  Occipital artery
	  Posterior auricular artery
	  Superior thyroid artery
	N **External Carotid Artery, Left**
	  See M *External Carotid Artery, Right*
	P **Vertebral Artery, Right**
	  Anterior spinal artery
	  Posterior spinal artery
	Q **Vertebral Artery, Left**
	  See P *Vertebral Artery, Right*
	R **Face Artery**
	  Angular artery
	  Ascending palatine artery
	  External maxillary artery
	  Facial artery
	  Inferior labial artery
	  Submental artery
	  Superior labial artery
	S **Temporal Artery, Right**
	  Middle temporal artery
	  Superficial temporal artery
	  Transverse facial artery
	T **Temporal Artery, Left**
	  See S *Temporal Artery, Right*
	U **Thyroid Artery, Right**
	  Cricothyroid artery
	  Hyoid artery
	  Sternocleidomastoid artery
	  Superior laryngeal artery
	  Superior thyroid artery
	  Thyrocervical trunk
	V **Thyroid Artery, Left**
	  See U *Thyroid Artery, Right*
	Y **Upper Artery**
	  Aortic intercostal artery
	  Bronchial artery
	  Esophageal artery
	  Subcostal artery
		Ø Open
		3 Percutaneous
		4 Percutaneous Endoscopic
			Z No Device	**Z** No Qualifier

| NC | Noncovered Procedure | LC | Limited Coverage | QA | Questionable OB Admit | NT | New Tech Add-on   ⊞ Combination Member   ♂ Male   ♀ Female

ICD-10-PCS 2022

Ø35–Ø35

199

Ø   Medical and Surgical
3   Upper Arteries
7   Dilation

Definition: Expanding an orifice or the lumen of a tubular body part

Explanation: The orifice can be a natural orifice or an artificially created orifice. Accomplished by stretching a tubular body part using intraluminal pressure or by cutting part of the orifice or wall of the tubular body part.

Body Part Character 4		Approach Character 5	Device Character 6	Qualifier Character 7
Ø **Internal Mammary Artery, Right** Anterior intercostal artery Internal thoracic artery Musculophrenic artery Pericardiophrenic artery Superior epigastric artery 1 **Internal Mammary Artery, Left** *See Ø Internal Mammary Artery, Right* 2 **Innominate Artery** Brachiocephalic artery Brachiocephalic trunk 3 **Subclavian Artery, Right** Costocervical trunk Dorsal scapular artery Internal thoracic artery 4 **Subclavian Artery, Left** *See 3 Subclavian Artery, Right* 5 **Axillary Artery, Right** Anterior circumflex humeral artery Lateral thoracic artery Posterior circumflex humeral artery Subscapular artery Superior thoracic artery Thoracoacromial artery	6 **Axillary Artery, Left** *See 5 Axillary Artery, Right* 7 **Brachial Artery, Right** Inferior ulnar collateral artery Profunda brachii Superior ulnar collateral artery 8 **Brachial Artery, Left** *See 7 Brachial Artery, Right* 9 **Ulnar Artery, Right** Anterior ulnar recurrent artery Common interosseous artery Posterior ulnar recurrent artery A **Ulnar Artery, Left** *See 9 Ulnar Artery, Right* B **Radial Artery, Right** Radial recurrent artery C **Radial Artery, Left** *See B Radial Artery, Right*	Ø **Open** 3 **Percutaneous** 4 **Percutaneous Endoscopic**	4 **Intraluminal Device, Drug-eluting** 5 **Intraluminal Device, Drug-eluting, Two** 6 **Intraluminal Device, Drug-eluting, Three** 7 **Intraluminal Device, Drug-eluting, Four or More** E **Intraluminal Device, Two** F **Intraluminal Device, Three** G **Intraluminal Device, Four or More**	Z **No Qualifier**
Ø **Internal Mammary Artery, Right** Anterior intercostal artery Internal thoracic artery Musculophrenic artery Pericardiophrenic artery Superior epigastric artery 1 **Internal Mammary Artery, Left** *See Ø Internal Mammary Artery, Right* 2 **Innominate Artery** Brachiocephalic artery Brachiocephalic trunk 3 **Subclavian Artery, Right** Costocervical trunk Dorsal scapular artery Internal thoracic artery 4 **Subclavian Artery, Left** *See 3 Subclavian Artery, Right* 5 **Axillary Artery, Right** Anterior circumflex humeral artery Lateral thoracic artery Posterior circumflex humeral artery Subscapular artery Superior thoracic artery Thoracoacromial artery	6 **Axillary Artery, Left** *See 5 Axillary Artery, Right* 7 **Brachial Artery, Right** Inferior ulnar collateral artery Profunda brachii Superior ulnar collateral artery 8 **Brachial Artery, Left** *See 7 Brachial Artery, Right* 9 **Ulnar Artery, Right** Anterior ulnar recurrent artery Common interosseous artery Posterior ulnar recurrent artery A **Ulnar Artery, Left** *See 9 Ulnar Artery, Right* B **Radial Artery, Right** Radial recurrent artery C **Radial Artery, Left** *See B Radial Artery, Right*	Ø **Open** 3 **Percutaneous** 4 **Percutaneous Endoscopic**	D **Intraluminal Device** Z **No Device**	1 **Drug-Coated Balloon** Z **No Qualifier**

Ø37 Continued on next page

Ø   Medical and Surgical
3   Upper Arteries
7   Dilation

Ø37 Continued

Definition: Expanding an orifice or the lumen of a tubular body part

Explanation: The orifice can be a natural orifice or an artificially created orifice. Accomplished by stretching a tubular body part using intraluminal pressure or by cutting part of the orifice or wall of the tubular body part.

Body Part Character 4		Approach Character 5	Device Character 6	Qualifier Character 7

D Hand Artery, Right
Deep palmar arch
Princeps pollicis artery
Radialis indicis
Superficial palmar arch
F Hand Artery, Left
See D Hand Artery, Right
G Intracranial Artery NC
Anterior cerebral artery
Anterior choroidal artery
Anterior communicating artery
Basilar artery
Circle of Willis
Internal carotid artery,
   intracranial portion
Middle cerebral artery
Ophthalmic artery
Posterior cerebral artery
Posterior communicating
   artery
Posterior inferior cerebellar
   artery (PICA)
**H Common Carotid Artery,
Right**
J Common Carotid Artery, Left
K Internal Carotid Artery, Right
Caroticotympanic artery
Carotid sinus
L Internal Carotid Artery, Left
*See K Internal Carotid Artery,
Right*
M External Carotid Artery, Right
Ascending pharyngeal artery
Internal maxillary artery
Lingual artery
Maxillary artery
Occipital artery
Posterior auricular artery
Superior thyroid artery
	N External Carotid Artery, Left
	*See M External Carotid Artery,
	Right*
	P Vertebral Artery, Right
	Anterior spinal artery
	Posterior spinal artery
	Q Vertebral Artery, Left
	See P Vertebral Artery, Right
	R Face Artery
	Angular artery
	Ascending palatine artery
	External maxillary artery
	Facial artery
	Inferior labial artery
	Submental artery
	Superior labial artery
	S Temporal Artery, Right
	Middle temporal artery
	Superficial temporal artery
	Transverse facial artery
	T Temporal Artery, Left
	See S Temporal Artery, Right
	U Thyroid Artery, Right
	Cricothyroid artery
	Hyoid artery
	Sternocleidomastoid artery
	Superior laryngeal artery
	Superior thyroid artery
	Thyrocervical trunk
	V Thyroid Artery, Left
	See U Thyroid Artery, Right
	Y Upper Artery
	Aortic intercostal artery
	Bronchial artery
	Esophageal artery
	Subcostal artery
		Ø Open
		3 Percutaneous
		4 Percutaneous Endoscopic
			**4 Intraluminal Device,
			Drug-eluting**
			**5 Intraluminal Device, Drug-
			eluting, Two**
			**6 Intraluminal Device, Drug-
			eluting, Three**
			**7 Intraluminal Device, Drug-
			eluting, Four or More**
			D Intraluminal Device
			E Intraluminal Device, Two
			F Intraluminal Device, Three
			**G Intraluminal Device, Four
			or More**
			Z No Device
				Z No Qualifier

NC   Ø37G[3,4]ZZ

NC Noncovered Procedure   LC Limited Coverage   QA Questionable OB Admit   NT New Tech Add-on   ⊞ Combination Member   ♂ Male   ♀ Female

ICD-10-PCS 2022   201

037–037

Ø　**Medical and Surgical**
3　**Upper Arteries**
9　**Drainage**　　Definition: Taking or letting out fluids and/or gases from a body part
　　　　　　　　　Explanation: The qualifier DIAGNOSTIC is used to identify drainage procedures that are biopsies

Body Part Character 4		Approach Character 5	Device Character 6	Qualifier Character 7
Ø **Internal Mammary Artery, 　Right** 　Anterior intercostal artery 　Internal thoracic artery 　Musculophrenic artery 　Pericardiophrenic artery 　Superior epigastric artery 1 **Internal Mammary Artery, 　Left** 　*See* Ø *Internal Mammary Artery, 　　Right above* 2 **Innominate Artery** 　Brachiocephalic artery 　Brachiocephalic trunk 3 **Subclavian Artery, Right** 　Costocervical trunk 　Dorsal scapular artery 　Internal thoracic artery 4 **Subclavian Artery, Left** 　*See* 3 *Subclavian Artery, Right* 5 **Axillary Artery, Right** 　Anterior circumflex humeral 　　artery 　Lateral thoracic artery 　Posterior circumflex humeral 　　artery 　Subscapular artery 　Superior thoracic artery 　Thoracoacromial artery 6 **Axillary Artery, Left** 　*See* 5 *Axillary Artery, Right* 7 **Brachial Artery, Right** 　Inferior ulnar collateral artery 　Profunda brachii 　Superior ulnar collateral artery 8 **Brachial Artery, Left** 　*See* 7 *Brachial Artery, Right* 9 **Ulnar Artery, Right** 　Anterior ulnar recurrent artery 　Common interosseous artery 　Posterior ulnar recurrent artery A **Ulnar Artery, Left** 　*See* 9 *Ulnar Artery, Right* B **Radial Artery, Right** 　Radial recurrent artery C **Radial Artery, Left** 　*See* B *Radial Artery, Right* D **Hand Artery, Right** 　Deep palmar arch 　Princeps pollicis artery 　Radialis indicis 　Superficial palmar arch F **Hand Artery, Left** 　*See* D *Hand Artery, Right* G **Intracranial Artery** 　Anterior cerebral artery 　Anterior choroidal artery 　Anterior communicating artery 　Basilar artery 　Circle of Willis 　Internal carotid artery, 　　intracranial portion 　Middle cerebral artery 　Ophthalmic artery 　Posterior cerebral artery 　Posterior communicating artery 　Posterior inferior cerebellar 　　artery (PICA)	H **Common Carotid Artery, 　Right** J **Common Carotid Artery, Left** K **Internal Carotid Artery, Right** 　Caroticotympanic artery 　Carotid sinus L **Internal Carotid Artery, Left** 　*See* K *Internal Carotid Artery, 　　Right* M **External Carotid Artery, Right** 　Ascending pharyngeal artery 　Internal maxillary artery 　Lingual artery 　Maxillary artery 　Occipital artery 　Posterior auricular artery 　Superior thyroid artery N **External Carotid Artery, Left** 　*See* M *External Carotid Artery, 　　Right* P **Vertebral Artery, Right** 　Anterior spinal artery 　Posterior spinal artery Q **Vertebral Artery, Left** 　*See* P *Vertebral Artery, Right* R **Face Artery** 　Angular artery 　Ascending palatine artery 　External maxillary artery 　Facial artery 　Inferior labial artery 　Submental artery 　Superior labial artery S **Temporal Artery, Right** 　Middle temporal artery 　Superficial temporal artery 　Transverse facial artery T **Temporal Artery, Left** 　*See* S *Temporal Artery, Right* U **Thyroid Artery, Right** 　Cricothyroid artery 　Hyoid artery 　Sternocleidomastoid artery 　Superior laryngeal artery 　Superior thyroid artery 　Thyrocervical trunk V **Thyroid Artery, Left** 　*See* U *Thyroid Artery, Right* Y **Upper Artery** 　Aortic intercostal artery 　Bronchial artery 　Esophageal artery 　Subcostal artery	Ø **Open** 3 **Percutaneous** 4 **Percutaneous Endoscopic**	Ø **Drainage Device**	Z **No Qualifier**

Non-OR　Ø39[Ø,1,2,3,4,5,6,7,8,9,A,B,C,D,F,G,H,J,K,L,M,N,P,Q,R,S,T,U,V,Y][Ø,3,4]ØZ

Ø39 Continued on next page

Ø   **Medical and Surgical**   *Ø39 Continued*
3   **Upper Arteries**
9   **Drainage**   Definition: Taking or letting out fluids and/or gases from a body part

                       Explanation: The qualifier DIAGNOSTIC is used to identify drainage procedures that are biopsies

Body Part Character 4		Approach Character 5	Device Character 6	Qualifier Character 7
Ø **Internal Mammary Artery, Right** Anterior intercostal artery Internal thoracic artery Musculophrenic artery Pericardiophrenic artery Superior epigastric artery **1** **Internal Mammary Artery, Left** *See* Ø *Internal Mammary Artery, Right* **2** **Innominate Artery** Brachiocephalic artery Brachiocephalic trunk **3** **Subclavian Artery, Right** Costocervical trunk Dorsal scapular artery Internal thoracic artery **4** **Subclavian Artery, Left** *See* 3 *Subclavian Artery, Right* **5** **Axillary Artery, Right** Anterior circumflex humeral artery Lateral thoracic artery Posterior circumflex humeral artery Subscapular artery Superior thoracic artery Thoracoacromial artery **6** **Axillary Artery, Left** *See* 5 *Axillary Artery, Right* **7** **Brachial Artery, Right** Inferior ulnar collateral artery Profunda brachii Superior ulnar collateral artery **8** **Brachial Artery, Left** *See* 7 *Brachial Artery, Right* **9** **Ulnar Artery, Right** Anterior ulnar recurrent artery Common interosseous artery Posterior ulnar recurrent artery **A** **Ulnar Artery, Left** *See* 9 *Ulnar Artery, Right* **B** **Radial Artery, Right** Radial recurrent artery **C** **Radial Artery, Left** *See* B *Radial Artery, Right* **D** **Hand Artery, Right** Deep palmar arch Princeps pollicis artery Radialis indicis Superficial palmar arch **F** **Hand Artery, Left** *See* D *Hand Artery, Right* **G** **Intracranial Artery** Anterior cerebral artery Anterior choroidal artery Anterior communicating artery Basilar artery Circle of Willis Internal carotid artery, intracranial portion Middle cerebral artery Ophthalmic artery Posterior cerebral artery Posterior communicating artery Posterior inferior cerebellar artery (PICA)	**H** **Common Carotid Artery, Right** **J** **Common Carotid Artery, Left** **K** **Internal Carotid Artery, Right** Caroticotympanic artery Carotid sinus **L** **Internal Carotid Artery, Left** *See* K *Internal Carotid Artery, Right* **M** **External Carotid Artery, Right** Ascending pharyngeal artery Internal maxillary artery Lingual artery Maxillary artery Occipital artery Posterior auricular artery Superior thyroid artery **N** **External Carotid Artery, Left** *See* M *External Carotid Artery, Right* **P** **Vertebral Artery, Right** Anterior spinal artery Posterior spinal artery **Q** **Vertebral Artery, Left** *See* P *Vertebral Artery, Right* **R** **Face Artery** Angular artery Ascending palatine artery External maxillary artery Facial artery Inferior labial artery Submental artery Superior labial artery **S** **Temporal Artery, Right** Middle temporal artery Superficial temporal artery Transverse facial artery **T** **Temporal Artery, Left** *See* S *Temporal Artery, Right* **U** **Thyroid Artery, Right** Cricothyroid artery Hyoid artery Sternocleidomastoid artery Superior laryngeal artery Superior thyroid artery Thyrocervical trunk **V** **Thyroid Artery, Left** *See* U *Thyroid Artery, Right* **Y** **Upper Artery** Aortic intercostal artery Bronchial artery Esophageal artery Subcostal artery	**Ø** Open **3** Percutaneous **4** Percutaneous Endoscopic	**Z** No Device	**X** Diagnostic **Z** No Qualifier

Non-OR   Ø39[Ø,1,2,3,4,5,6,7,8,9,A,B,C,D,F,G,H,J,K,L,M,N,P,Q,R,S,T,U,V,Y]3ZX
Non-OR   Ø39[Ø,1,2,3,4,5,6,7,8,9,A,B,C,D,F,G,H,J,K,L,M,N,P,Q,R,S,T,U,V,Y][Ø,3,4]ZZ

NC Noncovered Procedure   **LC** Limited Coverage   **QA** Questionable OB Admit   **NT** New Tech Add-on   ⊞ Combination Member   ♂ Male   ♀ Female

ICD-10-PCS 2022   **203**

Ø39–Ø39

Upper Arteries

Ø Medical and Surgical
3 Upper Arteries
B Excision   Definition: Cutting out or off, without replacement, a portion of a body part
                    Explanation: The qualifier DIAGNOSTIC is used to identify excision procedures that are biopsies

Body Part Character 4	Approach Character 5	Device Character 6	Qualifier Character 7
Ø Internal Mammary Artery, Right Anterior intercostal artery Internal thoracic artery Musculophrenic artery Pericardiophrenic artery Superior epigastric artery **1 Internal Mammary Artery, Left** *See Ø Internal Mammary Artery, Right* **2 Innominate Artery** Brachiocephalic artery Brachiocephalic trunk **3 Subclavian Artery, Right** Costocervical trunk Dorsal scapular artery Internal thoracic artery **4 Subclavian Artery, Left** *See 3 Subclavian Artery, Right* **5 Axillary Artery, Right** Anterior circumflex humeral artery Lateral thoracic artery Posterior circumflex humeral artery Subscapular artery Superior thoracic artery Thoracoacromial artery **6 Axillary Artery, Left** *See 5 Axillary Artery, Right* **7 Brachial Artery, Right** Inferior ulnar collateral artery Profunda brachii Superior ulnar collateral artery **8 Brachial Artery, Left** *See 7 Brachial Artery, Right* **9 Ulnar Artery, Right** Anterior ulnar recurrent artery Common interosseous artery Posterior ulnar recurrent artery **A Ulnar Artery, Left** *See 9 Ulnar Artery, Right* **B Radial Artery, Right** Radial recurrent artery **C Radial Artery, Left** *See B Radial Artery, Right* **D Hand Artery, Right** Deep palmar arch Princeps pollicis artery Radialis indicis Superficial palmar arch **F Hand Artery, Left** *See D Hand Artery, Right* **G Intracranial Artery** Anterior cerebral artery Anterior choroidal artery Anterior communicating artery Basilar artery Circle of Willis Internal carotid artery, intracranial portion Middle cerebral artery Ophthalmic artery Posterior cerebral artery Posterior communicating artery Posterior inferior cerebellar artery (PICA) **H Common Carotid Artery, Right** **J Common Carotid Artery, Left** **K Internal Carotid Artery, Right** Caroticotympanic artery Carotid sinus **L Internal Carotid Artery, Left** *See K Internal Carotid Artery, Right* **M External Carotid Artery, Right** Ascending pharyngeal artery Internal maxillary artery Lingual artery Maxillary artery Occipital artery Posterior auricular artery Superior thyroid artery **N External Carotid Artery, Left** *See M External Carotid Artery, Right* **P Vertebral Artery, Right** Anterior spinal artery Posterior spinal artery **Q Vertebral Artery, Left** *See P Vertebral Artery, Right* **R Face Artery** Angular artery Ascending palatine artery External maxillary artery Facial artery Inferior labial artery Submental artery Superior labial artery **S Temporal Artery, Right** Middle temporal artery Superficial temporal artery Transverse facial artery **T Temporal Artery, Left** *See S Temporal Artery, Right* **U Thyroid Artery, Right** Cricothyroid artery Hyoid artery Sternocleidomastoid artery Superior laryngeal artery Superior thyroid artery Thyrocervical trunk **V Thyroid Artery, Left** *See U Thyroid Artery, Right* **Y Upper Artery** Aortic intercostal artery Bronchial artery Esophageal artery Subcostal artery	**Ø Open** **3 Percutaneous** **4 Percutaneous Endoscopic**	**Z No Device**	**X Diagnostic** **Z No Qualifier**

Ø   Medical and Surgical
3   Upper Arteries
C   Extirpation   Definition: Taking or cutting out solid matter from a body part

Explanation: The solid matter may be an abnormal byproduct of a biological function or a foreign body; it may be imbedded in a body part or in the lumen of a tubular body part. The solid matter may or may not have been previously broken into pieces.

Body Part Character 4		Approach Character 5	Device Character 6	Qualifier Character 7

Ø Internal Mammary Artery, Right
  Anterior intercostal artery
  Internal thoracic artery
  Musculophrenic artery
  Pericardiophrenic artery
  Superior epigastric artery
1 Internal Mammary Artery, Left
  See Ø Internal Mammary Artery, Right
2 Innominate Artery
  Brachiocephalic artery
  Brachiocephalic trunk
3 Subclavian Artery, Right
  Costocervical trunk
  Dorsal scapular artery
  Internal thoracic artery
4 Subclavian Artery, Left
  See 3 Subclavian Artery, Right
5 Axillary Artery, Right
  Anterior circumflex humeral artery
  Lateral thoracic artery
  Posterior circumflex humeral artery
  Subscapular artery
  Superior thoracic artery
  Thoracoacromial artery
6 Axillary Artery, Left
  See 5 Axillary Artery, Right
7 Brachial Artery, Right
  Inferior ulnar collateral artery
  Profunda brachii
  Superior ulnar collateral artery
8 Brachial Artery, Left
  See 7 Brachial Artery, Right
9 Ulnar Artery, Right
  Anterior ulnar recurrent artery
  Common interosseous artery
  Posterior ulnar recurrent artery
	A Ulnar Artery, Left
	  See 9 Ulnar Artery, Right
	B Radial Artery, Right
	  Radial recurrent artery
	C Radial Artery, Left
	  See B Radial Artery, Right
	D Hand Artery, Right
	  Deep palmar arch
	  Princeps pollicis artery
	  Radialis indicis
	  Superficial palmar arch
	F Hand Artery, Left
	  See D Hand Artery, Right
	R Face Artery
	  Angular artery
	  Ascending palatine artery
	  External maxillary artery
	  Facial artery
	  Inferior labial artery
	  Submental artery
	  Superior labial artery
	S Temporal Artery, Right
	  Middle temporal artery
	  Superficial temporal artery
	  Transverse facial artery
	T Temporal Artery, Left
	  See S Temporal Artery, Right
	U Thyroid Artery, Right
	  Cricothyroid artery
	  Hyoid artery
	  Sternocleidomastoid artery
	  Superior laryngeal artery
	  Superior thyroid artery
	  Thyrocervical trunk
	V Thyroid Artery, Left
	  See U Thyroid Artery, Right
	Y Upper Artery
	  Aortic intercostal artery
	  Bronchial artery
	  Esophageal artery
	  Subcostal artery
		Ø Open
		3 Percutaneous
		4 Percutaneous Endoscopic
			Z No Device	**Z No Qualifier**

G Intracranial Artery
  Anterior cerebral artery
  Anterior choroidal artery
  Anterior communicating artery
  Basilar artery
  Circle of Willis
  Internal carotid artery, intracranial portion
  Middle cerebral artery
  Ophthalmic artery
  Posterior cerebral artery
  Posterior communicating artery
  Posterior inferior cerebellar artery (PICA)
H Common Carotid Artery, Right
J Common Carotid Artery, Left
K Internal Carotid Artery, Right
  Caroticotympanic artery
  Carotid sinus
	L Internal Carotid Artery, Left
	  See K Internal Carotid Artery, Right
	M External Carotid Artery, Right
	  Ascending pharyngeal artery
	  Internal maxillary artery
	  Lingual artery
	  Maxillary artery
	  Occipital artery
	  Posterior auricular artery
	  Superior thyroid artery
	N External Carotid Artery, Left
	  See M External Carotid Artery, Right
	P Vertebral Artery, Right
	  Anterior spinal artery
	  Posterior spinal artery
	Q Vertebral Artery, Left
	  See P Vertebral Artery, Right
		Ø Open
		4 Percutaneous Endoscopic
			Z No Device	**Z No Qualifier**

Ø3C Continued on next page

NC Noncovered Procedure   **LC** Limited Coverage   **QA** Questionable OB Admit   **NT** New Tech Add-on   ⊞ Combination Member   ♂ Male   ♀ Female

ICD-10-PCS 2022   **205**

Ø3C–Ø3C

Upper Arteries

0 Medical and Surgical
3 Upper Arteries
C Extirpation   Definition: Taking or cutting out solid matter from a body part

Explanation: The solid matter may be an abnormal byproduct of a biological function or a foreign body; it may be imbedded in a body part or in the lumen of a tubular body part. The solid matter may or may not have been previously broken into pieces.

Body Part Character 4		Approach Character 5	Device Character 6	Qualifier Character 7
G Intracranial Artery	**L Internal Carotid Artery, Left**	**3 Percutaneous**	**Z No Device**	**7 Stent Retriever**
Anterior cerebral artery	*See K Internal Carotid Artery, Right*			**Z No Qualifier**
Anterior choroidal artery	**M External Carotid Artery, Right**			
Anterior communicating artery	Ascending pharyngeal artery			
Basilar artery	Internal maxillary artery			
Circle of Willis	Lingual artery			
Internal carotid artery, intracranial portion	Maxillary artery			
Middle cerebral artery	Occipital artery			
Ophthalmic artery	Posterior auricular artery			
Posterior cerebral artery	Superior thyroid artery			
Posterior communicating artery	**N External Carotid Artery, Left**			
Posterior inferior cerebellar artery (PICA)	*See M External Carotid Artery, Right*			
H Common Carotid Artery, Right	**P Vertebral Artery, Right**			
	Anterior spinal artery			
	Posterior spinal artery			
J Common Carotid Artery, Left	**Q Vertebral Artery, Left**			
K Internal Carotid Artery, Right	*See P Vertebral Artery, Right*			
Caroticotympanic artery				
Carotid sinus				

0 Medical and Surgical
3 Upper Arteries
F Fragmentation   Definition: Breaking solid matter in a body part into pieces

Explanation: Physical force (e.g., manual, ultrasonic) applied directly or indirectly is used to break the solid matter into pieces. The solid matter may be an abnormal byproduct of a biological function or a foreign body. The pieces of solid matter are not taken out.

Body Part Character 4		Approach Character 5	Device Character 6	Qualifier Character 7
2 Innominate Artery	**9 Ulnar Artery, Right**	**3 Percutaneous**	**Z No Device**	**0 Ultrasonic**
Brachiocephalic artery	Anterior ulnar recurrent artery			**Z No Qualifier**
Brachiocephalic trunk	Common interosseous artery			
3 Subclavian Artery, Right	Posterior ulnar recurrent artery			
Costocervical trunk	**A Ulnar Artery, Left**			
Dorsal scapular artery	*See 9 Ulnar Artery, Right*			
Internal thoracic artery	**B Radial Artery, Right**			
4 Subclavian Artery, Left	Radial recurrent artery			
See 3 Subclavian Artery, Right	**C Radial Artery, Left**			
5 Axillary Artery, Right	*See B Radial Artery, Right*			
Anterior circumflex humeral artery	**G Intracranial Artery**			
	Anterior cerebral artery			
Lateral thoracic artery	Anterior choroidal artery			
Posterior circumflex humeral artery	Anterior communicating artery			
	Basilar artery			
Subscapular artery	Circle of Willis			
Superior thoracic artery	Internal carotid artery, intracranial portion			
Thoracoacromial artery	Middle cerebral artery			
6 Axillary Artery, Left	Ophthalmic artery			
See 5 Axillary Artery, Right	Posterior cerebral artery			
7 Brachial Artery, Right	Posterior communicating artery			
Inferior ulnar collateral artery	Posterior inferior cerebellar artery (PICA)			
Profunda brachii				
Superior ulnar collateral artery	**Y Upper Artery**			
8 Brachial Artery, Left	Aortic intercostal artery			
See 7 Brachial Artery, Right	Bronchial artery			
	Esophageal artery			
	Subcostal artery			

Ø   **Medical and Surgical**
3   **Upper Arteries**
H   **Insertion**   Definition: Putting in a nonbiological appliance that monitors, assists, performs, or prevents a physiological function but does not physically take the place of a body part

Explanation: None

Body Part — Character 4		Approach — Character 5	Device — Character 6	Qualifier — Character 7
Ø **Internal Mammary Artery, Right** Anterior intercostal artery Internal thoracic artery Musculophrenic artery Pericardiophrenic artery Superior epigastric artery **1** **Internal Mammary Artery, Left** *See Ø Internal Mammary Artery, Right* **2** **Innominate Artery** Brachiocephalic artery Brachiocephalic trunk **3** **Subclavian Artery, Right** Costocervical trunk Dorsal scapular artery Internal thoracic artery **4** **Subclavian Artery, Left** *See 3 Subclavian Artery, Right* **5** **Axillary Artery, Right** Anterior circumflex humeral artery Lateral thoracic artery Posterior circumflex humeral artery Subscapular artery Superior thoracic artery Thoracoacromial artery **6** **Axillary Artery, Left** *See 5 Axillary Artery, Right* **7** **Brachial Artery, Right** Inferior ulnar collateral artery Profunda brachii Superior ulnar collateral artery **8** **Brachial Artery, Left** *See 7 Brachial Artery, Right* **9** **Ulnar Artery, Right** Anterior ulnar recurrent artery Common interosseous artery Posterior ulnar recurrent artery **A** **Ulnar Artery, Left** *See 9 Ulnar Artery, Right* **B** **Radial Artery, Right** Radial recurrent artery **C** **Radial Artery, Left** *See B Radial Artery, Right* **D** **Hand Artery, Right** Deep palmar arch Princeps pollicis artery Radialis indicis Superficial palmar arch **F** **Hand Artery, Left** *See D Hand Artery, Right*	**G** **Intracranial Artery** Anterior cerebral artery Anterior choroidal artery Anterior communicating artery Basilar artery Circle of Willis Internal carotid artery, intracranial portion Middle cerebral artery Ophthalmic artery Posterior cerebral artery Posterior communicating artery Posterior inferior cerebellar artery (PICA) **H** **Common Carotid Artery, Right** **J** **Common Carotid Artery, Left** **M** **External Carotid Artery, Right** Ascending pharyngeal artery Internal maxillary artery Lingual artery Maxillary artery Occipital artery Posterior auricular artery Superior thyroid artery **N** **External Carotid Artery, Left** *See M External Carotid Artery, Right* **P** **Vertebral Artery, Right** Anterior spinal artery Posterior spinal artery **Q** **Vertebral Artery, Left** *See P Vertebral Artery, Right* **R** **Face Artery** Angular artery Ascending palatine artery External maxillary artery Facial artery Inferior labial artery Submental artery Superior labial artery **S** **Temporal Artery, Right** Middle temporal artery Superficial temporal artery Transverse facial artery **T** **Temporal Artery, Left** *See S Temporal Artery, Right* **U** **Thyroid Artery, Right** Cricothyroid artery Hyoid artery Sternocleidomastoid artery Superior laryngeal artery Superior thyroid artery Thyrocervical trunk **V** **Thyroid Artery, Left** *See U Thyroid Artery, Right*	**Ø** Open **3** Percutaneous **4** Percutaneous Endoscopic	**3** Infusion Device **D** Intraluminal Device	**Z** No Qualifier
K **Internal Carotid Artery, Right** Caroticotympanic artery Carotid sinus **L** **Internal Carotid Artery, Left** *See K Internal Carotid Artery, Right*		**Ø** Open **3** Percutaneous **4** Percutaneous Endoscope	**3** Infusion Device **D** Intraluminal Device **M** Stimulator Lead [NT]	**Z** No Qualifier
Y **Upper Artery** Aortic intercostal artery Bronchial artery Esophageal artery Subcostal artery		**Ø** Open **3** Percutaneous **4** Percutaneous Endoscopic	**2** Monitoring Device **3** Infusion Device **D** Intraluminal Device **Y** Other Device	**Z** No Qualifier

Non-OR	03H[Ø,1,2,3,4,5,6,7,8,9,A,B,C,D,F,G,H,J,M,N,P,Q,R,S,T,U,V][Ø,3,4]3Z
Non-OR	03H[K,L][Ø,3,4]3Z
Non-OR	03HY[Ø,3,4]3Z
Non-OR	03HY32Z
Non-OR	03HY[3,4]YZ
NT	03HK3MZ or 03HL3MZ in combination with ØJH6ØMZ *See Appendix H for applicable device trade name*

[NC] Noncovered Procedure   [LC] Limited Coverage   [QA] Questionable OB Admit   [NT] New Tech Add-on   ⊞ Combination Member   ♂ Male   ♀ Female

Ø   Medical and Surgical
3   Upper Arteries
J   Inspection   Definition: Visually and/or manually exploring a body part
                             Explanation: Visual exploration may be performed with or without optical instrumentation. Manual exploration may be performed directly or
                             through intervening body layers.

Body Part Character 4	Approach Character 5	Device Character 6	Qualifier Character 7

Y Upper Artery
   Aortic intercostal artery
   Bronchial artery
   Esophageal artery
   Subcostal artery
	Ø Open
	3 Percutaneous
	4 Percutaneous Endoscopic
	X External
		Z No Device	**Z** No Qualifier

Non-OR   Ø3JY[3,4,X]ZZ

Ø **Medical and Surgical**
3 **Upper Arteries**
L **Occlusion**   Definition: Completely closing an orifice or the lumen of a tubular body part
                Explanation: The orifice can be a natural orifice or an artificially created orifice

Body Part Character 4		Approach Character 5	Device Character 6	Qualifier Character 7
Ø **Internal Mammary Artery, Right** Anterior intercostal artery Internal thoracic artery Musculophrenic artery Pericardiophrenic artery Superior epigastric artery 1 **Internal Mammary Artery, Left** *See Ø Internal Mammary Artery, Left* 2 **Innominate Artery** Brachiocephalic artery Brachiocephalic trunk 3 **Subclavian Artery, Right** Costocervical trunk Dorsal scapular artery Internal thoracic artery 4 **Subclavian Artery, Left** *See 3 Subclavian Artery, Right* 5 **Axillary Artery, Right** Anterior circumflex humeral artery Lateral thoracic artery Posterior circumflex humeral artery Subscapular artery Superior thoracic artery Thoracoacromial artery 6 **Axillary Artery, Left** *See 5 Axillary Artery, Right* 7 **Brachial Artery, Right** Inferior ulnar collateral artery Profunda brachii Superior ulnar collateral artery 8 **Brachial Artery, Left** *See 7 Brachial Artery, Right* 9 **Ulnar Artery, Right** Anterior ulnar recurrent artery Common interosseous artery Posterior ulnar recurrent artery	A **Ulnar Artery, Left** *See 9 Ulnar Artery, Right* B **Radial Artery, Right** Radial recurrent artery C **Radial Artery, Left** *See B Radial Artery, Right* D **Hand Artery, Right** Deep palmar arch Princeps pollicis artery Radialis indicis Superficial palmar arch F **Hand Artery, Left** *See D Hand Artery, Right* R **Face Artery** Angular artery Ascending palatine artery External maxillary artery Facial artery Inferior labial artery Submental artery Superior labial artery S **Temporal Artery, Right** Middle temporal artery Superficial temporal artery Transverse facial artery T **Temporal Artery, Left** *See S Temporal Artery, Right* U **Thyroid Artery, Right** Cricothyroid artery Hyoid artery Sternocleidomastoid artery Superior laryngeal artery Superior thyroid artery Thyrocervical trunk V **Thyroid Artery, Left** *See U Thyroid Artery, Right* Y **Upper Artery** Aortic intercostal artery Bronchial artery Esophageal artery Subcostal artery	Ø **Open** 3 **Percutaneous** 4 **Percutaneous Endoscopic**	C **Extraluminal Device** D **Intraluminal Device** Z **No Device**	Z **No Qualifier**
G **Intracranial Artery** Anterior cerebral artery Anterior choroidal artery Anterior communicating artery Basilar artery Circle of Willis Internal carotid artery, intracranial portion Middle cerebral artery Ophthalmic artery Posterior cerebral artery Posterior communicating artery Posterior inferior cerebellar artery (PICA) H **Common Carotid Artery, Right** J **Common Carotid Artery, Left** K **Internal Carotid Artery, Right** Caroticotympanic artery Carotid sinus	L **Internal Carotid Artery, Left** *See K Internal Carotid Artery, Right* M **External Carotid Artery, Right** Ascending pharyngeal artery Internal maxillary artery Lingual artery Maxillary artery Occipital artery Posterior auricular artery Superior thyroid artery N **External Carotid Artery, Left** *See M External Carotid Artery, Right* P **Vertebral Artery, Right** Anterior spinal artery Posterior spinal artery Q **Vertebral Artery, Left** *See P Vertebral Artery, Right*	Ø **Open** 3 **Percutaneous** 4 **Percutaneous Endoscopic**	B **Intraluminal Device, Bioactive** C **Extraluminal Device** D **Intraluminal Device** Z **No Device**	Z **No Qualifier**

NC Noncovered Procedure   LC Limited Coverage   QA Questionable OB Admit   NT New Tech Add-on   ⊞ Combination Member   ♂ Male   ♀ Female

ICD-10-PCS 2022

209

03L–03L

Ø   Medical and Surgical
3   Upper Arteries
N   Release   Definition: Freeing a body part from an abnormal physical constraint by cutting or by the use of force
                       Explanation: Some of the restraining tissue may be taken out but none of the body part is taken out

Body Part Character 4		Approach Character 5	Device Character 6	Qualifier Character 7
Ø Internal Mammary Artery, Right	**H Common Carotid Artery, Right**	**Ø Open**	**Z No Device**	**Z No Qualifier**
Anterior intercostal artery	**J Common Carotid Artery, Left**	**3 Percutaneous**		
Internal thoracic artery	**K Internal Carotid Artery, Right**	**4 Percutaneous Endoscopic**		
Musculophrenic artery	Caroticotympanic artery			
Pericardiophrenic artery	Carotid sinus			
Superior epigastric artery	**L Internal Carotid Artery, Left**			
1 Internal Mammary Artery, Left	*See K Internal Carotid Artery, Right*			
See Ø Internal Mammary Artery, Right	**M External Carotid Artery, Right**			
2 Innominate Artery	Ascending pharyngeal artery			
Brachiocephalic artery	Internal maxillary artery			
Brachiocephalic trunk	Lingual artery			
3 Subclavian Artery, Right	Maxillary artery			
Costocervical trunk	Occipital artery			
Dorsal scapular artery	Posterior auricular artery			
Internal thoracic artery	Superior thyroid artery			
4 Subclavian Artery, Left	**N External Carotid Artery, Left**			
See 3 Subclavian Artery, Right	*See M External Carotid Artery, Right*			
5 Axillary Artery, Right	**P Vertebral Artery, Right**			
Anterior circumflex humeral artery	Anterior spinal artery			
Lateral thoracic artery	Posterior spinal artery			
Posterior circumflex humeral artery	**Q Vertebral Artery, Left**			
Subscapular artery	*See P Vertebral Artery, Right*			
Superior thoracic artery	**R Face Artery**			
Thoracoacromial artery	Angular artery			
6 Axillary Artery, Left	Ascending palatine artery			
See 5 Axillary Artery, Right	External maxillary artery			
7 Brachial Artery, Right	Facial artery			
Inferior ulnar collateral artery	Inferior labial artery			
Profunda brachii	Submental artery			
Superior ulnar collateral artery	Superior labial artery			
8 Brachial Artery, Left	**S Temporal Artery, Right**			
See 7 Brachial Artery, Right	Middle temporal artery			
9 Ulnar Artery, Right	Superficial temporal artery			
Anterior ulnar recurrent artery	Transverse facial artery			
Common interosseous artery	**T Temporal Artery, Left**			
Posterior ulnar recurrent artery	*See S Temporal Artery, Right*			
A Ulnar Artery, Left	**U Thyroid Artery, Right**			
See 9 Ulnar Artery, Right	Cricothyroid artery			
B Radial Artery, Right	Hyoid artery			
Radial recurrent artery	Sternocleidomastoid artery			
C Radial Artery, Left	Superior laryngeal artery			
See B Radial Artery, Right	Superior thyroid artery			
D Hand Artery, Right	Thyrocervical trunk			
Deep palmar arch	**V Thyroid Artery, Left**			
Princeps pollicis artery	*See U Thyroid Artery, Right*			
Radialis indicis	**Y Upper Artery**			
Superficial palmar arch	Aortic intercostal artery			
F Hand Artery, Left	Bronchial artery			
See D Hand Artery, Right	Esophageal artery			
G Intracranial Artery	Subcostal artery			
Anterior cerebral artery				
Anterior choroidal artery				
Anterior communicating artery				
Basilar artery				
Circle of Willis				
Internal carotid artery, intracranial portion				
Middle cerebral artery				
Ophthalmic artery				
Posterior cerebral artery				
Posterior communicating artery				
Posterior inferior cerebellar artery (PICA)				

Ø   Medical and Surgical
3   Upper Arteries
P   Removal   Definition: Taking out or off a device from a body part

Explanation: If a device is taken out and a similar device put in without cutting or puncturing the skin or mucous membrane, the procedure is coded to the root operation CHANGE. Otherwise, the procedure for taking out a device is coded to the root operation REMOVAL.

Body Part Character 4	Approach Character 5	Device Character 6	Qualifier Character 7
Y Upper Artery Aortic intercostal artery Bronchial artery Esophageal artery Subcostal artery	**Ø Open** **3 Percutaneous** **4 Percutaneous Endoscopic**	**Ø Drainage Device** **2 Monitoring Device** **3 Infusion Device** **7 Autologous Tissue Substitute** **C Extraluminal Device** **D Intraluminal Device** **J Synthetic Substitute** **K Nonautologous Tissue Substitute** **M Stimulator Lead** **Y Other Device**	**Z No Qualifier**
Y Upper Artery Aortic intercostal artery Bronchial artery Esophageal artery Subcostal artery	**X External**	**Ø Drainage Device** **2 Monitoring Device** **3 Infusion Device** **D Intraluminal Device** **M Stimulator Lead**	**Z No Qualifier**

Non-OR   Ø3PY3[Ø,2,3,D]Z
Non-OR   Ø3PY[3,4]YZ
Non-OR   Ø3PYX[Ø,2,3,D,M]Z

NC Noncovered Procedure   LC Limited Coverage   QA Questionable OB Admit   NT New Tech Add-on   ⊞ Combination Member   ♂ Male   ♀ Female

ICD-10-PCS 2022   211

Upper Arteries

0   **Medical and Surgical**
3   **Upper Arteries**
Q   **Repair**   Definition: Restoring, to the extent possible, a body part to its normal anatomic structure and function
                     Explanation: Used only when the method to accomplish the repair is not one of the other root operations

Body Part Character 4		Approach Character 5	Device Character 6	Qualifier Character 7

0 **Internal Mammary Artery, Right**
   Anterior intercostal artery
   Internal thoracic artery
   Musculophrenic artery
   Pericardiophrenic artery
   Superior epigastric artery
1 **Internal Mammary Artery, Left**
   See 0 Internal Mammary Artery, Right
2 **Innominate Artery**
   Brachiocephalic artery
   Brachiocephalic trunk
3 **Subclavian Artery, Right**
   Costocervical trunk
   Dorsal scapular artery
   Internal thoracic artery
4 **Subclavian Artery, Left**
   See 3 Subclavian Artery, Right
5 **Axillary Artery, Right**
   Anterior circumflex humeral artery
   Lateral thoracic artery
   Posterior circumflex humeral artery
   Subscapular artery
   Superior thoracic artery
   Thoracoacromial artery
6 **Axillary Artery, Left**
   See 5 Axillary Artery, Right
7 **Brachial Artery, Right**
   Inferior ulnar collateral artery
   Profunda brachii
   Superior ulnar collateral artery
8 **Brachial Artery, Left**
   See 7 Brachial Artery, Right
9 **Ulnar Artery, Right**
   Anterior ulnar recurrent artery
   Common interosseous artery
   Posterior ulnar recurrent artery
A **Ulnar Artery, Left**
   See 9 Ulnar Artery, Right
B **Radial Artery, Right**
   Radial recurrent artery
C **Radial Artery, Left**
   See B Radial Artery, Right
D **Hand Artery, Right**
   Deep palmar arch
   Princeps pollicis artery
   Radialis indicis
   Superficial palmar arch
F **Hand Artery, Left**
   See D Hand Artery, Right
G **Intracranial Artery**
   Anterior cerebral artery
   Anterior choroidal artery
   Anterior communicating artery
   Basilar artery
   Circle of Willis
   Internal carotid artery, intracranial portion
   Middle cerebral artery
   Ophthalmic artery
   Posterior cerebral artery
   Posterior communicating artery
   Posterior inferior cerebellar artery (PICA)
	H **Common Carotid Artery, Right**
	J **Common Carotid Artery, Left**
	K **Internal Carotid Artery, Right**
	   Caroticotympanic artery
	   Carotid sinus
	L **Internal Carotid Artery, Left**
	   See K Internal Carotid Artery, Right
	M **External Carotid Artery, Right**
	   Ascending pharyngeal artery
	   Internal maxillary artery
	   Lingual artery
	   Maxillary artery
	   Occipital artery
	   Posterior auricular artery
	   Superior thyroid artery
	N **External Carotid Artery, Left**
	   See M External Carotid Artery, Right
	P **Vertebral Artery, Right**
	   Anterior spinal artery
	   Posterior spinal artery
	Q **Vertebral Artery, Left**
	   See P Vertebral Artery, Right
	R **Face Artery**
	   Angular artery
	   Ascending palatine artery
	   External maxillary artery
	   Facial artery
	   Inferior labial artery
	   Submental artery
	   Superior labial artery
	S **Temporal Artery, Right**
	   Middle temporal artery
	   Superficial temporal artery
	   Transverse facial artery
	T **Temporal Artery, Left**
	   See S Temporal Artery, Right
	U **Thyroid Artery, Right**
	   Cricothyroid artery
	   Hyoid artery
	   Sternocleidomastoid artery
	   Superior laryngeal artery
	   Superior thyroid artery
	   Thyrocervical trunk
	V **Thyroid Artery, Left**
	   See U Thyroid Artery, Right
	Y **Upper Artery**
	   Aortic intercostal artery
	   Bronchial artery
	   Esophageal artery
	   Subcostal artery
		0 Open
		3 Percutaneous
		4 Percutaneous Endoscopic
			Z No Device	**Z** No Qualifier

Ø Medical and Surgical
3 Upper Arteries
R Replacement   Definition: Putting in or on biological or synthetic material that physically takes the place and/or function of all or a portion of a body part

Explanation: The body part may have been taken out or replaced, or may be taken out, physically eradicated, or rendered nonfunctional during the REPLACEMENT procedure. A REMOVAL procedure is coded for taking out the device used in a previous replacement procedure.

Body Part Character 4		Approach Character 5	Device Character 6	Qualifier Character 7
Ø Internal Mammary Artery, Right Anterior intercostal artery Internal thoracic artery Musculophrenic artery Pericardiophrenic artery Superior epigastric artery **1 Internal Mammary Artery, Left** *See Ø Internal Mammary Artery, Right* **2 Innominate Artery** Brachiocephalic artery Brachiocephalic trunk **3 Subclavian Artery, Right** Costocervical trunk Dorsal scapular artery Internal thoracic artery **4 Subclavian Artery, Left** *See 3 Subclavian Artery, Right* **5 Axillary Artery, Right** Anterior circumflex humeral artery Lateral thoracic artery Posterior circumflex humeral artery Subscapular artery Superior thoracic artery Thoracoacromial artery **6 Axillary Artery, Left** *See 5 Axillary Artery, Right* **7 Brachial Artery, Right** Inferior ulnar collateral artery Profunda brachii Superior ulnar collateral artery **8 Brachial Artery, Left** *See 7 Brachial Artery, Right* **9 Ulnar Artery, Right** Anterior ulnar recurrent artery Common interosseous artery Posterior ulnar recurrent artery **A Ulnar Artery, Left** *See 9 Ulnar Artery, Right* **B Radial Artery, Right** Radial recurrent artery **C Radial Artery, Left** *See B Radial Artery, Right* **D Hand Artery, Right** Deep palmar arch Princeps pollicis artery Radialis indicis Superficial palmar arch **F Hand Artery, Left** *See D Hand Artery, Right* **G Intracranial Artery** Anterior cerebral artery Anterior choroidal artery Anterior communicating artery Basilar artery Circle of Willis Internal carotid artery, intracranial portion Middle cerebral artery Ophthalmic artery Posterior cerebral artery Posterior communicating artery Posterior inferior cerebellar artery (PICA)	**H Common Carotid Artery, Right** **J Common Carotid Artery, Left** **K Internal Carotid Artery, Right** Caroticotympanic artery Carotid sinus **L Internal Carotid Artery, Left** *See K Internal Carotid Artery, Right* **M External Carotid Artery, Right** Ascending pharyngeal artery Internal maxillary artery Lingual artery Maxillary artery Occipital artery Posterior auricular artery Superior thyroid artery **N External Carotid Artery, Left** *See M External Carotid Artery, Right* **P Vertebral Artery, Right** Anterior spinal artery Posterior spinal artery **Q Vertebral Artery, Left** *See P Vertebral Artery, Right* **R Face Artery** Angular artery Ascending palatine artery External maxillary artery Facial artery Inferior labial artery Submental artery Superior labial artery **S Temporal Artery, Right** Middle temporal artery Superficial temporal artery Transverse facial artery **T Temporal Artery, Left** *See S Temporal Artery, Right* **U Thyroid Artery, Right** Cricothyroid artery Hyoid artery Sternocleidomastoid artery Superior laryngeal artery Superior thyroid artery Thyrocervical trunk **V Thyroid Artery, Left** *See U Thyroid Artery, Right* **Y Upper Artery** Aortic intercostal artery Bronchial artery Esophageal artery Subcostal artery	**Ø Open** **4 Percutaneous Endoscopic**	**7 Autologous Tissue Substitute** **J Synthetic Substitute** **K Nonautologous Tissue Substitute**	**Z No Qualifier**

NC Noncovered Procedure   LC Limited Coverage   QA Questionable OB Admit   NT New Tech Add-on   ⊞ Combination Member   ♂ Male   ♀ Female

Upper Arteries

0   Medical and Surgical
3   Upper Arteries
S   Reposition   Definition: Moving to its normal location, or other suitable location, all or a portion of a body part

Explanation: The body part is moved to a new location from an abnormal location, or from a normal location where it is not functioning correctly. The body part may or may not be cut out or off to be moved to the new location.

Body Part Character 4		Approach Character 5	Device Character 6	Qualifier Character 7
0 Internal Mammary Artery, Right Anterior intercostal artery Internal thoracic artery Musculophrenic artery Pericardiophrenic artery Superior epigastric artery **1 Internal Mammary Artery, Left** *See 0 Internal Mammary Artery, Right* **2 Innominate Artery** Brachiocephalic artery Brachiocephalic trunk **3 Subclavian Artery, Right** Costocervical trunk Dorsal scapular artery Internal thoracic artery **4 Subclavian Artery, Left** *See 3 Subclavian Artery, Right* **5 Axillary Artery, Right** Anterior circumflex humeral artery Lateral thoracic artery Posterior circumflex humeral artery Subscapular artery Superior thoracic artery Thoracoacromial artery **6 Axillary Artery, Left** *See 5 Axillary Artery, Right* **7 Brachial Artery, Right** Inferior ulnar collateral artery Profunda brachii Superior ulnar collateral artery **8 Brachial Artery, Left** *See 7 Brachial Artery, Right* **9 Ulnar Artery, Right** Anterior ulnar recurrent artery Common interosseous artery Posterior ulnar recurrent artery **A Ulnar Artery, Left** *See 9 Ulnar Artery, Right* **B Radial Artery, Right** Radial recurrent artery **C Radial Artery, Left** *See B Radial Artery, Right* **D Hand Artery, Right** Deep palmar arch Princeps pollicis artery Radialis indicis Superficial palmar arch **F Hand Artery, Left** *See D Hand Artery, Right* **G Intracranial Artery** Anterior cerebral artery Anterior choroidal artery Anterior communicating artery Basilar artery Circle of Willis Internal carotid artery, intracranial portion Middle cerebral artery Ophthalmic artery Posterior cerebral artery Posterior communicating artery Posterior inferior cerebellar artery (PICA)	**H Common Carotid Artery, Right** **J Common Carotid Artery, Left** **K Internal Carotid Artery, Right** Caroticotympanic artery Carotid sinus **L Internal Carotid Artery, Left** *See K Internal Carotid Artery, Right* **M External Carotid Artery, Right** Ascending pharyngeal artery Internal maxillary artery Lingual artery Maxillary artery Occipital artery Posterior auricular artery Superior thyroid artery **N External Carotid Artery, Left** *See M External Carotid Artery, Right* **P Vertebral Artery, Right** Anterior spinal artery Posterior spinal artery **Q Vertebral Artery, Left** *See P Vertebral Artery, Right* **R Face Artery** Angular artery Ascending palatine artery External maxillary artery Facial artery Inferior labial artery Submental artery Superior labial artery **S Temporal Artery, Right** Middle temporal artery Superficial temporal artery Transverse facial artery **T Temporal Artery, Left** *See S Temporal Artery, Right* **U Thyroid Artery, Right** Cricothyroid artery Hyoid artery Sternocleidomastoid artery Superior laryngeal artery Superior thyroid artery Thyrocervical trunk **V Thyroid Artery, Left** *See U Thyroid Artery, Right* **Y Upper Artery** Aortic intercostal artery Bronchial artery Esophageal artery Subcostal artery	**0 Open** **3 Percutaneous** **4 Percutaneous Endoscopic**	**Z No Device**	**Z No Qualifier**

0   Medical and Surgical
3   Upper Arteries
U   Supplement   Definition: Putting in or on biological or synthetic material that physically reinforces and/or augments the function of a portion of a body part

Explanation: The biological material is non-living, or is living and from the same individual. The body part may have been previously replaced, and the SUPPLEMENT procedure is performed to physically reinforce and/or augment the function of the replaced body part.

Body Part Character 4		Approach Character 5	Device Character 6	Qualifier Character 7
0 **Internal Mammary Artery, Right** Anterior intercostal artery Internal thoracic artery Musculophrenic artery Pericardiophrenic artery Superior epigastric artery **1** **Internal Mammary Artery, Left** *See 0 Internal Mammary Artery, Right* **2** **Innominate Artery** Brachiocephalic artery Brachiocephalic trunk **3** **Subclavian Artery, Right** Costocervical trunk Dorsal scapular artery Internal thoracic artery **4** **Subclavian Artery, Left** *See 3 Subclavian Artery, Right* **5** **Axillary Artery, Right** Anterior circumflex humeral artery Lateral thoracic artery Posterior circumflex humeral artery Subscapular artery Superior thoracic artery Thoracoacromial artery **6** **Axillary Artery, Left** *See 5 Axillary Artery, Right* **7** **Brachial Artery, Right** Inferior ulnar collateral artery Profunda brachii Superior ulnar collateral artery **8** **Brachial Artery, Left** *See 7 Brachial Artery, Right* **9** **Ulnar Artery, Right** Anterior ulnar recurrent artery Common interosseous artery Posterior ulnar recurrent artery **A** **Ulnar Artery, Left** *See 9 Ulnar Artery, Right* **B** **Radial Artery, Right** Radial recurrent artery **C** **Radial Artery, Left** *See B Radial Artery, Right* **D** **Hand Artery, Right** Deep palmar arch Princeps pollicis artery Radialis indicis Superficial palmar arch **F** **Hand Artery, Left** *See D Hand Artery, Right* **G** **Intracranial Artery** Anterior cerebral artery Anterior choroidal artery Anterior communicating artery Basilar artery Circle of Willis Internal carotid artery, intracranial portion Middle cerebral artery Ophthalmic artery Posterior cerebral artery Posterior communicating artery Posterior inferior cerebellar artery (PICA)	**H** **Common Carotid Artery, Right** **J** **Common Carotid Artery, Left** **K** **Internal Carotid Artery, Right** Caroticotympanic artery Carotid sinus **L** **Internal Carotid Artery, Left** *See K Internal Carotid Artery, Right* **M** **External Carotid Artery, Right** Ascending pharyngeal artery Internal maxillary artery Lingual artery Maxillary artery Occipital artery Posterior auricular artery Superior thyroid artery **N** **External Carotid Artery, Left** *See M External Carotid Artery, Right* **P** **Vertebral Artery, Right** Anterior spinal artery Posterior spinal artery **Q** **Vertebral Artery, Left** *See P Vertebral Artery, Right* **R** **Face Artery** Angular artery Ascending palatine artery External maxillary artery Facial artery Inferior labial artery Submental artery Superior labial artery **S** **Temporal Artery, Right** Middle temporal artery Superficial temporal artery Transverse facial artery **T** **Temporal Artery, Left** *See S Temporal Artery, Right* **U** **Thyroid Artery, Right** Cricothyroid artery Hyoid artery Sternocleidomastoid artery Superior laryngeal artery Superior thyroid artery Thyrocervical trunk **V** **Thyroid Artery, Left** *See U Thyroid Artery, Right* **Y** **Upper Artery** Aortic intercostal artery Bronchial artery Esophageal artery Subcostal artery	**0** Open **3** Percutaneous **4** Percutaneous Endoscopic	**7** Autologous Tissue Substitute **J** Synthetic Substitute **K** Nonautologous Tissue Substitute	**Z** No Qualifier

NC Noncovered Procedure   **LC** Limited Coverage   **QA** Questionable OB Admit   **NT** New Tech Add-on   ⊞ Combination Member   ♂ Male   ♀ Female

ICD-10-PCS 2022   215

0   Medical and Surgical
3   Upper Arteries
V   Restriction   Definition: Partially closing an orifice or the lumen of a tubular body part
                              Explanation: The orifice can be a natural orifice or an artificially created orifice

Body Part Character 4		Approach Character 5	Device Character 6	Qualifier Character 7
0 Internal Mammary Artery, Right Anterior intercostal artery Internal thoracic artery Musculophrenic artery Pericardiophrenic artery Superior epigastric artery **1 Internal Mammary Artery, Left** *See 0 Internal Mammary Artery, Right* **2 Innominate Artery** Brachiocephalic artery Brachiocephalic trunk **3 Subclavian Artery, Right** Costocervical trunk Dorsal scapular artery Internal thoracic artery **4 Subclavian Artery, Left** *See 3 Subclavian Artery, Right* **5 Axillary Artery, Right** Anterior circumflex humeral artery Lateral thoracic artery Posterior circumflex humeral artery Subscapular artery Superior thoracic artery Thoracoacromial artery **6 Axillary Artery, Left** *See 5 Axillary Artery, Right* **7 Brachial Artery, Right** Inferior ulnar collateral artery Profunda brachii Superior ulnar collateral artery **8 Brachial Artery, Left** *See 7 Brachial Artery, Right* **9 Ulnar Artery, Right** Anterior ulnar recurrent artery Common interosseous artery Posterior ulnar recurrent artery **A Ulnar Artery, Left** *See 9 Ulnar Artery, Right*	**B Radial Artery, Right** Radial recurrent artery **C Radial Artery, Left** *See B Radial Artery, Right* **D Hand Artery, Right** Deep palmar arch Princeps pollicis artery Radialis indicis Superficial palmar arch **F Hand Artery, Left** *See D Hand Artery, Right* **R Face Artery** Angular artery Ascending palatine artery External maxillary artery Facial artery Inferior labial artery Submental artery Superior labial artery **S Temporal Artery, Right** Middle temporal artery Superficial temporal artery Transverse facial artery **T Temporal Artery, Left** *See S Temporal Artery, Right* **U Thyroid Artery, Right** Cricothyroid artery Hyoid artery Sternocleidomastoid artery Superior laryngeal artery Superior thyroid artery Thyrocervical trunk **V Thyroid Artery, Left** *See U Thyroid Artery, Right* **Y Upper Artery** Aortic intercostal artery Bronchial artery Esophageal artery Subcostal artery	**0 Open** **3 Percutaneous** **4 Percutaneous Endoscopic**	**C Extraluminal Device** **D Intraluminal Device** **Z No Device**	**Z No Qualifier**
G Intracranial Artery Anterior cerebral artery Anterior choroidal artery Anterior communicating artery Basilar artery Circle of Willis Internal carotid artery, intracranial portion Middle cerebral artery Ophthalmic artery Posterior cerebral artery Posterior communicating artery Posterior inferior cerebellar artery (PICA) **H Common Carotid Artery, Right** **J Common Carotid Artery, Left** **K Internal Carotid Artery, Right** Caroticotympanic artery Carotid sinus	**L Internal Carotid Artery, Left** *See K Internal Carotid Artery, Right* **M External Carotid Artery, Right** Ascending pharyngeal artery Internal maxillary artery Lingual artery Maxillary artery Occipital artery Posterior auricular artery Superior thyroid artery **N External Carotid Artery, Left** *See M External Carotid Artery, Right* **P Vertebral Artery, Right** Anterior spinal artery Posterior spinal artery **Q Vertebral Artery, Left** *See P Vertebral Artery, Right*	**0 Open** **3 Percutaneous** **4 Percutaneous Endoscopic**	**B Intraluminal Device, Bioactive** **C Extraluminal Device** **D Intraluminal Device** **H Intraluminal Device, Flow Diverter** **Z No Device**	**Z No Qualifier**

Ø   **Medical and Surgical**
3   **Upper Arteries**
W   **Revision**   Definition: Correcting, to the extent possible, a portion of a malfunctioning device or the position of a displaced device

Explanation: Revision can include correcting a malfunctioning or displaced device by taking out or putting in components of the device such as a screw or pin

Body Part Character 4	Approach Character 5	Device Character 6	Qualifier Character 7
Y **Upper Artery** Aortic intercostal artery Bronchial artery Esophageal artery Subcostal artery	**Ø** Open **3** Percutaneous **4** Percutaneous Endoscopic	**Ø** Drainage Device **2** Monitoring Device **3** Infusion Device **7** Autologous Tissue Substitute **C** Extraluminal Device **D** Intraluminal Device **J** Synthetic Substitute **K** Nonautologous Tissue Substitute **M** Stimulator Lead **Y** Other Device	**Z** No Qualifier
Y **Upper Artery** Aortic intercostal artery Bronchial artery Esophageal artery Subcostal artery	**X** External	**Ø** Drainage Device **2** Monitoring Device **3** Infusion Device **7** Autologous Tissue Substitute **C** Extraluminal Device **D** Intraluminal Device **J** Synthetic Substitute **K** Nonautologous Tissue Substitute **M** Stimulator Lead	**Z** No Qualifier

Non-OR	Ø3WY3[Ø,2,3,D]Z
Non-OR	Ø3WY[3,4]YZ
Non-OR	Ø3WYX[Ø,2,3,7,C,D,J,K,M]Z

NC Noncovered Procedure   **LC** Limited Coverage   **QA** Questionable OB Admit   **NT** New Tech Add-on   ⊞ Combination Member   ♂ Male   ♀ Female

ICD-10-PCS 2022   **217**

Ø3W–Ø3W

Lower Arteries Ø41–Ø4W

Character Meanings

This Character Meaning table is provided as a guide to assist the user in the identification of character members that may be found in this section of code tables. It **SHOULD NOT** be used to build a PCS code.

Operation–Character 3	Body Part–Character 4	Approach–Character 5	Device–Character 6	Qualifier–Character 7
1 Bypass	Ø Abdominal Aorta	Ø Open	Ø Drainage Device	Ø Abdominal Aorta OR Ultrasonic
5 Destruction	1 Celiac Artery	3 Percutaneous	1 Radioactive Element	1 Celiac Artery OR Drug-Coated Balloon
7 Dilation	2 Gastric Artery	4 Percutaneous Endoscopic	2 Monitoring Device	2 Mesenteric Artery
9 Drainage	3 Hepatic Artery	X External	3 Infusion Device	3 Renal Artery, Right
B Excision	4 Splenic Artery		4 Intraluminal Device, Drug-eluting	4 Renal Artery, Left
C Extirpation	5 Superior Mesenteric Artery		5 Intraluminal Device, Drug-eluting, Two	5 Renal Artery, Bilateral
F Fragmentation	6 Colic Artery, Right		6 Intraluminal Device, Drug-eluting, Three	6 Common Iliac Artery, Right
H Insertion	7 Colic Artery, Left		7 Intraluminal Device, Drug-eluting, Four or More OR Autologous Tissue Substitute	7 Common Iliac Artery, Left
J Inspection	8 Colic Artery, Middle		9 Autologous Venous Tissue	8 Common Iliac Arteries, Bilateral
L Occlusion	9 Renal Artery, Right		A Autologous Arterial Tissue	9 Internal Iliac Artery, Right
N Release	A Renal Artery, Left		C Extraluminal Device	B Internal Iliac Artery, Left
P Removal	B Inferior Mesenteric Artery		D Intraluminal Device	C Internal Iliac Arteries, Bilateral
Q Repair	C Common Iliac Artery, Right		E Intraluminal Device, Two OR Intraluminal Device, Branched or Fenestrated, One or Two Arteries	D External Iliac Artery, Right
R Replacement	D Common Iliac Artery, Left		F Intraluminal Device, Three OR Intraluminal Device, Branched or Fenestrated, Three or More Arteries	F External Iliac Artery, Left
S Reposition	E Internal Iliac Artery, Right		G Intraluminal Device, Four or More	G External Iliac Arteries, Bilateral
U Supplement	F Internal Iliac Artery, Left		J Synthetic Substitute	H Femoral Artery, Right
V Restriction	H External Iliac Artery, Right		K Nonautologous Tissue Substitute	J Femoral Artery, Left OR Temporary
W Revision	J External Iliac Artery, Left		Y Other Device	K Femoral Arteries, Bilateral
	K Femoral Artery, Right		Z No Device	L Popliteal Artery
	L Femoral Artery, Left			M Peroneal Artery
	M Popliteal Artery, Right			N Posterior Tibial Artery
	N Popliteal Artery, Left			P Foot Artery
	P Anterior Tibial Artery, Right			Q Lower Extremity Artery
	Q Anterior Tibial Artery, Left			R Lower Artery
	R Posterior Tibial Artery, Right			S Lower Extremity Vein
	S Posterior Tibial Artery, Left			T Uterine Artery, Right
	T Peroneal Artery, Right			U Uterine Artery, Left
	U Peroneal Artery, Left			X Diagnostic
	V Foot Artery, Right			Z No Qualifier
	W Foot Artery, Left			
	Y Lower Artery			

Lower Arteries *(side tab)*

AHA Coding Clinic for table Ø41

2019, 1Q, 23	Endovascular repair of shaggy aorta and deployment of chimney stent grafts
2018, 3Q, 25	Femoral artery to tibioperoneal trunk bypass
2017, 4Q, 46-47	New and revised body part values - Bypass hepatic artery to renal artery
2017, 3Q, 5	Femoral artery to posterior tibial artery bypass using autologous and synthetic grafts
2017, 3Q, 16	Abdominal aortic debranching with bypass of external iliac artery to bilateral renal arteries and superior mesenteric artery
2017, 1Q, 32	Peroneal artery to dorsalis pedis artery bypass using saphenous vein graft
2016, 2Q, 18	Femoral-tibial artery bypass and saphenous vein graft
2015, 3Q, 28	Bilateral renal artery bypass

AHA Coding Clinic for table Ø47

2020, 4Q, 50	Intravascular lithotripsy
2019, 4Q, 27	Bifurcation Qualifier
2019, 2Q, 14	Revision of occluded femoral-popliteal bypass graft
2018, 2Q, 24	Coronary artery bifurcation
2016, 4Q, 86	Peripheral artery, number of stents
2016, 4Q, 86-88	Coronary and peripheral artery bifurcation
2016, 3Q, 39	Infrarenal abdominal aortic aneurysm repair with iliac graft extension
2015, 4Q, 4-7, 15	Drug-coated balloon angioplasty in peripheral vessels
2015, 3Q, 9	Aborted endovascular stenting of superficial femoral artery

AHA Coding Clinic for table Ø4C

2021, 1Q, 15	Iliofemoral endarterectomy and furthest point of entry
2019, 4Q, 27	Bifurcation Qualifier
2019, 1Q, 23	Endovascular repair of shaggy aorta and deployment of chimney stent grafts
2018, 2Q, 24	Coronary artery bifurcation
2017, 2Q, 23	Thrombectomy via Fogarty catheter
2016, 4Q, 86-88	Coronary and peripheral artery bifurcation
2016, 1Q, 31	Iliofemoral endarterectomy with patch repair
2015, 1Q, 29	Discontinued carotid endarterectomy
2015, 1Q, 36	Percutaneous mechanical thrombectomy of femoropopliteal bypass graft

AHA Coding Clinic for table Ø4F

2020, 4Q, 45-49	New fragmentation tables
2020, 4Q, 49-50	Intravascular ultrasound assisted thrombolysis
2020, 4Q, 50-51	Intravascular lithotripsy

AHA Coding Clinic for table Ø4H

2019, 3Q, 20	Removal and revision of ECMO component
2019, 1Q, 23	Endovascular repair of shaggy aorta and deployment of chimney stent grafts
2017, 1Q, 30	Insertion of umbilical artery catheter

AHA Coding Clinic for table Ø4L

2020, 3Q, 43	Staged laparoscopic gastric conduit and placement of feeding tube
2018, 2Q, 18	Transverse rectus abdominis myocutaneous (TRAM) delay
2017, 4Q, 31	Resuscitative endovascular balloon occlusion of the aorta
2015, 2Q, 27	Uterine artery embolization using Gelfoam
2014, 3Q, 26	Coil embolization of gastroduodenal artery with chemoembolization of hepatic artery
2014, 1Q, 24	Endovascular embolization for gastrointestinal bleeding

AHA Coding Clinic for table Ø4N

2015, 2Q, 28	Release and replacement of celiac artery

AHA Coding Clinic for table Ø4P

2019, 3Q, 20	Removal and revision of ECMO component

AHA Coding Clinic for table Ø4Q

2014, 1Q, 21	Repair of femoral artery pseudoaneurysm

AHA Coding Clinic for table Ø4R

2019, 1Q, 22	Abdominal aortic aneurysm repair using tube graft
2015, 2Q, 28	Release and replacement of celiac artery

AHA Coding Clinic for table Ø4U

2019, 1Q, 22	Abdominal aortic aneurysm repair using tube graft
2016, 2Q, 18	Femoral-tibial artery bypass and saphenous vein graft
2016, 1Q, 31	Iliofemoral endarterectomy with patch repair
2014, 4Q, 37	Bovine patch arterioplasty
2014, 1Q, 22	Repair of pseudoaneurysm of femoral-popliteal bypass graft

AHA Coding Clinic for table Ø4V

2019, 4Q, 27	Bifurcation Qualifier
2019, 1Q, 22	Abdominal aortic aneurysm repair using tube graft
2018, 2Q, 24	Coronary artery bifurcation
2016, 4Q, 86-87	Coronary and peripheral artery bifurcation
2016, 4Q, 89-93	Branched and fenestrated endograft repair of aneurysms
2016, 3Q, 39	Infrarenal abdominal aortic aneurysm repair with iliac graft extension
2014, 1Q, 9	Endovascular repair of abdominal aortic aneurysm

AHA Coding Clinic for table Ø4W

2020, 3Q, 5	Types of endoleaks following endovascular aneurysm repair
2019, 2Q, 14	Revision of occluded femoral-popliteal bypass graft
2015, 1Q, 36	Revision of femoropopliteal bypass graft
2014, 1Q, 9	Endovascular repair of endoleak
2014, 1Q, 22	Repair of pseudoaneurysm of femoral-popliteal bypass graft

Lower Arteries

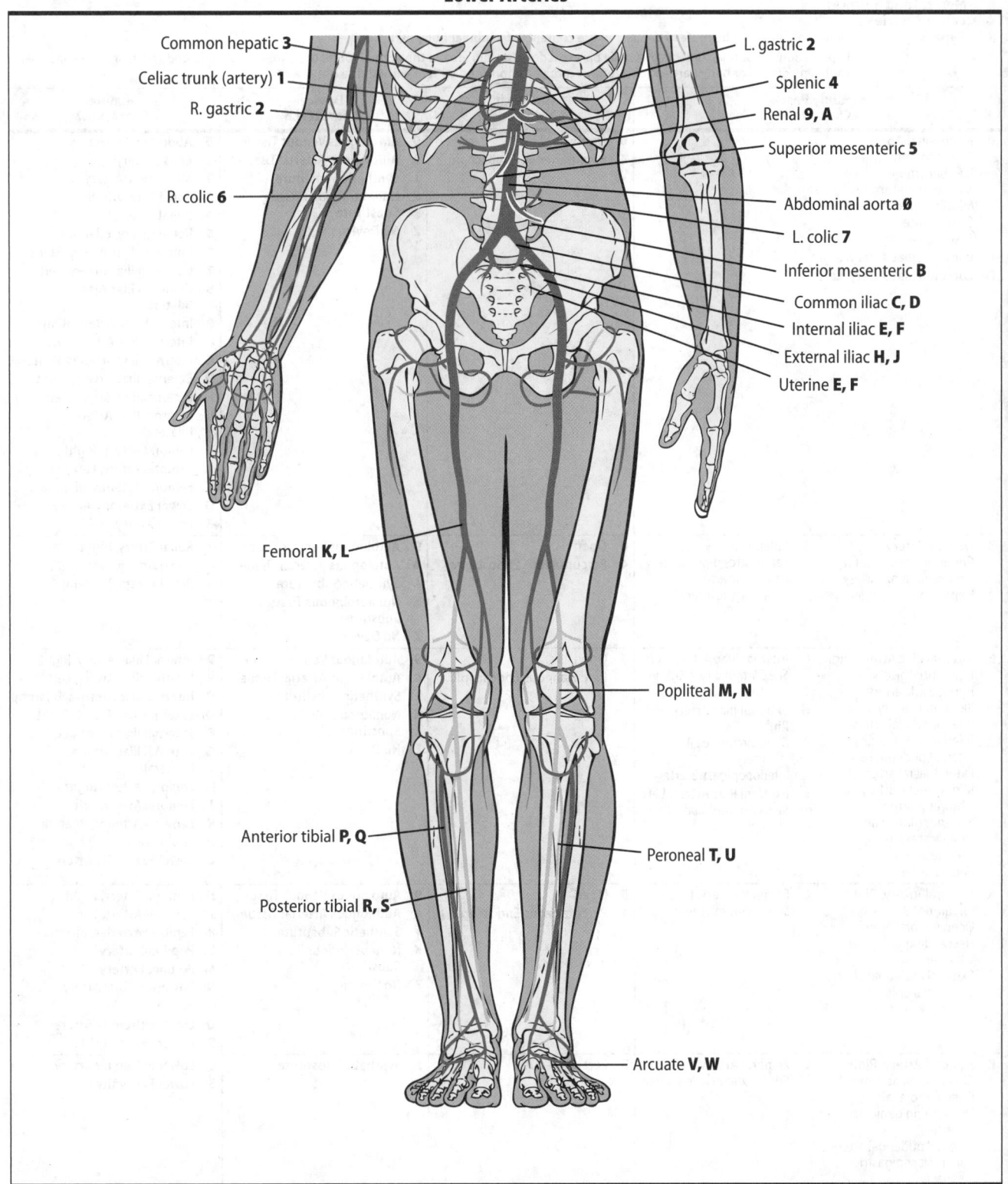

Common hepatic **3**
Celiac trunk (artery) **1**
R. gastric **2**
R. colic **6**

L. gastric **2**
Splenic **4**
Renal **9, A**
Superior mesenteric **5**
Abdominal aorta **Ø**
L. colic **7**
Inferior mesenteric **B**
Common iliac **C, D**
Internal iliac **E, F**
External iliac **H, J**
Uterine **E, F**

Femoral **K, L**

Popliteal **M, N**

Anterior tibial **P, Q**
Peroneal **T, U**

Posterior tibial **R, S**

Arcuate **V, W**

Lower Arteries

041–041

0   Medical and Surgical
4   Lower Arteries
1   Bypass   Definition: Altering the route of passage of the contents of a tubular body part

Explanation: Rerouting contents of a body part to a downstream area of the normal route, to a similar route and body part, or to an abnormal route and dissimilar body part. Includes one or more anastomoses, with or without the use of a device.

Body Part Character 4		Approach Character 5	Device Character 6	Qualifier Character 7
0 Abdominal Aorta Inferior phrenic artery Lumbar artery Median sacral artery Middle suprarenal artery Ovarian artery Testicular artery **C Common Iliac Artery, Right** **D Common Iliac Artery, Left**		**0 Open** **4 Percutaneous Endoscopic**	**9 Autologous Venous Tissue** **A Autologous Arterial Tissue** **J Synthetic Substitute** **K Nonautologous Tissue Substitute** **Z No Device**	**0 Abdominal Aorta** **1 Celiac Artery** **2 Mesenteric Artery** **3 Renal Artery, Right** **4 Renal Artery, Left** **5 Renal Artery, Bilateral** **6 Common Iliac Artery, Right** **7 Common Iliac Artery, Left** **8 Common Iliac Arteries, Bilateral** **9 Internal Iliac Artery, Right** **B Internal Iliac Artery, Left** **C Internal Iliac Arteries, Bilateral** **D External Iliac Artery, Right** **F External Iliac Artery, Left** **G External Iliac Arteries, Bilateral** **H Femoral Artery, Right** **J Femoral Artery, Left** **K Femoral Arteries, Bilateral** **Q Lower Extremity Artery** **R Lower Artery**
3 Hepatic Artery Common hepatic artery Gastroduodenal artery Hepatic artery proper	**4 Splenic Artery** Left gastroepiploic artery Pancreatic artery Short gastric artery	**0 Open** **4 Percutaneous Endoscopic**	**9 Autologous Venous Tissue** **A Autologous Arterial Tissue** **J Synthetic Substitute** **K Nonautologous Tissue Substitute** **Z No Device**	**3 Renal Artery, Right** **4 Renal Artery, Left** **5 Renal Artery, Bilateral**
E Internal Iliac Artery, Right Deferential artery Hypogastric artery Iliolumbar artery Inferior gluteal artery Inferior vesical artery Internal pudendal artery Lateral sacral artery Middle rectal artery Obturator artery Superior gluteal artery Umbilical artery Uterine artery Vaginal artery	**F Internal Iliac Artery, Left** *See E Internal Iliac Artery, Right* **H External Iliac Artery, Right** Deep circumflex iliac artery Inferior epigastric artery **J External Iliac Artery, Left** *See H External Iliac Artery, Right*	**0 Open** **4 Percutaneous Endoscopic**	**9 Autologous Venous Tissue** **A Autologous Arterial Tissue** **J Synthetic Substitute** **K Nonautologous Tissue Substitute** **Z No Device**	**9 Internal Iliac Artery, Right** **B Internal Iliac Artery, Left** **C Internal Iliac Arteries, Bilateral** **D External Iliac Artery, Right** **F External Iliac Artery, Left** **G External Iliac Arteries, Bilateral** **H Femoral Artery, Right** **J Femoral Artery, Left** **K Femoral Arteries, Bilateral** **P Foot Artery** **Q Lower Extremity Artery**
K Femoral Artery, Right Circumflex iliac artery Deep femoral artery Descending genicular artery External pudendal artery Superficial epigastric artery	**L Femoral Artery, Left** *See K Femoral Artery, Right*	**0 Open** **4 Percutaneous Endoscopic**	**9 Autologous Venous Tissue** **A Autologous Arterial Tissue** **J Synthetic Substitute** **K Nonautologous Tissue Substitute** **Z No Device**	**H Femoral Artery, Right** **J Femoral Artery, Left** **K Femoral Arteries, Bilateral** **L Popliteal Artery** **M Peroneal Artery** **N Posterior Tibial Artery** **P Foot Artery** **Q Lower Extremity Artery** **S Lower Extremity Vein**
K Femoral Artery, Right Circumflex iliac artery Deep femoral artery Descending genicular artery External pudendal artery Superficial epigastric artery	**L Femoral Artery, Left** *See K Femoral Artery, Right*	**3 Percutaneous**	**J Synthetic Substitute**	**Q Lower Extremity Artery** **S Lower Extremity Vein**
M Popliteal Artery, Right Inferior genicular artery Middle genicular artery Superior genicular artery Sural artery Tibioperoneal trunk	**N Popliteal Artery, Left** *See M Popliteal Artery, Right*	**0 Open** **4 Percutaneous Endoscopic**	**9 Autologous Venous Tissue** **A Autologous Arterial Tissue** **J Synthetic Substitute** **K Nonautologous Tissue Substitute** **Z No Device**	**L Popliteal Artery** **M Peroneal Artery** **P Foot Artery** **Q Lower Extremity Artery** **S Lower Extremity Vein**

041 Continued on next page

Ø   Medical and Surgical
4   Lower Arteries
1   Bypass   Definition: Altering the route of passage of the contents of a tubular body part

Ø41 Continued

Explanation: Rerouting contents of a body part to a downstream area of the normal route, to a similar route and body part, or to an abnormal route and dissimilar body part. Includes one or more anastomoses, with or without the use of a device.

Body Part Character 4	Approach Character 5	Device Character 6	Qualifier Character 7
M **Popliteal Artery, Right** Inferior genicular artery Middle genicular artery Superior genicular artery Sural artery Tibioperoneal trunk **N** **Popliteal Artery, Left** *See* M Popliteal Artery, Right	**3** Percutaneous	**J** Synthetic Substitute	**Q** Lower Extremity Artery **S** Lower Extremity Vein
P **Anterior Tibial Artery, Right** Anterior lateral malleolar artery Anterior medial malleolar artery Anterior tibial recurrent artery Dorsalis pedis artery Posterior tibial recurrent artery **Q** **Anterior Tibial Artery, Left** *See* P Anterior Tibial Artery, Right **R** **Posterior Tibial Artery, Right** **S** **Posterior Tibial Artery, Left**	**Ø** Open **3** Percutaneous **4** Percutaneous Endoscopic	**J** Synthetic Substitute	**Q** Lower Extremity Artery **S** Lower Extremity Vein
T **Peroneal Artery, Right** Fibular artery **U** **Peroneal Artery, Left** *See* T Peroneal Artery, Right **V** **Foot Artery, Right** Arcuate artery Dorsal metatarsal artery Lateral plantar artery Lateral tarsal artery Medial plantar artery **W** **Foot Artery, Left** *See* V Foot Artery, Right	**Ø** Open **4** Percutaneous Endoscopic	**9** Autologous Venous Tissue **A** Autologous Arterial Tissue **J** Synthetic Substitute **K** Nonautologous Tissue Substitute **Z** No Device	**P** Foot Artery **Q** Lower Extremity Artery **S** Lower Extremity Vein
T **Peroneal Artery, Right** Fibular artery **U** **Peroneal Artery, Left** *See* T Peroneal Artery, Right **V** **Foot Artery, Right** Arcuate artery Dorsal metatarsal artery Lateral plantar artery Lateral tarsal artery Medial plantar artery **W** **Foot Artery, Left** *See* V Foot Artery, Right	**3** Percutaneous	**J** Synthetic Substitute	**Q** Lower Extremity Artery **S** Lower Extremity Vein

NC Noncovered Procedure   LC Limited Coverage   QA Questionable OB Admit   NT New Tech Add-on   ⊞ Combination Member   ♂ Male   ♀ Female

ICD-10-PCS 2022   223

041–041

Lower Arteries

Ø   Medical and Surgical
4   Lower Arteries
5   Destruction   Definition: Physical eradication of all or a portion of a body part by the direct use of energy, force, or a destructive agent
Explanation: None of the body part is physically taken out

Body Part Character 4		Approach Character 5	Device Character 6	Qualifier Character 7

Ø Abdominal Aorta
Inferior phrenic artery
Lumbar artery
Median sacral artery
Middle suprarenal artery
Ovarian artery
Testicular artery
1 Celiac Artery
Celiac trunk
2 Gastric Artery
Left gastric artery
Right gastric artery
3 Hepatic Artery
Common hepatic artery
Gastroduodenal artery
Hepatic artery proper
4 Splenic Artery
Left gastroepiploic artery
Pancreatic artery
Short gastric artery
5 Superior Mesenteric Artery
Ileal artery
Ileocolic artery
Inferior pancreaticoduodenal
   artery
Jejunal artery
6 Colic Artery, Right
7 Colic Artery, Left
8 Colic Artery, Middle
9 Renal Artery, Right
Inferior suprarenal artery
Renal segmental artery
A Renal Artery, Left
See 9 Renal Artery, Right
B Inferior Mesenteric Artery
Sigmoid artery
Superior rectal artery
C Common Iliac Artery, Right
D Common Iliac Artery, Left
E Internal Iliac Artery, Right
Deferential artery
Hypogastric artery
Iliolumbar artery
Inferior gluteal artery
Inferior vesical artery
Internal pudendal artery
Lateral sacral artery
Middle rectal artery
Obturator artery
Superior gluteal artery
Umbilical artery
Uterine artery
Vaginal artery
	F Internal Iliac Artery, Left
	See E Internal Iliac Artery, Right
	H External Iliac Artery, Right
	Deep circumflex iliac artery
	Inferior epigastric artery
	J External Iliac Artery, Left
	See H External Iliac Artery, Right
	K Femoral Artery, Right
	Circumflex iliac artery
	Deep femoral artery
	Descending genicular artery
	External pudendal artery
	Superficial epigastric artery
	L Femoral Artery, Left
	See K Femoral Artery, Right
	M Popliteal Artery, Right
	Inferior genicular artery
	Middle genicular artery
	Superior genicular artery
	Sural artery
	Tibioperoneal trunk
	N Popliteal Artery, Left
	See M Popliteal Artery, Right
	P Anterior Tibial Artery, Right
	Anterior lateral malleolar
	   artery
	Anterior medial malleolar
	   artery
	Anterior tibial recurrent artery
	Dorsalis pedis artery
	Posterior tibial recurrent artery
	Q Anterior Tibial Artery, Left
	See P Anterior Tibial Artery,
	   Right
	R Posterior Tibial Artery, Right
	S Posterior Tibial Artery, Left
	T Peroneal Artery, Right
	Fibular artery
	U Peroneal Artery, Left
	See T Peroneal Artery, Right
	V Foot Artery, Right
	Arcuate artery
	Dorsal metatarsal artery
	Lateral plantar artery
	Lateral tarsal artery
	Medial plantar artery
	W Foot Artery, Left
	See V Foot Artery, Right
	Y Lower Artery
	Umbilical artery
		Ø Open
		3 Percutaneous
		4 Percutaneous Endoscopic
			Z No Device	**Z No Qualifier**

Ø Medical and Surgical
4 Lower Arteries
7 Dilation   Definition: Expanding an orifice or the lumen of a tubular body part
Explanation: The orifice can be a natural orifice or an artificially created orifice. Accomplished by stretching a tubular body part using intraluminal pressure or by cutting part of the orifice or wall of the tubular body part.

Body Part Character 4		Approach Character 5	Device Character 6	Qualifier Character 7

Ø Abdominal Aorta
Inferior phrenic artery
Lumbar artery
Median sacral artery
Middle suprarenal artery
Ovarian artery
Testicular artery
1 Celiac Artery
Celiac trunk
2 Gastric Artery
Left gastric artery
Right gastric artery
3 Hepatic Artery
Common hepatic artery
Gastroduodenal artery
Hepatic artery proper
4 Splenic Artery
Left gastroepiploic artery
Pancreatic artery
Short gastric artery
5 Superior Mesenteric Artery
Ileal artery
Ileocolic artery
Inferior pancreaticoduodenal
  artery
Jejunal artery
6 Colic Artery, Right
7 Colic Artery, Left
8 Colic Artery, Middle
9 Renal Artery, Right
Inferior suprarenal artery
Renal segmental artery
A Renal Artery, Left
See 9 Renal Artery, Right
B Inferior Mesenteric Artery
Sigmoid artery
Superior rectal artery
C Common Iliac Artery, Right
D Common Iliac Artery, Left
E Internal Iliac Artery, Right
Deferential artery
Hypogastric artery
Iliolumbar artery
Inferior gluteal artery
Inferior vesical artery
Internal pudendal artery
Lateral sacral artery
Middle rectal artery
Obturator artery
Superior gluteal artery
Umbilical artery
Uterine artery
Vaginal artery
	F Internal Iliac Artery, Left
	See E Internal Iliac Artery, Right
	H External Iliac Artery, Right
	Deep circumflex iliac artery
	Inferior epigastric artery
	J External Iliac Artery, Left
	See H External Iliac Artery, Right
	K Femoral Artery, Right
	Circumflex iliac artery
	Deep femoral artery
	Descending genicular artery
	External pudendal artery
	Superficial epigastric artery
	L Femoral Artery, Left
	See K Femoral Artery, Right
	M Popliteal Artery, Right
	Inferior genicular artery
	Middle genicular artery
	Superior genicular artery
	Sural artery
	Tibioperoneal trunk
	N Popliteal Artery, Left
	See M Popliteal Artery, Right
	P Anterior Tibial Artery, Right
	Anterior lateral malleolar
	  artery
	Anterior medial malleolar
	  artery
	Anterior tibial recurrent artery
	Dorsalis pedis artery
	Posterior tibial recurrent artery
	Q Anterior Tibial Artery, Left
	See P Anterior Tibial Artery,
	Right
	R Posterior Tibial Artery, Right
	S Posterior Tibial Artery, Left
	T Peroneal Artery, Right
	Fibular artery
	U Peroneal Artery, Left
	See T Peroneal Artery, Right
	V Foot Artery, Right
	Arcuate artery
	Dorsal metatarsal artery
	Lateral plantar artery
	Lateral tarsal artery
	Medial plantar artery
	W Foot Artery, Left
	See V Foot Artery, Right
	Y Lower Artery
	Umbilical artery
		Ø Open
		3 Percutaneous
		4 Percutaneous Endoscopic
			4 Intraluminal Device,
			  Drug-eluting
			D Intraluminal Device
			Z No Device
				1 Drug-Coated Balloon
				Z No Qualifier

Ø47 Continued on next page

NC Noncovered Procedure   **LC** Limited Coverage   **QA** Questionable OB Admit   **NT** New Tech Add-on   ⊞ Combination Member   ♂ Male   ♀ Female

ICD-10-PCS 2022   225

047–047

Ø   **Medical and Surgical**
4   **Lower Arteries**
7   **Dilation**   Definition: Expanding an orifice or the lumen of a tubular body part

047 Continued

Explanation: The orifice can be a natural orifice or an artificially created orifice. Accomplished by stretching a tubular body part using intraluminal pressure or by cutting part of the orifice or wall of the tubular body part.

Body Part Character 4		Approach Character 5	Device Character 6	Qualifier Character 7
Ø **Abdominal Aorta**	**F** **Internal Iliac Artery, Left**	**Ø** Open	**5** Intraluminal Device, Drug-eluting, Two	**Z** No Qualifier
Inferior phrenic artery	*See E Internal Iliac Artery, Right*	**3** Percutaneous	**6** Intraluminal Device, Drug-eluting, Three	
Lumbar artery	**H** **External Iliac Artery, Right**	**4** Percutaneous Endoscopic	**7** Intraluminal Device, Drug-eluting, Four or More	
Median sacral artery	Deep circumflex iliac artery		**E** Intraluminal Device, Two	
Middle suprarenal artery	Inferior epigastric artery		**F** Intraluminal Device, Three	
Ovarian artery	**J** **External Iliac Artery, Left**		**G** Intraluminal Device, Four or More	
Testicular artery	*See H External Iliac Artery, Right*			
1 **Celiac Artery**	**K** **Femoral Artery, Right**			
Celiac trunk	Circumflex iliac artery			
2 **Gastric Artery**	Deep femoral artery			
Left gastric artery	Descending genicular artery			
Right gastric artery	External pudendal artery			
3 **Hepatic Artery**	Superficial epigastric artery			
Common hepatic artery	**L** **Femoral Artery, Left**			
Gastroduodenal artery	*See K Femoral Artery, Right*			
Hepatic artery proper	**M** **Popliteal Artery, Right**			
4 **Splenic Artery**	Inferior genicular artery			
Left gastroepiploic artery	Middle genicular artery			
Pancreatic artery	Superior genicular artery			
Short gastric artery	Sural artery			
5 **Superior Mesenteric Artery**	Tibioperoneal trunk			
Ileal artery	**N** **Popliteal Artery, Left**			
Ileocolic artery	*See M Popliteal Artery, Right*			
Inferior pancreaticoduodenal artery	**P** **Anterior Tibial Artery, Right**			
Jejunal artery	Anterior lateral malleolar artery			
6 **Colic Artery, Right**	Anterior medial malleolar artery			
7 **Colic Artery, Left**	Anterior tibial recurrent artery			
8 **Colic Artery, Middle**	Dorsalis pedis artery			
9 **Renal Artery, Right**	Posterior tibial recurrent artery			
Inferior suprarenal artery	**Q** **Anterior Tibial Artery, Left**			
Renal segmental artery	*See P Anterior Tibial Artery, Right*			
A **Renal Artery, Left**	**R** **Posterior Tibial Artery, Right**			
See 9 Renal Artery, Right	**S** **Posterior Tibial Artery, Left**			
B **Inferior Mesenteric Artery**	**T** **Peroneal Artery, Right**			
Sigmoid artery	Fibular artery			
Superior rectal artery	**U** **Peroneal Artery, Left**			
C **Common Iliac Artery, Right**	*See T Peroneal Artery, Right*			
D **Common Iliac Artery, Left**	**V** **Foot Artery, Right**			
E **Internal Iliac Artery, Right**	Arcuate artery			
Deferential artery	Dorsal metatarsal artery			
Hypogastric artery	Lateral plantar artery			
Iliolumbar artery	Lateral tarsal artery			
Inferior gluteal artery	Medial plantar artery			
Inferior vesical artery	**W** **Foot Artery, Left**			
Internal pudendal artery	*See V Foot Artery, Right*			
Lateral sacral artery	**Y** **Lower Artery**			
Middle rectal artery	Umbilical artery			
Obturator artery				
Superior gluteal artery				
Umbilical artery				
Uterine artery				
Vaginal artery				

Ø   Medical and Surgical
4   Lower Arteries
9   Drainage   Definition: Taking or letting out fluids and/or gases from a body part
                    Explanation: The qualifier DIAGNOSTIC is used to identify drainage procedures that are biopsies

Body Part Character 4		Approach Character 5	Device Character 6	Qualifier Character 7

Ø **Abdominal Aorta**
 Inferior phrenic artery
 Lumbar artery
 Median sacral artery
 Middle suprarenal artery
 Ovarian artery
 Testicular artery
 1 **Celiac Artery**
 Celiac trunk
 2 **Gastric Artery**
 Left gastric artery
 Right gastric artery
 3 **Hepatic Artery**
 Common hepatic artery
 Gastroduodenal artery
 Hepatic artery proper
 4 **Splenic Artery**
 Left gastroepiploic artery
 Pancreatic artery
 Short gastric artery
 5 **Superior Mesenteric Artery**
 Ileal artery
 Ileocolic artery
 Inferior pancreaticoduodenal
     artery
 Jejunal artery
 6 **Colic Artery, Right**
 7 **Colic Artery, Left**
 8 **Colic Artery, Middle**
 9 **Renal Artery, Right**
 Inferior suprarenal artery
 Renal segmental artery
 A **Renal Artery, Left**
 See 9 Renal Artery, Right
 B **Inferior Mesenteric Artery**
 Sigmoid artery
 Superior rectal artery
 C **Common Iliac Artery, Right**
 D **Common Iliac Artery, Left**
 E **Internal Iliac Artery, Right**
 Deferential artery
 Hypogastric artery
 Iliolumbar artery
 Inferior gluteal artery
 Inferior vesical artery
 Internal pudendal artery
 Lateral sacral artery
 Middle rectal artery
 Obturator artery
 Superior gluteal artery
 Umbilical artery
 Uterine artery
 Vaginal artery
	F **Internal Iliac Artery, Left**
	 See E Internal Iliac Artery, Right
	 H **External Iliac Artery, Right**
	 Deep circumflex iliac artery
	 Inferior epigastric artery
	 J **External Iliac Artery, Left**
	 See H External Iliac Artery, Right
	 K **Femoral Artery, Right**
	 Circumflex iliac artery
	 Deep femoral artery
	 Descending genicular artery
	 External pudendal artery
	 Superficial epigastric artery
	 L **Femoral Artery, Left**
	 See K Femoral Artery, Right
	 M **Popliteal Artery, Right**
	 Inferior genicular artery
	 Middle genicular artery
	 Superior genicular artery
	 Sural artery
	 Tibioperoneal trunk
	 N **Popliteal Artery, Left**
	 See M Popliteal Artery, Right
	 P **Anterior Tibial Artery, Right**
	 Anterior lateral malleolar
	     artery
	 Anterior medial malleolar
	     artery
	 Anterior tibial recurrent artery
	 Dorsalis pedis artery
	 Posterior tibial recurrent artery
	 Q **Anterior Tibial Artery, Left**
	 See P Anterior Tibial Artery,
	 Right
	 R **Posterior Tibial Artery, Right**
	 S **Posterior Tibial Artery, Left**
	 T **Peroneal Artery, Right**
	 Fibular artery
	 U **Peroneal Artery, Left**
	 See T Peroneal Artery, Right
	 V **Foot Artery, Right**
	 Arcuate artery
	 Dorsal metatarsal artery
	 Lateral plantar artery
	 Lateral tarsal artery
	 Medial plantar artery
	 W **Foot Artery, Left**
	 See V Foot Artery, Right
	 Y **Lower Artery**
	 Umbilical artery
		Ø Open
		 3 Percutaneous
		 4 Percutaneous Endoscopic
			Ø Drainage Device	Z No Qualifier

Non-OR   049[Ø,1,2,3,4,5,6,7,8,9,A,B,C,D,E,F,H,J,K,L,M,N,P,Q,R,S,T,U,V,W,Y][Ø,3,4]ØZ

049 Continued on next page

Ø **Medical and Surgical**
4 **Lower Arteries**
9 **Drainage**

Definition: Taking or letting out fluids and/or gases from a body part
Explanation: The qualifier DIAGNOSTIC is used to identify drainage procedures that are biopsies

Body Part Character 4		Approach Character 5	Device Character 6	Qualifier Character 7
Ø **Abdominal Aorta**	**F** **Internal Iliac Artery, Left**	**Ø** Open	**Z** No Device	**X** Diagnostic
Inferior phrenic artery	*See E Internal Iliac Artery, Right*	**3** Percutaneous		**Z** No Qualifier
Lumbar artery	**H** **External Iliac Artery, Right**	**4** Percutaneous Endoscopic		
Median sacral artery	Deep circumflex iliac artery			
Middle suprarenal artery	Inferior epigastric artery			
Ovarian artery	**J** **External Iliac Artery, Left**			
Testicular artery	*See H External Iliac Artery, Right*			
1 **Celiac Artery**	**K** **Femoral Artery, Right**			
Celiac trunk	Circumflex iliac artery			
2 **Gastric Artery**	Deep femoral artery			
Left gastric artery	Descending genicular artery			
Right gastric artery	External pudendal artery			
3 **Hepatic Artery**	Superficial epigastric artery			
Common hepatic artery	**L** **Femoral Artery, Left**			
Gastroduodenal artery	*See K Femoral Artery, Right*			
Hepatic artery proper	**M** **Popliteal Artery, Right**			
4 **Splenic Artery**	Inferior genicular artery			
Left gastroepiploic artery	Middle genicular artery			
Pancreatic artery	Superior genicular artery			
Short gastric artery	Sural artery			
5 **Superior Mesenteric Artery**	Tibioperoneal trunk			
Ileal artery	**N** **Popliteal Artery, Left**			
Ileocolic artery	*See M Popliteal Artery, Right*			
Inferior pancreaticoduodenal artery	**P** **Anterior Tibial Artery, Right**			
Jejunal artery	Anterior lateral malleolar artery			
6 **Colic Artery, Right**	Anterior medial malleolar artery			
7 **Colic Artery, Left**	Anterior tibial recurrent artery			
8 **Colic Artery, Middle**	Dorsalis pedis artery			
9 **Renal Artery, Right**	Posterior tibial recurrent artery			
Inferior suprarenal artery	**Q** **Anterior Tibial Artery, Left**			
Renal segmental artery	*See P Anterior Tibial Artery, Right*			
A **Renal Artery, Left**	**R** **Posterior Tibial Artery, Right**			
See 9 Renal Artery, Right	**S** **Posterior Tibial Artery, Left**			
B **Inferior Mesenteric Artery**	**T** **Peroneal Artery, Right**			
Sigmoid artery	Fibular artery			
Superior rectal artery	**U** **Peroneal Artery, Left**			
C **Common Iliac Artery, Right**	*See T Peroneal Artery, Right*			
D **Common Iliac Artery, Left**	**V** **Foot Artery, Right**			
E **Internal Iliac Artery, Right**	Arcuate artery			
Deferential artery	Dorsal metatarsal artery			
Hypogastric artery	Lateral plantar artery			
Iliolumbar artery	Lateral tarsal artery			
Inferior gluteal artery	Medial plantar artery			
Inferior vesical artery	**W** **Foot Artery, Left**			
Internal pudendal artery	*See V Foot Artery, Right*			
Lateral sacral artery	**Y** **Lower Artery**			
Middle rectal artery	Umbilical artery			
Obturator artery				
Superior gluteal artery				
Umbilical artery				
Uterine artery				
Vaginal artery				

Non-OR 049[Ø,1,2,3,4,5,6,7,8,9,A,B,C,D,E,F,H,J,K,L,M,N,P,Q,R,S,T,U,V,W,Y]3ZX
Non-OR 049[Ø,1,2,3,4,5,6,7,8,9,A,B,C,D,E,F,H,J,K,L,M,N,P,Q,R,S,T,U,V,W,Y][Ø,3,4]ZZ

Ø   **Medical and Surgical**
4   **Lower Arteries**
B   **Excision**   Definition: Cutting out or off, without replacement, a portion of a body part

Explanation: The qualifier DIAGNOSTIC is used to identify excision procedures that are biopsies

Body Part Character 4		Approach Character 5	Device Character 6	Qualifier Character 7

Ø Abdominal Aorta
Inferior phrenic artery
Lumbar artery
Median sacral artery
Middle suprarenal artery
Ovarian artery
Testicular artery
1 Celiac Artery
Celiac trunk
2 Gastric Artery
Left gastric artery
Right gastric artery
3 Hepatic Artery
Common hepatic artery
Gastroduodenal artery
Hepatic artery proper
4 Splenic Artery
Left gastroepiploic artery
Pancreatic artery
Short gastric artery
5 Superior Mesenteric Artery
Ileal artery
Ileocolic artery
Inferior pancreaticoduodenal
   artery
Jejunal artery
6 Colic Artery, Right
7 Colic Artery, Left
8 Colic Artery, Middle
9 Renal Artery, Right
Inferior suprarenal artery
Renal segmental artery
A Renal Artery, Left
See 9 Renal Artery, Right
B Inferior Mesenteric Artery
Sigmoid artery
Superior rectal artery
C Common Iliac Artery, Right
D Common Iliac Artery, Left
E Internal Iliac Artery, Right
Deferential artery
Hypogastric artery
Iliolumbar artery
Inferior gluteal artery
Inferior vesical artery
Internal pudendal artery
Lateral sacral artery
Middle rectal artery
Obturator artery
Superior gluteal artery
Umbilical artery
Uterine artery
Vaginal artery
	F Internal Iliac Artery, Left
	See E Internal Iliac Artery, Right
	H External Iliac Artery, Right
	Deep circumflex iliac artery
	Inferior epigastric artery
	J External Iliac Artery, Left
	See H External Iliac Artery, Right
	K Femoral Artery, Right
	Circumflex iliac artery
	Deep femoral artery
	Descending genicular artery
	External pudendal artery
	Superficial epigastric artery
	L Femoral Artery, Left
	See K Femoral Artery, Right
	M Popliteal Artery, Right
	Inferior genicular artery
	Middle genicular artery
	Superior genicular artery
	Sural artery
	Tibioperoneal trunk
	N Popliteal Artery, Left
	See M Popliteal Artery, Right
	P Anterior Tibial Artery, Right
	Anterior lateral malleolar
	   artery
	Anterior medial malleolar
	   artery
	Anterior tibial recurrent artery
	Dorsalis pedis artery
	Posterior tibial recurrent artery
	Q Anterior Tibial Artery, Left
	*See P Anterior Tibial Artery,
	   Right*
	R Posterior Tibial Artery, Right
	S Posterior Tibial Artery, Left
	T Peroneal Artery, Right
	Fibular artery
	U Peroneal Artery, Left
	See T Peroneal Artery, Right
	V Foot Artery, Right
	Arcuate artery
	Dorsal metatarsal artery
	Lateral plantar artery
	Lateral tarsal artery
	Medial plantar artery
	W Foot Artery, Left
	See V Foot Artery, Right
	Y Lower Artery
	Umbilical artery
		Ø Open
		3 Percutaneous
		4 Percutaneous Endoscopic
			Z No Device	**X Diagnostic**
				Z No Qualifier

NC Noncovered Procedure   LC Limited Coverage   QA Questionable OB Admit   NT New Tech Add-on   ⊞ Combination Member   ♂Male   ♀Female

ICD-10-PCS 2022   **229**

04B–04B

Lower Arteries

Ø   **Medical and Surgical**
4   **Lower Arteries**
C   **Extirpation**   Definition: Taking or cutting out solid matter from a body part

Explanation: The solid matter may be an abnormal byproduct of a biological function or a foreign body; it may be imbedded in a body part or in the lumen of a tubular body part. The solid matter may or may not have been previously broken into pieces.

Body Part Character 4		Approach Character 5	Device Character 6	Qualifier Character 7
Ø **Abdominal Aorta** Inferior phrenic artery Lumbar artery Median sacral artery Middle suprarenal artery Ovarian artery Testicular artery **1** **Celiac Artery** Celiac trunk **2** **Gastric Artery** Left gastric artery Right gastric artery **3** **Hepatic Artery** Common hepatic artery Gastroduodenal artery Hepatic artery proper **4** **Splenic Artery** Left gastroepiploic artery Pancreatic artery Short gastric artery **5** **Superior Mesenteric Artery** Ileal artery Ileocolic artery Inferior pancreaticoduodenal artery Jejunal artery **6** **Colic Artery, Right** **7** **Colic Artery, Left** **8** **Colic Artery, Middle** **9** **Renal Artery, Right** Inferior suprarenal artery Renal segmental artery **A** **Renal Artery, Left** *See 9 Renal Artery, Right* **B** **Inferior Mesenteric Artery** Sigmoid artery Superior rectal artery **C** **Common Iliac Artery, Right** **D** **Common Iliac Artery, Left** **E** **Internal Iliac Artery, Right** Deferential artery Hypogastric artery Iliolumbar artery Inferior gluteal artery Inferior vesical artery Internal pudendal artery Lateral sacral artery Middle rectal artery Obturator artery Superior gluteal artery Umbilical artery Uterine artery Vaginal artery	**F** **Internal Iliac Artery, Left** *See E Internal Iliac Artery, Right* **H** **External Iliac Artery, Right** Deep circumflex iliac artery Inferior epigastric artery **J** **External Iliac Artery, Left** *See H External Iliac Artery, Right* **K** **Femoral Artery, Right** Circumflex iliac artery Deep femoral artery Descending genicular artery External pudendal artery Superficial epigastric artery **L** **Femoral Artery, Left** *See K Femoral Artery, Right* **M** **Popliteal Artery, Right** Inferior genicular artery Middle genicular artery Superior genicular artery Sural artery Tibioperoneal trunk **N** **Popliteal Artery, Left** *See M Popliteal Artery, Right* **P** **Anterior Tibial Artery, Right** Anterior lateral malleolar artery Anterior medial malleolar artery Anterior tibial recurrent artery Dorsalis pedis artery Posterior tibial recurrent artery **Q** **Anterior Tibial Artery, Left** *See P Anterior Tibial Artery,* *Right* **R** **Posterior Tibial Artery, Right** **S** **Posterior Tibial Artery, Left** **T** **Peroneal Artery, Right** Fibular artery **U** **Peroneal Artery, Left** *See T Peroneal Artery, Right* **V** **Foot Artery, Right** Arcuate artery Dorsal metatarsal artery Lateral plantar artery Lateral tarsal artery Medial plantar artery **W** **Foot Artery, Left** *See V Foot Artery, Right* **Y** **Lower Artery** Umbilical artery	**Ø** Open **3** Percutaneous **4** Percutaneous Endoscopic	**Z** No Device	**Z** No Qualifier

Ø   **Medical and Surgical**
4   **Lower Arteries**
F   **Fragmentation**   Definition: Breaking solid matter in a body part into pieces

         Explanation: Physical force (e.g., manual, ultrasonic) applied directly or indirectly is used to break the solid matter into pieces. The solid matter may be an abnormal byproduct of a biological function or a foreign body. The pieces of solid matter are not taken out.

Body Part Character 4	Approach Character 5	Device Character 6	Qualifier Character 7
C **Common Iliac Artery, Right**	**3** Percutaneous	**Z** No Device	**Ø** Ultrasonic
D **Common Iliac Artery, Left**			**Z** No Qualifier
E **Internal Iliac Artery, Right**			
Deferential artery			
Hypogastric artery			
Iliolumbar artery			
Inferior gluteal artery			
Inferior vesical artery			
Internal pudendal artery			
Lateral sacral artery			
Middle rectal artery			
Obturator artery			
Superior gluteal artery			
Umbilical artery			
Uterine artery			
Vaginal artery			
F **Internal Iliac Artery, Left**			
See E Internal Iliac Artery, Right			
H **External Iliac Artery, Right**			
Deep circumflex iliac artery			
Inferior epigastric artery			
J **External Iliac Artery, Left**			
See H External Iliac Artery, Right			
K **Femoral Artery, Right**			
Circumflex iliac artery			
Deep femoral artery			
Descending genicular artery			
External pudendal artery			
Superficial epigastric artery			
L **Femoral Artery, Left**			
See K Femoral Artery, Right			
M **Popliteal Artery, Right**			
Inferior genicular artery			
Middle genicular artery			
Superior genicular artery			
Sural artery			
Tibioperoneal trunk			
N **Popliteal Artery, Left**			
See M Popliteal Artery, Right			
P **Anterior Tibial Artery, Right**			
Anterior lateral malleolar artery			
Anterior medial malleolar artery			
Anterior tibial recurrent artery			
Dorsalis pedis artery			
Posterior tibial recurrent artery			
Q **Anterior Tibial Artery, Left**			
See P Anterior Tibial Artery, Right			
R **Posterior Tibial Artery, Right**			
S **Posterior Tibial Artery, Left**			
T **Peroneal Artery, Right**			
Fibular artery			
U **Peroneal Artery, Left**			
See T Peroneal Artery, Right			
Y **Lower Artery**			
Umbilical artery			

NC Noncovered Procedure   **LC** Limited Coverage   **QA** Questionable OB Admit   **NT** New Tech Add-on   ⊞ Combination Member   ♂ Male   ♀ Female

ICD-10-PCS 2022   231

04F–04F

Lower Arteries

Ø   **Medical and Surgical**
4   **Lower Arteries**
H   **Insertion**   Definition: Putting in a nonbiological appliance that monitors, assists, performs, or prevents a physiological function but does not physically take the place of a body part
           Explanation: None

Body Part Character 4		Approach Character 5	Device Character 6	Qualifier Character 7
Ø **Abdominal Aorta** Inferior phrenic artery Lumbar artery Median sacral artery Middle suprarenal artery Ovarian artery Testicular artery		**Ø** Open **3** Percutaneous **4** Percutaneous Endoscopic	**2** Monitoring Device **3** Infusion Device **D** Intraluminal Device	**Z** No Qualifier
1 **Celiac Artery** Celiac trunk **2** **Gastric Artery** Left gastric artery Right gastric artery **3** **Hepatic Artery** Common hepatic artery Gastroduodenal artery Hepatic artery proper **4** **Splenic Artery** Left gastroepiploic artery Pancreatic artery Short gastric artery **5** **Superior Mesenteric Artery** Ileal artery Ileocolic artery Inferior pancreaticoduodenal artery Jejunal artery **6** **Colic Artery, Right** **7** **Colic Artery, Left** **8** **Colic Artery, Middle** **9** **Renal Artery, Right** Inferior suprarenal artery Renal segmental artery **A** **Renal Artery, Left** *See 9 Renal Artery, Right* **B** **Inferior Mesenteric Artery** Sigmoid artery Superior rectal artery **C** **Common Iliac Artery, Right** **D** **Common Iliac Artery, Left** **E** **Internal Iliac Artery, Right** Deferential artery Hypogastric artery Iliolumbar artery Inferior gluteal artery Inferior vesical artery Internal pudendal artery Lateral sacral artery Middle rectal artery Obturator artery Superior gluteal artery Umbilical artery Uterine artery Vaginal artery	**F** **Internal Iliac Artery, Left** *See E Internal Iliac Artery, Right* **H** **External Iliac Artery, Right** Deep circumflex iliac artery Inferior epigastric artery **J** **External Iliac Artery, Left** *See H External Iliac Artery, Right* **K** **Femoral Artery, Right** Circumflex iliac artery Deep femoral artery Descending genicular artery External pudendal artery Superficial epigastric artery **L** **Femoral Artery, Left** *See K Femoral Artery, Right* **M** **Popliteal Artery, Right** Inferior genicular artery Middle genicular artery Superior genicular artery Sural artery Tibioperoneal trunk **N** **Popliteal Artery, Left** *See M Popliteal Artery, Right* **P** **Anterior Tibial Artery, Right** Anterior lateral malleolar artery Anterior medial malleolar artery Anterior tibial recurrent artery Dorsalis pedis artery Posterior tibial recurrent artery **Q** **Anterior Tibial Artery, Left** *See P Anterior Tibial Artery, Right* **R** **Posterior Tibial Artery, Right** **S** **Posterior Tibial Artery, Left** **T** **Peroneal Artery, Right** Fibular artery **U** **Peroneal Artery, Left** *See T Peroneal Artery, Right* **V** **Foot Artery, Right** Arcuate artery Dorsal metatarsal artery Lateral plantar artery Lateral tarsal artery Medial plantar artery **W** **Foot Artery, Left** *See V Foot Artery, Right*	**Ø** Open **3** Percutaneous **4** Percutaneous Endoscopic	**3** Infusion Device **D** Intraluminal Device	**Z** No Qualifier
Y **Lower Artery** Umbilical artery		**Ø** Open **3** Percutaneous **4** Percutaneous Endoscopic	**2** Monitoring Device **3** Infusion Device **D** Intraluminal Device **Y** Other Device	**Z** No Qualifier

Non-OR   04HØ[Ø,3,4][2,3]Z
Non-OR   04H[1,2,3,4,5,6,7,8,9,A,B,C,D,E,F,H,J,K,L,M,N,P,Q,R,S,T,U,V,W][Ø,3,4]3Z
Non-OR   04HY32Z
Non-OR   04HY[Ø,3,4]3Z
Non-OR   04HY[3,4]YZ

Ø   **Medical and Surgical**
4   **Lower Arteries**
J   **Inspection**   Definition: Visually and/or manually exploring a body part

Explanation: Visual exploration may be performed with or without optical instrumentation. Manual exploration may be performed directly or through intervening body layers.

Body Part Character 4	Approach Character 5	Device Character 6	Qualifier Character 7
Y Lower Artery Umbilical artery	**Ø** Open **3** Percutaneous **4** Percutaneous Endoscopic **X** External	**Z** No Device	**Z** No Qualifier

Non-OR   Ø4JY[3,4,X]ZZ

Ø   **Medical and Surgical**
4   **Lower Arteries**
L   **Occlusion**   Definition: Completely closing an orifice or the lumen of a tubular body part

Explanation: The orifice can be a natural orifice or an artificially created orifice

Body Part Character 4	Approach Character 5	Device Character 6	Qualifier Character 7

Ø   **Abdominal Aorta**
    Inferior phrenic artery
    Lumbar artery
    Median sacral artery
    Middle suprarenal artery
    Ovarian artery
    Testicular artery
	Ø Open
	4 Percutaneous Endoscopic
		C Extraluminal Device
		D Intraluminal Device
		Z No Device
			Z No Qualifier

Ø   **Abdominal Aorta**
    Inferior phrenic artery
    Lumbar artery
    Median sacral artery
    Middle suprarenal artery
    Ovarian artery
    Testicular artery
	3 Percutaneous	**C** Extraluminal Device
		Z No Device
			Z No Qualifier

Ø   **Abdominal Aorta**
    Inferior phrenic artery
    Lumbar artery
    Median sacral artery
    Middle suprarenal artery
    Ovarian artery
    Testicular artery
	3 Percutaneous	**D** Intraluminal Device	**J** Temporary
			Z No Qualifier

Ø4L Continued on next page

0   Medical and Surgical   *04L Continued*
4   Lower Arteries
L   Occlusion   Definition: Completely closing an orifice or the lumen of a tubular body part
                       Explanation: The orifice can be a natural orifice or an artificially created orifice

Body Part Character 4		Approach Character 5	Device Character 6	Qualifier Character 7

1 Celiac Artery
Celiac trunk
2 Gastric Artery
Left gastric artery
Right gastric artery
3 Hepatic Artery
Common hepatic artery
Gastroduodenal artery
Hepatic artery proper
4 Splenic Artery
Left gastroepiploic artery
Pancreatic artery
Short gastric artery
5 Superior Mesenteric Artery
Ileal artery
Ileocolic artery
Inferior pancreaticoduodenal
   artery
Jejunal artery
6 Colic Artery, Right
7 Colic Artery, Left
8 Colic Artery, Middle
9 Renal Artery, Right
Inferior suprarenal artery
Renal segmental artery
A Renal Artery, Left
  See 9 Renal Artery, Right
B Inferior Mesenteric Artery
Sigmoid artery
Superior rectal artery
C Common Iliac Artery, Right
D Common Iliac Artery, Left
H External Iliac Artery, Right
Deep circumflex iliac artery
Inferior epigastric artery
J External Iliac Artery, Left
  See H External Iliac Artery, Right
	K Femoral Artery, Right
	Circumflex iliac artery
	Deep femoral artery
	Descending genicular artery
	External pudendal artery
	Superficial epigastric artery
	L Femoral Artery, Left
	  See K Femoral Artery, Right
	M Popliteal Artery, Right
	Inferior genicular artery
	Middle genicular artery
	Superior genicular artery
	Sural artery
	Tibioperoneal trunk
	N Popliteal Artery, Left
	  See M Popliteal Artery, Right
	P Anterior Tibial Artery, Right
	Anterior lateral malleolar
	   artery
	Anterior medial malleolar
	   artery
	Anterior tibial recurrent artery
	Dorsalis pedis artery
	Posterior tibial recurrent artery
	Q Anterior Tibial Artery, Left
	  See P Anterior Tibial Artery,
	   Right
	R Posterior Tibial Artery, Right
	S Posterior Tibial Artery, Left
	T Peroneal Artery, Right
	Fibular artery
	U Peroneal Artery, Left
	  See T Peroneal Artery, Right
	V Foot Artery, Right
	Arcuate artery
	Dorsal metatarsal artery
	Lateral plantar artery
	Lateral tarsal artery
	Medial plantar artery
	W Foot Artery, Left
	  See V Foot Artery, Right
	Y Lower Artery
	Umbilical artery
		0 Open
		3 Percutaneous
		4 Percutaneous Endoscopic
			C Extraluminal Device
			D Intraluminal Device
			Z No Device
				Z No Qualifier

E Internal Iliac Artery, Right Deferential artery Hypogastric artery Iliolumbar artery Inferior gluteal artery Inferior vesical artery Internal pudendal artery Lateral sacral artery Middle rectal artery Obturator artery Superior gluteal artery Umbilical artery Uterine artery Vaginal artery		**0 Open** **3 Percutaneous** **4 Percutaneous Endoscopic**	**C Extraluminal Device** **D Intraluminal Device** **Z No Device**	**T Uterine Artery, Right** ♀ **Z No Qualifier**
F Internal Iliac Artery, Left Deferential artery Hypogastric artery Iliolumbar artery Inferior gluteal artery Inferior vesical artery Internal pudendal artery Lateral sacral artery Middle rectal artery Obturator artery Superior gluteal artery Umbilical artery Uterine Artery Vaginal artery		**0 Open** **3 Percutaneous** **4 Percutaneous Endoscopic**	**C Extraluminal Device** **D Intraluminal Device** **Z No Device**	**U Uterine Artery, Left** ♀ **Z No Qualifier**

♀   04LE[0,3,4][C,D,Z]T
♀   04LF[0,3,4][C,D,Z]U

Ø   Medical and Surgical
4   Lower Arteries
N   Release   Definition: Freeing a body part from an abnormal physical constraint by cutting or by the use of force
                         Explanation: Some of the restraining tissue may be taken out but none of the body part is taken out

Body Part Character 4		Approach Character 5	Device Character 6	Qualifier Character 7

Ø Abdominal Aorta
Inferior phrenic artery
Lumbar artery
Median sacral artery
Middle suprarenal artery
Ovarian artery
Testicular artery
1 Celiac Artery
Celiac trunk
2 Gastric Artery
Left gastric artery
Right gastric artery
3 Hepatic Artery
Common hepatic artery
Gastroduodenal artery
Hepatic artery proper
4 Splenic Artery
Left gastroepiploic artery
Pancreatic artery
Short gastric artery
5 Superior Mesenteric Artery
Ileal artery
Ileocolic artery
Inferior pancreaticoduodenal artery
Jejunal artery
6 Colic Artery, Right
7 Colic Artery, Left
8 Colic Artery, Middle
9 Renal Artery, Right
Inferior suprarenal artery
Renal segmental artery
A Renal Artery, Left
See 9 Renal Artery, Right
B Inferior Mesenteric Artery
Sigmoid artery
Superior rectal artery
C Common Iliac Artery, Right
D Common Iliac Artery, Left
E Internal Iliac Artery, Right
Deferential artery
Hypogastric artery
Iliolumbar artery
Inferior gluteal artery
Inferior vesical artery
Internal pudendal artery
Lateral sacral artery
Middle rectal artery
Obturator artery
Superior gluteal artery
Umbilical artery
Uterine artery
Vaginal artery
	F Internal Iliac Artery, Left
	See E Internal Iliac Artery, Right
	H External Iliac Artery, Right
	Deep circumflex iliac artery
	Inferior epigastric artery
	J External Iliac Artery, Left
	See H External Iliac Artery, Right
	K Femoral Artery, Right
	Circumflex iliac artery
	Deep femoral artery
	Descending genicular artery
	External pudendal artery
	Superficial epigastric artery
	L Femoral Artery, Left
	See K Femoral Artery, Right
	M Popliteal Artery, Right
	Inferior genicular artery
	Middle genicular artery
	Superior genicular artery
	Sural artery
	Tibioperoneal trunk
	N Popliteal Artery, Left
	See M Popliteal Artery, Right
	P Anterior Tibial Artery, Right
	Anterior lateral malleolar
	  artery
	Anterior medial malleolar
	  artery
	Anterior tibial recurrent
	  artery
	Dorsalis pedis artery
	Posterior tibial recurrent
	  artery
	Q Anterior Tibial Artery, Left
	See P Anterior Tibial Artery, Right
	R Posterior Tibial Artery, Right
	S Posterior Tibial Artery, Left
	T Peroneal Artery, Right
	Fibular artery
	U Peroneal Artery, Left
	See T Peroneal Artery, Right
	V Foot Artery, Right
	Arcuate artery
	Dorsal metatarsal artery
	Lateral plantar artery
	Lateral tarsal artery
	Medial plantar artery
	W Foot Artery, Left
	See V Foot Artery, Right
	Y Lower Artery
	Umbilical artery
		Ø Open
		3 Percutaneous
		4 Percutaneous Endoscopic
			Z No Device	**Z No Qualifier**

NC Noncovered Procedure   **LC** Limited Coverage   **QA** Questionable OB Admit   **NT** New Tech Add-on   ⊞ Combination Member   ♂ Male   ♀ Female

ICD-10-PCS 2022   **235**

Ø4N–Ø4N

Ø　Medical and Surgical
4　Lower Arteries
P　Removal

Definition: Taking out or off a device from a body part

Explanation: If a device is taken out and a similar device put in without cutting or puncturing the skin or mucous membrane, the procedure is coded to the root operation CHANGE. Otherwise, the procedure for taking out a device is coded to the root operation REMOVAL.

Body Part Character 4	Approach Character 5	Device Character 6	Qualifier Character 7
Y Lower Artery Umbilical artery	**Ø** Open **3** Percutaneous **4** Percutaneous Endoscopic	**Ø** Drainage Device **2** Monitoring Device **3** Infusion Device **7** Autologous Tissue Substitute **C** Extraluminal Device **D** Intraluminal Device **J** Synthetic Substitute **K** Nonautologous Tissue Substitute **Y** Other Device	**Z** No Qualifier
Y Lower Artery Umbilical artery	**X** External	**Ø** Drainage Device **1** Radioactive Element **2** Monitoring Device **3** Infusion Device **D** Intraluminal Device	**Z** No Qualifier

Non-OR	04PY3[Ø,2,3,D]Z
Non-OR	04PY[3,4]YZ
Non-OR	04PYX[Ø,1,2,3,D]Z

0   **Medical and Surgical**
4   **Lower Arteries**
Q   **Repair**   Definition: Restoring, to the extent possible, a body part to its normal anatomic structure and function
                   Explanation: Used only when the method to accomplish the repair is not one of the other root operations

Body Part Character 4		Approach Character 5	Device Character 6	Qualifier Character 7
0 **Abdominal Aorta**	**F** **Internal Iliac Artery, Left**	**0** **Open**	**Z** **No Device**	**Z** **No Qualifier**
Inferior phrenic artery	*See E Internal Iliac Artery,*	**3** **Percutaneous**		
Lumbar artery	*Right*	**4** **Percutaneous Endoscopic**		
Median sacral artery	**H** **External Iliac Artery, Right**			
Middle suprarenal artery	Deep circumflex iliac artery			
Ovarian artery	Inferior epigastric artery			
Testicular artery	**J** **External Iliac Artery, Left**			
1 **Celiac Artery**	*See H External Iliac Artery,*			
Celiac trunk	*Right*			
2 **Gastric Artery**	**K** **Femoral Artery, Right**			
Left gastric artery	Circumflex iliac artery			
Right gastric artery	Deep femoral artery			
3 **Hepatic Artery**	Descending genicular artery			
Common hepatic artery	External pudendal artery			
Gastroduodenal artery	Superficial epigastric artery			
Hepatic artery proper	**L** **Femoral Artery, Left**			
4 **Splenic Artery**	*See K Femoral Artery, Right*			
Left gastroepiploic artery	**M** **Popliteal Artery, Right**			
Pancreatic artery	Inferior genicular artery			
Short gastric artery	Middle genicular artery			
5 **Superior Mesenteric Artery**	Superior genicular artery			
Ileal artery	Sural artery			
Ileocolic artery	Tibioperoneal trunk			
Inferior pancreaticoduodenal	**N** **Popliteal Artery, Left**			
artery	*See M Popliteal Artery, Right*			
Jejunal artery	**P** **Anterior Tibial Artery, Right**			
6 **Colic Artery, Right**	Anterior lateral malleolar			
7 **Colic Artery, Left**	artery			
8 **Colic Artery, Middle**	Anterior medial malleolar			
9 **Renal Artery, Right**	artery			
Inferior suprarenal artery	Anterior tibial recurrent			
Renal segmental artery	artery			
A **Renal Artery, Left**	Dorsalis pedis artery			
See 9 Renal Artery, Right	Posterior tibial recurrent			
B **Inferior Mesenteric Artery**	artery			
Sigmoid artery	**Q** **Anterior Tibial Artery, Left**			
Superior rectal artery	*See P Anterior Tibial Artery,*			
C **Common Iliac Artery, Right**	*Right*			
D **Common Iliac Artery, Left**	**R** **Posterior Tibial Artery,**			
E **Internal Iliac Artery, Right**	**Right**			
Deferential artery	**S** **Posterior Tibial Artery, Left**			
Hypogastric artery	**T** **Peroneal Artery, Right**			
Iliolumbar artery	Fibular artery			
Inferior gluteal artery	**U** **Peroneal Artery, Left**			
Inferior vesical artery	*See T Peroneal Artery, Right*			
Internal pudendal artery	**V** **Foot Artery, Right**			
Lateral sacral artery	Arcuate artery			
Middle rectal artery	Dorsal metatarsal artery			
Obturator artery	Lateral plantar artery			
Superior gluteal artery	Lateral tarsal artery			
Umbilical artery	Medial plantar artery			
Uterine artery	**W** **Foot Artery, Left**			
Vaginal artery	*See V Foot Artery, Right*			
	Y **Lower Artery**			
	Umbilical artery			

NC Noncovered Procedure   **LC** Limited Coverage   **QA** Questionable OB Admit   **NT** New Tech Add-on   ➕ Combination Member   ♂ Male   ♀ Female

ICD-10-PCS 2022   **237**

Ø　Medical and Surgical
4　Lower Arteries
R　Replacement　　Definition: Putting in or on biological or synthetic material that physically takes the place and/or function of all or a portion of a body part
　　　　　　　　　　Explanation: The body part may have been taken out or replaced, or may be taken out, physically eradicated, or rendered nonfunctional during
　　　　　　　　　　the REPLACEMENT procedure. A REMOVAL procedure is coded for taking out the device used in a previous replacement procedure.

Body Part Character 4		Approach Character 5	Device Character 6	Qualifier Character 7
Ø　Abdominal Aorta 　　Inferior phrenic artery 　　Lumbar artery 　　Median sacral artery 　　Middle suprarenal artery 　　Ovarian artery 　　Testicular artery **1　Celiac Artery** 　　Celiac trunk **2　Gastric Artery** 　　Left gastric artery 　　Right gastric artery **3　Hepatic Artery** 　　Common hepatic artery 　　Gastroduodenal artery 　　Hepatic artery proper **4　Splenic Artery** 　　Left gastroepiploic artery 　　Pancreatic artery 　　Short gastric artery **5　Superior Mesenteric Artery** 　　Ileal artery 　　Ileocolic artery 　　Inferior pancreaticoduodenal 　　　artery 　　Jejunal artery **6　Colic Artery, Right** **7　Colic Artery, Left** **8　Colic Artery, Middle** **9　Renal Artery, Right** 　　Inferior suprarenal artery 　　Renal segmental artery **A　Renal Artery, Left** 　　*See 9 Renal Artery, Right* **B　Inferior Mesenteric Artery** 　　Sigmoid artery 　　Superior rectal artery **C　Common Iliac Artery, Right** **D　Common Iliac Artery, Left** **E　Internal Iliac Artery, Right** 　　Deferential artery 　　Hypogastric artery 　　Iliolumbar artery 　　Inferior gluteal artery 　　Inferior vesical artery 　　Internal pudendal artery 　　Lateral sacral artery 　　Middle rectal artery 　　Obturator artery 　　Superior gluteal artery 　　Umbilical artery 　　Uterine artery 　　Vaginal artery	**F　Internal Iliac Artery, Left** 　　*See E Internal Iliac Artery, Right* **H　External Iliac Artery, Right** 　　Deep circumflex iliac artery 　　Inferior epigastric artery **J　External Iliac Artery, Left** 　　*See H External Iliac Artery, Right* **K　Femoral Artery, Right** 　　Circumflex iliac artery 　　Deep femoral artery 　　Descending genicular artery 　　External pudendal artery 　　Superficial epigastric artery **L　Femoral Artery, Left** 　　*See K Femoral Artery, Right* **M　Popliteal Artery, Right** 　　Inferior genicular artery 　　Middle genicular artery 　　Superior genicular artery 　　Sural artery 　　Tibioperoneal trunk **N　Popliteal Artery, Left** 　　*See M Popliteal Artery, Right* **P　Anterior Tibial Artery, Right** 　　Anterior lateral malleolar 　　　artery 　　Anterior medial malleolar 　　　artery 　　Anterior tibial recurrent artery 　　Dorsalis pedis artery 　　Posterior tibial recurrent artery **Q　Anterior Tibial Artery, Left** 　　*See P Anterior Tibial Artery,* 　　　*Right* **R　Posterior Tibial Artery, Right** **S　Posterior Tibial Artery, Left** **T　Peroneal Artery, Right** 　　Fibular artery **U　Peroneal Artery, Left** 　　*See T Peroneal Artery, Right* **V　Foot Artery, Right** 　　Arcuate artery 　　Dorsal metatarsal artery 　　Lateral plantar artery 　　Lateral tarsal artery 　　Medial plantar artery **W　Foot Artery, Left** 　　*See V Foot Artery, Right* **Y　Lower Artery** 　　Umbilical artery	**Ø　Open** **4　Percutaneous Endoscopic**	**7　Autologous Tissue** 　　**Substitute** **J　Synthetic Substitute** **K　Nonautologous Tissue** 　　**Substitute**	**Z　No Qualifier**

Ø   **Medical and Surgical**
4   **Lower Arteries**
S   **Reposition**   Definition: Moving to its normal location, or other suitable location, all or a portion of a body part
                Explanation: The body part is moved to a new location from an abnormal location, or from a normal location where it is not functioning correctly. The body part may or may not be cut out or off to be moved to the new location.

Body Part Character 4		Approach Character 5	Device Character 6	Qualifier Character 7
Ø **Abdominal Aorta**	**F** **Internal Iliac Artery, Left**	**Ø** **Open**	**Z** **No Device**	**Z** **No Qualifier**
Inferior phrenic artery	*See E Internal Iliac Artery, Right*	**3** **Percutaneous**		
Lumbar artery	**H** **External Iliac Artery, Right**	**4** **Percutaneous Endoscopic**		
Median sacral artery	Deep circumflex iliac artery			
Middle suprarenal artery	Inferior epigastric artery			
Ovarian artery	**J** **External Iliac Artery, Left**			
Testicular artery	*See H External Iliac Artery, Right*			
1 **Celiac Artery**	**K** **Femoral Artery, Right**			
Celiac trunk	Circumflex iliac artery			
2 **Gastric Artery**	Deep femoral artery			
Left gastric artery	Descending genicular artery			
Right gastric artery	External pudendal artery			
3 **Hepatic Artery**	Superficial epigastric artery			
Common hepatic artery	**L** **Femoral Artery, Left**			
Gastroduodenal artery	*See K Femoral Artery, Right*			
Hepatic artery proper	**M** **Popliteal Artery, Right**			
4 **Splenic Artery**	Inferior genicular artery			
Left gastroepiploic artery	Middle genicular artery			
Pancreatic artery	Superior genicular artery			
Short gastric artery	Sural artery			
5 **Superior Mesenteric Artery**	Tibioperoneal trunk			
Ileal artery	**N** **Popliteal Artery, Left**			
Ileocolic artery	*See M Popliteal Artery, Right*			
Inferior pancreaticoduodenal	**P** **Anterior Tibial Artery, Right**			
artery	Anterior lateral malleolar			
Jejunal artery	artery			
6 **Colic Artery, Right**	Anterior medial malleolar			
7 **Colic Artery, Left**	artery			
8 **Colic Artery, Middle**	Anterior tibial recurrent artery			
9 **Renal Artery, Right**	Dorsalis pedis artery			
Inferior suprarenal artery	Posterior tibial recurrent artery			
Renal segmental artery	**Q** **Anterior Tibial Artery, Left**			
A **Renal Artery, Left**	*See P Anterior Tibial Artery,*			
See 9 Renal Artery, Right	*Right*			
B **Inferior Mesenteric Artery**	**R** **Posterior Tibial Artery, Right**			
Sigmoid artery	**S** **Posterior Tibial Artery, Left**			
Superior rectal artery	**T** **Peroneal Artery, Right**			
C **Common Iliac Artery, Right**	Fibular artery			
D **Common Iliac Artery, Left**	**U** **Peroneal Artery, Left**			
E **Internal Iliac Artery, Right**	*See T Peroneal Artery, Right*			
Deferential artery	**V** **Foot Artery, Right**			
Hypogastric artery	Arcuate artery			
Iliolumbar artery	Dorsal metatarsal artery			
Inferior gluteal artery	Lateral plantar artery			
Inferior vesical artery	Lateral tarsal artery			
Internal pudendal artery	Medial plantar artery			
Lateral sacral artery	**W** **Foot Artery, Left**			
Middle rectal artery	*See V Foot Artery, Right*			
Obturator artery	**Y** **Lower Artery**			
Superior gluteal artery	Umbilical artery			
Umbilical artery				
Uterine artery				
Vaginal artery				

NC Noncovered Procedure   **LC** Limited Coverage   **QA** Questionable OB Admit   **NT** New Tech Add-on   ⊞ Combination Member   ♂ Male   ♀ Female

ICD-10-PCS 2022   **239**

04S–04S

Ø   Medical and Surgical
4   Lower Arteries
U   Supplement   Definition: Putting in or on biological or synthetic material that physically reinforces and/or augments the function of a portion of a body part
                             Explanation: The biological material is non-living, or is living and from the same individual. The body part may have been previously replaced, and the SUPPLEMENT procedure is performed to physically reinforce and/or augment the function of the replaced body part.

Body Part Character 4		Approach Character 5	Device Character 6	Qualifier Character 7
Ø **Abdominal Aorta** Inferior phrenic artery Lumbar artery Median sacral artery Middle suprarenal artery Ovarian artery Testicular artery **1** **Celiac Artery** Celiac trunk **2** **Gastric Artery** Left gastric artery Right gastric artery **3** **Hepatic Artery** Common hepatic artery Gastroduodenal artery Hepatic artery proper **4** **Splenic Artery** Left gastroepiploic artery Pancreatic artery Short gastric artery **5** **Superior Mesenteric Artery** Ileal artery Ileocolic artery Inferior pancreaticoduodenal artery Jejunal artery **6** **Colic Artery, Right** **7** **Colic Artery, Left** **8** **Colic Artery, Middle** **9** **Renal Artery, Right** Inferior suprarenal artery Renal segmental artery **A** **Renal Artery, Left** *See 9 Renal Artery, Right* **B** **Inferior Mesenteric Artery** Sigmoid artery Superior rectal artery **C** **Common Iliac Artery, Right** **D** **Common Iliac Artery, Left** **E** **Internal Iliac Artery, Right** Deferential artery Hypogastric artery Iliolumbar artery Inferior gluteal artery Inferior vesical artery Internal pudendal artery Lateral sacral artery Middle rectal artery Obturator artery Superior gluteal artery Umbilical artery Uterine artery Vaginal artery	**F** **Internal Iliac Artery, Left** *See E Internal Iliac Artery, Right* **H** **External Iliac Artery, Right** Deep circumflex iliac artery Inferior epigastric artery **J** **External Iliac Artery, Left** *See H External Iliac Artery, Right* **K** **Femoral Artery, Right** Circumflex iliac artery Deep femoral artery Descending genicular artery External pudendal artery Superficial epigastric artery **L** **Femoral Artery, Left** *See K Femoral Artery, Right* **M** **Popliteal Artery, Right** Inferior genicular artery Middle genicular artery Superior genicular artery Sural artery Tibioperoneal trunk **N** **Popliteal Artery, Left** *See M Popliteal Artery, Right* **P** **Anterior Tibial Artery, Right** Anterior lateral malleolar artery Anterior medial malleolar artery Anterior tibial recurrent artery Dorsalis pedis artery Posterior tibial recurrent artery **Q** **Anterior Tibial Artery, Left** *See P Anterior Tibial Artery, Right* **R** **Posterior Tibial Artery, Right** **S** **Posterior Tibial Artery, Left** **T** **Peroneal Artery, Right** Fibular artery **U** **Peroneal Artery, Left** *See T Peroneal Artery, Right* **V** **Foot Artery, Right** Arcuate artery Dorsal metatarsal artery Lateral plantar artery Lateral tarsal artery Medial plantar artery **W** **Foot Artery, Left** *See V Foot Artery, Right* **Y** **Lower Artery** Umbilical artery	**Ø** Open **3** Percutaneous **4** Percutaneous Endoscopic	**7** Autologous Tissue Substitute **J** Synthetic Substitute **K** Nonautologous Tissue Substitute	**Z** No Qualifier

Ø   Medical and Surgical
4   Lower Arteries
V   Restriction   Definition: Partially closing an orifice or the lumen of a tubular body part

Explanation: The orifice can be a natural orifice or an artificially created orifice

Body Part Character 4		Approach Character 5	Device Character 6	Qualifier Character 7
Ø Abdominal Aorta Inferior phrenic artery Lumbar artery Median sacral artery Middle suprarenal artery Ovarian artery Testicular artery		**Ø** Open **3** Percutaneous **4** Percutaneous Endoscopic	**C** Extraluminal Device **E** Intraluminal Device, Branched or Fenestrated, One or Two Arteries **F** Intraluminal Device, Branched or Fenestrated, Three or More Arteries **Z** No Device	**Z** No Qualifier
Ø Abdominal Aorta Inferior phrenic artery Lumbar artery Median sacral artery Middle suprarenal artery Ovarian artery Testicular artery		**Ø** Open **3** Percutaneous **4** Percutaneous Endoscopic	**D** Intraluminal Device	**J** Temporary **Z** No Qualifier
1 Celiac Artery Celiac trunk **2 Gastric Artery** Left gastric artery Right gastric artery **3 Hepatic Artery** Common hepatic artery Gastroduodenal artery Hepatic artery proper **4 Splenic Artery** Left gastroepiploic artery Pancreatic artery Short gastric artery **5 Superior Mesenteric Artery** Ileal artery Ileocolic artery Inferior pancreaticoduodenal artery Jejunal artery **6 Colic Artery, Right** **7 Colic Artery, Left** **8 Colic Artery, Middle** **9 Renal Artery, Right** Inferior suprarenal artery Renal segmental artery **A Renal Artery, Left** *See 9 Renal Artery, Right* **B Inferior Mesenteric Artery** Sigmoid artery Superior rectal artery **E Internal Iliac Artery, Right** Deferential artery Hypogastric artery Iliolumbar artery Inferior gluteal artery Inferior vesical artery Internal pudendal artery Lateral sacral artery Middle rectal artery Obturator artery Superior gluteal artery Umbilical artery Uterine artery Vaginal artery **F Internal Iliac Artery, Left** *See E Internal Iliac Artery, Right*	**H External Iliac Artery, Right** Deep circumflex iliac artery Inferior epigastric artery **J External Iliac Artery, Left** *See H External Iliac Artery, Right* **K Femoral Artery, Right** Circumflex iliac artery Deep femoral artery Descending genicular artery External pudendal artery Superficial epigastric artery **L Femoral Artery, Left** *See K Femoral Artery, Right* **M Popliteal Artery, Right** Inferior genicular artery Middle genicular artery Superior genicular artery Sural artery Tibioperoneal trunk **N Popliteal Artery, Left** *See M Popliteal Artery, Right* **P Anterior Tibial Artery, Right** Anterior lateral malleolar artery Anterior medial malleolar artery Anterior tibial recurrent artery Dorsalis pedis artery Posterior tibial recurrent artery **Q Anterior Tibial Artery, Left** *See P Anterior Tibial Artery, Right* **R Posterior Tibial Artery, Right** **S Posterior Tibial Artery, Left** **T Peroneal Artery, Right** Fibular artery **U Peroneal Artery, Left** *See T Peroneal Artery, Right* **V Foot Artery, Right** Arcuate artery Dorsal metatarsal artery Lateral plantar artery Lateral tarsal artery Medial plantar artery **W Foot Artery, Left** *See V Foot Artery, Right* **Y Lower Artery** Umbilical artery	**Ø** Open **3** Percutaneous **4** Percutaneous Endoscopic	**C** Extraluminal Device **D** Intraluminal Device **Z** No Device	**Z** No Qualifier
C Common Iliac Artery, Right **D Common Iliac Artery, Left**		**Ø** Open **3** Percutaneous **4** Percutaneous Endoscopic	**C** Extraluminal Device **D** Intraluminal Device **E** Intraluminal Device, Branched or Fenestrated, One or Two Arteries **Z** No Device	**Z** No Qualifier

NC Noncovered Procedure   LC Limited Coverage   QA Questionable OB Admit   NT New Tech Add-on   ⊞ Combination Member   ♂ Male   ♀ Female

ICD-10-PCS 2022   241

Ø4V–Ø4V

Ø   Medical and Surgical
4   Lower Arteries
W   Revision

Definition: Correcting, to the extent possible, a portion of a malfunctioning device or the position of a displaced device

Explanation: Revision can include correcting a malfunctioning or displaced device by taking out or putting in components of the device such as a screw or pin

Body Part Character 4	Approach Character 5	Device Character 6	Qualifier Character 7
Y Lower Artery Umbilical artery	**Ø** Open **3** Percutaneous **4** Percutaneous Endoscopic	**Ø** Drainage Device **2** Monitoring Device **3** Infusion Device **7** Autologous Tissue Substitute **C** Extraluminal Device **D** Intraluminal Device **J** Synthetic Substitute **K** Nonautologous Tissue Substitute **Y** Other Device	**Z** No Qualifier
Y Lower Artery Umbilical artery	**X** External	**Ø** Drainage Device **2** Monitoring Device **3** Infusion Device **7** Autologous Tissue Substitute **C** Extraluminal Device **D** Intraluminal Device **J** Synthetic Substitute **K** Nonautologous Tissue Substitute	**Z** No Qualifier

Non-OR	Ø4WY3[Ø,2,3,D]Z
Non-OR	Ø4WY[3,4]YZ
Non-OR	Ø4WYX[Ø,2,3,7,C,D,J,K]Z

Non-OR Procedure   DRG Non-OR Procedure   Valid OR Procedure   HAC Associated Procedure   Combination Only   New/Revised GREEN

Upper Veins Ø51–Ø5W

Character Meanings

This Character Meaning table is provided as a guide to assist the user in the identification of character members that may be found in this section of code tables. It **SHOULD NOT** be used to build a PCS code.

Operation–Character 3	Body Part–Character 4	Approach–Character 5	Device–Character 6	Qualifier–Character 7
1 Bypass	Ø Azygos Vein	Ø Open	Ø Drainage Device	Ø Ultrasonic
5 Destruction	1 Hemiazygos Vein	3 Percutaneous	2 Monitoring Device	1 Drug-Coated Balloon
7 Dilation	3 Innominate Vein, Right	4 Percutaneous Endoscopic	3 Infusion Device	X Diagnostic
9 Drainage	4 Innominate Vein, Left	X External	7 Autologous Tissue Substitute	Y Upper Vein
B Excision	5 Subclavian Vein, Right		9 Autologous Venous Tissue	Z No Qualifier
C Extirpation	6 Subclavian Vein, Left		A Autologous Arterial Tissue	
D Extraction	7 Axillary Vein, Right		C Extraluminal Device	
F Fragmentation	8 Axillary Vein, Left		D Intraluminal Device	
H Insertion	9 Brachial Vein, Right		J Synthetic Substitute	
J Inspection	A Brachial Vein, Left		K Nonautologous Tissue Substitute	
L Occlusion	B Basilic Vein, Right		M Neurostimulator Lead	
N Release	C Basilic Vein, Left		Y Other Device	
P Removal	D Cephalic Vein, Right		Z No Device	
Q Repair	F Cephalic Vein, Left			
R Replacement	G Hand Vein, Right			
S Reposition	H Hand Vein, Left			
U Supplement	L Intracranial Vein			
V Restriction	M Internal Jugular Vein, Right			
W Revision	N Internal Jugular Vein, Left			
	P External Jugular Vein, Right			
	Q External Jugular Vein, Left			
	R Vertebral Vein, Right			
	S Vertebral Vein, Left			
	T Face Vein, Right			
	V Face Vein, Left			
	Y Upper Vein			

AHA Coding Clinic for table Ø51
2020, 1Q, 28   Free flap microvascular breast reconstruction
2017, 3Q, 15   Bypass of innominate vein to atrial appendage

AHA Coding Clinic for table Ø57
2020, 3Q, 38   Thrombectomy of arteriovenous fistula with angioplasty and stent placement

AHA Coding Clinic for table Ø59
2018, 3Q, 7   Catheter placement for treatment of congestive heart failure

AHA Coding Clinic for table Ø5B
2021, 2Q, 15   Excision of pituitary macroadenoma within cavernous sinus
2020, 3Q, 40   Excision of ulceration of arteriovenous fistula
2020, 1Q, 24   Resection of vascular malformation, likely cavernoma
2016, 2Q, 12   Resection of malignant neoplasm of infratemporal fossa

AHA Coding Clinic for table Ø5C
2020, 3Q, 37   Repair of aneurysm of arteriovenous fistula with endovenectomy
2020, 3Q, 38   Thrombectomy of arteriovenous fistula with angioplasty and stent placement

AHA Coding Clinic for table Ø5F
2020, 4Q, 45-49   New fragmentation tables
2020, 4Q, 49-50   Intravascular ultrasound assisted thrombolysis
2020, 4Q, 50   Intravascular lithotripsy

AHA Coding Clinic for table Ø5H
2016, 4Q, 97-98   Phrenic neurostimulator

AHA Coding Clinic for table Ø5P
2016, 4Q, 97-98   Phrenic neurostimulator

AHA Coding Clinic for table Ø5Q
2017, 3Q, 15   Bypass of innominate vein to atrial appendage

AHA Coding Clinic for table Ø5S
2013, 4Q, 125   Stage II cephalic vein transposition (superficialization) of arteriovenous fistula

AHA Coding Clinic for table Ø5V
2020, 3Q, 37   Repair of aneurysm of arteriovenous fistula with endovenectomy

AHA Coding Clinic for table Ø5W
2016, 4Q, 97-98   Phrenic neurostimulator

Head and Neck Veins

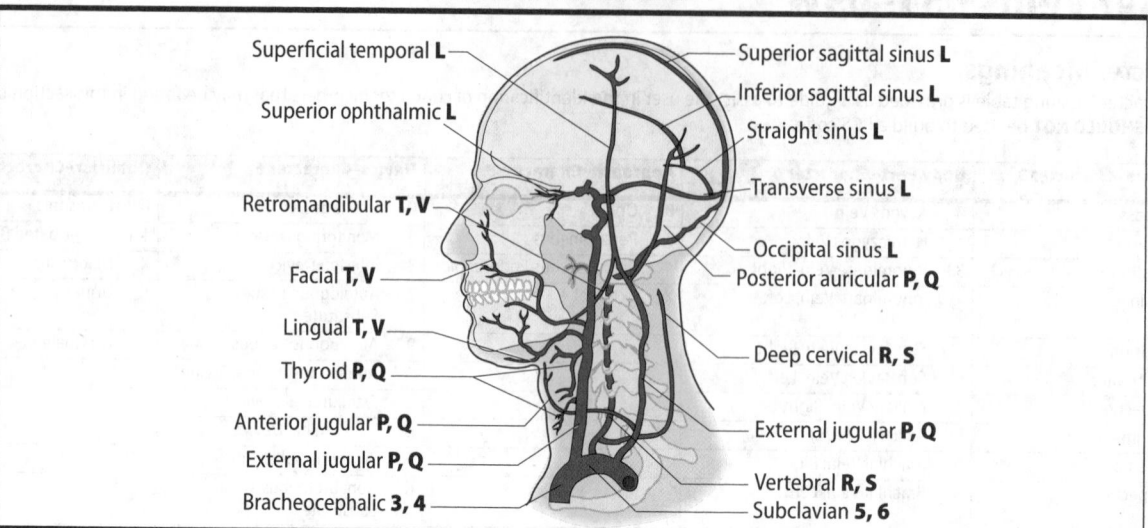

Superficial temporal **L**

Superior ophthalmic **L**

Retromandibular **T, V**

Facial **T, V**

Lingual **T, V**

Thyroid **P, Q**

Anterior jugular **P, Q**

External jugular **P, Q**

Bracheocephalic **3, 4**

Superior sagittal sinus **L**

Inferior sagittal sinus **L**

Straight sinus **L**

Transverse sinus **L**

Occipital sinus **L**

Posterior auricular **P, Q**

Deep cervical **R, S**

External jugular **P, Q**

Vertebral **R, S**

Subclavian **5, 6**

Upper Veins

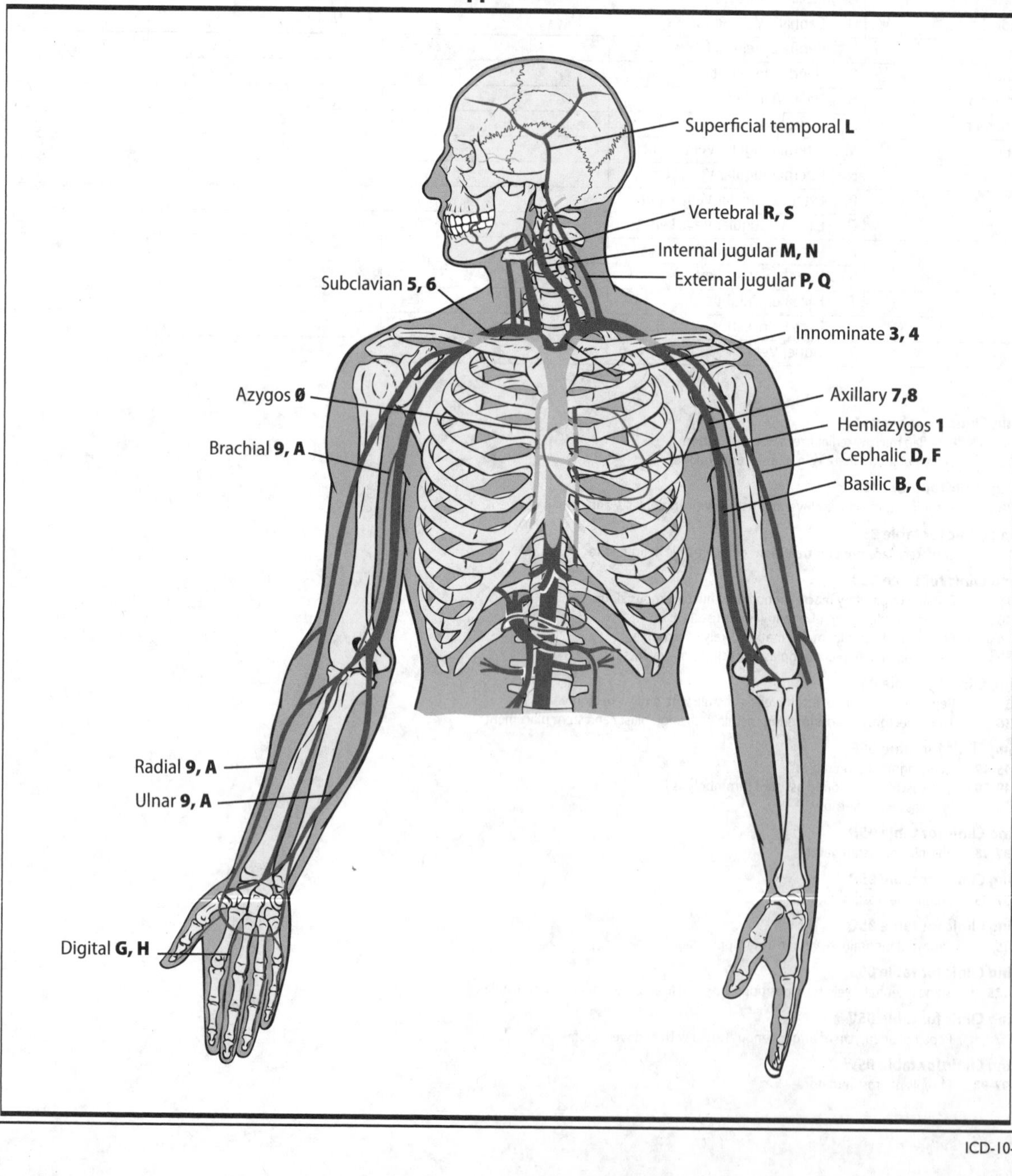

Superficial temporal **L**

Vertebral **R, S**

Internal jugular **M, N**

External jugular **P, Q**

Subclavian **5, 6**

Innominate **3, 4**

Azygos **Ø**

Axillary **7,8**

Hemiazygos **1**

Brachial **9, A**

Cephalic **D, F**

Basilic **B, C**

Radial **9, A**

Ulnar **9, A**

Digital **G, H**

Ø   Medical and Surgical
5   Upper Veins
1   Bypass   Definition: Altering the route of passage of the contents of a tubular body part

Explanation: Rerouting contents of a body part to a downstream area of the normal route, to a similar route and body part, or to an abnormal route and dissimilar body part. Includes one or more anastomoses, with or without the use of a device.

Body Part Character 4	Approach Character 5	Device Character 6	Qualifier Character 7

Ø   Azygos Vein
    Right ascending lumbar vein
    Right subcostal vein
1   Hemiazygos Vein
    Left ascending lumbar vein
    Left subcostal vein
3   Innominate Vein, Right
    Brachiocephalic vein
    Inferior thyroid vein
4   Innominate Vein, Left
    See 3 *Innominate Vein, Right*
5   Subclavian Vein, Right
6   Subclavian Vein, Left
7   Axillary Vein, Right
8   Axillary Vein, Left
9   Brachial Vein, Right
    Radial vein
    Ulnar vein
A   Brachial Vein, Left
    See 9 *Brachial Vein, Right*
B   Basilic Vein, Right
    Median antebrachial vein
    Median cubital vein
C   Basilic Vein, Left
    See B *Basilic Vein, Right*
D   Cephalic Vein, Right
    Accessory cephalic vein
F   Cephalic Vein, Left
    See D *Cephalic Vein, Right*
G   Hand Vein, Right
    Dorsal metacarpal vein
    Palmar (volar) digital vein
    Palmar (volar) metacarpal vein
    Superficial palmar venous arch
    Volar (palmar) digital vein
    Volar (palmar) metacarpal vein
H   Hand Vein, Left
    See G *Hand Vein, Right*
L   Intracranial Vein
    Anterior cerebral vein
    Basal (internal) cerebral vein
    Dural venous sinus
    Great cerebral vein
    Inferior cerebellar vein
    Inferior cerebral vein
    Internal (basal) cerebral vein
    Middle cerebral vein
    Ophthalmic vein
    Superior cerebellar vein
    Superior cerebral vein
M   Internal Jugular Vein, Right
N   Internal Jugular Vein, Left
P   External Jugular Vein, Right
    Posterior auricular vein
Q   External Jugular Vein, Left
    See P *External Jugular Vein, Right*
R   Vertebral Vein, Right
    Deep cervical vein
    Suboccipital venous plexus
S   Vertebral Vein, Left
    See R *Vertebral Vein, Right*
T   Face Vein, Right
    Angular vein
    Anterior facial vein
    Common facial vein
    Deep facial vein
    Frontal vein
    Posterior facial (retromandibular) vein
    Supraorbital vein
V   Face Vein, Left
    See T *Face Vein, Right*
	Ø Open
	4 Percutaneous Endoscopic
		7 Autologous Tissue Substitute
		9 Autologous Venous Tissue
		A Autologous Arterial Tissue
		J Synthetic Substitute
		K Nonautologous Tissue Substitute
		Z No Device
			Y Upper Vein

NC Noncovered Procedure   LC Limited Coverage   QA Questionable OB Admit   NT New Tech Add-on   ⊞ Combination Member   ♂ Male   ♀ Female

ICD-10-PCS 2022   **245**

Upper Veins

Ø   **Medical and Surgical**
5   **Upper Veins**
5   **Destruction**   Definition: Physical eradication of all or a portion of a body part by the direct use of energy, force, or a destructive agent
                        Explanation: None of the body part is physically taken out

Body Part Character 4	Approach Character 5	Device Character 6	Qualifier Character 7
Ø Azygos Vein Right ascending lumbar vein Right subcostal vein **1 Hemiazygos Vein** Left ascending lumbar vein Left subcostal vein **3 Innominate Vein, Right** Brachiocephalic vein Inferior thyroid vein **4 Innominate Vein, Left** *See 3 Innominate Vein, Right* **5 Subclavian Vein, Right** **6 Subclavian Vein, Left** **7 Axillary Vein, Right** **8 Axillary Vein, Left** **9 Brachial Vein, Right** Radial vein Ulnar vein **A Brachial Vein, Left** *See 9 Brachial Vein, Right* **B Basilic Vein, Right** Median antebrachial vein Median cubital vein **C Basilic Vein, Left** *See B Basilic Vein, Right* **D Cephalic Vein, Right** Accessory cephalic vein **F Cephalic Vein, Left** *See D Cephalic Vein, Right* **G Hand Vein, Right** Dorsal metacarpal vein Palmar (volar) digital vein Palmar (volar) metacarpal vein Superficial palmar venous arch Volar (palmar) digital vein Volar (palmar) metacarpal vein **H Hand Vein, Left** *See G Hand Vein, Right* **L Intracranial Vein** Anterior cerebral vein Basal (internal) cerebral vein Dural venous sinus Great cerebral vein Inferior cerebellar vein Inferior cerebral vein Internal (basal) cerebral vein Middle cerebral vein Ophthalmic vein Superior cerebellar vein Superior cerebral vein **M Internal Jugular Vein, Right** **N Internal Jugular Vein, Left** **P External Jugular Vein, Right** Posterior auricular vein **Q External Jugular Vein, Left** *See P External Jugular Vein, Right* **R Vertebral Vein, Right** Deep cervical vein Suboccipital venous plexus **S Vertebral Vein, Left** *See R Vertebral Vein, Right* **T Face Vein, Right** Angular vein Anterior facial vein Common facial vein Deep facial vein Frontal vein Posterior facial (retromandibular) vein Supraorbital vein **V Face Vein, Left** *See T Face Vein, Right* **Y Upper Vein**	**Ø Open** **3 Percutaneous** **4 Percutaneous Endoscopic**	**Z No Device**	**Z No Qualifier**

Non-OR Procedure   DRG Non-OR Procedure   Valid OR Procedure   HAC Associated Procedure   Combination Only   New/Revised GREEN

Ø   Medical and Surgical
5   Upper Veins
7   Dilation   Definition: Expanding an orifice or the lumen of a tubular body part

                Explanation: The orifice can be a natural orifice or an artificially created orifice. Accomplished by stretching a tubular body part using intraluminal pressure or by cutting part of the orifice or wall of the tubular body part.

Body Part Character 4	Approach Character 5	Device Character 6	Qualifier Character 7

Ø   Azygos Vein
    Right ascending lumbar vein
    Right subcostal vein
1   Hemiazygos Vein
    Left ascending lumbar vein
    Left subcostal vein
G   Hand Vein, Right
    Dorsal metacarpal vein
    Palmar (volar) digital vein
    Palmar (volar) metacarpal vein
    Superficial palmar venous arch
    Volar (palmar) digital vein
    Volar (palmar) metacarpal vein
H   Hand Vein, Left
    See G Hand Vein, Right
L   Intracranial Vein   NC
    Anterior cerebral vein
    Basal (internal) cerebral vein
    Dural venous sinus
    Great cerebral vein
    Inferior cerebellar vein
    Inferior cerebral vein
    Internal (basal) cerebral vein
    Middle cerebral vein
    Ophthalmic vein
    Superior cerebellar vein
    Superior cerebral vein
M   Internal Jugular Vein, Right
N   Internal Jugular Vein, Left
P   External Jugular Vein, Right
    Posterior auricular vein
Q   External Jugular Vein, Left
    See P External Jugular Vein, Right
R   Vertebral Vein, Right
    Deep cervical vein
    Suboccipital venous plexus
S   Vertebral Vein, Left
    See R Vertebral Vein, Right
T   Face Vein, Right
    Angular vein
    Anterior facial vein
    Common facial vein
    Deep facial vein
    Frontal vein
    Posterior facial (retromandibular) vein
    Supraorbital vein
V   Face Vein, Left
    See T Face Vein, Right
Y   Upper Vein
	Ø Open
	3 Percutaneous
	4 Percutaneous Endoscopic
		D Intraluminal Device
		Z No Device
			Z No Qualifier

3   Innominate Vein, Right
    Brachiocephalic vein
    Inferior thyroid vein
4   Innominate Vein, Left
    See 3 Innominate Vein, Right
5   Subclavian Vein, Right
6   Subclavian Vein, Left
7   Axillary Vein, Right
8   Axillary Vein, Left
9   Brachial Vein, Right
    Radial vein
    Ulnar vein
A   Brachial Vein, Left
    See 9 Brachial Vein, Right
B   Basilic Vein, Right
    Median antebrachial vein
    Median cubital vein
C   Basilic Vein, Left
    See B Basilic Vein, Right
D   Cephalic Vein, Right
    Accessory cephalic vein
F   Cephalic Vein, Left
    See D Cephalic Vein, Right
	Ø Open
	3 Percutaneous
	4 Percutaneous Endoscopic
		D Intraluminal Device
		Z No Device
			1 Drug-Coated Balloon
			Z No Qualifier

NC   Ø57L[3,4]ZZ

NC Noncovered Procedure   LC Limited Coverage   QA Questionable OB Admit   NT New Tech Add-on   ⊞ Combination Member   ♂ Male   ♀ Female

ICD-10-PCS 2022   **247**

Ø57–Ø57

Ø Medical and Surgical
5 Upper Veins
9 Drainage Definition: Taking or letting out fluids and/or gases from a body part
Explanation: The qualifier DIAGNOSTIC is used to identify drainage procedures that are biopsies

Body Part Character 4		Approach Character 5	Device Character 6	Qualifier Character 7
Ø Azygos Vein Right ascending lumbar vein Right subcostal vein **1 Hemiazygos Vein** Left ascending lumbar vein Left subcostal vein **3 Innominate Vein, Right** Brachiocephalic vein Inferior thyroid vein **4 Innominate Vein, Left** *See 3 Innominate Vein, Right* **5 Subclavian Vein, Right** **6 Subclavian Vein, Left** **7 Axillary Vein, Right** **8 Axillary Vein, Left** **9 Brachial Vein, Right** Radial vein Ulnar vein **A Brachial Vein, Left** *See 9 Brachial Vein, Right* **B Basilic Vein, Right** Median antebrachial vein Median cubital vein **C Basilic Vein, Left** *See B Basilic Vein, Right* **D Cephalic Vein, Right** Accessory cephalic vein **F Cephalic Vein, Left** *See D Cephalic Vein, Right* **G Hand Vein, Right** Dorsal metacarpal vein Palmar (volar) digital vein Palmar (volar) metacarpal vein Superficial palmar venous arch Volar (palmar) digital vein Volar (palmar) metacarpal vein	**H Hand Vein, Left** *See G Hand Vein, Right* **L Intracranial Vein** Anterior cerebral vein Basal (internal) cerebral vein Dural venous sinus Great cerebral vein Inferior cerebellar vein Inferior cerebral vein Internal (basal) cerebral vein Middle cerebral vein Ophthalmic vein Superior cerebellar vein Superior cerebral vein **M Internal Jugular Vein, Right** **N Internal Jugular Vein, Left** **P External Jugular Vein, Right** Posterior auricular vein **Q External Jugular Vein, Left** *See P External Jugular Vein, Right* **R Vertebral Vein, Right** Deep cervical vein Suboccipital venous plexus **S Vertebral Vein, Left** *See R Vertebral Vein, Right* **T Face Vein, Right** Angular vein Anterior facial vein Common facial vein Deep facial vein Frontal vein Posterior facial (retromandibular) vein Supraorbital vein **V Face Vein, Left** *See T Face Vein, Right* **Y Upper Vein**	**Ø Open** **3 Percutaneous** **4 Percutaneous Endoscopic**	**Ø Drainage Device**	**Z No Qualifier**
Ø Azygos Vein Right ascending lumbar vein Right subcostal vein **1 Hemiazygos Vein** Left ascending lumbar vein Left subcostal vein **3 Innominate Vein, Right** Brachiocephalic vein Inferior thyroid vein **4 Innominate Vein, Left** *See 3 Innominate Vein, Right* **5 Subclavian Vein, Right** **6 Subclavian Vein, Left** **7 Axillary Vein, Right** **8 Axillary Vein, Left** **9 Brachial Vein, Right** Radial vein Ulnar vein **A Brachial Vein, Left** *See 9 Brachial Vein, Right* **B Basilic Vein, Right** Median antebrachial vein Median cubital vein **C Basilic Vein, Left** *See B Basilic Vein, Right* **D Cephalic Vein, Right** Accessory cephalic vein **F Cephalic Vein, Left** *See D Cephalic Vein, Right* **G Hand Vein, Right** Dorsal metacarpal vein Palmar (volar) digital vein Palmar (volar) metacarpal vein Superficial palmar venous arch Volar (palmar) digital vein Volar (palmar) metacarpal vein	**H Hand Vein, Left** *See G Hand Vein, Right* **L Intracranial Vein** Anterior cerebral vein Basal (internal) cerebral vein Dural venous sinus Great cerebral vein Inferior cerebellar vein Inferior cerebral vein Internal (basal) cerebral vein Middle cerebral vein Ophthalmic vein Superior cerebellar vein Superior cerebral vein **M Internal Jugular Vein, Right** **N Internal Jugular Vein, Left** **P External Jugular Vein, Right** Posterior auricular vein **Q External Jugular Vein, Left** *See P External Jugular Vein, Right* **R Vertebral Vein, Right** Deep cervical vein Suboccipital venous plexus **S Vertebral Vein, Left** *See R Vertebral Vein, Right* **T Face Vein, Right** Angular vein Anterior facial vein Common facial vein Deep facial vein Frontal vein Posterior facial (retromandibular) vein Supraorbital vein **V Face Vein, Left** *See T Face Vein, Right* **Y Upper Vein**	**Ø Open** **3 Percutaneous** **4 Percutaneous Endoscopic**	**Z No Device**	**X Diagnostic** **Z No Qualifier**

Non-OR Ø59[Ø,1,3,4,5,6,7,8,9,A,B,C,D,F,G,H,L,M,N,P,Q,R,S,T,V,Y][Ø,3,4]ØZ
Non-OR Ø59[Ø,1,3,4,5,6,7,8,9,A,B,C,D,F,G,H,L,M,N,P,Q,R,S,T,V,Y]3ZX
Non-OR Ø59[Ø,1,3,4,5,6,7,8,9,A,B,C,D,F,G,H,L,M,N,P,Q,R,S,T,V,Y][Ø,3,4]ZZ

Ø   **Medical and Surgical**
5   **Upper Veins**
B   **Excision**   Definition: Cutting out or off, without replacement, a portion of a body part

                         Explanation: The qualifier DIAGNOSTIC is used to identify excision procedures that are biopsies

Body Part Character 4	Approach Character 5	Device Character 6	Qualifier Character 7

Ø **Azygos Vein**
   Right ascending lumbar vein
   Right subcostal vein
1 **Hemiazygos Vein**
   Left ascending lumbar vein
   Left subcostal vein
3 **Innominate Vein, Right**
   Brachiocephalic vein
   Inferior thyroid vein
4 **Innominate Vein, Left**
   See 3 Innominate Vein, Right
5 **Subclavian Vein, Right**
6 **Subclavian Vein, Left**
7 **Axillary Vein, Right**
8 **Axillary Vein, Left**
9 **Brachial Vein, Right**
   Radial vein
   Ulnar vein
A **Brachial Vein, Left**
   See 9 Brachial Vein, Right
B **Basilic Vein, Right**
   Median antebrachial vein
   Median cubital vein
C **Basilic Vein, Left**
   See B Basilic Vein, Right
D **Cephalic Vein, Right**
   Accessory cephalic vein
F **Cephalic Vein, Left**
   See D Cephalic Vein, Right
G **Hand Vein, Right**
   Dorsal metacarpal vein
   Palmar (volar) digital vein
   Palmar (volar) metacarpal vein
   Superficial palmar venous arch
   Volar (palmar) digital vein
   Volar (palmar) metacarpal vein
H **Hand Vein, Left**
   See G Hand Vein, Right
L **Intracranial Vein**
   Anterior cerebral vein
   Basal (internal) cerebral vein
   Dural venous sinus
   Great cerebral vein
   Inferior cerebellar vein
   Inferior cerebral vein
   Internal (basal) cerebral vein
   Middle cerebral vein
   Ophthalmic vein
   Superior cerebellar vein
   Superior cerebral vein
M **Internal Jugular Vein, Right**
N **Internal Jugular Vein, Left**
P **External Jugular Vein, Right**
   Posterior auricular vein
Q **External Jugular Vein, Left**
   See P External Jugular Vein, Right
R **Vertebral Vein, Right**
   Deep cervical vein
   Suboccipital venous plexus
S **Vertebral Vein, Left**
   See R Vertebral Vein, Right
T **Face Vein, Right**
   Angular vein
   Anterior facial vein
   Common facial vein
   Deep facial vein
   Frontal vein
   Posterior facial (retromandibular) vein
   Supraorbital vein
V **Face Vein, Left**
   See T Face Vein, Right
Y **Upper Vein**
	Ø Open
	3 Percutaneous
	4 Percutaneous Endoscopic
		Z No Device	**X** Diagnostic
			Z No Qualifier

NC Noncovered Procedure   **LC** Limited Coverage   **QA** Questionable OB Admit   **NT** New Tech Add-on   ⊞ Combination Member   ♂ Male   ♀ Female

ICD-10-PCS 2022   **249**

05B–05B

0   Medical and Surgical
5   Upper Veins
C   Extirpation   Definition: Taking or cutting out solid matter from a body part

Explanation: The solid matter may be an abnormal byproduct of a biological function or a foreign body; it may be imbedded in a body part or in the lumen of a tubular body part. The solid matter may or may not have been previously broken into pieces.

Body Part Character 4	Approach Character 5	Device Character 6	Qualifier Character 7

0   Azygos Vein
    Right ascending lumbar vein
    Right subcostal vein
1   Hemiazygos Vein
    Left ascending lumbar vein
    Left subcostal vein
3   Innominate Vein, Right
    Brachiocephalic vein
    Inferior thyroid vein
4   Innominate Vein, Left
    See 3 Innominate Vein, Right
5   Subclavian Vein, Right
6   Subclavian Vein, Left
7   Axillary Vein, Right
8   Axillary Vein, Left
9   Brachial Vein, Right
    Radial vein
    Ulnar vein
A   Brachial Vein, Left
    See 9 Brachial Vein, Right
B   Basilic Vein, Right
    Median antebrachial vein
    Median cubital vein
C   Basilic Vein, Left
    See B Basilic Vein, Right
D   Cephalic Vein, Right
    Accessory cephalic vein
F   Cephalic Vein, Left
    See D Cephalic Vein, Right
G   Hand Vein, Right
    Dorsal metacarpal vein
    Palmar (volar) digital vein
    Palmar (volar) metacarpal vein
    Superficial palmar venous arch
    Volar (palmar) digital vein
    Volar (palmar) metacarpal vein
H   Hand Vein, Left
    See G Hand Vein, Right
L   Intracranial Vein
    Anterior cerebral vein
    Basal (internal) cerebral vein
    Dural venous sinus
    Great cerebral vein
    Inferior cerebellar vein
    Inferior cerebral vein
    Internal (basal) cerebral vein
    Middle cerebral vein
    Ophthalmic vein
    Superior cerebellar vein
    Superior cerebral vein
M   Internal Jugular Vein, Right
N   Internal Jugular Vein, Left
P   External Jugular Vein, Right
    Posterior auricular vein
Q   External Jugular Vein, Left
    See P External Jugular Vein, Right
R   Vertebral Vein, Right
    Deep cervical vein
    Suboccipital venous plexus
S   Vertebral Vein, Left
    See R Vertebral Vein, Right
T   Face Vein, Right
    Angular vein
    Anterior facial vein
    Common facial vein
    Deep facial vein
    Frontal vein
    Posterior facial (retromandibular) vein
    Supraorbital vein
V   Face Vein, Left
    See T Face Vein, Right
Y   Upper Vein
	0 Open
	3 Percutaneous
	4 Percutaneous Endoscopic
		Z No Device	**Z No Qualifier**

0   **Medical and Surgical**
5   **Upper Veins**
D   **Extraction**   Definition: Pulling or stripping out or off all or a portion of a body part by the use of force

                 Explanation: The qualifier DIAGNOSTIC is used to identify extraction procedures that are biopsies

Body Part Character 4	Approach Character 5	Device Character 6	Qualifier Character 7

9 **Brachial Vein, Right**
    Radial vein
    Ulnar vein
A **Brachial Vein, Left**
    See 9 Brachial Vein, Right
B **Basilic Vein, Right**
    Median antebrachial vein
    Median cubital vein
C **Basilic Vein, Left**
    See B Basilic Vein, Right
D **Cephalic Vein, Right**
    Accessory cephalic vein
F **Cephalic Vein, Left**
    See D Cephalic Vein, Right
G **Hand Vein, Right**
    Dorsal metacarpal vein
    Palmar (volar) digital vein
    Palmar (volar) metacarpal vein
    Superficial palmar venous arch
    Volar (palmar) digital vein
    Volar (palmar) metacarpal vein
H **Hand Vein, Left**
    See G Hand Vein, Right
Y **Upper Vein**
	0 Open
	3 Percutaneous
		Z No Device	**Z** No Qualifier

0   **Medical and Surgical**
5   **Upper Veins**
F   **Fragmentation**   Definition: Breaking solid matter in a body part into pieces

                 Explanation: Physical force (e.g., manual, ultrasonic) applied directly or indirectly is used to break the solid matter into pieces. The solid matter may be an abnormal byproduct of a biological function or a foreign body. The pieces of solid matter are not taken out.

Body Part Character 4	Approach Character 5	Device Character 6	Qualifier Character 7

3 **Innominate Vein, Right**
    Brachiocephalic vein
    Inferior thyroid vein
4 **Innominate Vein, Left**
    See 3 Innominate Vein, Right
5 **Subclavian Vein, Right**
6 **Subclavian Vein, Left**
7 **Axillary Vein, Right**
8 **Axillary Vein, Left**
9 **Brachial Vein, Right**
    Radial vein
    Ulnar vein
A **Brachial Vein, Left**
    See 9 Brachial Vein, Right
B **Basilic Vein, Right**
    Median antebrachial vein
    Median cubital vein
C **Basilic Vein, Left**
    See B Basilic Vein, Right
D **Cephalic Vein, Right**
    Accessory cephalic vein
F **Cephalic Vein, Left**
    See D Cephalic Vein, Right
Y **Upper Vein**
	3 Percutaneous	**Z** No Device	**0** Ultrasonic
			Z No Qualifier

NC Noncovered Procedure   LC Limited Coverage   QA Questionable OB Admit   NT New Tech Add-on   ⊞ Combination Member   ♂ Male   ♀ Female

ICD-10-PCS 2022   **251**

05D–05F

Ø Medical and Surgical
5 Upper Veins
H Insertion

Definition: Putting in a nonbiological appliance that monitors, assists, performs, or prevents a physiological function but does not physically take the place of a body part

Explanation: None

Body Part Character 4		Approach Character 5	Device Character 6	Qualifier Character 7
Ø Azygos Vein ⊞ Right ascending lumbar vein Right subcostal vein		**Ø** Open **3** Percutaneous **4** Percutaneous Endoscopic	**2** Monitoring Device **3** Infusion Device **D** Intraluminal Device **M** Neurostimulator Lead	**Z** No Qualifier
1 Hemiazygos Vein Left ascending lumbar vein Left subcostal vein **5 Subclavian Vein, Right** **6 Subclavian Vein, Left** **7 Axillary Vein, Right** **8 Axillary Vein, Left** **9 Brachial Vein, Right** Radial vein Ulnar vein **A Brachial Vein, Left** *See 9 Brachial Vein, Right* **B Basilic Vein, Right** Median antebrachial vein Median cubital vein **C Basilic Vein, Left** *See B Basilic Vein, Right* **D Cephalic Vein, Right** Accessory cephalic vein **F Cephalic Vein, Left** *See D Cephalic Vein, Right* **G Hand Vein, Right** Dorsal metacarpal vein Palmar (volar) digital vein Palmar (volar) metacarpal vein Superficial palmar venous arch Volar (palmar) digital vein Volar (palmar) metacarpal vein **H Hand Vein, Left** *See G Hand Vein, Right*	**L Intracranial Vein** Anterior cerebral vein Basal (internal) cerebral vein Dural venous sinus Great cerebral vein Inferior cerebellar vein Inferior cerebral vein Internal (basal) cerebral vein Middle cerebral vein Ophthalmic vein Superior cerebellar vein Superior cerebral vein **M Internal Jugular Vein, Right** **N Internal Jugular Vein, Left** **P External Jugular Vein, Right** Posterior auricular vein **Q External Jugular Vein, Left** *See P External Jugular Vein, Right* **R Vertebral Vein, Right** Deep cervical vein Suboccipital venous plexus **S Vertebral Vein, Left** *See R Vertebral Vein, Right* **T Face Vein, Right** Angular vein Anterior facial vein Common facial vein Deep facial vein Frontal vein Posterior facial (retromandibular) vein Supraorbital vein **V Face Vein, Left** *See T Face Vein, Right*	**Ø** Open **3** Percutaneous **4** Percutaneous Endoscopic	**3** Infusion Device **D** Intraluminal Device	**Z** No Qualifier
3 Innominate Vein, Right ⊞ Brachiocephalic vein Inferior thyroid vein **4 Innominate Vein, Left** ⊞ *See 3 Innominate Vein, Right*		**Ø** Open **3** Percutaneous **4** Percutaneous Endoscopic	**3** Infusion Device **D** Intraluminal Device **M** Neurostimulator Lead	**Z** No Qualifier
Y Upper Vein		**Ø** Open **3** Percutaneous **4** Percutaneous Endoscopic	**2** Monitoring Device **3** Infusion Device **D** Intraluminal Device **Y** Other Device	**Z** No Qualifier

Non-OR	Ø5HØ[Ø,3,4]3Z
Non-OR	Ø5H[1,5,6,7,8,9,A,B,C,D,F,G,H,L,M,N,P,Q,R,S,T,V][Ø,3,4]3Z
Non-OR	Ø5H[3,4][Ø,3,4]3Z
Non-OR	Ø5HY[Ø,3,4]3Z
Non-OR	Ø5HY32Z
Non-OR	Ø5HY[3,4]YZ
HAC	Ø5HØ[3,4]3Z when reported with SDx J95.811
HAC	Ø5H[1,5,6][3,4]3Z when reported with SDx J95.811
HAC	Ø5H[M,N,P,Q]33Z when reported with SDx J95.811
HAC	Ø5H[3,4][3,4]3Z when reported with SDx J95.811

See Appendix L for Procedure Combinations
⊞ Ø5HØ[Ø,3,4]MZ
⊞ Ø5H[3,4][Ø,3,4]MZ

Ø Medical and Surgical
5 Upper Veins
J Inspection

Definition: Visually and/or manually exploring a body part

Explanation: Visual exploration may be performed with or without optical instrumentation. Manual exploration may be performed directly or through intervening body layers.

Body Part Character 4	Approach Character 5	Device Character 6	Qualifier Character 7
Y Upper Vein	**Ø** Open **3** Percutaneous **4** Percutaneous Endoscopic **X** External	**Z** No Device	**Z** No Qualifier

| Non-OR | Ø5JY[3,X]ZZ |

Ø   Medical and Surgical
5   Upper Veins
L   Occlusion   Definition: Completely closing an orifice or the lumen of a tubular body part
                 Explanation: The orifice can be a natural orifice or an artificially created orifice

Body Part Character 4	Approach Character 5	Device Character 6	Qualifier Character 7

Ø   Azygos Vein
    Right ascending lumbar vein
    Right subcostal vein
	Ø Open
	3 Percutaneous
	4 Percutaneous Endoscopic
		C Extraluminal Device
		D Intraluminal Device
		Z No Device
			Z No Qualifier

1   Hemiazygos Vein
    Left ascending lumbar vein
    Left subcostal vein			

3   Innominate Vein, Right
    Brachiocephalic vein
    Inferior thyroid vein			

4 Innominate Vein, Left *See 3 Innominate Vein, Right*			
5 Subclavian Vein, Right			
6 Subclavian Vein, Left			
7 Axillary Vein, Right			
8 Axillary Vein, Left			

9   Brachial Vein, Right
    Radial vein
    Ulnar vein			

A Brachial Vein, Left *See 9 Brachial Vein, Right*			

B   Basilic Vein, Right
    Median antebrachial vein
    Median cubital vein			

C Basilic Vein, Left *See B Basilic Vein, Right*			
D Cephalic Vein, Right Accessory cephalic vein			
F Cephalic Vein, Left *See D Cephalic Vein, Right*			

G   Hand Vein, Right
    Dorsal metacarpal vein
    Palmar (volar) digital vein
    Palmar (volar) metacarpal vein
    Superficial palmar venous arch
    Volar (palmar) digital vein
    Volar (palmar) metacarpal vein			

H Hand Vein, Left *See G Hand Vein, Right*			

L   Intracranial Vein
    Anterior cerebral vein
    Basal (internal) cerebral vein
    Dural venous sinus
    Great cerebral vein
    Inferior cerebellar vein
    Inferior cerebral vein
    Internal (basal) cerebral vein
    Middle cerebral vein
    Ophthalmic vein
    Superior cerebellar vein
    Superior cerebral vein			

M Internal Jugular Vein, Right			
N Internal Jugular Vein, Left			
P External Jugular Vein, Right Posterior auricular vein			
Q External Jugular Vein, Left *See P External Jugular Vein, Right*			

R   Vertebral Vein, Right
    Deep cervical vein
    Suboccipital venous plexus			

S Vertebral Vein, Left *See R Vertebral Vein, Right*			

T   Face Vein, Right
    Angular vein
    Anterior facial vein
    Common facial vein
    Deep facial vein
    Frontal vein
    Posterior facial (retromandibular) vein
    Supraorbital vein			

V Face Vein, Left *See T Face Vein, Right*			
Y Upper Vein			

NC Noncovered Procedure   **LC** Limited Coverage   **QA** Questionable OB Admit   **NT** New Tech Add-on   ✚ Combination Member   ♂ Male   ♀ Female

ICD-10-PCS 2022   253

Ø Medical and Surgical
5 Upper Veins
N Release Definition: Freeing a body part from an abnormal physical constraint by cutting or by the use of force
Explanation: Some of the restraining tissue may be taken out but none of the body part is taken out

Body Part Character 4	Approach Character 5	Device Character 6	Qualifier Character 7
Ø Azygos Vein Right ascending lumbar vein Right subcostal vein	**Ø Open** **3 Percutaneous** **4 Percutaneous Endoscopic**	**Z No Device**	**Z No Qualifier**
1 Hemiazygos Vein Left ascending lumbar vein Left subcostal vein			
3 Innominate Vein, Right Brachiocephalic vein Inferior thyroid vein			
4 Innominate Vein, Left *See 3 Innominate Vein, Right*			
5 Subclavian Vein, Right			
6 Subclavian Vein, Left			
7 Axillary Vein, Right			
8 Axillary Vein, Left			
9 Brachial Vein, Right Radial vein Ulnar vein			
A Brachial Vein, Left *See 9 Brachial Vein, Right*			
B Basilic Vein, Right Median antebrachial vein Median cubital vein			
C Basilic Vein, Left *See B Basilic Vein, Right*			
D Cephalic Vein, Right Accessory cephalic vein			
F Cephalic Vein, Left *See D Cephalic Vein, Right*			
G Hand Vein, Right Dorsal metacarpal vein Palmar (volar) digital vein Palmar (volar) metacarpal vein Superficial palmar venous arch Volar (palmar) digital vein Volar (palmar) metacarpal vein			
H Hand Vein, Left *See G Hand Vein, Right*			
L Intracranial Vein Anterior cerebral vein Basal (internal) cerebral vein Dural venous sinus Great cerebral vein Inferior cerebellar vein Inferior cerebral vein Internal (basal) cerebral vein Middle cerebral vein Ophthalmic vein Superior cerebellar vein Superior cerebral vein			
M Internal Jugular Vein, Right			
N Internal Jugular Vein, Left			
P External Jugular Vein, Right Posterior auricular vein			
Q External Jugular Vein, Left *See P External Jugular Vein, Right*			
R Vertebral Vein, Right Deep cervical vein Suboccipital venous plexus			
S Vertebral Vein, Left *See R Vertebral Vein, Right*			
T Face Vein, Right Angular vein Anterior facial vein Common facial vein Deep facial vein Frontal vein Posterior facial (retromandibular) vein Supraorbital vein			
V Face Vein, Left *See T Face Vein, Right*			
Y Upper Vein			

Non-OR Procedure   DRG Non-OR Procedure   Valid OR Procedure   HAC Associated Procedure   Combination Only   New/Revised GREEN

Ø   **Medical and Surgical**
5   **Upper Veins**
P   **Removal**   Definition: Taking out or off a device from a body part

                  Explanation: If a device is taken out and a similar device put in without cutting or puncturing the skin or mucous membrane, the procedure is coded to the root operation CHANGE. Otherwise, the procedure for taking out a device is coded to the root operation REMOVAL.

Body Part Character 4	Approach Character 5	Device Character 6	Qualifier Character 7
Ø **Azygos Vein** Right ascending lumbar vein Right subcostal vein	**Ø** Open **3** Percutaneous **4** Percutaneous Endoscopic **X** External	**2** Monitoring Device **M** Neurostimulator Lead	**Z** No Qualifier
3 **Innominate Vein, Right** Brachiocephalic vein Inferior thyroid vein **4** **Innominate Vein, Left** *See 3 Innominate Vein, Right*	**Ø** Open **3** Percutaneous **4** Percutaneous Endoscopic **X** External	**M** Neurostimulator Lead	**Z** No Qualifier
Y **Upper Vein**	**Ø** Open **3** Percutaneous **4** Percutaneous Endoscopic	**Ø** Drainage Device **2** Monitoring Device **3** Infusion Device **7** Autologous Tissue Substitute **C** Extraluminal Device **D** Intraluminal Device **J** Synthetic Substitute **K** Nonautologous Tissue Substitute **Y** Other Device	**Z** No Qualifier
Y **Upper Vein**	**X** External	**Ø** Drainage Device **2** Monitoring Device **3** Infusion Device **D** Intraluminal Device	**Z** No Qualifier

Non-OR	05PØ[Ø,3,4,X]2Z
Non-OR	05PY3[Ø,2,3]Z
Non-OR	05PY[3,4]YZ
Non-OR	05PYX[Ø,2,3,D]Z

NC Noncovered Procedure   **LC** Limited Coverage   **QA** Questionable OB Admit   **NT** New Tech Add-on   **⊞** Combination Member   ♂ Male   ♀ Female

ICD-10-PCS 2022   **255**

Ø   Medical and Surgical
5   Upper Veins
Q   Repair   Definition: Restoring, to the extent possible, a body part to its normal anatomic structure and function
                      Explanation: Used only when the method to accomplish the repair is not one of the other root operations

Body Part Character 4	Approach Character 5	Device Character 6	Qualifier Character 7
Ø Azygos Vein Right ascending lumbar vein Right subcostal vein **1 Hemiazygos Vein** Left ascending lumbar vein Left subcostal vein **3 Innominate Vein, Right** Brachiocephalic vein Inferior thyroid vein **4 Innominate Vein, Left** *See 3 Innominate Vein, Right* **5 Subclavian Vein, Right** **6 Subclavian Vein, Left** **7 Axillary Vein, Right** **8 Axillary Vein, Left** **9 Brachial Vein, Right** Radial vein Ulnar vein **A Brachial Vein, Left** *See 9 Brachial Vein, Right* **B Basilic Vein, Right** Median antebrachial vein Median cubital vein **C Basilic Vein, Left** *See B Basilic Vein, Right* **D Cephalic Vein, Right** Accessory cephalic vein **F Cephalic Vein, Left** *See D Cephalic Vein, Right* **G Hand Vein, Right** Dorsal metacarpal vein Palmar (volar) digital vein Palmar (volar) metacarpal vein Superficial palmar venous arch Volar (palmar) digital vein Volar (palmar) metacarpal vein **H Hand Vein, Left** *See G Hand Vein, Right* **L Intracranial Vein** Anterior cerebral vein Basal (internal) cerebral vein Dural venous sinus Great cerebral vein Inferior cerebellar vein Inferior cerebral vein Internal (basal) cerebral vein Middle cerebral vein Ophthalmic vein Superior cerebellar vein Superior cerebral vein **M Internal Jugular Vein, Right** **N Internal Jugular Vein, Left** **P External Jugular Vein, Right** Posterior auricular vein **Q External Jugular Vein, Left** *See P External Jugular Vein, Right* **R Vertebral Vein, Right** Deep cervical vein Suboccipital venous plexus **S Vertebral Vein, Left** *See R Vertebral Vein, Right* **T Face Vein, Right** Angular vein Anterior facial vein Common facial vein Deep facial vein Frontal vein Posterior facial (retromandibular) vein Supraorbital vein **V Face Vein, Left** *See T Face Vein, Right* **Y Upper Vein**	**Ø Open** **3 Percutaneous** **4 Percutaneous Endoscopic**	**Z No Device**	**Z No Qualifier**

Ø   Medical and Surgical
5   Upper Veins
R   Replacement   Definition: Putting in or on biological or synthetic material that physically takes the place and/or function of all or a portion of a body part

Explanation: The body part may have been taken out or replaced, or may be taken out, physically eradicated, or rendered nonfunctional during the REPLACEMENT procedure. A REMOVAL procedure is coded for taking out the device used in a previous replacement procedure.

Body Part Character 4	Approach Character 5	Device Character 6	Qualifier Character 7
Ø Azygos Vein Right ascending lumbar vein Right subcostal vein **1 Hemiazygos Vein** Left ascending lumbar vein Left subcostal vein **3 Innominate Vein, Right** Brachiocephalic vein Inferior thyroid vein **4 Innominate Vein, Left** *See 3 Innominate Vein, Right* **5 Subclavian Vein, Right** **6 Subclavian Vein, Left** **7 Axillary Vein, Right** **8 Axillary Vein, Left** **9 Brachial Vein, Right** Radial vein Ulnar vein **A Brachial Vein, Left** *See 9 Brachial Vein, Right* **B Basilic Vein, Right** Median antebrachial vein Median cubital vein **C Basilic Vein, Left** *See B Basilic Vein, Right* **D Cephalic Vein, Right** Accessory cephalic vein **F Cephalic Vein, Left** *See D Cephalic Vein, Right* **G Hand Vein, Right** Dorsal metacarpal vein Palmar (volar) digital vein Palmar (volar) metacarpal vein Superficial palmar venous arch Volar (palmar) digital vein Volar (palmar) metacarpal vein **H Hand Vein, Left** *See G Hand Vein, Right* **L Intracranial Vein** Anterior cerebral vein Basal (internal) cerebral vein Dural venous sinus Great cerebral vein Inferior cerebellar vein Inferior cerebral vein Internal (basal) cerebral vein Middle cerebral vein Ophthalmic vein Superior cerebellar vein Superior cerebral vein **M Internal Jugular Vein, Right** **N Internal Jugular Vein, Left** **P External Jugular Vein, Right** Posterior auricular vein **Q External Jugular Vein, Left** *See P External Jugular Vein, Right* **R Vertebral Vein, Right** Deep cervical vein Suboccipital venous plexus **S Vertebral Vein, Left** *See R Vertebral Vein, Right* **T Face Vein, Right** Angular vein Anterior facial vein Common facial vein Deep facial vein Frontal vein Posterior facial (retromandibular) vein Supraorbital vein **V Face Vein, Left** *See T Face Vein, Right* **Y Upper Vein**	**Ø Open** **4 Percutaneous Endoscopic**	**7 Autologous Tissue Substitute** **J Synthetic Substitute** **K Nonautologous Tissue Substitute**	**Z No Qualifier**

NC Noncovered Procedure   **LC** Limited Coverage   **QA** Questionable OB Admit   **NT** New Tech Add-on   ⊞ Combination Member   ♂ Male   ♀ Female

ICD-10-PCS 2022   257

Ø5R–Ø5R

Ø   **Medical and Surgical**
5   **Upper Veins**
S   **Reposition**   Definition: Moving to its normal location, or other suitable location, all or a portion of a body part

Explanation: The body part is moved to a new location from an abnormal location, or from a normal location where it is not functioning correctly. The body part may or may not be cut out or off to be moved to the new location.

Body Part Character 4	Approach Character 5	Device Character 6	Qualifier Character 7

Ø **Azygos Vein**
    Right ascending lumbar vein
    Right subcostal vein
1 **Hemiazygos Vein**
    Left ascending lumbar vein
    Left subcostal vein
3 **Innominate Vein, Right**
    Brachiocephalic vein
    Inferior thyroid vein
4 **Innominate Vein, Left**
    See 3 Innominate Vein, Right
5 **Subclavian Vein, Right**
6 **Subclavian Vein, Left**
7 **Axillary Vein, Right**
8 **Axillary Vein, Left**
9 **Brachial Vein, Right**
    Radial vein
    Ulnar vein
A **Brachial Vein, Left**
    See 9 Brachial Vein, Right
B **Basilic Vein, Right**
    Median antebrachial vein
    Median cubital vein
C **Basilic Vein, Left**
    See B Basilic Vein, Right
D **Cephalic Vein, Right**
    Accessory cephalic vein
F **Cephalic Vein, Left**
    See D Cephalic Vein, Right
G **Hand Vein, Right**
    Dorsal metacarpal vein
    Palmar (volar) digital vein
    Palmar (volar) metacarpal vein
    Superficial palmar venous arch
    Volar (palmar) digital vein
    Volar (palmar) metacarpal vein
H **Hand Vein, Left**
    See G Hand Vein, Right
L **Intracranial Vein**
    Anterior cerebral vein
    Basal (internal) cerebral vein
    Dural venous sinus
    Great cerebral vein
    Inferior cerebellar vein
    Inferior cerebral vein
    Internal (basal) cerebral vein
    Middle cerebral vein
    Ophthalmic vein
    Superior cerebellar vein
    Superior cerebral vein
M **Internal Jugular Vein, Right**
N **Internal Jugular Vein, Left**
P **External Jugular Vein, Right**
    Posterior auricular vein
Q **External Jugular Vein, Left**
    See P External Jugular Vein, Right
R **Vertebral Vein, Right**
    Deep cervical vein
    Suboccipital venous plexus
S **Vertebral Vein, Left**
    See R Vertebral Vein, Right
T **Face Vein, Right**
    Angular vein
    Anterior facial vein
    Common facial vein
    Deep facial vein
    Frontal vein
    Posterior facial (retromandibular) vein
    Supraorbital vein
V **Face Vein, Left**
    See T Face Vein, Right
Y **Upper Vein**
	Ø Open
	3 Percutaneous
	4 Percutaneous Endoscopic
		Z No Device	**Z** No Qualifier

Ø   Medical and Surgical
5   Upper Veins
U   Supplement   Definition: Putting in or on biological or synthetic material that physically reinforces and/or augments the function of a portion of a body part
                    Explanation: The biological material is non-living, or is living and from the same individual. The body part may have been previously replaced, and the SUPPLEMENT procedure is performed to physically reinforce and/or augment the function of the replaced body part.

Body Part Character 4	Approach Character 5	Device Character 6	Qualifier Character 7
Ø Azygos Vein Right ascending lumbar vein Right subcostal vein	**Ø** Open **3** Percutaneous **4** Percutaneous Endoscopic	**7** Autologous Tissue Substitute **J** Synthetic Substitute **K** Nonautologous Tissue Substitute	**Z** No Qualifier
1 Hemiazygos Vein Left ascending lumbar vein Left subcostal vein			
3 Innominate Vein, Right Brachiocephalic vein Inferior thyroid vein			
4 Innominate Vein, Left *See 3 Innominate Vein, Right*			
5 Subclavian Vein, Right			
6 Subclavian Vein, Left			
7 Axillary Vein, Right			
8 Axillary Vein, Left			
9 Brachial Vein, Right Radial vein Ulnar vein			
A Brachial Vein, Left *See 9 Brachial Vein, Right*			
B Basilic Vein, Right Median antebrachial vein Median cubital vein			
C Basilic Vein, Left *See B Basilic Vein, Right*			
D Cephalic Vein, Right Accessory cephalic vein			
F Cephalic Vein, Left *See D Cephalic Vein, Right*			
G Hand Vein, Right Dorsal metacarpal vein Palmar (volar) digital vein Palmar (volar) metacarpal vein Superficial palmar venous arch Volar (palmar) digital vein Volar (palmar) metacarpal vein			
H Hand Vein, Left *See G Hand Vein, Right*			
L Intracranial Vein Anterior cerebral vein Basal (internal) cerebral vein Dural venous sinus Great cerebral vein Inferior cerebellar vein Inferior cerebral vein Internal (basal) cerebral vein Middle cerebral vein Ophthalmic vein Superior cerebellar vein Superior cerebral vein			
M Internal Jugular Vein, Right			
N Internal Jugular Vein, Left			
P External Jugular Vein, Right Posterior auricular vein			
Q External Jugular Vein, Left *See P External Jugular Vein, Right*			
R Vertebral Vein, Right Deep cervical vein Suboccipital venous plexus			
S Vertebral Vein, Left *See R Vertebral Vein, Right*			
T Face Vein, Right Angular vein Anterior facial vein Common facial vein Deep facial vein Frontal vein Posterior facial (retromandibular) vein Supraorbital vein			
V Face Vein, Left *See T Face Vein, Right*			
Y Upper Vein			

NC Noncovered Procedure   LC Limited Coverage   QA Questionable OB Admit   NT New Tech Add-on   ✛ Combination Member   ♂ Male   ♀ Female

ICD-10-PCS 2022   259

Ø5U–Ø5U

Ø Medical and Surgical
5 Upper Veins
V Restriction   Definition: Partially closing an orifice or the lumen of a tubular body part
                           Explanation: The orifice can be a natural orifice or an artificially created orifice

Body Part Character 4	Approach Character 5	Device Character 6	Qualifier Character 7
Ø Azygos Vein Right ascending lumbar vein Right subcostal vein	**Ø Open** **3 Percutaneous** **4 Percutaneous Endoscopic**	**C Extraluminal Device** **D Intraluminal Device** **Z No Device**	**Z No Qualifier**
1 Hemiazygos Vein Left ascending lumbar vein Left subcostal vein			
3 Innominate Vein, Right Brachiocephalic vein Inferior thyroid vein			
4 Innominate Vein, Left *See 3 Innominate Vein, Right*			
5 Subclavian Vein, Right			
6 Subclavian Vein, Left			
7 Axillary Vein, Right			
8 Axillary Vein, Left			
9 Brachial Vein, Right Radial vein Ulnar vein			
A Brachial Vein, Left *See 9 Brachial Vein, Right*			
B Basilic Vein, Right Median antebrachial vein Median cubital vein			
C Basilic Vein, Left *See B Basilic Vein, Right*			
D Cephalic Vein, Right Accessory cephalic vein			
F Cephalic Vein, Left *See D Cephalic Vein, Right*			
G Hand Vein, Right Dorsal metacarpal vein Palmar (volar) digital vein Palmar (volar) metacarpal vein Superficial palmar venous arch Volar (palmar) digital vein Volar (palmar) metacarpal vein			
H Hand Vein, Left *See G Hand Vein, Right*			
L Intracranial Vein Anterior cerebral vein Basal (internal) cerebral vein Dural venous sinus Great cerebral vein Inferior cerebellar vein Inferior cerebral vein Internal (basal) cerebral vein Middle cerebral vein Ophthalmic vein Superior cerebellar vein Superior cerebral vein			
M Internal Jugular Vein, Right			
N Internal Jugular Vein, Left			
P External Jugular Vein, Right Posterior auricular vein			
Q External Jugular Vein, Left *See P External Jugular Vein, Right*			
R Vertebral Vein, Right Deep cervical vein Suboccipital venous plexus			
S Vertebral Vein, Left *See R Vertebral Vein, Right*			
T Face Vein, Right Angular vein Anterior facial vein Common facial vein Deep facial vein Frontal vein Posterior facial (retromandibular) vein Supraorbital vein			
V Face Vein, Left *See T Face Vein, Right*			
Y Upper Vein			

Ø   Medical and Surgical
5   Upper Veins
W   Revision   Definition: Correcting, to the extent possible, a portion of a malfunctioning device or the position of a displaced device
                       Explanation: Revision can include correcting a malfunctioning or displaced device by taking out or putting in components of the device such as a screw or pin

Body Part Character 4	Approach Character 5	Device Character 6	Qualifier Character 7
Ø Azygos Vein Right ascending lumbar vein Right subcostal vein	**Ø** Open **3** Percutaneous **4** Percutaneous Endoscopic **X** External	**2** Monitoring Device **M** Neurostimulator Lead	**Z** No Qualifier
3 Innominate Vein, Right Brachiocephalic vein Inferior thyroid vein **4 Innominate Vein, Left** *See 3 Innominate Vein, Right*	**Ø** Open **3** Percutaneous **4** Percutaneous Endoscopic **X** External	**M** Neurostimulator Lead	**Z** No Qualifier
Y Upper Vein	**Ø** Open **3** Percutaneous **4** Percutaneous Endoscopic	**Ø** Drainage Device **2** Monitoring Device **3** Infusion Device **7** Autologous Tissue Substitute **C** Extraluminal Device **D** Intraluminal Device **J** Synthetic Substitute **K** Nonautologous Tissue Substitute **Y** Other Device	**Z** No Qualifier
Y Upper Vein	**X** External	**Ø** Drainage Device **2** Monitoring Device **3** Infusion Device **7** Autologous Tissue Substitute **C** Extraluminal Device **D** Intraluminal Device **J** Synthetic Substitute **K** Nonautologous Tissue Substitute	**Z** No Qualifier

Non-OR	Ø5WØXMZ
Non-OR	Ø5W[3,4]XMZ
Non-OR	Ø5WY3[Ø,2,3,D]Z
Non-OR	Ø5WY[3,4]YZ
Non-OR	Ø5WYX[Ø,2,3,7,C,D,J,K]Z

Lower Veins Ø61–Ø6W

Character Meanings

This Character Meaning table is provided as a guide to assist the user in the identification of character members that may be found in this section of code tables. It **SHOULD NOT** be used to build a PCS code.

Operation–Character 3		Body Part–Character 4		Approach–Character 5		Device–Character 6		Qualifier–Character 7	
1	Bypass	Ø	Inferior Vena Cava	Ø	Open	Ø	Drainage Device	Ø	Ultrasonic
5	Destruction	1	Splenic Vein	3	Percutaneous	2	Monitoring Device	4	Hepatic Vein
7	Dilation	2	Gastric Vein	4	Percutaneous Endoscopic	3	Infusion Device	5	Superior Mesenteric Vein
9	Drainage	3	Esophageal Vein	7	Via Natural or Artificial Opening	7	Autologous Tissue Substitute	6	Inferior Mesenteric Vein
B	Excision	4	Hepatic Vein	8	Via Natural or Artificial Opening Endoscopic	9	Autologous Venous Tissue	9	Renal Vein, Right
C	Extirpation	5	Superior Mesenteric Vein	X	External	A	Autologous Arterial Tissue	B	Renal Vein, Left
D	Extraction	6	Inferior Mesenteric Vein			C	Extraluminal Device	C	Hemorrhoidal Plexus
F	Fragmentation	7	Colic Vein			D	Intraluminal Device	P	Pulmonary Trunk
H	Insertion	8	Portal Vein			J	Synthetic Substitute	Q	Pulmonary Artery, Right
J	Inspection	9	Renal Vein, Right			K	Nonautologous Tissue Substitute	R	Pulmonary Artery, Left
L	Occlusion	B	Renal Vein, Left			Y	Other Device	T	Via Umbilical Vein
N	Release	C	Common Iliac Vein, Right			Z	No Device	X	Diagnostic
P	Removal	D	Common Iliac Vein, Left					Y	Lower Vein
Q	Repair	F	External Iliac Vein, Right					Z	No Qualifier
R	Replacement	G	External Iliac Vein, Left						
S	Reposition	H	Hypogastric Vein, Right						
U	Supplement	J	Hypogastric Vein, Left						
V	Restriction	M	Femoral Vein, Right						
W	Revision	N	Femoral Vein, Left						
		P	Saphenous Vein, Right						
		Q	Saphenous Vein, Left						
		T	Foot Vein, Right						
		V	Foot Vein, Left						
		Y	Lower Vein						

AHA Coding Clinic for table Ø61
2017, 4Q, 36-38   Fontan completion procedure
2017, 4Q, 66-67   New qualifier values - Portal to hepatic shunt

AHA Coding Clinic for table Ø6B
2020, 1Q, 28   Free flap microvascular breast reconstruction
2017, 3Q, 5   Femoral artery to posterior tibial artery bypass using autologous and synthetic grafts
2017, 1Q, 31   Left to right common carotid artery bypass
2017, 1Q, 32   Peroneal artery to dorsalis pedis artery bypass using saphenous vein graft
2016, 3Q, 31   Femoral to peroneal artery bypass with in-situ saphenous vein graft and lysis of valves
2016, 2Q, 18   Femoral-tibial artery bypass and saphenous vein graft
2016, 1Q, 27   Aortocoronary bypass graft utilizing Y-graft
2014, 3Q, 8   Excision of saphenous vein for coronary artery bypass graft
2014, 3Q, 20   MAZE procedure performed with coronary artery bypass graft
2014, 1Q, 10   Repair of thoracic aortic aneurysm & coronary artery bypass graft

AHA Coding Clinic for table Ø6F
2020, 4Q, 45-49   New fragmentation tables
2020, 4Q, 49-50   Intravascular ultrasound assisted thrombolysis
2020, 4Q, 50   Intravascular lithotripsy

AHA Coding Clinic for table Ø6H
2017, 3Q, 11   Placement of peripherally inserted central catheter using 3CG ECG technology
2017, 1Q, 31   Umbilical vein catheterization
2017, 1Q, 31   Central catheter placement in femoral vein
2013, 3Q, 18   Heart transplant surgery

AHA Coding Clinic for table Ø6L
2020, 3Q, 44   Cardiophrenic vein embolization
2019, 4Q, 28   Transorifice occlusion of gastric varices
2018, 2Q, 18   Transverse rectus abdominis myocutaneous (TRAM) delay
2017, 4Q, 57-58   Added approach values - Transorifice esophageal vein banding
2013, 4Q, 112   Endoscopic banding of esophageal varices

AHA Coding Clinic for table Ø6V
2018, 3Q, 11   Transvenous transcatheter placement of valve in inferior vena cava
2018, 1Q, 10   Revision of transjugular intrahepatic portosystemic shunt

AHA Coding Clinic for table Ø6W
2019, 2Q, 39   Transjugular intrahepatic portosystemic shunt revision
2018, 1Q, 10   Revision of transjugular intrahepatic portosystemic shunt
2014, 3Q, 25   Revision of transjugular intrahepatic portosystemic shunt (TIPS)

Lower Veins

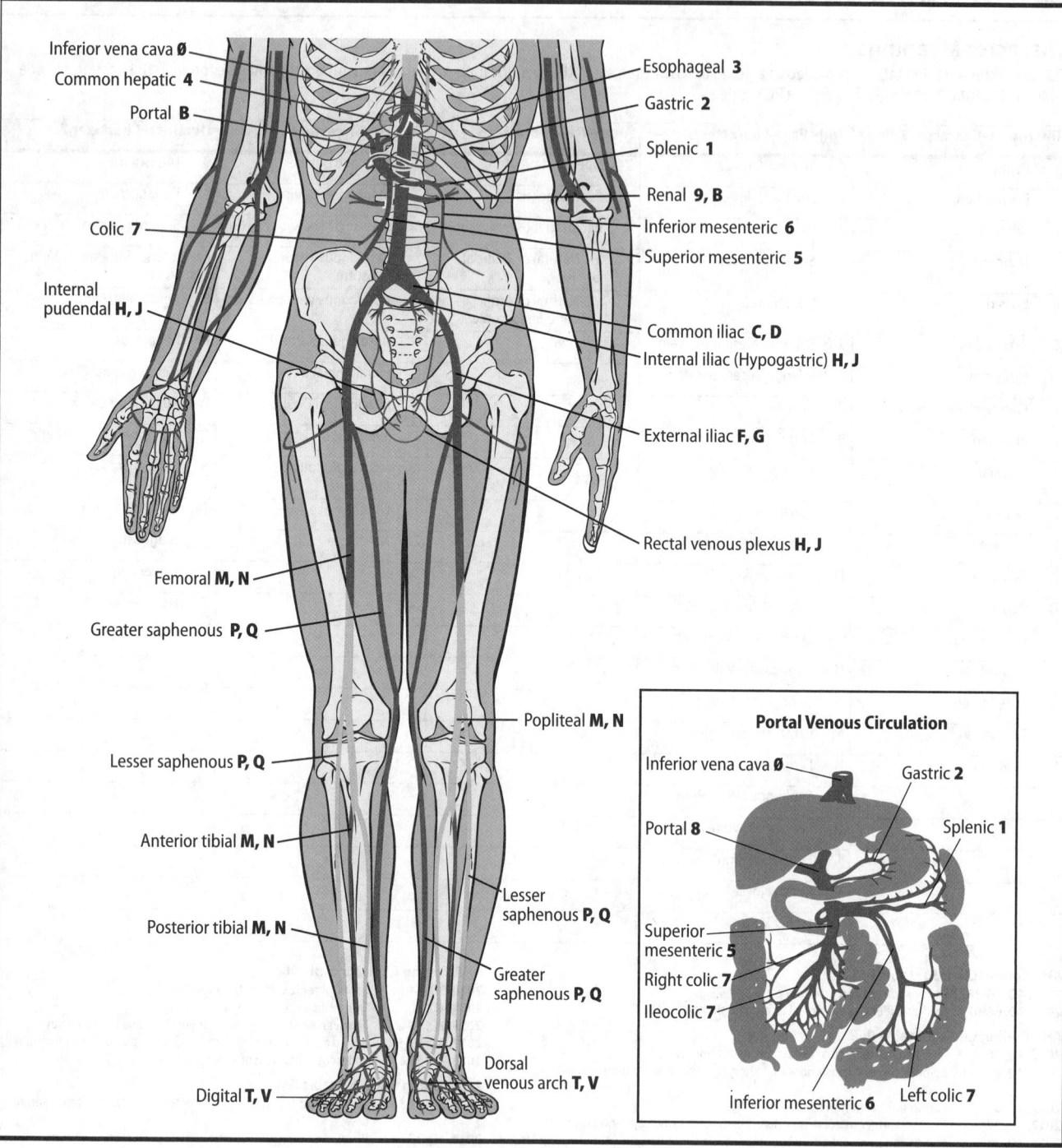

Inferior vena cava **Ø**
Common hepatic **4**
Portal **B**

Colic **7**

Internal
pudendal **H, J**

Femoral **M, N**

Greater saphenous **P, Q**

Lesser saphenous **P, Q**

Anterior tibial **M, N**

Posterior tibial **M, N**

Digital **T, V**

Esophageal **3**
Gastric **2**
Splenic **1**

Renal **9, B**
Inferior mesenteric **6**
Superior mesenteric **5**

Common iliac **C, D**
Internal iliac (Hypogastric) **H, J**

External iliac **F, G**

Rectal venous plexus **H, J**

Popliteal **M, N**

Lesser
saphenous **P, Q**

Greater
saphenous **P, Q**

Dorsal
venous arch **T, V**

Portal Venous Circulation

Inferior vena cava **Ø**
Portal **8**

Superior
mesenteric **5**
Right colic **7**
Ileocolic **7**

Gastric **2**
Splenic **1**

Inferior mesenteric **6**   Left colic **7**

0 Medical and Surgical
6 Lower Veins
1 Bypass Definition: Altering the route of passage of the contents of a tubular body part

Explanation: Rerouting contents of a body part to a downstream area of the normal route, to a similar route and body part, or to an abnormal route and dissimilar body part. Includes one or more anastomoses, with or without the use of a device.

Body Part Character 4		Approach Character 5	Device Character 6	Qualifier Character 7
0 Inferior Vena Cava Postcava Right inferior phrenic vein Right ovarian vein Right second lumbar vein Right suprarenal vein Right testicular vein		**0 Open** **4 Percutaneous Endoscopic**	**7 Autologous Tissue Substitute** **9 Autologous Venous Tissue** **A Autologous Arterial Tissue** **J Synthetic Substitute** **K Nonautologous Tissue Substitute** **Z No Device**	**5 Superior Mesenteric Vein** **6 Inferior Mesenteric Vein** **P Pulmonary Trunk** **Q Pulmonary Artery, Right** **R Pulmonary Artery, Left** **Y Lower Vein**
1 Splenic Vein Left gastroepiploic vein Pancreatic vein		**0 Open** **4 Percutaneous Endoscopic**	**7 Autologous Tissue Substitute** **9 Autologous Venous Tissue** **A Autologous Arterial Tissue** **J Synthetic Substitute** **K Nonautologous Tissue Substitute** **Z No Device**	**9 Renal Vein, Right** **B Renal Vein, Left** **Y Lower Vein**
2 Gastric Vein **3 Esophageal Vein** **4 Hepatic Vein** **5 Superior Mesenteric Vein** Right gastroepiploic vein **6 Inferior Mesenteric Vein** Sigmoid vein Superior rectal vein **7 Colic Vein** Ileocolic vein Left colic vein Middle colic vein Right colic vein **9 Renal Vein, Right** **B Renal Vein, Left** Left inferior phrenic vein Left ovarian vein Left second lumbar vein Left suprarenal vein Left testicular vein **C Common Iliac Vein, Right** **D Common Iliac Vein, Left** **F External Iliac Vein, Right** **G External Iliac Vein, Left** **H Hypogastric Vein, Right** Gluteal vein Internal iliac vein Internal pudendal vein Lateral sacral vein Middle hemorrhoidal vein Obturator vein Uterine vein Vaginal vein Vesical vein	**J Hypogastric Vein, Left** *See H Hypogastric Vein, Right* **M Femoral Vein, Right** Deep femoral (profunda femoris) vein Popliteal vein Profunda femoris (deep femoral) vein **N Femoral Vein, Left** *See M Femoral Vein, Right* **P Saphenous Vein, Right** External pudendal vein Great(er) saphenous vein Lesser saphenous vein Small saphenous vein Superficial circumflex iliac vein Superficial epigastric vein **Q Saphenous Vein, Left** *See P Saphenous Vein, Right* **T Foot Vein, Right** Common digital vein Dorsal metatarsal vein Dorsal venous arch Plantar digital vein Plantar metatarsal vein Plantar venous arch **V Foot Vein, Left** *See T Foot Vein, Right*	**0 Open** **4 Percutaneous Endoscopic**	**7 Autologous Tissue Substitute** **9 Autologous Venous Tissue** **A Autologous Arterial Tissue** **J Synthetic Substitute** **K Nonautologous Tissue Substitute** **Z No Device**	**Y Lower Vein**
8 Portal Vein Hepatic portal vein		**0 Open**	**7 Autologous Tissue Substitute** **9 Autologous Venous Tissue** **A Autologous Arterial Tissue** **J Synthetic Substitute** **K Nonautologous Tissue Substitute** **Z No Device**	**9 Renal Vein, Right** **B Renal Vein, Left** **Y Lower Vein**
8 Portal Vein Hepatic portal vein		**3 Percutaneous**	**J Synthetic Substitute**	**4 Hepatic Vein** **Y Lower Vein**
8 Portal Vein Hepatic portal vein		**4 Percutaneous Endoscopic**	**7 Autologous Tissue Substitute** **9 Autologous Venous Tissue** **A Autologous Arterial Tissue** **K Nonautologous Tissue Substitute** **Z No Device**	**9 Renal Vein, Right** **B Renal Vein, Left** **Y Lower Vein**
8 Portal Vein Hepatic portal vein		**4 Percutaneous Endoscopic**	**J Synthetic Substitute**	**4 Hepatic Vein** **9 Renal Vein, Right** **B Renal Vein, Left** **Y Lower Vein**

NC Noncovered Procedure   LC Limited Coverage   QA Questionable OB Admit   NT New Tech Add-on   ⊞ Combination Member   ♂ Male   ♀ Female

ICD-10-PCS 2022   265

061–061

Ø   **Medical and Surgical**
6   **Lower Veins**
5   **Destruction**   Definition: Physical eradication of all or a portion of a body part by the direct use of energy, force, or a destructive agent
                         Explanation: None of the body part is physically taken out

Body Part Character 4	Approach Character 5	Device Character 6	Qualifier Character 7
Ø **Inferior Vena Cava** Postcava Right inferior phrenic vein Right ovarian vein Right second lumbar vein Right suprarenal vein Right testicular vein	**Ø** Open **3** Percutaneous **4** Percutaneous Endoscopic	**Z** No Device	**Z** No Qualifier
1 **Splenic Vein** Left gastroepiploic vein Pancreatic vein			
2 **Gastric Vein**			
3 **Esophageal Vein**			
4 **Hepatic Vein**			
5 **Superior Mesenteric Vein** Right gastroepiploic vein			
6 **Inferior Mesenteric Vein** Sigmoid vein Superior rectal vein			
7 **Colic Vein** Ileocolic vein Left colic vein Middle colic vein Right colic vein			
8 **Portal Vein** Hepatic portal vein			
9 **Renal Vein, Right**			
B **Renal Vein, Left** Left inferior phrenic vein Left ovarian vein Left second lumbar vein Left suprarenal vein Left testicular vein			
C **Common Iliac Vein, Right**			
D **Common Iliac Vein, Left**			
F **External Iliac Vein, Right**			
G **External Iliac Vein, Left**			
H **Hypogastric Vein, Right** Gluteal vein Internal iliac vein Internal pudendal vein Lateral sacral vein Middle hemorrhoidal vein Obturator vein Uterine vein Vaginal vein Vesical vein			
J **Hypogastric Vein, Left** *See H Hypogastric Vein, Right*			
M **Femoral Vein, Right** Deep femoral (profunda femoris) vein Popliteal vein Profunda femoris (deep femoral) vein			
N **Femoral Vein, Left** *See M Femoral Vein, Right*			
P **Saphenous Vein, Right** External pudendal vein Great(er) saphenous vein Lesser saphenous vein Small saphenous vein Superficial circumflex iliac vein Superficial epigastric vein			
Q **Saphenous Vein, Left** *See P Saphenous Vein, Right*			
T **Foot Vein, Right** Common digital vein Dorsal metatarsal vein Dorsal venous arch Plantar digital vein Plantar metatarsal vein Plantar venous arch			
V **Foot Vein, Left** *See T Foot Vein, Right*			
Y **Lower Vein**	**Ø** Open **3** Percutaneous **4** Percutaneous Endoscopic	**Z** No Device	**C** Hemorrhoidal Plexus **Z** No Qualifier

Ø　**Medical and Surgical**
6　**Lower Veins**
7　**Dilation**　　　Definition: Expanding an orifice or the lumen of a tubular body part

Explanation: The orifice can be a natural orifice or an artificially created orifice. Accomplished by stretching a tubular body part using intraluminal pressure or by cutting part of the orifice or wall of the tubular body part.

Body Part Character 4	Approach Character 5	Device Character 6	Qualifier Character 7
Ø Inferior Vena Cava 　Postcava 　Right inferior phrenic vein 　Right ovarian vein 　Right second lumbar vein 　Right suprarenal vein 　Right testicular vein **1 Splenic Vein** 　Left gastroepiploic vein 　Pancreatic vein **2 Gastric Vein** **3 Esophageal Vein** **4 Hepatic Vein** **5 Superior Mesenteric Vein** 　Right gastroepiploic vein **6 Inferior Mesenteric Vein** 　Sigmoid vein 　Superior rectal vein **7 Colic Vein** 　Ileocolic vein 　Left colic vein 　Middle colic vein 　Right colic vein **8 Portal Vein** 　Hepatic portal vein **9 Renal Vein, Right** **B Renal Vein, Left** 　Left inferior phrenic vein 　Left ovarian vein 　Left second lumbar vein 　Left suprarenal vein 　Left testicular vein **C Common Iliac Vein, Right** **D Common Iliac Vein, Left** **F External Iliac Vein, Right** **G External Iliac Vein, Left** **H Hypogastric Vein, Right** 　Gluteal vein 　Internal iliac vein 　Internal pudendal vein 　Lateral sacral vein 　Middle hemorrhoidal vein 　Obturator vein 　Uterine vein 　Vaginal vein 　Vesical vein **J Hypogastric Vein, Left** 　*See H Hypogastric Vein, Right* **M Femoral Vein, Right** 　Deep femoral (profunda femoris) vein 　Popliteal vein 　Profunda femoris (deep femoral) vein **N Femoral Vein, Left** 　*See M Femoral Vein, Right* **P Saphenous Vein, Right** 　External pudendal vein 　Great(er) saphenous vein 　Lesser saphenous vein 　Small saphenous vein 　Superficial circumflex iliac vein 　Superficial epigastric vein **Q Saphenous Vein, Left** 　*See P Saphenous Vein, Right* **T Foot Vein, Right** 　Common digital vein 　Dorsal metatarsal vein 　Dorsal venous arch 　Plantar digital vein 　Plantar metatarsal vein 　Plantar venous arch **V Foot Vein, Left** 　*See T Foot Vein, Right* **Y Lower Vein**	**Ø Open** **3 Percutaneous** **4 Percutaneous Endoscopic**	**D Intraluminal Device** **Z No Device**	**Z No Qualifier**

NC Noncovered Procedure　　LC Limited Coverage　　QA Questionable OB Admit　　NT New Tech Add-on　　⊞ Combination Member　　♂ Male　　♀ Female

ICD-10-PCS 2022

267

Ø67–Ø67

Ø Medical and Surgical
6 Lower Veins
9 Drainage Definition: Taking or letting out fluids and/or gases from a body part
Explanation: The qualifier DIAGNOSTIC is used to identify drainage procedures that are biopsies

Body Part Character 4	Approach Character 5	Device Character 6	Qualifier Character 7
Ø Inferior Vena Cava Postcava Right inferior phrenic vein Right ovarian vein Right second lumbar vein Right suprarenal vein Right testicular vein 1 Splenic Vein Left gastroepiploic vein Pancreatic vein 2 Gastric Vein 3 Esophageal Vein 4 Hepatic Vein 5 Superior Mesenteric Vein Right gastroepiploic vein 6 Inferior Mesenteric Vein Sigmoid vein Superior rectal vein 7 Colic Vein Ileocolic vein Left colic vein Middle colic vein Right colic vein 8 Portal Vein Hepatic portal vein 9 Renal Vein, Right B Renal Vein, Left Left inferior phrenic vein Left ovarian vein Left second lumbar vein Left suprarenal vein Left testicular vein C Common Iliac Vein, Right D Common Iliac Vein, Left F External Iliac Vein, Right G External Iliac Vein, Left H Hypogastric Vein, Right Gluteal vein Internal iliac vein Internal pudendal vein Lateral sacral vein Middle hemorrhoidal vein Obturator vein Uterine vein Vaginal vein Vesical vein J Hypogastric Vein, Left *See H Hypogastric Vein, Right* M Femoral Vein, Right Deep femoral (profunda femoris) vein Popliteal vein Profunda femoris (deep femoral) vein N Femoral Vein, Left *See M Femoral Vein, Right* P Saphenous Vein, Right External pudendal vein Great(er) saphenous vein Lesser saphenous vein Small saphenous vein Superficial circumflex iliac vein Superficial epigastric vein Q Saphenous Vein, Left *See P Saphenous Vein, Right* T Foot Vein, Right Common digital vein Dorsal metatarsal vein Dorsal venous arch Plantar digital vein Plantar metatarsal vein Plantar venous arch V Foot Vein, Left *See T Foot Vein, Right* Y Lower Vein	Ø Open 3 Percutaneous 4 Percutaneous Endoscopic	Ø Drainage Device	Z No Qualifier

Non-OR Ø69[Ø,1,2,4,5,6,7,8,9,B,C,D,F,G,H,J,M,N,P,Q,T,V,Y][Ø,3,4]ØZ
Non-OR Ø6933ØZ

Ø69 Continued on next page

Ø   **Medical and Surgical**   *Ø69 Continued*
6   **Lower Veins**
9   **Drainage**   Definition: Taking or letting out fluids and/or gases from a body part
                           Explanation: The qualifier DIAGNOSTIC is used to identify drainage procedures that are biopsies

Body Part Character 4	Approach Character 5	Device Character 6	Qualifier Character 7

Ø **Inferior Vena Cava**
   Postcava
   Right inferior phrenic vein
   Right ovarian vein
   Right second lumbar vein
   Right suprarenal vein
   Right testicular vein
	Ø Open
	3 Percutaneous
	4 Percutaneous Endoscopic
		Z No Device	**X** Diagnostic
			Z No Qualifier

1 **Splenic Vein**
   Left gastroepiploic vein
   Pancreatic vein			

2 **Gastric Vein**			
3 **Esophageal Vein**			
4 **Hepatic Vein**			
5 **Superior Mesenteric Vein** Right gastroepiploic vein			

6 **Inferior Mesenteric Vein**
   Sigmoid vein
   Superior rectal vein			

7 **Colic Vein**
   Ileocolic vein
   Left colic vein
   Middle colic vein
   Right colic vein			

8 **Portal Vein** Hepatic portal vein			
9 **Renal Vein, Right**			

B **Renal Vein, Left**
   Left inferior phrenic vein
   Left ovarian vein
   Left second lumbar vein
   Left suprarenal vein
   Left testicular vein			

C **Common Iliac Vein, Right**			
D **Common Iliac Vein, Left**			
F **External Iliac Vein, Right**			
G **External Iliac Vein, Left**			

H **Hypogastric Vein, Right**
   Gluteal vein
   Internal iliac vein
   Internal pudendal vein
   Lateral sacral vein
   Middle hemorrhoidal vein
   Obturator vein
   Uterine vein
   Vaginal vein
   Vesical vein			

J **Hypogastric Vein, Left** *See H Hypogastric Vein, Right*			

M **Femoral Vein, Right**
   Deep femoral (profunda femoris) vein
   Popliteal vein
   Profunda femoris (deep femoral) vein			

N **Femoral Vein, Left** *See M Femoral Vein, Right*			

P **Saphenous Vein, Right**
   External pudendal vein
   Great(er) saphenous vein
   Lesser saphenous vein
   Small saphenous vein
   Superficial circumflex iliac vein
   Superficial epigastric vein			

Q **Saphenous Vein, Left** *See P Saphenous Vein, Right*			

T **Foot Vein, Right**
   Common digital vein
   Dorsal metatarsal vein
   Dorsal venous arch
   Plantar digital vein
   Plantar metatarsal vein
   Plantar venous arch			

V **Foot Vein, Left** *See T Foot Vein, Right*			
Y **Lower Vein**			

Non-OR   Ø69[Ø,1,2,3,4,5,6,7,8,9,B,C,D,F,G,H,J,M,N,P,Q,T,V,Y]3ZX
Non-OR   Ø69[Ø,1,2,4,5,6,7,8,9,B,C,D,F,G,H,J,M,N,P,Q,T,V,Y][Ø,3,4]ZZ
Non-OR   Ø6933ZZ

NC Noncovered Procedure   LC Limited Coverage   QA Questionable OB Admit   NT New Tech Add-on   ⊞ Combination Member   ♂ Male   ♀ Female

Lower Veins

0 Medical and Surgical
6 Lower Veins
B Excision   Definition: Cutting out or off, without replacement, a portion of a body part
                  Explanation: The qualifier DIAGNOSTIC is used to identify excision procedures that are biopsies

Body Part Character 4	Approach Character 5	Device Character 6	Qualifier Character 7

0 Inferior Vena Cava
   Postcava
   Right inferior phrenic vein
   Right ovarian vein
   Right second lumbar vein
   Right suprarenal vein
   Right testicular vein
1 Splenic Vein
   Left gastroepiploic vein
   Pancreatic vein
2 Gastric Vein
3 Esophageal Vein
4 Hepatic Vein
5 Superior Mesenteric Vein
   Right gastroepiploic vein
6 Inferior Mesenteric Vein
   Sigmoid vein
   Superior rectal vein
7 Colic Vein
   Ileocolic vein
   Left colic vein
   Middle colic vein
   Right colic vein
8 Portal Vein
   Hepatic portal vein
9 Renal Vein, Right
B Renal Vein, Left
   Left inferior phrenic vein
   Left ovarian vein
   Left second lumbar vein
   Left suprarenal vein
   Left testicular vein
C Common Iliac Vein, Right
D Common Iliac Vein, Left
F External Iliac Vein, Right
G External Iliac Vein, Left
H Hypogastric Vein, Right
   Gluteal vein
   Internal iliac vein
   Internal pudendal vein
   Lateral sacral vein
   Middle hemorrhoidal vein
   Obturator vein
   Uterine vein
   Vaginal vein
   Vesical vein
J Hypogastric Vein, Left
   See H Hypogastric Vein, Right
M Femoral Vein, Right
   Deep femoral (profunda femoris) vein
   Popliteal vein
   Profunda femoris (deep femoral) vein
N Femoral Vein, Left
   See M Femoral Vein, Right
P Saphenous Vein, Right
   External pudendal vein
   Great(er) saphenous vein
   Lesser saphenous vein
   Small saphenous vein
   Superficial circumflex iliac vein
   Superficial epigastric vein
Q Saphenous Vein, Left
   See P Saphenous Vein, Right
T Foot Vein, Right
   Common digital vein
   Dorsal metatarsal vein
   Dorsal venous arch
   Plantar digital vein
   Plantar metatarsal vein
   Plantar venous arch
V Foot Vein, Left
   See T Foot Vein, Right
	0 Open
	3 Percutaneous
	4 Percutaneous Endoscopic
		Z No Device	**X** Diagnostic
			Z No Qualifier

Y Lower Vein	**0** Open **3** Percutaneous **4** Percutaneous Endoscopic	**Z** No Device	**C** Hemorrhoidal Plexus **X** Diagnostic **Z** No Qualifier

Ø   **Medical and Surgical**
6   **Lower Veins**
C   **Extirpation**   Definition: Taking or cutting out solid matter from a body part

Explanation: The solid matter may be an abnormal byproduct of a biological function or a foreign body; it may be imbedded in a body part or in the lumen of a tubular body part. The solid matter may or may not have been previously broken into pieces.

Body Part Character 4	Approach Character 5	Device Character 6	Qualifier Character 7

Ø **Inferior Vena Cava**
   Postcava
   Right inferior phrenic vein
   Right ovarian vein
   Right second lumbar vein
   Right suprarenal vein
   Right testicular vein
	Ø Open
	3 Percutaneous
	4 Percutaneous Endoscopic
		Z No Device	**Z** No Qualifier

1 **Splenic Vein**
   Left gastroepiploic vein
   Pancreatic vein			

2 **Gastric Vein**			
3 **Esophageal Vein**			
4 **Hepatic Vein**			
5 **Superior Mesenteric Vein** Right gastroepiploic vein			

6 **Inferior Mesenteric Vein**
   Sigmoid vein
   Superior rectal vein			

7 **Colic Vein**
   Ileocolic vein
   Left colic vein
   Middle colic vein
   Right colic vein			

8 **Portal Vein** Hepatic portal vein			
9 **Renal Vein, Right**			

B **Renal Vein, Left**
   Left inferior phrenic vein
   Left ovarian vein
   Left second lumbar vein
   Left suprarenal vein
   Left testicular vein			

C **Common Iliac Vein, Right**			
D **Common Iliac Vein, Left**			
F **External Iliac Vein, Right**			
G **External Iliac Vein, Left**			

H **Hypogastric Vein, Right**
   Gluteal vein
   Internal iliac vein
   Internal pudendal vein
   Lateral sacral vein
   Middle hemorrhoidal vein
   Obturator vein
   Uterine vein
   Vaginal vein
   Vesical vein			

J **Hypogastric Vein, Left** *See H Hypogastric Vein, Right*			

M **Femoral Vein, Right**
   Deep femoral (profunda femoris) vein
   Popliteal vein
   Profunda femoris (deep femoral) vein			

N **Femoral Vein, Left** *See M Femoral Vein, Right*			

P **Saphenous Vein, Right**
   External pudendal vein
   Great(er) saphenous vein
   Lesser saphenous vein
   Small saphenous vein
   Superficial circumflex iliac vein
   Superficial epigastric vein			

Q **Saphenous Vein, Left** *See P Saphenous Vein, Right*			

T **Foot Vein, Right**
   Common digital vein
   Dorsal metatarsal vein
   Dorsal venous arch
   Plantar digital vein
   Plantar metatarsal vein
   Plantar venous arch			

V **Foot Vein, Left** *See T Foot Vein, Right*			
Y **Lower Vein**			

NC Noncovered Procedure   LC Limited Coverage   QA Questionable OB Admit   NT New Tech Add-on   ⊞ Combination Member   ♂ Male   ♀ Female

Ø   Medical and Surgical
6   Lower Veins
D   Extraction   Definition: Pulling or stripping out or off all or a portion of a body part by the use of force
                       Explanation: The qualifier DIAGNOSTIC is used to identify extraction procedures that are biopsies

Body Part Character 4	Approach Character 5	Device Character 6	Qualifier Character 7

M Femoral Vein, Right
  Deep femoral (profunda femoris) vein
  Popliteal vein
  Profunda femoris (deep femoral) vein
N Femoral Vein, Left
  See M Femoral Vein, Right
P Saphenous Vein, Right
  External pudendal vein
  Great(er) saphenous vein
  Lesser saphenous vein
  Small saphenous vein
  Superficial circumflex iliac vein
  Superficial epigastric vein
Q Saphenous Vein, Left
  See P Saphenous Vein, Right
T Foot Vein, Right
  Common digital vein
  Dorsal metatarsal vein
  Dorsal venous arch
  Plantar digital vein
  Plantar metatarsal vein
  Plantar venous arch
V Foot Vein, Left
  See T Foot Vein, Right
Y Lower Vein
	Ø Open
	3 Percutaneous
	4 Percutaneous Endoscopic
		Z No Device	**Z** No Qualifier

Ø   Medical and Surgical
6   Lower Veins
F   Fragmentation   Definition: Breaking solid matter in a body part into pieces
                          Explanation: Physical force (e.g., manual, ultrasonic) applied directly or indirectly is used to break the solid matter into pieces. The solid matter may be an abnormal byproduct of a biological function or a foreign body. The pieces of solid matter are not taken out.

Body Part Character 4	Approach Character 5	Device Character 6	Qualifier Character 7

C Common Iliac Vein, Right
D Common Iliac Vein, Left
F External Iliac Vein, Right
G External Iliac Vein, Left
H Hypogastric Vein, Right
  Gluteal vein
  Internal iliac vein
  Internal pudendal vein
  Lateral sacral vein
  Middle hemorrhoidal vein
  Obturator vein
  Uterine vein
  Vaginal vein
  Vesical vein
J Hypogastric Vein, Left
  See H Hypogastric Vein, Right
M Femoral Vein, Right
  Deep femoral (profunda femoris) vein
  Popliteal vein
  Profunda femoris (deep femoral) vein
N Femoral Vein, Left
  See M Femoral Vein, Right
P Saphenous Vein, Right
  External pudendal vein
  Great(er) saphenous vein
  Lesser saphenous vein
  Small saphenous vein
  Superficial circumflex iliac vein
  Superficial epigastric vein
Q Saphenous Vein, Left
  See P Saphenous Vein, Right
Y Lower Vein
	3 Percutaneous	**Z** No Device	**Ø** Ultrasonic
			Z No Qualifier

Non-OR Procedure   DRG Non-OR Procedure   Valid OR Procedure   HAC Associated Procedure   Combination Only   New/Revised GREEN
272   ICD-10-PCS 2022

Ø6D–Ø6F

Ø   Medical and Surgical
6   Lower Veins
H   Insertion   Definition: Putting in a nonbiological appliance that monitors, assists, performs, or prevents a physiological function but does not physically take the place of a body part
             Explanation: None

Body Part Character 4		Approach Character 5	Device Character 6	Qualifier Character 7

Ø   Inferior Vena Cava
   Postcava
   Right inferior phrenic vein
   Right ovarian vein
   Right second lumbar vein
   Right suprarenal vein
   Right testicular vein
		Ø Open
		3 Percutaneous
			3 Infusion Device	**T Via Umbilical Vein**
				Z No Qualifier

Ø   Inferior Vena Cava
   Postcava
   Right inferior phrenic vein
   Right ovarian vein
   Right second lumbar vein
   Right suprarenal vein
   Right testicular vein
		Ø Open
		3 Percutaneous
			D Intraluminal Device	**Z No Qualifier**

Ø   Inferior Vena Cava
   Postcava
   Right inferior phrenic vein
   Right ovarian vein
   Right second lumbar vein
   Right suprarenal vein
   Right testicular vein
		4 Percutaneous Endoscopic	**3 Infusion Device**
			D Intraluminal Device
				Z No Qualifier

1   Splenic Vein
   Left gastroepiploic vein
   Pancreatic vein
2   Gastric Vein
3   Esophageal Vein
4   Hepatic Vein
5   Superior Mesenteric Vein
   Right gastroepiploic vein
6   Inferior Mesenteric Vein
   Sigmoid vein
   Superior rectal vein
7   Colic Vein
   Ileocolic vein
   Left colic vein
   Middle colic vein
   Right colic vein
8   Portal Vein
   Hepatic portal vein
9   Renal Vein, Right
B   Renal Vein, Left
   Left inferior phrenic vein
   Left ovarian vein
   Left second lumbar vein
   Left suprarenal vein
   Left testicular vein
C   Common Iliac Vein, Right
D   Common Iliac Vein, Left
F   External Iliac Vein, Right
G   External Iliac Vein, Left
	H Hypogastric Vein, Right
	   Gluteal vein
	   Internal iliac vein
	   Internal pudendal vein
	   Lateral sacral vein
	   Middle hemorrhoidal vein
	   Obturator vein
	   Uterine vein
	   Vaginal vein
	   Vesical vein
	J Hypogastric Vein, Left
	   See H Hypogastric Vein, Right
	M Femoral Vein, Right
	   Deep femoral (profunda femoris) vein
	   Popliteal vein
	   Profunda femoris (deep femoral) vein
	N Femoral Vein, Left
	   See M Femoral Vein, Right
	P Saphenous Vein, Right
	   External pudendal vein
	   Great(er) saphenous vein
	   Lesser saphenous vein
	   Small saphenous vein
	   Superficial circumflex iliac vein
	   Superficial epigastric vein
	Q Saphenous Vein, Left
	   See P Saphenous Vein, Right
	T Foot Vein, Right
	   Common digital vein
	   Dorsal metatarsal vein
	   Dorsal venous arch
	   Plantar digital vein
	   Plantar metatarsal vein
	   Plantar venous arch
	V Foot Vein, Left
	   See T Foot Vein, Right
		Ø Open
		3 Percutaneous
		4 Percutaneous Endoscopic
			3 Infusion Device
			D Intraluminal Device
				Z No Qualifier

Y Lower Vein		**Ø Open** **3 Percutaneous** **4 Percutaneous Endoscopic**	**2 Monitoring Device** **3 Infusion Device** **D Intraluminal Device** **Y Other Device**	**Z No Qualifier**

Non-OR	06HØ[Ø,3]3[T,Z]
Non-OR	06HØ3DZ
Non-OR	06HØ43Z
Non-OR	06H[1,2,3,4,5,6,7,8,9,B,C,D,F,G,H,J,M,N,P,Q,T,V][Ø,3,4]3Z
Non-OR	06HY[Ø,3,4]3Z
Non-OR	06HY32Z
Non-OR	06HY[3,4]YZ

NC Noncovered Procedure   **LC** Limited Coverage   **QA** Questionable OB Admit   **NT** New Tech Add-on   ✛ Combination Member   ♂ Male   ♀ Female

ICD-10-PCS 2022   273

06H–06H

0 Medical and Surgical
6 Lower Veins
J Inspection   Definition: Visually and/or manually exploring a body part

Explanation: Visual exploration may be performed with or without optical instrumentation. Manual exploration may be performed directly or through intervening body layers.

Body Part Character 4	Approach Character 5	Device Character 6	Qualifier Character 7
Y Lower Vein	0 Open 3 Percutaneous 4 Percutaneous Endoscopic X External	Z No Device	Z No Qualifier

Non-OR   06JY[3,X]ZZ

---

0 Medical and Surgical
6 Lower Veins
L Occlusion   Definition: Completely closing an orifice or the lumen of a tubular body part

Explanation: The orifice can be a natural orifice or an artificially created orifice

Body Part Character 4	Approach Character 5	Device Character 6	Qualifier Character 7

0 Inferior Vena Cava
  Postcava
  Right inferior phrenic vein
  Right ovarian vein
  Right second lumbar vein
  Right suprarenal vein
  Right testicular vein
1 Splenic Vein
  Left gastroepiploic vein
  Pancreatic vein
4 Hepatic Vein
5 Superior Mesenteric Vein
  Right gastroepiploic vein
6 Inferior Mesenteric Vein
  Sigmoid vein
  Superior rectal vein
7 Colic Vein
  Ileocolic vein
  Left colic vein
  Middle colic vein
  Right colic vein
8 Portal Vein
  Hepatic portal vein
9 Renal Vein, Right
B Renal Vein, Left
  Left inferior phrenic vein
  Left ovarian vein
  Left second lumbar vein
  Left suprarenal vein
  Left testicular vein
C Common Iliac Vein, Right
D Common Iliac Vein, Left
F External Iliac Vein, Right
G External Iliac Vein, Left
	H Hypogastric Vein, Right
	  Gluteal vein
	  Internal iliac vein
	  Internal pudendal vein
	  Lateral sacral vein
	  Middle hemorrhoidal vein
	  Obturator vein
	  Uterine vein
	  Vaginal vein
	  Vesical vein
	J Hypogastric Vein, Left
	  See H Hypogastric Vein, Right
	M Femoral Vein, Right
	  Deep femoral (profunda femoris) vein
	  Popliteal vein
	  Profunda femoris (deep femoral) vein
	N Femoral Vein, Left
	  See M Femoral Vein, Right
	P Saphenous Vein, Right
	  External pudendal vein
	  Great(er) saphenous vein
	  Lesser saphenous vein
	  Small saphenous vein
	  Superficial circumflex iliac vein
	  Superficial epigastric vein
	Q Saphenous Vein, Left
	  See P Saphenous Vein, Right
	T Foot Vein, Right
	  Common digital vein
	  Dorsal metatarsal vein
	  Dorsal venous arch
	  Plantar digital vein
	  Plantar metatarsal vein
	  Plantar venous arch
	V Foot Vein, Left
	  See T Foot Vein, Right
		0 Open
		3 Percutaneous
		4 Percutaneous Endoscopic
			C Extraluminal Device
			D Intraluminal Device
			Z No Device
				Z No Qualifier

2 Gastric Vein 3 Esophageal Vein		0 Open 3 Percutaneous 4 Percutaneous Endoscopic 7 Via Natural or Artificial Opening 8 Via Natural or Artificial Opening Endoscopic	C Extraluminal Device D Intraluminal Device Z No Device	Z No Qualifier
Y Lower Vein		0 Open 3 Percutaneous 4 Percutaneous Endoscopic 7 Via Natural or Artificial Opening 8 Via Natural or Artificial Opening Endoscopic	C Extraluminal Device D Intraluminal Device Z No Device	C Hemorrhoidal Plexus Z No Qualifier

Non-OR   06L2[7,8][C,D,Z]Z
Non-OR   06L3[3,4,7,8][C,D,Z]Z

Ø Medical and Surgical
6 Lower Veins
N Release　　　Definition: Freeing a body part from an abnormal physical constraint by cutting or by the use of force

Explanation: Some of the restraining tissue may be taken out but none of the body part is taken out

Body Part Character 4		Approach Character 5	Device Character 6	Qualifier Character 7
Ø Inferior Vena Cava Postcava Right inferior phrenic vein Right ovarian vein Right second lumbar vein Right suprarenal vein Right testicular vein **1 Splenic Vein** Left gastroepiploic vein Pancreatic vein **2 Gastric Vein** **3 Esophageal Vein** **4 Hepatic Vein** **5 Superior Mesenteric Vein** Right gastroepiploic vein **6 Inferior Mesenteric Vein** Sigmoid vein Superior rectal vein **7 Colic Vein** Ileocolic vein Left colic vein Middle colic vein Right colic vein **8 Portal Vein** Hepatic portal vein **9 Renal Vein, Right** **B Renal Vein, Left** Left inferior phrenic vein Left ovarian vein Left second lumbar vein Left suprarenal vein Left testicular vein **C Common Iliac Vein, Right** **D Common Iliac Vein, Left** **F External Iliac Vein, Right** **G External Iliac Vein, Left**	**H Hypogastric Vein, Right** Gluteal vein Internal iliac vein Internal pudendal vein Lateral sacral vein Middle hemorrhoidal vein Obturator vein Uterine vein Vaginal vein Vesical vein **J Hypogastric Vein, Left** *See H Hypogastric Vein, Right* **M Femoral Vein, Right** Deep femoral (profunda femoris) vein Popliteal vein Profunda femoris (deep femoral) vein **N Femoral Vein, Left** *See M Femoral Vein, Right* **P Saphenous Vein, Right** External pudendal vein Great(er) saphenous vein Lesser saphenous vein Small saphenous vein Superficial circumflex iliac vein Superficial epigastric vein **Q Saphenous Vein, Left** *See P Saphenous Vein, Right* **T Foot Vein, Right** Common digital vein Dorsal metatarsal vein Dorsal venous arch Plantar digital vein Plantar metatarsal vein Plantar venous arch **V Foot Vein, Left** *See T Foot Vein, Right* **Y Lower Vein**	**Ø Open** **3 Percutaneous** **4 Percutaneous Endoscopic**	**Z No Device**	**Z No Qualifier**

Ø Medical and Surgical
6 Lower Veins
P Removal　　　Definition: Taking out or off a device from a body part

Explanation: If a device is taken out and a similar device put in without cutting or puncturing the skin or mucous membrane, the procedure is coded to the root operation CHANGE. Otherwise, the procedure for taking out a device is coded to the root operation REMOVAL.

Body Part Character 4	Approach Character 5	Device Character 6	Qualifier Character 7
Y Lower Vein	**Ø Open** **3 Percutaneous** **4 Percutaneous Endoscopic**	**Ø Drainage Device** **2 Monitoring Device** **3 Infusion Device** **7 Autologous Tissue Substitute** **C Extraluminal Device** **D Intraluminal Device** **J Synthetic Substitute** **K Nonautologous Tissue Substitute** **Y Other Device**	**Z No Qualifier**
Y Lower Vein	**X External**	**Ø Drainage Device** **2 Monitoring Device** **3 Infusion Device** **D Intraluminal Device**	**Z No Qualifier**

Non-OR	Ø6PY3[Ø,2,3]Z
Non-OR	Ø6PY[3,4]YZ
Non-OR	Ø6PYX[Ø,2,3,D]Z

NC Noncovered Procedure　　LC Limited Coverage　　QA Questionable OB Admit　　NT New Tech Add-on　　⊞ Combination Member　　♂ Male　　♀ Female

ICD-10-PCS 2022　　　　　　　　　　　　　　　　　　　　　　　　　　　　　　　　　　275

Ø Medical and Surgical
6 Lower Veins
Q Repair   Definition: Restoring, to the extent possible, a body part to its normal anatomic structure and function
                       Explanation: Used only when the method to accomplish the repair is not one of the other root operations

Body Part Character 4	Approach Character 5	Device Character 6	Qualifier Character 7
Ø Inferior Vena Cava Postcava Right inferior phrenic vein Right ovarian vein Right second lumbar vein Right suprarenal vein Right testicular vein	**Ø Open** **3 Percutaneous** **4 Percutaneous Endoscopic**	**Z No Device**	**Z No Qualifier**
1 Splenic Vein Left gastroepiploic vein Pancreatic vein			
2 Gastric Vein			
3 Esophageal Vein			
4 Hepatic Vein			
5 Superior Mesenteric Vein Right gastroepiploic vein			
6 Inferior Mesenteric Vein Sigmoid vein Superior rectal vein			
7 Colic Vein Ileocolic vein Left colic vein Middle colic vein Right colic vein			
8 Portal Vein Hepatic portal vein			
9 Renal Vein, Right			
B Renal Vein, Left Left inferior phrenic vein Left ovarian vein Left second lumbar vein Left suprarenal vein Left testicular vein			
C Common Iliac Vein, Right			
D Common Iliac Vein, Left			
F External Iliac Vein, Right			
G External Iliac Vein, Left			
H Hypogastric Vein, Right Gluteal vein Internal iliac vein Internal pudendal vein Lateral sacral vein Middle hemorrhoidal vein Obturator vein Uterine vein Vaginal vein Vesical vein			
J Hypogastric Vein, Left *See H Hypogastric Vein, Right*			
M Femoral Vein, Right Deep femoral (profunda femoris) vein Popliteal vein Profunda femoris (deep femoral) vein			
N Femoral Vein, Left *See M Femoral Vein, Right*			
P Saphenous Vein, Right External pudendal vein Great(er) saphenous vein Lesser saphenous vein Small saphenous vein Superficial circumflex iliac vein Superficial epigastric vein			
Q Saphenous Vein, Left *See P Saphenous Vein, Right*			
T Foot Vein, Right Common digital vein Dorsal metatarsal vein Dorsal venous arch Plantar digital vein Plantar metatarsal vein Plantar venous arch			
V Foot Vein, Left *See T Foot Vein, Right*			
Y Lower Vein			

Ø Medical and Surgical
6 Lower Veins
R Replacement   Definition: Putting in or on biological or synthetic material that physically takes the place and/or function of all or a portion of a body part

Explanation: The body part may have been taken out or replaced, or may be taken out, physically eradicated, or rendered nonfunctional during the REPLACEMENT procedure. A REMOVAL procedure is coded for taking out the device used in a previous replacement procedure.

Body Part Character 4	Approach Character 5	Device Character 6	Qualifier Character 7

Ø Inferior Vena Cava
   Postcava
   Right inferior phrenic vein
   Right ovarian vein
   Right second lumbar vein
   Right suprarenal vein
   Right testicular vein
	Ø Open
	4 Percutaneous Endoscopic
		7 Autologous Tissue Substitute
		J Synthetic Substitute
		K Nonautologous Tissue Substitute
			Z No Qualifier

1 Splenic Vein
   Left gastroepiploic vein
   Pancreatic vein			

2 Gastric Vein			
3 Esophageal Vein			
4 Hepatic Vein			
5 Superior Mesenteric Vein Right gastroepiploic vein			

6 Inferior Mesenteric Vein
   Sigmoid vein
   Superior rectal vein			

7 Colic Vein
   Ileocolic vein
   Left colic vein
   Middle colic vein
   Right colic vein			

8 Portal Vein Hepatic portal vein			
9 Renal Vein, Right			

B Renal Vein, Left
   Left inferior phrenic vein
   Left ovarian vein
   Left second lumbar vein
   Left suprarenal vein
   Left testicular vein			

C Common Iliac Vein, Right			
D Common Iliac Vein, Left			
F External Iliac Vein, Right			
G External Iliac Vein, Left			

H Hypogastric Vein, Right
   Gluteal vein
   Internal iliac vein
   Internal pudendal vein
   Lateral sacral vein
   Middle hemorrhoidal vein
   Obturator vein
   Uterine vein
   Vaginal vein
   Vesical vein			

J Hypogastric Vein, Left *See H Hypogastric Vein, Right*			

M Femoral Vein, Right
   Deep femoral (profunda femoris) vein
   Popliteal vein
   Profunda femoris (deep femoral) vein			

N Femoral Vein, Left *See M Femoral Vein, Right*			

P Saphenous Vein, Right
   External pudendal vein
   Great(er) saphenous vein
   Lesser saphenous vein
   Small saphenous vein
   Superficial circumflex iliac vein
   Superficial epigastric vein			

Q Saphenous Vein, Left *See P Saphenous Vein, Right*			

T Foot Vein, Right
   Common digital vein
   Dorsal metatarsal vein
   Dorsal venous arch
   Plantar digital vein
   Plantar metatarsal vein
   Plantar venous arch			

V Foot Vein, Left *See T Foot Vein, Right*			
Y Lower Vein			

☒ Noncovered Procedure   ☒ Limited Coverage   ☒ Questionable OB Admit   ☒ New Tech Add-on   ⊞ Combination Member   ♂ Male   ♀ Female

ICD-10-PCS 2022   277

06R–06R

Lower Veins *(side tab)*

0   **Medical and Surgical**
6   **Lower Veins**
S   **Reposition**   Definition: Moving to its normal location, or other suitable location, all or a portion of a body part

Explanation: The body part is moved to a new location from an abnormal location, or from a normal location where it is not functioning correctly. The body part may or may not be cut out or off to be moved to the new location.

Body Part Character 4	Approach Character 5	Device Character 6	Qualifier Character 7

0 **Inferior Vena Cava**
   Postcava
   Right inferior phrenic vein
   Right ovarian vein
   Right second lumbar vein
   Right suprarenal vein
   Right testicular vein
1 **Splenic Vein**
   Left gastroepiploic vein
   Pancreatic vein
2 **Gastric Vein**
3 **Esophageal Vein**
4 **Hepatic Vein**
5 **Superior Mesenteric Vein**
   Right gastroepiploic vein
6 **Inferior Mesenteric Vein**
   Sigmoid vein
   Superior rectal vein
7 **Colic Vein**
   Ileocolic vein
   Left colic vein
   Middle colic vein
   Right colic vein
8 **Portal Vein**
   Hepatic portal vein
9 **Renal Vein, Right**
B **Renal Vein, Left**
   Left inferior phrenic vein
   Left ovarian vein
   Left second lumbar vein
   Left suprarenal vein
   Left testicular vein
C **Common Iliac Vein, Right**
D **Common Iliac Vein, Left**
F **External Iliac Vein, Right**
G **External Iliac Vein, Left**
H **Hypogastric Vein, Right**
   Gluteal vein
   Internal iliac vein
   Internal pudendal vein
   Lateral sacral vein
   Middle hemorrhoidal vein
   Obturator vein
   Uterine vein
   Vaginal vein
   Vesical vein
J **Hypogastric Vein, Left**
   See H Hypogastric Vein, Right
M **Femoral Vein, Right**
   Deep femoral (profunda femoris) vein
   Popliteal vein
   Profunda femoris (deep femoral) vein
N **Femoral Vein, Left**
   See M Femoral Vein, Right
P **Saphenous Vein, Right**
   External pudendal vein
   Great(er) saphenous vein
   Lesser saphenous vein
   Small saphenous vein
   Superficial circumflex iliac vein
   Superficial epigastric vein
Q **Saphenous Vein, Left**
   See P Saphenous Vein, Right
T **Foot Vein, Right**
   Common digital vein
   Dorsal metatarsal vein
   Dorsal venous arch
   Plantar digital vein
   Plantar metatarsal vein
   Plantar venous arch
V **Foot Vein, Left**
   See T Foot Vein, Right
Y **Lower Vein**
	0 Open
	3 Percutaneous
	4 Percutaneous Endoscopic
		Z No Device	**Z** No Qualifier

Lower Veins

0   **Medical and Surgical**
6   **Lower Veins**
U   **Supplement**   Definition: Putting in or on biological or synthetic material that physically reinforces and/or augments the function of a portion of a body part
              Explanation: The biological material is non-living, or is living and from the same individual. The body part may have been previously replaced, and the SUPPLEMENT procedure is performed to physically reinforce and/or augment the function of the replaced body part.

Body Part Character 4	Approach Character 5	Device Character 6	Qualifier Character 7
0 **Inferior Vena Cava** Postcava Right inferior phrenic vein Right ovarian vein Right second lumbar vein Right suprarenal vein Right testicular vein	**0** Open **3** Percutaneous **4** Percutaneous Endoscopic	**7** Autologous Tissue Substitute **J** Synthetic Substitute **K** Nonautologous Tissue Substitute	**Z** No Qualifier
1 **Splenic Vein** Left gastroepiploic vein Pancreatic vein			
2 **Gastric Vein**			
3 **Esophageal Vein**			
4 **Hepatic Vein**			
5 **Superior Mesenteric Vein** Right gastroepiploic vein			
6 **Inferior Mesenteric Vein** Sigmoid vein Superior rectal vein			
7 **Colic Vein** Ileocolic vein Left colic vein Middle colic vein Right colic vein			
8 **Portal Vein** Hepatic portal vein			
9 **Renal Vein, Right**			
B **Renal Vein, Left** Left inferior phrenic vein Left ovarian vein Left second lumbar vein Left suprarenal vein Left testicular vein			
C **Common Iliac Vein, Right**			
D **Common Iliac Vein, Left**			
F **External Iliac Vein, Right**			
G **External Iliac Vein, Left**			
H **Hypogastric Vein, Right** Gluteal vein Internal iliac vein Internal pudendal vein Lateral sacral vein Middle hemorrhoidal vein Obturator vein Uterine vein Vaginal vein Vesical vein			
J **Hypogastric Vein, Left** *See H Hypogastric Vein, Right*			
M **Femoral Vein, Right** Deep femoral (profunda femoris) vein Popliteal vein Profunda femoris (deep femoral) vein			
N **Femoral Vein, Left** *See M Femoral Vein, Right*			
P **Saphenous Vein, Right** External pudendal vein Great(er) saphenous vein Lesser saphenous vein Small saphenous vein Superficial circumflex iliac vein Superficial epigastric vein			
Q **Saphenous Vein, Left** *See P Saphenous Vein, Right*			
T **Foot Vein, Right** Common digital vein Dorsal metatarsal vein Dorsal venous arch Plantar digital vein Plantar metatarsal vein Plantar venous arch			
V **Foot Vein, Left** *See T Foot Vein, Right*			
Y **Lower Vein**			

0   **Medical and Surgical**
6   **Lower Veins**
V   **Restriction**   Definition: Partially closing an orifice or the lumen of a tubular body part
                          Explanation: The orifice can be a natural orifice or an artificially created orifice

Body Part Character 4	Approach Character 5	Device Character 6	Qualifier Character 7

0   **Inferior Vena Cava**
    Postcava
    Right inferior phrenic vein
    Right ovarian vein
    Right second lumbar vein
    Right suprarenal vein
    Right testicular vein
1   **Splenic Vein**
    Left gastroepiploic vein
    Pancreatic vein
2   **Gastric Vein**
3   **Esophageal Vein**
4   **Hepatic Vein**
5   **Superior Mesenteric Vein**
    Right gastroepiploic vein
6   **Inferior Mesenteric Vein**
    Sigmoid vein
    Superior rectal vein
7   **Colic Vein**
    Ileocolic vein
    Left colic vein
    Middle colic vein
    Right colic vein
8   **Portal Vein**
    Hepatic portal vein
9   **Renal Vein, Right**
B   **Renal Vein, Left**
    Left inferior phrenic vein
    Left ovarian vein
    Left second lumbar vein
    Left suprarenal vein
    Left testicular vein
C   **Common Iliac Vein, Right**
D   **Common Iliac Vein, Left**
F   **External Iliac Vein, Right**
G   **External Iliac Vein, Left**
H   **Hypogastric Vein, Right**
    Gluteal vein
    Internal iliac vein
    Internal pudendal vein
    Lateral sacral vein
    Middle hemorrhoidal vein
    Obturator vein
    Uterine vein
    Vaginal vein
    Vesical vein
J   **Hypogastric Vein, Left**
    See H Hypogastric Vein, Right
M   **Femoral Vein, Right**
    Deep femoral (profunda femoris) vein
    Popliteal vein
    Profunda femoris (deep femoral) vein
N   **Femoral Vein, Left**
    See M Femoral Vein, Right
P   **Saphenous Vein, Right**
    External pudendal vein
    Great(er) saphenous vein
    Lesser saphenous vein
    Small saphenous vein
    Superficial circumflex iliac vein
    Superficial epigastric vein
Q   **Saphenous Vein, Left**
    See P Saphenous Vein, Right
T   **Foot Vein, Right**
    Common digital vein
    Dorsal metatarsal vein
    Dorsal venous arch
    Plantar digital vein
    Plantar metatarsal vein
    Plantar venous arch
V   **Foot Vein, Left**
    See T Foot Vein, Right
Y   **Lower Vein**
	0 Open
	3 Percutaneous
	4 Percutaneous Endoscopic
		C Extraluminal Device
		D Intraluminal Device
		Z No Device
			Z No Qualifier

Ø   Medical and Surgical
6   Lower Veins
W   Revision   Definition: Correcting, to the extent possible, a portion of a malfunctioning device or the position of a displaced device

Explanation: Revision can include correcting a malfunctioning or displaced device by taking out or putting in components of the device such as a screw or pin

Body Part Character 4	Approach Character 5	Device Character 6	Qualifier Character 7
Y Lower Vein	Ø Open 3 Percutaneous 4 Percutaneous Endoscopic	Ø Drainage Device 2 Monitoring Device 3 Infusion Device 7 Autologous Tissue Substitute C Extraluminal Device D Intraluminal Device J Synthetic Substitute K Nonautologous Tissue Substitute Y Other Device	Z No Qualifier
Y Lower Vein	X External	Ø Drainage Device 2 Monitoring Device 3 Infusion Device 7 Autologous Tissue Substitute C Extraluminal Device D Intraluminal Device J Synthetic Substitute K Nonautologous Tissue Substitute	Z No Qualifier

Non-OR	06WY3[Ø,2,3,D]Z
Non-OR	06WY[3,4]YZ
Non-OR	06WYX[Ø,2,3,7,C,D,J,K]Z

NC Noncovered Procedure   LC Limited Coverage   QA Questionable OB Admit   NT New Tech Add-on   ⊞ Combination Member   ♂ Male   ♀ Female

ICD-10-PCS 2022   281

Lymphatic and Hemic Systems Ø72–Ø7Y

Character Meanings*

This Character Meaning table is provided as a guide to assist the user in the identification of character members that may be found in this section of code tables. It **SHOULD NOT** be used to build a PCS code.

Operation–Character 3		Body Part–Character 4		Approach–Character 5		Device–Character 6		Qualifier–Character 7	
2	Change	Ø	Lymphatic, Head	Ø	Open	Ø	Drainage Device	Ø	Allogeneic
5	Destruction	1	Lymphatic, Right Neck	3	Percutaneous	1	Radioactive Element	1	Syngeneic
9	Drainage	2	Lymphatic, Left Neck	4	Percutaneous Endoscopic	3	Infusion Device	2	Zooplastic
B	Excision	3	Lymphatic, Right Upper Extremity	8	Via Natural or Artificial Opening Endoscopic	7	Autologous Tissue Substitute	X	Diagnostic
C	Extirpation	4	Lymphatic, Left Upper Extremity	X	External	C	Extraluminal Device	Z	No Qualifier
D	Extraction	5	Lymphatic, Right Axillary			D	Intraluminal Device		
H	Insertion	6	Lymphatic, Left Axillary			J	Synthetic Substitute		
J	Inspection	7	Lymphatic, Thorax			K	Nonautologous Tissue Substitute		
L	Occlusion	8	Lymphatic, Internal Mammary, Right			Y	Other Device		
N	Release	9	Lymphatic, Internal Mammary, Left			Z	No Device		
P	Removal	B	Lymphatic, Mesenteric						
Q	Repair	C	Lymphatic, Pelvis						
S	Reposition	D	Lymphatic, Aortic						
T	Resection	F	Lymphatic, Right Lower Extremity						
U	Supplement	G	Lymphatic, Left Lower Extremity						
V	Restriction	H	Lymphatic, Right Inguinal						
W	Revision	J	Lymphatic, Left Inguinal						
Y	Transplantation	K	Thoracic Duct						
		L	Cisterna Chyli						
		M	Thymus						
		N	Lymphatic						
		P	Spleen						
		Q	Bone Marrow, Sternum						
		R	Bone Marrow, Iliac						
		S	Bone Marrow, Vertebral						
		T	Bone Marrow						

* Includes lymph vessels and lymph nodes.

AHA Coding Clinic for table Ø79

2018, 4Q, 84	Fine needle aspiration biopsy of lymphatic tissue
2017, 1Q, 34	Lymphovenous bypass following mastectomy
2014, 1Q, 26	Transbronchial needle aspiration lymph node biopsy
2013, 4Q, 111	Transbronchial needle aspiration lymph node biopsy

AHA Coding Clinic for table Ø7B

2019, 1Q, 3-8	Whipple procedure
2018, 4Q, 84	Fine needle aspiration biopsy of lymphatic tissue
2018, 1Q, 22	Resection of lymph node chains
2016, 1Q, 30	Axillary lymph node resection with modified radical mastectomy
2014, 3Q, 10	Selective excision of paratracheal lymph nodes
2014, 1Q, 20	Fiducial marker placement
2014, 1Q, 26	Transbronchial endoscopic lymph node aspiration biopsy

AHA Coding Clinic for table Ø7D

2018, 4Q, 84	Fine needle aspiration biopsy of lymphatic tissue
2013, 4Q, 111	Root operation for bone marrow biopsy

AHA Coding Clinic for table Ø7H

2020, 4Q, 43-44	Insertion of radioactive element
2020, 4Q, 53	Bone marrow body part

AHA Coding Clinic for table Ø7Q

2017, 1Q, 34	Lymphovenous bypass following mastectomy

AHA Coding Clinic for table Ø7S

2019, 3Q, 29	Thymus transplant for T-Cell production

AHA Coding Clinic for table Ø7T

2018, 1Q, 22	Resection of lymph node chains
2016, 2Q, 12	Resection of malignant neoplasm of infratemporal fossa
2016, 1Q, 30	Axillary lymph node resection with modified radical mastectomy
2015, 4Q, 13	New Section X codes—New Technology procedures
2014, 3Q, 9	Radical resection of level I lymph nodes
2014, 3Q, 16	Repair of Tetralogy of Fallot

AHA Coding Clinic for table Ø7Y

2019, 3Q, 29	Thymus transplant for T-Cell production

Lymphatic System

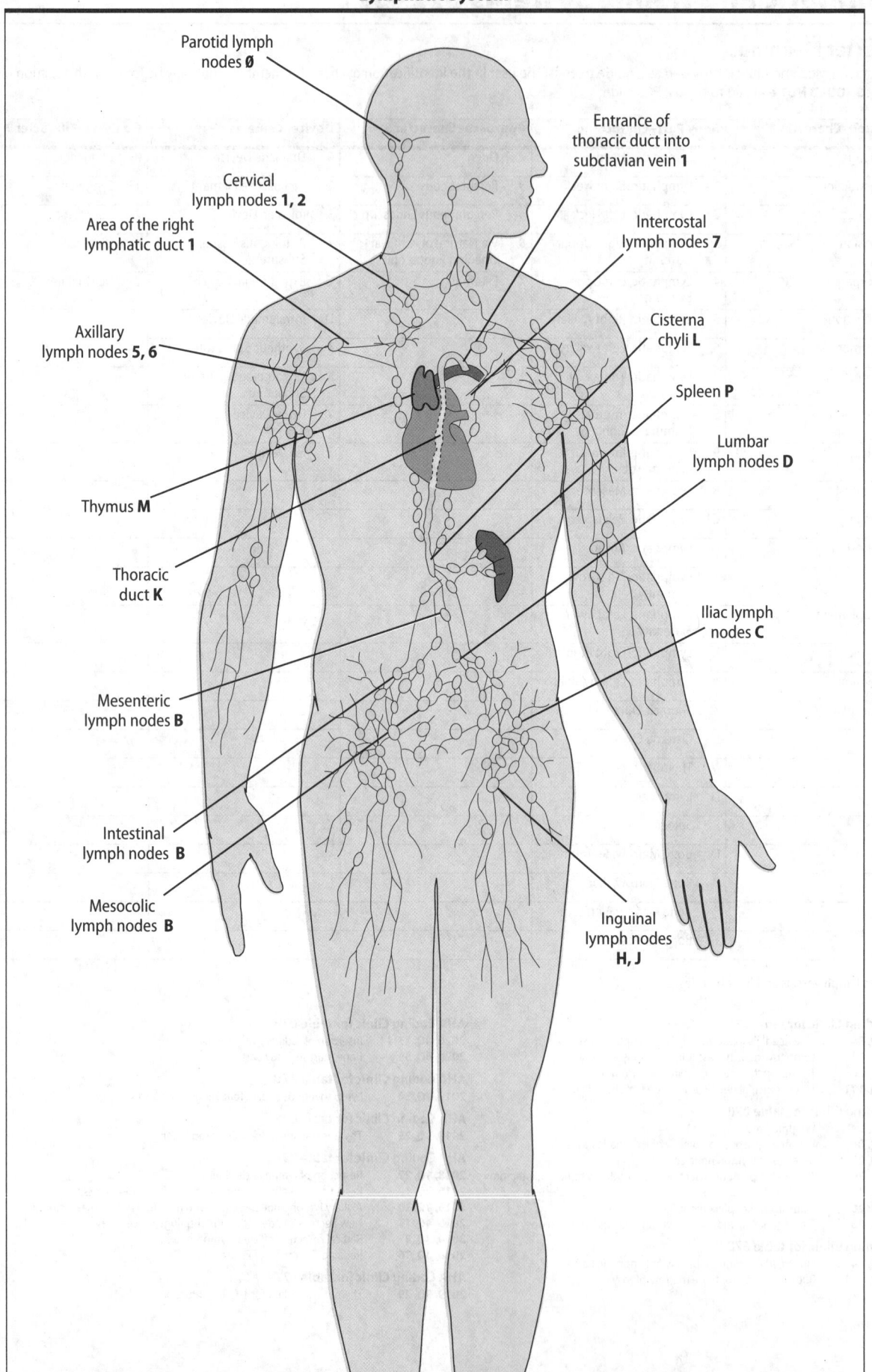

Parotid lymph nodes **Ø**

Entrance of thoracic duct into subclavian vein **1**

Cervical lymph nodes **1, 2**

Area of the right lymphatic duct **1**

Intercostal lymph nodes **7**

Axillary lymph nodes **5, 6**

Cisterna chyli **L**

Spleen **P**

Lumbar lymph nodes **D**

Thymus **M**

Thoracic duct **K**

Iliac lymph nodes **C**

Mesenteric lymph nodes **B**

Intestinal lymph nodes **B**

Mesocolic lymph nodes **B**

Inguinal lymph nodes **H, J**

Ø **Medical and Surgical**
7 **Lymphatic and Hemic Systems**
2 **Change**   Definition: Taking out or off a device from a body part and putting back an identical or similar device in or on the same body part without cutting or puncturing the skin or a mucous membrane

               Explanation: All CHANGE procedures are coded using the approach EXTERNAL

Body Part Character 4		Approach Character 5	Device Character 6	Qualifier Character 7

K **Thoracic Duct**
  Left jugular trunk
  Left subclavian trunk
L **Cisterna Chyli**
  Intestinal lymphatic trunk
  Lumbar lymphatic trunk
	M **Thymus**
	  Thymus gland
	N **Lymphatic**
	P **Spleen**
	  Accessory spleen
	T **Bone Marrow**
		X External	Ø Drainage Device
			Y Other Device
				Z No Qualifier

> **Non-OR**   All body part, approach, device, and qualifier values

Ø **Medical and Surgical**
7 **Lymphatic and Hemic Systems**
5 **Destruction**   Definition: Physical eradication of all or a portion of a body part by the direct use of energy, force, or a destructive agent

               Explanation: None of the body part is physically taken out

Body Part Character 4		Approach Character 5	Device Character 6	Qualifier Character 7

Ø **Lymphatic, Head**
  Buccinator lymph node
  Infraauricular lymph node
  Infraparotid lymph node
  Parotid lymph node
  Preauricular lymph node
  Submandibular lymph node
  Submaxillary lymph node
  Submental lymph node
  Subparotid lymph node
  Suprahyoid lymph node
1 **Lymphatic, Right Neck**
  Cervical lymph node
  Jugular lymph node
  Mastoid (postauricular) lymph node
  Occipital lymph node
  Postauricular (mastoid) lymph node
  Retropharyngeal lymph node
  Right jugular trunk
  Right lymphatic duct
  Right subclavian trunk
  Supraclavicular (Virchow's) lymph node
  Virchow's (supraclavicular) lymph node
2 **Lymphatic, Left Neck**
  Cervical lymph node
  Jugular lymph node
  Mastoid (postauricular) lymph node
  Occipital lymph node
  Postauricular (mastoid) lymph node
  Retropharyngeal lymph node
  Supraclavicular (Virchow's) lymph node
  Virchow's (supraclavicular) lymph node
3 **Lymphatic, Right Upper Extremity**
  Cubital lymph node
  Deltopectoral (infraclavicular) lymph
    node
  Epitrochlear lymph node
  Infraclavicular (deltopectoral) lymph
    node
  Supratrochlear lymph node
4 **Lymphatic, Left Upper Extremity**
  See 3 Lymphatic, Right Upper Extremity
5 **Lymphatic, Right Axillary**
  Anterior (pectoral) lymph node
  Apical (subclavicular) lymph node
  Brachial (lateral) lymph node
  Central axillary lymph node
  Lateral (brachial) lymph node
  Pectoral (anterior) lymph node
  Posterior (subscapular) lymph node
  Subclavicular (apical) lymph node
  Subscapular (posterior) lymph node
	6 **Lymphatic, Left Axillary**
	  See 5 Lymphatic, Right Axillary
	7 **Lymphatic, Thorax**
	  Intercostal lymph node
	  Mediastinal lymph node
	  Parasternal lymph node
	  Paratracheal lymph node
	  Tracheobronchial lymph node
	8 **Lymphatic, Internal Mammary, Right**
	9 **Lymphatic, Internal Mammary, Left**
	B **Lymphatic, Mesenteric**
	  Inferior mesenteric lymph node
	  Pararectal lymph node
	  Superior mesenteric lymph node
	C **Lymphatic, Pelvis**
	  Common iliac (subaortic) lymph node
	  Gluteal lymph node
	  Iliac lymph node
	  Inferior epigastric lymph node
	  Obturator lymph node
	  Sacral lymph node
	  Subaortic (common iliac) lymph node
	  Suprainguinal lymph node
	D **Lymphatic, Aortic**
	  Celiac lymph node
	  Gastric lymph node
	  Hepatic lymph node
	  Lumbar lymph node
	  Pancreaticosplenic lymph node
	  Paraaortic lymph node
	  Retroperitoneal lymph node
	F **Lymphatic, Right Lower Extremity**
	  Femoral lymph node
	  Popliteal lymph node
	G **Lymphatic, Left Lower Extremity**
	  See F Lymphatic, Right Lower Extremity
	H **Lymphatic, Right Inguinal**
	J **Lymphatic, Left Inguinal**
	K **Thoracic Duct**
	  Left jugular trunk
	  Left subclavian trunk
	L **Cisterna Chyli**
	  Intestinal lymphatic trunk
	  Lumbar lymphatic trunk
	M **Thymus**
	  Thymus gland
	P **Spleen**
	  Accessory spleen
		Ø Open
		3 Percutaneous
		4 Percutaneous
		   Endoscopic
			Z No Device	Z No Qualifier

Ø Medical and Surgical
7 Lymphatic and Hemic Systems
9 Drainage 　　Definition: Taking or letting out fluids and/or gases from a body part
　　　　　　　　　Explanation: The qualifier DIAGNOSTIC is used to identify drainage procedures that are biopsies

Body Part Character 4		Approach Character 5	Device Character 6	Qualifier Character 7
Ø Lymphatic, Head 　Buccinator lymph node 　Infraauricular lymph node 　Infraparotid lymph node 　Parotid lymph node 　Preauricular lymph node 　Submandibular lymph node 　Submaxillary lymph node 　Submental lymph node 　Subparotid lymph node 　Suprahyoid lymph node **1 Lymphatic, Right Neck** 　Cervical lymph node 　Jugular lymph node 　Mastoid (postauricular) lymph node 　Occipital lymph node 　Postauricular (mastoid) lymph node 　Retropharyngeal lymph node 　Right jugular trunk 　Right lymphatic duct 　Right subclavian trunk 　Supraclavicular (Virchow's) lymph 　　node 　Virchow's (supraclavicular) lymph 　　node **2 Lymphatic, Left Neck** 　Cervical lymph node 　Jugular lymph node 　Mastoid (postauricular) lymph node 　Occipital lymph node 　Postauricular (mastoid) lymph node 　Retropharyngeal lymph node 　Supraclavicular (Virchow's) lymph 　　node 　Virchow's (supraclavicular) lymph 　　node **3 Lymphatic, Right Upper Extremity** 　Cubital lymph node 　Deltopectoral (infraclavicular) lymph 　　node 　Epitrochlear lymph node 　Infraclavicular (deltopectoral) lymph 　　node 　Supratrochlear lymph node **4 Lymphatic, Left Upper Extremity** 　*See 3 Lymphatic, Right Upper Extremity* **5 Lymphatic, Right Axillary** 　Anterior (pectoral) lymph node 　Apical (subclavicular) lymph node 　Brachial (lateral) lymph node 　Central axillary lymph node 　Lateral (brachial) lymph node 　Pectoral (anterior) lymph node 　Posterior (subscapular) lymph node 　Subclavicular (apical) lymph node 　Subscapular (posterior) lymph node	**6 Lymphatic, Left Axillary** 　*See 5 Lymphatic, Right Axillary* **7 Lymphatic, Thorax** 　Intercostal lymph node 　Mediastinal lymph node 　Parasternal lymph node 　Paratracheal lymph node 　Tracheobronchial lymph node **8 Lymphatic, Internal Mammary, Right** **9 Lymphatic, Internal Mammary, Left** **B Lymphatic, Mesenteric** 　Inferior mesenteric lymph node 　Pararectal lymph node 　Superior mesenteric lymph node **C Lymphatic, Pelvis** 　Common iliac (subaortic) lymph node 　Gluteal lymph node 　Iliac lymph node 　Inferior epigastric lymph node 　Obturator lymph node 　Sacral lymph node 　Subaortic (common iliac) lymph node 　Suprainguinal lymph node **D Lymphatic, Aortic** 　Celiac lymph node 　Gastric lymph node 　Hepatic lymph node 　Lumbar lymph node 　Pancreaticosplenic lymph node 　Paraaortic lymph node 　Retroperitoneal lymph node **F Lymphatic, Right Lower Extremity** 　Femoral lymph node 　Popliteal lymph node **G Lymphatic, Left Lower Extremity** 　*See F Lymphatic, Right Lower Extremity* **H Lymphatic, Right Inguinal** **J Lymphatic, Left Inguinal** **K Thoracic Duct** 　Left jugular trunk 　Left subclavian trunk **L Cisterna Chyli** 　Intestinal lymphatic trunk 　Lumbar lymphatic trunk	**Ø Open** **3 Percutaneous** **4 Percutaneous 　Endoscopic** **8 Via Natural or 　Artificial Opening 　Endoscopic**	**Ø Drainage Device**	**Z No Qualifier**

Non-OR　　　Ø79[Ø,1,2,3,4,5,6,7,8,9,B,C,D,F,G,H,J,K,L][3,8]ØZ

Ø79 Continued on next page

Ø79 Continued

Ø   **Medical and Surgical**
7   **Lymphatic and Hemic Systems**
9   **Drainage**   Definition: Taking or letting out fluids and/or gases from a body part
               Explanation: The qualifier DIAGNOSTIC is used to identify drainage procedures that are biopsies

Body Part Character 4		Approach Character 5	Device Character 6	Qualifier Character 7

Ø   **Lymphatic, Head**
    Buccinator lymph node
    Infraauricular lymph node
    Infraparotid lymph node
    Parotid lymph node
    Preauricular lymph node
    Submandibular lymph node
    Submaxillary lymph node
    Submental lymph node
    Subparotid lymph node
    Suprahyoid lymph node
1   **Lymphatic, Right Neck**
    Cervical lymph node
    Jugular lymph node
    Mastoid (postauricular) lymph node
    Occipital lymph node
    Postauricular (mastoid) lymph node
    Retropharyngeal lymph node
    Right jugular trunk
    Right lymphatic duct
    Right subclavian trunk
    Supraclavicular (Virchow's) lymph
       node
    Virchow's (supraclavicular) lymph
       node
2   **Lymphatic, Left Neck**
    Cervical lymph node
    Jugular lymph node
    Mastoid (postauricular) lymph node
    Occipital lymph node
    Postauricular (mastoid) lymph node
    Retropharyngeal lymph node
    Supraclavicular (Virchow's) lymph
       node
    Virchow's (supraclavicular) lymph
       node
3   **Lymphatic, Right Upper Extremity**
    Cubital lymph node
    Deltopectoral (infraclavicular) lymph
       node
    Epitrochlear lymph node
    Infraclavicular (deltopectoral) lymph
       node
    Supratrochlear lymph node
4   **Lymphatic, Left Upper Extremity**
    See 3 Lymphatic, Right Upper Extremity
5   **Lymphatic, Right Axillary**
    Anterior (pectoral) lymph node
    Apical (subclavicular) lymph node
    Brachial (lateral) lymph node
    Central axillary lymph node
    Lateral (brachial) lymph node
    Pectoral (anterior) lymph node
    Posterior (subscapular) lymph node
    Subclavicular (apical) lymph node
    Subscapular (posterior) lymph node
	6 **Lymphatic, Left Axillary**
	    See 5 Lymphatic, Right Axillary
	7 **Lymphatic, Thorax**
	    Intercostal lymph node
	    Mediastinal lymph node
	    Parasternal lymph node
	    Paratracheal lymph node
	    Tracheobronchial lymph node
	8 **Lymphatic, Internal Mammary, Right**
	9 **Lymphatic, Internal Mammary, Left**
	B **Lymphatic, Mesenteric**
	    Inferior mesenteric lymph node
	    Pararectal lymph node
	    Superior mesenteric lymph node
	C **Lymphatic, Pelvis**
	    Common iliac (subaortic) lymph node
	    Gluteal lymph node
	    Iliac lymph node
	    Inferior epigastric lymph node
	    Obturator lymph node
	    Sacral lymph node
	    Subaortic (common iliac) lymph node
	    Suprainguinal lymph node
	D **Lymphatic, Aortic**
	    Celiac lymph node
	    Gastric lymph node
	    Hepatic lymph node
	    Lumbar lymph node
	    Pancreaticosplenic lymph node
	    Paraaortic lymph node
	    Retroperitoneal lymph node
	F **Lymphatic, Right Lower Extremity**
	    Femoral lymph node
	    Popliteal lymph node
	G **Lymphatic, Left Lower Extremity**
	    See F Lymphatic, Right Lower Extremity
	H **Lymphatic, Right Inguinal**
	J **Lymphatic, Left Inguinal**
	K **Thoracic Duct**
	    Left jugular trunk
	    Left subclavian trunk
	L **Cisterna Chyli**
	    Intestinal lymphatic trunk
	    Lumbar lymphatic trunk
		Ø Open
		3 Percutaneous
		4 Percutaneous
		    Endoscopic
		8 Via Natural or
		    Artificial Opening
		    Endoscopic
			Z No Device	**X** Diagnostic
				Z No Qualifier

M   **Thymus**
    Thymus gland
P   **Spleen**
    Accessory spleen
T   **Bone Marrow**
		Ø Open
		3 Percutaneous
		4 Percutaneous
		    Endoscopic
			Ø Drainage Device	**Z** No Qualifier

M   **Thymus**
    Thymus gland
P   **Spleen**
    Accessory spleen
T   **Bone Marrow**
		Ø Open
		3 Percutaneous
		4 Percutaneous
		    Endoscopic
			Z No Device	**X** Diagnostic
				Z No Qualifier

    Non-OR   Ø79[Ø,1,2,3,4,5,6,7,8,9,B,C,D,F,G,H,J,K,L]8ZX
    Non-OR   Ø79[Ø,1,2,3,4,5,6,7,8,9,B,C,D,F,G,H,J,K,L][3,8]ZZ
    Non-OR   Ø79M3ØZ
    Non-OR   Ø79P[3,4]ØZ
    Non-OR   Ø79T[Ø,3,4]ØZ
    Non-OR   Ø79M3ZZ
    Non-OR   Ø79P[3,4]Z[X,Z]
    Non-OR   Ø79T[Ø,3,4]Z[X,Z]

NC Noncovered Procedure   **LC** Limited Coverage   **QA** Questionable OB Admit   **NT** New Tech Add-on   ⊞ Combination Member   ♂ Male   ♀ Female

ICD-10-PCS 2022   287

Ø   Medical and Surgical
7   Lymphatic and Hemic Systems
B   Excision   Definition: Cutting out or off, without replacement, a portion of a body part
                          Explanation: The qualifier DIAGNOSTIC is used to identify excision procedures that are biopsies

Body Part Character 4		Approach Character 5	Device Character 6	Qualifier Character 7
Ø Lymphatic, Head Buccinator lymph node Infraauricular lymph node Infraparotid lymph node Parotid lymph node Preauricular lymph node Submandibular lymph node Submaxillary lymph node Submental lymph node Subparotid lymph node Suprahyoid lymph node **1 Lymphatic, Right Neck** Cervical lymph node Jugular lymph node Mastoid (postauricular) lymph node Occipital lymph node Postauricular (mastoid) lymph node Retropharyngeal lymph node Right jugular trunk Right lymphatic duct Right subclavian trunk Supraclavicular (Virchow's) lymph node Virchow's (supraclavicular) lymph node **2 Lymphatic, Left Neck** Cervical lymph node Jugular lymph node Mastoid (postauricular) lymph node Occipital lymph node Postauricular (mastoid) lymph node Retropharyngeal lymph node Supraclavicular (Virchow's) lymph node Virchow's (supraclavicular) lymph node **3 Lymphatic, Right Upper Extremity** Cubital lymph node Deltopectoral (infraclavicular) lymph node Epitrochlear lymph node Infraclavicular (deltopectoral) lymph node Supratrochlear lymph node **4 Lymphatic, Left Upper Extremity** See 3 Lymphatic, Right Upper Extremity **5 Lymphatic, Right Axillary** Anterior (pectoral) lymph node Apical (subclavicular) lymph node Brachial (lateral) lymph node Central axillary lymph node Lateral (brachial) lymph node Pectoral (anterior) lymph node Posterior (subscapular) lymph node Subclavicular (apical) lymph node Subscapular (posterior) lymph node	**6 Lymphatic, Left Axillary** See 5 Lymphatic, Right Axillary **7 Lymphatic, Thorax** Intercostal lymph node Mediastinal lymph node Parasternal lymph node Paratracheal lymph node Tracheobronchial lymph node **8 Lymphatic, Internal Mammary, Right** **9 Lymphatic, Internal Mammary, Left** **B Lymphatic, Mesenteric** Inferior mesenteric lymph node Pararectal lymph node Superior mesenteric lymph node **C Lymphatic, Pelvis** Common iliac (subaortic) lymph node Gluteal lymph node Iliac lymph node Inferior epigastric lymph node Obturator lymph node Sacral lymph node Subaortic (common iliac) lymph node Suprainguinal lymph node **D Lymphatic, Aortic** Celiac lymph node Gastric lymph node Hepatic lymph node Lumbar lymph node Pancreaticosplenic lymph node Paraaortic lymph node Retroperitoneal lymph node **F Lymphatic, Right Lower Extremity** Femoral lymph node Popliteal lymph node **G Lymphatic, Left Lower Extremity** See F Lymphatic, Right Lower Extremity **H Lymphatic, Right Inguinal** ⊞ **J Lymphatic, Left Inguinal** ⊞ **K Thoracic Duct** Left jugular trunk Left subclavian trunk **L Cisterna Chyli** Intestinal lymphatic trunk Lumbar lymphatic trunk **M Thymus** Thymus gland **P Spleen** Accessory spleen	**Ø Open** **3 Percutaneous** **4 Percutaneous Endoscopic**	**Z No Device**	**X Diagnostic** **Z No Qualifier**

Non-OR   07BP[3,4]ZX

See Appendix L for Procedure Combinations
⊞   07B[H,J][Ø,4]ZZ

Ø Medical and Surgical
7 Lymphatic and Hemic Systems
C Extirpation   Definition: Taking or cutting out solid matter from a body part

Explanation: The solid matter may be an abnormal byproduct of a biological function or a foreign body; it may be imbedded in a body part or in the lumen of a tubular body part. The solid matter may or may not have been previously broken into pieces.

Body Part Character 4		Approach Character 5	Device Character 6	Qualifier Character 7
Ø Lymphatic, Head Buccinator lymph node Infraauricular lymph node Infraparotid lymph node Parotid lymph node Preauricular lymph node Submandibular lymph node Submaxillary lymph node Submental lymph node Subparotid lymph node Suprahyoid lymph node **1 Lymphatic, Right Neck** Cervical lymph node Jugular lymph node Mastoid (postauricular) lymph node Occipital lymph node Postauricular (mastoid) lymph node Retropharyngeal lymph node Right jugular trunk Right lymphatic duct Right subclavian trunk Supraclavicular (Virchow's) lymph node Virchow's (supraclavicular) lymph node **2 Lymphatic, Left Neck** Cervical lymph node Jugular lymph node Mastoid (postauricular) lymph node Occipital lymph node Postauricular (mastoid) lymph node Retropharyngeal lymph node Supraclavicular (Virchow's) lymph node Virchow's (supraclavicular) lymph node **3 Lymphatic, Right Upper Extremity** Cubital lymph node Deltopectoral (infraclavicular) lymph node Epitrochlear lymph node Infraclavicular (deltopectoral) lymph node Supratrochlear lymph node **4 Lymphatic, Left Upper Extremity** *See 3 Lymphatic, Right Upper Extremity* **5 Lymphatic, Right Axillary** Anterior (pectoral) lymph node Apical (subclavicular) lymph node Brachial (lateral) lymph node Central axillary lymph node Lateral (brachial) lymph node Pectoral (anterior) lymph node Posterior (subscapular) lymph node Subclavicular (apical) lymph node Subscapular (posterior) lymph node	**6 Lymphatic, Left Axillary** *See 5 Lymphatic, Right Axillary* **7 Lymphatic, Thorax** Intercostal lymph node Mediastinal lymph node Parasternal lymph node Paratracheal lymph node Tracheobronchial lymph node **8 Lymphatic, Internal Mammary, Right** **9 Lymphatic, Internal Mammary, Left** **B Lymphatic, Mesenteric** Inferior mesenteric lymph node Pararectal lymph node Superior mesenteric lymph node **C Lymphatic, Pelvis** Common iliac (subaortic) lymph node Gluteal lymph node Iliac lymph node Inferior epigastric lymph node Obturator lymph node Sacral lymph node Subaortic (common iliac) lymph node Suprainguinal lymph node **D Lymphatic, Aortic** Celiac lymph node Gastric lymph node Hepatic lymph node Lumbar lymph node Pancreaticosplenic lymph node Paraaortic lymph node Retroperitoneal lymph node **F Lymphatic, Right Lower Extremity** Femoral lymph node Popliteal lymph node **G Lymphatic, Left Lower Extremity** *See F Lymphatic, Right Lower Extremity* **H Lymphatic, Right Inguinal** **J Lymphatic, Left Inguinal** **K Thoracic Duct** Left jugular trunk Left subclavian trunk **L Cisterna Chyli** Intestinal lymphatic trunk Lumbar lymphatic trunk **M Thymus** Thymus gland **P Spleen** Accessory spleen	**Ø Open** **3 Percutaneous** **4 Percutaneous Endoscopic**	**Z No Device**	**Z No Qualifier**

Non-OR   Ø7CP[3,4]ZZ

Lymphatic and Hemic Systems

0   **Medical and Surgical**
7   **Lymphatic and Hemic Systems**
D   **Extraction**   Definition: Pulling or stripping out or off all or a portion of a body part by the use of force
         Explanation: The qualifier DIAGNOSTIC is used to identify extraction procedures that are biopsies

Body Part Character 4		Approach Character 5	Device Character 6	Qualifier Character 7

0   **Lymphatic, Head**
Buccinator lymph node
Infraauricular lymph node
Infraparotid lymph node
Parotid lymph node
Preauricular lymph node
Submandibular lymph node
Submaxillary lymph node
Submental lymph node
Subparotid lymph node
Suprahyoid lymph node
1   **Lymphatic, Right Neck**
Cervical lymph node
Jugular lymph node
Mastoid (postauricular) lymph
   node
Occipital lymph node
Postauricular (mastoid) lymph
   node
Retropharyngeal lymph node
Right jugular trunk
Right lymphatic duct
Right subclavian trunk
Supraclavicular (Virchow's)
   lymph node
Virchow's (supraclavicular)
   lymph node
2   **Lymphatic, Left Neck**
Cervical lymph node
Jugular lymph node
Mastoid (postauricular) lymph
   node
Occipital lymph node
Postauricular (mastoid) lymph
   node
Retropharyngeal lymph node
Supraclavicular (Virchow's)
   lymph node
Virchow's (supraclavicular)
   lymph node
3   **Lymphatic, Right Upper**
   Extremity
Cubital lymph node
Deltopectoral (infraclavicular)
   lymph node
Epitrochlear lymph node
Infraclavicular (deltopectoral)
   lymph node
Supratrochlear lymph node
4   **Lymphatic, Left Upper**
   Extremity
See 3 Lymphatic, Right Upper
   Extremity
5   **Lymphatic, Right Axillary**
Anterior (pectoral) lymph node
Apical (subclavicular) lymph
   node
Brachial (lateral) lymph node
Central axillary lymph node
Lateral (brachial) lymph node
Pectoral (anterior) lymph node
Posterior (subscapular) lymph
   node
Subclavicular (apical) lymph
   node
Subscapular (posterior) lymph
   node
	6 **Lymphatic, Left Axillary**
	See 5 Lymphatic, Right Axillary
	7 **Lymphatic, Thorax**
	Intercostal lymph node
	Mediastinal lymph node
	Parasternal lymph node
	Paratracheal lymph node
	Tracheobronchial lymph node
	8 **Lymphatic, Internal**
	   Mammary, Right
	9 **Lymphatic, Internal**
	   Mammary, Left
	B **Lymphatic, Mesenteric**
	Inferior mesenteric lymph
	   node
	Pararectal lymph node
	Superior mesenteric lymph
	   node
	C **Lymphatic, Pelvis**
	Common iliac (subaortic)
	   lymph node
	Gluteal lymph node
	Iliac lymph node
	Inferior epigastric lymph node
	Obturator lymph node
	Sacral lymph node
	Subaortic (common iliac)
	   lymph node
	Suprainguinal lymph node
	D **Lymphatic, Aortic**
	Celiac lymph node
	Gastric lymph node
	Hepatic lymph node
	Lumbar lymph node
	Pancreaticosplenic lymph
	   node
	Paraaortic lymph node
	Retroperitoneal lymph node
	F **Lymphatic, Right Lower**
	   Extremity
	Femoral lymph node
	Popliteal lymph node
	G **Lymphatic, Left Lower**
	   Extremity
	See F Lymphatic, Right Lower
	   Extremity
	H **Lymphatic, Right Inguinal**
	J **Lymphatic, Left Inguinal**
	K **Thoracic Duct**
	Left jugular trunk
	Left subclavian trunk
	L **Cisterna Chyli**
	Intestinal lymphatic trunk
	Lumbar lymphatic trunk
		3 Percutaneous
		4 Percutaneous Endoscopic
		8 Via Natural or Artificial
		   Opening Endoscopic
			Z No Device	**X** Diagnostic

M **Thymus** Thymus gland **P** **Spleen** Accessory spleen		**3** Percutaneous **4** Percutaneous Endoscopic	**Z** No Device	**X** Diagnostic
Q **Bone Marrow, Sternum** **R** **Bone Marrow, Iliac** **S** **Bone Marrow, Vertebral** **T** **Bone Marrow**		**0** Open **3** Percutaneous	**Z** No Device	**X** Diagnostic **Z** No Qualifier

Non-OR   All body part, approach, device, and qualifier values

Non-OR Procedure   DRG Non-OR Procedure   Valid OR Procedure   HAC Associated Procedure   Combination Only   New/Revised GREEN

0   **Medical and Surgical**
7   **Lymphatic and Hemic Systems**
H   **Insertion**   Definition: Putting in a nonbiological appliance that monitors, assists, performs, or prevents a physiological function but does not physically take the place of a body part

                                  Explanation: None

Body Part Character 4	Approach Character 5	Device Character 6	Qualifier Character 7

K Thoracic Duct
    Left jugular trunk
    Left subclavian trunk
L Cisterna Chyli
    Intestinal lymphatic trunk
    Lumbar lymphatic trunk
M Thymus
    Thymus gland
N Lymphatic
P Spleen
    Accessory spleen
T Bone Marrow
	0 Open
	3 Percutaneous
	4 Percutaneous Endoscopic
		1 Radioactive Element
		3 Infusion Device
		Y Other Device
			Z No Qualifier

Non-OR	07H[K,L,M,N,P][0,4]3Z
Non-OR	07H[K,L,M,N,P,T]3[1,3,Y]Z
Non-OR	07H[N,P]4YZ
Non-OR	07HT[0,4][1,3,Y]Z

0   **Medical and Surgical**
7   **Lymphatic and Hemic Systems**
J   **Inspection**   Definition: Visually and/or manually exploring a body part

                                  Explanation: Visual exploration may be performed with or without optical instrumentation. Manual exploration may be performed directly or through intervening body layers.

Body Part Character 4	Approach Character 5	Device Character 6	Qualifier Character 7

K Thoracic Duct
    Left jugular trunk
    Left subclavian trunk
L Cisterna Chyli
    Intestinal lymphatic trunk
    Lumbar lymphatic trunk
M Thymus
    Thymus gland
T Bone Marrow
	0 Open
	3 Percutaneous
	4 Percutaneous Endoscopic
		Z No Device	**Z** No Qualifier

N Lymphatic	**0** Open **3** Percutaneous **4** Percutaneous Endoscopic **8** Via Natural or Artificial Opening Endoscopic **X** External	**Z** No Device	**Z** No Qualifier
P Spleen Accessory spleen	**0** Open **3** Percutaneous **4** Percutaneous Endoscopic **X** External	**Z** No Device	**Z** No Qualifier

Non-OR	07J[K,L,M]3ZZ
Non-OR	07JT[0,3,4]ZZ
Non-OR	07JN[3,8,X]ZZ
Non-OR	07JP[3,4,X]ZZ

NC Noncovered Procedure   **LC** Limited Coverage   **QA** Questionable OB Admit   **NT** New Tech Add-on   ⊞ Combination Member   ♂ Male   ♀ Female

ICD-10-PCS 2022   291

Ø   Medical and Surgical
7   Lymphatic and Hemic Systems
L   Occlusion   Definition: Completely closing an orifice or the lumen of a tubular body part
                     Explanation: The orifice can be a natural orifice or an artificially created orifice

Body Part Character 4		Approach Character 5	Device Character 6	Qualifier Character 7

Ø Lymphatic, Head
 Buccinator lymph node
 Infraauricular lymph node
 Infraparotid lymph node
 Parotid lymph node
 Preauricular lymph node
 Submandibular lymph node
 Submaxillary lymph node
 Submental lymph node
 Subparotid lymph node
 Suprahyoid lymph node
 1 Lymphatic, Right Neck
 Cervical lymph node
 Jugular lymph node
 Mastoid (postauricular) lymph node
 Occipital lymph node
 Postauricular (mastoid) lymph node
 Retropharyngeal lymph node
 Right jugular trunk
 Right lymphatic duct
 Right subclavian trunk
 Supraclavicular (Virchow's) lymph
     node
 Virchow's (supraclavicular) lymph
     node
 2 Lymphatic, Left Neck
 Cervical lymph node
 Jugular lymph node
 Mastoid (postauricular) lymph node
 Occipital lymph node
 Postauricular (mastoid) lymph node
 Retropharyngeal lymph node
 Supraclavicular (Virchow's) lymph
     node
 Virchow's (supraclavicular) lymph
     node
 3 Lymphatic, Right Upper Extremity
 Cubital lymph node
 Deltopectoral (infraclavicular) lymph
     node
 Epitrochlear lymph node
 Infraclavicular (deltopectoral) lymph
     node
 Supratrochlear lymph node
 4 Lymphatic, Left Upper Extremity
 See 3 Lymphatic, Right Upper Extremity
 5 Lymphatic, Right Axillary
 Anterior (pectoral) lymph node
 Apical (subclavicular) lymph node
 Brachial (lateral) lymph node
 Central axillary lymph node
 Lateral (brachial) lymph node
 Pectoral (anterior) lymph node
 Posterior (subscapular) lymph node
 Subclavicular (apical) lymph node
 Subscapular (posterior) lymph node
	6 Lymphatic, Left Axillary
	 See 5 Lymphatic, Right Axillary
	 7 Lymphatic, Thorax
	 Intercostal lymph node
	 Mediastinal lymph node
	 Parasternal lymph node
	 Paratracheal lymph node
	 Tracheobronchial lymph node
	 8 Lymphatic, Internal Mammary, Right
	 9 Lymphatic, Internal Mammary, Left
	 B Lymphatic, Mesenteric
	 Inferior mesenteric lymph node
	 Pararectal lymph node
	 Superior mesenteric lymph node
	 C Lymphatic, Pelvis
	 Common iliac (subaortic) lymph node
	 Gluteal lymph node
	 Iliac lymph node
	 Inferior epigastric lymph node
	 Obturator lymph node
	 Sacral lymph node
	 Subaortic (common iliac) lymph node
	 Suprainguinal lymph node
	 D Lymphatic, Aortic
	 Celiac lymph node
	 Gastric lymph node
	 Hepatic lymph node
	 Lumbar lymph node
	 Pancreaticosplenic lymph node
	 Paraaortic lymph node
	 Retroperitoneal lymph node
	 F Lymphatic, Right Lower Extremity
	 Femoral lymph node
	 Popliteal lymph node
	 G Lymphatic, Left Lower Extremity
	 See F Lymphatic, Right Lower Extremity
	 H Lymphatic, Right Inguinal
	 J Lymphatic, Left Inguinal
	 K Thoracic Duct
	 Left jugular trunk
	 Left subclavian trunk
	 L Cisterna Chyli
	 Intestinal lymphatic trunk
	 Lumbar lymphatic trunk
		Ø Open
		 3 Percutaneous
		 4 Percutaneous Endoscopic
			C Extraluminal Device
			 D Intraluminal Device
			 Z No Device
				Z No Qualifier

0   **Medical and Surgical**
7   **Lymphatic and Hemic Systems**
N   **Release**   Definition: Freeing a body part from an abnormal physical constraint by cutting or by the use of force
                       Explanation: Some of the restraining tissue may be taken out but none of the body part is taken out

Body Part Character 4		Approach Character 5	Device Character 6	Qualifier Character 7

0 Lymphatic, Head
  Buccinator lymph node
  Infraauricular lymph node
  Infraparotid lymph node
  Parotid lymph node
  Preauricular lymph node
  Submandibular lymph node
  Submaxillary lymph node
  Submental lymph node
  Subparotid lymph node
  Suprahyoid lymph node
1 Lymphatic, Right Neck
  Cervical lymph node
  Jugular lymph node
  Mastoid (postauricular) lymph node
  Occipital lymph node
  Postauricular (mastoid) lymph node
  Retropharyngeal lymph node
  Right jugular trunk
  Right lymphatic duct
  Right subclavian trunk
  Supraclavicular (Virchow's) lymph
    node
  Virchow's (supraclavicular) lymph
    node
2 Lymphatic, Left Neck
  Cervical lymph node
  Jugular lymph node
  Mastoid (postauricular) lymph node
  Occipital lymph node
  Postauricular (mastoid) lymph node
  Retropharyngeal lymph node
  Supraclavicular (Virchow's) lymph
    node
  Virchow's (supraclavicular) lymph
    node
3 Lymphatic, Right Upper Extremity
  Cubital lymph node
  Deltopectoral (infraclavicular) lymph
    node
  Epitrochlear lymph node
  Infraclavicular (deltopectoral) lymph
    node
  Supratrochlear lymph node
4 Lymphatic, Left Upper Extremity
  See 3 Lymphatic, Right Upper Extremity
5 Lymphatic, Right Axillary
  Anterior (pectoral) lymph node
  Apical (subclavicular) lymph node
  Brachial (lateral) lymph node
  Central axillary lymph node
  Lateral (brachial) lymph node
  Pectoral (anterior) lymph node
  Posterior (subscapular) lymph node
  Subclavicular (apical) lymph node
  Subscapular (posterior) lymph node
	6 Lymphatic, Left Axillary
	  See 5 Lymphatic, Right Axillary
	7 Lymphatic, Thorax
	  Intercostal lymph node
	  Mediastinal lymph node
	  Parasternal lymph node
	  Paratracheal lymph node
	  Tracheobronchial lymph node
	8 Lymphatic, Internal Mammary, Right
	9 Lymphatic, Internal Mammary, Left
	B Lymphatic, Mesenteric
	  Inferior mesenteric lymph node
	  Pararectal lymph node
	  Superior mesenteric lymph node
	C Lymphatic, Pelvis
	  Common iliac (subaortic) lymph node
	  Gluteal lymph node
	  Iliac lymph node
	  Inferior epigastric lymph node
	  Obturator lymph node
	  Sacral lymph node
	  Subaortic (common iliac) lymph node
	  Suprainguinal lymph node
	D Lymphatic, Aortic
	  Celiac lymph node
	  Gastric lymph node
	  Hepatic lymph node
	  Lumbar lymph node
	  Pancreaticosplenic lymph node
	  Paraaortic lymph node
	  Retroperitoneal lymph node
	F Lymphatic, Right Lower Extremity
	  Femoral lymph node
	  Popliteal lymph node
	G Lymphatic, Left Lower Extremity
	  See F Lymphatic, Right Lower Extremity
	H Lymphatic, Right Inguinal
	J Lymphatic, Left Inguinal
	K Thoracic Duct
	  Left jugular trunk
	  Left subclavian trunk
	L Cisterna Chyli
	  Intestinal lymphatic trunk
	  Lumbar lymphatic trunk
	M Thymus
	  Thymus gland
	P Spleen
	  Accessory spleen
		0 Open
		3 Percutaneous
		**4 Percutaneous
		  Endoscopic**
			Z No Device	**Z No Qualifier**

NC Noncovered Procedure   **LC** Limited Coverage   **QA** Questionable OB Admit   **NT** New Tech Add-on   ⊞ Combination Member   ♂ Male   ♀ Female

ICD-10-PCS 2022   293

07N–07N

Ø   **Medical and Surgical**
7   **Lymphatic and Hemic Systems**
P   **Removal**   Definition: Taking out or off a device from a body part

Explanation: If a device is taken out and a similar device put in without cutting or puncturing the skin or mucous membrane, the procedure is coded to the root operation CHANGE. Otherwise, the procedure for taking out a device is coded to the root operation REMOVAL.

Body Part Character 4	Approach Character 5	Device Character 6	Qualifier Character 7
K Thoracic Duct Left jugular trunk Left subclavian trunk **L** Cisterna Chyli Intestinal lymphatic trunk Lumbar lymphatic trunk **N** Lymphatic	**Ø** Open **3** Percutaneous **4** Percutaneous Endoscopic	**Ø** Drainage Device **3** Infusion Device **7** Autologous Tissue Substitute **C** Extraluminal Device **D** Intraluminal Device **J** Synthetic Substitute **K** Nonautologous Tissue Substitute **Y** Other Device	**Z** No Qualifier
K Thoracic Duct Left jugular trunk Left subclavian trunk **L** Cisterna Chyli Intestinal lymphatic trunk Lumbar lymphatic trunk **N** Lymphatic	**X** External	**Ø** Drainage Device **3** Infusion Device **D** Intraluminal Device	**Z** No Qualifier
M Thymus Thymus gland **P** Spleen Accessory spleen	**Ø** Open **3** Percutaneous **4** Percutaneous Endoscopic	**Ø** Drainage Device **3** Infusion Device **Y** Other Device	**Z** No Qualifier
M Thymus Thymus gland **P** Spleen Accessory spleen	**X** External	**Ø** Drainage Device **3** Infusion Device	**Z** No Qualifier
T Bone Marrow	**Ø** Open **3** Percutaneous **4** Percutaneous Endoscopic **X** External	**Ø** Drainage Device	**Z** No Qualifier

Non-OR	Ø7P[K,L,N][3,4]YZ
Non-OR	Ø7P[K,L,N]X[Ø,3,D]Z
Non-OR	Ø7P[M,P][3,4]YZ
Non-OR	Ø7P[M,P]X[Ø,3]Z
Non-OR	Ø7PT[Ø,3,4,X]ØZ

0   **Medical and Surgical**
7   **Lymphatic and Hemic Systems**
Q   **Repair**   Definition: Restoring, to the extent possible, a body part to its normal anatomic structure and function
                    Explanation: Used only when the method to accomplish the repair is not one of the other root operations

Body Part Character 4		Approach Character 5	Device Character 6	Qualifier Character 7

0 Lymphatic, Head
 Buccinator lymph node
 Infraauricular lymph node
 Infraparotid lymph node
 Parotid lymph node
 Preauricular lymph node
 Submandibular lymph node
 Submaxillary lymph node
 Submental lymph node
 Subparotid lymph node
 Suprahyoid lymph node
 1 Lymphatic, Right Neck
 Cervical lymph node
 Jugular lymph node
 Mastoid (postauricular) lymph node
 Occipital lymph node
 Postauricular (mastoid) lymph node
 Retropharyngeal lymph node
 Right jugular trunk
 Right lymphatic duct
 Right subclavian trunk
 Supraclavicular (Virchow's) lymph
    node
 Virchow's (supraclavicular) lymph
    node
 2 Lymphatic, Left Neck
 Cervical lymph node
 Jugular lymph node
 Mastoid (postauricular) lymph node
 Occipital lymph node
 Postauricular (mastoid) lymph node
 Retropharyngeal lymph node
 Supraclavicular (Virchow's) lymph
    node
 Virchow's (supraclavicular) lymph
    node
 3 Lymphatic, Right Upper Extremity
 Cubital lymph node
 Deltopectoral (infraclavicular) lymph
    node
 Epitrochlear lymph node
 Infraclavicular (deltopectoral) lymph
    node
 Supratrochlear lymph node
 4 Lymphatic, Left Upper Extremity
 See 3 Lymphatic, Right Upper Extremity
 5 Lymphatic, Right Axillary
 Anterior (pectoral) lymph node
 Apical (subclavicular) lymph node
 Brachial (lateral) lymph node
 Central axillary lymph node
 Lateral (brachial) lymph node
 Pectoral (anterior) lymph node
 Posterior (subscapular) lymph node
 Subclavicular (apical) lymph node
 Subscapular (posterior) lymph node
	6 Lymphatic, Left Axillary
	 See 5 Lymphatic, Right Axillary
	 7 Lymphatic, Thorax
	 Intercostal lymph node
	 Mediastinal lymph node
	 Parasternal lymph node
	 Paratracheal lymph node
	 Tracheobronchial lymph node
	 8 Lymphatic, Internal Mammary, Right
	 9 Lymphatic, Internal Mammary, Left
	 B Lymphatic, Mesenteric
	 Inferior mesenteric lymph node
	 Pararectal lymph node
	 Superior mesenteric lymph node
	 C Lymphatic, Pelvis
	 Common iliac (subaortic) lymph node
	 Gluteal lymph node
	 Iliac lymph node
	 Inferior epigastric lymph node
	 Obturator lymph node
	 Sacral lymph node
	 Subaortic (common iliac) lymph node
	 Suprainguinal lymph node
	 D Lymphatic, Aortic
	 Celiac lymph node
	 Gastric lymph node
	 Hepatic lymph node
	 Lumbar lymph node
	 Pancreaticosplenic lymph node
	 Paraaortic lymph node
	 Retroperitoneal lymph node
	 F Lymphatic, Right Lower Extremity
	 Femoral lymph node
	 Popliteal lymph node
	 G Lymphatic, Left Lower Extremity
	 See F Lymphatic, Right Lower Extremity
	 H Lymphatic, Right Inguinal
	 J Lymphatic, Left Inguinal
	 K Thoracic Duct
	 Left jugular trunk
	 Left subclavian trunk
	 L Cisterna Chyli
	 Intestinal lymphatic trunk
	 Lumbar lymphatic trunk
		0 Open
		 3 Percutaneous
		 4 Percutaneous Endoscopic
		 8 Via Natural or Artificial Opening Endoscopic
			Z No Device	**Z** No Qualifier

M Thymus Thymus gland **P Spleen** Accessory spleen		**0** Open **3** Percutaneous **4** Percutaneous Endoscopic	**Z** No Device	**Z** No Qualifier

Lymphatic and Hemic Systems

Ø   **Medical and Surgical**
7   **Lymphatic and Hemic Systems**
S   **Reposition**   Definition: Moving to its normal location, or other suitable location, all or a portion of a body part

Explanation: The body part is moved to a new location from an abnormal location, or from a normal location where it is not functioning correctly. The body part may or may not be cut out or off to be moved to the new location.

Body Part Character 4	Approach Character 5	Device Character 6	Qualifier Character 7

M   Thymus
     Thymus gland
P   Spleen
     Accessory spleen
	Ø Open	**Z** No Device	**Z** No Qualifier

Ø   **Medical and Surgical**
7   **Lymphatic and Hemic Systems**
T   **Resection**   Definition: Cutting out or off, without replacement, all of a body part

Explanation: None

Body Part Character 4		Approach Character 5	Device Character 6	Qualifier Character 7

Ø   Lymphatic, Head
     Buccinator lymph node
     Infraauricular lymph node
     Infraparotid lymph node
     Parotid lymph node
     Preauricular lymph node
     Submandibular lymph node
     Submaxillary lymph node
     Submental lymph node
     Subparotid lymph node
     Suprahyoid lymph node
1   Lymphatic, Right Neck
     Cervical lymph node
     Jugular lymph node
     Mastoid (postauricular) lymph node
     Occipital lymph node
     Postauricular (mastoid) lymph node
     Retropharyngeal lymph node
     Right jugular trunk
     Right lymphatic duct
     Right subclavian trunk
     Supraclavicular (Virchow's) lymph
       node
     Virchow's (supraclavicular) lymph
       node
2   Lymphatic, Left Neck
     Cervical lymph node
     Jugular lymph node
     Mastoid (postauricular) lymph node
     Occipital lymph node
     Postauricular (mastoid) lymph node
     Retropharyngeal lymph node
     Supraclavicular (Virchow's) lymph
       node
     Virchow's (supraclavicular) lymph
       node
3   Lymphatic, Right Upper Extremity
     Cubital lymph node
     Deltopectoral (infraclavicular) lymph
       node
     Epitrochlear lymph node
     Infraclavicular (deltopectoral) lymph
       node
     Supratrochlear lymph node
4   Lymphatic, Left Upper Extremity
     See 3 Lymphatic, Right Upper Extremity
5   Lymphatic, Right Axillary ⊞
     Anterior (pectoral) lymph node
     Apical (subclavicular) lymph node
     Brachial (lateral) lymph node
     Central axillary lymph node
     Lateral (brachial) lymph node
     Pectoral (anterior) lymph node
     Posterior (subscapular) lymph node
     Subclavicular (apical) lymph node
     Subscapular (posterior) lymph node
	6 Lymphatic, Left Axillary ⊞
	     See 5 Lymphatic, Right Axillary
	7 Lymphatic, Thorax ⊞
	     Intercostal lymph node
	     Mediastinal lymph node
	     Parasternal lymph node
	     Paratracheal lymph node
	     Tracheobronchial lymph node
	8 Lymphatic, Internal ⊞
	     Mammary, Right
	9 Lymphatic, Internal ⊞
	     Mammary, Left
	B Lymphatic, Mesenteric
	     Inferior mesenteric lymph node
	     Pararectal lymph node
	     Superior mesenteric lymph node
	C Lymphatic, Pelvis
	     Common iliac (subaortic) lymph node
	     Gluteal lymph node
	     Iliac lymph node
	     Inferior epigastric lymph node
	     Obturator lymph node
	     Sacral lymph node
	     Subaortic (common iliac) lymph node
	     Suprainguinal lymph node
	D Lymphatic, Aortic
	     Celiac lymph node
	     Gastric lymph node
	     Hepatic lymph node
	     Lumbar lymph node
	     Pancreaticosplenic lymph node
	     Paraaortic lymph node
	     Retroperitoneal lymph node
	F Lymphatic, Right Lower Extremity
	     Femoral lymph node
	     Popliteal lymph node
	G Lymphatic, Left Lower Extremity
	     See F Lymphatic, Right Lower Extremity
	H Lymphatic, Right Inguinal
	J Lymphatic, Left Inguinal
	K Thoracic Duct
	     Left jugular trunk
	     Left subclavian trunk
	L Cisterna Chyli
	     Intestinal lymphatic trunk
	     Lumbar lymphatic trunk
	M Thymus
	     Thymus gland
	P Spleen
	     Accessory spleen
		Ø Open
		4 Percutaneous
		     Endoscopic
			Z No Device	**Z** No Qualifier

See Appendix L for Procedure Combinations
⊞   07T[5,6,7,8,9]ØZZ

0̸ Medical and Surgical
7 Lymphatic and Hemic Systems
U Supplement   Definition: Putting in or on biological or synthetic material that physically reinforces and/or augments the function of a portion of a body part

Explanation: The biological material is non-living, or is living and from the same individual. The body part may have been previously replaced, and the SUPPLEMENT procedure is performed to physically reinforce and/or augment the function of the replaced body part.

Body Part Character 4		Approach Character 5	Device Character 6	Qualifier Character 7
0̸ Lymphatic, Head Buccinator lymph node Infraauricular lymph node Infraparotid lymph node Parotid lymph node Preauricular lymph node Submandibular lymph node Submaxillary lymph node Submental lymph node Subparotid lymph node Suprahyoid lymph node **1 Lymphatic, Right Neck** Cervical lymph node Jugular lymph node Mastoid (postauricular) lymph node Occipital lymph node Postauricular (mastoid) lymph node Retropharyngeal lymph node Right jugular trunk Right lymphatic duct Right subclavian trunk Supraclavicular (Virchow's) lymph node Virchow's (supraclavicular) lymph node **2 Lymphatic, Left Neck** Cervical lymph node Jugular lymph node Mastoid (postauricular) lymph node Occipital lymph node Postauricular (mastoid) lymph node Retropharyngeal lymph node Supraclavicular (Virchow's) lymph node Virchow's (supraclavicular) lymph node **3 Lymphatic, Right Upper Extremity** Cubital lymph node Deltopectoral (infraclavicular) lymph node Epitrochlear lymph node Infraclavicular (deltopectoral) lymph node Supratrochlear lymph node **4 Lymphatic, Left Upper Extremity** *See 3 Lymphatic, Right Upper Extremity* **5 Lymphatic, Right Axillary** Anterior (pectoral) lymph node Apical (subclavicular) lymph node Brachial (lateral) lymph node Central axillary lymph node Lateral (brachial) lymph node Pectoral (anterior) lymph node Posterior (subscapular) lymph node Subclavicular (apical) lymph node Subscapular (posterior) lymph node	**6 Lymphatic, Left Axillary** *See 5 Lymphatic, Right Axillary* **7 Lymphatic, Thorax** Intercostal lymph node Mediastinal lymph node Parasternal lymph node Paratracheal lymph node Tracheobronchial lymph node **8 Lymphatic, Internal Mammary, Right** **9 Lymphatic, Internal Mammary, Left** **B Lymphatic, Mesenteric** Inferior mesenteric lymph node Pararectal lymph node Superior mesenteric lymph node **C Lymphatic, Pelvis** Common iliac (subaortic) lymph node Gluteal lymph node Iliac lymph node Inferior epigastric lymph node Obturator lymph node Sacral lymph node Subaortic (common iliac) lymph node Suprainguinal lymph node **D Lymphatic, Aortic** Celiac lymph node Gastric lymph node Hepatic lymph node Lumbar lymph node Pancreaticosplenic lymph node Paraaortic lymph node Retroperitoneal lymph node **F Lymphatic, Right Lower Extremity** Femoral lymph node Popliteal lymph node **G Lymphatic, Left Lower Extremity** *See F Lymphatic, Right Lower Extremity* **H Lymphatic, Right Inguinal** **J Lymphatic, Left Inguinal** **K Thoracic Duct** Left jugular trunk Left subclavian trunk **L Cisterna Chyli** Intestinal lymphatic trunk Lumbar lymphatic trunk	**0̸ Open** **4 Percutaneous Endoscopic**	**7 Autologous Tissue Substitute** **J Synthetic Substitute** **K Nonautologous Tissue Substitute**	**Z No Qualifier**

NC Noncovered Procedure   LC Limited Coverage   QA Questionable OB Admit   NT New Tech Add-on   ⊞ Combination Member   ♂ Male   ♀ Female

ICD-10-PCS 2022   297

Lymphatic and Hemic Systems

Ø   **Medical and Surgical**
7   **Lymphatic and Hemic Systems**
V   **Restriction**   Definition: Partially closing an orifice or the lumen of a tubular body part
                   Explanation: The orifice can be a natural orifice or an artificially created orifice

Body Part Character 4		Approach Character 5	Device Character 6	Qualifier Character 7

Ø **Lymphatic, Head**
  Buccinator lymph node
  Infraauricular lymph node
  Infraparotid lymph node
  Parotid lymph node
  Preauricular lymph node
  Submandibular lymph node
  Submaxillary lymph node
  Submental lymph node
  Subparotid lymph node
  Suprahyoid lymph node
1 **Lymphatic, Right Neck**
  Cervical lymph node
  Jugular lymph node
  Mastoid (postauricular) lymph node
  Occipital lymph node
  Postauricular (mastoid) lymph node
  Retropharyngeal lymph node
  Right jugular trunk
  Right lymphatic duct
  Right subclavian trunk
  Supraclavicular (Virchow's) lymph
    node
  Virchow's (supraclavicular) lymph
    node
2 **Lymphatic, Left Neck**
  Cervical lymph node
  Jugular lymph node
  Mastoid (postauricular) lymph node
  Occipital lymph node
  Postauricular (mastoid) lymph node
  Retropharyngeal lymph node
  Supraclavicular (Virchow's) lymph
    node
  Virchow's (supraclavicular) lymph
    node
3 **Lymphatic, Right Upper Extremity**
  Cubital lymph node
  Deltopectoral (infraclavicular) lymph
    node
  Epitrochlear lymph node
  Infraclavicular (deltopectoral) lymph
    node
  Supratrochlear lymph node
4 **Lymphatic, Left Upper Extremity**
  See 3 Lymphatic, Right Upper Extremity
5 **Lymphatic, Right Axillary**
  Anterior (pectoral) lymph node
  Apical (subclavicular) lymph node
  Brachial (lateral) lymph node
  Central axillary lymph node
  Lateral (brachial) lymph node
  Pectoral (anterior) lymph node
  Posterior (subscapular) lymph node
  Subclavicular (apical) lymph node
  Subscapular (posterior) lymph node
	6 **Lymphatic, Left Axillary**
	  See 5 Lymphatic, Right Axillary
	7 **Lymphatic, Thorax**
	  Intercostal lymph node
	  Mediastinal lymph node
	  Parasternal lymph node
	  Paratracheal lymph node
	  Tracheobronchial lymph node
	8 **Lymphatic, Internal Mammary, Right**
	9 **Lymphatic, Internal Mammary, Left**
	B **Lymphatic, Mesenteric**
	  Inferior mesenteric lymph node
	  Pararectal lymph node
	  Superior mesenteric lymph node
	C **Lymphatic, Pelvis**
	  Common iliac (subaortic) lymph node
	  Gluteal lymph node
	  Iliac lymph node
	  Inferior epigastric lymph node
	  Obturator lymph node
	  Sacral lymph node
	  Subaortic (common iliac) lymph node
	  Suprainguinal lymph node
	D **Lymphatic, Aortic**
	  Celiac lymph node
	  Gastric lymph node
	  Hepatic lymph node
	  Lumbar lymph node
	  Pancreaticosplenic lymph node
	  Paraaortic lymph node
	  Retroperitoneal lymph node
	F **Lymphatic, Right Lower Extremity**
	  Femoral lymph node
	  Popliteal lymph node
	G **Lymphatic, Left Lower Extremity**
	  See F Lymphatic, Right Lower Extremity
	H **Lymphatic, Right Inguinal**
	J **Lymphatic, Left Inguinal**
	K **Thoracic Duct**
	  Left jugular trunk
	  Left subclavian trunk
	L **Cisterna Chyli**
	  Intestinal lymphatic trunk
	  Lumbar lymphatic trunk
		Ø Open
		3 Percutaneous
		4 Percutaneous
		    Endoscopic
			C Extraluminal Device
			D Intraluminal Device
			Z No Device
				Z No Qualifier

0   Medical and Surgical
7   Lymphatic and Hemic Systems
W   Revision   Definition: Correcting, to the extent possible, a portion of a malfunctioning device or the position of a displaced device

Explanation: Revision can include correcting a malfunctioning or displaced device by taking out or putting in components of the device such as a screw or pin

Body Part Character 4	Approach Character 5	Device Character 6	Qualifier Character 7

K   Thoracic Duct
     Left jugular trunk
     Left subclavian trunk
L   Cisterna Chyli
     Intestinal lymphatic trunk
     Lumbar lymphatic trunk
N   Lymphatic
	0 Open
	3 Percutaneous
	4 Percutaneous Endoscopic
		0 Drainage Device
		3 Infusion Device
		7 Autologous Tissue
		     Substitute
		C Extraluminal Device
		D Intraluminal Device
		J Synthetic Substitute
		K Nonautologous Tissue
		     Substitute
		Y Other Device
			Z No Qualifier

K   Thoracic Duct
     Left jugular trunk
     Left subclavian trunk
L   Cisterna Chyli
     Intestinal lymphatic trunk
     Lumbar lymphatic trunk
N   Lymphatic
	X External	0 Drainage Device
		3 Infusion Device
		7 Autologous Tissue
		     Substitute
		C Extraluminal Device
		D Intraluminal Device
		J Synthetic Substitute
		K Nonautologous Tissue
		     Substitute
			Z No Qualifier

M   Thymus
     Thymus gland
P   Spleen
     Accessory spleen
	0 Open
	3 Percutaneous
	4 Percutaneous Endoscopic
		0 Drainage Device
		3 Infusion Device
		Y Other Device
			Z No Qualifier

M   Thymus
     Thymus gland
P   Spleen
     Accessory spleen
	X External	0 Drainage Device
		3 Infusion Device
			Z No Qualifier

T Bone Marrow	0 Open 3 Percutaneous 4 Percutaneous Endoscopic X External	0 Drainage Device	Z No Qualifier

Non-OR	07W[K,L,N][3,4]YZ
Non-OR	07W[K,L,N]X[0,3,7,C,D,J,K]Z
Non-OR	07W[M,P][3,4]YZ
Non-OR	07W[M,P]X[0,3]Z
Non-OR	07WT[0,3,4,X]0Z

0   Medical and Surgical
7   Lymphatic and Hemic Systems
Y   Transplantation   Definition: Putting in or on all or a portion of a living body part taken from another individual or animal to physically take the place and/or function of all or a portion of a similar body part

Explanation: The native body part may or may not be taken out, and the transplanted body part may take over all or a portion of its function

Body Part Character 4	Approach Character 5	Device Character 6	Qualifier Character 7

M   Thymus
     Thymus gland
P   Spleen
     Accessory spleen
	0 Open	Z No Device	0 Allogeneic
			1 Syngeneic
			2 Zooplastic

NC Noncovered Procedure   LC Limited Coverage   QA Questionable OB Admit   NT New Tech Add-on   ⊞ Combination Member   ♂ Male   ♀ Female

ICD-10-PCS 2022   299

Eye Ø8Ø–Ø8X

Character Meanings

This Character Meaning table is provided as a guide to assist the user in the identification of character members that may be found in this section of code tables. It **SHOULD NOT** be used to build a PCS code.

Operation–Character 3	Body Part–Character 4	Approach–Character 5	Device–Character 6	Qualifier–Character 7
Ø Alteration	Ø Eye, Right	Ø Open	Ø Drainage Device OR Synthetic Substitute, Intraocular Telescope	3 Nasal Cavity
1 Bypass	1 Eye, Left	3 Percutaneous	1 Radioactive Element	4 Sclera
2 Change	2 Anterior Chamber, Right	7 Via Natural or Artificial Opening	3 Infusion Device	X Diagnostic
5 Destruction	3 Anterior Chamber, Left	8 Via Natural or Artificial Opening Endoscopic	5 Epiretinal Visual Prosthesis	Z No Qualifier
7 Dilation	4 Vitreous, Right	X External	7 Autologous Tissue Substitute	
9 Drainage	5 Vitreous, Left		C Extraluminal Device	
B Excision	6 Sclera, Right		D Intraluminal Device	
C Extirpation	7 Sclera, Left		J Synthetic Substitute	
D Extraction	8 Cornea, Right		K Nonautologous Tissue Substitute	
F Fragmentation	9 Cornea, Left		Y Other Device	
H Insertion	A Choroid, Right		Z No Device	
J Inspection	B Choroid, Left			
L Occlusion	C Iris, Right			
M Reattachment	D Iris, Left			
N Release	E Retina, Right			
P Removal	F Retina, Left			
Q Repair	G Retinal Vessel, Right			
R Replacement	H Retinal Vessel, Left			
S Reposition	J Lens, Right			
T Resection	K Lens, Left			
U Supplement	L Extraocular Muscle, Right			
V Restriction	M Extraocular Muscle, Left			
W Revision	N Upper Eyelid, Right			
X Transfer	P Upper Eyelid, Left			
	Q Lower Eyelid, Right			
	R Lower Eyelid, Left			
	S Conjunctiva, Right			
	T Conjunctiva, Left			
	V Lacrimal Gland, Right			
	W Lacrimal Gland, Left			
	X Lacrimal Duct, Right			
	Y Lacrimal Duct, Left			

AHA Coding Clinic for table Ø81
2019, 1Q, 27   Glaucoma tube shunt

AHA Coding Clinic for table Ø89
2016, 2Q, 21   Laser trabeculoplasty

AHA Coding Clinic for table Ø8B
2014, 4Q, 35   Vitrectomy with air/fluid exchange
2014, 4Q, 36   Pars plans vitrectomy without mention of instillation of oil, air or fluid

AHA Coding Clinic for table Ø8J
2015, 1Q, 35   Attempted removal of foreign body from cornea

AHA Coding Clinic for table Ø8N
2015, 2Q, 24   Penetrating keratoplasty and anterior segment reconstruction

AHA Coding Clinic for table Ø8Q
2018, 3Q, 13   Repair of ruptured globe

AHA Coding Clinic for table Ø8R
2015, 2Q, 24   Penetrating keratoplasty and anterior segment reconstruction
2015, 2Q, 25   Penetrating keratoplasty and placement of viscoelastic eye with paracentesis

AHA Coding Clinic for table Ø8T
2015, 2Q, 12   Orbital exenteration

AHA Coding Clinic for table Ø8U
2014, 3Q, 31   Corneal amniotic membrane transplantation

Eye

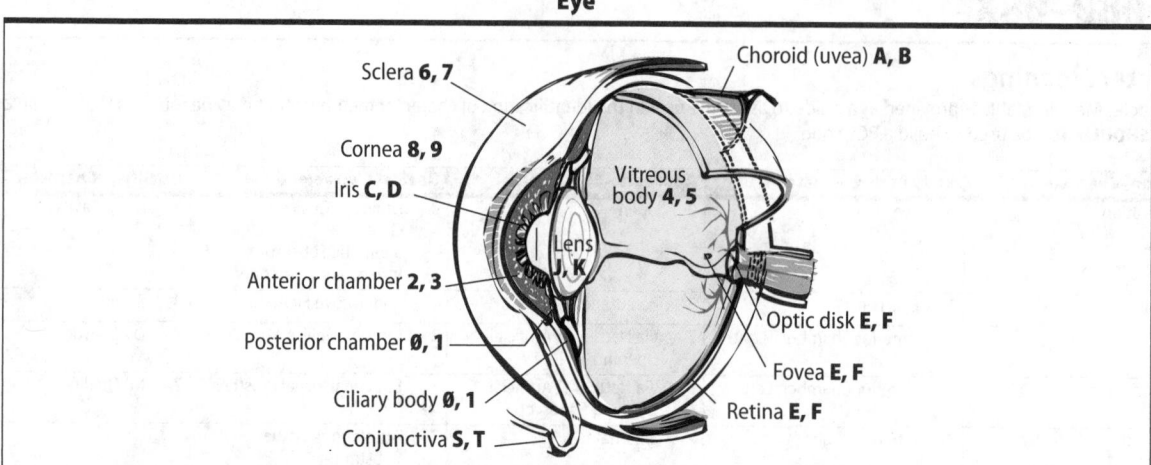

Sclera **6, 7**
Choroid (uvea) **A, B**
Cornea **8, 9**
Iris **C, D**
Vitreous body **4, 5**
Lens **J, K**
Anterior chamber **2, 3**
Posterior chamber **Ø, 1**
Optic disk **E, F**
Fovea **E, F**
Ciliary body **Ø, 1**
Retina **E, F**
Conjunctiva **S, T**

Eye Musculature

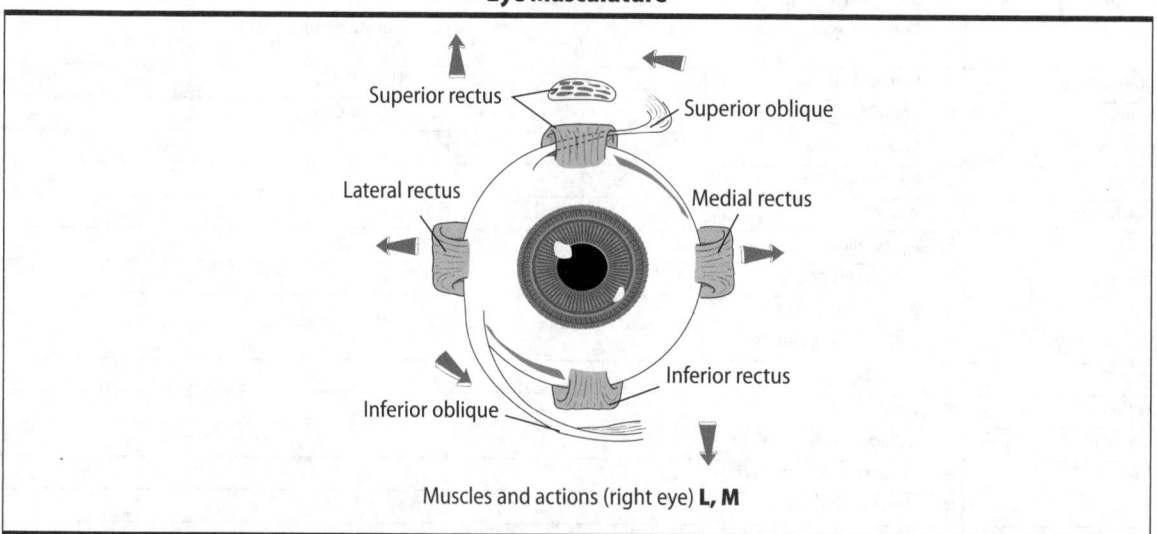

Superior rectus
Superior oblique
Lateral rectus
Medial rectus
Inferior oblique
Inferior rectus

Muscles and actions (right eye) **L, M**

Lacrimal System

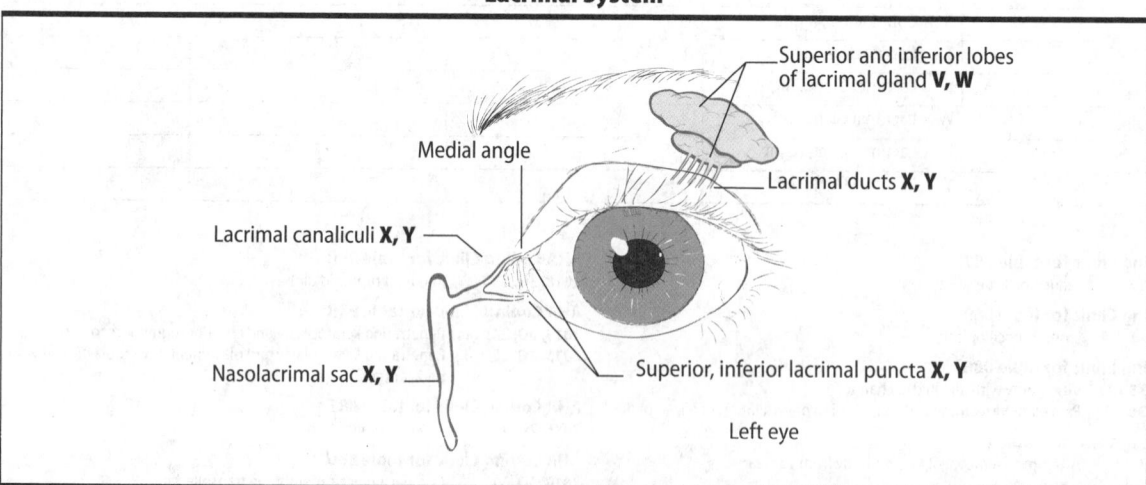

Superior and inferior lobes of lacrimal gland **V, W**
Medial angle
Lacrimal ducts **X, Y**
Lacrimal canaliculi **X, Y**
Nasolacrimal sac **X, Y**
Superior, inferior lacrimal puncta **X, Y**

Left eye

Ø   Medical and Surgical
8   Eye
Ø   Alteration   Definition: Modifying the anatomic structure of a body part without affecting the function of the body part

                       Explanation: Principal purpose is to improve appearance

Body Part Character 4	Approach Character 5	Device Character 6	Qualifier Character 7

N Upper Eyelid, Right
   Lateral canthus
   Levator palpebrae superioris muscle
   Orbicularis oculi muscle
   Superior tarsal plate
P Upper Eyelid, Left
   See N Upper Eyelid, Right
Q Lower Eyelid, Right
   Inferior tarsal plate
   Medial canthus
R Lower Eyelid, Left
   See Q Lower Eyelid, Right
	Ø Open
	3 Percutaneous
	X External
		7 Autologous Tissue Substitute
		J Synthetic Substitute
		K Nonautologous Tissue Substitute
		Z No Device
			Z No Qualifier

Non-OR   All body part, approach, device, and qualifier values

---

Ø   Medical and Surgical
8   Eye
1   Bypass   Definition: Altering the route of passage of the contents of a tubular body part

                       Explanation: Rerouting contents of a body part to a downstream area of the normal route, to a similar route and body part, or to an abnormal route and dissimilar body part. Includes one or more anastomoses, with or without the use of a device.

Body Part Character 4	Approach Character 5	Device Character 6	Qualifier Character 7

2 Anterior Chamber, Right
   Aqueous humour
3 Anterior Chamber, Left
   See 2 Anterior Chamber, Right
	3 Percutaneous	**J** Synthetic Substitute
		K Nonautologous Tissue Substitute
		Z No Device
			4 Sclera

X Lacrimal Duct, Right
   Lacrimal canaliculus
   Lacrimal punctum
   Lacrimal sac
   Nasolacrimal duct
Y Lacrimal Duct, Left
   See X Lacrimal Duct, Right
	Ø Open
	3 Percutaneous
		J Synthetic Substitute
		K Nonautologous Tissue Substitute
		Z No Device
			3 Nasal Cavity

Ø   Medical and Surgical
8   Eye
2   Change   Definition: Taking out or off a device from a body part and putting back an identical or similar device in or on the same body part without cutting or puncturing the skin or a mucous membrane

                       Explanation: All CHANGE procedures are coded using the approach EXTERNAL

Body Part Character 4	Approach Character 5	Device Character 6	Qualifier Character 7

Ø Eye, Right
   Ciliary body
   Posterior chamber
1 Eye, Left
   See Ø Eye, Right
	X External	**Ø** Drainage Device
		Y Other Device
			Z No Qualifier

Non-OR   All body part, approach, device, and qualifier values

---

NC Noncovered Procedure   **LC** Limited Coverage   **QA** Questionable OB Admit   **NT** New Tech Add-on   ⊞ Combination Member   ♂ Male   ♀ Female

Ø   Medical and Surgical
8   Eye
5   Destruction   Definition: Physical eradication of all or a portion of a body part by the direct use of energy, force, or a destructive agent

Explanation: None of the body part is physically taken out

Body Part Character 4		Approach Character 5	Device Character 6	Qualifier Character 7

Ø   Eye, Right
    Ciliary body
    Posterior chamber
1   Eye, Left
    See Ø Eye, Right
6   Sclera, Right
7   Sclera, Left
	8 Cornea, Right
	9 Cornea, Left
	S Conjunctiva, Right
	    Plica semilunaris
	T Conjunctiva, Left
	    See S Conjunctiva, Right
		X External	Z No Device	Z No Qualifier

2   Anterior Chamber, Right
    Aqueous humour
3   Anterior Chamber, Left
    See 2 Anterior Chamber, Right
4   Vitreous, Right
    Vitreous body
5   Vitreous, Left
    See 4 Vitreous, Right
C   Iris, Right
D   Iris, Left
	E Retina, Right
	    Fovea
	    Macula
	    Optic disc
	F Retina, Left
	    See E Retina, Right
	G Retinal Vessel, Right
	H Retinal Vessel, Left
	J Lens, Right
	    Zonule of Zinn
	K Lens, Left
	    See J Lens, Right
		3 Percutaneous	Z No Device	Z No Qualifier

A   Choroid, Right
B   Choroid, Left
L   Extraocular Muscle, Right
    Inferior oblique muscle
    Inferior rectus muscle
    Lateral rectus muscle
    Medial rectus muscle
    Superior oblique muscle
    Superior rectus muscle
	M Extraocular Muscle, Left
	    See L Extraocular Muscle, Right
	V Lacrimal Gland, Right
	W Lacrimal Gland, Left
		Ø Open
		3 Percutaneous
			Z No Device	Z No Qualifier

N   Upper Eyelid, Right
    Lateral canthus
    Levator palpebrae superioris
      muscle
    Orbicularis oculi muscle
    Superior tarsal plate
P   Upper Eyelid, Left
    See N Upper Eyelid, Right
	Q Lower Eyelid, Right
	    Inferior tarsal plate
	    Medial canthus
	R Lower Eyelid, Left
	    See Q Lower Eyelid, Right
		Ø Open
		3 Percutaneous
		X External
			Z No Device	Z No Qualifier

X   Lacrimal Duct, Right
    Lacrimal canaliculus
    Lacrimal punctum
    Lacrimal sac
    Nasolacrimal duct
	Y Lacrimal Duct, Left
	    See X Lacrimal Duct, Right
		Ø Open
		3 Percutaneous
		7 Via Natural or Artificial
		    Opening
		8 Via Natural or Artificial
		    Opening Endoscopic
			Z No Device	Z No Qualifier

Non-OR	Ø85[E,F]3ZZ

Ø   Medical and Surgical
8   Eye
7   Dilation   Definition: Expanding an orifice or the lumen of a tubular body part

Explanation: The orifice can be a natural orifice or an artificially created orifice. Accomplished by stretching a tubular body part using intraluminal pressure or by cutting part of the orifice or wall of the tubular body part.

Body Part Character 4	Approach Character 5	Device Character 6	Qualifier Character 7

X   Lacrimal Duct, Right
    Lacrimal canaliculus
    Lacrimal punctum
    Lacrimal sac
    Nasolacrimal duct
Y   Lacrimal Duct, Left
    See X Lacrimal Duct, Right
	Ø Open
	3 Percutaneous
	7 Via Natural or Artificial
	    Opening
	8 Via Natural or Artificial
	    Opening Endoscopic
		D Intraluminal Device
		Z No Device
			Z No Qualifier

Ø Medical and Surgical
8 Eye
9 Drainage   Definition: Taking or letting out fluids and/or gases from a body part
                 Explanation: The qualifier DIAGNOSTIC is used to identify drainage procedures that are biopsies

Body Part Character 4		Approach Character 5	Device Character 6	Qualifier Character 7

Ø Eye, Right
  Ciliary body
  Posterior chamber
1 Eye, Left
  See Ø Eye, Right
6 Sclera, Right
7 Sclera, Left
	8 Cornea, Right
	9 Cornea, Left
	S Conjunctiva, Right
	  Plica semilunaris
	T Conjunctiva, Left
	  See S Conjunctiva, Right
		X External	Ø Drainage Device	Z No Qualifier

Ø Eye, Right
  Ciliary body
  Posterior chamber
1 Eye, Left
  See Ø Eye, Right
6 Sclera, Right
7 Sclera, Left
	8 Cornea, Right
	9 Cornea, Left
	S Conjunctiva, Right
	  Plica semilunaris
	T Conjunctiva, Left
	  See S Conjunctiva, Right
		X External	Z No Device	X Diagnostic
				Z No Qualifier

2 Anterior Chamber, Right
  Aqueous humour
3 Anterior Chamber, Left
  See 2 Anterior Chamber, Right
4 Vitreous, Right
  Vitreous body
5 Vitreous, Left
  See 4 Vitreous, Right
C Iris, Right
D Iris, Left
	E Retina, Right
	  Fovea
	  Macula
	  Optic disc
	F Retina, Left
	  See E Retina, Right
	G Retinal Vessel, Right
	H Retinal Vessel, Left
	J Lens, Right
	  Zonule of Zinn
	K Lens, Left
	  See J Lens, Right
		3 Percutaneous	Ø Drainage Device	Z No Qualifier

2 Anterior Chamber, Right
  Aqueous humour
3 Anterior Chamber, Left
  See 2 Anterior Chamber, Right
4 Vitreous, Right
  Vitreous body
5 Vitreous, Left
  See 4 Vitreous, Right
C Iris, Right
D Iris, Left
	E Retina, Right
	  Fovea
	  Macula
	  Optic disc
	F Retina, Left
	  See E Retina, Right
	G Retinal Vessel, Right
	H Retinal Vessel, Left
	J Lens, Right
	  Zonule of Zinn
	K Lens, Left
	  See J Lens, Right
		3 Percutaneous	Z No Device	X Diagnostic
				Z No Qualifier

A Choroid, Right
B Choroid, Left
L Extraocular Muscle, Right
  Inferior oblique muscle
  Inferior rectus muscle
  Lateral rectus muscle
  Medial rectus muscle
  Superior oblique muscle
  Superior rectus muscle
	M Extraocular Muscle, Left
	  See L Extraocular Muscle, Right
	V Lacrimal Gland, Right
	W Lacrimal Gland, Left
		Ø Open
		3 Percutaneous
			Ø Drainage Device	Z No Qualifier

A Choroid, Right
B Choroid, Left
L Extraocular Muscle, Right
  Inferior oblique muscle
  Inferior rectus muscle
  Lateral rectus muscle
  Medial rectus muscle
  Superior oblique muscle
  Superior rectus muscle
	M Extraocular Muscle, Left
	  See L Extraocular Muscle, Right
	V Lacrimal Gland, Right
	W Lacrimal Gland, Left
		Ø Open
		3 Percutaneous
			Z No Device	X Diagnostic
				Z No Qualifier

N Upper Eyelid, Right
  Lateral canthus
  Levator palpebrae superioris
    muscle
  Orbicularis oculi muscle
  Superior tarsal plate
P Upper Eyelid, Left
  See N Upper Eyelid, Right
	Q Lower Eyelid, Right
	  Inferior tarsal plate
	  Medial canthus
	R Lower Eyelid, Left
	  See Q Lower Eyelid, Right
		Ø Open
		3 Percutaneous
		X External
			Ø Drainage Device	Z No Qualifier

Non-OR   Ø89[Ø,1,6,7,8,9,S,T]XZ[X,Z]
Non-OR   Ø89[N,P,Q,R][Ø,3,X]ØZ

Ø89 Continued on next page

NC Noncovered Procedure   **LC** Limited Coverage   **QA** Questionable OB Admit   **NT** New Tech Add-on   ⊞ Combination Member   ♂ Male   ♀ Female

Ø Medical and Surgical
8 Eye
9 Drainage

Ø89 Continued

Definition: Taking or letting out fluids and/or gases from a body part

Explanation: The qualifier DIAGNOSTIC is used to identify drainage procedures that are biopsies

Body Part Character 4		Approach Character 5	Device Character 6	Qualifier Character 7
N Upper Eyelid, Right Lateral canthus Levator palpebrae superioris muscle Orbicularis oculi muscle Superior tarsal plate **P** Upper Eyelid, Left *See N Upper Eyelid, Right*	**Q** Lower Eyelid, Right Inferior tarsal plate Medial canthus **R** Lower Eyelid, Left *See Q Lower Eyelid, Right*	**Ø** Open **3** Percutaneous **X** External	**Z** No Device	**X** Diagnostic **Z** No Qualifier
X Lacrimal Duct, Right Lacrimal canaliculus Lacrimal punctum Lacrimal sac Nasolacrimal duct	**Y** Lacrimal Duct, Left *See X Lacrimal Duct, Right*	**Ø** Open **3** Percutaneous **7** Via Natural or Artificial Opening **8** Via Natural or Artificial Opening Endoscopic	**Ø** Drainage Device	**Z** No Qualifier
X Lacrimal Duct, Right Lacrimal canaliculus Lacrimal punctum Lacrimal sac Nasolacrimal duct	**Y** Lacrimal Duct, Left *See X Lacrimal Duct, Right*	**Ø** Open **3** Percutaneous **7** Via Natural or Artificial Opening **8** Via Natural or Artificial Opening Endoscopic	**Z** No Device	**X** Diagnostic **Z** No Qualifier

Non-OR Ø89[N,P,Q,R]ØZZ
Non-OR Ø89[N,P,Q,R][3,X]Z[X,Z]

Ø Medical and Surgical
8 Eye
B Excision

Definition: Cutting out or off, without replacement, a portion of a body part

Explanation: The qualifier DIAGNOSTIC is used to identify excision procedures that are biopsies

Body Part Character 4		Approach Character 5	Device Character 6	Qualifier Character 7
Ø Eye, Right Ciliary body Posterior chamber **1** Eye, Left *See Ø Eye, Right* **N** Upper Eyelid, Right Lateral canthus Levator palpebrae superioris muscle Orbicularis oculi muscle Superior tarsal plate	**P** Upper Eyelid, Left *See N Upper Eyelid, Right* **Q** Lower Eyelid, Right Inferior tarsal plate Medial canthus **R** Lower Eyelid, Left *See Q Lower Eyelid, Right*	**Ø** Open **3** Percutaneous **X** External	**Z** No Device	**X** Diagnostic **Z** No Qualifier
4 Vitreous, Right Vitreous body **5** Vitreous, Left *See 4 Vitreous, Right* **C** Iris, Right **D** Iris, Left **E** Retina, Right Fovea Macula Optic disc	**F** Retina, Left *See E Retina, Right* **J** Lens, Right Zonule of Zinn **K** Lens, Left *See J Lens, Right*	**3** Percutaneous	**Z** No Device	**X** Diagnostic **Z** No Qualifier
6 Sclera, Right **7** Sclera, Left **8** Cornea, Right **9** Cornea, Left	**S** Conjunctiva, Right Plica semilunaris **T** Conjunctiva, Left *See S Conjunctiva, Right*	**X** External	**Z** No Device	**X** Diagnostic **Z** No Qualifier
A Choroid, Right **B** Choroid, Left **L** Extraocular Muscle, Right Inferior oblique muscle Inferior rectus muscle Lateral rectus muscle Medial rectus muscle Superior oblique muscle Superior rectus muscle	**M** Extraocular Muscle, Left *See L Extraocular Muscle, Right* **V** Lacrimal Gland, Right **W** Lacrimal Gland, Left	**Ø** Open **3** Percutaneous	**Z** No Device	**X** Diagnostic **Z** No Qualifier
X Lacrimal Duct, Right Lacrimal canaliculus Lacrimal punctum Lacrimal sac Nasolacrimal duct	**Y** Lacrimal Duct, Left *See X Lacrimal Duct, Right*	**Ø** Open **3** Percutaneous **7** Via Natural or Artificial Opening **8** Via Natural or Artificial Opening Endoscopic	**Z** No Device	**X** Diagnostic **Z** No Qualifier

Ø Medical and Surgical
8 Eye
C Extirpation   Definition: Taking or cutting out solid matter from a body part

Explanation: The solid matter may be an abnormal byproduct of a biological function or a foreign body; it may be imbedded in a body part or in the lumen of a tubular body part. The solid matter may or may not have been previously broken into pieces.

Body Part Character 4	Approach Character 5	Device Character 6	Qualifier Character 7
Ø Eye, Right Ciliary body Posterior chamber **1 Eye, Left** *See Ø Eye, Right* **6 Sclera, Right** **7 Sclera, Left** **8 Cornea, Right** **9 Cornea, Left** **S Conjunctiva, Right** Plica semilunaris **T Conjunctiva, Left** *See S Conjunctiva, Right*	**X** External	**Z** No Device	**Z** No Qualifier
2 Anterior Chamber, Right Aqueous humour **3 Anterior Chamber, Left** *See 2 Anterior Chamber, Right* **4 Vitreous, Right** Vitreous body **5 Vitreous, Left** *See 4 Vitreous, Right* **C Iris, Right** **D Iris, Left** **E Retina, Right** Fovea Macula Optic disc **F Retina, Left** *See E Retina, Right* **G Retinal Vessel, Right** **H Retinal Vessel, Left** **J Lens, Right** Zonule of Zinn **K Lens, Left** *See J Lens, Right*	**3** Percutaneous **X** External	**Z** No Device	**Z** No Qualifier
A Choroid, Right **B Choroid, Left** **L Extraocular Muscle, Right** Inferior oblique muscle Inferior rectus muscle Lateral rectus muscle Medial rectus muscle Superior oblique muscle Superior rectus muscle **M Extraocular Muscle, Left** *See L Extraocular Muscle, Right* **N Upper Eyelid, Right** Lateral canthus Levator palpebrae superioris muscle Orbicularis oculi muscle Superior tarsal plate **P Upper Eyelid, Left** *See N Upper Eyelid, Right* **Q Lower Eyelid, Right** Inferior tarsal plate Medial canthus **R Lower Eyelid, Left** *See Q Lower Eyelid, Right* **V Lacrimal Gland, Right** **W Lacrimal Gland, Left**	**Ø** Open **3** Percutaneous **X** External	**Z** No Device	**Z** No Qualifier
X Lacrimal Duct, Right Lacrimal canaliculus Lacrimal punctum Lacrimal sac Nasolacrimal duct **Y Lacrimal Duct, Left** *See X Lacrimal Duct, Right*	**Ø** Open **3** Percutaneous **7** Via Natural or Artificial Opening **8** Via Natural or Artificial Opening Endoscopic	**Z** No Device	**Z** No Qualifier

Non-OR   Ø8C[Ø,1,6,7,S,T]XZZ
Non-OR   Ø8C[2,3]XZZ
Non-OR   Ø8C[N,P,Q,R][Ø,3,X]ZZ

NC Noncovered Procedure   LC Limited Coverage   QA Questionable OB Admit   NT New Tech Add-on   ⊞ Combination Member   ♂ Male   ♀ Female

Ø   Medical and Surgical
8   Eye
D   Extraction   Definition: Pulling or stripping out or off all or a portion of a body part by the use of force
                        Explanation: The qualifier DIAGNOSTIC is used to identify extraction procedures that are biopsies

Body Part Character 4	Approach Character 5	Device Character 6	Qualifier Character 7
8 Cornea, Right 9 Cornea, Left	X External	Z No Device	X Diagnostic Z No Qualifier
J Lens, Right Zonule of Zinn K Lens, Left *See J Lens, Right*	3 Percutaneous	Z No Device	Z No Qualifier

Ø   Medical and Surgical
8   Eye
F   Fragmentation   Definition: Breaking solid matter in a body part into pieces
                        Explanation: Physical force (e.g., manual, ultrasonic) applied directly or indirectly is used to break the solid matter into pieces. The solid matter may be an abnormal byproduct of a biological function or a foreign body. The pieces of solid matter are not taken out.

Body Part Character 4	Approach Character 5	Device Character 6	Qualifier Character 7
4 Vitreous, Right NC Vitreous body 5 Vitreous, Left NC *See 4 Vitreous, Right*	3 Percutaneous X External	Z No Device	Z No Qualifier

Non-OR	Ø8F[4,5]XZZ
NC	Ø8F[4,5]XZZ

Ø   Medical and Surgical
8   Eye
H   Insertion   Definition: Putting in a nonbiological appliance that monitors, assists, performs, or prevents a physiological function but does not physically take the place of a body part
                        Explanation: None

Body Part Character 4	Approach Character 5	Device Character 6	Qualifier Character 7
Ø Eye, Right Ciliary body Posterior chamber 1 Eye, Left *See Ø Eye, Right*	Ø Open	5 Epiretinal Visual Prosthesis Y Other Device	Z No Qualifier
Ø Eye, Right Ciliary body Posterior chamber 1 Eye, Left *See Ø Eye, Right*	3 Percutaneous	1 Radioactive Element 3 Infusion Device Y Other Device	Z No Qualifier
Ø Eye, Right Ciliary body Posterior chamber 1 Eye, Left *See Ø Eye, Right*	7 Via Natural or Artificial Opening 8 Via Natural or Artificial Opening Endoscopic	Y Other Device	Z No Qualifier
Ø Eye, Right Ciliary body Posterior chamber 1 Eye, Left *See Ø Eye, Right*	X External	1 Radioactive Element 3 Infusion Device	Z No Qualifier

Non-OR	Ø8H[Ø,1]3YZ
Non-OR	Ø8H[Ø,1][7,8]YZ

0   **Medical and Surgical**
8   **Eye**
J   **Inspection**   Definition: Visually and/or manually exploring a body part

                   Explanation: Visual exploration may be performed with or without optical instrumentation. Manual exploration may be performed directly or through intervening body layers.

Body Part Character 4	Approach Character 5	Device Character 6	Qualifier Character 7

0   **Eye, Right**
    Ciliary body
    Posterior chamber
1   **Eye, Left**
    See 0 Eye, Right
J   **Lens, Right**
    Zonule of Zinn
K   **Lens, Left**
    See J Lens, Right
	X External	**Z** No Device	**Z** No Qualifier

L   **Extraocular Muscle, Right**
    Inferior oblique muscle
    Inferior rectus muscle
    Lateral rectus muscle
    Medial rectus muscle
    Superior oblique muscle
    Superior rectus muscle
M   **Extraocular Muscle, Left**
    See L Extraocular Muscle, Right
	0 Open
	X External
		Z No Device	**Z** No Qualifier

Non-OR   08J[0,1,J,K]XZZ
Non-OR   08J[L,M]XZZ

0   **Medical and Surgical**
8   **Eye**
L   **Occlusion**   Definition: Completely closing an orifice or the lumen of a tubular body part

                   Explanation: The orifice can be a natural orifice or an artificially created orifice

Body Part Character 4	Approach Character 5	Device Character 6	Qualifier Character 7

X   **Lacrimal Duct, Right**
    Lacrimal canaliculus
    Lacrimal punctum
    Lacrimal sac
    Nasolacrimal duct
Y   **Lacrimal Duct, Left**
    See X Lacrimal Duct, Right
	0 Open
	3 Percutaneous
		C Extraluminal Device
		D Intraluminal Device
		Z No Device
			Z No Qualifier

X   **Lacrimal Duct, Right**
    Lacrimal canaliculus
    Lacrimal punctum
    Lacrimal sac
    Nasolacrimal duct
Y   **Lacrimal Duct, Left**
    See X Lacrimal Duct, Right
	7 Via Natural or Artificial Opening
	8 Via Natural or Artificial Opening Endoscopic
		D Intraluminal Device
		Z No Device
			Z No Qualifier

0   **Medical and Surgical**
8   **Eye**
M   **Reattachment**   Definition: Putting back in or on all or a portion of a separated body part to its normal location or other suitable location

                   Explanation: Vascular circulation and nervous pathways may or may not be reestablished

Body Part Character 4	Approach Character 5	Device Character 6	Qualifier Character 7

N   **Upper Eyelid, Right**
    Lateral canthus
    Levator palpebrae superioris muscle
    Orbicularis oculi muscle
    Superior tarsal plate
P   **Upper Eyelid, Left**
    See N Upper Eyelid, Right
Q   **Lower Eyelid, Right**
    Inferior tarsal plate
    Medial canthus
R   **Lower Eyelid, Left**
    See Q Lower Eyelid, Right
	X External	**Z** No Device	**Z** No Qualifier

NC Noncovered Procedure   **LC** Limited Coverage   **QA** Questionable OB Admit   **NT** New Tech Add-on   ✚ Combination Member   ♂ Male   ♀ Female

ICD-10-PCS 2022

309

08J–08M

Ø   **Medical and Surgical**
8   **Eye**
N   **Release**   Definition: Freeing a body part from an abnormal physical constraint by cutting or by the use of force
                     Explanation: Some of the restraining tissue may be taken out but none of the body part is taken out

Body Part Character 4	Approach Character 5	Device Character 6	Qualifier Character 7
Ø **Eye, Right** Ciliary body Posterior chamber **1** **Eye, Left** *See Ø Eye, Right* **6** **Sclera, Right** **7** **Sclera, Left** **8** **Cornea, Right** **9** **Cornea, Left** **S** **Conjunctiva, Right** Plica semilunaris **T** **Conjunctiva, Left** *See S Conjunctiva, Right*	**X** External	**Z** No Device	**Z** No Qualifier
2 **Anterior Chamber, Right** Aqueous humour **3** **Anterior Chamber, Left** *See 2 Anterior Chamber, Right* **4** **Vitreous, Right** Vitreous body **5** **Vitreous, Left** *See 4 Vitreous, Right* **C** **Iris, Right** **D** **Iris, Left** **E** **Retina, Right** Fovea Macula Optic disc **F** **Retina, Left** *See E Retina, Right* **G** **Retinal Vessel, Right** **H** **Retinal Vessel, Left** **J** **Lens, Right** Zonule of Zinn **K** **Lens, Left** *See J Lens, Right*	**3** Percutaneous	**Z** No Device	**Z** No Qualifier
A **Choroid, Right** **B** **Choroid, Left** **L** **Extraocular Muscle, Right** Inferior oblique muscle Inferior rectus muscle Lateral rectus muscle Medial rectus muscle Superior oblique muscle Superior rectus muscle **M** **Extraocular Muscle, Left** *See L Extraocular Muscle, Right* **V** **Lacrimal Gland, Right** **W** **Lacrimal Gland, Left**	**Ø** Open **3** Percutaneous	**Z** No Device	**Z** No Qualifier
N **Upper Eyelid, Right** Lateral canthus Levator palpebrae superioris muscle Orbicularis oculi muscle Superior tarsal plate **P** **Upper Eyelid, Left** *See N Upper Eyelid, Right* **Q** **Lower Eyelid, Right** Inferior tarsal plate Medial canthus **R** **Lower Eyelid, Left** *See Q Lower Eyelid, Right*	**Ø** Open **3** Percutaneous **X** External	**Z** No Device	**Z** No Qualifier
X **Lacrimal Duct, Right** Lacrimal canaliculus Lacrimal punctum Lacrimal sac Nasolacrimal duct **Y** **Lacrimal Duct, Left** *See X Lacrimal Duct, Right*	**Ø** Open **3** Percutaneous **7** Via Natural or Artificial Opening **8** Via Natural or Artificial Opening Endoscopic	**Z** No Device	**Z** No Qualifier

Ø   **Medical and Surgical**
8   **Eye**
P   **Removal**   Definition: Taking out or off a device from a body part

Explanation: If a device is taken out and a similar device put in without cutting or puncturing the skin or mucous membrane, the procedure is coded to the root operation CHANGE. Otherwise, the procedure for taking out a device is coded to the root operation REMOVAL.

Body Part Character 4	Approach Character 5	Device Character 6	Qualifier Character 7
Ø **Eye, Right** Ciliary body Posterior chamber **1** **Eye, Left** *See Ø Eye, Right*	**Ø** Open **3** Percutaneous **7** Via Natural or Artificial Opening **8** Via Natural or Artificial Opening Endoscopic	**Ø** Drainage Device **1** Radioactive Element **3** Infusion Device **7** Autologous Tissue Substitute **C** Extraluminal Device **D** Intraluminal Device **J** Synthetic Substitute **K** Nonautologous Tissue Substitute **Y** Other Device	**Z** No Qualifier
Ø **Eye, Right** Ciliary body Posterior chamber **1** **Eye, Left** *See Ø Eye, Right*	**X** External	**Ø** Drainage Device **1** Radioactive Element **3** Infusion Device **7** Autologous Tissue Substitute **C** Extraluminal Device **D** Intraluminal Device **J** Synthetic Substitute **K** Nonautologous Tissue Substitute	**Z** No Qualifier
J **Lens, Right** Zonule of Zinn **K** **Lens, Left** *See J Lens, Right*	**3** Percutaneous	**J** Synthetic Substitute **Y** Other Device	**Z** No Qualifier
L **Extraocular Muscle, Right** Inferior oblique muscle Inferior rectus muscle Lateral rectus muscle Medial rectus muscle Superior oblique muscle Superior rectus muscle **M** **Extraocular Muscle, Left** *See L Extraocular Muscle, Right*	**Ø** Open **3** Percutaneous	**Ø** Drainage Device **7** Autologous Tissue Substitute **J** Synthetic Substitute **K** Nonautologous Tissue Substitute **Y** Other Device	**Z** No Qualifier

Non-OR	08P[Ø,1]3YZ
Non-OR	08P[Ø,1][7,8][Ø,3,D,Y]Z
Non-OR	08P[Ø,1]X[Ø,1,3,C,D,J]Z
Non-OR	08P[J,K]3YZ
Non-OR	08P[L,M]3YZ

Ø Medical and Surgical
8 Eye
Q Repair   Definition: Restoring, to the extent possible, a body part to its normal anatomic structure and function
                Explanation: Used only when the method to accomplish the repair is not one of the other root operations

Body Part Character 4	Approach Character 5	Device Character 6	Qualifier Character 7

Ø Eye, Right
  Ciliary body
  Posterior chamber
1 Eye, Left
  See Ø Eye, Right
6 Sclera, Right
7 Sclera, Left
8 Cornea, Right   `NC`
9 Cornea, Left   `NC`
S Conjunctiva, Right
  Plica semilunaris
T Conjunctiva, Left
  See S Conjunctiva, Right
	X External	**Z No Device**	**Z No Qualifier**

2 Anterior Chamber, Right
  Aqueous humour
3 Anterior Chamber, Left
  See 2 Anterior Chamber, Right
4 Vitreous, Right
  Vitreous body
5 Vitreous, Left
  See 4 Vitreous, Right
C Iris, Right
D Iris, Left
E Retina, Right
  Fovea
  Macula
  Optic disc
F Retina, Left
  See E Retina, Right
G Retinal Vessel, Right
H Retinal Vessel, Left
J Lens, Right
  Zonule of Zinn
K Lens, Left
  See J Lens, Right
	3 Percutaneous	**Z No Device**	**Z No Qualifier**

A Choroid, Right
B Choroid, Left
L Extraocular Muscle, Right
  Inferior oblique muscle
  Inferior rectus muscle
  Lateral rectus muscle
  Medial rectus muscle
  Superior oblique muscle
  Superior rectus muscle
M Extraocular Muscle, Left
  See L Extraocular Muscle, Right
V Lacrimal Gland, Right
W Lacrimal Gland, Left
	Ø Open
	3 Percutaneous
		Z No Device	**Z No Qualifier**

N Upper Eyelid, Right
  Lateral canthus
  Levator palpebrae superioris muscle
  Orbicularis oculi muscle
  Superior tarsal plate
P Upper Eyelid, Left
  See N Upper Eyelid, Right
Q Lower Eyelid, Right
  Inferior tarsal plate
  Medial canthus
R Lower Eyelid, Left
  See Q Lower Eyelid, Right
	Ø Open
	3 Percutaneous
	X External
		Z No Device	**Z No Qualifier**

X Lacrimal Duct, Right
  Lacrimal canaliculus
  Lacrimal punctum
  Lacrimal sac
  Nasolacrimal duct
Y Lacrimal Duct, Left
  See X Lacrimal Duct, Right
	Ø Open
	3 Percutaneous
	7 Via Natural or Artificial Opening
	8 Via Natural or Artificial Opening Endoscopic
		Z No Device	**Z No Qualifier**

Non-OR   Ø8Q[N,P,Q,R][Ø,3,X]ZZ
`NC`   Ø8Q[8,9]XZZ

Non-OR Procedure   DRG Non-OR Procedure   Valid OR Procedure   HAC Associated Procedure   Combination Only   New/Revised GREEN

Ø　Medical and Surgical
8　Eye
R　Replacement　Definition: Putting in or on biological or synthetic material that physically takes the place and/or function of all or a portion of a body part

Explanation: The body part may have been taken out or replaced, or may be taken out, physically eradicated, or rendered nonfunctional during the REPLACEMENT procedure. A REMOVAL procedure is coded for taking out the device used in a previous replacement procedure.

Body Part Character 4	Approach Character 5	Device Character 6	Qualifier Character 7
Ø　Eye, Right 　　Ciliary body 　　Posterior chamber 1　Eye, Left 　　See Ø Eye, Right A　Choroid, Right B　Choroid, Left	Ø　Open 3　Percutaneous	7　Autologous Tissue Substitute J　Synthetic Substitute K　Nonautologous Tissue Substitute	Z　No Qualifier
4　Vitreous, Right 　　Vitreous body 5　Vitreous, Left 　　See 4 Vitreous, Right C　Iris, Right D　Iris, Left G　Retinal Vessel, Right H　Retinal Vessel, Left	3　Percutaneous	7　Autologous Tissue Substitute J　Synthetic Substitute K　Nonautologous Tissue Substitute	Z　No Qualifier
6　Sclera, Right 7　Sclera, Left S　Conjunctiva, Right 　　Plica semilunaris T　Conjunctiva, Left 　　See S Conjunctiva, Right	X　External	7　Autologous Tissue Substitute J　Synthetic Substitute K　Nonautologous Tissue Substitute	Z　No Qualifier
8　Cornea, Right 9　Cornea, Left	3　Percutaneous X　External	7　Autologous Tissue Substitute J　Synthetic Substitute K　Nonautologous Tissue Substitute	Z　No Qualifier
J　Lens, Right 　　Zonule of Zinn K　Lens, Left 　　See J Lens, Right	3　Percutaneous	Ø　Synthetic Substitute, Intraocular Telescope 7　Autologous Tissue Substitute J　Synthetic Substitute K　Nonautologous Tissue Substitute	Z　No Qualifier
N　Upper Eyelid, Right 　　Lateral canthus 　　Levator palpebrae superioris muscle 　　Orbicularis oculi muscle 　　Superior tarsal plate P　Upper Eyelid, Left 　　See N Upper Eyelid, Right Q　Lower Eyelid, Right 　　Inferior tarsal plate 　　Medial canthus R　Lower Eyelid, Left 　　See Q Lower Eyelid, Right	Ø　Open 3　Percutaneous X　External	7　Autologous Tissue Substitute J　Synthetic Substitute K　Nonautologous Tissue Substitute	Z　No Qualifier
X　Lacrimal Duct, Right 　　Lacrimal canaliculus 　　Lacrimal punctum 　　Lacrimal sac 　　Nasolacrimal duct Y　Lacrimal Duct, Left 　　See X Lacrimal Duct, Right	Ø　Open 3　Percutaneous 7　Via Natural or Artificial Opening 8　Via Natural or Artificial Opening Endoscopic	7　Autologous Tissue Substitute J　Synthetic Substitute K　Nonautologous Tissue Substitute	Z　No Qualifier

NC Noncovered Procedure　　LC Limited Coverage　　QA Questionable OB Admit　　NT New Tech Add-on　　⊞ Combination Member　　♂ Male　　♀ Female

ICD-10-PCS 2022　　　　　　　　　　　　　　　　　　　　　　　　　　　　　　　　313

08R–08R

Ø   Medical and Surgical
8   Eye
S   Reposition   Definition: Moving to its normal location, or other suitable location, all or a portion of a body part

Explanation: The body part is moved to a new location from an abnormal location, or from a normal location where it is not functioning correctly. The body part may or may not be cut out or off to be moved to the new location.

Body Part Character 4	Approach Character 5	Device Character 6	Qualifier Character 7

C Iris, Right
D Iris, Left
G Retinal Vessel, Right
H Retinal Vessel, Left
J Lens, Right
  Zonule of Zinn
K Lens, Left
  See J Lens, Right
	3 Percutaneous	**Z** No Device	**Z** No Qualifier

L Extraocular Muscle, Right
  Inferior oblique muscle
  Inferior rectus muscle
  Lateral rectus muscle
  Medial rectus muscle
  Superior oblique muscle
  Superior rectus muscle
M Extraocular Muscle, Left
  See L Extraocular Muscle, Right
V Lacrimal Gland, Right
W Lacrimal Gland, Left
	Ø Open
	3 Percutaneous
		Z No Device	**Z** No Qualifier

N Upper Eyelid, Right
  Lateral canthus
  Levator palpebrae superioris muscle
  Orbicularis oculi muscle
  Superior tarsal plate
P Upper Eyelid, Left
  See N Upper Eyelid, Right
Q Lower Eyelid, Right
  Inferior tarsal plate
  Medial canthus
R Lower Eyelid, Left
  See Q Lower Eyelid, Right
	Ø Open
	3 Percutaneous
	X External
		Z No Device	**Z** No Qualifier

X Lacrimal Duct, Right
  Lacrimal canaliculus
  Lacrimal punctum
  Lacrimal sac
  Nasolacrimal duct
Y Lacrimal Duct, Left
  See X Lacrimal Duct, Right
	Ø Open
	3 Percutaneous
	7 Via Natural or Artificial Opening
	8 Via Natural or Artificial Opening Endoscopic
		Z No Device	**Z** No Qualifier

Non-OR Procedure   DRG Non-OR Procedure   Valid OR Procedure   HAC Associated Procedure   Combination Only   New/Revised GREEN
314   ICD-10-PCS 2022

08S–08S

0 Medical and Surgical
8 Eye
T Resection　　Definition: Cutting out or off, without replacement, all of a body part
　　　　　　Explanation: None

Body Part Character 4	Approach Character 5	Device Character 6	Qualifier Character 7
0 Eye, Right 　Ciliary body 　Posterior chamber **1** Eye, Left 　*See 0 Eye, Right* **8** Cornea, Right **9** Cornea, Left	**X** External	**Z** No Device	**Z** No Qualifier
4 Vitreous, Right 　Vitreous body **5** Vitreous, Left 　*See 4 Vitreous, Right* **C** Iris, Right **D** Iris, Left **J** Lens, Right 　Zonule of Zinn **K** Lens, Left 　*See J Lens, Right*	**3** Percutaneous	**Z** No Device	**Z** No Qualifier
L Extraocular Muscle, Right 　Inferior oblique muscle 　Inferior rectus muscle 　Lateral rectus muscle 　Medial rectus muscle 　Superior oblique muscle 　Superior rectus muscle **M** Extraocular Muscle, Left 　*See L Extraocular Muscle, Right* **V** Lacrimal Gland, Right **W** Lacrimal Gland, Left	**0** Open **3** Percutaneous	**Z** No Device	**Z** No Qualifier
N Upper Eyelid, Right 　Lateral canthus 　Levator palpebrae superioris muscle 　Orbicularis oculi muscle 　Superior tarsal plate **P** Upper Eyelid, Left 　*See N Upper Eyelid, Right* **Q** Lower Eyelid, Right 　Inferior tarsal plate 　Medial canthus **R** Lower Eyelid, Left 　*See Q Lower Eyelid, Right*	**0** Open **X** External	**Z** No Device	**Z** No Qualifier
X Lacrimal Duct, Right 　Lacrimal canaliculus 　Lacrimal punctum 　Lacrimal sac 　Nasolacrimal duct **Y** Lacrimal Duct, Left 　*See X Lacrimal Duct, Right*	**0** Open **3** Percutaneous **7** Via Natural or Artificial Opening **8** Via Natural or Artificial Opening Endoscopic	**Z** No Device	**Z** No Qualifier

NC Noncovered Procedure　　LC Limited Coverage　　OA Questionable OB Admit　　NT New Tech Add-on　　⊞ Combination Member　　♂ Male　　♀ Female

ICD-10-PCS 2022　　　　　315

08T–08T

Ø Medical and Surgical
8 Eye
U Supplement Definition: Putting in or on biological or synthetic material that physically reinforces and/or augments the function of a portion of a body part

Explanation: The biological material is non-living, or is living and from the same individual. The body part may have been previously replaced, and the SUPPLEMENT procedure is performed to physically reinforce and/or augment the function of the replaced body part.

Body Part Character 4	Approach Character 5	Device Character 6	Qualifier Character 7
Ø Eye, Right Ciliary body Posterior chamber 1 Eye, Left See Ø Eye, Right C Iris, Right D Iris, Left E Retina, Right Fovea Macula Optic disc F Retina, Left See E Retina, Right G Retinal Vessel, Right H Retinal Vessel, Left L Extraocular Muscle, Right Inferior oblique muscle Inferior rectus muscle Lateral rectus muscle Medial rectus muscle Superior oblique muscle Superior rectus muscle M Extraocular Muscle, Left See L Extraocular Muscle, Right	Ø Open 3 Percutaneous	7 Autologous Tissue Substitute J Synthetic Substitute K Nonautologous Tissue Substitute	Z No Qualifier
8 Cornea, Right **NC** 9 Cornea, Left **NC** N Upper Eyelid, Right Lateral canthus Levator palpebrae superioris muscle Orbicularis oculi muscle Superior tarsal plate P Upper Eyelid, Left See N Upper Eyelid, Right Q Lower Eyelid, Right Inferior tarsal plate Medial canthus R Lower Eyelid, Left See Q Lower Eyelid, Right	Ø Open 3 Percutaneous X External	7 Autologous Tissue Substitute J Synthetic Substitute K Nonautologous Tissue Substitute	Z No Qualifier
X Lacrimal Duct, Right Lacrimal canaliculus Lacrimal punctum Lacrimal sac Nasolacrimal duct Y Lacrimal Duct, Left See X Lacrimal Duct, Right	Ø Open 3 Percutaneous 7 Via Natural or Artificial Opening 8 Via Natural or Artificial Opening Endoscopic	7 Autologous Tissue Substitute J Synthetic Substitute K Nonautologous Tissue Substitute	Z No Qualifier

NC Ø8U[8,9][Ø,3,X]KZ

Ø Medical and Surgical
8 Eye
V Restriction Definition: Partially closing an orifice or the lumen of a tubular body part

Explanation: The orifice can be a natural orifice or an artificially created orifice

Body Part Character 4	Approach Character 5	Device Character 6	Qualifier Character 7
X Lacrimal Duct, Right Lacrimal canaliculus Lacrimal punctum Lacrimal sac Nasolacrimal duct Y Lacrimal Duct, Left See X Lacrimal Duct, Right	Ø Open 3 Percutaneous	C Extraluminal Device D Intraluminal Device Z No Device	Z No Qualifier
X Lacrimal Duct, Right Lacrimal canaliculus Lacrimal punctum Lacrimal sac Nasolacrimal duct Y Lacrimal Duct, Left See X Lacrimal Duct, Right	7 Via Natural or Artificial Opening 8 Via Natural or Artificial Opening Endoscopic	D Intraluminal Device Z No Device	Z No Qualifier

0   **Medical and Surgical**
8   **Eye**
W   **Revision**   Definition: Correcting, to the extent possible, a portion of a malfunctioning device or the position of a displaced device

                 Explanation: Revision can include correcting a malfunctioning or displaced device by taking out or putting in components of the device such as a screw or pin

Body Part Character 4	Approach Character 5	Device Character 6	Qualifier Character 7

0 Eye, Right
  Ciliary body
  Posterior chamber
1 Eye, Left
  See 0 Eye, Right
	0 Open
	3 Percutaneous
	7 Via Natural or Artificial Opening
	8 Via Natural or Artificial Opening Endoscopic
		0 Drainage Device
		3 Infusion Device
		7 Autologous Tissue Substitute
		C Extraluminal Device
		D Intraluminal Device
		J Synthetic Substitute
		K Nonautologous Tissue Substitute
		Y Other Device
			Z No Qualifier

0 Eye, Right
  Ciliary body
  Posterior chamber
1 Eye, Left
  See 0 Eye, Right
	X External	**0** Drainage Device
		3 Infusion Device
		7 Autologous Tissue Substitute
		C Extraluminal Device
		D Intraluminal Device
		J Synthetic Substitute
		K Nonautologous Tissue Substitute
			Z No Qualifier

J Lens, Right
  Zonule of Zinn
K Lens, Left
  See J Lens, Right
	3 Percutaneous	**J** Synthetic Substitute
		Y Other Device
			Z No Qualifier

J Lens, Right
  Zonule of Zinn
K Lens, Left
  See J Lens, Right
	X External	**J** Synthetic Substitute	**Z** No Qualifier

L Extraocular Muscle, Right
  Inferior oblique muscle
  Inferior rectus muscle
  Lateral rectus muscle
  Medial rectus muscle
  Superior oblique muscle
  Superior rectus muscle
M Extraocular Muscle, Left
  See L Extraocular Muscle, Right
	0 Open
	3 Percutaneous
		0 Drainage Device
		7 Autologous Tissue Substitute
		J Synthetic Substitute
		K Nonautologous Tissue Substitute
		Y Other Device
			Z No Qualifier

Non-OR	08W[0,1][3,7,8]YZ
Non-OR	08W[0,1]X[0,3,7,C,D,J,K]Z
Non-OR	08W[J,K]3YZ
Non-OR	08W[J,K]XJZ
Non-OR	08W[L,M]3YZ

0   **Medical and Surgical**
8   **Eye**
X   **Transfer**   Definition: Moving, without taking out, all or a portion of a body part to another location to take over the function of all or a portion of a body part

                 Explanation: The body part transferred remains connected to its vascular and nervous supply

Body Part Character 4	Approach Character 5	Device Character 6	Qualifier Character 7

L Extraocular Muscle, Right
  Inferior oblique muscle
  Inferior rectus muscle
  Lateral rectus muscle
  Medial rectus muscle
  Superior oblique muscle
  Superior rectus muscle
M Extraocular Muscle, Left
  See L Extraocular Muscle, Right
	0 Open
	3 Percutaneous
		Z No Device	**Z** No Qualifier

Ear, Nose, Sinus Ø9Ø–Ø9W

Character Meanings*

This Character Meaning table is provided as a guide to assist the user in the identification of character members that may be found in this section of code tables. It **SHOULD NOT** be used to build a PCS code.

Operation–Character 3		Body Part–Character 4		Approach–Character 5		Device–Character 6		Qualifier–Character 7	
Ø	Alteration	Ø	External Ear, Right	Ø	Open	Ø	Drainage Device	Ø	Endolymphatic
1	Bypass	1	External Ear, Left	3	Percutaneous	1	Radioactive Element	X	Diagnostic
2	Change	2	External Ear, Bilateral	4	Percutaneous Endoscopic	4	Hearing Device, Bone Conduction	Z	No Qualifier
3	Control	3	External Auditory Canal, Right	7	Via Natural or Artificial Opening	5	Hearing Device, Single Channel Cochlear Prosthesis		
5	Destruction	4	External Auditory Canal, Left	8	Via Natural or Artificial Opening Endoscopic	6	Hearing Device, Multiple Channel Cochlear Prosthesis		
7	Dilation	5	Middle Ear, Right	X	External	7	Autologous Tissue Substitute		
8	Division	6	Middle Ear, Left			B	Intraluminal Device, Airway		
9	Drainage	7	Tympanic Membrane, Right			D	Intraluminal Device		
B	Excision	8	Tympanic Membrane, Left			J	Synthetic Substitute		
C	Extirpation	9	Auditory Ossicle, Right			K	Nonautologous Tissue Substitute		
D	Extraction	A	Auditory Ossicle, Left			S	Hearing Device		
H	Insertion	B	Mastoid Sinus, Right			Y	Other Device		
J	Inspection	C	Mastoid Sinus, Left			Z	No Device		
M	Reattachment	D	Inner Ear, Right						
N	Release	E	Inner Ear, Left						
P	Removal	F	Eustachian Tube, Right						
Q	Repair	G	Eustachian Tube, Left						
R	Replacement	H	Ear, Right						
S	Reposition	J	Ear, Left						
T	Resection	K	Nasal Mucosa and Soft Tissue						
U	Supplement	L	Nasal Turbinate						
W	Revision	M	Nasal Septum						
		N	Nasopharynx						
		P	Accessory Sinus						
		Q	Maxillary Sinus, Right						
		R	Maxillary Sinus, Left						
		S	Frontal Sinus, Right						
		T	Frontal Sinus, Left						
		U	Ethmoid Sinus, Right						
		V	Ethmoid Sinus, Left						
		W	Sphenoid Sinus, Right						
		X	Sphenoid Sinus, Left						
		Y	Sinus						

* Includes sinus ducts.

AHA Coding Clinic for table Ø93
2018, 4Q, 38   Control of epistaxis

AHA Coding Clinic for table Ø95
2018, 1Q, 19   Control of epistaxis via silver nitrate cauterization

AHA Coding Clinic for table Ø9H
2020, 4Q, 43-44   Insertion of radioactive element

AHA Coding Clinic for table Ø9Q
2018, 1Q, 19   Control of epistaxis via silver nitrate cauterization
2017, 4Q, 106   Control of bleeding of external naris using suture
2014, 4Q, 20   Control of epistaxis
2014, 3Q, 22   Transsphenoidal removal of pituitary tumor and fat graft placement
2013, 4Q, 114   Balloon sinuplasty

AHA Coding Clinic for table Ø9U
2019, 4Q, 28-29   Sinus supplement

Ear Anatomy

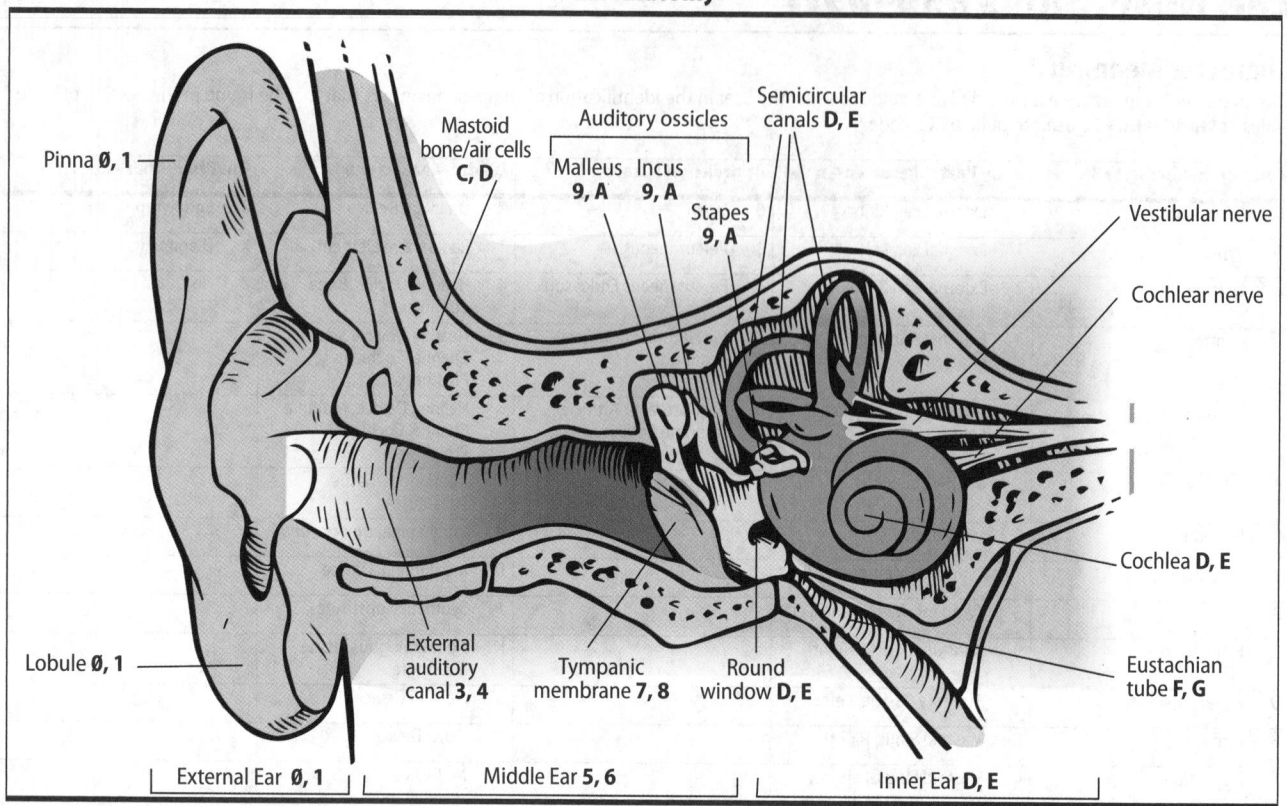

Pinna Ø, 1

Mastoid bone/air cells **C, D**

Auditory ossicles

Malleus **9, A**

Incus **9, A**

Stapes **9, A**

Semicircular canals **D, E**

Vestibular nerve

Cochlear nerve

Lobule Ø, 1

External auditory canal **3, 4**

Tympanic membrane **7, 8**

Round window **D, E**

Cochlea **D, E**

Eustachian tube **F, G**

External Ear Ø, 1

Middle Ear 5, 6

Inner Ear **D, E**

Nasal Turbinates

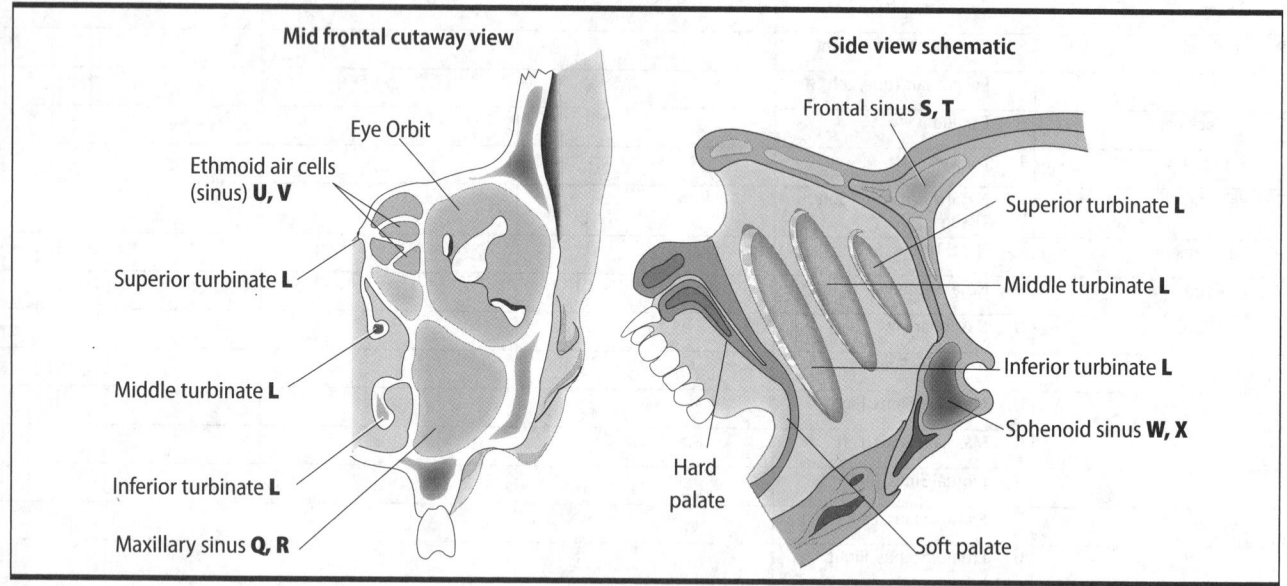

Mid frontal cutaway view

Eye Orbit

Ethmoid air cells (sinus) **U, V**

Superior turbinate **L**

Middle turbinate **L**

Inferior turbinate **L**

Maxillary sinus **Q, R**

Side view schematic

Frontal sinus **S, T**

Superior turbinate **L**

Middle turbinate **L**

Inferior turbinate **L**

Sphenoid sinus **W, X**

Hard palate

Soft palate

Paranasal Sinuses

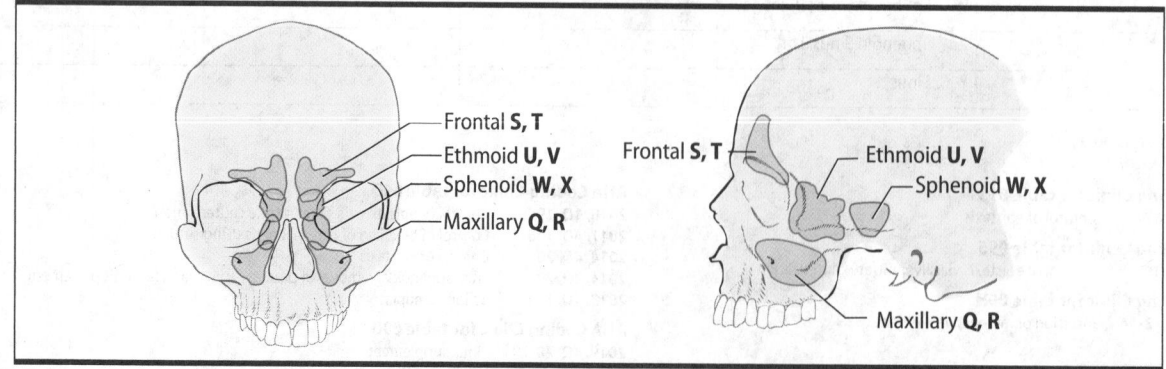

Frontal **S, T**

Ethmoid **U, V**

Sphenoid **W, X**

Maxillary **Q, R**

Frontal **S, T**

Ethmoid **U, V**

Sphenoid **W, X**

Maxillary **Q, R**

Ø   Medical and Surgical
9   Ear, Nose, Sinus
Ø   Alteration   Definition: Modifying the anatomic structure of a body part without affecting the function of the body part

                  Explanation: Principal purpose is to improve appearance

Body Part Character 4		Approach Character 5	Device Character 6	Qualifier Character 7

Ø External Ear, Right
Antihelix
Antitragus
Auricle
Earlobe
Helix
Pinna
Tragus
1 External Ear, Left
See Ø External Ear, Right
	2 External Ear, Bilateral
	See Ø External Ear, Right
	K Nasal Mucosa and Soft Tissue
	Columella
	External naris
	Greater alar cartilage
	Internal naris
	Lateral nasal cartilage
	Lesser alar cartilage
	Nasal cavity
	Nostril
		Ø Open
		3 Percutaneous
		4 Percutaneous Endoscopic
		X External
			**7 Autologous Tissue
			   Substitute**
			J Synthetic Substitute
			**K Nonautologous Tissue
			   Substitute**
			Z No Device
				Z No Qualifier

Ø   Medical and Surgical
9   Ear, Nose, Sinus
1   Bypass   Definition: Altering the route of passage of the contents of a tubular body part

                  Explanation: Rerouting contents of a body part to a downstream area of the normal route, to a similar route and body part, or to an abnormal route and dissimilar body part. Includes one or more anastomoses, with or without the use of a device.

Body Part Character 4	Approach Character 5	Device Character 6	Qualifier Character 7

D Inner Ear, Right
Bony labyrinth
Bony vestibule
Cochlea
Round window
Semicircular canal
E Inner Ear, Left
See D Inner Ear, Right
	Ø Open	**7 Autologous Tissue
		   Substitute**
		J Synthetic Substitute
		**K Nonautologous Tissue
		   Substitute**
		Z No Device
			Ø Endolymphatic

Ø   Medical and Surgical
9   Ear, Nose, Sinus
2   Change   Definition: Taking out or off a device from a body part and putting back an identical or similar device in or on the same body part without cutting or puncturing the skin or a mucous membrane

                  Explanation: All CHANGE procedures are coded using the approach EXTERNAL

Body Part Character 4	Approach Character 5	Device Character 6	Qualifier Character 7
H Ear, Right **J Ear, Left** **K Nasal Mucosa and Soft Tissue** Columella External naris Greater alar cartilage Internal naris Lateral nasal cartilage Lesser alar cartilage Nasal cavity Nostril **Y Sinus**	**X External**	**Ø Drainage Device** **Y Other Device**	**Z No Qualifier**

Non-OR   All body part, approach, device, and qualifier values

Ø   Medical and Surgical
9   Ear, Nose, Sinus
3   Control   Definition: Stopping, or attempting to stop, postprocedural or other acute bleeding

                  Explanation: None

Body Part Character 4	Approach Character 5	Device Character 6	Qualifier Character 7

K Nasal Mucosa and Soft Tissue
Columella
External naris
Greater alar cartilage
Internal naris
Lateral nasal cartilage
Lesser alar cartilage
Nasal cavity
Nostril
	**7 Via Natural or Artificial
	   Opening**
	**8 Via Natural or Artificial
	   Opening Endoscopic**
		Z No Device	**Z No Qualifier**

Non-OR   093K[7,8]ZZ

Ear, Nose, Sinus

Ø   **Medical and Surgical**
9   **Ear, Nose, Sinus**
5   **Destruction**   Definition: Physical eradication of all or a portion of a body part by the direct use of energy, force, or a destructive agent
                    Explanation: None of the body part is physically taken out

Body Part Character 4		Approach Character 5	Device Character 6	Qualifier Character 7
Ø **External Ear, Right** Antihelix Antitragus Auricle Earlobe Helix Pinna Tragus	1 **External Ear, Left** *See Ø External Ear, Right*	Ø Open 3 Percutaneous 4 Percutaneous Endoscopic X External	Z No Device	Z No Qualifier
3 **External Auditory Canal, Right** External auditory meatus	4 **External Auditory Canal, Left** *See 3 External Auditory Canal, Right*	Ø Open 3 Percutaneous 4 Percutaneous Endoscopic 7 Via Natural or Artificial Opening 8 Via Natural or Artificial Opening Endoscopic X External	Z No Device	Z No Qualifier
5 **Middle Ear, Right** Oval window Tympanic cavity 6 **Middle Ear, Left** *See 5 Middle Ear, Right* 9 **Auditory Ossicle, Right** Incus Malleus Stapes A **Auditory Ossicle, Left** *See 9 Auditory Ossicle, Right*	D **Inner Ear, Right** Bony labyrinth Bony vestibule Cochlea Round window Semicircular canal E **Inner Ear, Left** *See D Inner Ear, Right*	Ø Open 8 Via Natural or Artificial Opening Endoscopic	Z No Device	Z No Qualifier
7 **Tympanic Membrane, Right** Pars flaccida 8 **Tympanic Membrane, Left** *See 7 Tympanic Membrane, Right* F **Eustachian Tube, Right** Auditory tube Pharyngotympanic tube G **Eustachian Tube, Left** *See F Eustachian Tube, Right*	L **Nasal Turbinate** Inferior turbinate Middle turbinate Nasal concha Superior turbinate N **Nasopharynx** Choana Fossa of Rosenmuller Pharyngeal recess Rhinopharynx	Ø Open 3 Percutaneous 4 Percutaneous Endoscopic 7 Via Natural or Artificial Opening 8 Via Natural or Artificial Opening Endoscopic	Z No Device	Z No Qualifier
B **Mastoid Sinus, Right** Mastoid air cells C **Mastoid Sinus, Left** *See B Mastoid Sinus, Right* M **Nasal Septum** Quadrangular cartilage Septal cartilage Vomer bone P **Accessory Sinus** Q **Maxillary Sinus, Right** Antrum of Highmore	R **Maxillary Sinus, Left** *See Q Maxillary Sinus, Right* S **Frontal Sinus, Right** T **Frontal Sinus, Left** U **Ethmoid Sinus, Right** Ethmoidal air cell V **Ethmoid Sinus, Left** *See U Ethmoid Sinus, Right* W **Sphenoid Sinus, Right** X **Sphenoid Sinus, Left**	Ø Open 3 Percutaneous 4 Percutaneous Endoscopic 8 Via Natural or Artificial Opening Endoscopic	Z No Device	Z No Qualifier
K **Nasal Mucosa and Soft Tissue** Columella External naris Greater alar cartilage Internal naris Lateral nasal cartilage Lesser alar cartilage Nasal cavity Nostril		Ø Open 3 Percutaneous 4 Percutaneous Endoscopic 8 Via Natural or Artificial Opening Endoscopic X External	Z No Device	Z No Qualifier

Non-OR   Ø95[Ø,1][Ø,3,4,X]ZZ
Non-OR   Ø95[3,4][Ø,3,4,7,8,X]ZZ
Non-OR   Ø95[F,G][Ø,3,4,7,8]ZZ
Non-OR   Ø95M[Ø,3,4,8]ZZ
Non-OR   Ø95K[Ø,3,4,8,X]ZZ

Ø   **Medical and Surgical**
9   **Ear, Nose, Sinus**
7   **Dilation**   Definition: Expanding an orifice or the lumen of a tubular body part

Explanation: The orifice can be a natural orifice or an artificially created orifice. Accomplished by stretching a tubular body part using intraluminal pressure or by cutting part of the orifice or wall of the tubular body part.

Body Part Character 4	Approach Character 5	Device Character 6	Qualifier Character 7

F Eustachian Tube, Right
   Auditory tube
   Pharyngotympanic tube
G Eustachian Tube, Left
   See F Eustachian Tube, Right
	Ø Open
	7 Via Natural or Artificial Opening
	8 Via Natural or Artificial Opening
	   Endoscopic
		D Intraluminal Device
		Z No Device
			Z No Qualifier

F Eustachian Tube, Right
   Auditory tube
   Pharyngotympanic tube
G Eustachian Tube, Left
   See F Eustachian Tube, Right
	3 Percutaneous
	4 Percutaneous Endoscopic
		Z No Device	**Z** No Qualifier

Non-OR   All body part, approach, device, and qualifier values

Ø   **Medical and Surgical**
9   **Ear, Nose, Sinus**
8   **Division**   Definition: Cutting into a body part, without draining fluids and/or gases from the body part, in order to separate or transect a body part

Explanation: All or a portion of the body part is separated into two or more portions

Body Part Character 4	Approach Character 5	Device Character 6	Qualifier Character 7

L Nasal Turbinate
   Inferior turbinate
   Middle turbinate
   Nasal concha
   Superior turbinate
	Ø Open
	3 Percutaneous
	4 Percutaneous Endoscopic
	7 Via Natural or Artificial Opening
	8 Via Natural or Artificial Opening
	   Endoscopic
		Z No Device	**Z** No Qualifier

Ear, Nose, Sinus

Ø   **Medical and Surgical**
9   **Ear, Nose, Sinus**
9   **Drainage**   Definition: Taking or letting out fluids and/or gases from a body part
                       Explanation: The qualifier DIAGNOSTIC is used to identify drainage procedures that are biopsies

Body Part Character 4		Approach Character 5	Device Character 6	Qualifier Character 7

Ø **External Ear, Right**
  Antihelix
  Antitragus
  Auricle
  Earlobe
  Helix
  Pinna
  Tragus
	1 **External Ear, Left**
	  See Ø External Ear, Right
		Ø Open
		3 Percutaneous
		4 Percutaneous Endoscopic
		X External
			Ø Drainage Device	Z No Qualifier

Ø **External Ear, Right**
  Antihelix
  Antitragus
  Auricle
  Earlobe
  Helix
  Pinna
  Tragus
	1 **External Ear, Left**
	  See Ø External Ear, Right
		Ø Open
		3 Percutaneous
		4 Percutaneous Endoscopic
		X External
			Z No Device	X Diagnostic
				Z No Qualifier

3 **External Auditory Canal, Right**
  External auditory meatus
4 **External Auditory Canal, Left**
  See 3 External Auditory Canal, Right
	K **Nasal Mucosa and Soft Tissue**
	  Columella
	  External naris
	  Greater alar cartilage
	  Internal naris
	  Lateral nasal cartilage
	  Lesser alar cartilage
	  Nasal cavity
	  Nostril
		Ø Open
		3 Percutaneous
		4 Percutaneous Endoscopic
		7 Via Natural or Artificial Opening
		8 Via Natural or Artificial Opening Endoscopic
		X External
			Ø Drainage Device	Z No Qualifier

3 **External Auditory Canal, Right**
  External auditory meatus
4 **External Auditory Canal, Left**
  See 3 External Auditory Canal, Right
	K **Nasal Mucosa and Soft Tissue**
	  Columella
	  External naris
	  Greater alar cartilage
	  Internal naris
	  Lateral nasal cartilage
	  Lesser alar cartilage
	  Nasal cavity
	  Nostril
		Ø Open
		3 Percutaneous
		4 Percutaneous Endoscopic
		7 Via Natural or Artificial Opening
		8 Via Natural or Artificial Opening Endoscopic
		X External
			Z No Device	X Diagnostic
				Z No Qualifier

5 **Middle Ear, Right**
  Oval window
  Tympanic cavity
6 **Middle Ear, Left**
  See 5 Middle Ear, Right
9 **Auditory Ossicle, Right**
  Incus
  Malleus
  Stapes
	A **Auditory Ossicle, Left**
	  See 9 Auditory Ossicle, Right
	D **Inner Ear, Right**
	  Bony labyrinth
	  Bony vestibule
	  Cochlea
	  Round window
	  Semicircular canal
	E **Inner Ear, Left**
	  See D Inner Ear, Right
		Ø Open
		7 Via Natural or Artificial Opening
		8 Via Natural or Artificial Opening Endoscopic
			Ø Drainage Device	Z No Qualifier

5 **Middle Ear, Right**
  Oval window
  Tympanic cavity
6 **Middle Ear, Left**
  See 5 Middle Ear, Right
9 **Auditory Ossicle, Right**
  Incus
  Malleus
  Stapes
	A **Auditory Ossicle, Left**
	  See 9 Auditory Ossicle, Right
	D **Inner Ear, Right**
	  Bony labyrinth
	  Bony vestibule
	  Cochlea
	  Round window
	  Semicircular canal
	E **Inner Ear, Left**
	  See D Inner Ear, Right
		Ø Open
		7 Via Natural or Artificial Opening
		8 Via Natural or Artificial Opening Endoscopic
			Z No Device	X Diagnostic
				Z No Qualifier

Non-OR   Ø99[Ø,1][Ø,3,4,X]ØZ
Non-OR   Ø99[Ø,1][Ø,3,4,X]Z[X,Z]
Non-OR   Ø99[3,4,K][Ø,3,4,7,8,X]ØZ
Non-OR   Ø99[3,4,K][Ø,3,4,7,8,X]Z[X,Z]
Non-OR   Ø99[5,6]8ØZ
Non-OR   Ø99[9,A,D,E][7,8]ØZ
Non-OR   Ø99[5,6]ØZZ
Non-OR   Ø99[5,6,9,A,D,E][7,8]Z[X,Z]

Ø99 Continued on next page

Ø **Medical and Surgical**
9 **Ear, Nose, Sinus**
9 **Drainage** Definition: Taking or letting out fluids and/or gases from a body part

Ø99 Continued

Explanation: The qualifier DIAGNOSTIC is used to identify drainage procedures that are biopsies

Body Part Character 4		Approach Character 5	Device Character 6	Qualifier Character 7
7 Tympanic Membrane, Right Pars flaccida 8 Tympanic Membrane, Left *See 7 Tympanic Membrane, Right* B Mastoid Sinus, Right Mastoid air cells C Mastoid Sinus, Left *See B Mastoid Sinus, Right* F Eustachian Tube, Right Auditory tube Pharyngotympanic tube G Eustachian Tube, Left *See F Eustachian Tube, Right* L Nasal Turbinate Inferior turbinate Middle turbinate Nasal concha Superior turbinate M Nasal Septum Quadrangular cartilage Septal cartilage Vomer bone	N Nasopharynx Choana Fossa of Rosenmuller Pharyngeal recess Rhinopharynx P Accessory Sinus Q Maxillary Sinus, Right Antrum of Highmore R Maxillary Sinus, Left *See Q Maxillary Sinus, Right* S Frontal Sinus, Right T Frontal Sinus, Left U Ethmoid Sinus, Right Ethmoidal air cell V Ethmoid Sinus, Left *See U Ethmoid Sinus, Right* W Sphenoid Sinus, Right X Sphenoid Sinus, Left	Ø Open 3 Percutaneous 4 Percutaneous Endoscopic 7 Via Natural or Artificial Opening 8 Via Natural or Artificial Opening Endoscopic	Ø Drainage Device	Z No Qualifier
7 Tympanic Membrane, Right Pars flaccida 8 Tympanic Membrane, Left *See 7 Tympanic Membrane, Right* B Mastoid Sinus, Right Mastoid air cells C Mastoid Sinus, Left *See B Mastoid Sinus, Right* F Eustachian Tube, Right Auditory tube Pharyngotympanic tube G Eustachian Tube, Left *See F Eustachian Tube, Right* L Nasal Turbinate Inferior turbinate Middle turbinate Nasal concha Superior turbinate M Nasal Septum Quadrangular cartilage Septal cartilage Vomer bone	N Nasopharynx Choana Fossa of Rosenmuller Pharyngeal recess Rhinopharynx P Accessory Sinus Q Maxillary Sinus, Right Antrum of Highmore R Maxillary Sinus, Left *See Q Maxillary Sinus, Right* S Frontal Sinus, Right T Frontal Sinus, Left U Ethmoid Sinus, Right Ethmoidal air cell V Ethmoid Sinus, Left *See U Ethmoid Sinus, Right* W Sphenoid Sinus, Right X Sphenoid Sinus, Left	Ø Open 3 Percutaneous 4 Percutaneous Endoscopic 7 Via Natural or Artificial Opening 8 Via Natural or Artificial Opening Endoscopic	Z No Device	X Diagnostic Z No Qualifier

Non-OR	Ø99[B,C][3,7,8]ØZ
Non-OR	Ø99[F,G,L,M][Ø,3,4,7,8]ØZ
Non-OR	Ø99N3ØZ
Non-OR	Ø99[P,Q,R,S,T,U,V,W,X][3,4,7,8]ØZ
Non-OR	Ø99[7,8][Ø,3,4,7,8]ZZ
Non-OR	Ø99[7,8][7,8]ZX
Non-OR	Ø99[B,C]3ZZ
Non-OR	Ø99[B,C][7,8]Z[X,Z]
Non-OR	Ø99[F,G][Ø,3,4,7,8]ZZ
Non-OR	Ø99[F,G][7,8]ZX
Non-OR	Ø99[L,M][Ø,3,4,7,8]Z[X,Z]
Non-OR	Ø99N[Ø,3,4,7,8]ZX
Non-OR	Ø99N3ZZ
Non-OR	Ø99[P,Q,R,S,T,U,V,W,X][3,4,7,8]Z[X,Z]

Ear, Nose, Sinus

0   Medical and Surgical
9   Ear, Nose, Sinus
B   Excision   Definition: Cutting out or off, without replacement, a portion of a body part
                         Explanation: The qualifier DIAGNOSTIC is used to identify excision procedures that are biopsies

Body Part Character 4		Approach Character 5	Device Character 6	Qualifier Character 7

0 External Ear, Right
   Antihelix
   Antitragus
   Auricle
   Earlobe
   Helix
   Pinna
   Tragus
	1 External Ear, Left
	   See 0 External Ear, Right
		0 Open
		3 Percutaneous
		4 Percutaneous Endoscopic
		X External
			Z No Device	**X Diagnostic**
				Z No Qualifier

3 External Auditory Canal, Right
   External auditory meatus
	4 External Auditory Canal, Left
	   See 3 External Auditory Canal, Right
		0 Open
		3 Percutaneous
		4 Percutaneous Endoscopic
		7 Via Natural or Artificial Opening
		8 Via Natural or Artificial Opening Endoscopic
		X External
			Z No Device	**X Diagnostic**
				Z No Qualifier

5 Middle Ear, Right
   Oval window
   Tympanic cavity
6 Middle Ear, Left
   See 5 Middle Ear, Right
9 Auditory Ossicle, Right
   Incus
   Malleus
   Stapes
	A Auditory Ossicle, Left
	   See 9 Auditory Ossicle, Right
	D Inner Ear, Right
	   Bony labyrinth
	   Bony vestibule
	   Cochlea
	   Round window
	   Semicircular canal
	E Inner Ear, Left
	   See D Inner Ear, Right
		0 Open
		8 Via Natural or Artificial Opening Endoscopic
			Z No Device	**X Diagnostic**
				Z No Qualifier

7 Tympanic Membrane, Right
   Pars flaccida
8 Tympanic Membrane, Left
   See 7 Tympanic Membrane, Right
F Eustachian Tube, Right
   Auditory tube
   Pharyngotympanic tube
G Eustachian Tube, Left
   See F Eustachian Tube, Right
	L Nasal Turbinate
	   Inferior turbinate
	   Middle turbinate
	   Nasal concha
	   Superior turbinate
	N Nasopharynx
	   Choana
	   Fossa of Rosenmuller
	   Pharyngeal recess
	   Rhinopharynx
		0 Open
		3 Percutaneous
		4 Percutaneous Endoscopic
		7 Via Natural or Artificial Opening
		8 Via Natural or Artificial Opening Endoscopic
			Z No Device	**X Diagnostic**
				Z No Qualifier

B Mastoid Sinus, Right
   Mastoid air cells
C Mastoid Sinus, Left
   See B Mastoid Sinus, Right
M Nasal Septum
   Quadrangular cartilage
   Septal cartilage
   Vomer bone
P Accessory Sinus
Q Maxillary Sinus, Right
   Antrum of Highmore
	R Maxillary Sinus, Left
	   See Q Maxillary Sinus, Right
	S Frontal Sinus, Right
	T Frontal Sinus, Left
	U Ethmoid Sinus, Right
	   Ethmoidal air cell
	V Ethmoid Sinus, Left
	   See U Ethmoid Sinus, Right
	W Sphenoid Sinus, Right
	X Sphenoid Sinus, Left
		0 Open
		3 Percutaneous
		4 Percutaneous Endoscopic
		8 Via Natural or Artificial Opening Endoscopic
			Z No Device	**X Diagnostic**
				Z No Qualifier

K Nasal Mucosa and Soft Tissue
   Columella
   External naris
   Greater alar cartilage
   Internal naris
   Lateral nasal cartilage
   Lesser alar cartilage
   Nasal cavity
   Nostril
		0 Open
		3 Percutaneous
		4 Percutaneous Endoscopic
		8 Via Natural or Artificial Opening Endoscopic
		X External
			Z No Device	**X Diagnostic**
				Z No Qualifier

Non-OR   09B[0,1][0,3,4,X]Z[X,Z]
Non-OR   09B[3,4][0,3,4,7,8,X]Z[X,Z]
Non-OR   09B[F,G,L,N][0,3,4,7,8]Z[X,Z]
Non-OR   09BM[0,3,4,8]ZX
Non-OR   09B[P,Q,R,S,T,U,V,W,X][3,4,8]ZX
Non-OR   09BK8Z[X,Z]

Ø   Medical and Surgical
9   Ear, Nose, Sinus
C   Extirpation   Definition: Taking or cutting out solid matter from a body part

                 Explanation: The solid matter may be an abnormal byproduct of a biological function or a foreign body; it may be imbedded in a body part or in the lumen of a tubular body part. The solid matter may or may not have been previously broken into pieces.

Body Part Character 4		Approach Character 5	Device Character 6	Qualifier Character 7
Ø External Ear, Right Antihelix Antitragus Auricle Earlobe Helix Pinna Tragus	**1 External Ear, Left** *See Ø External Ear, Right*	**Ø** Open **3** Percutaneous **4** Percutaneous Endoscopic **X** External	**Z** No Device	**Z** No Qualifier
3 External Auditory Canal, Right External auditory meatus	**4 External Auditory Canal, Left** *See 3 External Auditory Canal, Right*	**Ø** Open **3** Percutaneous **4** Percutaneous Endoscopic **7** Via Natural or Artificial Opening **8** Via Natural or Artificial Opening Endoscopic **X** External	**Z** No Device	**Z** No Qualifier
5 Middle Ear, Right Oval window Tympanic cavity **6 Middle Ear, Left** *See 5 Middle Ear, Right* **9 Auditory Ossicle, Right** Incus Malleus Stapes	**A Auditory Ossicle, Left** *See 9 Auditory Ossicle, Right* **D Inner Ear, Right** Bony labyrinth Bony vestibule Cochlea Round window Semicircular canal **E Inner Ear, Left** *See D Inner Ear, Right*	**Ø** Open **8** Via Natural or Artificial Opening Endoscopic	**Z** No Device	**Z** No Qualifier
7 Tympanic Membrane, Right Pars flaccida **8 Tympanic Membrane, Left** *See 7 Tympanic Membrane, Right* **F Eustachian Tube, Right** Auditory tube Pharyngotympanic tube **G Eustachian Tube, Left** *See F Eustachian Tube, Right*	**L Nasal Turbinate** Inferior turbinate Middle turbinate Nasal concha Superior turbinate **N Nasopharynx** Choana Fossa of Rosenmuller Pharyngeal recess Rhinopharynx	**Ø** Open **3** Percutaneous **4** Percutaneous Endoscopic **7** Via Natural or Artificial Opening **8** Via Natural or Artificial Opening Endoscopic	**Z** No Device	**Z** No Qualifier
B Mastoid Sinus, Right Mastoid air cells **C Mastoid Sinus, Left** *See B Mastoid Sinus, Right* **M Nasal Septum** Quadrangular cartilage Septal cartilage Vomer bone **P Accessory Sinus** **Q Maxillary Sinus, Right** Antrum of Highmore	**R Maxillary Sinus, Left** *See Q Maxillary Sinus, Right* **S Frontal Sinus, Right** **T Frontal Sinus, Left** **U Ethmoid Sinus, Right** Ethmoidal air cell **V Ethmoid Sinus, Left** *See U Ethmoid Sinus, Right* **W Sphenoid Sinus, Right** **X Sphenoid Sinus, Left**	**Ø** Open **3** Percutaneous **4** Percutaneous Endoscopic **8** Via Natural or Artificial Opening Endoscopic	**Z** No Device	**Z** No Qualifier
K Nasal Mucosa and Soft Tissue Columella External naris Greater alar cartilage Internal naris Lateral nasal cartilage Lesser alar cartilage Nasal cavity Nostril		**Ø** Open **3** Percutaneous **4** Percutaneous Endoscopic **8** Via Natural or Artificial Opening Endoscopic **X** External	**Z** No Device	**Z** No Qualifier

Non-OR	09C[Ø,1][Ø,3,4,X]ZZ
Non-OR	09C[3,4][Ø,3,4,7,8,X]ZZ
Non-OR	09C[7,8,F,G,L][Ø,3,4,7,8]ZZ
Non-OR	09CM[Ø,3,4,8]ZZ
Non-OR	09CK8ZZ

NC Noncovered Procedure   **LC** Limited Coverage   **QA** Questionable OB Admit   **NT** New Tech Add-on   ⊞ Combination Member   ♂ Male   ♀ Female

ICD-10-PCS 2022   327

09C–09C

Ear, Nose, Sinus

Ø   **Medical and Surgical**
9   **Ear, Nose, Sinus**
D   **Extraction**   Definition: Pulling or stripping out or off all or a portion of a body part by the use of force

                       Explanation: The qualifier DIAGNOSTIC is used to identify extraction procedures that are biopsies

Body Part Character 4	Approach Character 5	Device Character 6	Qualifier Character 7

7 **Tympanic Membrane, Right**
   Pars flaccida
8 **Tympanic Membrane, Left**
   See 7 Tympanic Membrane, Right
L **Nasal Turbinate**
   Inferior turbinate
   Middle turbinate
   Nasal concha
   Superior turbinate
	Ø Open
	3 Percutaneous
	4 Percutaneous Endoscopic
	7 Via Natural or Artificial Opening
	8 Via Natural or Artificial Opening
	   Endoscopic
		Z No Device	**Z** No Qualifier

9 **Auditory Ossicle, Right**
   Incus
   Malleus
   Stapes
A **Auditory Ossicle, Left**
   See 9 Auditory Ossicle, Right
	Ø Open	**Z** No Device	**Z** No Qualifier

B **Mastoid Sinus, Right**
   Mastoid air cells
C **Mastoid Sinus, Left**
   See B Mastoid Sinus, Right
M **Nasal Septum**
   Quadrangular cartilage
   Septal cartilage
   Vomer bone
P **Accessory Sinus**
Q **Maxillary Sinus, Right**
   Antrum of Highmore
R **Maxillary Sinus, Left**
   See Q Maxillary Sinus, Right
S **Frontal Sinus, Right**
T **Frontal Sinus, Left**
U **Ethmoid Sinus, Right**
   Ethmoidal air cell
V **Ethmoid Sinus, Left**
   See U Ethmoid Sinus, Right
W **Sphenoid Sinus, Right**
X **Sphenoid Sinus, Left**
	Ø Open
	3 Percutaneous
	4 Percutaneous Endoscopic
		Z No Device	**Z** No Qualifier

Ø   **Medical and Surgical**
9   **Ear, Nose, Sinus**
H   **Insertion**   Definition: Putting in a nonbiological appliance that monitors, assists, performs, or prevents a physiological function but does not physically take the place of a body part

                     Explanation: None

Body Part Character 4	Approach Character 5	Device Character 6	Qualifier Character 7

D **Inner Ear, Right**
   Bony labyrinth
   Bony vestibule
   Cochlea
   Round window
   Semicircular canal
E **Inner Ear, Left**
   See D Inner Ear, Right
	Ø Open
	3 Percutaneous
	4 Percutaneous Endoscopic
		1 Radioactive Element
		4 Hearing Device, Bone Conduction
		5 Hearing Device, Single Channel
		   Cochlear Prosthesis
		6 Hearing Device, Multiple Channel
		   Cochlear Prosthesis
		S Hearing Device
			Z No Qualifier

H **Ear, Right**
J **Ear, Left**
K **Nasal Mucosa and Soft Tissue**
   Columella
   External naris
   Greater alar cartilage
   Internal naris
   Lateral nasal cartilage
   Lesser alar cartilage
   Nasal cavity
   Nostril
Y **Sinus**
	Ø Open
	3 Percutaneous
	4 Percutaneous Endoscopic
	7 Via Natural or Artificial Opening
	8 Via Natural or Artificial Opening
	   Endoscopic
		1 Radioactive Element
		Y Other Device
			Z No Qualifier

N **Nasopharynx**
   Choana
   Fossa of Rosenmuller
   Pharyngeal recess
   Rhinopharynx
	7 Via Natural or Artificial Opening
	8 Via Natural or Artificial Opening
	   Endoscopic
		1 Radioactive Element
		B Intraluminal Device, Airway
			Z No Qualifier

Non-OR Ø9H[H,J,K]Ø1Z		**Non-OR** Ø9H[H,J,K,Y][3,4,7,8][1,Y]Z	
Non-OR Ø9HKØYZ		**Non-OR** Ø9HN[7,8][1,B]Z	

Non-OR Procedure   DRG Non-OR Procedure   Valid OR Procedure   HAC Associated Procedure   Combination Only   New/Revised GREEN

Ø   Medical and Surgical
9   Ear, Nose, Sinus
J   Inspection   Definition: Visually and/or manually exploring a body part

Explanation: Visual exploration may be performed with or without optical instrumentation. Manual exploration may be performed directly or through intervening body layers.

Body Part Character 4	Approach Character 5	Device Character 6	Qualifier Character 7
7 Tympanic Membrane, Right Pars flaccida **8 Tympanic Membrane, Left** *See 7 Tympanic Membrane, Right* **H Ear, Right** **J Ear, Left**	Ø Open 3 Percutaneous 4 Percutaneous Endoscopic 7 Via Natural or Artificial Opening 8 Via Natural or Artificial Opening Endoscopic X External	Z No Device	Z No Qualifier
D Inner Ear, Right Bony labyrinth Bony vestibule Cochlea Round window Semicircular canal **E Inner Ear, Left** *See D Inner Ear, Right* **K Nasal Mucosa and Soft Tissue** Columella External naris Greater alar cartilage Internal naris Lateral nasal cartilage Lesser alar cartilage Nasal cavity Nostril **Y Sinus**	Ø Open 3 Percutaneous 4 Percutaneous Endoscopic 8 Via Natural or Artificial Opening Endoscopic X External	Z No Device	Z No Qualifier

Non-OR	09J[7,8][3,7,8,X]ZZ
Non-OR	09J[H,J][0,3,4,7,8,X]ZZ
Non-OR	09J[D,E][3,8,X]ZZ
Non-OR	09J[K,Y][0,3,4,8,X]ZZ

Ø   Medical and Surgical
9   Ear, Nose, Sinus
M   Reattachment   Definition: Putting back in or on all or a portion of a separated body part to its normal location or other suitable location

Explanation: Vascular circulation and nervous pathways may or may not be reestablished

Body Part Character 4	Approach Character 5	Device Character 6	Qualifier Character 7
Ø External Ear, Right Antihelix Antitragus Auricle Earlobe Helix Pinna Tragus **1 External Ear, Left** *See Ø External Ear, Right* **K Nasal Mucosa and Soft Tissue** Columella External naris Greater alar cartilage Internal naris Lateral nasal cartilage Lesser alar cartilage Nasal cavity Nostril	X External	Z No Device	Z No Qualifier

NC Noncovered Procedure   LC Limited Coverage   QA Questionable OB Admit   NT New Tech Add-on   ⊞ Combination Member   ♂ Male   ♀ Female

ICD-10-PCS 2022   329

Ø Medical and Surgical
9 Ear, Nose, Sinus
N Release   Definition: Freeing a body part from an abnormal physical constraint by cutting or by the use of force
Explanation: Some of the restraining tissue may be taken out but none of the body part is taken out

Body Part Character 4		Approach Character 5	Device Character 6	Qualifier Character 7
Ø External Ear, Right Antihelix Antitragus Auricle Earlobe Helix Pinna Tragus	**1 External Ear, Left** *See Ø External Ear, Right*	**Ø** Open **3** Percutaneous **4** Percutaneous Endoscopic **X** External	**Z** No Device	**Z** No Qualifier
3 External Auditory Canal, Right External auditory meatus	**4 External Auditory Canal, Left** *See 3 External Auditory Canal, Right*	**Ø** Open **3** Percutaneous **4** Percutaneous Endoscopic **7** Via Natural or Artificial Opening **8** Via Natural or Artificial Opening Endoscopic **X** External	**Z** No Device	**Z** No Qualifier
5 Middle Ear, Right Oval window Tympanic cavity **6 Middle Ear, Left** *See 5 Middle Ear, Right* **9 Auditory Ossicle, Right** Incus Malleus Stapes	**A Auditory Ossicle, Left** *See 9 Auditory Ossicle, Right* **D Inner Ear, Right** Bony labyrinth Bony vestibule Cochlea Round window Semicircular canal **E Inner Ear, Left** *See D Inner Ear, Right*	**Ø** Open **8** Via Natural or Artificial Opening Endoscopic	**Z** No Device	**Z** No Qualifier
7 Tympanic Membrane, Right Pars flaccida **8 Tympanic Membrane, Left** *See 7 Tympanic Membrane, Right* **F Eustachian Tube, Right** Auditory tube Pharyngotympanic tube **G Eustachian Tube, Left** *See F Eustachian Tube, Right*	**L Nasal Turbinate** Inferior turbinate Middle turbinate Nasal concha Superior turbinate **N Nasopharynx** Choana Fossa of Rosenmuller Pharyngeal recess Rhinopharynx	**Ø** Open **3** Percutaneous **4** Percutaneous Endoscopic **7** Via Natural or Artificial Opening **8** Via Natural or Artificial Opening Endoscopic	**Z** No Device	**Z** No Qualifier
B Mastoid Sinus, Right Mastoid air cells **C Mastoid Sinus, Left** *See B Mastoid Sinus, Right* **M Nasal Septum** Quadrangular cartilage Septal cartilage Vomer bone **P Accessory Sinus** **Q Maxillary Sinus, Right** Antrum of Highmore	**R Maxillary Sinus, Left** *See Q Maxillary Sinus, Right* **S Frontal Sinus, Right** **T Frontal Sinus, Left** **U Ethmoid Sinus, Right** Ethmoidal air cell **V Ethmoid Sinus, Left** *See U Ethmoid Sinus, Right* **W Sphenoid Sinus, Right** **X Sphenoid Sinus, Left**	**Ø** Open **3** Percutaneous **4** Percutaneous Endoscopic **8** Via Natural or Artificial Opening Endoscopic	**Z** No Device	**Z** No Qualifier
K Nasal Mucosa and Soft Tissue Columella External naris Greater alar cartilage Internal naris Lateral nasal cartilage Lesser alar cartilage Nasal cavity Nostril		**Ø** Open **3** Percutaneous **4** Percutaneous Endoscopic **8** Via Natural or Artificial Opening Endoscopic **X** External	**Z** No Device	**Z** No Qualifier

Non-OR	Ø9N[Ø,1]XZZ
Non-OR	Ø9N[3,4]XZZ
Non-OR	Ø9N[F,G,L][Ø,3,4,7,8]ZZ
Non-OR	Ø9NM[Ø,3,4,8]ZZ
Non-OR	Ø9NK[Ø,3,4,8,X]ZZ

0   Medical and Surgical
9   Ear, Nose, Sinus
P   Removal   Definition: Taking out or off a device from a body part

Explanation: If a device is taken out and a similar device put in without cutting or puncturing the skin or mucous membrane, the procedure is coded to the root operation CHANGE. Otherwise, the procedure for taking out a device is coded to the root operation REMOVAL.

Body Part Character 4	Approach Character 5	Device Character 6	Qualifier Character 7

7   Tympanic Membrane, Right
    Pars flaccida
8   Tympanic Membrane, Left
    See 7 Tympanic Membrane, Right
	0 Open
	7 Via Natural or Artificial Opening
	8 Via Natural or Artificial Opening Endoscopic
	X External
		0 Drainage Device	**Z No Qualifier**

D   Inner Ear, Right
    Bony labyrinth
    Bony vestibule
    Cochlea
    Round window
    Semicircular canal
E   Inner Ear, Left
    See D Inner Ear, Right
	0 Open
	7 Via Natural or Artificial Opening
	8 Via Natural or Artificial Opening Endoscopic
		S Hearing Device	**Z No Qualifier**

H   Ear, Right
J   Ear, Left
K   Nasal Mucosa and Soft Tissue
    Columella
    External naris
    Greater alar cartilage
    Internal naris
    Lateral nasal cartilage
    Lesser alar cartilage
    Nasal cavity
    Nostril
	0 Open
	3 Percutaneous
	4 Percutaneous Endoscopic
	7 Via Natural or Artificial Opening
	8 Via Natural or Artificial Opening Endoscopic
		0 Drainage Device
		7 Autologous Tissue Substitute
		D Intraluminal Device
		J Synthetic Substitute
		K Nonautologous Tissue Substitute
		Y Other Device
			Z No Qualifier

H   Ear, Right
J   Ear, Left
K   Nasal Mucosa and Soft Tissue
    Columella
    External naris
    Greater alar cartilage
    Internal naris
    Lateral nasal cartilage
    Lesser alar cartilage
    Nasal cavity
    Nostril
	X External	**0 Drainage Device**
		7 Autologous Tissue Substitute
		D Intraluminal Device
		J Synthetic Substitute
		K Nonautologous Tissue Substitute
			Z No Qualifier

Y Sinus	**0 Open** **3 Percutaneous** **4 Percutaneous Endoscopic**	**0 Drainage Device** **Y Other Device**	**Z No Qualifier**
Y Sinus	**7 Via Natural or Artificial Opening** **8 Via Natural or Artificial Opening Endoscopic**	**Y Other Device**	**Z No Qualifier**
Y Sinus	**X External**	**0 Drainage Device**	**Z No Qualifier**

Non-OR	09P[7,8][0,7,8,X]0Z
Non-OR	09P[H,J][3,4][0,J,K,Y]Z
Non-OR	09P[H,J][7,8][0,D,Y]Z
Non-OR	09PK[0,3,4,7,8][0,7,D,J,K,Y]Z
Non-OR	09P[H,J]X[0,7,D,J,K]Z
Non-OR	09PKX[0,7,D,J,K]Z
Non-OR	09PY[3,4]YZ
Non-OR	09PY[7,8]YZ
Non-OR	09PYX0Z

0　Medical and Surgical
9　Ear, Nose, Sinus
Q　Repair　　Definition: Restoring, to the extent possible, a body part to its normal anatomic structure and function
　　　　　　　　Explanation: Used only when the method to accomplish the repair is not one of the other root operations

Body Part Character 4		Approach Character 5	Device Character 6	Qualifier Character 7
0 External Ear, Right Antihelix Antitragus Auricle Earlobe Helix Pinna Tragus	**1 External Ear, Left** *See 0 External Ear, Right* **2 External Ear, Bilateral** *See 0 External Ear, Right*	**0** Open **3** Percutaneous **4** Percutaneous Endoscopic **X** External	**Z** No Device	**Z** No Qualifier
3 External Auditory Canal, Right External auditory meatus **4 External Auditory Canal, Left** *See 3 External Auditory Canal, Right*	**F Eustachian Tube, Right** Auditory tube Pharyngotympanic tube **G Eustachian Tube, Left** *See F Eustachian Tube, Right*	**0** Open **3** Percutaneous **4** Percutaneous Endoscopic **7** Via Natural or Artificial Opening **8** Via Natural or Artificial Opening Endoscopic **X** External	**Z** No Device	**Z** No Qualifier
5 Middle Ear, Right Oval window Tympanic cavity **6 Middle Ear, Left** *See 5 Middle Ear, Right* **9 Auditory Ossicle, Right** Incus Malleus Stapes	**A Auditory Ossicle, Left** *See 9 Auditory Ossicle, Right* **D Inner Ear, Right** Bony labyrinth Bony vestibule Cochlea Round window Semicircular canal **E Inner Ear, Left** *See D Inner Ear, Right*	**0** Open **8** Via Natural or Artificial Opening Endoscopic	**Z** No Device	**Z** No Qualifier
7 Tympanic Membrane, Right Pars flaccida **8 Tympanic Membrane, Left** *See 7 Tympanic Membrane, Right* **L Nasal Turbinate** Inferior turbinate Middle turbinate Nasal concha Superior turbinate	**N Nasopharynx** Choana Fossa of Rosenmuller Pharyngeal recess Rhinopharynx	**0** Open **3** Percutaneous **4** Percutaneous Endoscopic **7** Via Natural or Artificial Opening **8** Via Natural or Artificial Opening Endoscopic	**Z** No Device	**Z** No Qualifier
B Mastoid Sinus, Right Mastoid air cells **C Mastoid Sinus, Left** *See B Mastoid Sinus, Right* **M Nasal Septum** Quadrangular cartilage Septal cartilage Vomer bone **P Accessory Sinus** **Q Maxillary Sinus, Right** Antrum of Highmore	**R Maxillary Sinus, Left** *See Q Maxillary Sinus, Right* **S Frontal Sinus, Right** **T Frontal Sinus, Left** **U Ethmoid Sinus, Right** Ethmoidal air cell **V Ethmoid Sinus, Left** *See U Ethmoid Sinus, Right* **W Sphenoid Sinus, Right** **X Sphenoid Sinus, Left**	**0** Open **3** Percutaneous **4** Percutaneous Endoscopic **8** Via Natural or Artificial Opening Endoscopic	**Z** No Device	**Z** No Qualifier
K Nasal Mucosa and Soft Tissue Columella External naris Greater alar cartilage Internal naris Lateral nasal cartilage Lesser alar cartilage Nasal cavity Nostril		**0** Open **3** Percutaneous **4** Percutaneous Endoscopic **8** Via Natural or Artificial Opening Endoscopic **X** External	**Z** No Device	**Z** No Qualifier

Non-OR	09Q[0,1,2]XZZ
Non-OR	09Q[3,4]XZZ
Non-OR	09Q[F,G][0,3,4,7,8,X]ZZ
Non-OR	09QKXZZ

Ø   Medical and Surgical
9   Ear, Nose, Sinus
R   Replacement   Definition: Putting in or on biological or synthetic material that physically takes the place and/or function of all or a portion of a body part

Explanation: The body part may have been taken out or replaced, or may be taken out, physically eradicated, or rendered nonfunctional during the REPLACEMENT procedure. A REMOVAL procedure is coded for taking out the device used in a previous replacement procedure.

Body Part Character 4	Approach Character 5	Device Character 6	Qualifier Character 7

Ø   External Ear, Right
  Antihelix
  Antitragus
  Auricle
  Earlobe
  Helix
  Pinna
  Tragus
1   External Ear, Left
  See Ø External Ear, Right
2   External Ear, Bilateral
  See Ø External Ear, Right
K   Nasal Mucosa and Soft Tissue
  Columella
  External naris
  Greater alar cartilage
  Internal naris
  Lateral nasal cartilage
  Lesser alar cartilage
  Nasal cavity
  Nostril
	Ø Open
	X External
		7 Autologous Tissue Substitute
		J Synthetic Substitute
		K Nonautologous Tissue Substitute
			Z No Qualifier

5   Middle Ear, Right
  Oval window
  Tympanic cavity
6   Middle Ear, Left
  See 5 Middle Ear, Right
9   Auditory Ossicle, Right
  Incus
  Malleus
  Stapes
A   Auditory Ossicle, Left
  See 9 Auditory Ossicle, Right
D   Inner Ear, Right
  Bony labyrinth
  Bony vestibule
  Cochlea
  Round window
  Semicircular canal
E   Inner Ear, Left
  See D Inner Ear, Right
	Ø Open	**7 Autologous Tissue Substitute**
		J Synthetic Substitute
		K Nonautologous Tissue Substitute
			Z No Qualifier

7   Tympanic Membrane, Right
  Pars flaccida
8   Tympanic Membrane, Left
  See 7 Tympanic Membrane, Right
N   Nasopharynx
  Choana
  Fossa of Rosenmuller
  Pharyngeal recess
  Rhinopharynx
	Ø Open
	7 Via Natural or Artificial Opening
	8 Via Natural or Artificial Opening Endoscopic
		7 Autologous Tissue Substitute
		J Synthetic Substitute
		K Nonautologous Tissue Substitute
			Z No Qualifier

L   Nasal Turbinate
  Inferior turbinate
  Middle turbinate
  Nasal concha
  Superior turbinate
	Ø Open
	3 Percutaneous
	4 Percutaneous Endoscopic
	7 Via Natural or Artificial Opening
	8 Via Natural or Artificial Opening Endoscopic
		7 Autologous Tissue Substitute
		J Synthetic Substitute
		K Nonautologous Tissue Substitute
			Z No Qualifier

M   Nasal Septum
  Quadrangular cartilage
  Septal cartilage
  Vomer bone
	Ø Open
	3 Percutaneous
	4 Percutaneous Endoscopic
		7 Autologous Tissue Substitute
		J Synthetic Substitute
		K Nonautologous Tissue Substitute
			Z No Qualifier

NC Noncovered Procedure   LC Limited Coverage   QA Questionable OB Admit   NT New Tech Add-on   ⊞ Combination Member   ♂ Male   ♀ Female

ICD-10-PCS 2022   333

Ø9R–Ø9R

Ear, Nose, Sinus

0   **Medical and Surgical**
9   **Ear, Nose, Sinus**
S   **Reposition**   Definition: Moving to its normal location, or other suitable location, all or a portion of a body part

Explanation: The body part is moved to a new location from an abnormal location, or from a normal location where it is not functioning correctly. The body part may or may not be cut out or off to be moved to the new location.

Body Part Character 4	Approach Character 5	Device Character 6	Qualifier Character 7

0   **External Ear, Right**
    Antihelix
    Antitragus
    Auricle
    Earlobe
    Helix
    Pinna
    Tragus
1   **External Ear, Left**
    See 0 External Ear, Right
2   **External Ear, Bilateral**
    See 0 External Ear, Right
K   **Nasal Mucosa and Soft Tissue**
    Columella
    External naris
    Greater alar cartilage
    Internal naris
    Lateral nasal cartilage
    Lesser alar cartilage
    Nasal cavity
    Nostril
	0 Open
	4 Percutaneous Endoscopic
	X External
		Z No Device	**Z** No Qualifier

7   **Tympanic Membrane, Right**
    Pars flaccida
8   **Tympanic Membrane, Left**
    See 7 Tympanic Membrane, Right
F   Eustachian Tube, Right
    Auditory tube
    Pharyngotympanic tube
G   Eustachian Tube, Left
    See F Eustachian Tube, Right
L   **Nasal Turbinate**
    Inferior turbinate
    Middle turbinate
    Nasal concha
    Superior turbinate
	0 Open
	4 Percutaneous Endoscopic
	7 Via Natural or Artificial Opening
	8 Via Natural or Artificial Opening
	    Endoscopic
		Z No Device	**Z** No Qualifier

9   **Auditory Ossicle, Right**
    Incus
    Malleus
    Stapes
A   **Auditory Ossicle, Left**
    See 9 Auditory Ossicle, Right
M   **Nasal Septum**
    Quadrangular cartilage
    Septal cartilage
    Vomer bone
	0 Open
	4 Percutaneous Endoscopic
		Z No Device	**Z** No Qualifier

Non-OR   09S[F,G][0,4,7,8]ZZ

0   Medical and Surgical
9   Ear, Nose, Sinus
T   Resection   Definition: Cutting out or off, without replacement, all of a body part
                Explanation: None

Body Part Character 4		Approach Character 5	Device Character 6	Qualifier Character 7
0 External Ear, Right Antihelix Antitragus Auricle Earlobe Helix Pinna Tragus	**1 External Ear, Left** *See 0 External Ear, Right*	**0 Open** **4 Percutaneous Endoscopic** **X External**	**Z No Device**	**Z No Qualifier**
5 Middle Ear, Right Oval window Tympanic cavity **6 Middle Ear, Left** *See 5 Middle Ear, Right* **9 Auditory Ossicle, Right** Incus Malleus Stapes	**A Auditory Ossicle, Left** *See 9 Auditory Ossicle, Right* **D Inner Ear, Right** Bony labyrinth Bony vestibule Cochlea Round window Semicircular canal **E Inner Ear, Left** *See D Inner Ear, Right*	**0 Open** **8 Via Natural or Artificial Opening Endoscopic**	**Z No Device**	**Z No Qualifier**
7 Tympanic Membrane, Right Pars flaccida **8 Tympanic Membrane, Left** *See 7 Tympanic Membrane, Right* **F Eustachian Tube, Right** Auditory tube Pharyngotympanic tube **G Eustachian Tube, Left** *See F Eustachian Tube, Right*	**L Nasal Turbinate** Inferior turbinate Middle turbinate Nasal concha Superior turbinate **N Nasopharynx** Choana Fossa of Rosenmuller Pharyngeal recess Rhinopharynx	**0 Open** **4 Percutaneous Endoscopic** **7 Via Natural or Artificial Opening** **8 Via Natural or Artificial Opening Endoscopic**	**Z No Device**	**Z No Qualifier**
B Mastoid Sinus, Right Mastoid air cells **C Mastoid Sinus, Left** *See B Mastoid Sinus, Right* **M Nasal Septum** Quadrangular cartilage Septal cartilage Vomer bone **P Accessory Sinus** **Q Maxillary Sinus, Right** Antrum of Highmore	**R Maxillary Sinus, Left** *See Q Maxillary Sinus, Right* **S Frontal Sinus, Right** **T Frontal Sinus, Left** **U Ethmoid Sinus, Right** Ethmoidal air cell **V Ethmoid Sinus, Left** *See U Ethmoid Sinus, Right* **W Sphenoid Sinus, Right** **X Sphenoid Sinus, Left**	**0 Open** **4 Percutaneous Endoscopic** **8 Via Natural or Artificial Opening Endoscopic**	**Z No Device**	**Z No Qualifier**
K Nasal Mucosa and Soft Tissue Columella External naris Greater alar cartilage Internal naris Lateral nasal cartilage Lesser alar cartilage Nasal cavity Nostril		**0 Open** **4 Percutaneous Endoscopic** **8 Via Natural or Artificial Opening Endoscopic** **X External**	**Z No Device**	**Z No Qualifier**

Non-OR 09T[F,G][0,4,7,8]ZZ

NC Noncovered Procedure   **LC** Limited Coverage   **UA** Questionable OB Admit   **NT** New Tech Add-on   ⊞ Combination Member   ♂ Male   ♀ Female

ICD-10-PCS 2022   **335**

Ear, Nose, Sinus

Ø   **Medical and Surgical**
9   **Ear, Nose, Sinus**
U   **Supplement**   Definition: Putting in or on biological or synthetic material that physically reinforces and/or augments the function of a portion of a body part
                           Explanation: The biological material is non-living, or is living and from the same individual. The body part may have been previously replaced, and the SUPPLEMENT procedure is performed to physically reinforce and/or augment the function of the replaced body part.

Body Part Character 4		Approach Character 5	Device Character 6	Qualifier Character 7

Ø   **External Ear, Right**
    Antihelix
    Antitragus
    Auricle
    Earlobe
    Helix
    Pinna
    Tragus
	1 **External Ear, Left**
	    See Ø External Ear, Right
	2 **External Ear, Bilateral**
	    See Ø External Ear, Right
		Ø Open
		X External
			7 Autologous Tissue
			    Substitute
			J Synthetic Substitute
			K Nonautologous Tissue
			    Substitute
				Z No Qualifier

5   **Middle Ear, Right**
    Oval window
    Tympanic cavity
6   **Middle Ear, Left**
    See 5 Middle Ear, Right
9   **Auditory Ossicle, Right**
    Incus
    Malleus
    Stapes
A   **Auditory Ossicle, Left**
    See 9 Auditory Ossicle, Right
	D **Inner Ear, Right**
	    Bony labyrinth
	    Bony vestibule
	    Cochlea
	    Round window
	    Semicircular canal
	E **Inner Ear, Left**
	    See D Inner Ear, Right
		Ø Open
		8 Via Natural or Artificial
		    Opening Endoscopic
			7 Autologous Tissue
			    Substitute
			J Synthetic Substitute
			K Nonautologous Tissue
			    Substitute
				Z No Qualifier

7   **Tympanic Membrane, Right**
    Pars flaccida
8   **Tympanic Membrane, Left**
    See 7 Tympanic Membrane,
    Right
	N **Nasopharynx**
	    Choana
	    Fossa of Rosenmuller
	    Pharyngeal recess
	    Rhinopharynx
		Ø Open
		7 Via Natural or Artificial
		    Opening
		8 Via Natural or Artificial
		    Opening Endoscopic
			7 Autologous Tissue
			    Substitute
			J Synthetic Substitute
			K Nonautologous Tissue
			    Substitute
				Z No Qualifier

B   **Mastoid Sinus, Right**
    Mastoid air cells
C   **Mastoid Sinus, Left**
    See B Mastoid Sinus, Right
L   **Nasal Turbinate**
    Inferior turbinate
    Middle turbinate
    Nasal concha
    Superior turbinate
P   **Accessory Sinus**
Q   **Maxillary Sinus, Right**
    Antrum of Highmore
	R **Maxillary Sinus, Left**
	    See Q Maxillary Sinus, Right
	S **Frontal Sinus, Right**
	T **Frontal Sinus, Left**
	U **Ethmoid Sinus, Right**
	    Ethmoidal air cell
	V **Ethmoid Sinus, Left**
	    See U Ethmoid Sinus, Right
	W **Sphenoid Sinus, Right**
	X **Sphenoid Sinus, Left**
		Ø Open
		3 Percutaneous
		4 Percutaneous Endoscopic
		7 Via Natural or Artificial
		    Opening
		8 Via Natural or Artificial
		    Opening Endoscopic
			7 Autologous Tissue
			    Substitute
			J Synthetic Substitute
			K Nonautologous Tissue
			    Substitute
				Z No Qualifier

K   **Nasal Mucosa and Soft Tissue**
    Columella
    External naris
    Greater alar cartilage
    Internal naris
    Lateral nasal cartilage
    Lesser alar cartilage
    Nasal cavity
    Nostril
		Ø Open
		8 Via Natural or Artificial
		    Opening Endoscopic
		X External
			7 Autologous Tissue
			    Substitute
			J Synthetic Substitute
			K Nonautologous Tissue
			    Substitute
				Z No Qualifier

M   **Nasal Septum**
    Quadrangular cartilage
    Septal cartilage
    Vomer bone
		Ø Open
		3 Percutaneous
		4 Percutaneous Endoscopic
		8 Via Natural or Artificial
		    Opening Endoscopic
			7 Autologous Tissue
			    Substitute
			J Synthetic Substitute
			K Nonautologous Tissue
			    Substitute
				Z No Qualifier

Ø Medical and Surgical
9 Ear, Nose, Sinus
W Revision   Definition: Correcting, to the extent possible, a portion of a malfunctioning device or the position of a displaced device
           Explanation: Revision can include correcting a malfunctioning or displaced device by taking out or putting in components of the device such as a screw or pin

Body Part Character 4	Approach Character 5	Device Character 6	Qualifier Character 7
7 Tympanic Membrane, Right Pars flaccida **8 Tympanic Membrane, Left** *See 7 Tympanic Membrane, Right* **9 Auditory Ossicle, Right** Incus Malleus Stapes **A Auditory Ossicle, Left** *See 9 Auditory Ossicle, Right*	**Ø** Open **7** Via Natural or Artificial Opening **8** Via Natural or Artificial Opening Endoscopic	**7** Autologous Tissue Substitute **J** Synthetic Substitute **K** Nonautologous Tissue Substitute	**Z** No Qualifier
D Inner Ear, Right Bony labyrinth Bony vestibule Cochlea Round window Semicircular canal **E Inner Ear, Left** *See D Inner Ear, Right*	**Ø** Open **7** Via Natural or Artificial Opening **8** Via Natural or Artificial Opening Endoscopic	**S** Hearing Device	**Z** No Qualifier
H Ear, Right **J Ear, Left** **K Nasal Mucosa and Soft Tissue** Columella External naris Greater alar cartilage Internal naris Lateral nasal cartilage Lesser alar cartilage Nasal cavity Nostril	**Ø** Open **3** Percutaneous **4** Percutaneous Endoscopic **7** Via Natural or Artificial Opening **8** Via Natural or Artificial Opening Endoscopic	**Ø** Drainage Device **7** Autologous Tissue Substitute **D** Intraluminal Device **J** Synthetic Substitute **K** Nonautologous Tissue Substitute **Y** Other Device	**Z** No Qualifier
H Ear, Right **J Ear, Left** **K Nasal Mucosa and Soft Tissue** Columella External naris Greater alar cartilage Internal naris Lateral nasal cartilage Lesser alar cartilage Nasal cavity Nostril	**X** External	**Ø** Drainage Device **7** Autologous Tissue Substitute **D** Intraluminal Device **J** Synthetic Substitute **K** Nonautologous Tissue Substitute	**Z** No Qualifier
Y Sinus	**Ø** Open **3** Percutaneous **4** Percutaneous Endoscopic	**Ø** Drainage Device **Y** Other Device	**Z** No Qualifier
Y Sinus	**7** Via Natural or Artificial Opening **8** Via Natural or Artificial Opening Endoscopic	**Y** Other Device	**Z** No Qualifier
Y Sinus	**X** External	**Ø** Drainage Device	**Z** No Qualifier

Non-OR Ø9W[H,J][3,4][J,K,Y]Z
Non-OR Ø9W[H,J][7,8][D,Y]Z
Non-OR Ø9WK[Ø,3,4,7,8][Ø,7,D,J,K,Y]Z
Non-OR Ø9W[H,J,K]X[Ø,7,D,J,K]Z
Non-OR Ø9WY[3,4]YZ
Non-OR Ø9WY[7,8]YZ
Non-OR Ø9WYXØZ

NC Noncovered Procedure   **LC** Limited Coverage   **QA** Questionable OB Admit   **NT** New Tech Add-on   ⊞ Combination Member   ♂ Male   ♀ Female

Respiratory System ØB1–ØBY

Character Meanings

This Character Meaning table is provided as a guide to assist the user in the identification of character members that may be found in this section of code tables. It **SHOULD NOT** be used to build a PCS code.

Operation–Character 3	Body Part–Character 4	Approach–Character 5	Device–Character 6	Qualifier–Character 7
1 Bypass	Ø Tracheobronchial Tree	Ø Open	Ø Drainage Device	Ø Allogeneic
2 Change	1 Trachea	3 Percutaneous	1 Radioactive Element	1 Syngeneic
5 Destruction	2 Carina	4 Percutaneous Endoscopic	2 Monitoring Device	2 Zooplastic
7 Dilation	3 Main Bronchus, Right	7 Via Natural or Artificial Opening	3 Infusion Device	4 Cutaneous
9 Drainage	4 Upper Lobe Bronchus, Right	8 Via Natural or Artificial Opening Endoscopic	7 Autologous Tissue Substitute	6 Esophagus
B Excision	5 Middle Lobe Bronchus, Right	X External	C Extraluminal Device	X Diagnostic
C Extirpation	6 Lower Lobe Bronchus, Right		D Intraluminal Device	Z No Qualifier
D Extraction	7 Main Bronchus, Left		E Intraluminal Device, Endotracheal Airway	
F Fragmentation	8 Upper Lobe Bronchus, Left		F Tracheostomy Device	
H Insertion	9 Lingula Bronchus		G Intraluminal Device, Endobronchial Valve	
J Inspection	B Lower Lobe Bronchus, Left		J Synthetic Substitute	
L Occlusion	C Upper Lung Lobe, Right		K Nonautologous Tissue Substitute	
M Reattachment	D Middle Lung Lobe, Right		M Diaphragmatic Pacemaker Lead	
N Release	F Lower Lung Lobe, Right		Y Other Device	
P Removal	G Upper Lung Lobe, Left		Z No Device	
Q Repair	H Lung Lingula			
R Replacement	J Lower Lung Lobe, Left			
S Reposition	K Lung, Right			
T Resection	L Lung, Left			
U Supplement	M Lungs, Bilateral			
V Restriction	N Pleura, Right			
W Revision	P Pleura, Left			
Y Transplantation	Q Pleura			
	T Diaphragm			

AHA Coding Clinic for table ØB5
| 2016, 2Q, 17 | Photodynamic therapy for treatment of malignant mesothelioma |
| 2015, 2Q, 31 | Thoracoscopic talc pleurodesis |

AHA Coding Clinic for table ØB7
| 2020, 3Q, 43 | Tracheobronchomalacia with placement of tracheobronchial stent |

AHA Coding Clinic for table ØB9
2017, 3Q, 15	Bronchoscopy with suctioning for removal of retained secretions
2017, 1Q, 51	Bronchoalveolar lavage
2016, 1Q, 26	Bronchoalveolar lavage, endobronchial biopsy and transbronchial biopsy
2016, 1Q, 27	Fiberoptic bronchoscopy with brushings and bronchoalveolar lavage

AHA Coding Clinic for table ØBB
2016, 1Q, 26	Bronchoalveolar lavage, endobronchial biopsy and transbronchial biopsy
2016, 1Q, 27	Fiberoptic bronchoscopy with brushings and bronchoalveolar lavage
2014, 1Q, 20	Fiducial marker placement

AHA Coding Clinic for table ØBC
| 2017, 3Q, 14 | Bronchoscopy with suctioning and washings for removal of mucus plug |

AHA Coding Clinic for table ØBD
| 2020, 3Q, 40 | Transbronchial cryobiopsy of upper, middle and lower lobes of lung |
| 2018, 3Q, 28 | Lung decortication for empyema |

AHA Coding Clinic for table ØBH
| 2019, 3Q, 33 | Insertion of endobronchial valve |
| 2014, 4Q, 3-10 | Mechanical ventilation |

AHA Coding Clinic for table ØBJ
| 2015, 2Q, 31 | Thoracoscopic talc pleurodesis |
| 2014, 1Q, 20 | Fiducial marker placement |

AHA Coding Clinic for table ØBL
| 2019, 3Q, 33 | Insertion of endobronchial valve |

AHA Coding Clinic for table ØBN
2019, 2Q, 20	Pericardiectomy for constrictive pericarditis
2018, 3Q, 28	Lung decortication
2018, 3Q, 28	Lung decortication for empyema
2015, 3Q, 15	Vascular ring surgery with release of esophagus and trachea

AHA Coding Clinic for table ØBQ
2020, 3Q, 41	Plication of diaphragm
2016, 2Q, 22	Esophageal lengthening Collis gastroplasty with Nissen fundoplication and hiatal hernia
2014, 3Q, 28	Laparoscopic Nissen fundoplication and diaphragmatic hernia repair

AHA Coding Clinic for table ØBU
| 2020, 3Q, 43 | Tracheobronchomalacia with placement of tracheobronchial stent |
| 2015, 1Q, 28 | Repair of bronchopleural fistula using omental pedicle graft |

AHA Coding Clinic for table ØBV
| 2020, 3Q, 41 | Plication of diaphragm |

Respiratory System

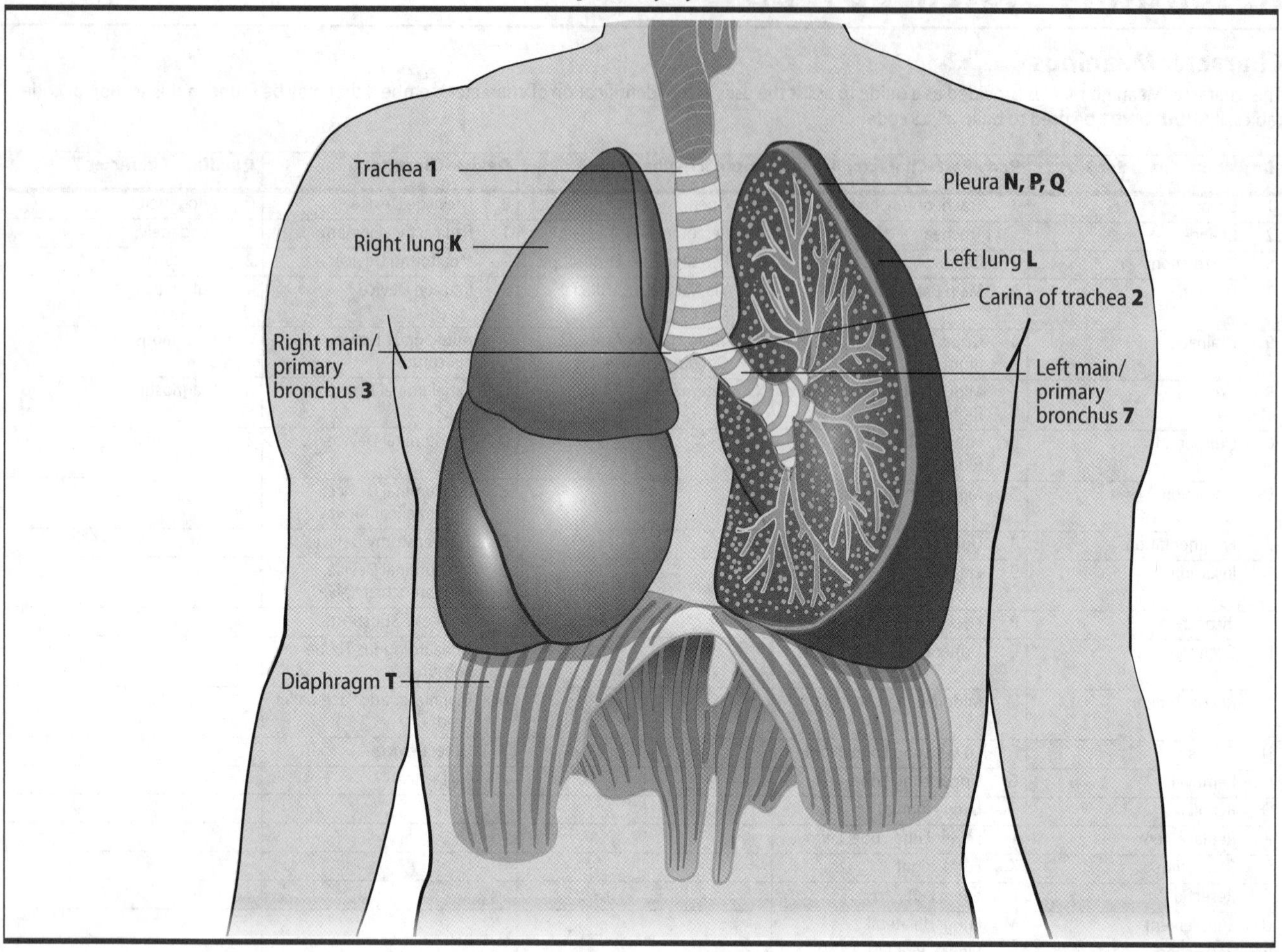

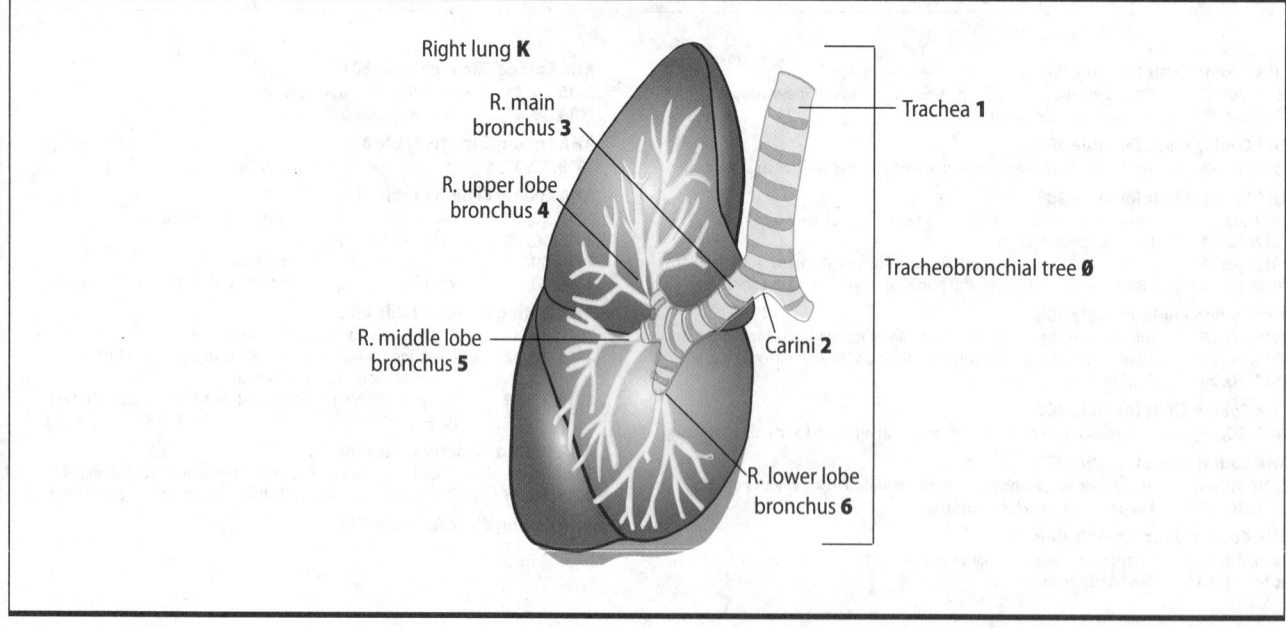

Trachea **1**

Right lung **K**

Right main/ primary bronchus **3**

Diaphragm **T**

Pleura **N, P, Q**

Left lung **L**

Carina of trachea **2**

Left main/ primary bronchus **7**

Right Lung Bronchi

Right lung **K**

R. main bronchus **3**

R. upper lobe bronchus **4**

R. middle lobe bronchus **5**

R. lower lobe bronchus **6**

Trachea **1**

Tracheobronchial tree **Ø**

Carini **2**

0   **Medical and Surgical**
B   **Respiratory System**
1   **Bypass**   Definition: Altering the route of passage of the contents of a tubular body part

                         Explanation: Rerouting contents of a body part to a downstream area of the normal route, to a similar route and body part, or to an abnormal route and dissimilar body part. Includes one or more anastomoses, with or without the use of a device.

Body Part Character 4	Approach Character 5	Device Character 6	Qualifier Character 7
1 Trachea Cricoid cartilage	**0** Open	**D** Intraluminal Device	**6** Esophagus
1 Trachea Cricoid cartilage	**0** Open	**F** Tracheostomy Device **Z** No Device	**4** Cutaneous
1 Trachea Cricoid cartilage	**3** Percutaneous **4** Percutaneous Endoscopic	**F** Tracheostomy Device **Z** No Device	**4** Cutaneous

DRG Non-OR   0B113[F,Z]4
Non-OR   0B110D6

---

0   **Medical and Surgical**
B   **Respiratory System**
2   **Change**   Definition: Taking out or off a device from a body part and putting back an identical or similar device in or on the same body part without cutting or puncturing the skin or a mucous membrane

                         Explanation: All CHANGE procedures are coded using the approach EXTERNAL

Body Part Character 4	Approach Character 5	Device Character 6	Qualifier Character 7
0 Tracheobronchial Tree **K** Lung, Right **L** Lung, Left **Q** Pleura **T** Diaphragm	**X** External	**0** Drainage Device **Y** Other Device	**Z** No Qualifier
1 Trachea Cricoid cartilage	**X** External	**0** Drainage Device **E** Intraluminal Device, Endotracheal Airway **F** Tracheostomy Device **Y** Other Device	**Z** No Qualifier

Non-OR   All body part, approach, device, and qualifier values

---

0   **Medical and Surgical**
B   **Respiratory System**
5   **Destruction**   Definition: Physical eradication of all or a portion of a body part by the direct use of energy, force, or a destructive agent

                         Explanation: None of the body part is physically taken out

Body Part Character 4	Approach Character 5	Device Character 6	Qualifier Character 7

1   Trachea
    Cricoid cartilage
2   Carina
3   Main Bronchus, Right
    Bronchus intermedius
    Intermediate bronchus
4   Upper Lobe Bronchus, Right
5   Middle Lobe Bronchus, Right
6   Lower Lobe Bronchus, Right
7   Main Bronchus, Left
8   Upper Lobe Bronchus, Left
9   Lingula Bronchus
B   Lower Lobe Bronchus, Left
C   Upper Lung Lobe, Right
D   Middle Lung Lobe, Right
F   Lower Lung Lobe, Right
G   Upper Lung Lobe, Left
H   Lung Lingula
J   Lower Lung Lobe, Left
K   Lung, Right
L   Lung, Left
M   Lungs, Bilateral
	0 Open
	3 Percutaneous
	4 Percutaneous Endoscopic
	7 Via Natural or Artificial Opening
	8 Via Natural or Artificial Opening Endoscopic
		Z No Device	**Z** No Qualifier

N Pleura, Right **P** Pleura, Left **T** Diaphragm	**0** Open **3** Percutaneous **4** Percutaneous Endoscopic	**Z** No Device	**Z** No Qualifier

Non-OR   0B5[3,4,5,6,7,8,9,B][4,8]ZZ
Non-OR   0B5[C,D,F,G,H,J,K,L,M]8ZZ

NC Noncovered Procedure   **LC** Limited Coverage   **QA** Questionable OB Admit   **NT** New Tech Add-on   ⊞ Combination Member   ♂ Male   ♀ Female

ICD-10-PCS 2022   **341**

Respiratory System

Ø   Medical and Surgical
B   Respiratory System
7   Dilation   Definition: Expanding an orifice or the lumen of a tubular body part

                Explanation: The orifice can be a natural orifice or an artificially created orifice. Accomplished by stretching a tubular body part using intraluminal pressure or by cutting part of the orifice or wall of the tubular body part.

Body Part Character 4	Approach Character 5	Device Character 6	Qualifier Character 7

1 Trachea
   Cricoid cartilage
2 Carina
3 Main Bronchus, Right
   Bronchus intermedius
   Intermediate bronchus
4 Upper Lobe Bronchus, Right
5 Middle Lobe Bronchus, Right
6 Lower Lobe Bronchus, Right
7 Main Bronchus, Left
8 Upper Lobe Bronchus, Left
9 Lingula Bronchus
B Lower Lobe Bronchus, Left
	Ø Open
	3 Percutaneous
	4 Percutaneous Endoscopic
	7 Via Natural or Artificial
	   Opening
	8 Via Natural or Artificial
	   Opening Endoscopic
		D Intraluminal Device
		Z No Device
			Z No Qualifier

     Non-OR   ØB7[3,4,5,6,7,8,9,B][Ø,3,4,7,8][D,Z]Z

Ø   Medical and Surgical
B   Respiratory System
9   Drainage   Definition: Taking or letting out fluids and/or gases from a body part

                Explanation: The qualifier DIAGNOSTIC is used to identify drainage procedures that are biopsies

Body Part Character 4	Approach Character 5	Device Character 6	Qualifier Character 7

1 Trachea
   Cricoid cartilage
2 Carina
3 Main Bronchus, Right
   Bronchus intermedius
   Intermediate bronchus
4 Upper Lobe Bronchus, Right
5 Middle Lobe Bronchus, Right
6 Lower Lobe Bronchus, Right
7 Main Bronchus, Left   8 Upper Lobe Bronchus, Left
9 Lingula Bronchus
B Lower Lobe Bronchus, Left
C Upper Lung Lobe, Right
D Middle Lung Lobe, Right
F Lower Lung Lobe, Right
G Upper Lung Lobe, Left
H Lung Lingula
J Lower Lung Lobe, Left
K Lung, Right
L Lung, Left
M Lungs, Bilateral
	Ø Open
	3 Percutaneous
	4 Percutaneous Endoscopic
	7 Via Natural or Artificial
	   Opening
	8 Via Natural or Artificial
	   Opening Endoscopic
		Ø Drainage Device	Z No Qualifier

1 Trachea
   Cricoid cartilage
2 Carina
3 Main Bronchus, Right
   Bronchus intermedius
   Intermediate bronchus
4 Upper Lobe Bronchus, Right
5 Middle Lobe Bronchus, Right
6 Lower Lobe Bronchus, Right
7 Main Bronchus, Left   8 Upper Lobe Bronchus, Left
9 Lingula Bronchus
B Lower Lobe Bronchus, Left
C Upper Lung Lobe, Right
D Middle Lung Lobe, Right
F Lower Lung Lobe, Right
G Upper Lung Lobe, Left
H Lung Lingula
J Lower Lung Lobe, Left
K Lung, Right
L Lung, Left
M Lungs, Bilateral
	Ø Open
	3 Percutaneous
	4 Percutaneous Endoscopic
	7 Via Natural or Artificial
	   Opening
	8 Via Natural or Artificial
	   Opening Endoscopic
		Z No Device	X Diagnostic
			Z No Qualifier

N Pleura, Right P Pleura, Left	Ø Open 3 Percutaneous 4 Percutaneous Endoscopic 8 Via Natural or Artificial Opening Endoscopic	Ø Drainage Device	Z No Qualifier
N Pleura, Right P Pleura, Left	Ø Open 3 Percutaneous 4 Percutaneous Endoscopic 8 Via Natural or Artificial Opening Endoscopic	Z No Device	X Diagnostic Z No Qualifier
T Diaphragm	Ø Open 3 Percutaneous 4 Percutaneous Endoscopic	Ø Drainage Device	Z No Qualifier
T Diaphragm	Ø Open 3 Percutaneous 4 Percutaneous Endoscopic	Z No Device	X Diagnostic Z No Qualifier

     Non-OR   ØB9[1,2,3,4,5,6,7,8,9,B][7,8]ØZ
     Non-OR   ØB9[1,2,3,4,5,6,7,8,9,B][3,4]ZX
     Non-OR   ØB9[1,2,3,4,5,6,7,8,9,B][7,8]Z[X,Z]
     Non-OR   ØB9[C,D,F,G,H,J,K,L,M][3,4,7]ZX
     Non-OR   ØB9[C,D,F,G,H,J,K,L,M]8Z[X,Z]
     Non-OR   ØB9[N,P][Ø,3,8]ØZ
     Non-OR   ØB9[N,P][Ø,3,8]Z[X,Z]
     Non-OR   ØB9[N,P]4ZX
     Non-OR   ØB9T[3,4]ØZ
     Non-OR   ØB9T[3,4]Z[X,Z]

Ø   Medical and Surgical
B   Respiratory System
B   Excision   Definition: Cutting out or off, without replacement, a portion of a body part

                   Explanation: The qualifier DIAGNOSTIC is used to identify excision procedures that are biopsies

Body Part Character 4	Approach Character 5	Device Character 6	Qualifier Character 7

1 Trachea
    Cricoid cartilage
2 Carina
3 Main Bronchus, Right
    Bronchus intermedius
    Intermediate bronchus
4 Upper Lobe Bronchus, Right
5 Middle Lobe Bronchus, Right
6 Lower Lobe Bronchus, Right
7 Main Bronchus, Left
8 Upper Lobe Bronchus, Left
9 Lingula Bronchus
B Lower Lobe Bronchus, Left
C Upper Lung Lobe, Right
D Middle Lung Lobe, Right
F Lower Lung Lobe, Right
G Upper Lung Lobe, Left
H Lung Lingula
J Lower Lung Lobe, Left
K Lung, Right
L Lung, Left
M Lungs, Bilateral
	Ø Open
	3 Percutaneous
	4 Percutaneous Endoscopic
	7 Via Natural or Artificial Opening
	8 Via Natural or Artificial Opening
	    Endoscopic
		Z No Device	**X** Diagnostic
			Z No Qualifier

N Pleura, Right **P** Pleura, Left	**Ø** Open **3** Percutaneous **4** Percutaneous Endoscopic **8** Via Natural or Artificial Opening Endoscopic	**Z** No Device	**X** Diagnostic **Z** No Qualifier
T Diaphragm	**Ø** Open **3** Percutaneous **4** Percutaneous Endoscopic	**Z** No Device	**X** Diagnostic **Z** No Qualifier

Non-OR   ØBB[1,2,3,4,5,6,7,8,9,B][3,4,7,8]ZX
Non-OR   ØBB[3,4,5,6,7,8,9,B,M][4,8]ZZ
Non-OR   ØBB[C,D,F,G,H,J,K,L,M]3ZX
Non-OR   ØBB[C,D,F,G,H,J,K,L]8ZZ
Non-OR   ØBB[N,P][Ø,3]ZX

Ø   Medical and Surgical
B   Respiratory System
C   Extirpation   Definition: Taking or cutting out solid matter from a body part

                   Explanation: The solid matter may be an abnormal byproduct of a biological function or a foreign body; it may be imbedded in a body part or in
                   the lumen of a tubular body part. The solid matter may or may not have been previously broken into pieces.

Body Part Character 4	Approach Character 5	Device Character 6	Qualifier Character 7

1 Trachea
    Cricoid cartilage
2 Carina
3 Main Bronchus, Right
    Bronchus intermedius
    Intermediate bronchus
4 Upper Lobe Bronchus, Right
5 Middle Lobe Bronchus, Right
6 Lower Lobe Bronchus, Right
7 Main Bronchus, Left
8 Upper Lobe Bronchus, Left
9 Lingula Bronchus
B Lower Lobe Bronchus, Left
C Upper Lung Lobe, Right
D Middle Lung Lobe, Right
F Lower Lung Lobe, Right
G Upper Lung Lobe, Left
H Lung Lingula
J Lower Lung Lobe, Left
K Lung, Right
L Lung, Left
M Lungs, Bilateral
	Ø Open
	3 Percutaneous
	4 Percutaneous Endoscopic
	7 Via Natural or Artificial Opening
	8 Via Natural or Artificial Opening
	    Endoscopic
		Z No Device	**Z** No Qualifier

N Pleura, Right **P** Pleura, Left **T** Diaphragm	**Ø** Open **3** Percutaneous **4** Percutaneous Endoscopic	**Z** No Device	**Z** No Qualifier

Non-OR   ØBC[1,2,3,4,5,6,7,8,9,B][7,8]ZZ
Non-OR   ØBC[N,P]3ZZ

NC Noncovered Procedure   **LC** Limited Coverage   **QA** Questionable OB Admit   **NT** New Tech Add-on   ⊞ Combination Member   ♂ Male   ♀ Female

Ø   **Medical and Surgical**
B   **Respiratory System**
D   **Extraction**   Definition: Pulling or stripping out or off all or a portion of a body part by the use of force

                       Explanation: The qualifier DIAGNOSTIC is used to identify extraction procedures that are biopsies

Body Part Character 4	Approach Character 5	Device Character 6	Qualifier Character 7

1   Trachea
     Cricoid cartilage
2   Carina
3   Main Bronchus, Right
     Bronchus intermedius
     Intermediate bronchus
4   Upper Lobe Bronchus, Right
5   Middle Lobe Bronchus, Right
6   Lower Lobe Bronchus, Right
7   Main Bronchus, Left
8   Upper Lobe Bronchus, Left
9   Lingula Bronchus
B   Lower Lobe Bronchus, Left
C   Upper Lung Lobe, Right
D   Middle Lung Lobe, Right
F   Lower Lung Lobe, Right
G   Upper Lung Lobe, Left
H   Lung Lingula
J   Lower Lung Lobe, Left
K   Lung, Right
L   Lung, Left
M   Lungs, Bilateral
	4 Percutaneous Endoscopic
	8 Via Natural or Artificial Opening
	     Endoscopic
		Z No Device	X Diagnostic

N Pleura, Right P Pleura, Left	Ø Open 3 Percutaneous 4 Percutaneous Endoscopic	Z No Device	X Diagnostic Z No Qualifier

Non-OR   ØBD[1,2,3,4,5,6,7,8,9,B,C,D,F,G,H,J,K,L,M][4,8]ZX

Ø   **Medical and Surgical**
B   **Respiratory System**
F   **Fragmentation**   Definition: Breaking solid matter in a body part into pieces

                     Explanation: Physical force (e.g., manual, ultrasonic) applied directly or indirectly is used to break the solid matter into pieces. The solid matter may be an abnormal byproduct of a biological function or a foreign body. The pieces of solid matter are not taken out.

Body Part Character 4	Approach Character 5	Device Character 6	Qualifier Character 7

1   Trachea   NC
     Cricoid cartilage
2   Carina   NC
3   Main Bronchus, Right   NC
     Bronchus intermedius
     Intermediate bronchus
4   Upper Lobe Bronchus, Right   NC
5   Middle Lobe Bronchus, Right   NC
6   Lower Lobe Bronchus, Right   NC
7   Main Bronchus, Left   NC
8   Upper Lobe Bronchus, Left   NC
9   Lingula Bronchus   NC
B   Lower Lobe Bronchus, Left   NC
	Ø Open
	3 Percutaneous
	4 Percutaneous Endoscopic
	7 Via Natural or Artificial Opening
	8 Via Natural or Artificial Opening
	     Endoscopic
	X External
		Z No Device	Z No Qualifier

Non-OR   ØBF[1,2,3,4,5,6,7,8,9,B]XZZ
Non-OR   ØBF[3,4,5,6,7,8,9,B][7,8]ZZ
NC   ØBF[1,2,3,4,5,6,7,8,9,B]XZZ

Ø   **Medical and Surgical**
B   **Respiratory System**
H   **Insertion**   Definition: Putting in a nonbiological appliance that monitors, assists, performs, or prevents a physiological function but does not physically take the place of a body part
                   Explanation: None

Body Part Character 4	Approach Character 5	Device Character 6	Qualifier Character 7
Ø Tracheobronchial Tree	**Ø** Open **3** Percutaneous **4** Percutaneous Endoscopic **7** Via Natural or Artificial Opening **8** Via Natural or Artificial Opening Endoscopic	**1** Radioactive Element **2** Monitoring Device **3** Infusion Device **D** Intraluminal Device **Y** Other Device	**Z** No Qualifier
1 Trachea Cricoid cartilage	**Ø** Open	**2** Monitoring Device **D** Intraluminal Device **Y** Other Device	**Z** No Qualifier
1 Trachea Cricoid cartilage	**3** Percutaneous	**D** Intraluminal Device **E** Intraluminal Device, Endotracheal Airway **Y** Other Device	**Z** No Qualifier
1 Trachea Cricoid cartilage	**4** Percutaneous Endoscopic	**D** Intraluminal Device **Y** Other Device	**Z** No Qualifier
1 Trachea Cricoid cartilage	**7** Via Natural or Artificial Opening **8** Via Natural or Artificial Opening Endoscopic	**2** Monitoring Device **D** Intraluminal Device **E** Intraluminal Device, Endotracheal Airway **Y** Other Device	**Z** No Qualifier

3 Main Bronchus, Right
     Bronchus intermedius
     Intermediate bronchus
4 Upper Lobe Bronchus, Right
5 Middle Lobe Bronchus, Right
6 Lower Lobe Bronchus, Right
7 Main Bronchus, Left
8 Upper Lobe Bronchus, Left
9 Lingula Bronchus
B Lower Lobe Bronchus, Left
	Ø Open
	3 Percutaneous
	4 Percutaneous Endoscopic
	7 Via Natural or Artificial Opening
	8 Via Natural or Artificial Opening Endoscopic
		G Intraluminal Device, Endobronchial Valve	**Z** No Qualifier

K Lung, Right **L** Lung, Left	**Ø** Open **3** Percutaneous **4** Percutaneous Endoscopic **7** Via Natural or Artificial Opening **8** Via Natural or Artificial Opening Endoscopic	**1** Radioactive Element **2** Monitoring Device **3** Infusion Device **Y** Other Device	**Z** No Qualifier
Q Pleura	**Ø** Open **3** Percutaneous **4** Percutaneous Endoscopic **7** Via Natural or Artificial Opening **8** Via Natural or Artificial Opening Endoscopic	**Y** Other Device	**Z** No Qualifier
T Diaphragm	**Ø** Open **3** Percutaneous **4** Percutaneous Endoscopic	**2** Monitoring Device **M** Diaphragmatic Pacemaker Lead **Y** Other Device	**Z** No Qualifier
T Diaphragm	**7** Via Natural or Artificial Opening **8** Via Natural or Artificial Opening Endoscopic	**Y** Other Device	**Z** No Qualifier

DRG Non-OR	ØBH[3,4,5,6,7,8,9,B]8GZ
Non-OR	ØBH03YZ
Non-OR	ØBHØ[7,8][2,3,D,Y]Z
Non-OR	ØBH13[E,Y]Z
Non-OR	ØBH1[7,8][2,D,E,Y]Z
Non-OR	ØBH[K,L]3YZ
Non-OR	ØBH[K,L]7[2,3,Y]Z
Non-OR	ØBH[K,L]8[2,3]Z
Non-OR	ØBHQ[3,7]YZ
Non-OR	ØBHT3YZ
Non-OR	ØBHT[7,8]YZ

NC Noncovered Procedure   **LC** Limited Coverage   **QA** Questionable OB Admit   **NT** New Tech Add-on   ⊞ Combination Member   ♂ Male   ♀ Female

ICD-10-PCS 2022   **345**

ØBH–ØBH

Ø   **Medical and Surgical**
B   **Respiratory System**
J   **Inspection**   Definition: Visually and/or manually exploring a body part

Explanation: Visual exploration may be performed with or without optical instrumentation. Manual exploration may be performed directly or through intervening body layers.

Body Part Character 4	Approach Character 5	Device Character 6	Qualifier Character 7

Ø   Tracheobronchial Tree
1   Trachea
     Cricoid cartilage
K   Lung, Right
L   Lung, Left
Q   Pleura
T   Diaphragm
	Ø Open
	3 Percutaneous
	4 Percutaneous Endoscopic
	7 Via Natural or Artificial Opening
	8 Via Natural or Artificial Opening
	     Endoscopic
	X External
		Z No Device	Z No Qualifier

Non-OR   ØBJ[Ø,K,L,Q,T][3,7,8,X]ZZ
Non-OR   ØBJ1[3,4,7,8,X]ZZ

Ø   **Medical and Surgical**
B   **Respiratory System**
L   **Occlusion**   Definition: Completely closing an orifice or the lumen of a tubular body part

Explanation: The orifice can be a natural orifice or an artificially created orifice

Body Part Character 4	Approach Character 5	Device Character 6	Qualifier Character 7

1   Trachea
     Cricoid cartilage
2   Carina
3   Main Bronchus, Right
     Bronchus intermedius
     Intermediate bronchus
4   Upper Lobe Bronchus, Right
5   Middle Lobe Bronchus, Right
6   Lower Lobe Bronchus, Right
7   Main Bronchus, Left
8   Upper Lobe Bronchus, Left
9   Lingula Bronchus
B   Lower Lobe Bronchus, Left
	Ø Open
	3 Percutaneous
	4 Percutaneous Endoscopic
		C Extraluminal Device
		D Intraluminal Device
		Z No Device
			Z No Qualifier

1   Trachea
     Cricoid cartilage
2   Carina
3   Main Bronchus, Right
     Bronchus intermedius
     Intermediate bronchus
4   Upper Lobe Bronchus, Right
5   Middle Lobe Bronchus, Right
6   Lower Lobe Bronchus, Right
7   Main Bronchus, Left
8   Upper Lobe Bronchus, Left
9   Lingula Bronchus
B   Lower Lobe Bronchus, Left
	7 Via Natural or Artificial Opening
	8 Via Natural or Artificial Opening
	     Endoscopic
		D Intraluminal Device
		Z No Device
			Z No Qualifier

Ø   Medical and Surgical
B   Respiratory System
M   Reattachment   Definition: Putting back in or on all or a portion of a separated body part to its normal location or other suitable location

                        Explanation: Vascular circulation and nervous pathways may or may not be reestablished

Body Part Character 4	Approach Character 5	Device Character 6	Qualifier Character 7

1   Trachea
     Cricoid cartilage
2   Carina
3   Main Bronchus, Right
     Bronchus intermedius
     Intermediate bronchus
4   Upper Lobe Bronchus, Right
5   Middle Lobe Bronchus, Right
6   Lower Lobe Bronchus, Right
7   Main Bronchus, Left
8   Upper Lobe Bronchus, Left
9   Lingula Bronchus
B   Lower Lobe Bronchus, Left
C   Upper Lung Lobe, Right
D   Middle Lung Lobe, Right
F   Lower Lung Lobe, Right
G   Upper Lung Lobe, Left
H   Lung Lingula
J   Lower Lung Lobe, Left
K   Lung, Right
L   Lung, Left
T   Diaphragm
	Ø Open	**Z** No Device	**Z** No Qualifier

Ø   Medical and Surgical
B   Respiratory System
N   Release   Definition: Freeing a body part from an abnormal physical constraint by cutting or by the use of force

                 Explanation: Some of the restraining tissue may be taken out but none of the body part is taken out

Body Part Character 4	Approach Character 5	Device Character 6	Qualifier Character 7

1   Trachea
     Cricoid cartilage
2   Carina
3   Main Bronchus, Right
     Bronchus intermedius
     Intermediate bronchus
4   Upper Lobe Bronchus, Right
5   Middle Lobe Bronchus, Right
6   Lower Lobe Bronchus, Right
7   Main Bronchus, Left
8   Upper Lobe Bronchus, Left
9   Lingula Bronchus
B   Lower Lobe Bronchus, Left
C   Upper Lung Lobe, Right
D   Middle Lung Lobe, Right
F   Lower Lung Lobe, Right
G   Upper Lung Lobe, Left
H   Lung Lingula
J   Lower Lung Lobe, Left
K   Lung, Right
L   Lung, Left
M   Lungs, Bilateral
	Ø Open
	3 Percutaneous
	4 Percutaneous Endoscopic
	7 Via Natural or Artificial Opening
	8 Via Natural or Artificial Opening
	     Endoscopic
		Z No Device	**Z** No Qualifier

N Pleura, Right **P** Pleura, Left **T** Diaphragm	**Ø** Open **3** Percutaneous **4** Percutaneous Endoscopic	**Z** No Device	**Z** No Qualifier

NC Noncovered Procedure   **LC** Limited Coverage   **QA** Questionable OB Admit   **NT** New Tech Add-on   ⊞ Combination Member   ♂ Male   ♀ Female

ICD-10-PCS 2022   **347**

Respiratory System

Ø   Medical and Surgical
B   Respiratory System
P   Removal   Definition: Taking out or off a device from a body part

Explanation: If a device is taken out and a similar device put in without cutting or puncturing the skin or mucous membrane, the procedure is coded to the root operation CHANGE. Otherwise, the procedure for taking out a device is coded to the root operation REMOVAL.

Body Part Character 4	Approach Character 5	Device Character 6	Qualifier Character 7
Ø Tracheobronchial Tree	Ø Open 3 Percutaneous 4 Percutaneous Endoscopic 7 Via Natural or Artificial Opening 8 Via Natural or Artificial Opening Endoscopic	Ø Drainage Device 1 Radioactive Element 2 Monitoring Device 3 Infusion Device 7 Autologous Tissue Substitute C Extraluminal Device D Intraluminal Device J Synthetic Substitute K Nonautologous Tissue Substitute Y Other Device	Z No Qualifier
Ø Tracheobronchial Tree	X External	Ø Drainage Device 1 Radioactive Element 2 Monitoring Device 3 Infusion Device D Intraluminal Device	Z No Qualifier

1   Trachea
    Cricoid cartilage
	Ø Open
	3 Percutaneous
	4 Percutaneous Endoscopic
	7 Via Natural or Artificial Opening
	8 Via Natural or Artificial Opening
	    Endoscopic
		Ø Drainage Device
		2 Monitoring Device
		7 Autologous Tissue Substitute
		C Extraluminal Device
		D Intraluminal Device
		F Tracheostomy Device
		J Synthetic Substitute
		K Nonautologous Tissue Substitute
			Z No Qualifier

1 Trachea Cricoid cartilage	X External	Ø Drainage Device 2 Monitoring Device D Intraluminal Device F Tracheostomy Device	Z No Qualifier
K Lung, Right L Lung, Left	Ø Open 3 Percutaneous 4 Percutaneous Endoscopic 7 Via Natural or Artificial Opening 8 Via Natural or Artificial Opening Endoscopic	Ø Drainage Device 1 Radioactive Element 2 Monitoring Device 3 Infusion Device Y Other Device	Z No Qualifier
K Lung, Right L Lung, Left	X External	Ø Drainage Device 1 Radioactive Element 2 Monitoring Device 3 Infusion Device	Z No Qualifier
Q Pleura	Ø Open 3 Percutaneous 4 Percutaneous Endoscopic 7 Via Natural or Artificial Opening 8 Via Natural or Artificial Opening Endoscopic	Ø Drainage Device 1 Radioactive Element 2 Monitoring Device Y Other Device	Z No Qualifier
Q Pleura	X External	Ø Drainage Device 1 Radioactive Element 2 Monitoring Device	Z No Qualifier
T Diaphragm	Ø Open 3 Percutaneous 4 Percutaneous Endoscopic 7 Via Natural or Artificial Opening 8 Via Natural or Artificial Opening Endoscopic	Ø Drainage Device 2 Monitoring Device 7 Autologous Tissue Substitute J Synthetic Substitute K Nonautologous Tissue Substitute M Diaphragmatic Pacemaker Lead Y Other Device	Z No Qualifier
T Diaphragm	X External	Ø Drainage Device 2 Monitoring Device M Diaphragmatic Pacemaker Lead	Z No Qualifier

Non-OR	ØBPØ[3,4]YZ	**Non-OR**	ØBPL7[Ø,2,3,Y]Z
Non-OR	ØBPØ[7,8][Ø,2,3,D,Y]Z	**Non-OR**	ØBPL8[Ø,2,3]Z
Non-OR	ØBPØX[Ø,1,2,3,D]Z	**Non-OR**	ØBP[K,L]X[Ø,1,2,3]Z
Non-OR	ØBP1[Ø,3,4]FZ	**Non-OR**	ØBPQ[Ø,3,4,7,8][Ø,1,2,]Z
Non-OR	ØBP1[7,8][Ø,2,D,F]Z	**Non-OR**	ØBPQ[3,7]YZ
Non-OR	ØBP1X[Ø,2,D,F]Z	**Non-OR**	ØBPQX[Ø,1,2]Z
Non-OR	ØBP[K,L]3YZ	**Non-OR**	ØBPT3YZ
Non-OR	ØBPK7[Ø,1,2,3,Y]Z	**Non-OR**	ØBPT[7,8][Ø,2,Y]Z
Non-OR	ØBPK8[Ø,1,2,3]Z	**Non-OR**	ØBPTX[Ø,2,M]Z

Non-OR Procedure   DRG Non-OR Procedure   Valid OR Procedure   HAC Associated Procedure   Combination Only   New/Revised GREEN

Ø   Medical and Surgical
B   Respiratory System
Q   Repair   Definition: Restoring, to the extent possible, a body part to its normal anatomic structure and function

                      Explanation: Used only when the method to accomplish the repair is not one of the other root operations

Body Part Character 4	Approach Character 5	Device Character 6	Qualifier Character 7

1 Trachea
     Cricoid cartilage
2 Carina
3 Main Bronchus, Right
     Bronchus intermedius
     Intermediate bronchus
4 Upper Lobe Bronchus, Right
5 Middle Lobe Bronchus, Right
6 Lower Lobe Bronchus, Right
7 Main Bronchus, Left
8 Upper Lobe Bronchus, Left
9 Lingula Bronchus
B Lower Lobe Bronchus, Left
C Upper Lung Lobe, Right
D Middle Lung Lobe, Right
F Lower Lung Lobe, Right
G Upper Lung Lobe, Left
H Lung Lingula
J Lower Lung Lobe, Left
K Lung, Right
L Lung, Left
M Lungs, Bilateral
	Ø Open
	3 Percutaneous
	4 Percutaneous Endoscopic
	7 Via Natural or Artificial Opening
	8 Via Natural or Artificial Opening
	     Endoscopic
		Z No Device	**Z** No Qualifier

N Pleura, Right **P** Pleura, Left **T** Diaphragm	**Ø** Open **3** Percutaneous **4** Percutaneous Endoscopic	**Z** No Device	**Z** No Qualifier

NC Noncovered Procedure   **LC** Limited Coverage   **QA** Questionable OB Admit   **NT** New Tech Add-on   ⊞ Combination Member   ♂ Male   ♀ Female

ICD-10-PCS 2022   **349**

Respiratory System

Ø   **Medical and Surgical**
B   **Respiratory System**
R   **Replacement**   Definition: Putting in or on biological or synthetic material that physically takes the place and/or function of all or a portion of a body part

Explanation: The body part may have been taken out or replaced, or may be taken out, physically eradicated, or rendered nonfunctional during the REPLACEMENT procedure. A REMOVAL procedure is coded for taking out the device used in a previous replacement procedure.

Body Part Character 4	Approach Character 5	Device Character 6	Qualifier Character 7

1   Trachea
    Cricoid cartilage
2   Carina
3   Main Bronchus, Right
    Bronchus intermedius
    Intermediate bronchus
4   Upper Lobe Bronchus, Right
5   Middle Lobe Bronchus, Right
6   Lower Lobe Bronchus, Right
7   Main Bronchus, Left
8   Upper Lobe Bronchus, Left
9   Lingula Bronchus
B   Lower Lobe Bronchus, Left
T   Diaphragm
	Ø Open
	4 Percutaneous Endoscopic
		7 Autologous Tissue Substitute
		J Synthetic Substitute
		K Nonautologous Tissue Substitute
			Z No Qualifier

Ø   **Medical and Surgical**
B   **Respiratory System**
S   **Reposition**   Definition: Moving to its normal location, or other suitable location, all or a portion of a body part

Explanation: The body part is moved to a new location from an abnormal location, or from a normal location where it is not functioning correctly. The body part may or may not be cut out or off to be moved to the new location.

Body Part Character 4	Approach Character 5	Device Character 6	Qualifier Character 7

1   Trachea
    Cricoid cartilage
2   Carina
3   Main Bronchus, Right
    Bronchus intermedius
    Intermediate bronchus
4   Upper Lobe Bronchus, Right
5   Middle Lobe Bronchus, Right
6   Lower Lobe Bronchus, Right
7   Main Bronchus, Left
8   Upper Lobe Bronchus, Left
9   Lingula Bronchus
B   Lower Lobe Bronchus, Left
C   Upper Lung Lobe, Right
D   Middle Lung Lobe, Right
F   Lower Lung Lobe, Right
G   Upper Lung Lobe, Left
H   Lung Lingula
J   Lower Lung Lobe, Left
K   Lung, Right
L   Lung, Left
T   Diaphragm
	Ø Open	Z No Device	Z No Qualifier

Ø   **Medical and Surgical**
B   **Respiratory System**
T   **Resection**   Definition: Cutting out or off, without replacement, all of a body part
                    Explanation: None

Body Part Character 4	Approach Character 5	Device Character 6	Qualifier Character 7

1 Trachea
    Cricoid cartilage
2 Carina
3 Main Bronchus, Right
    Bronchus intermedius
    Intermediate bronchus
4 Upper Lobe Bronchus, Right
5 Middle Lobe Bronchus, Right
6 Lower Lobe Bronchus, Right
7 Main Bronchus, Left
8 Upper Lobe Bronchus, Left
9 Lingula Bronchus
B Lower Lobe Bronchus, Left
C Upper Lung Lobe, Right
D Middle Lung Lobe, Right
F Lower Lung Lobe, Right
G Upper Lung Lobe, Left
H Lung Lingula
J Lower Lung Lobe, Left
K Lung, Right
L Lung, Left
M Lungs, Bilateral
T Diaphragm
	Ø Open
	4 Percutaneous Endoscopic
		Z No Device	**Z** No Qualifier

Ø   **Medical and Surgical**
B   **Respiratory System**
U   **Supplement**   Definition: Putting in or on biological or synthetic material that physically reinforces and/or augments the function of a portion of a body part
                    Explanation: The biological material is non-living, or is living and from the same individual. The body part may have been previously replaced, and the SUPPLEMENT procedure is performed to physically reinforce and/or augment the function of the replaced body part.

Body Part Character 4	Approach Character 5	Device Character 6	Qualifier Character 7

1 Trachea
    Cricoid cartilage
2 Carina
3 Main Bronchus, Right
    Bronchus intermedius
    Intermediate bronchus
4 Upper Lobe Bronchus, Right
5 Middle Lobe Bronchus, Right
6 Lower Lobe Bronchus, Right
7 Main Bronchus, Left
8 Upper Lobe Bronchus, Left
9 Lingula Bronchus
B Lower Lobe Bronchus, Left
	Ø Open
	4 Percutaneous Endoscopic
	8 Via Natural or Artificial Opening
	    Endoscopic
		7 Autologous Tissue Substitute
		J Synthetic Substitute
		K Nonautologous Tissue Substitute
			Z No Qualifier

T Diaphragm	**Ø** Open **4** Percutaneous Endoscopic	**7** Autologous Tissue Substitute **J** Synthetic Substitute **K** Nonautologous Tissue Substitute	**Z** No Qualifier

NC Noncovered Procedure   LC Limited Coverage   QA Questionable OB Admit   NT New Tech Add-on   ⊞ Combination Member   ♂ Male   ♀ Female

ICD-10-PCS 2022   351

Ø Medical and Surgical
B Respiratory System
V Restriction   Definition: Partially closing an orifice or the lumen of a tubular body part
                     Explanation: The orifice can be a natural orifice or an artificially created orifice

Body Part Character 4	Approach Character 5	Device Character 6	Qualifier Character 7

1 Trachea
    Cricoid cartilage
2 Carina
3 Main Bronchus, Right
    Bronchus intermedius
    Intermediate bronchus
4 Upper Lobe Bronchus, Right
5 Middle Lobe Bronchus, Right
6 Lower Lobe Bronchus, Right
7 Main Bronchus, Left
8 Upper Lobe Bronchus, Left
9 Lingula Bronchus
B Lower Lobe Bronchus, Left
	Ø Open
	3 Percutaneous
	4 Percutaneous Endoscopic
		C Extraluminal Device
		D Intraluminal Device
		Z No Device
			Z No Qualifier

1 Trachea
    Cricoid cartilage
2 Carina
3 Main Bronchus, Right
    Bronchus intermedius
    Intermediate bronchus
4 Upper Lobe Bronchus, Right
5 Middle Lobe Bronchus, Right
6 Lower Lobe Bronchus, Right
7 Main Bronchus, Left
8 Upper Lobe Bronchus, Left
9 Lingula Bronchus
B Lower Lobe Bronchus, Left
	7 Via Natural or Artificial Opening
	8 Via Natural or Artificial Opening Endoscopic
		D Intraluminal Device
		Z No Device
			Z No Qualifier

Ø   Medical and Surgical
B   Respiratory System
W   Revision   Definition: Correcting, to the extent possible, a portion of a malfunctioning device or the position of a displaced device

                 Explanation: Revision can include correcting a malfunctioning or displaced device by taking out or putting in components of the device such as a screw or pin

Body Part Character 4	Approach Character 5	Device Character 6	Qualifier Character 7
Ø Tracheobronchial Tree	**Ø** Open **3** Percutaneous **4** Percutaneous Endoscopic **7** Via Natural or Artificial Opening **8** Via Natural or Artificial Opening Endoscopic	**Ø** Drainage Device **2** Monitoring Device **3** Infusion Device **7** Autologous Tissue Substitute **C** Extraluminal Device **D** Intraluminal Device **J** Synthetic Substitute **K** Nonautologous Tissue Substitute **Y** Other Device	**Z** No Qualifier
Ø Tracheobronchial Tree	**X** External	**Ø** Drainage Device **2** Monitoring Device **3** Infusion Device **7** Autologous Tissue Substitute **C** Extraluminal Device **D** Intraluminal Device **J** Synthetic Substitute **K** Nonautologous Tissue Substitute	**Z** No Qualifier
1 Trachea Cricoid cartilage	**Ø** Open **3** Percutaneous **4** Percutaneous Endoscopic **7** Via Natural or Artificial Opening **8** Via Natural or Artificial Opening Endoscopic **X** External	**Ø** Drainage Device **2** Monitoring Device **7** Autologous Tissue Substitute **C** Extraluminal Device **D** Intraluminal Device **F** Tracheostomy Device **J** Synthetic Substitute **K** Nonautologous Tissue Substitute	**Z** No Qualifier
K Lung, Right **L** Lung, Left	**Ø** Open **3** Percutaneous **4** Percutaneous Endoscopic **7** Via Natural or Artificial Opening **8** Via Natural or Artificial Opening Endoscopic	**Ø** Drainage Device **2** Monitoring Device **3** Infusion Device **Y** Other Device	**Z** No Qualifier
K Lung, Right **L** Lung, Left	**X** External	**Ø** Drainage Device **2** Monitoring Device **3** Infusion Device	**Z** No Qualifier
Q Pleura	**Ø** Open **3** Percutaneous **4** Percutaneous Endoscopic **7** Via Natural or Artificial Opening **8** Via Natural or Artificial Opening Endoscopic	**Ø** Drainage Device **2** Monitoring Device **Y** Other Device	**Z** No Qualifier
Q Pleura	**X** External	**Ø** Drainage Device **2** Monitoring Device	**Z** No Qualifier
T Diaphragm	**Ø** Open **3** Percutaneous **4** Percutaneous Endoscopic **7** Via Natural or Artificial Opening **8** Via Natural or Artificial Opening Endoscopic	**Ø** Drainage Device **2** Monitoring Device **7** Autologous Tissue Substitute **J** Synthetic Substitute **K** Nonautologous Tissue Substitute **M** Diaphragmatic Pacemaker Lead **Y** Other Device	**Z** No Qualifier
T Diaphragm	**X** External	**Ø** Drainage Device **2** Monitoring Device **7** Autologous Tissue Substitute **J** Synthetic Substitute **K** Nonautologous Tissue Substitute **M** Diaphragmatic Pacemaker Lead	**Z** No Qualifier

Non-OR	ØBWØ[3,4]YZ
Non-OR	ØBWØ[7,8][2,3,D,Y]Z
Non-OR	ØBWØX[Ø,2,3,7,C,D,J,K]Z
Non-OR	ØBW1X[Ø,2,7,C,D,F,J,K]Z
Non-OR	ØBW[K,L]3YZ
Non-OR	ØBW[K,L]7[Ø,2,3,Y]Z
Non-OR	ØBW[K,L]8[Ø,2,3]Z
Non-OR	ØBW[K,L]X[Ø,2,3]Z
Non-OR	ØBWQ[Ø,3,4,7,8][Ø,2]Z
Non-OR	ØBWQ[Ø,3,7]YZ
Non-OR	ØBWQX[Ø,2]Z
Non-OR	ØBWT[3,7,8]YZ
Non-OR	ØBWTX[Ø,2,7,J,K,M]Z

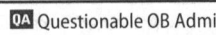

NC Noncovered Procedure   **LC** Limited Coverage   **QA** Questionable OB Admit   **NT** New Tech Add-on   ⊞ Combination Member   ♂ Male   ♀ Female

Ø   **Medical and Surgical**
B   **Respiratory System**
Y   **Transplantation**   Definition: Putting in or on all or a portion of a living body part taken from another individual or animal to physically take the place and/or function of all or a portion of a similar body part

Explanation: The native body part may or may not be taken out, and the transplanted body part may take over all or a portion of its function

Body Part Character 4		Approach Character 5	Device Character 6	Qualifier Character 7
C Upper Lung Lobe, Right LC D Middle Lung Lobe, Right LC F Lower Lung Lobe, Right LC G Upper Lung Lobe, Left LC H Lung Lingula LC J Lower Lung Lobe, Left LC K Lung, Right LC L Lung, Left LC M Lungs, Bilateral LC		Ø Open	Z No Device	Ø Allogeneic 1 Syngeneic 2 Zooplastic

LC   ØBY[C,D,F,G,H,J,K,L,M]ØZ[Ø,1,2]

Mouth and Throat 0C0–0CX

Character Meanings

This Character Meaning table is provided as a guide to assist the user in the identification of character members that may be found in this section of code tables. It **SHOULD NOT** be used to build a PCS code.

Operation–Character 3		Body Part–Character 4		Approach–Character 5		Device–Character 6		Qualifier–Character 7	
0	Alteration	0	Upper Lip	0	Open	0	Drainage Device	0	Single
2	Change	1	Lower Lip	3	Percutaneous	1	Radioactive Element	1	Multiple
5	Destruction	2	Hard Palate	4	Percutaneous Endoscopic	5	External Fixation Device	2	All
7	Dilation	3	Soft Palate	7	Via Natural or Artificial Opening	7	Autologous Tissue Substitute	X	Diagnostic
9	Drainage	4	Buccal Mucosa	8	Via Natural or Artificial Opening Endoscopic	B	Intraluminal Device, Airway	Z	No Qualifier
B	Excision	5	Upper Gingiva	X	External	C	Extraluminal Device		
C	Extirpation	6	Lower Gingiva			D	Intraluminal Device		
D	Extraction	7	Tongue			J	Synthetic Substitute		
F	Fragmentation	8	Parotid Gland, Right			K	Nonautologous Tissue Substitute		
H	Insertion	9	Parotid Gland, Left			Y	Other Device		
J	Inspection	A	Salivary Gland			Z	No Device		
L	Occlusion	B	Parotid Duct, Right						
M	Reattachment	C	Parotid Duct, Left						
N	Release	D	Sublingual Gland, Right						
P	Removal	F	Sublingual Gland, Left						
Q	Repair	G	Submaxillary Gland, Right						
R	Replacement	H	Submaxillary Gland, Left						
S	Reposition	J	Minor Salivary Gland						
T	Resection	M	Pharynx						
U	Supplement	N	Uvula						
V	Restriction	P	Tonsils						
W	Revision	Q	Adenoids						
X	Transfer	R	Epiglottis						
		S	Larynx						
		T	Vocal Cord, Right						
		V	Vocal Cord, Left						
		W	Upper Tooth						
		X	Lower Tooth						
		Y	Mouth and Throat						

AHA Coding Clinic for table 0C9
2017, 2Q, 16   Incision and drainage of floor of mouth

AHA Coding Clinic for table 0CB
2017, 2Q, 16   Excision of floor of mouth
2016, 3Q, 28   Lingual tonsillectomy, tongue base excision and epiglottopexy
2016, 2Q, 19   Biopsy of the base of tongue
2014, 3Q, 21   Superficial parotidectomy

AHA Coding Clinic for table 0CC
2016, 2Q, 20   Sialendoscopy with stone removal

AHA Coding Clinic for table 0CH
2020, 4Q, 43-44   Insertion of radioactive element

AHA Coding Clinic for table 0CQ
2017, 1Q, 20   Preparatory nasal adhesion repair before definitive cleft palate repair

AHA Coding Clinic for table 0CR
2014, 3Q, 25   Excision of soft palate with placement of surgical obturator
2014, 2Q, 5   Oasis acellular matrix graft
2014, 2Q, 6   Composite grafting (synthetic versus nonautologous tissue substitute)

AHA Coding Clinic for table 0CS
2016, 3Q, 28   Lingual tonsillectomy, tongue base excision and epiglottopexy

AHA Coding Clinic for table 0CT
2016, 2Q, 12   Resection of malignant neoplasm of infratemporal fossa
2014, 3Q, 21   Superficial parotidectomy
2014, 3Q, 23   Le Fort I osteotomy

Salivary Glands

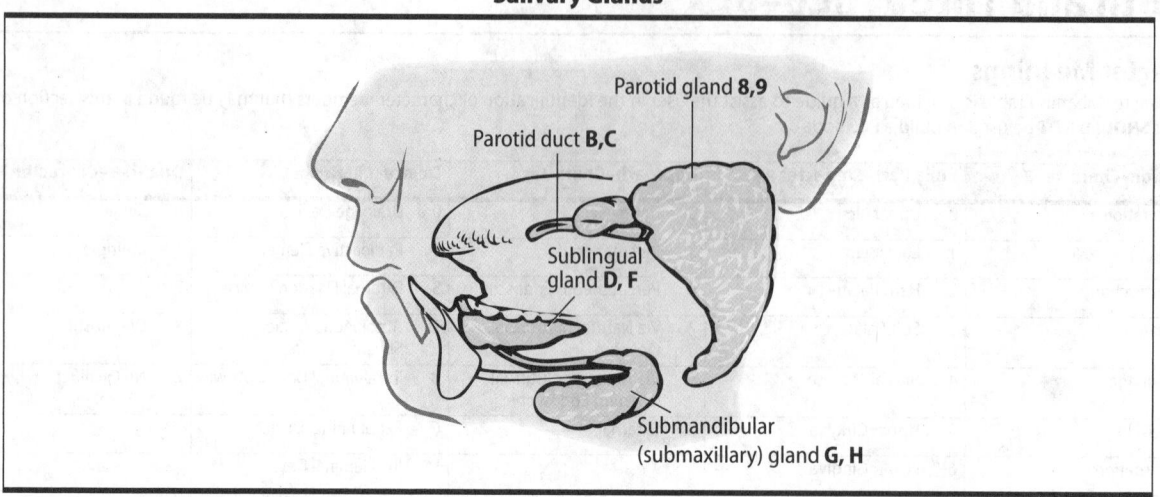

Parotid gland **8,9**

Parotid duct **B,C**

Sublingual gland **D, F**

Submandibular (submaxillary) gland **G, H**

Oral Anatomy

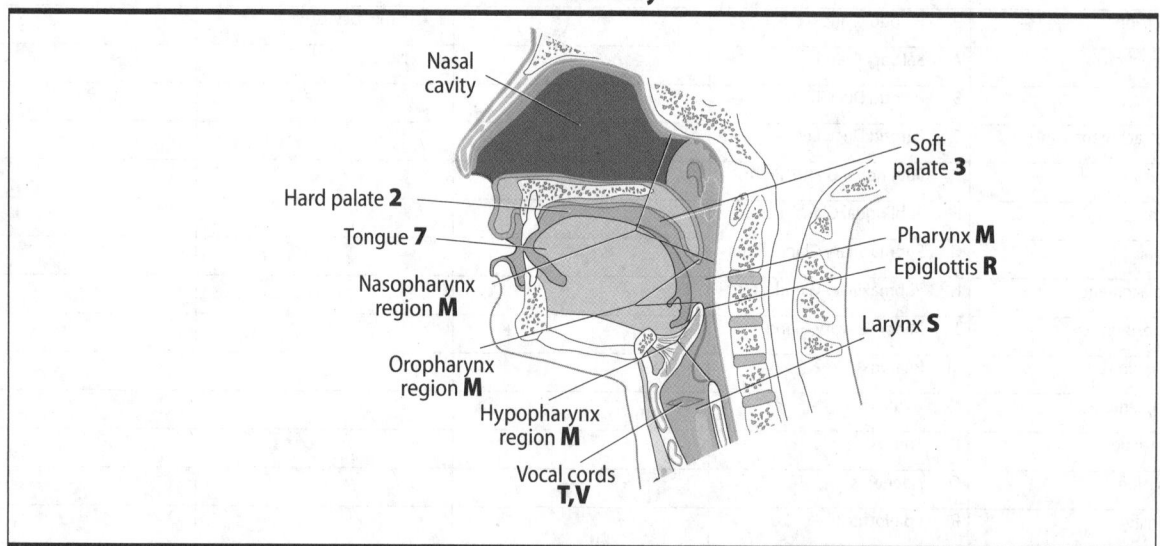

Nasal cavity

Soft palate **3**

Hard palate **2**

Tongue **7**

Pharynx **M**

Epiglottis **R**

Nasopharynx region **M**

Larynx **S**

Oropharynx region **M**

Hypopharynx region **M**

Vocal cords **T,V**

Mouth Frontal View (Upper)

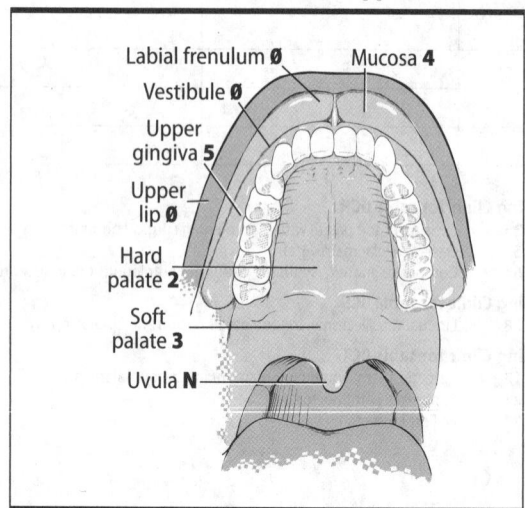

Labial frenulum **Ø**

Mucosa **4**

Vestibule **Ø**

Upper gingiva **5**

Upper lip **Ø**

Hard palate **2**

Soft palate **3**

Uvula **N**

Mouth Frontal View (Lower)

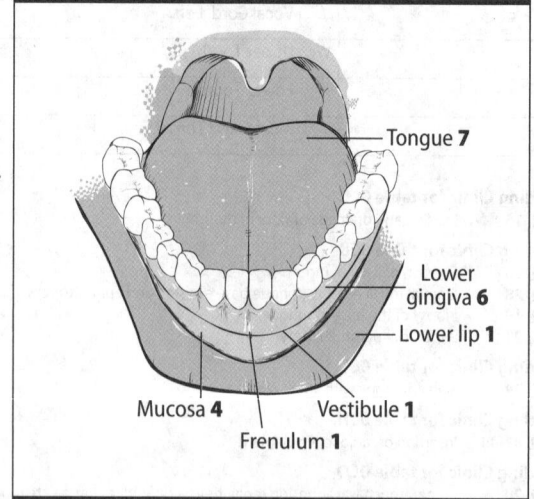

Tongue **7**

Lower gingiva **6**

Lower lip **1**

Mucosa **4**

Vestibule **1**

Frenulum **1**

0   **Medical and Surgical**
C   **Mouth and Throat**
0   **Alteration**   Definition: Modifying the anatomic structure of a body part without affecting the function of the body part

                         Explanation: Principal purpose is to improve appearance

Body Part Character 4	Approach Character 5	Device Character 6	Qualifier Character 7

0 Upper Lip
   Frenulum labii superioris
   Labial gland
   Vermilion border
1 Lower Lip
   Frenulum labii inferioris
   Labial gland
   Vermilion border
	X External	**7** Autologous Tissue Substitute
		J Synthetic Substitute
		K Nonautologous Tissue Substitute
		Z No Device
			Z No Qualifier

0   **Medical and Surgical**
C   **Mouth and Throat**
2   **Change**   Definition: Taking out or off a device from a body part and putting back an identical or similar device in or on the same body part without cutting or puncturing the skin or a mucous membrane

                         Explanation: All CHANGE procedures are coded using the approach EXTERNAL

Body Part Character 4	Approach Character 5	Device Character 6	Qualifier Character 7

A Salivary Gland
S Larynx
   Aryepiglottic fold
   Arytenoid cartilage
   Corniculate cartilage
   Cuneiform cartilage
   False vocal cord
   Glottis
   Rima glottidis
   Thyroid cartilage
   Ventricular fold
Y Mouth and Throat
	X External	**0** Drainage Device
		Y Other Device
			Z No Qualifier

     Non-OR   All body part, approach, device, and qualifier values

NC Noncovered Procedure   **LC** Limited Coverage   **QA** Questionable OB Admit   **NT** New Tech Add-on   ⊞ Combination Member   ♂ Male   ♀ Female

ICD-10-PCS 2022   **357**

Mouth and Throat

Ø   **Medical and Surgical**
C   **Mouth and Throat**
5   **Destruction**   Definition: Physical eradication of all or a portion of a body part by the direct use of energy, force, or a destructive agent
                        Explanation: None of the body part is physically taken out

Body Part Character 4		Approach Character 5	Device Character 6	Qualifier Character 7

Ø **Upper Lip**
  Frenulum labii superioris
  Labial gland
  Vermilion border
1 **Lower Lip**
  Frenulum labii inferioris
  Labial gland
  Vermilion border
2 **Hard Palate**
3 **Soft Palate**
4 **Buccal Mucosa**
  Buccal gland
  Molar gland
  Palatine gland
	5 **Upper Gingiva**
	6 **Lower Gingiva**
	7 **Tongue**
	  Frenulum linguae
	N **Uvula**
	  Palatine uvula
	P **Tonsils**
	  Palatine tonsil
	Q **Adenoids**
	  Pharyngeal tonsil
		Ø Open
		3 Percutaneous
		X External
			Z No Device	Z No Qualifier

8 **Parotid Gland, Right**
9 **Parotid Gland, Left**
B **Parotid Duct, Right**
  Stensen's duct
C **Parotid Duct, Left**
  See B Parotid Duct, Right
D **Sublingual Gland, Right**
	F **Sublingual Gland, Left**
	G **Submaxillary Gland, Right**
	  Submandibular gland
	H **Submaxillary Gland, Left**
	  See G Submaxillary Gland, Right
	J **Minor Salivary Gland**
	  Anterior lingual gland
		Ø Open
		3 Percutaneous
			Z No Device	Z No Qualifier

M **Pharynx**
  Base of tongue
  Hypopharynx
  Laryngopharynx
  Lingual tonsil
  Oropharynx
  Piriform recess (sinus)
  Tongue, base of
R **Epiglottis**
  Glossoepiglottic fold
	S **Larynx**
	  Aryepiglottic fold
	  Arytenoid cartilage
	  Corniculate cartilage
	  Cuneiform cartilage
	  False vocal cord
	  Glottis
	  Rima glottidis
	  Thyroid cartilage
	  Ventricular fold
	T **Vocal Cord, Right**
	  Vocal fold
	V **Vocal Cord, Left**
	  See T Vocal Cord, Right
		Ø Open
		3 Percutaneous
		4 Percutaneous Endoscopic
		7 Via Natural or Artificial Opening
		8 Via Natural or Artificial Opening Endoscopic
			Z No Device	Z No Qualifier

W **Upper Tooth** X **Lower Tooth**		Ø Open X External	Z No Device	Ø Single 1 Multiple 2 All

Non-OR   ØC5[5,6][Ø,3,X]ZZ
Non-OR   ØC5[W,X][Ø,X]Z[Ø,1,2]

Ø   **Medical and Surgical**
C   **Mouth and Throat**
7   **Dilation**   Definition: Expanding an orifice or the lumen of a tubular body part
               Explanation: The orifice can be a natural orifice or an artificially created orifice. Accomplished by stretching a tubular body part using intraluminal pressure or by cutting part of the orifice or wall of the tubular body part.

Body Part Character 4	Approach Character 5	Device Character 6	Qualifier Character 7

B **Parotid Duct, Right**
  Stensen's duct
C **Parotid Duct, Left**
  See B Parotid Duct, Right
	Ø Open
	3 Percutaneous
	7 Via Natural or Artificial Opening
		D Intraluminal Device
		Z No Device
			Z No Qualifier

M **Pharynx**
  Base of tongue
  Hypopharynx
  Laryngopharynx
  Lingual tonsil
  Oropharynx
  Piriform recess (sinus)
  Tongue, base of
	7 Via Natural or Artificial Opening
	8 Via Natural or Artificial Opening Endoscopic
		D Intraluminal Device
		Z No Device
			Z No Qualifier

S **Larynx**
  Aryepiglottic fold
  Arytenoid cartilage
  Corniculate cartilage
  Cuneiform cartilage
  False vocal cord
  Glottis
  Rima glottidis
  Thyroid cartilage
  Ventricular fold
	Ø Open
	3 Percutaneous
	4 Percutaneous Endoscopic
	7 Via Natural or Artificial Opening
	8 Via Natural or Artificial Opening Endoscopic
		D Intraluminal Device
		Z No Device
			Z No Qualifier

Non-OR   ØC7[B,C][Ø,3,7][D,Z]Z
Non-OR   ØC7M[7,8][D,Z]Z

Non-OR Procedure   DRG Non-OR Procedure   Valid OR Procedure   HAC Associated Procedure   Combination Only   New/Revised GREEN

0   **Medical and Surgical**
C   **Mouth and Throat**
9   **Drainage**   Definition: Taking or letting out fluids and/or gases from a body part

Explanation: The qualifier DIAGNOSTIC is used to identify drainage procedures that are biopsies

Body Part Character 4		Approach Character 5	Device Character 6	Qualifier Character 7
0 **Upper Lip** Frenulum labii superioris Labial gland Vermilion border **1** **Lower Lip** Frenulum labii inferioris Labial gland Vermilion border **2** **Hard Palate** **3** **Soft Palate** **4** **Buccal Mucosa** Buccal gland Molar gland Palatine gland	**5** **Upper Gingiva** **6** **Lower Gingiva** **7** **Tongue** Frenulum linguae **N** **Uvula** Palatine uvula **P** **Tonsils** Palatine tonsil **Q** **Adenoids** Pharyngeal tonsil	**0** Open **3** Percutaneous **X** External	**0** Drainage Device	**Z** No Qualifier
0 **Upper Lip** Frenulum labii superioris Labial gland Vermilion border **1** **Lower Lip** Frenulum labii inferioris Labial gland Vermilion border **2** **Hard Palate** **3** **Soft Palate** **4** **Buccal Mucosa** Buccal gland Molar gland Palatine gland	**5** **Upper Gingiva** **6** **Lower Gingiva** **7** **Tongue** Frenulum linguae **N** **Uvula** Palatine uvula **P** **Tonsils** Palatine tonsil **Q** **Adenoids** Pharyngeal tonsil	**0** Open **3** Percutaneous **X** External	**Z** No Device	**X** Diagnostic **Z** No Qualifier
8 **Parotid Gland, Right** **9** **Parotid Gland, Left** **B** **Parotid Duct, Right** Stensen's duct **C** **Parotid Duct, Left** See B Parotid Duct, Right **D** **Sublingual Gland, Right**	**F** **Sublingual Gland, Left** **G** **Submaxillary Gland, Right** Submandibular gland **H** **Submaxillary Gland, Left** See G Submaxillary Gland, Right **J** **Minor Salivary Gland** Anterior lingual gland	**0** Open **3** Percutaneous	**0** Drainage Device	**Z** No Qualifier
8 **Parotid Gland, Right** **9** **Parotid Gland, Left** **B** **Parotid Duct, Right** Stensen's duct **C** **Parotid Duct, Left** See B Parotid Duct, Right	**D** **Sublingual Gland, Right** **F** **Sublingual Gland, Left** **G** **Submaxillary Gland, Right** Submandibular gland **H** **Submaxillary Gland, Left** See G Submaxillary Gland, Right **J** **Minor Salivary Gland** Anterior lingual gland	**0** Open **3** Percutaneous	**Z** No Device	**X** Diagnostic **Z** No Qualifier

M **Pharynx**
Base of tongue
Hypopharynx
Laryngopharynx
Lingual tonsil
Oropharynx
Piriform recess (sinus)
Tongue, base of
R **Epiglottis**
Glossoepiglottic fold
	S **Larynx**
	Aryepiglottic fold
	Arytenoid cartilage
	Corniculate cartilage
	Cuneiform cartilage
	False vocal cord
	Glottis
	Rima glottidis
	Thyroid cartilage
	Ventricular fold
	T **Vocal Cord, Right**
	Vocal fold
	V **Vocal Cord, Left**
	See T Vocal Cord, Right
		0 Open
		3 Percutaneous
		4 Percutaneous Endoscopic
		7 Via Natural or Artificial
		    Opening
		8 Via Natural or Artificial
		    Opening Endoscopic
			0 Drainage Device	**Z** No Qualifier

Non-OR	0C9[0,1,2,3,4,7,N,P,Q]30Z
Non-OR	0C9[5,6][0,3,X]0Z
Non-OR	0C9[0,1,4][0,3,X]ZX
Non-OR	0C9[0,1,2,3,4,7,N,P,Q]3ZZ
Non-OR	0C9[5,6][0,3,X]Z[X,Z]
Non-OR	0C97[3,X]ZX
Non-OR	0C9[8,9,B,C,D,F,G,H,J][0,3]0Z
Non-OR	0C9[8,9,B,C,D,F,G,H,J]3ZX
Non-OR	0C9[8,9,G,H]3ZZ
Non-OR	0C9[B,C,D, F,J][0,3]ZZ
Non-OR	0C9[M,R,S,T,V]30Z

0C9 Continued on next page

NC Noncovered Procedure   **LC** Limited Coverage   **QA** Questionable OB Admit   **NT** New Tech Add-on   ⊞ Combination Member   ♂Male   ♀Female

0 **Medical and Surgical**
C **Mouth and Throat**
9 **Drainage**

0C9 Continued

Definition: Taking or letting out fluids and/or gases from a body part
Explanation: The qualifier DIAGNOSTIC is used to identify drainage procedures that are biopsies

Body Part Character 4		Approach Character 5	Device Character 6	Qualifier Character 7

M Pharynx
  Base of tongue
  Hypopharynx
  Laryngopharynx
  Lingual tonsil
  Oropharynx
  Piriform recess (sinus)
  Tongue, base of
R Epiglottis
  Glossoepiglottic fold
	S Larynx
	  Aryepiglottic fold
	  Arytenoid cartilage
	  Corniculate cartilage
	  Cuneiform cartilage
	  False vocal cord
	  Glottis
	  Rima glottidis
	  Thyroid cartilage
	  Ventricular fold
	T Vocal Cord, Right
	  Vocal fold
	V Vocal Cord, Left
	  See T Vocal Cord, Right
		0 Open
		3 Percutaneous
		4 Percutaneous Endoscopic
		7 Via Natural or Artificial Opening
		8 Via Natural or Artificial Opening Endoscopic
			Z No Device	**X** Diagnostic
				Z No Qualifier

W Upper Tooth **X** Lower Tooth		**0** Open **X** External	**0** Drainage Device **Z** No Device	**0** Single **1** Multiple **2** All

Non-OR	0C9M[0,3,4,7,8]ZX
Non-OR	0C9[M,R,S,T,V]3ZZ
Non-OR	0C9[R,S,T,V][3,4,7,8]ZX
Non-OR	0C9[W,X][0,X][0,Z][0,1,2]

0 **Medical and Surgical**
C **Mouth and Throat**
B **Excision**

Definition: Cutting out or off, without replacement, a portion of a body part
Explanation: The qualifier DIAGNOSTIC is used to identify excision procedures that are biopsies

Body Part Character 4		Approach Character 5	Device Character 6	Qualifier Character 7

0 Upper Lip
  Frenulum labii superioris
  Labial gland
  Vermilion border
1 Lower Lip
  Frenulum labii inferioris
  Labial gland
  Vermilion border
2 Hard Palate
3 Soft Palate
4 Buccal Mucosa
  Buccal gland
  Molar gland
  Palatine gland
	5 Upper Gingiva
	6 Lower Gingiva
	7 Tongue
	  Frenulum linguae
	N Uvula
	  Palatine uvula
	P Tonsils
	  Palatine tonsil
	Q Adenoids
	  Pharyngeal tonsil
		0 Open
		3 Percutaneous
		X External
			Z No Device	**X** Diagnostic
				Z No Qualifier

8 Parotid Gland, Right
9 Parotid Gland, Left
B Parotid Duct, Right
  Stensen's duct
C Parotid Duct, Left
  See B Parotid Duct, Right
D Sublingual Gland, Right
	F Sublingual Gland, Left
	G Submaxillary Gland, Right
	  Submandibular gland
	H Submaxillary Gland, Left
	  See G Submaxillary Gland, Right
	J Minor Salivary Gland
	  Anterior lingual gland
		0 Open
		3 Percutaneous
			Z No Device	**X** Diagnostic
				Z No Qualifier

M Pharynx
  Base of tongue
  Hypopharynx
  Laryngopharynx
  Lingual tonsil
  Oropharynx
  Piriform recess (sinus)
  Tongue, base of
R Epiglottis
  Glossoepiglottic fold
	S Larynx
	  Aryepiglottic fold
	  Arytenoid cartilage
	  Corniculate cartilage
	  Cuneiform cartilage
	  False vocal cord
	  Glottis
	  Rima glottidis
	  Thyroid cartilage
	  Ventricular fold
	T Vocal Cord, Right
	  Vocal fold
	V Vocal Cord, Left
	  See T Vocal Cord, Right
		0 Open
		3 Percutaneous
		4 Percutaneous Endoscopic
		7 Via Natural or Artificial Opening
		8 Via Natural or Artificial Opening Endoscopic
			Z No Device	**X** Diagnostic
				Z No Qualifier

W Upper Tooth **X** Lower Tooth		**0** Open **X** External	**Z** No Device	**0** Single **1** Multiple **2** All

Non-OR	0CB[0,1,4][0,3,X]ZX	**Non-OR**	0CBM[0,3,4,7,8]ZX
Non-OR	0CB[5,6][0,3,X]Z[X,Z]	**Non-OR**	0CB[R,S,T,V][3,4,7,8]ZX
Non-OR	0CB7[3,X]ZX	**Non-OR**	0CB[W,X][0,X]Z[0,1,2]
Non-OR	0CB[8,9,B,C,D,F,G,H,J]3ZX		

Ø **Medical and Surgical**
C **Mouth and Throat**
C **Extirpation**   Definition: Taking or cutting out solid matter from a body part

Explanation: The solid matter may be an abnormal byproduct of a biological function or a foreign body; it may be imbedded in a body part or in the lumen of a tubular body part. The solid matter may or may not have been previously broken into pieces.

Body Part Character 4		Approach Character 5	Device Character 6	Qualifier Character 7
Ø **Upper Lip** Frenulum labii superioris Labial gland Vermilion border 1 **Lower Lip** Frenulum labii inferioris Labial gland Vermilion border 2 **Hard Palate** 3 **Soft Palate** 4 **Buccal Mucosa** Buccal gland Molar gland Palatine gland	5 **Upper Gingiva** 6 **Lower Gingiva** 7 **Tongue** Frenulum linguae N **Uvula** Palatine uvula P **Tonsils** Palatine tonsil Q **Adenoids** Pharyngeal tonsil	Ø Open 3 Percutaneous X External	Z No Device	Z No Qualifier
8 **Parotid Gland, Right** 9 **Parotid Gland, Left** B **Parotid Duct, Right** Stensen's duct C **Parotid Duct, Left** *See B Parotid Duct, Right* D **Sublingual Gland, Right**	F **Sublingual Gland, Left** G **Submaxillary Gland, Right** Submandibular gland H **Submaxillary Gland, Left** *See G Submaxillary Gland, Right* J **Minor Salivary Gland** Anterior lingual gland	Ø Open 3 Percutaneous	Z No Device	Z No Qualifier
M **Pharynx** Base of tongue Hypopharynx Laryngopharynx Lingual tonsil Oropharynx Piriform recess (sinus) Tongue, base of R **Epiglottis** Glossoepiglottic fold	S **Larynx** Aryepiglottic fold Arytenoid cartilage Corniculate cartilage Cuneiform cartilage False vocal cord Glottis Rima glottidis Thyroid cartilage Ventricular fold T **Vocal Cord, Right** Vocal fold V **Vocal Cord, Left** *See T Vocal Cord, Right*	Ø Open 3 Percutaneous 4 Percutaneous Endoscopic 7 Via Natural or Artificial Opening 8 Via Natural or Artificial Opening Endoscopic	Z No Device	Z No Qualifier
W **Upper Tooth** X **Lower Tooth**		Ø Open X External	Z No Device	Ø Single 1 Multiple 2 All

Non-OR	ØCC[Ø,1,2,3,4,7,N,P,Q]XZZ
Non-OR	ØCC[5,6][Ø,3,X]ZZ
Non-OR	ØCC[8,9,G,H]3ZZ
Non-OR	ØCC[B,C,D, F,J][Ø,3]ZZ
Non-OR	ØCC[M,S][7,8]ZZ
Non-OR	ØCC[W,X][Ø,X]Z[Ø,1,2]

Ø **Medical and Surgical**
C **Mouth and Throat**
D **Extraction**   Definition: Pulling or stripping out or off all or a portion of a body part by the use of force

Explanation: The qualifier DIAGNOSTIC is used to identify extraction procedures that are biopsies

Body Part Character 4	Approach Character 5	Device Character 6	Qualifier Character 7
T **Vocal Cord, Right** Vocal fold V **Vocal Cord, Left** *See T Vocal Cord, Right*	Ø Open 3 Percutaneous 4 Percutaneous Endoscopic 7 Via Natural or Artificial Opening 8 Via Natural or Artificial Opening Endoscopic	Z No Device	Z No Qualifier
W **Upper Tooth** X **Lower Tooth**	X External	Z No Device	Ø Single 1 Multiple 2 All

Non-OR	ØCD[W,X]XZ[Ø,1,2]

NC Noncovered Procedure   LC Limited Coverage   QA Questionable OB Admit   NT New Tech Add-on   ⊞ Combination Member   ♂ Male   ♀ Female

ICD-10-PCS 2022   **361**

0 **Medical and Surgical**
C **Mouth and Throat**
F **Fragmentation**   Definition: Breaking solid matter in a body part into pieces

Explanation: Physical force (e.g., manual, ultrasonic) applied directly or indirectly is used to break the solid matter into pieces. The solid matter may be an abnormal byproduct of a biological function or a foreign body. The pieces of solid matter are not taken out.

Body Part Character 4	Approach Character 5	Device Character 6	Qualifier Character 7

B Parotid Duct, Right `NC`
   Stensen's duct
C Parotid Duct, Left `NC`
   See B Parotid Duct, Right
	Ø Open
	3 Percutaneous
	7 Via Natural or Artificial Opening
	X External
		Z No Device	**Z** No Qualifier

Non-OR `NC`	All body part, approach, device, and qualifier values 0CF[B,C]XZZ

0 **Medical and Surgical**
C **Mouth and Throat**
H **Insertion**   Definition: Putting in a nonbiological appliance that monitors, assists, performs, or prevents a physiological function but does not physically take the place of a body part

Explanation: None

Body Part Character 4	Approach Character 5	Device Character 6	Qualifier Character 7
7 Tongue Frenulum linguae	**Ø** Open **3** Percutaneous **X** External	**1** Radioactive Element	**Z** No Qualifier

A Salivary Gland
S Larynx
   Aryepiglottic fold
   Arytenoid cartilage
   Corniculate cartilage
   Cuneiform cartilage
   False vocal cord
   Glottis
   Rima glottidis
   Thyroid cartilage
   Ventricular fold
	Ø Open
	3 Percutaneous
	7 Via Natural or Artificial Opening
	8 Via Natural or Artificial Opening Endoscopic
		1 Radioactive Element
		Y Other Device
			Z No Qualifier

Y Mouth and Throat	**Ø** Open **3** Percutaneous	**1** Radioactive Element **Y** Other Device	**Z** No Qualifier
Y Mouth and Throat	**7** Via Natural or Artificial Opening **8** Via Natural or Artificial Opening Endoscopic	**1** Radioactive Element **B** Intraluminal Device, Airway **Y** Other Device	**Z** No Qualifier

Non-OR	0CH[A,S]01Z
Non-OR	0CHS0YZ
Non-OR	0CH[A,S][3,7,8][1,Y]Z
Non-OR	0CHY[0,3][1,Y]Z
Non-OR	0CHY[7,8][1,B,Y]Z

0 **Medical and Surgical**
C **Mouth and Throat**
J **Inspection**   Definition: Visually and/or manually exploring a body part

Explanation: Visual exploration may be performed with or without optical instrumentation. Manual exploration may be performed directly or through intervening body layers.

Body Part Character 4	Approach Character 5	Device Character 6	Qualifier Character 7
A Salivary Gland	**Ø** Open **3** Percutaneous **X** External	**Z** No Device	**Z** No Qualifier

S Larynx
   Aryepiglottic fold
   Arytenoid cartilage
   Corniculate cartilage
   Cuneiform cartilage
   False vocal cord
   Glottis
   Rima glottidis
   Thyroid cartilage
   Ventricular fold
Y Mouth and Throat
	Ø Open
	3 Percutaneous
	4 Percutaneous Endoscopic
	7 Via Natural or Artificial Opening
	8 Via Natural or Artificial Opening Endoscopic
	X External
		Z No Device	**Z** No Qualifier

Non-OR	All body part, approach, device, and qualifier values

Ø   **Medical and Surgical**
C   **Mouth and Throat**
L   **Occlusion**   Definition: Completely closing an orifice or the lumen of a tubular body part
                    Explanation: The orifice can be a natural orifice or an artificially created orifice

Body Part Character 4	Approach Character 5	Device Character 6	Qualifier Character 7

B Parotid Duct, Right
   Stensen's duct
C Parotid Duct, Left
   See B Parotid Duct, Right
	Ø Open
	3 Percutaneous
	4 Percutaneous Endoscopic
		C Extraluminal Device
		D Intraluminal Device
		Z No Device
			Z No Qualifier

B Parotid Duct, Right
   Stensen's duct
C Parotid Duct, Left
   See B Parotid Duct, Right
	7 Via Natural or Artificial Opening
	8 Via Natural or Artificial Opening
	   Endoscopic
		D Intraluminal Device
		Z No Device
			Z No Qualifier

Ø   **Medical and Surgical**
C   **Mouth and Throat**
M   **Reattachment**   Definition: Putting back in or on all or a portion of a separated body part to its normal location or other suitable location
                       Explanation: Vascular circulation and nervous pathways may or may not be reestablished

Body Part Character 4	Approach Character 5	Device Character 6	Qualifier Character 7

Ø Upper Lip
   Frenulum labii superioris
   Labial gland
   Vermilion border
1 Lower Lip
   Frenulum labii inferioris
   Labial gland
   Vermilion border
3 Soft Palate
7 Tongue
   Frenulum linguae
N Uvula
   Palatine uvula
	Ø Open	**Z** No Device	**Z** No Qualifier

W Upper Tooth **X** Lower Tooth	**Ø** Open **X** External	**Z** No Device	**Ø** Single **1** Multiple **2** All

Non-OR   ØCM[W,X][Ø,X]Z[Ø,1,2]

Ø   Medical and Surgical
C   Mouth and Throat
N   Release   Definition: Freeing a body part from an abnormal physical constraint by cutting or by the use of force
                         Explanation: Some of the restraining tissue may be taken out but none of the body part is taken out

Body Part Character 4	Approach Character 5	Device Character 6	Qualifier Character 7

Ø   Upper Lip
    Frenulum labii superioris
    Labial gland
    Vermilion border
1   Lower Lip
    Frenulum labii inferioris
    Labial gland
    Vermilion border
2   Hard Palate
3   Soft Palate
4   Buccal Mucosa
    Buccal gland
    Molar gland
    Palatine gland
5   Upper Gingiva
6   Lower Gingiva
7   Tongue
    Frenulum linguae
N   Uvula
    Palatine uvula
P   Tonsils
    Palatine tonsil
Q   Adenoids
    Pharyngeal tonsil
	Ø Open
	3 Percutaneous
	X External
		Z No Device	**Z No Qualifier**

8   Parotid Gland, Right
9   Parotid Gland, Left
B   Parotid Duct, Right
    Stensen's duct
C   Parotid Duct, Left
    See B Parotid Duct, Right
D   Sublingual Gland, Right
F   Sublingual Gland, Left
G   Submaxillary Gland, Right
    Submandibular gland
H   Submaxillary Gland, Left
    See G Submaxillary Gland, Right
J   Minor Salivary Gland
    Anterior lingual gland
	Ø Open
	3 Percutaneous
		Z No Device	**Z No Qualifier**

M   Pharynx
    Base of tongue
    Hypopharynx
    Laryngopharynx
    Lingual tonsil
    Oropharynx
    Piriform recess (sinus)
    Tongue, base of
R   Epiglottis
    Glossoepiglottic fold
S   Larynx
    Aryepiglottic fold
    Arytenoid cartilage
    Corniculate cartilage
    Cuneiform cartilage
    False vocal cord
    Glottis
    Rima glottidis
    Thyroid cartilage
    Ventricular fold
T   Vocal Cord, Right
    Vocal fold
V   Vocal Cord, Left
    See T Vocal Cord, Right
	Ø Open
	3 Percutaneous
	4 Percutaneous Endoscopic
	7 Via Natural or Artificial Opening
	**8 Via Natural or Artificial Opening
	    Endoscopic**
		Z No Device	**Z No Qualifier**

W Upper Tooth **X Lower Tooth**	**Ø Open** **X External**	**Z No Device**	**Ø Single** **1 Multiple** **2 All**

Non-OR	ØCN[Ø,1,5,6,7][Ø,3,X]ZZ
Non-OR	ØCN[W,X][Ø,X]Z[Ø,1,2]

Ø   **Medical and Surgical**
C   **Mouth and Throat**
P   **Removal**   Definition: Taking out or off a device from a body part
                    Explanation: If a device is taken out and a similar device put in without cutting or puncturing the skin or mucous membrane, the procedure is coded to the root operation CHANGE. Otherwise, the procedure for taking out a device is coded to the root operation REMOVAL.

Body Part Character 4	Approach Character 5	Device Character 6	Qualifier Character 7
A Salivary Gland	**Ø** Open **3** Percutaneous	**Ø** Drainage Device **C** Extraluminal Device **Y** Other Device	**Z** No Qualifier
A Salivary Gland	**7** Via Natural or Artificial Opening **8** Via Natural or Artificial Opening Endoscopic	**Y** Other Device	**Z** No Qualifier

S Larynx
    Aryepiglottic fold
    Arytenoid cartilage
    Corniculate cartilage
    Cuneiform cartilage
    False vocal cord
    Glottis
    Rima glottidis
    Thyroid cartilage
    Ventricular fold
	Ø Open
	3 Percutaneous
	7 Via Natural or Artificial Opening
	8 Via Natural or Artificial Opening Endoscopic
		Ø Drainage Device
		7 Autologous Tissue Substitute
		D Intraluminal Device
		J Synthetic Substitute
		K Nonautologous Tissue Substitute
		Y Other Device
			Z No Qualifier

S Larynx
    Aryepiglottic fold
    Arytenoid cartilage
    Corniculate cartilage
    Cuneiform cartilage
    False vocal cord
    Glottis
    Rima glottidis
    Thyroid cartilage
    Ventricular fold
	X External	**Ø** Drainage Device
		7 Autologous Tissue Substitute
		D Intraluminal Device
		J Synthetic Substitute
		K Nonautologous Tissue Substitute
			Z No Qualifier

Y Mouth and Throat	**Ø** Open **3** Percutaneous **7** Via Natural or Artificial Opening **8** Via Natural or Artificial Opening Endoscopic	**Ø** Drainage Device **1** Radioactive Element **7** Autologous Tissue Substitute **D** Intraluminal Device **J** Synthetic Substitute **K** Nonautologous Tissue Substitute **Y** Other Device	**Z** No Qualifier
Y Mouth and Throat	**X** External	**Ø** Drainage Device **1** Radioactive Element **7** Autologous Tissue Substitute **D** Intraluminal Device **J** Synthetic Substitute **K** Nonautologous Tissue Substitute	**Z** No Qualifier

Non-OR   ØCPA[Ø,3][Ø,C,Y]Z
Non-OR   ØCPA[7,8]YZ
Non-OR   ØCPS3YZ
Non-OR   ØCPS[7,8][Ø,D,Y]Z
Non-OR   ØCPSX[Ø,7,D,J,K]Z
Non-OR   ØCPY3YZ
Non-OR   ØCPY[7,8][Ø,D,Y]Z
Non-OR   ØCPYX[Ø,1,7,D,J,K]Z

Mouth and Throat

Ø **Medical and Surgical**
C **Mouth and Throat**
Q **Repair**   Definition: Restoring, to the extent possible, a body part to its normal anatomic structure and function
                  Explanation: Used only when the method to accomplish the repair is not one of the other root operations

Body Part Character 4	Approach Character 5	Device Character 6	Qualifier Character 7

Ø **Upper Lip**
  Frenulum labii superioris
  Labial gland
  Vermilion border
1 **Lower Lip**
  Frenulum labii inferioris
  Labial gland
  Vermilion border
2 **Hard Palate**
3 **Soft Palate**
4 **Buccal Mucosa**
  Buccal gland
  Molar gland
  Palatine gland
5 **Upper Gingiva**
6 **Lower Gingiva**
7 **Tongue**
  Frenulum linguae
N **Uvula**
  Palatine uvula
P **Tonsils**
  Palatine tonsil
Q **Adenoids**
  Pharyngeal tonsil
	Ø Open
	3 Percutaneous
	X External
		Z No Device	Z No Qualifier

8 **Parotid Gland, Right**
9 **Parotid Gland, Left**
B **Parotid Duct, Right**
  Stensen's duct
C **Parotid Duct, Left**
  See B Parotid Duct, Right
D **Sublingual Gland, Right**
F **Sublingual Gland, Left**
G **Submaxillary Gland, Right**
  Submandibular gland
H **Submaxillary Gland, Left**
  See G Submaxillary Gland, Right
J **Minor Salivary Gland**
  Anterior lingual gland
	Ø Open
	3 Percutaneous
		Z No Device	Z No Qualifier

M **Pharynx**
  Base of tongue
  Hypopharynx
  Laryngopharynx
  Lingual tonsil
  Oropharynx
  Piriform recess (sinus)
  Tongue, base of
R **Epiglottis**
  Glossoepiglottic fold
S **Larynx**
  Aryepiglottic fold
  Arytenoid cartilage
  Corniculate cartilage
  Cuneiform cartilage
  False vocal cord
  Glottis
  Rima glottidis
  Thyroid cartilage
  Ventricular fold
T **Vocal Cord, Right**
  Vocal fold
V **Vocal Cord, Left**
  See T Vocal Cord, Right
	Ø Open
	3 Percutaneous
	4 Percutaneous Endoscopic
	7 Via Natural or Artificial Opening
	8 Via Natural or Artificial Opening
	   Endoscopic
		Z No Device	Z No Qualifier

W **Upper Tooth** X **Lower Tooth**	Ø Open X External	Z No Device	Ø Single 1 Multiple 2 All

Non-OR	ØCQ[Ø,1,4,7]XZZ
Non-OR	ØCQ[5,6][Ø,3,X]ZZ
Non-OR	ØCQ[W,X][Ø,X]Z[Ø,1,2]

Ø   **Medical and Surgical**
C   **Mouth and Throat**
R   **Replacement**   Definition: Putting in or on biological or synthetic material that physically takes the place and/or function of all or a portion of a body part

                        Explanation: The body part may have been taken out or replaced, or may be taken out, physically eradicated, or rendered nonfunctional during the REPLACEMENT procedure. A REMOVAL procedure is coded for taking out the device used in a previous replacement procedure.

Body Part Character 4	Approach Character 5	Device Character 6	Qualifier Character 7

Ø **Upper Lip**
    Frenulum labii superioris
    Labial gland
    Vermilion border
1 **Lower Lip**
    Frenulum labii inferioris
    Labial gland
    Vermilion border
2 **Hard Palate**
3 **Soft Palate**
4 **Buccal Mucosa**
    Buccal gland
    Molar gland
    Palatine gland
5 **Upper Gingiva**
6 **Lower Gingiva**
7 **Tongue**
    Frenulum linguae
N **Uvula**
    Palatine uvula
	Ø Open
	3 Percutaneous
	X External
		7 Autologous Tissue Substitute
		J Synthetic Substitute
		K Nonautologous Tissue Substitute
			Z No Qualifier

B **Parotid Duct, Right**
    Stensen's duct
C **Parotid Duct, Left**
    See B Parotid Duct, Right
	Ø Open
	3 Percutaneous
		7 Autologous Tissue Substitute
		J Synthetic Substitute
		K Nonautologous Tissue Substitute
			Z No Qualifier

M **Pharynx**
    Base of tongue
    Hypopharynx
    Laryngopharynx
    Lingual tonsil
    Oropharynx
    Piriform recess (sinus)
    Tongue, base of
R **Epiglottis**
    Glossoepiglottic fold
S **Larynx**
    Aryepiglottic fold
    Arytenoid cartilage
    Corniculate cartilage
    Cuneiform cartilage
    False vocal cord
    Glottis
    Rima glottidis
    Thyroid cartilage
    Ventricular fold
T **Vocal Cord, Right**
    Vocal fold
V **Vocal Cord, Left**
    See T Vocal Cord, Right
	Ø Open
	7 Via Natural or Artificial Opening
	8 Via Natural or Artificial Opening Endoscopic
		7 Autologous Tissue Substitute
		J Synthetic Substitute
		K Nonautologous Tissue Substitute
			Z No Qualifier

W **Upper Tooth** **X** **Lower Tooth**	**Ø** Open **X** External	**7** Autologous Tissue Substitute **J** Synthetic Substitute **K** Nonautologous Tissue Substitute	**Ø** Single **1** Multiple **2** All

Non-OR   ØCR[W,X][Ø,X][7,J,K][Ø,1,2]

Mouth and Throat

Ø   **Medical and Surgical**
C   **Mouth and Throat**
S   **Reposition**   Definition: Moving to its normal location, or other suitable location, all or a portion of a body part

Explanation: The body part is moved to a new location from an abnormal location, or from a normal location where it is not functioning correctly. The body part may or may not be cut out or off to be moved to the new location.

Body Part Character 4	Approach Character 5	Device Character 6	Qualifier Character 7
Ø **Upper Lip** Frenulum labii superioris Labial gland Vermilion border 1 **Lower Lip** Frenulum labii inferioris Labial gland Vermilion border 2 **Hard Palate** 3 **Soft Palate** 7 **Tongue** Frenulum linguae N **Uvula** Palatine uvula	Ø Open X External	Z No Device	Z No Qualifier
B **Parotid Duct, Right** Stensen's duct C **Parotid Duct, Left** *See B Parotid Duct, Right*	Ø Open 3 Percutaneous	Z No Device	Z No Qualifier
R **Epiglottis** Glossoepiglottic fold T **Vocal Cord, Right** Vocal fold V **Vocal Cord, Left** *See T Vocal Cord, Right*	Ø Open 7 Via Natural or Artificial Opening 8 Via Natural or Artificial Opening Endoscopic	Z No Device	Z No Qualifier
W **Upper Tooth** X **Lower Tooth**	Ø Open X External	5 External Fixation Device Z No Device	Ø Single 1 Multiple 2 All

Non-OR   ØCS[W,X][Ø,X][5,Z][Ø,1,2]

Ø Medical and Surgical
C Mouth and Throat
T Resection   Definition: Cutting out or off, without replacement, all of a body part
            Explanation: None

Body Part Character 4	Approach Character 5	Device Character 6	Qualifier Character 7

Ø Upper Lip
  Frenulum labii superioris
  Labial gland
  Vermilion border
1 Lower Lip
  Frenulum labii inferioris
  Labial gland
  Vermilion border
2 Hard Palate
3 Soft Palate
7 Tongue
  Frenulum linguae
N Uvula
  Palatine uvula
P Tonsils
  Palatine tonsil
Q Adenoids
  Pharyngeal tonsil
	Ø Open
	X External
		Z No Device	**Z No Qualifier**

8 Parotid Gland, Right
9 Parotid Gland, Left
B Parotid Duct, Right
  Stensen's duct
C Parotid Duct, Left
  See B Parotid Duct, Right
D Sublingual Gland, Right
F Sublingual Gland, Left
G Submaxillary Gland, Right
  Submandibular gland
H Submaxillary Gland, Left
  See G Submaxillary Gland, Right
J Minor Salivary Gland
  Anterior lingual gland
	Ø Open	**Z No Device**	**Z No Qualifier**

M Pharynx
  Base of tongue
  Hypopharynx
  Laryngopharynx
  Lingual tonsil
  Oropharynx
  Piriform recess (sinus)
  Tongue, base of
R Epiglottis
  Glossoepiglottic fold
S Larynx
  Aryepiglottic fold
  Arytenoid cartilage
  Corniculate cartilage
  Cuneiform cartilage
  False vocal cord
  Glottis
  Rima glottidis
  Thyroid cartilage
  Ventricular fold
T Vocal Cord, Right
  Vocal fold
V Vocal Cord, Left
  See T Vocal Cord, Right
	Ø Open
	4 Percutaneous Endoscopic
	7 Via Natural or Artificial Opening
	**8 Via Natural or Artificial Opening
	   Endoscopic**
		Z No Device	**Z No Qualifier**

W Upper Tooth **X Lower Tooth**	**Ø Open**	**Z No Device**	**Ø Single** **1 Multiple** **2 All**

Non-OR   ØCT[W,X]ØZ[Ø,1,2]

Mouth and Throat

Ø   **Medical and Surgical**
C   **Mouth and Throat**
U   **Supplement**   Definition: Putting in or on biological or synthetic material that physically reinforces and/or augments the function of a portion of a body part
                    Explanation: The biological material is non-living, or is living and from the same individual. The body part may have been previously replaced, and the SUPPLEMENT procedure is performed to physically reinforce and/or augment the function of the replaced body part.

Body Part Character 4	Approach Character 5	Device Character 6	Qualifier Character 7

Ø   **Upper Lip**
    Frenulum labii superioris
    Labial gland
    Vermilion border
1   **Lower Lip**
    Frenulum labii inferioris
    Labial gland
    Vermilion border
2   **Hard Palate**
3   **Soft Palate**
4   **Buccal Mucosa**
    Buccal gland
    Molar gland
    Palatine gland
5   **Upper Gingiva**
6   **Lower Gingiva**
7   **Tongue**
    Frenulum linguae
N   **Uvula**
    Palatine uvula
	Ø Open
	3 Percutaneous
	X External
		7 Autologous Tissue Substitute
		J Synthetic Substitute
		K Nonautologous Tissue Substitute
			Z No Qualifier

M   **Pharynx**
    Base of tongue
    Hypopharynx
    Laryngopharynx
    Lingual tonsil
    Oropharynx
    Piriform recess (sinus)
    Tongue, base of
R   **Epiglottis**
    Glossoepiglottic fold
S   **Larynx**
    Aryepiglottic fold
    Arytenoid cartilage
    Corniculate cartilage
    Cuneiform cartilage
    False vocal cord
    Glottis
    Rima glottidis
    Thyroid cartilage
    Ventricular fold
T   **Vocal Cord, Right**
    Vocal fold
V   **Vocal Cord, Left**
    See T Vocal Cord, Right
	Ø Open
	7 Via Natural or Artificial Opening
	8 Via Natural or Artificial Opening Endoscopic
		7 Autologous Tissue Substitute
		J Synthetic Substitute
		K Nonautologous Tissue Substitute
			Z No Qualifier

Non-OR   ØCU2[Ø,3]JZ

Ø   **Medical and Surgical**
C   **Mouth and Throat**
V   **Restriction**   Definition: Partially closing an orifice or the lumen of a tubular body part
                    Explanation: The orifice can be a natural orifice or an artificially created orifice

Body Part Character 4	Approach Character 5	Device Character 6	Qualifier Character 7

B   **Parotid Duct, Right**
    Stensen's duct
C   **Parotid Duct, Left**
    See B Parotid Duct, Right
	Ø Open
	3 Percutaneous
		C Extraluminal Device
		D Intraluminal Device
		Z No Device
			Z No Qualifier

B   **Parotid Duct, Right**
    Stensen's duct
C   **Parotid Duct, Left**
    See B Parotid Duct, Right
	7 Via Natural or Artificial Opening
	8 Via Natural or Artificial Opening Endoscopic
		D Intraluminal Device
		Z No Device
			Z No Qualifier

Ø   Medical and Surgical
C   Mouth and Throat
W   Revision   Definition: Correcting, to the extent possible, a portion of a malfunctioning device or the position of a displaced device

               Explanation: Revision can include correcting a malfunctioning or displaced device by taking out or putting in components of the device such as a screw or pin

Body Part Character 4	Approach Character 5	Device Character 6	Qualifier Character 7
A Salivary Gland	**Ø** Open **3** Percutaneous	**Ø** Drainage Device **C** Extraluminal Device **Y** Other Device	**Z** No Qualifier
A Salivary Gland	**7** Via Natural or Artificial Opening **8** Via Natural or Artificial Opening Endoscopic	**Y** Other Device	**Z** No Qualifier
A Salivary Gland	**X** External	**Ø** Drainage Device **C** Extraluminal Device	**Z** No Qualifier

S   Larynx
     Aryepiglottic fold
     Arytenoid cartilage
     Corniculate cartilage
     Cuneiform cartilage
     False vocal cord
     Glottis
     Rima glottidis
     Thyroid cartilage
     Ventricular fold
	Ø Open
	3 Percutaneous
	7 Via Natural or Artificial Opening
	8 Via Natural or Artificial Opening Endoscopic
		Ø Drainage Device
		7 Autologous Tissue Substitute
		D Intraluminal Device
		J Synthetic Substitute
		K Nonautologous Tissue Substitute
		Y Other Device
			Z No Qualifier

S   Larynx
     Aryepiglottic fold
     Arytenoid cartilage
     Corniculate cartilage
     Cuneiform cartilage
     False vocal cord
     Glottis
     Rima glottidis
     Thyroid cartilage
     Ventricular fold
	X External	**Ø** Drainage Device
		7 Autologous Tissue Substitute
		D Intraluminal Device
		J Synthetic Substitute
		K Nonautologous Tissue Substitute
			Z No Qualifier

Y Mouth and Throat	**Ø** Open **3** Percutaneous **7** Via Natural or Artificial Opening **8** Via Natural or Artificial Opening Endoscopic	**Ø** Drainage Device **1** Radioactive Element **7** Autologous Tissue Substitute **D** Intraluminal Device **J** Synthetic Substitute **K** Nonautologous Tissue Substitute **Y** Other Device	**Z** No Qualifier
Y Mouth and Throat	**X** External	**Ø** Drainage Device **1** Radioactive Element **7** Autologous Tissue Substitute **D** Intraluminal Device **J** Synthetic Substitute **K** Nonautologous Tissue Substitute	**Z** No Qualifier

Non-OR	ØCWA[Ø,3][Ø,C,Y]Z
Non-OR	ØCWA[7,8]YZ
Non-OR	ØCWAX[Ø,C]Z
Non-OR	ØCWS[3,7,8]YZ
Non-OR	ØCWSX[Ø,7,D,J,K]Z
Non-OR	ØCWYØ7Z
Non-OR	ØCWY[3,7,8]YZ
Non-OR	ØCWYX[Ø,1,7,D,J,K]Z

NC Noncovered Procedure   **LC** Limited Coverage   **QA** Questionable OB Admit   **NT** New Tech Add-on   ⊞ Combination Member   ♂ Male   ♀ Female

ICD-10-PCS 2022   371

Mouth and Throat

Ø   **Medical and Surgical**
C   **Mouth and Throat**
X   **Transfer**   Definition: Moving, without taking out, all or a portion of a body part to another location to take over the function of all or a portion of a body part
Explanation: The body part transferred remains connected to its vascular and nervous supply

Body Part Character 4	Approach Character 5	Device Character 6	Qualifier Character 7

Ø   **Upper Lip**
     Frenulum labii superioris
     Labial gland
     Vermilion border
1   **Lower Lip**
     Frenulum labii inferioris
     Labial gland
     Vermilion border
3   **Soft Palate**
4   **Buccal Mucosa**
     Buccal gland
     Molar gland
     Palatine gland
5   **Upper Gingiva**
6   **Lower Gingiva**
7   **Tongue**
     Frenulum linguae
	Ø Open
	X External
		Z No Device	Z No Qualifier

Gastrointestinal System ØD1–ØDY

Character Meanings

This Character Meaning table is provided as a guide to assist the user in the identification of character members that may be found in this section of code tables. It **SHOULD NOT** be used to build a PCS code.

Operation–Character 3		Body Part–Character 4		Approach–Character 5		Device–Character 6		Qualifier–Character 7	
1	Bypass	Ø	Upper Intestinal Tract	Ø	Open	Ø	Drainage Device	Ø	Allogeneic
2	Change	1	Esophagus, Upper	3	Percutaneous	1	Radioactive Element	1	Syngeneic
5	Destruction	2	Esophagus, Middle	4	Percutaneous Endoscopic	2	Monitoring Device	2	Zooplastic
7	Dilation	3	Esophagus, Lower	7	Via Natural or Artificial Opening	3	Infusion Device	3	Vertical
8	Division	4	Esophagogastric Junction	8	Via Natural or Artificial Opening Endoscopic	7	Autologous Tissue Substitute	4	Cutaneous
9	Drainage	5	Esophagus	F	Via Natural or Artificial Opening with Percutaneous Endoscopic Assistance	B	Intraluminal Device, Airway	5	Esophagus
B	Excision	6	Stomach	X	External	C	Extraluminal Device	6	Stomach
C	Extirpation	7	Stomach, Pylorus			D	Intraluminal Device	7	Vagina
D	Extraction	8	Small Intestine			J	Synthetic Substitute	8	Small Intestine
F	Fragmentation	9	Duodenum			K	Nonautologous Tissue Substitute	9	Duodenum
H	Insertion	A	Jejunum			L	Artificial Sphincter	A	Jejunum
J	Inspection	B	Ileum			M	Stimulator Lead	B	Ileum
L	Occlusion	C	Ileocecal Valve			U	Feeding Device	E	Large Intestine
M	Reattachment	D	Lower Intestinal Tract			Y	Other Device	H	Cecum
N	Release	E	Large Intestine			Z	No Device	K	Ascending Colon
P	Removal	F	Large Intestine, Right					L	Transverse Colon
Q	Repair	G	Large Intestine, Left					M	Descending Colon
R	Replacement	H	Cecum					N	Sigmoid Colon
S	Reposition	J	Appendix					P	Rectum
T	Resection	K	Ascending Colon					Q	Anus
U	Supplement	L	Transverse Colon					X	Diagnostic
V	Restriction	M	Descending Colon					Z	No Qualifier
W	Revision	N	Sigmoid Colon						
X	Transfer	P	Rectum						
Y	Transplantation	Q	Anus						
		R	Anal Sphincter						
		U	Omentum						
		V	Mesentery						
		W	Peritoneum						

AHA Coding Clinic for table 0D1

2021, 1Q, 19	Kock pouch revision surgery
2019, 4Q, 29	Intestinal bypass
2017, 2Q, 17	Billroth II (distal gastrectomy and gastrojejunostomy)
2016, 2Q, 31	Laparoscopic biliopancreatic diversion with duodenal switch
2014, 4Q, 41	Abdominoperineal resection (APR) with flap closure of perineum and colostomy

AHA Coding Clinic for table 0D2

2019, 1Q, 26	Exchange of clogged gastrojejunostomy tube

AHA Coding Clinic for table 0D5

2017, 1Q, 34	Debulking of tumor and peritoneum ablation

AHA Coding Clinic for table 0D7

2020, 3Q, 45	Dilation versus drainage of perirectal cyst
2017, 3Q, 23	Laparoscopic pyloromyotomy
2014, 4Q, 40	Dilation of gastrojejunostomy anastomosis stricture

AHA Coding Clinic for table 0D8

2019, 2Q, 15	Reversal of Roux-en-Y bypass
2017, 3Q, 22	Laparoscopic esophagomyotomy (Heller type) and Toupet fundoplication
2017, 3Q, 23	Laparoscopic pyloromyotomy

AHA Coding Clinic for table 0D9

2020, 3Q, 45	Dilation versus drainage of perirectal cyst
2015, 2Q, 29	Insertion of nasogastric tube for drainage and feeding

AHA Coding Clinic for table 0DB

2021, 2Q, 11	Serosal injury with excision of small intestine
2021, 1Q, 20	Rectal suction biopsy
2021, 1Q, 22	Total proctocolectomy with creation of J-pouch
2019, 2Q, 15	Reversal of Roux-en-Y bypass
2019, 1Q, 3-8	Whipple procedure
2019, 1Q, 27	Excision of pelvic sidewall mass
2017, 2Q, 17	Billroth II (distal gastrectomy and gastrojejunostomy)
2017, 1Q, 16	Hepatic flexure versus transverse colon
2016, 3Q, 3-7	Stoma creation & takedown procedures
2016, 2Q, 31	Laparoscopic biliopancreatic diversion with duodenal switch
2016, 1Q, 22	Perineal proctectomy
2016, 1Q, 24	Endoscopic brush biopsy of esophagus
2014, 4Q, 40	Abdominoperineal resection (APR) with flap closure of perineum and colostomy
2014, 3Q, 28	Ileostomy takedown and parastomal hernia repair
2014, 3Q, 32	Pyloric-sparing Whipple procedure

AHA Coding Clinic for table 0DD

2021, 1Q, 20	Rectal suction biopsy
2017, 4Q, 41-42	Extraction procedures

AHA Coding Clinic for table 0DH

2020, 4Q, 43-44	Insertion of radioactive element
2020, 3Q, 43	Staged laparoscopic gastric conduit and placement of feeding tube
2019, 2Q, 18	Endoscopic wound VAC placement
2016, 3Q, 26	Insertion of gastrostomy tube
2013, 4Q, 117	Percutaneous endoscopic placement of gastrostomy tube

AHA Coding Clinic for table 0DJ

2019, 1Q, 25	Laparoscopic appendectomy converted to open procedure
2019, 1Q, 25	Milking of inspissated material from ileum to colon
2017, 2Q, 15	Low anterior resection with sigmoidoscopy
2016, 2Q, 20	Capsule endoscopy of small intestine
2015, 3Q, 24	Esophagogastroduodenoscopy with epinephrine injection for control of bleeding

AHA Coding Clinic for table 0DL

2013, 4Q, 112	Endoscopic banding of esophageal varices

AHA Coding Clinic for table 0DN

2017, 4Q, 49-50	New and revised body part values - Repositioning of the intestine
2017, 1Q, 35	Lysis of omental and peritoneal adhesions
2015, 3Q, 15	Vascular ring surgery with release of esophagus and trachea
2015, 3Q, 16	Vascular ring surgery and double aortic arch

AHA Coding Clinic for table 0DP

2019, 2Q, 18	Removal of wound VAC

AHA Coding Clinic for table 0DQ

2019, 2Q, 15	Reversal of Roux-en-Y bypass
2018, 2Q, 25	Third and fourth degree obstetric lacerations
2018, 1Q, 11	Repair of internal hernia at Petersen space
2017, 3Q, 17	Posterior sagittal anorectoplasty
2016, 3Q, 3-7	Stoma creation & takedown procedures
2016, 3Q, 26	Insertion of gastrostomy tube
2016, 1Q, 7	Obstetrical perineal laceration repair
2016, 1Q, 8	Obstetrical perineal laceration repair
2014, 4Q, 20	Control of bleeding duodenal ulcer

AHA Coding Clinic for table 0DS

2019, 1Q, 30	Laparoscopic-assisted rectopexy with manual reduction of prolapse
2017, 4Q, 49-50	New and revised body part values - Repositioning of the intestine
2017, 3Q, 9	Ileocolic intussusception reduction via air enema
2017, 3Q, 17	Posterior sagittal anorectoplasty
2016, 3Q, 3-5	Stoma creation & takedown procedures

AHA Coding Clinic for table 0DT

2021, 1Q, 22	Total proctocolectomy with creation of J-pouch
2020, 4Q, 100	Robotic-assisted sigmoid colectomy with extension of incision for specimen removal
2019, 1Q, 3-8	Whipple procedure
2019, 1Q, 14	Esophagectomy with colon interposition
2017, 4Q, 49-50	New and revised body part values - Repositioning of the intestine
2014, 4Q, 40	Abdominoperineal resection (APR) with flap closure of perineum and colostomy
2014, 4Q, 42	Right colectomy with side-to-side functional end-to-end anastomosis
2014, 3Q, 6	Ileocecectomy including cecum, terminal ileum and appendix
2014, 3Q, 6	Right colectomy

AHA Coding Clinic for table 0DU

2021, 2Q, 20	Malone antegrade continence enema procedure
2021, 1Q, 22	Total proctocolectomy with creation of J-pouch
2019, 1Q, 30	Laparoscopic-assisted rectopexy with manual reduction of prolapse

AHA Coding Clinic for table 0DV

2017, 3Q, 22	Laparoscopic esophagomyotomy (Heller type) and Toupet fundoplication
2016, 2Q, 22	Esophageal lengthening Collis gastroplasty with Nissen fundoplication and hiatal hernia
2014, 3Q, 28	Laparoscopic Nissen fundoplication and diaphragmatic hernia repair

AHA Coding Clinic for table 0DW

2021, 1Q, 19	Kock pouch revision surgery
2018, 1Q, 20	Adjustment of gastric band

AHA Coding Clinic for table 0DX

2019, 4Q, 29-30	Transfer large intestine to vagina
2019, 1Q, 14	Esophagectomy with colon interposition
2017, 2Q, 18	Esophagectomy and esophagogastrectomy with cervical esophagogastrostomy
2016, 2Q, 22	Esophageal lengthening Collis gastroplasty with Nissen fundoplication and hiatal hernia
2015, 1Q, 28	Repair of bronchopleural fistula using omental pedicle graft

Upper Intestinal Tract (Ø) and Lower Intestinal Tract (D)

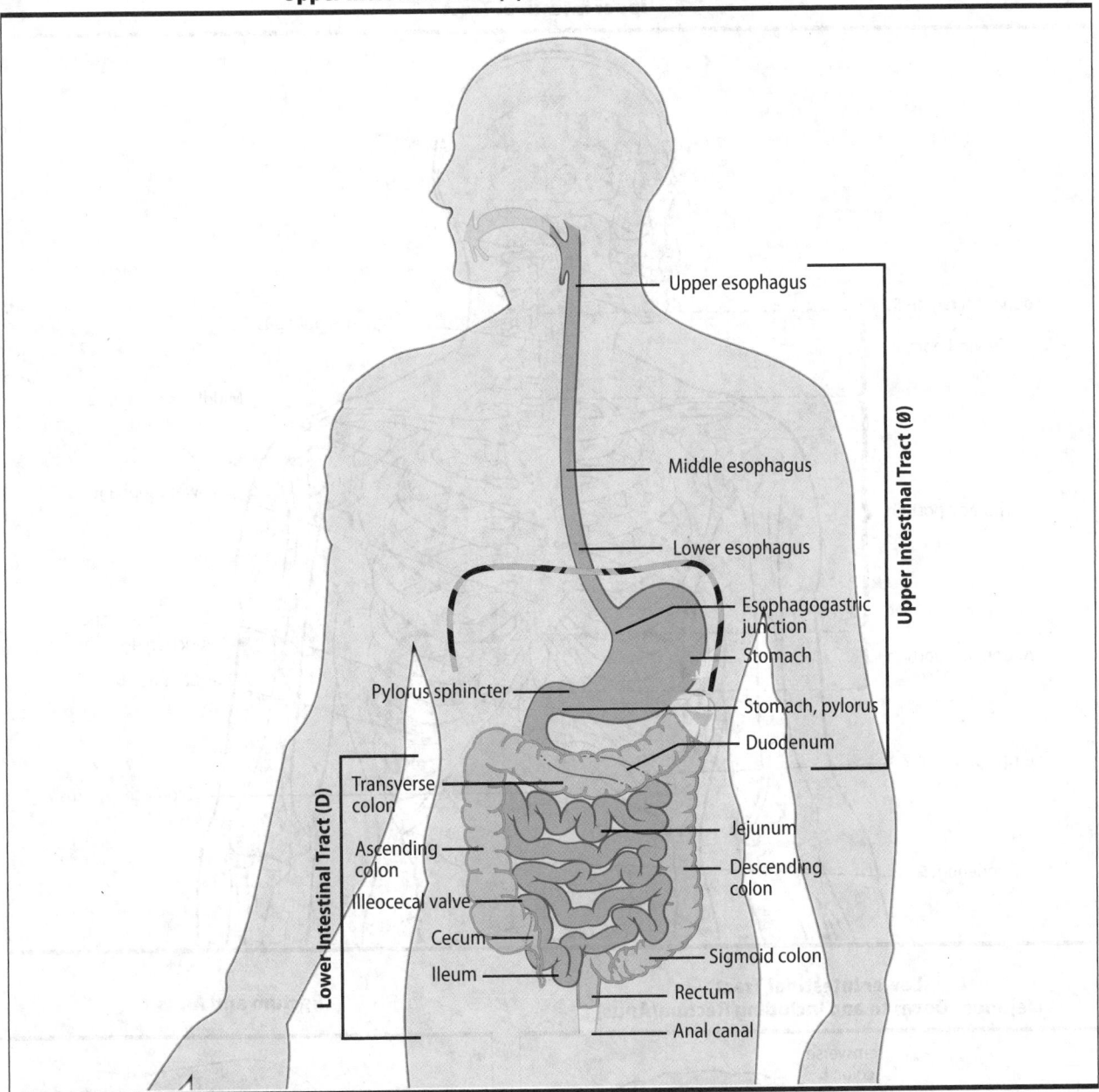

Upper Intestinal Tract

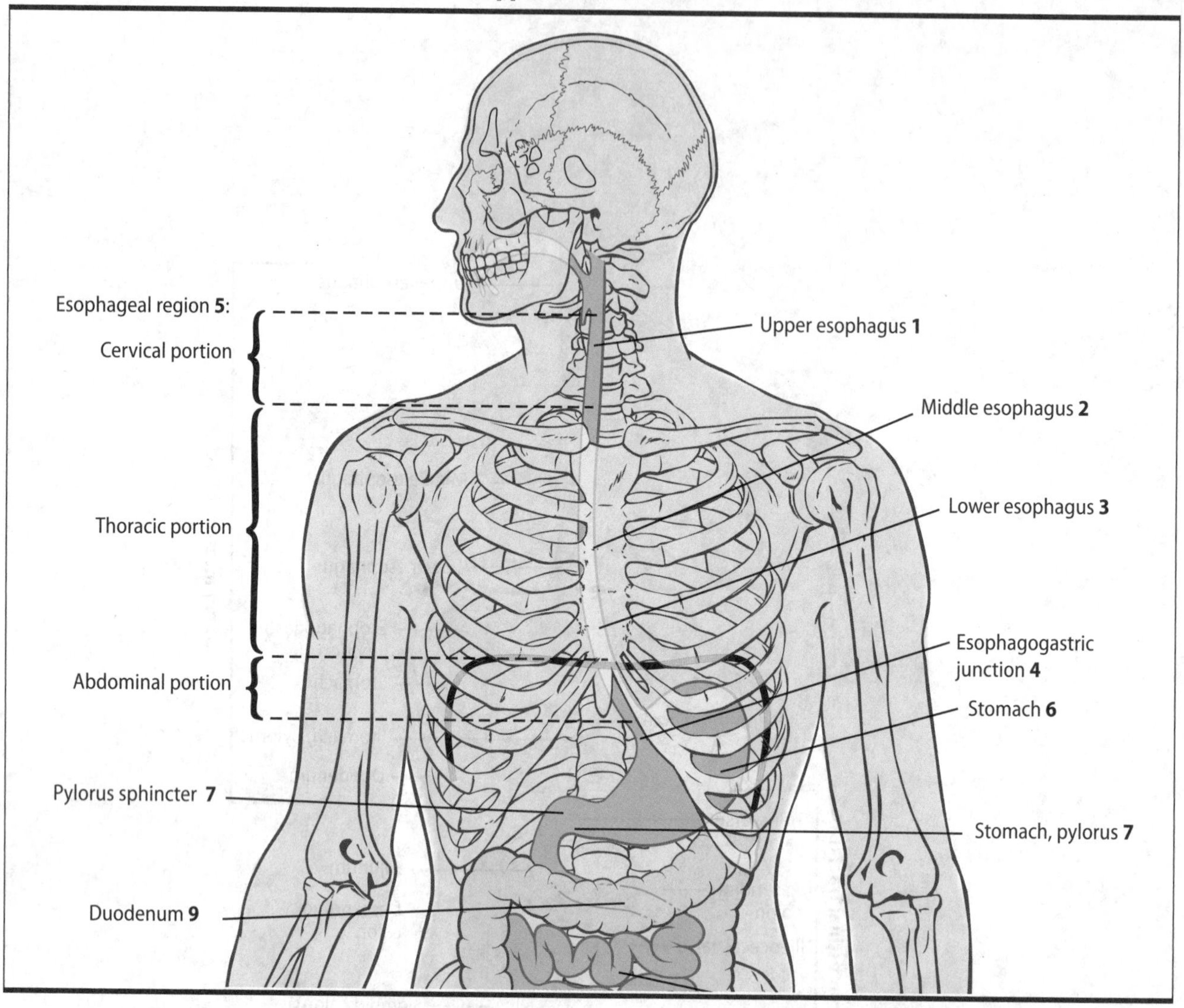

Esophageal region **5**:

Cervical portion

Thoracic portion

Abdominal portion

Pylorus sphincter **7**

Duodenum **9**

Upper esophagus **1**

Middle esophagus **2**

Lower esophagus **3**

Esophagogastric junction **4**

Stomach **6**

Stomach, pylorus **7**

Lower Intestinal Tract
(Jejunum Down to and Including Rectum/Anus)

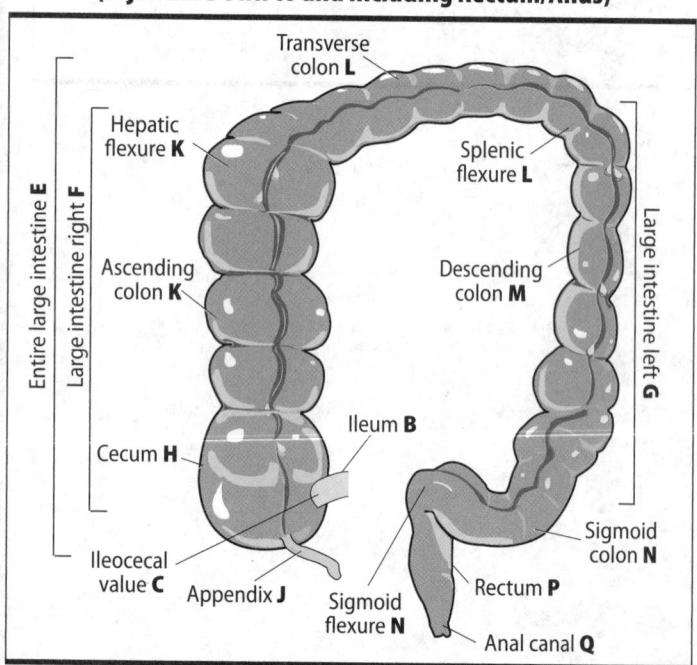

Transverse colon **L**

Hepatic flexure **K**

Splenic flexure **L**

Ascending colon **K**

Descending colon **M**

Entire large intestine **E**

Large intestine right **F**

Large intestine left **G**

Cecum **H**

Ileum **B**

Ileocecal value **C**

Appendix **J**

Sigmoid flexure **N**

Rectum **P**

Sigmoid colon **N**

Anal canal **Q**

Rectum and Anus

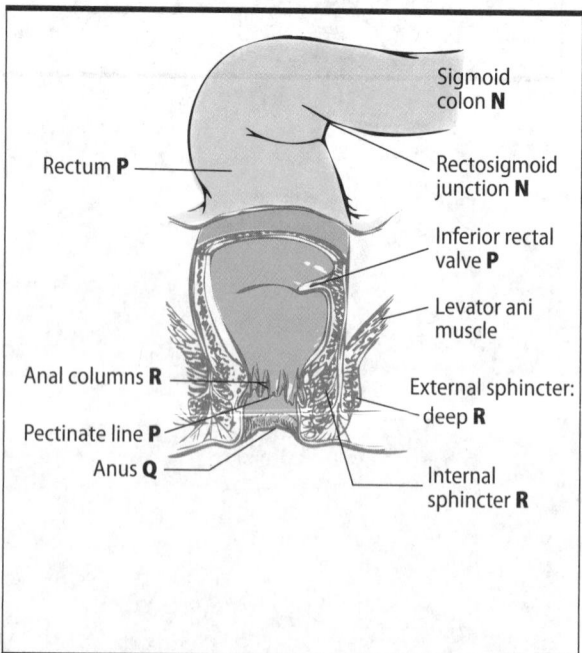

Sigmoid colon **N**

Rectum **P**

Rectosigmoid junction **N**

Inferior rectal valve **P**

Levator ani muscle

Anal columns **R**

Pectinate line **P**

Anus **Q**

External sphincter: deep **R**

Internal sphincter **R**

Ø Medical and Surgical
D Gastrointestinal System
1 Bypass   Definition: Altering the route of passage of the contents of a tubular body part
   Explanation: Rerouting contents of a body part to a downstream area of the normal route, to a similar route and body part, or to an abnormal route and dissimilar body part. Includes one or more anastomoses, with or without the use of a device.

Body Part Character 4	Approach Character 5	Device Character 6	Qualifier Character 7
1 Esophagus, Upper Cervical esophagus **2 Esophagus, Middle** Thoracic esophagus **3 Esophagus, Lower** Abdominal esophagus **5 Esophagus**	**Ø** Open **4** Percutaneous Endoscopic **8** Via Natural or Artificial Opening Endoscopic	**7** Autologous Tissue Substitute **J** Synthetic Substitute **K** Nonautologous Tissue Substitute **Z** No Device	**4** Cutaneous **6** Stomach **9** Duodenum **A** Jejunum **B** Ileum
1 Esophagus, Upper Cervical esophagus **2 Esophagus, Middle** Thoracic esophagus **3 Esophagus, Lower** Abdominal esophagus **5 Esophagus**	**3** Percutaneous	**J** Synthetic Substitute	**4** Cutaneous
6 Stomach **9 Duodenum**	**Ø** Open **4** Percutaneous Endoscopic **8** Via Natural or Artificial Opening Endoscopic	**7** Autologous Tissue Substitute **J** Synthetic Substitute **K** Nonautologous Tissue Substitute **Z** No Device	**4** Cutaneous **9** Duodenum **A** Jejunum **B** Ileum **L** Transverse Colon
6 Stomach **9 Duodenum**	**3** Percutaneous	**J** Synthetic Substitute	**4** Cutaneous
8 Small Intestine	**Ø** Open **4** Percutaneous Endoscopic **8** Via Natural or Artificial Opening Endoscopic	**7** Autologous Tissue Substitute **J** Synthetic Substitute **K** Nonautologous Tissue Substitute **Z** No Device	**4** Cutaneous **8** Small Intestine **H** Cecum **K** Ascending Colon **L** Transverse Colon **M** Descending Colon **N** Sigmoid Colon **P** Rectum **Q** Anus
A Jejunum Duodenojejunal flexure	**Ø** Open **4** Percutaneous Endoscopic **8** Via Natural or Artificial Opening Endoscopic	**7** Autologous Tissue Substitute **J** Synthetic Substitute **K** Nonautologous Tissue Substitute **Z** No Device	**4** Cutaneous **A** Jejunum **B** Ileum **H** Cecum **K** Ascending Colon **L** Transverse Colon **M** Descending Colon **N** Sigmoid Colon **P** Rectum **Q** Anus
A Jejunum Duodenojejunal flexure	**3** Percutaneous	**J** Synthetic Substitute	**4** Cutaneous
B Ileum	**Ø** Open **4** Percutaneous Endoscopic **8** Via Natural or Artificial Opening Endoscopic	**7** Autologous Tissue Substitute **J** Synthetic Substitute **K** Nonautologous Tissue Substitute **Z** No Device	**4** Cutaneous **B** Ileum **H** Cecum **K** Ascending Colon **L** Transverse Colon **M** Descending Colon **N** Sigmoid Colon **P** Rectum **Q** Anus
B Ileum	**3** Percutaneous	**J** Synthetic Substitute	**4** Cutaneous
E Large Intestine	**Ø** Open **4** Percutaneous Endoscopic **8** Via Natural or Artificial Opening Endoscopic	**7** Autologous Tissue Substitute **J** Synthetic Substitute **K** Nonautologous Tissue Substitute **Z** No Device	**4** Cutaneous **E** Large Intestine **P** Rectum
H Cecum	**Ø** Open **4** Percutaneous Endoscopic **8** Via Natural or Artificial Opening Endoscopic	**7** Autologous Tissue Substitute **J** Synthetic Substitute **K** Nonautologous Tissue Substitute **Z** No Device	**4** Cutaneous **H** Cecum **K** Ascending Colon **L** Transverse Colon **M** Descending Colon **N** Sigmoid Colon **P** Rectum
H Cecum	**3** Percutaneous	**J** Synthetic Substitute	**4** Cutaneous

Non-OR ØD16[Ø,4,8][7,J,K,Z]4
Non-OR ØD163J4
HAC ØD16[Ø,4,8][7,J,K,Z][9,A,B,L] when reported with PDx E66.Ø1 and SDx K68.11, K95.Ø1, K95.81 or T81.4Ø–T81.49 with 7th character A

ØD1 Continued on next page

NC Noncovered Procedure   **LC** Limited Coverage   **OA** Questionable OB Admit   **NT** New Tech Add-on   ⊞ Combination Member   ♂ Male   ♀ Female

ICD-10-PCS 2022   377

ØD1–ØD1

ØD1 Continued

Ø   Medical and Surgical
D   Gastrointestinal System
1   Bypass   Definition: Altering the route of passage of the contents of a tubular body part

Explanation: Rerouting contents of a body part to a downstream area of the normal route, to a similar route and body part, or to an abnormal route and dissimilar body part. Includes one or more anastomoses, with or without the use of a device.

Body Part Character 4	Approach Character 5	Device Character 6	Qualifier Character 7
K Ascending Colon	Ø Open 4 Percutaneous Endoscopic 8 Via Natural or Artificial Opening Endoscopic	7 Autologous Tissue Substitute J Synthetic Substitute K Nonautologous Tissue Substitute Z No Device	4 Cutaneous K Ascending Colon L Transverse Colon M Descending Colon N Sigmoid Colon P Rectum
K Ascending Colon	3 Percutaneous	J Synthetic Substitute	4 Cutaneous
L Transverse Colon Hepatic flexure Splenic flexure	Ø Open 4 Percutaneous Endoscopic 8 Via Natural or Artificial Opening Endoscopic	7 Autologous Tissue Substitute J Synthetic Substitute K Nonautologous Tissue Substitute Z No Device	4 Cutaneous L Transverse Colon M Descending Colon N Sigmoid Colon P Rectum
L Transverse Colon Hepatic flexure Splenic flexure	3 Percutaneous	J Synthetic Substitute	4 Cutaneous
M Descending Colon	Ø Open 4 Percutaneous Endoscopic 8 Via Natural or Artificial Opening Endoscopic	7 Autologous Tissue Substitute J Synthetic Substitute K Nonautologous Tissue Substitute Z No Device	4 Cutaneous M Descending Colon N Sigmoid Colon P Rectum
M Descending Colon	3 Percutaneous	J Synthetic Substitute	4 Cutaneous
N Sigmoid Colon Rectosigmoid junction Sigmoid flexure	Ø Open 4 Percutaneous Endoscopic 8 Via Natural or Artificial Opening Endoscopic	7 Autologous Tissue Substitute J Synthetic Substitute K Nonautologous Tissue Substitute Z No Device	4 Cutaneous N Sigmoid Colon P Rectum
N Sigmoid Colon Rectosigmoid junction Sigmoid flexure	3 Percutaneous	J Synthetic Substitute	4 Cutaneous

Ø   Medical and Surgical
D   Gastrointestinal System
2   Change   Definition: Taking out or off a device from a body part and putting back an identical or similar device in or on the same body part without cutting or puncturing the skin or a mucous membrane

Explanation: All CHANGE procedures are coded using the approach EXTERNAL

Body Part Character 4	Approach Character 5	Device Character 6	Qualifier Character 7
Ø Upper Intestinal Tract D Lower Intestinal Tract	X External	Ø Drainage Device U Feeding Device Y Other Device	Z No Qualifier
U Omentum Gastrocolic ligament Gastrocolic omentum Gastrohepatic omentum Gastrophrenic ligament Gastrosplenic ligament Greater Omentum Hepatogastric ligament Lesser Omentum V Mesentery Mesoappendix Mesocolon W Peritoneum Epiploic foramen	X External	Ø Drainage Device Y Other Device	Z No Qualifier

Non-OR   All body part, approach, device, and qualifier values

Ø   **Medical and Surgical**
D   **Gastrointestinal System**
5   **Destruction**   Definition: Physical eradication of all or a portion of a body part by the direct use of energy, force, or a destructive agent
                    Explanation: None of the body part is physically taken out

Body Part Character 4	Approach Character 5	Device Character 6	Qualifier Character 7

1 Esophagus, Upper
   Cervical esophagus
2 Esophagus, Middle
   Thoracic esophagus
3 Esophagus, Lower
   Abdominal esophagus
4 Esophagogastric Junction
   Cardia
   Cardioesophageal junction
   Gastroesophageal (GE) junction
5 Esophagus
6 Stomach
7 Stomach, Pylorus
   Pyloric antrum
   Pyloric canal
   Pyloric sphincter
8 Small Intestine
9 Duodenum
A Jejunum
   Duodenojejunal flexure
B Ileum
C Ileocecal Valve
E Large Intestine
F Large Intestine, Right
G Large Intestine, Left
H Cecum
J Appendix
   Vermiform appendix
K Ascending Colon
L Transverse Colon
   Hepatic flexure
   Splenic flexure
M Descending Colon
N Sigmoid Colon
   Rectosigmoid junction
   Sigmoid flexure
P Rectum
   Anorectal junction
	Ø Open
	3 Percutaneous
	4 Percutaneous Endoscopic
	7 Via Natural or Artificial Opening
	8 Via Natural or Artificial Opening Endoscopic
		Z No Device	**Z** No Qualifier

Q Anus Anal orifice	**Ø** Open **3** Percutaneous **4** Percutaneous Endoscopic **7** Via Natural or Artificial Opening **8** Via Natural or Artificial Opening Endoscopic **X** External	**Z** No Device	**Z** No Qualifier

R Anal Sphincter
   External anal sphincter
   Internal anal sphincter
U Omentum
   Gastrocolic ligament
   Gastrocolic omentum
   Gastrohepatic omentum
   Gastrophrenic ligament
   Gastrosplenic ligament
   Greater Omentum
   Hepatogastric ligament
   Lesser Omentum
V Mesentery
   Mesoappendix
   Mesocolon
W Peritoneum
   Epiploic foramen
	Ø Open
	3 Percutaneous
	4 Percutaneous Endoscopic
		Z No Device	**Z** No Qualifier

Non-OR   ØD5[1,2,3,4,5,6,7,9,E,F,G,H,K,L,M,N][4,8]ZZ
Non-OR   ØD5[8,A,B,C]8ZZ
Non-OR   ØD5P[Ø,3,4,7,8]ZZ
Non-OR   ØD5Q[4,8]ZZ
Non-OR   ØD5R4ZZ

NC Noncovered Procedure   **LC** Limited Coverage   **QA** Questionable OB Admit   **NT** New Tech Add-on   ⊞ Combination Member   ♂ Male   ♀ Female

ICD-10-PCS 2022   379

ØD5–ØD5

Ø   **Medical and Surgical**
D   **Gastrointestinal System**
7   **Dilation**   Definition: Expanding an orifice or the lumen of a tubular body part

Explanation: The orifice can be a natural orifice or an artificially created orifice. Accomplished by stretching a tubular body part using intraluminal pressure or by cutting part of the orifice or wall of the tubular body part.

Body Part Character 4	Approach Character 5	Device Character 6	Qualifier Character 7
1 Esophagus, Upper Cervical esophagus **2 Esophagus, Middle** Thoracic esophagus **3 Esophagus, Lower** Abdominal esophagus **4 Esophagogastric Junction** Cardia Cardioesophageal junction Gastroesophageal (GE) junction **5 Esophagus** **6 Stomach** **7 Stomach, Pylorus** Pyloric antrum Pyloric canal Pyloric sphincter **8 Small Intestine** **9 Duodenum** **A Jejunum** Duodenojejunal flexure **B Ileum** **C Ileocecal Valve** **E Large Intestine** **F Large Intestine, Right** **G Large Intestine, Left** **H Cecum** **K Ascending Colon** **L Transverse Colon** Hepatic flexure Splenic flexure **M Descending Colon** **N Sigmoid Colon** Rectosigmoid junction Sigmoid flexure **P Rectum** Anorectal junction **Q Anus** Anal orifice	**Ø Open** **3 Percutaneous** **4 Percutaneous Endoscopic** **7 Via Natural or Artificial Opening** **8 Via Natural or Artificial Opening Endoscopic**	**D Intraluminal Device** **Z No Device**	**Z No Qualifier**

Non-OR	ØD7[1,2,3,4,5,6,8,9,A,B,C,E,F,G,H,K,L,M,N,P,Q][7,8][D,Z]Z
Non-OR	ØD77[4,8]DZ
Non-OR	ØD777[D,Z]Z
Non-OR	ØD7[8,9,A,B,C,E,F,G,H,K,L,M,N][Ø,3,4]DZ

Ø   **Medical and Surgical**
D   **Gastrointestinal System**
8   **Division**   Definition: Cutting into a body part, without draining fluids and/or gases from the body part, in order to separate or transect a body part

Explanation: All or a portion of the body part is separated into two or more portions

Body Part Character 4	Approach Character 5	Device Character 6	Qualifier Character 7
4 Esophagogastric Junction Cardia Cardioesophageal junction Gastroesophageal (GE) junction **7 Stomach, Pylorus** Pyloric antrum Pyloric canal Pyloric sphincter	**Ø Open** **3 Percutaneous** **4 Percutaneous Endoscopic** **7 Via Natural or Artificial Opening** **8 Via Natural or Artificial Opening Endoscopic**	**Z No Device**	**Z No Qualifier**
R Anal Sphincter External anal sphincter Internal anal sphincter	**Ø Open** **3 Percutaneous**	**Z No Device**	**Z No Qualifier**

Ø   **Medical and Surgical**
D   **Gastrointestinal System**
9   **Drainage**   Definition: Taking or letting out fluids and/or gases from a body part
                        Explanation: The qualifier DIAGNOSTIC is used to identify drainage procedures that are biopsies

Body Part Character 4		Approach Character 5	Device Character 6	Qualifier Character 7

1 Esophagus, Upper
  Cervical esophagus
2 Esophagus, Middle
  Thoracic esophagus
3 Esophagus, Lower
  Abdominal esophagus
4 Esophagogastric
  Junction
  Cardia
  Cardioesophageal
    junction
  Gastroesophageal (GE)
    junction
5 Esophagus
6 Stomach
7 Stomach, Pylorus
  Pyloric antrum
  Pyloric canal
  Pyloric sphincter
8 Small Intestine
9 Duodenum
	A Jejunum
	  Duodenojejunal flexure
	B Ileum
	C Ileocecal Valve
	E Large Intestine
	F Large Intestine, Right
	G Large Intestine, Left
	H Cecum
	J Appendix
	  Vermiform appendix
	K Ascending Colon
	L Transverse Colon
	  Hepatic flexure
	  Splenic flexure
	M Descending Colon
	N Sigmoid Colon
	  Rectosigmoid junction
	  Sigmoid flexure
	P Rectum
	  Anorectal junction
		Ø Open
		3 Percutaneous
		4 Percutaneous Endoscopic
		7 Via Natural or Artificial
		  Opening
		8 Via Natural or Artificial
		  Opening Endoscopic
			Ø Drainage Device	**Z No Qualifier**

1 Esophagus, Upper
  Cervical esophagus
2 Esophagus, Middle
  Thoracic esophagus
3 Esophagus, Lower
  Abdominal esophagus
4 Esophagogastric
  Junction
  Cardia
  Cardioesophageal
    junction
  Gastroesophageal (GE)
    junction
5 Esophagus
6 Stomach
7 Stomach, Pylorus
  Pyloric antrum
  Pyloric canal
  Pyloric sphincter
8 Small Intestine
9 Duodenum
	A Jejunum
	  Duodenojejunal flexure
	B Ileum
	C Ileocecal Valve
	E Large Intestine
	F Large Intestine, Right
	G Large Intestine, Left
	H Cecum
	J Appendix
	  Vermiform appendix
	K Ascending Colon
	L Transverse Colon
	  Hepatic flexure
	  Splenic flexure
	M Descending Colon
	N Sigmoid Colon
	  Rectosigmoid junction
	  Sigmoid flexure
	P Rectum
	  Anorectal junction
		Ø Open
		3 Percutaneous
		4 Percutaneous Endoscopic
		7 Via Natural or Artificial
		  Opening
		8 Via Natural or Artificial
		  Opening Endoscopic
			Z No Device	**X Diagnostic**
				Z No Qualifier

Q Anus
  Anal orifice
		Ø Open
		3 Percutaneous
		4 Percutaneous Endoscopic
		7 Via Natural or Artificial
		  Opening
		8 Via Natural or Artificial
		  Opening Endoscopic
		X External
			Ø Drainage Device	**Z No Qualifier**

Q Anus
  Anal orifice
		Ø Open
		3 Percutaneous
		4 Percutaneous Endoscopic
		7 Via Natural or Artificial
		  Opening
		8 Via Natural or Artificial
		  Opening Endoscopic
		X External
			Z No Device	**X Diagnostic**
				Z No Qualifier

Non-OR   ØD9[1,2,3,4,5,C,J]3ØZ
Non-OR   ØD9[6,7,8,9,A,B,E,F,G,H,K,L,M,N,P][3,7,8]ØZ
Non-OR   ØD9[1,2,3,4,5,6,7,8,9,A,B,C,E,F,G,H,K,L,M,N,P][3,4,7,8]ZX
Non-OR   ØD9[1,2,3,4,5,6,7,8,9,A,B,C,E,F,G,H,J,K,L,M,N,P]3ZZ
Non-OR   ØD9Q3ØZ
Non-OR   ØD9Q[Ø,3,4,7,8,X]ZX
Non-OR   ØD9Q3ZZ

ØD9 Continued on next page

NC Noncovered Procedure   **LC** Limited Coverage   **QA** Questionable OB Admit   **NT** New Tech Add-on   ⊞ Combination Member   ♂ Male   ♀ Female

ICD-10-PCS 2022   **381**

Ø   **Medical and Surgical**
D   **Gastrointestinal System**
9   **Drainage**   Definition: Taking or letting out fluids and/or gases from a body part
                          Explanation: The qualifier DIAGNOSTIC is used to identify drainage procedures that are biopsies

Body Part Character 4	Approach Character 5	Device Character 6	Qualifier Character 7
R Anal Sphincter External anal sphincter Internal anal sphincter **U Omentum** Gastrocolic ligament Gastrocolic omentum Gastrohepatic omentum Gastrophrenic ligament Gastrosplenic ligament Greater Omentum Hepatogastric ligament Lesser Omentum **V Mesentery** Mesoappendix Mesocolon **W Peritoneum** Epiploic foramen	Ø Open 3 Percutaneous 4 Percutaneous Endoscopic	Ø Drainage Device	Z No Qualifier
R Anal Sphincter External anal sphincter Internal anal sphincter **U Omentum** Gastrocolic ligament Gastrocolic omentum Gastrohepatic omentum Gastrophrenic ligament Gastrosplenic ligament Greater Omentum Hepatogastric ligament Lesser Omentum **V Mesentery** Mesoappendix Mesocolon **W Peritoneum** Epiploic foramen	Ø Open 3 Percutaneous 4 Percutaneous Endoscopic	Z No Device	X Diagnostic Z No Qualifier

Non-OR	ØD9[R,W]3ØZ
Non-OR	ØD9[U,V][3,4]ØZ
Non-OR	ØD9[R,U,V,W]3Z[X,Z]
Non-OR	ØD9R[Ø,4]ZX
Non-OR	ØD9[U,V]4ZZ

Ø   **Medical and Surgical**
D   **Gastrointestinal System**
B   **Excision**   Definition: Cutting out or off, without replacement, a portion of a body part
                     Explanation: The qualifier DIAGNOSTIC is used to identify excision procedures that are biopsies

Body Part Character 4		Approach Character 5	Device Character 6	Qualifier Character 7
1 Esophagus, Upper Cervical esophagus **2 Esophagus, Middle** Thoracic esophagus **3 Esophagus, Lower** Abdominal esophagus **4 Esophagogastric Junction** Cardia Cardioesophageal junction Gastroesophageal (GE) junction **5 Esophagus** **7 Stomach, Pylorus** Pyloric antrum Pyloric canal Pyloric sphincter	**8 Small Intestine** **9 Duodenum** **A Jejunum** Duodenojejunal flexure **B Ileum** **C Ileocecal Valve** **E Large Intestine** **F Large Intestine, Right** **H Cecum** **J Appendix** Vermiform appendix **K Ascending Colon** **P Rectum** Anorectal junction	**Ø** Open **3** Percutaneous **4** Percutaneous Endoscopic **7** Via Natural or Artificial Opening **8** Via Natural or Artificial Opening Endoscopic	**Z** No Device	**X** Diagnostic **Z** No Qualifier
6 Stomach		**Ø** Open **3** Percutaneous **4** Percutaneous Endoscopic **7** Via Natural or Artificial Opening **8** Via Natural or Artificial Opening Endoscopic	**Z** No Device	**3** Vertical **X** Diagnostic **Z** No Qualifier
G Large Intestine, Left **L Transverse Colon** Hepatic flexure Splenic flexure **M Descending Colon** **N Sigmoid Colon** Rectosigmoid junction Sigmoid flexure		**Ø** Open **3** Percutaneous **4** Percutaneous Endoscopic **7** Via Natural or Artificial Opening **8** Via Natural or Artificial Opening Endoscopic	**Z** No Device	**X** Diagnostic **Z** No Qualifier
G Large Intestine, Left **L Transverse Colon** Hepatic flexure Splenic flexure **M Descending Colon** **N Sigmoid Colon** Rectosigmoid junction Sigmoid flexure		**F** Via Natural or Artificial Opening with Percutaneous Endoscopic Assistance	**Z** No Device	**Z** No Qualifier
Q Anus Anal orifi		**Ø** Open **3** Percutaneous **4** Percutaneous Endoscopic **7** Via Natural or Artificial Opening **8** Via Natural or Artificial Opening Endoscopic **X** External	**Z** No Device	**X** Diagnostic **Z** No Qualifier
R Anal Sphincter External anal sphincter Internal anal sphincter **U Omentum** Gastrocolic ligament Gastrocolic omentum Gastrohepatic omentum Gastrophrenic ligament Gastrosplenic ligament Greater Omentum Hepatogastric ligament Lesser Omentum **V Mesentery** Mesoappendix Mesocolon **W Peritoneum** Epiploic foramen		**Ø** Open **3** Percutaneous **4** Percutaneous Endoscopic	**Z** No Device	**X** Diagnostic **Z** No Qualifier

Non-OR ØDB[1,2,3,4,5,7,8,9,A,B,C,E,F,H,K,P][3,4,7,8]ZX **Non-OR** ØDB[1,2,3,5,7,9][4,8]ZZ **Non-OR** ØDB[4,E,F,H,K,P]8ZZ **Non-OR** ØDB6[3,7]ZX **Non-OR** ØDB68Z[X,Z] **Non-OR** ØDB[G,L,M,N][3,4,7,8]ZX	**Non-OR** ØDB[G,L,M,N]8ZZ **Non-OR** ØDBQ[Ø,3,4,7,8,X]ZX **Non-OR** ØDBQ8ZZ **Non-OR** ØDBR[Ø,3,4]ZX **Non-OR** ØDB[U,V,W][3,4]ZX

NC Noncovered Procedure   **LC** Limited Coverage   **QA** Questionable OB Admit   **NT** New Tech Add-on   ⊞ Combination Member   ♂ Male   ♀ Female

ICD-10-PCS 2022   **383**

Gastrointestinal System

Ø	Medical and Surgical
D	Gastrointestinal System
C	Extirpation

Definition: Taking or cutting out solid matter from a body part

Explanation: The solid matter may be an abnormal byproduct of a biological function or a foreign body; it may be imbedded in a body part or in the lumen of a tubular body part. The solid matter may or may not have been previously broken into pieces.

Body Part Character 4	Approach Character 5	Device Character 6	Qualifier Character 7

1 Esophagus, Upper
   Cervical esophagus
2 Esophagus, Middle
   Thoracic esophagus
3 Esophagus, Lower
   Abdominal esophagus
4 Esophagogastric Junction
   Cardia
   Cardioesophageal junction
   Gastroesophageal (GE) junction
5 Esophagus
6 Stomach
7 Stomach, Pylorus
   Pyloric antrum
   Pyloric canal
   Pyloric sphincter
8 Small Intestine
9 Duodenum
A Jejunum
   Duodenojejunal flexure
B Ileum
C Ileocecal Valve
E Large Intestine
F Large Intestine, Right
G Large Intestine, Left
H Cecum
J Appendix
   Vermiform appendix
K Ascending Colon
L Transverse Colon
   Hepatic flexure
   Splenic flexure
M Descending Colon
N Sigmoid Colon
   Rectosigmoid junction
   Sigmoid flexure
P Rectum
   Anorectal junction
	Ø Open
	3 Percutaneous
	4 Percutaneous Endoscopic
	7 Via Natural or Artificial Opening
	8 Via Natural or Artificial Opening
	   Endoscopic
		Z No Device	Z No Qualifier

Q Anus
   Anal orifice
	Ø Open
	3 Percutaneous
	4 Percutaneous Endoscopic
	7 Via Natural or Artificial Opening
	8 Via Natural or Artificial Opening
	   Endoscopic
	X External
		Z No Device	Z No Qualifier

R Anal Sphincter
   External anal sphincter
   Internal anal sphincter
U Omentum
   Gastrocolic ligament
   Gastrocolic omentum
   Gastrohepatic omentum
   Gastrophrenic ligament
   Gastrosplenic ligament
   Greater Omentum
   Hepatogastric ligament
   Lesser Omentum
V Mesentery
   Mesoappendix
   Mesocolon
W Peritoneum
   Epiploic foramen
	Ø Open
	3 Percutaneous
	4 Percutaneous Endoscopic
		Z No Device	Z No Qualifier

Non-OR	ØDC[1,2,3,4,5,6,7,8,9,A,B,C,E,F,G,H,K,L,M,N,P][7,8]ZZ
Non-OR	ØDCQ[7,8,X]ZZ

Ø   Medical and Surgical
D   Gastrointestinal System
D   Extraction   Definition: Pulling or stripping out or off all or a portion of a body part by the use of force
                      Explanation: The qualifier DIAGNOSTIC is used to identify extraction procedures that are biopsies

Body Part Character 4	Approach Character 5	Device Character 6	Qualifier Character 7

1 Esophagus, Upper
  Cervical esophagus
2 Esophagus, Middle
  Thoracic esophagus
3 Esophagus, Lower
  Abdominal esophagus
4 Esophagogastric Junction
  Cardia
  Cardioesophageal junction
  Gastroesophageal (GE) junction
5 Esophagus
6 Stomach
7 Stomach, Pylorus
  Pyloric antrum
  Pyloric canal
  Pyloric sphincter
8 Small Intestine
9 Duodenum
A Jejunum
  Duodenojejunal flexure
B Ileum
C Ileocecal Valve
E Large Intestine
F Large Intestine, Right
G Large Intestine, Left
H Cecum
J Appendix
  Vermiform appendix
K Ascending Colon
L Transverse Colon
  Hepatic flexure
  Splenic flexure
M Descending Colon
N Sigmoid Colon
  Rectosigmoid junction
  Sigmoid flexure
P Rectum
  Anorectal junction
	3 Percutaneous
	4 Percutaneous Endoscopic
	8 Via Natural or Artificial Opening
	   Endoscopic
		Z No Device	**X** Diagnostic

Q Anus
  Anal orifice
	3 Percutaneous
	4 Percutaneous Endoscopic
	8 Via Natural or Artificial Opening
	   Endoscopic
	X External
		Z No Device	**X** Diagnostic

Non-OR   ØDD[1,2,3,4,5,6,7,8,9,A,B,C,E,F,G,H,K,L,M,N,P][3,4,8]ZX
Non-OR   ØDDQ[3,4,8,X]ZX

Ø Medical and Surgical
D Gastrointestinal System
F Fragmentation Definition: Breaking solid matter in a body part into pieces

Explanation: Physical force (e.g., manual, ultrasonic) applied directly or indirectly is used to break the solid matter into pieces. The solid matter may be an abnormal byproduct of a biological function or a foreign body. The pieces of solid matter are not taken out.

Body Part Character 4	Approach Character 5	Device Character 6	Qualifier Character 7
5 Esophagus NC	Ø Open	Z No Device	Z No Qualifier
6 Stomach NC	3 Percutaneous		
8 Small Intestine NC	4 Percutaneous Endoscopic		
9 Duodenum NC	7 Via Natural or Artificial Opening		
A Jejunum NC	8 Via Natural or Artificial Opening Endoscopic		
Duodenojejunal flexure	X External		
B Ileum NC			
E Large Intestine NC			
F Large Intestine, Right NC			
G Large Intestine, Left NC			
H Cecum NC			
J Appendix NC			
Vermiform appendix			
K Ascending Colon NC			
L Transverse Colon NC			
Hepatic flexure			
Splenic flexure			
M Descending Colon NC			
N Sigmoid Colon NC			
Rectosigmoid junction			
Sigmoid flexure			
P Rectum NC			
Anorectal junction			
Q Anus NC			
Anal orifice			

Non-OR ØDF[5,6,8,9,A,B,E,F,G,H,J,K,L,M,N,P,Q]XZZ
NC ØDF[5,6,8,9,A,B,E,F,G,H,J,K,L,M,N,P,Q]XZZ

Ø   **Medical and Surgical**
D   **Gastrointestinal System**
H   **Insertion**   Definition: Putting in a nonbiological appliance that monitors, assists, performs, or prevents a physiological function but does not physically take the place of a body part

Explanation: None

Body Part Character 4	Approach Character 5	Device Character 6	Qualifier Character 7
Ø Upper Intestinal Tract **D** Lower Intestinal Tract	**Ø** Open **3** Percutaneous **4** Percutaneous Endoscopic **7** Via Natural or Artificial Opening **8** Via Natural or Artificial Opening Endoscopic	**Y** Other Device	**Z** No Qualifier
5 Esophagus	**Ø** Open **3** Percutaneous **4** Percutaneous Endoscopic	**1** Radioactive Element **2** Monitoring Device **3** Infusion Device **D** Intraluminal Device **U** Feeding Device **Y** Other Device	**Z** No Qualifier
5 Esophagus	**7** Via Natural or Artificial Opening **8** Via Natural or Artificial Opening Endoscopic	**1** Radioactive Element **2** Monitoring Device **3** Infusion Device **B** Intraluminal Device, Airway **D** Intraluminal Device **U** Feeding Device **Y** Other Device	**Z** No Qualifier
6 Stomach ⊞	**Ø** Open **3** Percutaneous **4** Percutaneous Endoscopic	**1** Radioactive Element **2** Monitoring Device **3** Infusion Device **D** Intraluminal Device **M** Stimulator Lead **U** Feeding Device **Y** Other Device	**Z** No Qualifier
6 Stomach	**7** Via Natural or Artificial Opening **8** Via Natural or Artificial Opening Endoscopic	**1** Radioactive Element **2** Monitoring Device **3** Infusion Device **D** Intraluminal Device **U** Feeding Device **Y** Other Device	**Z** No Qualifier
8 Small Intestine **9** Duodenum **A** Jejunum Duodenojejunal flexure **B** Ileum	**Ø** Open **3** Percutaneous **4** Percutaneous Endoscopic **7** Via Natural or Artificial Opening **8** Via Natural or Artificial Opening Endoscopic	**1** Radioactive Element **2** Monitoring Device **3** Infusion Device **D** Intraluminal Device **U** Feeding Device	**Z** No Qualifier
E Large Intestine **P** Rectum Anorectal junction	**Ø** Open **3** Percutaneous **4** Percutaneous Endoscopic **7** Via Natural or Artificial Opening **8** Via Natural or Artificial Opening Endoscopic	**1** Radioactive Element **D** Intraluminal Device	**Z** No Qualifier
Q Anus Anal orifice	**Ø** Open **3** Percutaneous **4** Percutaneous Endoscopic	**D** Intraluminal Device **L** Artificial Sphincter	**Z** No Qualifier
Q Anus Anal orifice	**7** Via Natural or Artificial Opening **8** Via Natural or Artificial Opening Endoscopic	**D** Intraluminal Device	**Z** No Qualifier

R Anal Sphincter
   External anal sphincter
   Internal anal sphincter
	Ø Open
	3 Percutaneous
	4 Percutaneous Endoscopic
		M Stimulator Lead	**Z** No Qualifier

Non-OR ØDH[Ø,D][Ø,3,4,7,8]YZ	
Non-OR ØDH5[Ø,3,4][D,U]Z	**See Appendix L for Procedure Combinations**
Non-OR ØDH5[3,4]YZ	⊞ ØDH6[Ø,3,4]MZ
Non-OR ØDH5[7,8][2,3,B,D,U,Y]Z	
Non-OR ØDH631Z	
Non-OR ØDH6[3,4][U,Y]Z	
Non-OR ØDH6[7,8][1,2,3,D,U,Y]Z	
Non-OR ØDH[8,9,A,B][Ø,3,4,7,8][1,D,U]Z	
Non-OR ØDH[8,9,A,B][7,8][2,3]Z	
Non-OR ØDHE[Ø,3,4,7,8][1,D]Z	
Non-OR ØDHP[Ø,3,4,7,8]DZ	

NC Noncovered Procedure   **LC** Limited Coverage   **QA** Questionable OB Admit   **NT** New Tech Add-on   ⊞ Combination Member   ♂ Male   ♀ Female

ICD-10-PCS 2022   **387**

ØDH–ØDH

Ø   **Medical and Surgical**
D   **Gastrointestinal System**
J   **Inspection**   Definition: Visually and/or manually exploring a body part

Explanation: Visual exploration may be performed with or without optical instrumentation. Manual exploration may be performed directly or through intervening body layers.

Body Part Character 4	Approach Character 5	Device Character 6	Qualifier Character 7
Ø Upper Intestinal Tract **6** Stomach **D** Lower Intestinal Tract	**Ø** Open **3** Percutaneous **4** Percutaneous Endoscopic **7** Via Natural or Artificial Opening **8** Via Natural or Artificial Opening Endoscopic **X** External	**Z** No Device	**Z** No Qualifier

U Omentum
    Gastrocolic ligament
    Gastrocolic omentum
    Gastrohepatic omentum
    Gastrophrenic ligament
    Gastrosplenic ligament
    Greater Omentum
    Hepatogastric ligament
    Lesser Omentum
V Mesentery
    Mesoappendix
    Mesocolon
W Peritoneum
    Epiploic foramen
	Ø Open
	3 Percutaneous
	4 Percutaneous Endoscopic
	X External
		Z No Device	**Z** No Qualifier

Non-OR	ØDJ[Ø,6,D][3,7,8,X]ZZ
Non-OR	ØDJ[U,V,W][3,X]ZZ

Ø   **Medical and Surgical**
D   **Gastrointestinal System**
L   **Occlusion**   Definition: Completely closing an orifice or the lumen of a tubular body part
                  Explanation: The orifice can be a natural orifice or an artificially created orifice

Body Part Character 4		Approach Character 5	Device Character 6	Qualifier Character 7
1 Esophagus, Upper Cervical esophagus **2 Esophagus, Middle** Thoracic esophagus **3 Esophagus, Lower** Abdominal esophagus **4 Esophagogastric Junction** Cardia Cardioesophageal junction Gastroesophageal (GE) junction **5 Esophagus** **6 Stomach** **7 Stomach, Pylorus** Pyloric antrum Pyloric canal Pyloric sphincter **8 Small Intestine**	**9 Duodenum** **A Jejunum** Duodenojejunal flexure **B Ileum** **C Ileocecal Valve** **E Large Intestine** **F Large Intestine, Right** **G Large Intestine, Left** **H Cecum** **K Ascending Colon** **L Transverse Colon** Hepatic flexure Splenic flexure **M Descending Colon** **N Sigmoid Colon** Rectosigmoid junction Sigmoid flexure **P Rectum** Anorectal junction	**Ø Open** **3 Percutaneous** **4 Percutaneous Endoscopic**	**C Extraluminal Device** **D Intraluminal Device** **Z No Device**	**Z No Qualifier**
1 Esophagus, Upper Cervical esophagus **2 Esophagus, Middle** Thoracic esophagus **3 Esophagus, Lower** Abdominal esophagus **4 Esophagogastric Junction** Cardia Cardioesophageal junction Gastroesophageal (GE) junction **5 Esophagus** **6 Stomach** **7 Stomach, Pylorus** Pyloric antrum Pyloric canal Pyloric sphincter **8 Small Intestine**	**9 Duodenum** **A Jejunum** Duodenojejunal flexure **B Ileum** **C Ileocecal Valve** **E Large Intestine** **F Large Intestine, Right** **G Large Intestine, Left** **H Cecum** **K Ascending Colon** **L Transverse Colon** Hepatic flexure Splenic flexure **M Descending Colon** **N Sigmoid Colon** Rectosigmoid junction Sigmoid flexure **P Rectum** Anorectal junction	**7 Via Natural or Artificial Opening** **8 Via Natural or Artificial Opening Endoscopic**	**D Intraluminal Device** **Z No Device**	**Z No Qualifier**
Q Anus Anal orifice		**Ø Open** **3 Percutaneous** **4 Percutaneous Endoscopic** **X External**	**C Extraluminal Device** **D Intraluminal Device** **Z No Device**	**Z No Qualifier**
Q Anus Anal orifice		**7 Via Natural or Artificial Opening** **8 Via Natural or Artificial Opening Endoscopic**	**D Intraluminal Device** **Z No Device**	**Z No Qualifier**

Non-OR   ØDL[1,2,3,4,5][Ø,3,4][C,D,Z]Z
Non-OR   ØDL[1,2,3,4,5][7,8][D,Z]Z

NC Noncovered Procedure   LC Limited Coverage   QA Questionable OB Admit   NT New Tech Add-on   ⊞ Combination Member   ♂ Male   ♀ Female

ICD-10-PCS 2022   **389**

Gastrointestinal System

Ø **Medical and Surgical**
D **Gastrointestinal System**
M **Reattachment**   Definition: Putting back in or on all or a portion of a separated body part to its normal location or other suitable location
               Explanation: Vascular circulation and nervous pathways may or may not be reestablished

Body Part Character 4	Approach Character 5	Device Character 6	Qualifier Character 7

5 Esophagus
6 Stomach
8 Small Intestine
9 Duodenum
A Jejunum
   Duodenojejunal flexure
B Ileum
E Large Intestine
F Large Intestine, Right
G Large Intestine, Left
H Cecum
K Ascending Colon
L Transverse Colon
   Hepatic flexure
   Splenic flexure
M Descending Colon
N Sigmoid Colon
   Rectosigmoid junction
   Sigmoid flexure
P Rectum
   Anorectal junction
	Ø Open
	4 Percutaneous Endoscopic
		Z No Device	Z No Qualifier

Ø **Medical and Surgical**
D **Gastrointestinal System**
N **Release**   Definition: Freeing a body part from an abnormal physical constraint by cutting or by the use of force
              Explanation: Some of the restraining tissue may be taken out but none of the body part is taken out

Body Part Character 4	Approach Character 5	Device Character 6	Qualifier Character 7

1 Esophagus, Upper
   Cervical esophagus
2 Esophagus, Middle
   Thoracic esophagus
3 Esophagus, Lower
   Abdominal esophagus
4 Esophagogastric Junction
   Cardia
   Cardioesophageal junction
   Gastroesophageal (GE) junction
5 Esophagus
6 Stomach
7 Stomach, Pylorus
   Pyloric antrum
   Pyloric canal
   Pyloric sphincter
8 Small Intestine
9 Duodenum
 	
A Jejunum
   Duodenojejunal flexure
B Ileum
C Ileocecal Valve
E Large Intestine
F Large Intestine, Right
G Large Intestine, Left
H Cecum
J Appendix
   Vermiform appendix
K Ascending Colon
L Transverse Colon
   Hepatic flexure
   Splenic flexure
M Descending Colon
N Sigmoid Colon
   Rectosigmoid junction
   Sigmoid flexure
P Rectum
   Anorectal junction
	Ø Open
	3 Percutaneous
	4 Percutaneous Endoscopic
	7 Via Natural or Artificial Opening
	8 Via Natural or Artificial Opening Endoscopic
		Z No Device	Z No Qualifier

Q Anus Anal orifice	Ø Open 3 Percutaneous 4 Percutaneous Endoscopic 7 Via Natural or Artificial Opening 8 Via Natural or Artificial Opening Endoscopic X External	Z No Device	Z No Qualifier

R Anal Sphincter
   External anal sphincter
   Internal anal sphincter
U Omentum
   Gastrocolic ligament
   Gastrocolic omentum
   Gastrohepatic omentum
   Gastrophrenic ligament
   Gastrosplenic ligament
   Greater Omentum
   Hepatogastric ligament
   Lesser Omentum
V Mesentery
   Mesoappendix
   Mesocolon
W Peritoneum
   Epiploic foramen
	Ø Open
	3 Percutaneous
	4 Percutaneous Endoscopic
		Z No Device	Z No Qualifier

Non-OR   ØDN[8,9,A,B,E,F,G,H,K,L,M,N][7,8]ZZ

Non-OR Procedure   DRG Non-OR Procedure   Valid OR Procedure   HAC Associated Procedure   Combination Only   New/Revised GREEN

Ø   Medical and Surgical
D   Gastrointestinal System
P   Removal   Definition: Taking out or off a device from a body part

Explanation: If a device is taken out and a similar device put in without cutting or puncturing the skin or mucous membrane, the procedure is coded to the root operation CHANGE. Otherwise, the procedure for taking out a device is coded to the root operation REMOVAL.

Body Part Character 4	Approach Character 5	Device Character 6	Qualifier Character 7
Ø Upper Intestinal Tract D Lower Intestinal Tract	Ø Open 3 Percutaneous 4 Percutaneous Endoscopic 7 Via Natural or Artificial Opening 8 Via Natural or Artificial Opening Endoscopic	Ø Drainage Device 2 Monitoring Device 3 Infusion Device 7 Autologous Tissue Substitute C Extraluminal Device D Intraluminal Device J Synthetic Substitute K Nonautologous Tissue Substitute U Feeding Device Y Other Device	Z No Qualifier
Ø Upper Intestinal Tract D Lower Intestinal Tract	X External	Ø Drainage Device 2 Monitoring Device 3 Infusion Device D Intraluminal Device U Feeding Device	Z No Qualifier
5 Esophagus	Ø Open 3 Percutaneous 4 Percutaneous Endoscopic	1 Radioactive Element 2 Monitoring Device 3 Infusion Device U Feeding Device Y Other Device	Z No Qualifier
5 Esophagus	7 Via Natural or Artificial Opening 8 Via Natural or Artificial Opening Endoscopic	1 Radioactive Element D Intraluminal Device Y Other Device	Z No Qualifier
5 Esophagus	X External	1 Radioactive Element 2 Monitoring Device 3 Infusion Device D Intraluminal Device U Feeding Device	Z No Qualifier
6 Stomach	Ø Open 3 Percutaneous 4 Percutaneous Endoscopic	Ø Drainage Device 2 Monitoring Device 3 Infusion Device 7 Autologous Tissue Substitute C Extraluminal Device D Intraluminal Device J Synthetic Substitute K Nonautologous Tissue Substitute M Stimulator Lead U Feeding Device Y Other Device	Z No Qualifier
6 Stomach	7 Via Natural or Artificial Opening 8 Via Natural or Artificial Opening Endoscopic	Ø Drainage Device 2 Monitoring Device 3 Infusion Device 7 Autologous Tissue Substitute C Extraluminal Device D Intraluminal Device J Synthetic Substitute K Nonautologous Tissue Substitute U Feeding Device Y Other Device	Z No Qualifier
6 Stomach	X External	Ø Drainage Device 2 Monitoring Device 3 Infusion Device D Intraluminal Device U Feeding Device	Z No Qualifier

Non-OR	ØDP[Ø,D][3,4]YZ
Non-OR	ØDP[Ø,D][7,8][Ø,2,3,D,U,Y]Z
Non-OR	ØDP[Ø,D]X[Ø,2,3,D,U]Z
Non-OR	ØDP5[3,4]YZ
Non-OR	ØDP5[7,8][1,D,Y]Z
Non-OR	ØDP5X[1,2,3,D,U]Z
Non-OR	ØDP6[3,4]YZ
Non-OR	ØDP6[7,8][Ø,2,3,D,U,Y]Z
Non-OR	ØDP6X[Ø,2,3,D,U]Z

ØDP Continued on next page

NC Noncovered Procedure   LC Limited Coverage   QA Questionable OB Admit   NT New Tech Add-on   ⊞ Combination Member   ♂ Male   ♀ Female

Ø   Medical and Surgical   *ØDP Continued*
D   Gastrointestinal System
P   Removal   Definition: Taking out or off a device from a body part

Explanation: If a device is taken out and a similar device put in without cutting or puncturing the skin or mucous membrane, the procedure is coded to the root operation CHANGE. Otherwise, the procedure for taking out a device is coded to the root operation REMOVAL.

Body Part Character 4	Approach Character 5	Device Character 6	Qualifier Character 7
P Rectum Anorectal junction	**Ø** Open **3** Percutaneous **4** Percutaneous Endoscopic **7** Via Natural or Artificial Opening **8** Via Natural or Artificial Opening Endoscopic **X** External	**1** Radioactive Element	**Z** No Qualifier
Q Anus Anal orifice	**Ø** Open **3** Percutaneous **4** Percutaneous Endoscopic **7** Via Natural or Artificial Opening **8** Via Natural or Artificial Opening Endoscopic	**L** Artificial Sphincter	**Z** No Qualifier
R Anal Sphincter External anal sphincter Internal anal sphincter	**Ø** Open **3** Percutaneous **4** Percutaneous Endoscopic	**M** Stimulator Lead	**Z** No Qualifier
U Omentum Gastrocolic ligament Gastrocolic omentum Gastrohepatic omentum Gastrophrenic ligament Gastrosplenic ligament Greater Omentum Hepatogastric ligament Lesser Omentum **V** Mesentery Mesoappendix Mesocolon **W** Peritoneum Epiploic foramen	**Ø** Open **3** Percutaneous **4** Percutaneous Endoscopic	**Ø** Drainage Device **1** Radioactive Element **7** Autologous Tissue Substitute **J** Synthetic Substitute **K** Nonautologous Tissue Substitute	**Z** No Qualifier

Non-OR   ØDPP[7,8,X]1Z

Ø   Medical and Surgical
D   Gastrointestinal System
Q   Repair   Definition: Restoring, to the extent possible, a body part to its normal anatomic structure and function
               Explanation: Used only when the method to accomplish the repair is not one of the other root operations

Body Part Character 4	Approach Character 5	Device Character 6	Qualifier Character 7

1   Esophagus, Upper
     Cervical esophagus
2   Esophagus, Middle
     Thoracic esophagus
3   Esophagus, Lower
     Abdominal esophagus
4   Esophagogastric Junction
     Cardia
     Cardioesophageal junction
     Gastroesophageal (GE) junction
5   Esophagus
6   Stomach
7   Stomach, Pylorus
     Pyloric antrum
     Pyloric canal
     Pyloric sphincter
8   Small Intestine ⊞
9   Duodenum ⊞
A   Jejunum ⊞
     Duodenojejunal flexure
B   Ileum ⊞
C   Ileocecal Valve
E   Large Intestine ⊞
F   Large Intestine, Right ⊞
G   Large Intestine, Left ⊞
H   Cecum ⊞
J   Appendix
     Vermiform appendix
K   Ascending Colon ⊞
L   Transverse Colon ⊞
     Hepatic flexure
     Splenic flexure
M   Descending Colon ⊞
N   Sigmoid Colon ⊞
     Rectosigmoid junction
     Sigmoid flexure
P   Rectum
     Anorectal junction
	Ø Open
	3 Percutaneous
	4 Percutaneous Endoscopic
	7 Via Natural or Artificial Opening
	8 Via Natural or Artificial Opening
	     Endoscopic
		Z No Device	Z No Qualifier

Q   Anus
     Anal orifice
	Ø Open
	3 Percutaneous
	4 Percutaneous Endoscopic
	7 Via Natural or Artificial Opening
	8 Via Natural or Artificial Opening
	     Endoscopic
	X External
		Z No Device	Z No Qualifier

R   Anal Sphincter
     External anal sphincter
     Internal anal sphincter
U   Omentum
     Gastrocolic ligament
     Gastrocolic omentum
     Gastrohepatic omentum
     Gastrophrenic ligament
     Gastrosplenic ligament
     Greater Omentum
     Hepatogastric ligament
     Lesser Omentum
V   Mesentery
     Mesoappendix
     Mesocolon
W   Peritoneum
     Epiploic foramen
	Ø Open
	3 Percutaneous
	4 Percutaneous Endoscopic
		Z No Device	Z No Qualifier

Non-OR   ØDQU[Ø,3,4]ZZ

See Appendix L for Procedure Combinations
    ⊞   ØDQ[8,9,A,B,E,F,G,H,K,L,M,N]ØZZ

NC Noncovered Procedure   LC Limited Coverage   QA Questionable OB Admit   NT New Tech Add-on   ⊞ Combination Member   ♂ Male   ♀ Female

Ø　**Medical and Surgical**
D　**Gastrointestinal System**
R　**Replacement**　　Definition: Putting in or on biological or synthetic material that physically takes the place and/or function of all or a portion of a body part
　　　　　　　　　　　Explanation: The body part may have been taken out or replaced, or may be taken out, physically eradicated, or rendered nonfunctional during the REPLACEMENT procedure. A REMOVAL procedure is coded for taking out the device used in a previous replacement procedure.

Body Part Character 4	Approach Character 5	Device Character 6	Qualifier Character 7
5 Esophagus	**Ø** Open **4** Percutaneous Endoscopic **7** Via Natural or Artificial Opening **8** Via Natural or Artificial Opening Endoscopic	**7** Autologous Tissue Substitute **J** Synthetic Substitute **K** Nonautologous Tissue Substitute	**Z** No Qualifier
R Anal Sphincter 　External anal sphincter 　Internal anal sphincter **U** Omentum 　Gastrocolic ligament 　Gastrocolic omentum 　Gastrohepatic omentum 　Gastrophrenic ligament 　Gastrosplenic ligament 　Greater Omentum 　Hepatogastric ligament 　Lesser Omentum **V** Mesentery 　Mesoappendix 　Mesocolon **W** Peritoneum 　Epiploic foramen	**Ø** Open **4** Percutaneous Endoscopic	**7** Autologous Tissue Substitute **J** Synthetic Substitute **K** Nonautologous Tissue Substitute	**Z** No Qualifier

Ø　**Medical and Surgical**
D　**Gastrointestinal System**
S　**Reposition**　　Definition: Moving to its normal location, or other suitable location, all or a portion of a body part
　　　　　　　　　　Explanation: The body part is moved to a new location from an abnormal location, or from a normal location where it is not functioning correctly. The body part may or may not be cut out or off to be moved to the new location.

Body Part Character 4	Approach Character 5	Device Character 6	Qualifier Character 7
5 Esophagus **6** Stomach **9** Duodenum **A** Jejunum 　Duodenojejunal flexure **B** Ileum **H** Cecum **K** Ascending Colon **L** Transverse Colon 　Hepatic flexure 　Splenic flexure **M** Descending Colon **N** Sigmoid Colon 　Rectosigmoid junction 　Sigmoid flexure **P** Rectum 　Anorectal junction **Q** Anus 　Anal orifice	**Ø** Open **4** Percutaneous Endoscopic **7** Via Natural or Artificial Opening **8** Via Natural or Artificial Opening Endoscopic **X** External	**Z** No Device	**Z** No Qualifier
8 Small Intestine **E** Large Intestine	**Ø** Open **4** Percutaneous Endoscopic **7** Via Natural or Artificial Opening **8** Via Natural or Artificial Opening Endoscopic	**Z** No Device	**Z** No Qualifier

Non-OR　ØDS[5,6,9,A,B,H,K,L,M,N,P,Q]XZZ

Ø   Medical and Surgical
D   Gastrointestinal System
T   Resection   Definition: Cutting out or off, without replacement, all of a body part
                  Explanation: None

Body Part Character 4	Approach Character 5	Device Character 6	Qualifier Character 7

1 Esophagus, Upper
   Cervical esophagus
2 Esophagus, Middle
   Thoracic esophagus
3 Esophagus, Lower
   Abdominal esophagus
4 Esophagogastric Junction
   Cardia
   Cardioesophageal junction
   Gastroesophageal (GE) junction
5 Esophagus
6 Stomach
7 Stomach, Pylorus
   Pyloric antrum
   Pyloric canal
   Pyloric sphincter
8 Small Intestine
9 Duodenum ⊞
A Jejunum
   Duodenojejunal flexure
B Ileum
C Ileocecal Valve
E Large Intestine
F Large Intestine, Right
H Cecum
J Appendix
   Vermiform appendix
K Ascending Colon
P Rectum
   Anorectal junction
Q Anus
   Anal orifice
	Ø Open
	4 Percutaneous Endoscopic
	7 Via Natural or Artificial Opening
	8 Via Natural or Artificial Opening
	    Endoscopic
		Z No Device	**Z** No Qualifier

G Large Intestine, Left
L Transverse Colon
   Hepatic flexure
   Splenic flexure
M Descending Colon
N Sigmoid Colon
   Rectosigmoid junction
   Sigmoid flexure
	Ø Open
	4 Percutaneous Endoscopic
	7 Via Natural or Artificial Opening
	8 Via Natural or Artificial Opening
	    Endoscopic
	F Via Natural or Artificial Opening
	    with Percutaneous Endoscopic
	    Assistance
		Z No Device	**Z** No Qualifier

R Anal Sphincter
   External anal sphincter
   Internal anal sphincter
U Omentum
   Gastrocolic ligament
   Gastrocolic omentum
   Gastrohepatic omentum
   Gastrophrenic ligament
   Gastrosplenic ligament
   Greater Omentum
   Hepatogastric ligament
   Lesser Omentum
	Ø Open
	4 Percutaneous Endoscopic
		Z No Device	**Z** No Qualifier

See Appendix L for Procedure Combinations
⊞   ØDT9ØZZ

Ø   Medical and Surgical
D   Gastrointestinal System
U   Supplement   Definition: Putting in or on biological or synthetic material that physically reinforces and/or augments the function of a portion of a body part
Explanation: The biological material is non-living, or is living and from the same individual. The body part may have been previously replaced, and the SUPPLEMENT procedure is performed to physically reinforce and/or augment the function of the replaced body part.

Body Part Character 4	Approach Character 5	Device Character 6	Qualifier Character 7
1 Esophagus, Upper Cervical esophagus **2 Esophagus, Middle** Thoracic esophagus **3 Esophagus, Lower** Abdominal esophagus **4 Esophagogastric Junction** Cardia Cardioesophageal junction Gastroesophageal (GE) junction **5 Esophagus** **6 Stomach** **7 Stomach, Pylorus** Pyloric antrum Pyloric canal Pyloric sphincter **8 Small Intestine** **9 Duodenum** **A Jejunum** Duodenojejunal flexure **B Ileum** **C Ileocecal Valve** **E Large Intestine** **F Large Intestine, Right** **G Large Intestine, Left** **H Cecum** **K Ascending Colon** **L Transverse Colon** Hepatic flexure Splenic flexure **M Descending Colon** **N Sigmoid Colon** Rectosigmoid junction Sigmoid flexure **P Rectum** Anorectal junction	**Ø Open** **4 Percutaneous Endoscopic** **7 Via Natural or Artificial Opening** **8 Via Natural or Artificial Opening Endoscopic**	**7 Autologous Tissue Substitute** **J Synthetic Substitute** **K Nonautologous Tissue Substitute**	**Z No Qualifier**
Q Anus Anal orifice	**Ø Open** **4 Percutaneous Endoscopic** **7 Via Natural or Artificial Opening** **8 Via Natural or Artificial Opening Endoscopic** **X External**	**7 Autologous Tissue Substitute** **J Synthetic Substitute** **K Nonautologous Tissue Substitute**	**Z No Qualifier**
R Anal Sphincter External anal sphincter Internal anal sphincter **U Omentum** Gastrocolic ligament Gastrocolic omentum Gastrohepatic omentum Gastrophrenic ligament Gastrosplenic ligament Greater Omentum Hepatogastric ligament Lesser Omentum **V Mesentery** Mesoappendix Mesocolon **W Peritoneum** Epiploic foramen	**Ø Open** **4 Percutaneous Endoscopic**	**7 Autologous Tissue Substitute** **J Synthetic Substitute** **K Nonautologous Tissue Substitute**	**Z No Qualifier**

Ø   Medical and Surgical
D   Gastrointestinal System
V   Restriction   Definition: Partially closing an orifice or the lumen of a tubular body part
                        Explanation: The orifice can be a natural orifice or an artificially created orifice

Body Part Character 4		Approach Character 5	Device Character 6	Qualifier Character 7

1 Esophagus, Upper
  Cervical esophagus
2 Esophagus, Middle
  Thoracic esophagus
3 Esophagus, Lower
  Abdominal esophagus
4 Esophagogastric
  Junction
  Cardia
  Cardioesophageal
    junction
  Gastroesophageal (GE)
    junction
5 Esophagus
6 Stomach
7 Stomach, Pylorus
  Pyloric antrum
  Pyloric canal
  Pyloric sphincter
8 Small Intestine
	9 Duodenum
	A Jejunum
	  Duodenojejunal flexure
	B Ileum
	C Ileocecal Valve
	E Large Intestine
	F Large Intestine, Right
	G Large Intestine, Left
	H Cecum
	K Ascending Colon
	L Transverse Colon
	  Hepatic flexure
	  Splenic flexure
	M Descending Colon
	N Sigmoid Colon
	  Rectosigmoid junction
	  Sigmoid flexure
	P Rectum
	  Anorectal junction
		Ø Open
		3 Percutaneous
		4 Percutaneous Endoscopic
			C Extraluminal Device
			D Intraluminal Device
			Z No Device
				Z No Qualifier

1 Esophagus, Upper
  Cervical esophagus
2 Esophagus, Middle
  Thoracic esophagus
3 Esophagus, Lower
  Abdominal esophagus
4 Esophagogastric
  Junction
  Cardia
  Cardioesophageal
    junction
  Gastroesophageal (GE)
    junction
5 Esophagus
6 Stomach **NC**
7 Stomach, Pylorus
  Pyloric antrum
  Pyloric canal
  Pyloric sphincter
8 Small Intestine
	9 Duodenum
	A Jejunum
	  Duodenojejunal flexure
	B Ileum
	C Ileocecal Valve
	E Large Intestine
	F Large Intestine, Right
	G Large Intestine, Left
	H Cecum
	K Ascending Colon
	L Transverse Colon
	  Hepatic flexure
	  Splenic flexure
	M Descending Colon
	N Sigmoid Colon
	  Rectosigmoid junction
	  Sigmoid flexure
	P Rectum
	  Anorectal junction
		7 Via Natural or Artificial
		  Opening
		8 Via Natural or Artificial
		  Opening Endoscopic
			D Intraluminal Device
			Z No Device
				Z No Qualifier

Q Anus Anal orifice		Ø Open 3 Percutaneous 4 Percutaneous Endoscopic X External	C Extraluminal Device D Intraluminal Device Z No Device	Z No Qualifier

Q Anus
  Anal orifice
		7 Via Natural or Artificial
		  Opening
		8 Via Natural or Artificial
		  Opening Endoscopic
			D Intraluminal Device
			Z No Device
				Z No Qualifier

Non-OR   ØDV6[7,8]DZ
HAC   ØDV64CZ when reported with PDx E66.Ø1 and SDx K68.11, K95.Ø1, K95.81, or T81.4Ø–T81.49 with 7th character A
NC   ØDV6[7,8]DZ

NC Noncovered Procedure   **LC** Limited Coverage   **QA** Questionable OB Admit   **NT** New Tech Add-on   ⊞ Combination Member   ♂Male   ♀Female

ICD-10-PCS 2022   397

ØDV–ØDV

Gastrointestinal System

Ø   Medical and Surgical
D   Gastrointestinal System
W   Revision   Definition: Correcting, to the extent possible, a portion of a malfunctioning device or the position of a displaced device
                          Explanation: Revision can include correcting a malfunctioning or displaced device by taking out or putting in components of the device such as a screw or pin

Body Part Character 4	Approach Character 5	Device Character 6	Qualifier Character 7
Ø Upper Intestinal Tract D Lower Intestinal Tract	Ø Open 3 Percutaneous 4 Percutaneous Endoscopic 7 Via Natural or Artificial Opening 8 Via Natural or Artificial Opening Endoscopic	Ø Drainage Device 2 Monitoring Device 3 Infusion Device 7 Autologous Tissue Substitute C Extraluminal Device D Intraluminal Device J Synthetic Substitute K Nonautologous Tissue Substitute U Feeding Device Y Other Device	Z No Qualifier
Ø Upper Intestinal Tract D Lower Intestinal Tract	X External	Ø Drainage Device 2 Monitoring Device 3 Infusion Device 7 Autologous Tissue Substitute C Extraluminal Device D Intraluminal Device J Synthetic Substitute K Nonautologous Tissue Substitute U Feeding Device	Z No Qualifier
5 Esophagus	Ø Open 3 Percutaneous 4 Percutaneous Endoscopic	Y Other Device	Z No Qualifier
5 Esophagus	7 Via Natural or Artificial Opening 8 Via Natural or Artificial Opening Endoscopic	D Intraluminal Device Y Other Device	Z No Qualifier
5 Esophagus	X External	D Intraluminal Device	Z No Qualifier
6 Stomach	Ø Open 3 Percutaneous 4 Percutaneous Endoscopic	Ø Drainage Device 2 Monitoring Device 3 Infusion Device 7 Autologous Tissue Substitute C Extraluminal Device D Intraluminal Device J Synthetic Substitute K Nonautologous Tissue Substitute M Stimulator Lead U Feeding Device Y Other Device	Z No Qualifier
6 Stomach	7 Via Natural or Artificial Opening 8 Via Natural or Artificial Opening Endoscopic	Ø Drainage Device 2 Monitoring Device 3 Infusion Device 7 Autologous Tissue Substitute C Extraluminal Device D Intraluminal Device J Synthetic Substitute K Nonautologous Tissue Substitute U Feeding Device Y Other Device	Z No Qualifier
6 Stomach	X External	Ø Drainage Device 2 Monitoring Device 3 Infusion Device 7 Autologous Tissue Substitute C Extraluminal Device D Intraluminal Device J Synthetic Substitute K Nonautologous Tissue Substitute U Feeding Device	Z No Qualifier

Non-OR	ØDW[Ø,D][3,4,7,8]YZ
Non-OR	ØDW[Ø,D]8UZ
Non-OR	ØDW[Ø,D]X[Ø,2,3,7,C,D,J,K,U]Z
Non-OR	ØDW5[Ø,3,4]YZ
Non-OR	ØDW5[7,8]YZ
Non-OR	ØDW5XDZ
Non-OR	ØDW6[3,4]YZ
Non-OR	ØDW68UZ
Non-OR	ØDW6[7,8]YZ
Non-OR	ØDW6X[Ø,2,3,7,C,D,J,K,U]Z

ØDW Continued on next page

ØDW Continued

Ø Medical and Surgical
D Gastrointestinal System
W Revision Definition: Correcting, to the extent possible, a portion of a malfunctioning device or the position of a displaced device

Explanation: Revision can include correcting a malfunctioning or displaced device by taking out or putting in components of the device such as a screw or pin

Body Part Character 4	Approach Character 5	Device Character 6	Qualifier Character 7
8 Small Intestine E Large Intestine	Ø Open 4 Percutaneous Endoscopic 7 Via Natural or Artificial Opening 8 Via Natural or Artificial Opening Endoscopic	7 Autologous Tissue Substitute J Synthetic Substitute K Nonautologous Tissue Substitute	Z No Qualifier
Q Anus Anal orifice	Ø Open 3 Percutaneous 4 Percutaneous Endoscopic 7 Via Natural or Artificial Opening 8 Via Natural or Artificial Opening Endoscopic	L Artificial Sphincter	Z No Qualifier
R Anal Sphincter External anal sphincter Internal anal sphincter	Ø Open 3 Percutaneous 4 Percutaneous Endoscopic	M Stimulator Lead	Z No Qualifier
U Omentum Gastrocolic ligament Gastrocolic omentum Gastrohepatic omentum Gastrophrenic ligament Gastrosplenic ligament Greater Omentum Hepatogastric ligament Lesser Omentum V Mesentery Mesoappendix Mesocolon W Peritoneum Epiploic foramen	Ø Open 3 Percutaneous 4 Percutaneous Endoscopic	Ø Drainage Device 7 Autologous Tissue Substitute J Synthetic Substitute K Nonautologous Tissue Substitute	Z No Qualifier

Non-OR ØDW[U,V,W][Ø,3,4]ØZ

Ø Medical and Surgical
D Gastrointestinal System
X Transfer Definition: Moving, without taking out, all or a portion of a body part to another location to take over the function of all or a portion of a body part

Explanation: The body part transferred remains connected to its vascular and nervous supply

Body Part Character 4	Approach Character 5	Device Character 6	Qualifier Character 7
6 Stomach 8 Small Intestine	Ø Open 4 Percutaneous Endoscopic	Z No Device	5 Esophagus
E Large Intestine	Ø Open 4 Percutaneous Endoscopic	Z No Device	5 Esophagus 7 Vagina ♀

♀ ØDXE[Ø,4]Z7

Ø Medical and Surgical
D Gastrointestinal System
Y Transplantation Definition: Putting in or on all or a portion of a living body part taken from another individual or animal to physically take the place and/or function of all or a portion of a similar body part

Explanation: The native body part may or may not be taken out, and the transplanted body part may take over all or a portion of its function

Body Part Character 4	Approach Character 5	Device Character 6	Qualifier Character 7
5 Esophagus 6 Stomach 8 Small Intestine LC E Large Intestine LC	Ø Open	Z No Device	Ø Allogeneic 1 Syngeneic 2 Zooplastic

Non-OR ØDY5ØZ[Ø,1,2]
LC ØDY[8,E]ØZ[Ø,1,2]

NC Noncovered Procedure   LC Limited Coverage   QA Questionable OB Admit   NT New Tech Add-on   ⊞ Combination Member   ♂ Male   ♀ Female

Hepatobiliary System and Pancreas ØF1–ØFY

Character Meanings

This Character Meaning table is provided as a guide to assist the user in the identification of character members that may be found in this section of code tables. It **SHOULD NOT** be used to build a PCS code.

Operation–Character 3	Body Part–Character 4	Approach–Character 5	Device–Character 6	Qualifier–Character 7
1 Bypass	Ø Liver	Ø Open	Ø Drainage Device	Ø Allogeneic
2 Change	1 Liver, Right Lobe	3 Percutaneous	1 Radioactive Element	1 Syngeneic
5 Destruction	2 Liver, Left Lobe	4 Percutaneous Endoscopic	2 Monitoring Device	2 Zooplastic
7 Dilation	4 Gallbladder	7 Via Natural or Artificial Opening	3 Infusion Device	3 Duodenum
8 Division	5 Hepatic Duct, Right	8 Via Natural or Artificial Opening Endoscopic	7 Autologous Tissue Substitute	4 Stomach
9 Drainage	6 Hepatic Duct, Left	X External	C Extraluminal Device	5 Hepatic Duct, Right
B Excision	7 Hepatic Duct, Common		D Intraluminal Device	6 Hepatic Duct, Left
C Extirpation	8 Cystic Duct		J Synthetic Substitute	7 Hepatic Duct, Caudate
D Extraction	9 Common Bile Duct		K Nonautologous Tissue Substitute	8 Cystic Duct
F Fragmentation	B Hepatobiliary Duct		Y Other Device	9 Common Bile Duct
H Insertion	C Ampulla of Vater		Z No Device	B Small Intestine
J Inspection	D Pancreatic Duct			C Large Intestine
L Occlusion	F Pancreatic Duct, Accessory			F Irreversible Electroporation
M Reattachment	G Pancreas			X Diagnostic
N Release				Z No Qualifier
P Removal				
Q Repair				
R Replacement				
S Reposition				
T Resection				
U Supplement				
V Restriction				
W Revision				
Y Transplantation				

AHA Coding Clinic for table ØF1
2020, 4Q, 53   Bypass pancreatic duct to stomach

AHA Coding Clinic for table ØF5
2018, 4Q, 39   Irreversible electroporation

AHA Coding Clinic for table ØF7
2016, 3Q, 27   Endoscopic retrograde cholangiopancreatography with sphincterotomy and insertion of pancreatic stent
2016, 1Q, 25   Endoscopic retrograde cholangiopancreatography with brush biopsy of pancreatic and common bile ducts
2015, 1Q, 32   Percutaneous transhepatic biliary drainage catheter placement
2014, 3Q, 15   Drainage of pancreatic pseudocyst

AHA Coding Clinic for table ØF9
2020, 3Q, 34   Cystogastrostomy with stent insertion
2015, 1Q, 32   Percutaneous transhepatic biliary drainage catheter placement
2014, 3Q, 15   Drainage of pancreatic pseudocyst

AHA Coding Clinic for table ØFB
2019, 1Q, 3-8   Whipple procedure
2016, 3Q, 41   Open cholecystectomy with needle biopsy of liver
2016, 1Q, 23   Endoscopic ultrasound with aspiration biopsy of common hepatic duct
2016, 1Q, 25   Endoscopic retrograde cholangiopancreatography with brush biopsy of pancreatic and common bile ducts
2014, 3Q, 32   Pyloric-sparing Whipple procedure

AHA Coding Clinic for table ØFC
2016, 3Q, 27   Endoscopic retrograde cholangiopancreatography with sphincterotomy and insertion of pancreatic stent

AHA Coding Clinic for table ØFH
2020, 4Q, 43-44   Insertion of radioactive element

AHA Coding Clinic for table ØFQ
2016, 3Q, 27   Revision of common bile duct anastomosis
2013, 4Q, 109   Separating conjoined twins

AHA Coding Clinic for table ØFT
2019, 1Q, 3-8   Whipple Procedure
2012, 4Q, 99   Domino liver transplant

AHA Coding Clinic for table ØFY
2014, 3Q, 13   Orthotopic liver transplant with end to side cavoplasty
2012, 4Q, 99   Domino liver transplant

Liver

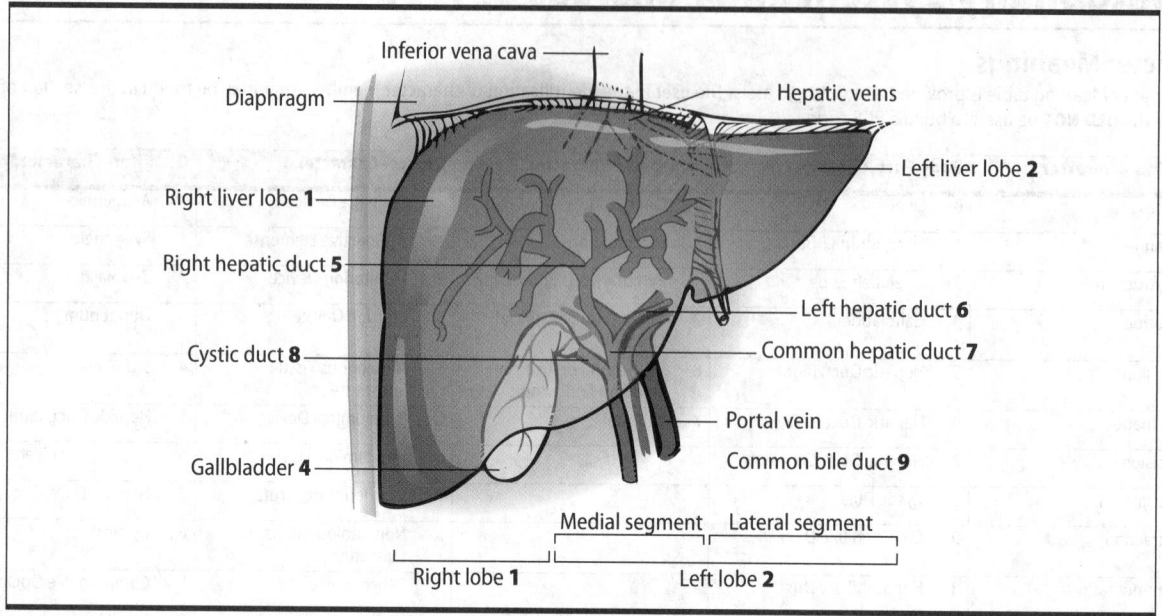

Inferior vena cava

Diaphragm

Hepatic veins

Left liver lobe **2**

Right liver lobe **1**

Right hepatic duct **5**

Left hepatic duct **6**

Cystic duct **8**

Common hepatic duct **7**

Portal vein

Gallbladder **4**

Common bile duct **9**

Medial segment — Lateral segment

Right lobe **1**

Left lobe **2**

Pancreas

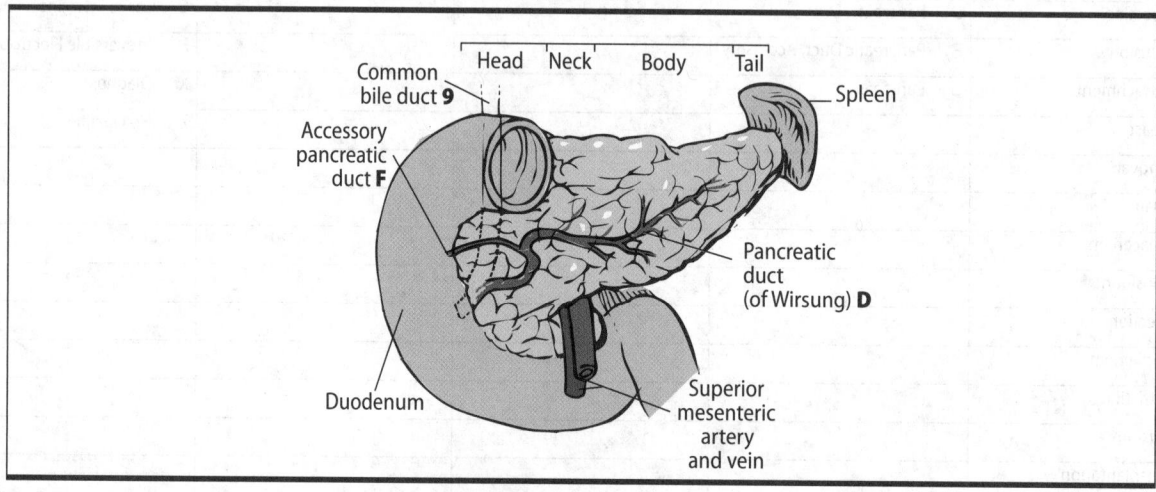

Head — Neck — Body — Tail

Common bile duct **9**

Spleen

Accessory pancreatic duct **F**

Pancreatic duct (of Wirsung) **D**

Duodenum

Superior mesenteric artery and vein

Gallbladder and Ducts

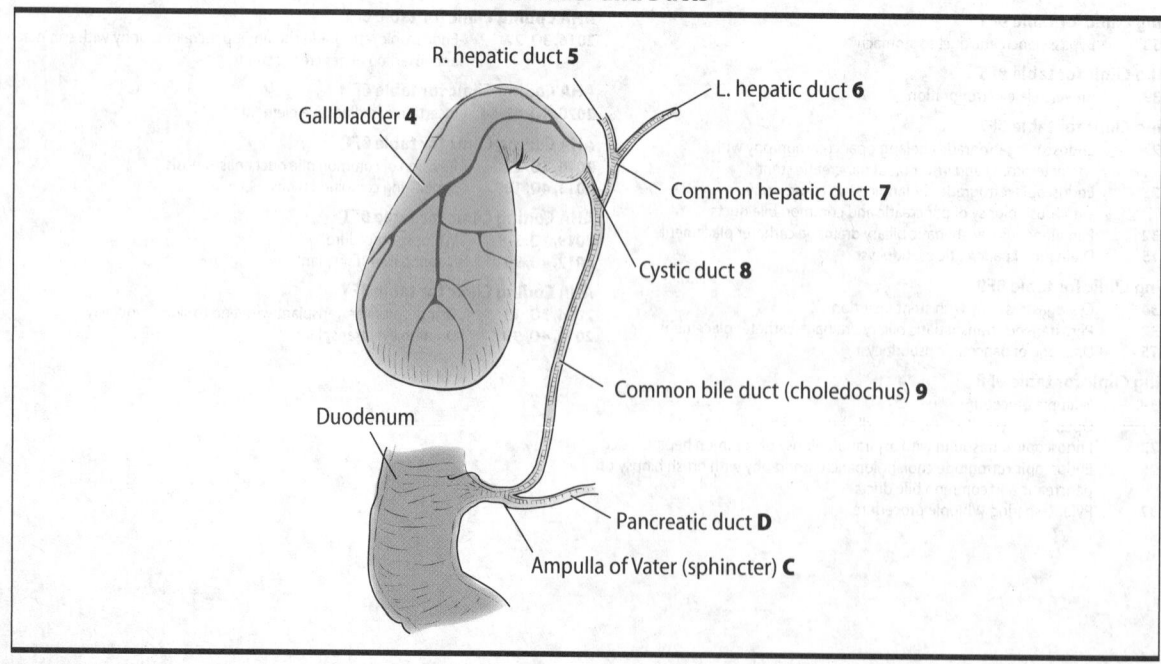

R. hepatic duct **5**

L. hepatic duct **6**

Gallbladder **4**

Common hepatic duct **7**

Cystic duct **8**

Common bile duct (choledochus) **9**

Duodenum

Pancreatic duct **D**

Ampulla of Vater (sphincter) **C**

Hepatobiliary System and Pancreas

Ø   Medical and Surgical
F   Hepatobiliary System and Pancreas
1   Bypass   Definition: Altering the route of passage of the contents of a tubular body part

Explanation: Rerouting contents of a body part to a downstream area of the normal route, to a similar route and body part, or to an abnormal route and dissimilar body part. Includes one or more anastomoses, with or without the use of a device.

Body Part Character 4	Approach Character 5	Device Character 6	Qualifier Character 7
4 Gallbladder 5 Hepatic Duct, Right 6 Hepatic Duct, Left 7 Hepatic Duct, Common 8 Cystic Duct 9 Common Bile Duct	Ø Open 4 Percutaneous Endoscopic	D Intraluminal Device Z No Device	3 Duodenum 4 Stomach 5 Hepatic Duct, Right 6 Hepatic Duct, Left 7 Hepatic Duct, Caudate 8 Cystic Duct 9 Common Bile Duct B Small Intestine
D Pancreatic Duct Duct of Wirsung	Ø Open 4 Percutaneous Endoscopic	D Intraluminal Device Z No Device	3 Duodenum 4 Stomach B Small Intestine C Large Intestine
F Pancreatic Duct, Accessory Duct of Santorini G Pancreas	Ø Open 4 Percutaneous Endoscopic	D Intraluminal Device Z No Device	3 Duodenum B Small Intestine C Large Intestine

Ø   Medical and Surgical
F   Hepatobiliary System and Pancreas
2   Change   Definition: Taking out or off a device from a body part and putting back an identical or similar device in or on the same body part without cutting or puncturing the skin or a mucous membrane

Explanation: All CHANGE procedures are coded using the approach EXTERNAL

Body Part Character 4	Approach Character 5	Device Character 6	Qualifier Character 7

Ø   Liver
     Quadrate lobe
4   Gallbladder
B   Hepatobiliary Duct
D   Pancreatic Duct
     Duct of Wirsung
G   Pancreas
	X External	Ø Drainage Device
		Y Other Device
			Z No Qualifier

Non-OR   All body part, approach, device, and qualifier values

Ø   Medical and Surgical
F   Hepatobiliary System and Pancreas
5   Destruction   Definition: Physical eradication of all or a portion of a body part by the direct use of energy, force, or a destructive agent

Explanation: None of the body part is physically taken out

Body Part Character 4	Approach Character 5	Device Character 6	Qualifier Character 7
Ø Liver Quadrate lobe 1 Liver, Right Lobe 2 Liver, Left Lobe	Ø Open 3 Percutaneous 4 Percutaneous Endoscopic	Z No Device	F Irreversible Electroporation Z No Qualifier
4 Gallbladder	Ø Open 3 Percutaneous 4 Percutaneous Endoscopic 8 Via Natural or Artificial Opening Endoscopic	Z No Device	Z No Qualifier

5   Hepatic Duct, Right
6   Hepatic Duct, Left
7   Hepatic Duct, Common
8   Cystic Duct
9   Common Bile Duct
C   Ampulla of Vater
     Duodenal ampulla
     Hepatopancreatic ampulla
D   Pancreatic Duct
     Duct of Wirsung
F   Pancreatic Duct, Accessory
     Duct of Santorini
	Ø Open
	3 Percutaneous
	4 Percutaneous Endoscopic
	7 Via Natural or Artificial Opening
	8 Via Natural or Artificial Opening
	     Endoscopic
		Z No Device	Z No Qualifier

G Pancreas	Ø Open 3 Percutaneous 4 Percutaneous Endoscopic	Z No Device	F Irreversible Electroporation Z No Qualifier
G Pancreas	8 Via Natural or Artificial Opening Endoscopic	Z No Device	Z No Qualifier

Non-OR   ØF5[5,6,7,8,9,C,D,F][4,8]ZZ
Non-OR   ØF5G4Z[F,Z]
Non-OR   ØF5G8ZZ

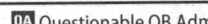 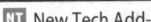

NC Noncovered Procedure   LC Limited Coverage   QA Questionable OB Admit   NT New Tech Add-on   ⊞ Combination Member   ♂ Male   ♀ Female

ICD-10-PCS 2022   **403**

ØF1–ØF5

Ø   Medical and Surgical
F   Hepatobiliary System and Pancreas
7   Dilation   Definition: Expanding an orifice or the lumen of a tubular body part

Explanation: The orifice can be a natural orifice or an artificially created orifice. Accomplished by stretching a tubular body part using intraluminal pressure or by cutting part of the orifice or wall of the tubular body part.

Body Part Character 4	Approach Character 5	Device Character 6	Qualifier Character 7

5   Hepatic Duct, Right
6   Hepatic Duct, Left
7   Hepatic Duct, Common
8   Cystic Duct
9   Common Bile Duct
C   Ampulla of Vater
     Duodenal ampulla
     Hepatopancreatic ampulla
D   Pancreatic Duct
     Duct of Wirsung
F   Pancreatic Duct, Accessory
     Duct of Santorini
	Ø Open
	3 Percutaneous
	4 Percutaneous Endoscopic
	7 Via Natural or Artificial Opening
	8 Via Natural or Artificial Opening
	     Endoscopic
		D Intraluminal Device
		Z No Device
			Z No Qualifier

Non-OR	ØF7[5,6,7,8,9][3,4,8][D,Z]Z
Non-OR	ØF7[5,6,7,8,9,D]]7DZ
Non-OR	ØF7C8[D,Z]Z
Non-OR	ØF7[D,F][4,8][D,Z]Z

Ø   Medical and Surgical
F   Hepatobiliary System and Pancreas
8   Division   Definition: Cutting into a body part, without draining fluids and/or gases from the body part, in order to separate or transect a body part

Explanation: All or a portion of the body part is separated into two or more portions

Body Part Character 4	Approach Character 5	Device Character 6	Qualifier Character 7
Ø Liver 1 Liver, Right Lobe 2 Liver, Left Lobe G Pancreas	Ø Open 3 Percutaneous 4 Percutaneous Endoscopic	Z No Device	Z No Qualifier

Non-OR	ØF8[Ø,1,2]3ZZ

Ø　Medical and Surgical
F　Hepatobiliary System and Pancreas
9　Drainage　　　　Definition: Taking or letting out fluids and/or gases from a body part
　　　　　　　　　　　Explanation: The qualifier DIAGNOSTIC is used to identify drainage procedures that are biopsies

Body Part Character 4	Approach Character 5	Device Character 6	Qualifier Character 7
Ø　Liver 　　Quadrate lobe **1　Liver, Right Lobe** **2　Liver, Left Lobe**	**Ø　Open** **3　Percutaneous** **4　Percutaneous Endoscopic**	**Ø　Drainage Device**	**Z　No Qualifier**
Ø　Liver 　　Quadrate lobe **1　Liver, Right Lobe** **2　Liver, Left Lobe**	**Ø　Open** **3　Percutaneous** **4　Percutaneous Endoscopic**	**Z　No Device**	**X　Diagnostic** **Z　No Qualifier**
4　Gallbladder **G　Pancreas**	**Ø　Open** **3　Percutaneous** **4　Percutaneous Endoscopic** **8　Via Natural or Artificial Opening Endoscopic**	**Ø　Drainage Device**	**Z　No Qualifier**
4　Gallbladder **G　Pancreas**	**Ø　Open** **3　Percutaneous** **4　Percutaneous Endoscopic** **8　Via Natural or Artificial Opening Endoscopic**	**Z　No Device**	**X　Diagnostic** **Z　No Qualifier**
5　Hepatic Duct, Right **6　Hepatic Duct, Left** **7　Hepatic Duct, Common** **8　Cystic Duct** **9　Common Bile Duct** **C　Ampulla of Vater** 　　Duodenal ampulla 　　Hepatopancreatic ampulla **D　Pancreatic Duct** 　　Duct of Wirsung **F　Pancreatic Duct, Accessory** 　　Duct of Santorini	**Ø　Open** **3　Percutaneous** **4　Percutaneous Endoscopic** **7　Via Natural or Artificial Opening** **8　Via Natural or Artificial Opening Endoscopic**	**Ø　Drainage Device**	**Z　No Qualifier**
5　Hepatic Duct, Right **6　Hepatic Duct, Left** **7　Hepatic Duct, Common** **8　Cystic Duct** **9　Common Bile Duct** **C　Ampulla of Vater** 　　Duodenal ampulla 　　Hepatopancreatic ampulla **D　Pancreatic Duct** 　　Duct of Wirsung **F　Pancreatic Duct, Accessory** 　　Duct of Santorini	**Ø　Open** **3　Percutaneous** **4　Percutaneous Endoscopic** **7　Via Natural or Artificial Opening** **8　Via Natural or Artificial Opening Endoscopic**	**Z　No Device**	**X　Diagnostic** **Z　No Qualifier**

Non-OR　ØF9[Ø,1,2][3,4]ØZ	**Non-OR**　ØF99[3,8]ØZ
Non-OR　ØF9[Ø,1,2][3,4]Z[X,Z]	**Non-OR**　ØF9C[3,4,8]ØZ
Non-OR　ØF9[4,G]8ØZ	**Non-OR**　ØF9[D,F][3,8]ØZ
Non-OR　ØF9G3ØZ	**Non-OR**　ØF9[5,6,8,9,C,D,F]3Z[X,Z]
Non-OR　ØF9[4,G]8Z[X,Z]	**Non-OR**　ØF9[5,6,8,9,C,D,F][4,7,8]ZX
Non-OR　ØF9G3Z[XZ]	**Non-OR**　ØF9[5,6,8,D,F]8ZZ
Non-OR　ØF9G4ZX	**Non-OR**　ØF97[3,4,7,8]Z[X,Z]
Non-OR　ØF9[5,6,8][3,8]ØZ	**Non-OR**　ØF99[4,7,8]ZZ
Non-OR　ØF97[3,4,7,8]ØZ	**Non-OR**　ØF9C[4,8]ZZ

NC Noncovered Procedure　　**LC** Limited Coverage　　**OA** Questionable OB Admit　　**NT** New Tech Add-on　　⊞ Combination Member　　♂ Male　　♀ Female

ICD-10-PCS 2022　　　　　　　　　　　　　　　　　　　　　　　　　　　　　　　　　　　　　　　**405**

Ø   Medical and Surgical
F   Hepatobiliary System and Pancreas
B   Excision   Definition: Cutting out or off, without replacement, a portion of a body part

Explanation: The qualifier DIAGNOSTIC is used to identify excision procedures that are biopsies

Body Part Character 4	Approach Character 5	Device Character 6	Qualifier Character 7
Ø Liver Quadrate lobe 1 Liver, Right Lobe 2 Liver, Left Lobe	Ø Open 3 Percutaneous 4 Percutaneous Endoscopic	Z No Device	X Diagnostic Z No Qualifier
4 Gallbladder G Pancreas	Ø Open 3 Percutaneous 4 Percutaneous Endoscopic 8 Via Natural or Artificial Opening Endoscopic	Z No Device	X Diagnostic Z No Qualifier

5 Hepatic Duct, Right
6 Hepatic Duct, Left
7 Hepatic Duct, Common
8 Cystic Duct
9 Common Bile Duct
C Ampulla of Vater
    Duodenal ampulla
    Hepatopancreatic ampulla
D Pancreatic Duct
    Duct of Wirsung
F Pancreatic Duct, Accessory
    Duct of Santorini
	Ø Open
	3 Percutaneous
	4 Percutaneous Endoscopic
	7 Via Natural or Artificial Opening
	8 Via Natural or Artificial Opening
	    Endoscopic
		Z No Device	X Diagnostic
			Z No Qualifier

Non-OR   ØFB[Ø,1,2]3ZX
Non-OR   ØFB[4,G][3,4,8]ZX
Non-OR   ØFB[5,6,7,8,9,C,D,F][3,4,7,8]ZX
Non-OR   ØFB[5,6,7,8,9,C,D,F][4,8]ZZ

Ø   Medical and Surgical
F   Hepatobiliary System and Pancreas
C   Extirpation   Definition: Taking or cutting out solid matter from a body part

Explanation: The solid matter may be an abnormal byproduct of a biological function or a foreign body; it may be imbedded in a body part or in the lumen of a tubular body part. The solid matter may or may not have been previously broken into pieces.

Body Part Character 4	Approach Character 5	Device Character 6	Qualifier Character 7
Ø Liver Quadrate lobe 1 Liver, Right Lobe 2 Liver, Left Lobe	Ø Open 3 Percutaneous 4 Percutaneous Endoscopic	Z No Device	Z No Qualifier
4 Gallbladder G Pancreas	Ø Open 3 Percutaneous 4 Percutaneous Endoscopic 8 Via Natural or Artificial Opening Endoscopic	Z No Device	Z No Qualifier

5 Hepatic Duct, Right
6 Hepatic Duct, Left
7 Hepatic Duct, Common
8 Cystic Duct
9 Common Bile Duct
C Ampulla of Vater
    Duodenal ampulla
    Hepatopancreatic ampulla
D Pancreatic Duct
    Duct of Wirsung
F Pancreatic Duct, Accessory
    Duct of Santorini
	Ø Open
	3 Percutaneous
	4 Percutaneous Endoscopic
	7 Via Natural or Artificial Opening
	8 Via Natural or Artificial Opening
	    Endoscopic
		Z No Device	Z No Qualifier

Non-OR   ØFC[5,6,7,8,9][3,4,7,8]ZZ
Non-OR   ØFCC[4,8]ZZ
Non-OR   ØFC[D,F][3,4,8]ZZ

Ø Medical and Surgical
F Hepatobiliary System and Pancreas
D Extraction   Definition: Pulling or stripping out or off all or a portion of a body part by the use of force

Explanation: The qualifier DIAGNOSTIC is used to identify extraction procedures that are biopsies

Body Part Character 4	Approach Character 5	Device Character 6	Qualifier Character 7
Ø Liver Quadrate lobe 1 Liver, Right Lobe 2 Liver, Left Lobe	3 Percutaneous 4 Percutaneous Endoscopic	Z No Device	X Diagnostic

4 Gallbladder
5 Hepatic Duct, Right
6 Hepatic Duct, Left
7 Hepatic Duct, Common
8 Cystic Duct
9 Common Bile Duct
C Ampulla of Vater
  Duodenal ampulla
  Hepatopancreatic ampulla
D Pancreatic Duct
  Duct of Wirsung
F Pancreatic Duct, Accessory
  Duct of Santorini
G Pancreas
	3 Percutaneous
	4 Percutaneous Endoscopic
	8 Via Natural or Artificial Opening Endoscopic
		Z No Device	X Diagnostic

Non-OR ØFD[Ø,1,2]3ZX
Non-OR ØFD[4,5,6,7,8,9,C,D,F,G][3,4,8]ZX

Ø Medical and Surgical
F Hepatobiliary System and Pancreas
F Fragmentation   Definition: Breaking solid matter in a body part into pieces

Explanation: Physical force (e.g., manual, ultrasonic) applied directly or indirectly is used to break the solid matter into pieces. The solid matter may be an abnormal byproduct of a biological function or a foreign body. The pieces of solid matter are not taken out.

Body Part Character 4	Approach Character 5	Device Character 6	Qualifier Character 7

4 Gallbladder NC
5 Hepatic Duct, Right NC
6 Hepatic Duct, Left NC
7 Hepatic Duct, Common
8 Cystic Duct NC
9 Common Bile Duct NC
C Ampulla of Vater NC
  Duodenal ampulla
  Hepatopancreatic ampulla
D Pancreatic Duct NC
  Duct of Wirsung
F Pancreatic Duct, Accessory NC
  Duct of Santorini
	Ø Open
	3 Percutaneous
	4 Percutaneous Endoscopic
	7 Via Natural or Artificial Opening
	8 Via Natural or Artificial Opening Endoscopic
	X External
		Z No Device	Z No Qualifier

Non-OR ØFF[4,5,6,7,8,9,C,D,F][8,X]ZZ
NC ØFF[4,5,6,8,9,C,D,F]XZZ

Ø Medical and Surgical
F Hepatobiliary System and Pancreas
H Insertion   Definition: Putting in a nonbiological appliance that monitors, assists, performs, or prevents a physiological function but does not physically take the place of a body part

Explanation: None

Body Part Character 4	Approach Character 5	Device Character 6	Qualifier Character 7
Ø Liver Quadrate lobe 4 Gallbladder G Pancreas	Ø Open 3 Percutaneous 4 Percutaneous Endoscopic	1 Radioactive Element 2 Monitoring Device 3 Infusion Device Y Other Device	Z No Qualifier
1 Liver, Right Lobe 2 Liver, Left Lobe	Ø Open 3 Percutaneous 4 Percutaneous Endoscopic	2 Monitoring Device 3 Infusion Device	Z No Qualifier
B Hepatobiliary Duct ⊞ D Pancreatic Duct Duct of Wirsung	Ø Open 3 Percutaneous 4 Percutaneous Endoscopic 7 Via Natural or Artificial Opening 8 Via Natural or Artificial Opening Endoscopic	1 Radioactive Element 2 Monitoring Device 3 Infusion Device D Intraluminal Device Y Other Device	Z No Qualifier

Non-OR ØFH[Ø,4,G]31Z
Non-OR ØFH[Ø,4,G][Ø,3,4]3Z
Non-OR ØFH[Ø,4,G][3,4]YZ
Non-OR ØFH[1,2][Ø,3,4]3Z

Non-OR ØFH[B,D][Ø,3,4]3Z
Non-OR ØFH[B,D][4,8]DZ
Non-OR ØFH[B,D][7,8][2,3]Z
Non-OR ØFH[B,D][3,4,7,8]YZ

See Appendix L for Procedure Combinations
 ⊞   ØFHB7DZ

NC Noncovered Procedure   LC Limited Coverage   QA Questionable OB Admit   NT New Tech Add-on   ⊞ Combination Member   ♂ Male   ♀ Female

Ø Medical and Surgical
F Hepatobiliary System and Pancreas
J Inspection   Definition: Visually and/or manually exploring a body part

Explanation: Visual exploration may be performed with or without optical instrumentation. Manual exploration may be performed directly or through intervening body layers.

Body Part Character 4	Approach Character 5	Device Character 6	Qualifier Character 7
Ø Liver Quadrate lobe	**Ø** Open **3** Percutaneous **4** Percutaneous Endoscopic **X** External	**Z** No Device	**Z** No Qualifier
4 Gallbladder **G Pancreas**	**Ø** Open **3** Percutaneous **4** Percutaneous Endoscopic **8** Via Natural or Artificial Opening Endoscopic **X** External	**Z** No Device	**Z** No Qualifier

B Hepatobiliary Duct
D Pancreatic Duct
   Duct of Wirsung
	Ø Open
	3 Percutaneous
	4 Percutaneous Endoscopic
	7 Via Natural or Artificial Opening
	8 Via Natural or Artificial Opening
	   Endoscopic
		Z No Device	**Z** No Qualifier

Non-OR	ØFJØ[3,X]ZZ
Non-OR	ØFJ[4,G][3,8,X]ZZ
Non-OR	ØFJ[B,D][3,7,8]ZZ

Ø Medical and Surgical
F Hepatobiliary System and Pancreas
L Occlusion   Definition: Completely closing an orifice or the lumen of a tubular body part

Explanation: The orifice can be a natural orifice or an artificially created orifice

Body Part Character 4	Approach Character 5	Device Character 6	Qualifier Character 7

5 Hepatic Duct, Right
6 Hepatic Duct, Left
7 Hepatic Duct, Common
8 Cystic Duct
9 Common Bile Duct
C Ampulla of Vater
   Duodenal ampulla
   Hepatopancreatic ampulla
D Pancreatic Duct
   Duct of Wirsung
F Pancreatic Duct, Accessory
   Duct of Santorini
	Ø Open
	3 Percutaneous
	4 Percutaneous Endoscopic
		C Extraluminal Device
		D Intraluminal Device
		Z No Device
			Z No Qualifier

5 Hepatic Duct, Right
6 Hepatic Duct, Left
7 Hepatic Duct, Common
8 Cystic Duct
9 Common Bile Duct
C Ampulla of Vater
   Duodenal ampulla
   Hepatopancreatic ampulla
D Pancreatic Duct
   Duct of Wirsung
F Pancreatic Duct, Accessory
   Duct of Santorini
	7 Via Natural or Artificial Opening
	8 Via Natural or Artificial Opening
	   Endoscopic
		D Intraluminal Device
		Z No Device
			Z No Qualifier

Non-OR	ØFL[5,6,7,8,9][3,4][C,D,Z]Z
Non-OR	ØFL[5,6,7,8,9][7,8][D,Z]Z

Ø   Medical and Surgical
F   Hepatobiliary System and Pancreas
M   Reattachment   Definition: Putting back in or on all or a portion of a separated body part to its normal location or other suitable location

                      Explanation: Vascular circulation and nervous pathways may or may not be reestablished

Body Part Character 4	Approach Character 5	Device Character 6	Qualifier Character 7

Ø   Liver
     Quadrate lobe
1   Liver, Right Lobe
2   Liver, Left Lobe
4   Gallbladder
5   Hepatic Duct, Right
6   Hepatic Duct, Left
7   Hepatic Duct, Common
8   Cystic Duct
9   Common Bile Duct
C   Ampulla of Vater
     Duodenal ampulla
     Hepatopancreatic ampulla
D   Pancreatic Duct
     Duct of Wirsung
F   Pancreatic Duct, Accessory
     Duct of Santorini
G   Pancreas
	Ø Open
	4 Percutaneous Endoscopic
		Z No Device	**Z** No Qualifier

Non-OR   ØFM[4,5,6,7,8,9]4ZZ

Ø   Medical and Surgical
F   Hepatobiliary System and Pancreas
N   Release   Definition: Freeing a body part from an abnormal physical constraint by cutting or by the use of force

                 Explanation: Some of the restraining tissue may be taken out but none of the body part is taken out

Body Part Character 4	Approach Character 5	Device Character 6	Qualifier Character 7
Ø Liver Quadrate lobe **1** Liver, Right Lobe **2** Liver, Left Lobe	**Ø** Open **3** Percutaneous **4** Percutaneous Endoscopic	**Z** No Device	**Z** No Qualifier
4 Gallbladder **G** Pancreas	**Ø** Open **3** Percutaneous **4** Percutaneous Endoscopic **8** Via Natural or Artificial Opening Endoscopic	**Z** No Device	**Z** No Qualifier

5   Hepatic Duct, Right
6   Hepatic Duct, Left
7   Hepatic Duct, Common
8   Cystic Duct
9   Common Bile Duct
C   Ampulla of Vater
     Duodenal ampulla
     Hepatopancreatic ampulla
D   Pancreatic Duct
     Duct of Wirsung
F   Pancreatic Duct, Accessory
     Duct of Santorini
	Ø Open
	3 Percutaneous
	4 Percutaneous Endoscopic
	7 Via Natural or Artificial Opening
	8 Via Natural or Artificial Opening
	     Endoscopic
		Z No Device	**Z** No Qualifier

Ø   Medical and Surgical
F   Hepatobiliary System and Pancreas
P   Removal   Definition: Taking out or off a device from a body part

Explanation: If a device is taken out and a similar device put in without cutting or puncturing the skin or mucous membrane, the procedure is coded to the root operation CHANGE. Otherwise, the procedure for taking out a device is coded to the root operation REMOVAL.

Body Part Character 4	Approach Character 5	Device Character 6	Qualifier Character 7
Ø Liver Quadrate lobe	**Ø** Open **3** Percutaneous **4** Percutaneous Endoscopic	**Ø** Drainage Device **2** Monitoring Device **3** Infusion Device **Y** Other Device	**Z** No Qualifier
Ø Liver Quadrate lobe	**X** External	**Ø** Drainage Device **2** Monitoring Device **3** Infusion Device	**Z** No Qualifier
4 Gallbladder **G** Pancreas	**Ø** Open **3** Percutaneous **4** Percutaneous Endoscopic	**Ø** Drainage Device **2** Monitoring Device **3** Infusion Device **D** Intraluminal Device **Y** Other Device	**Z** No Qualifier
4 Gallbladder **G** Pancreas	**X** External	**Ø** Drainage Device **2** Monitoring Device **3** Infusion Device **D** Intraluminal Device	**Z** No Qualifier
B Hepatobiliary Duct **D** Pancreatic Duct Duct of Wirsung	**Ø** Open **3** Percutaneous **4** Percutaneous Endoscopic **7** Via Natural or Artificial Opening **8** Via Natural or Artificial Opening Endoscopic	**Ø** Drainage Device **1** Radioactive Element **2** Monitoring Device **3** Infusion Device **7** Autologous Tissue Substitute **C** Extraluminal Device **D** Intraluminal Device **J** Synthetic Substitute **K** Nonautologous Tissue Substitute **Y** Other Device	**Z** No Qualifier
B Hepatobiliary Duct **D** Pancreatic Duct Duct of Wirsung	**X** External	**Ø** Drainage Device **1** Radioactive Element **2** Monitoring Device **3** Infusion Device **D** Intraluminal Device	**Z** No Qualifier

Non-OR ØFPØ[3,4]YZ		
Non-OR ØFPØX[Ø,2,3]Z	**See Appendix L for Procedure Combinations**	
Non-OR ØFPG3ØZ	**Combo-only** ØFP[B,D][7,8]DZ	
Non-OR ØFP[4,G][3,4]YZ	**Combo-only** ØFP[B,D]XDZ	
Non-OR ØFP4X[Ø,2,3,D]Z		
Non-OR ØFPGX[Ø,2,3]Z		
Non-OR ØFP[B,D][3,4]YZ		
Non-OR ØFP[B,D][7,8][Ø,2,3,D,Y]Z		
Non-OR ØFP[B,D]X[Ø,1,2,3,D]Z		

Hepatobiliary System and Pancreas

Ø   **Medical and Surgical**
F   **Hepatobiliary System and Pancreas**
Q   **Repair**   Definition: Restoring, to the extent possible, a body part to its normal anatomic structure and function

Explanation: Used only when the method to accomplish the repair is not one of the other root operations

Body Part Character 4	Approach Character 5	Device Character 6	Qualifier Character 7
Ø Liver Quadrate lobe 1 Liver, Right Lobe 2 Liver, Left Lobe	Ø Open 3 Percutaneous 4 Percutaneous Endoscopic	Z No Device	Z No Qualifier
4 Gallbladder G Pancreas	Ø Open 3 Percutaneous 4 Percutaneous Endoscopic 8 Via Natural or Artificial Opening Endoscopic	Z No Device	Z No Qualifier

5 Hepatic Duct, Right
6 Hepatic Duct, Left
7 Hepatic Duct, Common
8 Cystic Duct
9 Common Bile Duct
C Ampulla of Vater
   Duodenal ampulla
   Hepatopancreatic ampulla
D Pancreatic Duct
   Duct of Wirsung
F Pancreatic Duct, Accessory
   Duct of Santorini
	Ø Open
	3 Percutaneous
	4 Percutaneous Endoscopic
	7 Via Natural or Artificial Opening
	8 Via Natural or Artificial Opening Endoscopic
		Z No Device	Z No Qualifier

Ø   **Medical and Surgical**
F   **Hepatobiliary System and Pancreas**
R   **Replacement**   Definition: Putting in or on biological or synthetic material that physically takes the place and/or function of all or a portion of a body part

Explanation: The body part may have been taken out or replaced, or may be taken out, physically eradicated, or rendered nonfunctional during the REPLACEMENT procedure. A REMOVAL procedure is coded for taking out the device used in a previous replacement procedure.

Body Part Character 4	Approach Character 5	Device Character 6	Qualifier Character 7

5 Hepatic Duct, Right
6 Hepatic Duct, Left
7 Hepatic Duct, Common
8 Cystic Duct
9 Common Bile Duct
C Ampulla of Vater
   Duodenal ampulla
   Hepatopancreatic ampulla
D Pancreatic Duct
   Duct of Wirsung
F Pancreatic Duct, Accessory
   Duct of Santorini
	Ø Open
	4 Percutaneous Endoscopic
	8 Via Natural or Artificial Opening Endoscopic
		7 Autologous Tissue Substitute
		J Synthetic Substitute
		K Nonautologous Tissue Substitute
			Z No Qualifier

Ø   **Medical and Surgical**
F   **Hepatobiliary System and Pancreas**
S   **Reposition**   Definition: Moving to its normal location, or other suitable location, all or a portion of a body part

Explanation: The body part is moved to a new location from an abnormal location, or from a normal location where it is not functioning correctly. The body part may or may not be cut out or off to be moved to the new location.

Body Part Character 4	Approach Character 5	Device Character 6	Qualifier Character 7

Ø Liver
   Quadrate lobe
4 Gallbladder
5 Hepatic Duct, Right
6 Hepatic Duct, Left
7 Hepatic Duct, Common
8 Cystic Duct
9 Common Bile Duct
C Ampulla of Vater
   Duodenal ampulla
   Hepatopancreatic ampulla
D Pancreatic Duct
   Duct of Wirsung
F Pancreatic Duct, Accessory
   Duct of Santorini
G Pancreas
	Ø Open
	4 Percutaneous Endoscopic
		Z No Device	Z No Qualifier

NC Noncovered Procedure   **LC** Limited Coverage   **QA** Questionable OB Admit   **NT** New Tech Add-on   ⊞ Combination Member   ♂ Male   ♀ Female

ICD-10-PCS 2022   411

Ø Medical and Surgical
F Hepatobiliary System and Pancreas
T Resection   Definition: Cutting out or off, without replacement, all of a body part
                Explanation: None

Body Part Character 4	Approach Character 5	Device Character 6	Qualifier Character 7
Ø Liver Quadrate lobe **1** Liver, Right Lobe **2** Liver, Left Lobe **4** Gallbladder **G** Pancreas ⊞	**Ø** Open **4** Percutaneous Endoscopic	**Z** No Device	**Z** No Qualifier

5 Hepatic Duct, Right
6 Hepatic Duct, Left
7 Hepatic Duct, Common
8 Cystic Duct
9 Common Bile Duct
C Ampulla of Vater
    Duodenal ampulla
    Hepatopancreatic ampulla
D Pancreatic Duct
    Duct of Wirsung
F Pancreatic Duct, Accessory
    Duct of Santorini
	Ø Open
	4 Percutaneous Endoscopic
	7 Via Natural or Artificial Opening
	8 Via Natural or Artificial Opening
	    Endoscopic
		Z No Device	**Z** No Qualifier

Non-OR   ØFT[D,F][4,8]ZZ

See Appendix L for Procedure Combinations
⊞   ØFTGØZZ

Ø Medical and Surgical
F Hepatobiliary System and Pancreas
U Supplement   Definition: Putting in or on biological or synthetic material that physically reinforces and/or augments the function of a portion of a body part
                      Explanation: The biological material is non-living, or is living and from the same individual. The body part may have been previously replaced, and the SUPPLEMENT procedure is performed to physically reinforce and/or augment the function of the replaced body part.

Body Part Character 4	Approach Character 5	Device Character 6	Qualifier Character 7

5 Hepatic Duct, Right
6 Hepatic Duct, Left
7 Hepatic Duct, Common
8 Cystic Duct
9 Common Bile Duct
C Ampulla of Vater
    Duodenal ampulla
    Hepatopancreatic ampulla
D Pancreatic Duct
    Duct of Wirsung
F Pancreatic Duct, Accessory
    Duct of Santorini
	Ø Open
	3 Percutaneous
	4 Percutaneous Endoscopic
	8 Via Natural or Artificial Opening
	    Endoscopic
		7 Autologous Tissue Substitute
		J Synthetic Substitute
		K Nonautologous Tissue Substitute
			Z No Qualifier

Ø Medical and Surgical
F Hepatobiliary System and Pancreas
V Restriction   Definition: Partially closing an orifice or the lumen of a tubular body part
                 Explanation: The orifice can be a natural orifice or an artificially created orifice

Body Part Character 4	Approach Character 5	Device Character 6	Qualifier Character 7

5 Hepatic Duct, Right
6 Hepatic Duct, Left
7 Hepatic Duct, Common
8 Cystic Duct
9 Common Bile Duct
C Ampulla of Vater
   Duodenal ampulla
   Hepatopancreatic ampulla
D Pancreatic Duct
   Duct of Wirsung
F Pancreatic Duct, Accessory
   Duct of Santorini
	Ø Open
	3 Percutaneous
	4 Percutaneous Endoscopic
		C Extraluminal Device
		D Intraluminal Device
		Z No Device
			Z No Qualifier

5 Hepatic Duct, Right
6 Hepatic Duct, Left
7 Hepatic Duct, Common
8 Cystic Duct
9 Common Bile Duct
C Ampulla of Vater
   Duodenal ampulla
   Hepatopancreatic ampulla
D Pancreatic Duct
   Duct of Wirsung
F Pancreatic Duct, Accessory
   Duct of Santorini
	7 Via Natural or Artificial Opening
	8 Via Natural or Artificial Opening
	   Endoscopic
		D Intraluminal Device
		Z No Device
			Z No Qualifier

Non-OR   ØFV[5,6,7,8,9][3,4][C,D,Z]Z
Non-OR   ØFV[5,6,7,8,9][7,8][D,Z]Z

NC Noncovered Procedure   LC Limited Coverage   QA Questionable OB Admit   NT New Tech Add-on   ⊞ Combination Member   ♂ Male   ♀ Female

ICD-10-PCS 2022   413

Hepatobiliary System and Pancreas

Ø   **Medical and Surgical**
F   **Hepatobiliary System and Pancreas**
W   **Revision**   Definition: Correcting, to the extent possible, a portion of a malfunctioning device or the position of a displaced device

              Explanation: Revision can include correcting a malfunctioning or displaced device by taking out or putting in components of the device such as a screw or pin

Body Part Character 4		Approach Character 5		Device Character 6		Qualifier Character 7	
Ø	Liver Quadrate lobe	Ø 3 4	Open Percutaneous Percutaneous Endoscopic	Ø 2 3 Y	Drainage Device Monitoring Device Infusion Device Other Device	Z	No Qualifier
Ø	Liver Quadrate lobe	X	External	Ø 2 3	Drainage Device Monitoring Device Infusion Device	Z	No Qualifier
4 G	Gallbladder Pancreas	Ø 3 4	Open Percutaneous Percutaneous Endoscopic	Ø 2 3 D Y	Drainage Device Monitoring Device Infusion Device Intraluminal Device Other Device	Z	No Qualifier
4 G	Gallbladder Pancreas	X	External	Ø 2 3 D	Drainage Device Monitoring Device Infusion Device Intraluminal Device	Z	No Qualifier
B D	Hepatobiliary Duct Pancreatic Duct Duct of Wirsung	Ø 3 4 7 8	Open Percutaneous Percutaneous Endoscopic Via Natural or Artificial Opening Via Natural or Artificial Opening Endoscopic	Ø 2 3 7 C D J K Y	Drainage Device Monitoring Device Infusion Device Autologous Tissue Substitute Extraluminal Device Intraluminal Device Synthetic Substitute Nonautologous Tissue Substitute Other Device	Z	No Qualifier
B D	Hepatobiliary Duct Pancreatic Duct Duct of Wirsung	X	External	Ø 2 3 7 C D J K	Drainage Device Monitoring Device Infusion Device Autologous Tissue Substitute Extraluminal Device Intraluminal Device Synthetic Substitute Nonautologous Tissue Substitute	Z	No Qualifier

Non-OR	ØFWØ[3,4]YZ
Non-OR	ØFWØX[Ø,2,3]Z
Non-OR	ØFW[4,G][3,4]YZ
Non-OR	ØFW[4,G]X[Ø,2,3,D]Z
Non-OR	ØFW[B,D][3,4,7,8]YZ
Non-OR	ØFW[B,D]X[Ø,2,3,7,C,D,J,K]Z

Ø   **Medical and Surgical**
F   **Hepatobiliary System and Pancreas**
Y   **Transplantation**   Definition: Putting in or on all or a portion of a living body part taken from another individual or animal to physically take the place and/or function of all or a portion of a similar body part

                       Explanation: The native body part may or may not be taken out, and the transplanted body part may take over all or a portion of its function

Body Part Character 4		Approach Character 5		Device Character 6		Qualifier Character 7	
Ø	Liver **LC** Quadrate lobe G Pancreas **LC NC ⊞**	Ø	Open	Z	No Device	Ø 1 2	Allogeneic Syngeneic Zooplastic

LC	ØFYØØZ[Ø,1,2]	**See Appendix L for Procedure Combinations**
LC	ØFYGØZ[Ø,1]	⊞ ØFYGØZ[Ø,1,2]
NC	ØFYGØZ2	

NC	ØFYGØZ[Ø,1] If reported alone without one of the following procedures
	    ØTYØØZ[Ø,1,2], ØTY1ØZ[Ø,1,2] and without one of the following
	    diagnoses E1Ø.1Ø-E1Ø.9, E89.1	

Endocrine System ØG2–ØGW

Character Meanings

This Character Meaning table is provided as a guide to assist the user in the identification of character members that may be found in this section of code tables. It **SHOULD NOT** be used to build a PCS code.

Operation–Character 3	Body Part–Character 4	Approach–Character 5	Device–Character 6	Qualifier–Character 7
2 Change	Ø Pituitary Gland	Ø Open	Ø Drainage Device	X Diagnostic
5 Destruction	1 Pineal Body	3 Percutaneous	1 Radioactive Element	Z No Qualifier
8 Division	2 Adrenal Gland, Left	4 Percutaneous Endoscopic	2 Monitoring Device	
9 Drainage	3 Adrenal Gland, Right	X External	3 Infusion Device	
B Excision	4 Adrenal Glands, Bilateral		Y Other Device	
C Extirpation	5 Adrenal Gland		Z No Device	
H Insertion	6 Carotid Body, Left			
J Inspection	7 Carotid Body, Right			
M Reattachment	8 Carotid Bodies, Bilateral			
N Release	9 Para-aortic Body			
P Removal	B Coccygeal Glomus			
Q Repair	C Glomus Jugulare			
S Reposition	D Aortic Body			
T Resection	F Paraganglion Extremity			
W Revision	G Thyroid Gland Lobe, Left			
	H Thyroid Gland Lobe, Right			
	J Thyroid Gland Isthmus			
	K Thyroid Gland			
	L Superior Parathyroid Gland, Right			
	M Superior Parathyroid Gland, Left			
	N Inferior Parathyroid Gland, Right			
	P Inferior Parathyroid Gland, Left			
	Q Parathyroid Glands, Multiple			
	R Parathyroid Gland			
	S Endocrine Gland			

AHA Coding Clinic for table ØGB

2021, 2Q, 7	Infrarenal para-aortic paraganglioma with excision
2017, 2Q, 20	Near total thyroidectomy
2014, 3Q, 22	Transsphenoidal removal of pituitary tumor and fat graft placement

AHA Coding Clinic for table ØGH

2020, 4Q, 43-44	Insertion of radioactive element

AHA Coding Clinic for table ØGT

2017, 2Q, 20	Near total thyroidectomy

Endocrine System

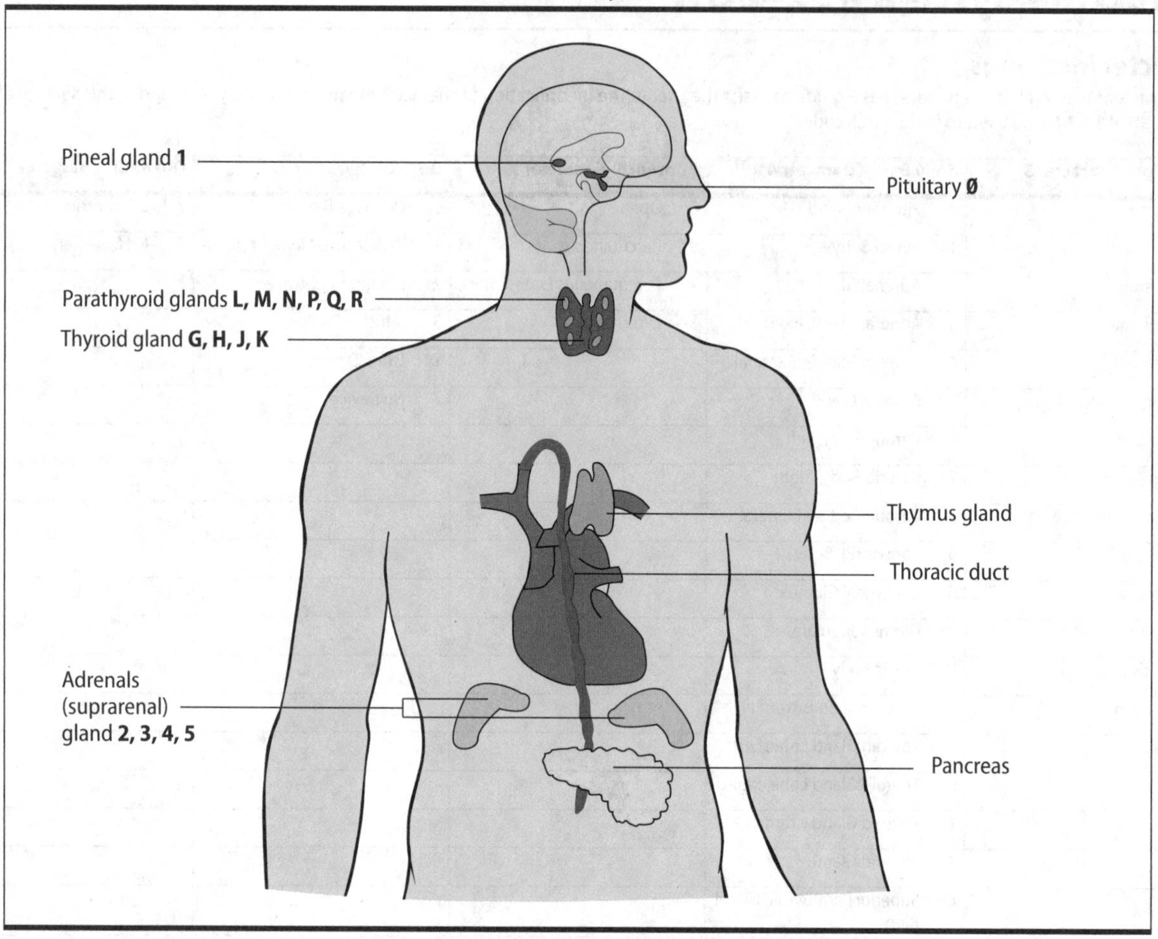

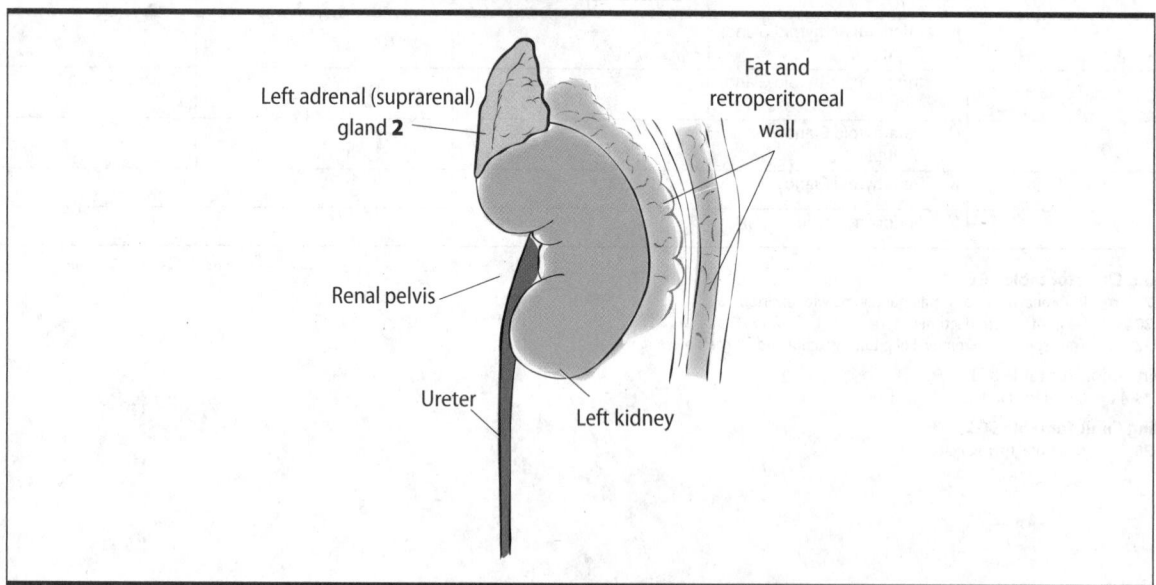

Left Adrenal Gland

Thyroid

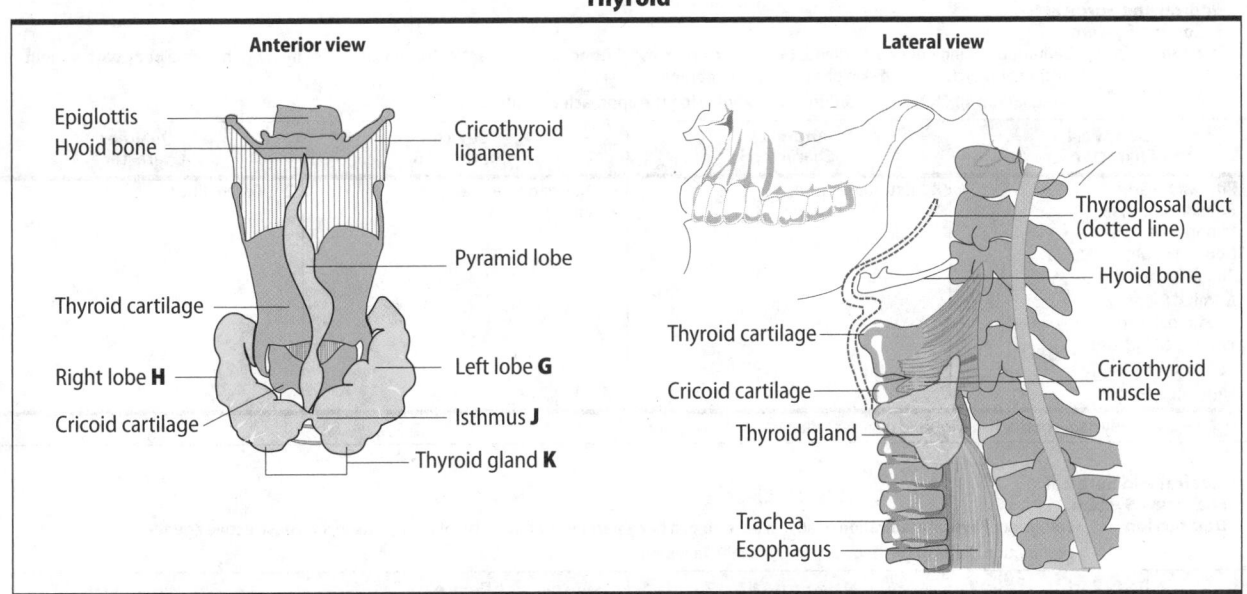

Anterior view

Epiglottis
Hyoid bone
Cricothyroid ligament
Pyramid lobe
Thyroid cartilage
Right lobe **H**
Left lobe **G**
Cricoid cartilage
Isthmus **J**
Thyroid gland **K**

Lateral view

Thyroglossal duct (dotted line)
Hyoid bone
Thyroid cartilage
Cricoid cartilage
Cricothyroid muscle
Thyroid gland
Trachea
Esophagus

Thyroid and Parathyroid Glands

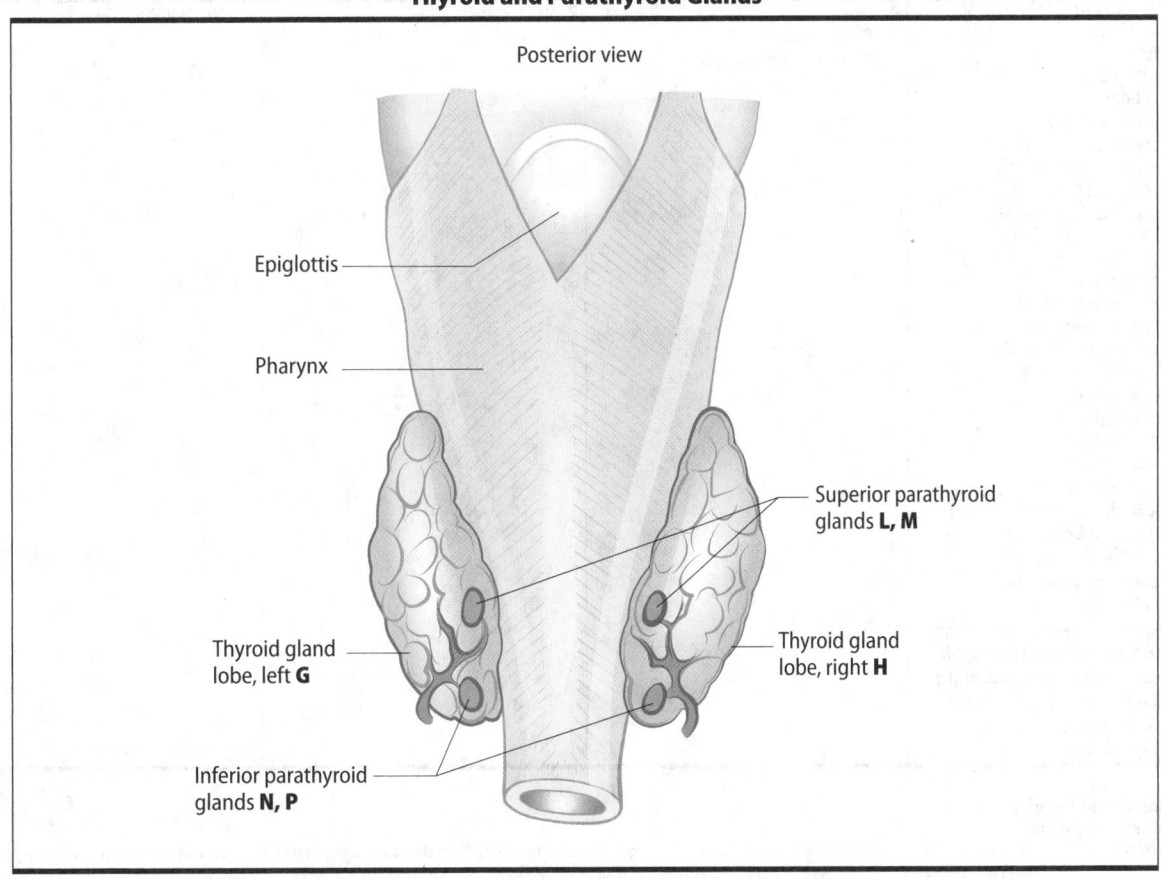

Posterior view

Epiglottis
Pharynx
Superior parathyroid glands **L, M**
Thyroid gland lobe, left **G**
Thyroid gland lobe, right **H**
Inferior parathyroid glands **N, P**

Ø Medical and Surgical
G Endocrine System
2 Change   Definition: Taking out or off a device from a body part and putting back an identical or similar device in or on the same body part without cutting or puncturing the skin or a mucous membrane

Explanation: All CHANGE procedures are coded using the approach EXTERNAL

Body Part Character 4	Approach Character 5	Device Character 6	Qualifier Character 7

Ø Pituitary Gland
  Adenohypophysis
  Hypophysis
  Neurohypophysis
1 Pineal Body
5 Adrenal Gland
  Suprarenal gland
K Thyroid Gland
R Parathyroid Gland
S Endocrine Gland
	X External	**Ø** Drainage Device
		Y Other Device
			Z No Qualifier

Non-OR All body part, approach, device, and qualifier values

Ø Medical and Surgical
G Endocrine System
5 Destruction   Definition: Physical eradication of all or a portion of a body part by the direct use of energy, force, or a destructive agent

Explanation: None of the body part is physically taken out

Body Part Character 4	Approach Character 5	Device Character 6	Qualifier Character 7

Ø Pituitary Gland
  Adenohypophysis
  Hypophysis
  Neurohypophysis
1 Pineal Body
2 Adrenal Gland, Left
  Suprarenal gland
3 Adrenal Gland, Right
  See 2 Adrenal Gland, Left
4 Adrenal Glands, Bilateral
  See 2 Adrenal Gland, Left
6 Carotid Body, Left
  Carotid glomus
7 Carotid Body, Right
  See 6 Carotid Body, Left
8 Carotid Bodies, Bilateral
  See 6 Carotid Body, Left
9 Para-aortic Body
B Coccygeal Glomus
  Coccygeal body
C Glomus Jugulare
  Jugular body
D Aortic Body
F Paraganglion Extremity
G Thyroid Gland Lobe, Left
H Thyroid Gland Lobe, Right
K Thyroid Gland
L Superior Parathyroid Gland, Right
M Superior Parathyroid Gland, Left
N Inferior Parathyroid Gland, Right
P Inferior Parathyroid Gland, Left
Q Parathyroid Glands, Multiple
R Parathyroid Gland
	Ø Open
	3 Percutaneous
	4 Percutaneous Endoscopic
		Z No Device	**Z** No Qualifier

Ø Medical and Surgical
G Endocrine System
8 Division   Definition: Cutting into a body part, without draining fluids and/or gases from the body part, in order to separate or transect a body part

Explanation: All or a portion of the body part is separated into two or more portions

Body Part Character 4	Approach Character 5	Device Character 6	Qualifier Character 7

Ø Pituitary Gland
  Adenohypophysis
  Hypophysis
  Neurohypophysis
J Thyroid Gland Isthmus
	Ø Open
	3 Percutaneous
	4 Percutaneous Endoscopic
		Z No Device	**Z** No Qualifier

0   **Medical and Surgical**
G   **Endocrine System**
9   **Drainage**   Definition: Taking or letting out fluids and/or gases from a body part
                       Explanation: The qualifier DIAGNOSTIC is used to identify drainage procedures that are biopsies

Body Part Character 4	Approach Character 5	Device Character 6	Qualifier Character 7

0 **Pituitary Gland**
    Adenohypophysis
    Hypophysis
    Neurohypophysis
1 **Pineal Body**
2 **Adrenal Gland, Left**
    Suprarenal gland
3 **Adrenal Gland, Right**
    See 2 Adrenal Gland, Left
4 **Adrenal Glands, Bilateral**
    See 2 Adrenal Gland, Left
6 **Carotid Body, Left**
    Carotid glomus
7 **Carotid Body, Right**
    See 6 Carotid Body, Left
8 **Carotid Bodies, Bilateral**
    See 6 Carotid Body, Left
9 **Para-aortic Body**
B **Coccygeal Glomus**
    Coccygeal body
C **Glomus Jugulare**
    Jugular body
D **Aortic Body**
F **Paraganglion Extremity**
G **Thyroid Gland Lobe, Left**
H **Thyroid Gland Lobe, Right**
K **Thyroid Gland**
L **Superior Parathyroid Gland, Right**
M **Superior Parathyroid Gland, Left**
N **Inferior Parathyroid Gland, Right**
P **Inferior Parathyroid Gland, Left**
Q **Parathyroid Glands, Multiple**
R **Parathyroid Gland**
	0 Open
	3 Percutaneous
	4 Percutaneous Endoscopic
		0 Drainage Device	**Z** No Qualifier

0 **Pituitary Gland**
    Adenohypophysis
    Hypophysis
    Neurohypophysis
1 **Pineal Body**
2 **Adrenal Gland, Left**
    Suprarenal gland
3 **Adrenal Gland, Right**
    See 2 Adrenal Gland, Left
4 **Adrenal Glands, Bilateral**
    See 2 Adrenal Gland, Left
6 **Carotid Body, Left**
    Carotid glomus
7 **Carotid Body, Right**
    See 6 Carotid Body, Left
8 **Carotid Bodies, Bilateral**
    See 6 Carotid Body, Left
9 **Para-aortic Body**
B **Coccygeal Glomus**
    Coccygeal body
C **Glomus Jugulare**
    Jugular body
D **Aortic Body**
F **Paraganglion Extremity**
G **Thyroid Gland Lobe, Left**
H **Thyroid Gland Lobe, Right**
K **Thyroid Gland**
L **Superior Parathyroid Gland, Right**
M **Superior Parathyroid Gland, Left**
N **Inferior Parathyroid Gland, Right**
P **Inferior Parathyroid Gland, Left**
Q **Parathyroid Glands, Multiple**
R **Parathyroid Gland**
	0 Open
	3 Percutaneous
	4 Percutaneous Endoscopic
		Z No Device	**X** Diagnostic
			Z No Qualifier

Non-OR	0G9[0,1,2,3,4,6,7,8,9,B,C,D,F,G,H,K,L,M,N,P,Q,R]30Z
Non-OR	0G9[G,H,K,L,M,N,P,Q,R]40Z
Non-OR	0G9[2,3,4,G,H,K][3,4]ZX
Non-OR	0G9[0,1,2,3,4,6,7,8,9,B,C,D,F,G,H,K,L,M,N,P,Q,R]3ZZ
Non-OR	0G9[G,H,K,L,M,N,P,Q,R]4ZZ

NC Noncovered Procedure   **LC** Limited Coverage   **QA** Questionable OB Admit   **NT** New Tech Add-on   ⊞ Combination Member   ♂ Male   ♀ Female

ICD-10-PCS 2022   **419**

0G9–0G9

Ø **Medical and Surgical**
G **Endocrine System**
B **Excision**   Definition: Cutting out or off, without replacement, a portion of a body part

Explanation: The qualifier DIAGNOSTIC is used to identify excision procedures that are biopsies

Body Part Character 4	Approach Character 5	Device Character 6	Qualifier Character 7
Ø **Pituitary Gland** Adenohypophysis Hypophysis Neurohypophysis 1 **Pineal Body** 2 **Adrenal Gland, Left** Suprarenal gland 3 **Adrenal Gland, Right** *See 2 Adrenal Gland, Left* 4 **Adrenal Glands, Bilateral** *See 2 Adrenal Gland, Left* 6 **Carotid Body, Left** Carotid glomus 7 **Carotid Body, Right** *See 6 Carotid Body, Left* 8 **Carotid Bodies, Bilateral** *See 6 Carotid Body, Left* 9 **Para-aortic Body** B **Coccygeal Glomus** Coccygeal body C **Glomus Jugulare** Jugular body D **Aortic Body** F **Paraganglion Extremity** G **Thyroid Gland Lobe, Left** H **Thyroid Gland Lobe, Right** J **Thyroid Gland Isthmus** L **Superior Parathyroid Gland, Right** M **Superior Parathyroid Gland, Left** N **Inferior Parathyroid Gland, Right** P **Inferior Parathyroid Gland, Left** Q **Parathyroid Glands, Multiple** R **Parathyroid Gland**	Ø **Open** 3 **Percutaneous** 4 **Percutaneous Endoscopic**	Z **No Device**	X **Diagnostic** Z **No Qualifier**

Non-OR   ØGB[2,3,4,G,H,J][3,4]ZX

Ø **Medical and Surgical**
G **Endocrine System**
C **Extirpation**   Definition: Taking or cutting out solid matter from a body part

Explanation: The solid matter may be an abnormal byproduct of a biological function or a foreign body; it may be imbedded in a body part or in the lumen of a tubular body part. The solid matter may or may not have been previously broken into pieces.

Body Part Character 4	Approach Character 5	Device Character 6	Qualifier Character 7
Ø **Pituitary Gland** Adenohypophysis Hypophysis Neurohypophysis 1 **Pineal Body** 2 **Adrenal Gland, Left** Suprarenal gland 3 **Adrenal Gland, Right** *See 2 Adrenal Gland, Left* 4 **Adrenal Glands, Bilateral** *See 2 Adrenal Gland, Left* 6 **Carotid Body, Left** Carotid glomus 7 **Carotid Body, Right** *See 6 Carotid Body, Left* 8 **Carotid Bodies, Bilateral** *See 6 Carotid Body, Left* 9 **Para-aortic Body** B **Coccygeal Glomus** Coccygeal body C **Glomus Jugulare** Jugular body D **Aortic Body** F **Paraganglion Extremity** G **Thyroid Gland Lobe, Left** H **Thyroid Gland Lobe, Right** K **Thyroid Gland** L **Superior Parathyroid Gland, Right** M **Superior Parathyroid Gland, Left** N **Inferior Parathyroid Gland, Right** P **Inferior Parathyroid Gland, Left** Q **Parathyroid Glands, Multiple** R **Parathyroid Gland**	Ø **Open** 3 **Percutaneous** 4 **Percutaneous Endoscopic**	Z **No Device**	Z **No Qualifier**

Ø   Medical and Surgical
G   Endocrine System
H   Insertion   Definition: Putting in a nonbiological appliance that monitors, assists, performs, or prevents a physiological function but does not physically take the place of a body part
                   Explanation: None

Body Part Character 4	Approach Character 5	Device Character 6	Qualifier Character 7
S Endocrine Gland	**Ø** Open **3** Percutaneous **4** Percutaneous Endoscopic	**1** Radioactive Element **2** Monitoring Device **3** Infusion Device **Y** Other Device	**Z** No Qualifier

Non-OR   ØGHS31Z
Non-OR   ØGHS[3,4]YZ

Ø   Medical and Surgical
G   Endocrine System
J   Inspection   Definition: Visually and/or manually exploring a body part
                   Explanation: Visual exploration may be performed with or without optical instrumentation. Manual exploration may be performed directly or through intervening body layers.

Body Part Character 4	Approach Character 5	Device Character 6	Qualifier Character 7

Ø Pituitary Gland
    Adenohypophysis
    Hypophysis
    Neurohypophysis
1 Pineal Body
5 Adrenal Gland
    Suprarenal gland
K Thyroid Gland
R Parathyroid Gland
S Endocrine Gland
	Ø Open
	3 Percutaneous
	4 Percutaneous Endoscopic
		Z No Device	**Z** No Qualifier

Non-OR   ØGJ[Ø,1,5,K,R,S]3ZZ

Ø   Medical and Surgical
G   Endocrine System
M   Reattachment   Definition: Putting back in or on all or a portion of a separated body part to its normal location or other suitable location
                      Explanation: Vascular circulation and nervous pathways may or may not be reestablished

Body Part Character 4	Approach Character 5	Device Character 6	Qualifier Character 7

2 Adrenal Gland, Left
    Suprarenal gland
3 Adrenal Gland, Right
    See 2 Adrenal Gland, Left
G Thyroid Gland Lobe, Left
H Thyroid Gland Lobe, Right
L Superior Parathyroid Gland, Right
M Superior Parathyroid Gland, Left
N Inferior Parathyroid Gland, Right
P Inferior Parathyroid Gland, Left
Q Parathyroid Glands, Multiple
R Parathyroid Gland
	Ø Open
	4 Percutaneous Endoscopic
		Z No Device	**Z** No Qualifier

Ø   Medical and Surgical
G   Endocrine System
N   Release   Definition: Freeing a body part from an abnormal physical constraint by cutting or by the use of force
                         Explanation: Some of the restraining tissue may be taken out but none of the body part is taken out

Body Part Character 4	Approach Character 5	Device Character 6	Qualifier Character 7
Ø Pituitary Gland Adenohypophysis Hypophysis Neurohypophysis **1** Pineal Body **2** Adrenal Gland, Left Suprarenal gland **3** Adrenal Gland, Right *See 2 Adrenal Gland, Left* **4** Adrenal Glands, Bilateral *See 2 Adrenal Gland, Left* **6** Carotid Body, Left Carotid glomus **7** Carotid Body, Right *See 6 Carotid Body, Left* **8** Carotid Bodies, Bilateral *See 6 Carotid Body, Left* **9** Para-aortic Body **B** Coccygeal Glomus Coccygeal body **C** Glomus Jugulare Jugular body **D** Aortic Body **F** Paraganglion Extremity **G** Thyroid Gland Lobe, Left **H** Thyroid Gland Lobe, Right **K** Thyroid Gland **L** Superior Parathyroid Gland, Right **M** Superior Parathyroid Gland, Left **N** Inferior Parathyroid Gland, Right **P** Inferior Parathyroid Gland, Left **Q** Parathyroid Glands, Multiple **R** Parathyroid Gland	**Ø** Open **3** Percutaneous **4** Percutaneous Endoscopic	**Z** No Device	**Z** No Qualifier

Non-OR   ØGN[6,7,8,9,B,C,D,F][Ø,3,4]ZZ

Ø   Medical and Surgical
G   Endocrine System
P   Removal   Definition: Taking out or off a device from a body part
                         Explanation: If a device is taken out and a similar device put in without cutting or puncturing the skin or mucous membrane, the procedure is
                         coded to the root operation CHANGE. Otherwise, the procedure for taking out a device is coded to the root operation REMOVAL.

Body Part Character 4	Approach Character 5	Device Character 6	Qualifier Character 7
Ø Pituitary Gland Adenohypophysis Hypophysis Neurohypophysis **1** Pineal Body **5** Adrenal Gland Suprarenal gland **K** Thyroid Gland **R** Parathyroid Gland	**Ø** Open **3** Percutaneous **4** Percutaneous Endoscopic **X** External	**Ø** Drainage Device	**Z** No Qualifier
S Endocrine Gland	**Ø** Open **3** Percutaneous **4** Percutaneous Endoscopic	**Ø** Drainage Device **2** Monitoring Device **3** Infusion Device **Y** Other Device	**Z** No Qualifier
S Endocrine Gland	**X** External	**Ø** Drainage Device **2** Monitoring Device **3** Infusion Device	**Z** No Qualifier

Non-OR   ØGP[Ø,1,5,K,R]XØZ
Non-OR   ØGPS[3,4]YZ
Non-OR   ØGPSX[Ø,2,3]Z

Ø   **Medical and Surgical**
G   **Endocrine System**
Q   **Repair**   Definition: Restoring, to the extent possible, a body part to its normal anatomic structure and function

Explanation: Used only when the method to accomplish the repair is not one of the other root operations

Body Part Character 4	Approach Character 5	Device Character 6	Qualifier Character 7

Ø Pituitary Gland
   Adenohypophysis
   Hypophysis
   Neurohypophysis
1 Pineal Body
2 Adrenal Gland, Left
   Suprarenal gland
3 Adrenal Gland, Right
   See 2 Adrenal Gland, Left
4 Adrenal Glands, Bilateral
   See 2 Adrenal Gland, Left
6 Carotid Body, Left
   Carotid glomus
7 Carotid Body, Right
   See 6 Carotid Body, Left
8 Carotid Bodies, Bilateral
   See 6 Carotid Body, Left
9 Para-aortic Body
B Coccygeal Glomus
   Coccygeal body
C Glomus Jugulare
   Jugular body
D Aortic Body
F Paraganglion Extremity
G Thyroid Gland Lobe, Left
H Thyroid Gland Lobe, Right
J Thyroid Gland Isthmus
K Thyroid Gland
L Superior Parathyroid Gland, Right
M Superior Parathyroid Gland, Left
N Inferior Parathyroid Gland, Right
P Inferior Parathyroid Gland, Left
Q Parathyroid Glands, Multiple
R Parathyroid Gland
	Ø Open
	3 Percutaneous
	4 Percutaneous Endoscopic
		Z No Device	**Z** No Qualifier

Ø   **Medical and Surgical**
G   **Endocrine System**
S   **Reposition**   Definition: Moving to its normal location, or other suitable location, all or a portion of a body part

Explanation: The body part is moved to a new location from an abnormal location, or from a normal location where it is not functioning correctly. The body part may or may not be cut out or off to be moved to the new location.

Body Part Character 4	Approach Character 5	Device Character 6	Qualifier Character 7

2 Adrenal Gland, Left
   Suprarenal gland
3 Adrenal Gland, Right
   See 2 Adrenal Gland, Left
G Thyroid Gland Lobe, Left
H Thyroid Gland Lobe, Right
L Superior Parathyroid Gland, Right
M Superior Parathyroid Gland, Left
N Inferior Parathyroid Gland, Right
P Inferior Parathyroid Gland, Left
Q Parathyroid Glands, Multiple
R Parathyroid Gland
	Ø Open
	4 Percutaneous Endoscopic
		Z No Device	**Z** No Qualifier

NC Noncovered Procedure   LC Limited Coverage   QA Questionable OB Admit   NT New Tech Add-on   ⊞ Combination Member   ♂ Male   ♀ Female

ICD-10-PCS 2022   **423**

ØGQ–ØGS

Ø   Medical and Surgical
G   Endocrine System
T   Resection   Definition: Cutting out or off, without replacement, all of a body part
                           Explanation: None

Body Part Character 4	Approach Character 5	Device Character 6	Qualifier Character 7

Ø   Pituitary Gland
    Adenohypophysis
    Hypophysis
    Neurohypophysis
1   Pineal Body
2   Adrenal Gland, Left
    Suprarenal gland
3   Adrenal Gland, Right
    See 2 Adrenal Gland, Left
4   Adrenal Glands, Bilateral
    See 2 Adrenal Gland, Left
6   Carotid Body, Left
    Carotid glomus
7   Carotid Body, Right
    See 6 Carotid Body, Left
8   Carotid Bodies, Bilateral
    See 6 Carotid Body, Left
9   Para-aortic Body
B   Coccygeal Glomus
    Coccygeal body
C   Glomus Jugulare
    Jugular body
D   Aortic Body
F   Paraganglion Extremity
G   Thyroid Gland Lobe, Left
H   Thyroid Gland Lobe, Right
J   Thyroid Gland Isthmus
K   Thyroid Gland
L   Superior Parathyroid Gland, Right
M   Superior Parathyroid Gland, Left
N   Inferior Parathyroid Gland, Right
P   Inferior Parathyroid Gland, Left
Q   Parathyroid Glands, Multiple
R   Parathyroid Gland
	Ø Open
	4 Percutaneous Endoscopic
		Z No Device	**Z No Qualifier**

Non-OR   ØGT[6,7,8,9,B,C,D,F][Ø,4]ZZ

Ø   Medical and Surgical
G   Endocrine System
W   Revision   Definition: Correcting, to the extent possible, a portion of a malfunctioning device or the position of a displaced device
                          Explanation: Revision can include correcting a malfunctioning or displaced device by taking out or putting in components of the device such as a screw or pin

Body Part Character 4	Approach Character 5	Device Character 6	Qualifier Character 7

Ø   Pituitary Gland
    Adenohypophysis
    Hypophysis
    Neurohypophysis
1   Pineal Body
5   Adrenal Gland
    Suprarenal gland
K   Thyroid Gland
R   Parathyroid Gland
	Ø Open
	3 Percutaneous
	4 Percutaneous Endoscopic
	X External
		Ø Drainage Device	**Z No Qualifier**

S Endocrine Gland	**Ø Open** **3 Percutaneous** **4 Percutaneous Endoscopic**	**Ø Drainage Device** **2 Monitoring Device** **3 Infusion Device** **Y Other Device**	**Z No Qualifier**
S Endocrine Gland	**X External**	**Ø Drainage Device** **2 Monitoring Device** **3 Infusion Device**	**Z No Qualifier**

Non-OR   ØGW[Ø,1,5,K,R]XØZ
Non-OR   ØGWS[3,4]YZ
Non-OR   ØGWSX[Ø,2,3]Z

Skin and Breast ØHØ–ØHX

Character Meanings*

This Character Meaning table is provided as a guide to assist the user in the identification of character members that may be found in this section of code tables. It **SHOULD NOT** be used to build a PCS code.

Operation–Character 3		Body Part–Character 4		Approach–Character 5		Device–Character 6		Qualifier–Character 7	
Ø	Alteration	Ø	Skin, Scalp	Ø	Open	Ø	Drainage Device	2	Cell Suspension Technique
2	Change	1	Skin, Face	3	Percutaneous	1	Radioactive Element	3	Full Thickness
5	Destruction	2	Skin, Right Ear	7	Via Natural or Artificial Opening	7	Autologous Tissue Substitute	4	Partial Thickness
8	Division	3	Skin, Left Ear	8	Via Natural or Artificial Opening Endoscopic	J	Synthetic Substitute	5	Latissimus Dorsi Myocutaneous Flap
9	Drainage	4	Skin, Neck	X	External	K	Nonautologous Tissue Substitute	6	Transverse Rectus Abdominis Myocutaneous Flap
B	Excision	5	Skin, Chest			N	Tissue Expander	7	Deep Inferior Epigastric Artery Perforator Flap
C	Extirpation	6	Skin, Back			Y	Other Device	8	Superficial Inferior Epigastric Artery Flap
D	Extraction	7	Skin, Abdomen			Z	No Device	9	Gluteal Artery Perforator Flap
H	Insertion	8	Skin, Buttock					D	Multiple
J	Inspection	9	Skin, Perineum					X	Diagnostic
M	Reattachment	A	Skin, Inguinal					Z	No Qualifier
N	Release	B	Skin, Right Upper Arm						
P	Removal	C	Skin, Left Upper Arm						
Q	Repair	D	Skin, Right Lower Arm						
R	Replacement	E	Skin, Left Lower Arm						
S	Reposition	F	Skin, Right Hand						
T	Resection	G	Skin, Left Hand						
U	Supplement	H	Skin, Right Upper Leg						
W	Revision	J	Skin, Left Upper Leg						
X	Transfer	K	Skin, Right Lower Leg						
		L	Skin, Left Lower Leg						
		M	Skin, Right Foot						
		N	Skin, Left Foot						
		P	Skin						
		Q	Finger Nail						
		R	Toe Nail						
		S	Hair						
		T	Breast, Right						
		U	Breast, Left						
		V	Breast, Bilateral						
		W	Nipple, Right						
		X	Nipple, Left						
		Y	Supernumerary Breast						

* Includes skin and breast glands and ducts.

Skin and Breast

AHA Coding Clinic for table ØHØ
2019, 4Q, 30-31   Breast procedures

AHA Coding Clinic for table ØH5
2019, 4Q, 30-31   Breast procedures

AHA Coding Clinic for table ØH9
2019, 4Q, 30-31   Breast procedures

AHA Coding Clinic for table ØHB
2020, 1Q, 31   Repair of buried penis
2019, 4Q, 30-31   Breast procedures
2018, 1Q, 14   Excisional debridement of breast tissue and skin
2016, 3Q, 29   Closure of bilateral alveolar clefts
2015, 3Q, 3-8   Excisional and nonexcisional debridement

AHA Coding Clinic for table ØHC
2019, 4Q, 30-31   Breast procedures

AHA Coding Clinic for table ØHD
2019, 4Q, 30-31   Breast procedures
2016, 1Q, 40   Nonexcisional debridement of skin and subcutaneous tissue
2015, 3Q, 3-8   Excisional and nonexcisional debridement

AHA Coding Clinic for table ØHH
2019, 4Q, 30-31   Breast procedures
2017, 4Q, 67   New qualifier values - Pedicle flap procedures
2014, 2Q, 12   Pedicle latissimus myocutaneous flap with placement of breast tissue expanders
2013, 4Q, 107   Breast tissue expander placement using acellular dermal matrix

AHA Coding Clinic for table ØHJ
2019, 4Q, 30-31   Breast procedures

AHA Coding Clinic for table ØHN
2019, 4Q, 30-31   Breast procedures

AHA Coding Clinic for table ØHP
2019, 4Q, 30-31   Breast procedures
2018, 3Q, 13   Deep inferior epigastric artery perforator flap breast reconstruction
2016, 2Q, 27   Removal of nonviable transverse rectus abdominis myocutaneous (TRAM) flaps

AHA Coding Clinic for table ØHQ
2019, 4Q, 30-31   Breast procedures
2018, 2Q, 25   Third and fourth degree obstetric lacerations
2016, 1Q, 7   Obstetrical perineal laceration repair
2014, 4Q, 31   Delayed wound closure following fracture treatment

AHA Coding Clinic for table ØHR
2020, 1Q, 27   Delayed reconstruction following mastectomy using gracilis musculocutaneous free flap
2020, 1Q, 28   Free flap microvascular breast reconstruction
2020, 1Q, 30   Polarity Skin TE™ application
2019, 4Q, 30-31   Breast procedures
2019, 4Q, 32   Cell suspension epithelial autograft
2019, 3Q, 32   Breast reconstruction with neurotization
2018, 3Q, 13   Deep inferior epigastric artery perforator flap breast reconstruction
2017, 1Q, 35   Epifix® allograft
2014, 3Q, 14   Application of TheraSkin® and excisional debridement

AHA Coding Clinic for table ØHT
2021, 2Q, 16   Goldilocks breast reconstruction
2018, 3Q, 13   Deep inferior epigastric artery perforator flap breast reconstruction
2014, 4Q, 34   Skin-sparing mastectomy

AHA Coding Clinic for table ØHU
2019, 4Q, 30-31   Breast procedures

AHA Coding Clinic for table ØHW
2019, 4Q, 30-31   Breast procedures

Integumentary Anatomy

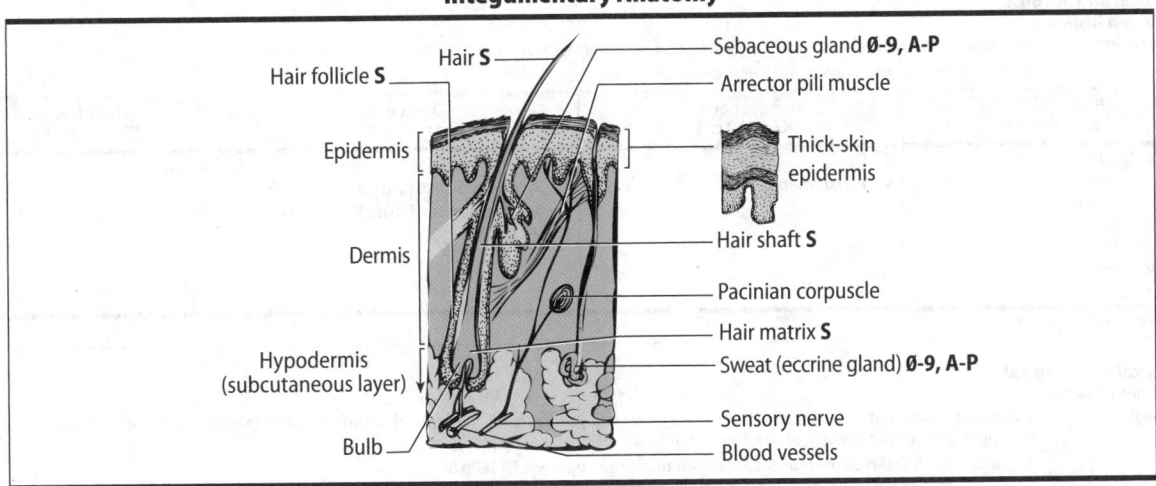

Nail Anatomy

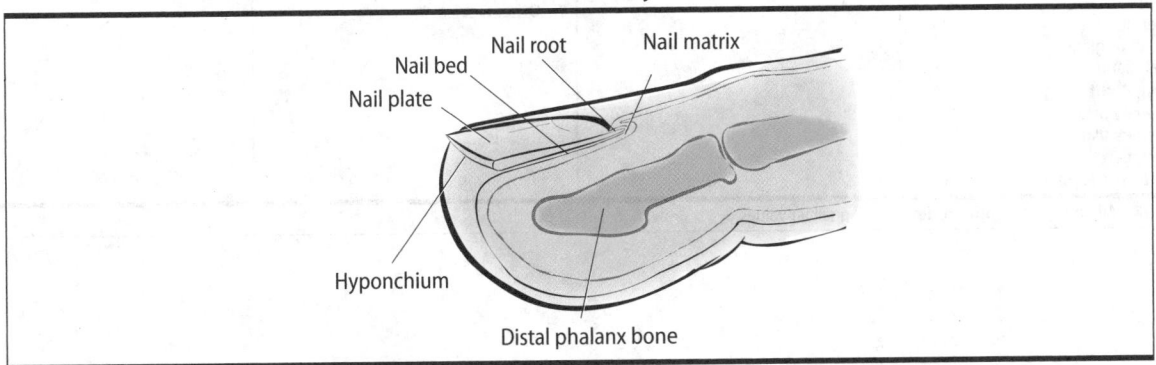

Breast

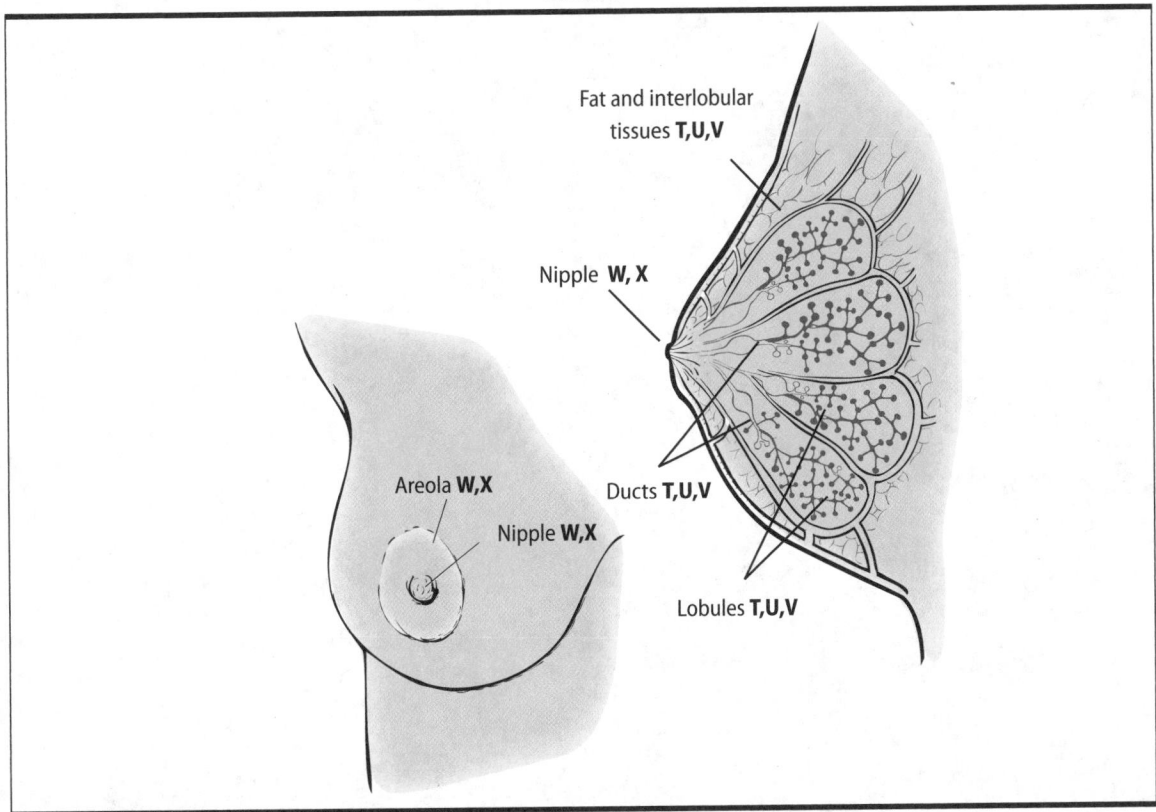

Skin and Breast

Ø **Medical and Surgical**
H **Skin and Breast**
Ø **Alteration** Definition: Modifying the anatomic structure of a body part without affecting the function of the body part
Explanation: Principal purpose is to improve appearance

Body Part Character 4	Approach Character 5	Device Character 6	Qualifier Character 7
T Breast, Right Mammary duct Mammary gland **U** Breast, Left *See* T Breast, Right **V** Breast, Bilateral *See* T Breast, Right	**Ø** Open **3** Percutaneous	**7** Autologous Tissue Substitute **J** Synthetic Substitute **K** Nonautologous Tissue Substitute **Z** No Device	**Z** No Qualifier

Non-OR ØHØ[T,U,V]3JZ

Ø **Medical and Surgical**
H **Skin and Breast**
2 **Change** Definition: Taking out or off a device from a body part and putting back an identical or similar device in or on the same body part without cutting or puncturing the skin or a mucous membrane
Explanation: All CHANGE procedures are coded using the approach EXTERNAL

Body Part Character 4	Approach Character 5	Device Character 6	Qualifier Character 7
P Skin Dermis Epidermis Sebaceous gland Sweat gland **T** Breast, Right Mammary duct Mammary gland **U** Breast, Left *See* T Breast, Right	**X** External	**Ø** Drainage Device **Y** Other Device	**Z** No Qualifier

Non-OR All body part, approach, device, and qualifier values

Ø   Medical and Surgical
H   Skin and Breast
5   Destruction   Definition: Physical eradication of all or a portion of a body part by the direct use of energy, force, or a destructive agent
                          Explanation: None of the body part is physically taken out

Body Part Character 4	Approach Character 5	Device Character 6	Qualifier Character 7
Ø Skin, Scalp 1 Skin, Face 2 Skin, Right Ear 3 Skin, Left Ear 4 Skin, Neck 5 Skin, Chest Breast procedures, skin only 6 Skin, Back 7 Skin, Abdomen 8 Skin, Buttock 9 Skin, Perineum A Skin, Inguinal B Skin, Right Upper Arm C Skin, Left Upper Arm D Skin, Right Lower Arm E Skin, Left Lower Arm F Skin, Right Hand G Skin, Left Hand H Skin, Right Upper Leg J Skin, Left Upper Leg K Skin, Right Lower Leg L Skin, Left Lower Leg M Skin, Right Foot N Skin, Left Foot	X External	Z No Device	D Multiple Z No Qualifier

Q   Finger Nail
     Nail bed
     Nail plate
R   Toe Nail
     See Q Finger Nail
	X External	Z No Device	Z No Qualifier

T   Breast, Right
     Mammary duct
     Mammary gland
U   Breast, Left
     See T Breast, Right
V   Breast, Bilateral
     See T Breast, Right
	Ø Open
	3 Percutaneous
	7 Via Natural or Artificial Opening
	8 Via Natural or Artificial Opening
	     Endoscopic
		Z No Device	Z No Qualifier

W   Nipple, Right
     Areola
X   Nipple, Left
     See W Nipple, Right
	Ø Open
	3 Percutaneous
	7 Via Natural or Artificial Opening
	8 Via Natural or Artificial Opening
	     Endoscopic
	X External
		Z No Device	Z No Qualifier

DRG Non-OR   ØH5[Ø,1,4,5,6,7,8,9,A,B,C,D,E,F,G,H,J,K,L,M,N]XZ[D,Z]
DRG Non-OR   ØH5[Q,R]XZZ
Non-OR   ØH5[2,3]XZ[D,Z]

Ø   **Medical and Surgical**
H   **Skin and Breast**
8   **Division**   Definition: Cutting into a body part, without draining fluids and/or gases from the body part, in order to separate or transect a body part
                   Explanation: All or a portion of the body part is separated into two or more portions

Body Part Character 4	Approach Character 5	Device Character 6	Qualifier Character 7
Ø Skin, Scalp	X External	Z No Device	Z No Qualifier
1 Skin, Face			
2 Skin, Right Ear			
3 Skin, Left Ear			
4 Skin, Neck			
5 Skin, Chest Breast procedures, skin only			
6 Skin, Back			
7 Skin, Abdomen			
8 Skin, Buttock			
9 Skin, Perineum			
A Skin, Inguinal			
B Skin, Right Upper Arm			
C Skin, Left Upper Arm			
D Skin, Right Lower Arm			
E Skin, Left Lower Arm			
F Skin, Right Hand			
G Skin, Left Hand			
H Skin, Right Upper Leg			
J Skin, Left Upper Leg			
K Skin, Right Lower Leg			
L Skin, Left Lower Leg			
M Skin, Right Foot			
N Skin, Left Foot			

Non-OR   All body part, approach, device, and qualifier values

Ø Medical and Surgical
H Skin and Breast
9 Drainage   Definition: Taking or letting out fluids and/or gases from a body part
                       Explanation: The qualifier DIAGNOSTIC is used to identify drainage procedures that are biopsies

Body Part — Character 4		Approach — Character 5	Device — Character 6	Qualifier — Character 7

Ø Skin, Scalp
1 Skin, Face
2 Skin, Right Ear
3 Skin, Left Ear
4 Skin, Neck
5 Skin, Chest
   Breast procedures, skin only
6 Skin, Back
7 Skin, Abdomen
8 Skin, Buttock
9 Skin, Perineum
A Skin, Inguinal
B Skin, Right Upper Arm
C Skin, Left Upper Arm
D Skin, Right Lower Arm
	E Skin, Left Lower Arm
	F Skin, Right Hand
	G Skin, Left Hand
	H Skin, Right Upper Leg
	J Skin, Left Upper Leg
	K Skin, Right Lower Leg
	L Skin, Left Lower Leg
	M Skin, Right Foot
	N Skin, Left Foot
	Q Finger Nail
	   Nail bed
	   Nail plate
	R Toe Nail
	   See Q Finger Nail
		X External	**Ø** Drainage Device	**Z** No Qualifier

Ø Skin, Scalp
1 Skin, Face
2 Skin, Right Ear
3 Skin, Left Ear
4 Skin, Neck
5 Skin, Chest
   Breast procedures, skin only
6 Skin, Back
7 Skin, Abdomen
8 Skin, Buttock
9 Skin, Perineum
A Skin, Inguinal
B Skin, Right Upper Arm
C Skin, Left Upper Arm
D Skin, Right Lower Arm
	E Skin, Left Lower Arm
	F Skin, Right Hand
	G Skin, Left Hand
	H Skin, Right Upper Leg
	J Skin, Left Upper Leg
	K Skin, Right Lower Leg
	L Skin, Left Lower Leg
	M Skin, Right Foot
	N Skin, Left Foot
	Q Finger Nail
	   Nail bed
	   Nail plate
	R Toe Nail
	   See Q Finger Nail
		X External	**Z** No Device	**X** Diagnostic
				Z No Qualifier

T Breast, Right
   Mammary duct
   Mammary gland
U Breast, Left
   See T Breast, Right
V Breast, Bilateral
   See T Breast, Right
		Ø Open
		3 Percutaneous
		7 Via Natural or Artificial Opening
		8 Via Natural or Artificial Opening Endoscopic
			Ø Drainage Device	**Z** No Qualifier

T Breast, Right
   Mammary duct
   Mammary gland
U Breast, Left
   See T Breast, Right
V Breast, Bilateral
   See T Breast, Right
		Ø Open
		3 Percutaneous
		7 Via Natural or Artificial Opening
		8 Via Natural or Artificial Opening Endoscopic
			Z No Device	**X** Diagnostic
				Z No Qualifier

W Nipple, Right
   Areola
X Nipple, Left
   See W Nipple, Right
		Ø Open
		3 Percutaneous
		7 Via Natural or Artificial Opening
		8 Via Natural or Artificial Opening Endoscopic
		X External
			Ø Drainage Device	**Z** No Qualifier

W Nipple, Right
   Areola
X Nipple, Left
   See W Nipple, Right
		Ø Open
		3 Percutaneous
		7 Via Natural or Artificial Opening
		8 Via Natural or Artificial Opening Endoscopic
		X External
			Z No Device	**X** Diagnostic
				Z No Qualifier

Non-OR ØH9[Ø,1,2,3,4,5,6,7,8,A,B,C,D,E,F,G,H,J,K,L,M,N,Q,R]XØZ
Non-OR ØH9[Ø,1,2,3,4,5,6,7,8,A,B,C,D,E,F,G,H,J,K,L,M,N,Q,R]XZ[X,Z]
Non-OR ØH99XZX
Non-OR ØH9[T,U,V][Ø,3,7,8]ØZ
Non-OR ØH9[T,U,V][3,7,8]Z[X,Z]
Non-OR ØH9[W,X][Ø,3,7,8,X]ØZ
Non-OR ØH9[W,X][3,7,8,X]Z[X,Z]

Ø Medical and Surgical
H Skin and Breast
B Excision   Definition: Cutting out or off, without replacement, a portion of a body part
                 Explanation: The qualifier DIAGNOSTIC is used to identify excision procedures that are biopsies

Body Part Character 4	Approach Character 5	Device Character 6	Qualifier Character 7

Ø Skin, Scalp
1 Skin, Face
2 Skin, Right Ear
3 Skin, Left Ear
4 Skin, Neck
5 Skin, Chest
    Breast procedures, skin only
6 Skin, Back
7 Skin, Abdomen
8 Skin, Buttock
9 Skin, Perineum
A Skin, Inguinal
B Skin, Right Upper Arm
C Skin, Left Upper Arm
D Skin, Right Lower Arm
E Skin, Left Lower Arm
F Skin, Right Hand
G Skin, Left Hand
H Skin, Right Upper Leg
J Skin, Left Upper Leg
K Skin, Right Lower Leg
L Skin, Left Lower Leg
M Skin, Right Foot
N Skin, Left Foot
Q Finger Nail
    Nail bed
    Nail plate
R Toe Nail
    See Q Finger Nail
	X External	**Z** No Device	**X** Diagnostic
			Z No Qualifier

T Breast, Right
    Mammary duct
    Mammary gland
U Breast, Left
    See T Breast, Right
V Breast, Bilateral
    See T Breast, Right
Y Supernumerary Breast
	Ø Open
	3 Percutaneous
	7 Via Natural or Artificial Opening
	8 Via Natural or Artificial Opening
	    Endoscopic
		Z No Device	**X** Diagnostic
			Z No Qualifier

W Nipple, Right
    Areola
X Nipple, Left
    See W Nipple, Right
	Ø Open
	3 Percutaneous
	7 Via Natural or Artificial Opening
	8 Via Natural or Artificial Opening
	    Endoscopic
	X External
		Z No Device	**X** Diagnostic
			Z No Qualifier

DRG Non-OR	ØHB9XZZ
Non-OR	ØHB[Ø,1,2,3,4,5,6,7,8,A,B,C,D,E,F,G,H,J,K,L,M,N,Q,R]XZ[X,Z]
Non-OR	ØHB9XZX
Non-OR	ØHB[T,U,V,Y][3,7,8]ZX
Non-OR	ØHB[W,X][3,7,8,X]ZX

Ø   Medical and Surgical
H   Skin and Breast
C   Extirpation   Definition: Taking or cutting out solid matter from a body part

Explanation: The solid matter may be an abnormal byproduct of a biological function or a foreign body; it may be imbedded in a body part or in the lumen of a tubular body part. The solid matter may or may not have been previously broken into pieces.

Body Part Character 4	Approach Character 5	Device Character 6	Qualifier Character 7

Ø Skin, Scalp
1 Skin, Face
2 Skin, Right Ear
3 Skin, Left Ear
4 Skin, Neck
5 Skin, Chest
   Breast procedures, skin only
6 Skin, Back
7 Skin, Abdomen
8 Skin, Buttock
9 Skin, Perineum
A Skin, Inguinal
B Skin, Right Upper Arm
C Skin, Left Upper Arm
D Skin, Right Lower Arm
E Skin, Left Lower Arm
F Skin, Right Hand
G Skin, Left Hand
H Skin, Right Upper Leg
J Skin, Left Upper Leg
K Skin, Right Lower Leg
L Skin, Left Lower Leg
M Skin, Right Foot
N Skin, Left Foot
Q Finger Nail
   Nail bed
   Nail plate
R Toe Nail
   See Q Finger Nail
	X External	**Z** No Device	**Z** No Qualifier

T Breast, Right
   Mammary duct
   Mammary gland
U Breast, Left
   See T Breast, Right
V Breast, Bilateral
   See T Breast, Right
	Ø Open
	3 Percutaneous
	7 Via Natural or Artificial Opening
	8 Via Natural or Artificial Opening Endoscopic
		Z No Device	**Z** No Qualifier

W Nipple, Right
   Areola
X Nipple, Left
   See W Nipple, Right
	Ø Open
	3 Percutaneous
	7 Via Natural or Artificial Opening
	8 Via Natural or Artificial Opening Endoscopic
	X External
		Z No Device	**Z** No Qualifier

Non-OR   ØHC[Ø,1,2,3,4,5,6,7,8,9,A,B,C,D,E,F,G,H,J,K,L,M,N,Q,R]XZZ
Non-OR   ØHC[T,U,V][3,7,8]ZZ
Non-OR   ØHC[W,X][3,7,8,X]ZZ

NC Noncovered Procedure   **LC** Limited Coverage   **QA** Questionable OB Admit   **NT** New Tech Add-on   ✚ Combination Member   ♂ Male   ♀ Female

ICD-10-PCS 2022   433

Skin and Breast

Ø   **Medical and Surgical**
H   **Skin and Breast**
D   **Extraction**   Definition: Pulling or stripping out or off all or a portion of a body part by the use of force
                        Explanation: The qualifier DIAGNOSTIC is used to identify extraction procedures that are biopsies

Body Part Character 4	Approach Character 5	Device Character 6	Qualifier Character 7

Ø Skin, Scalp
1 Skin, Face
2 Skin, Right Ear
3 Skin, Left Ear
4 Skin, Neck
5 Skin, Chest
     Breast procedures, skin only
6 Skin, Back
7 Skin, Abdomen
8 Skin, Buttock
9 Skin, Perineum
A Skin, Inguinal
B Skin, Right Upper Arm
C Skin, Left Upper Arm
D Skin, Right Lower Arm
E Skin, Left Lower Arm
F Skin, Right Hand
G Skin, Left Hand
H Skin, Right Upper Leg
J Skin, Left Upper Leg
K Skin, Right Lower Leg
L Skin, Left Lower Leg
M Skin, Right Foot
N Skin, Left Foot
Q Finger Nail
     Nail bed
     Nail plate
R Toe Nail
     See Q Finger Nail
S Hair
	X External	Z No Device	Z No Qualifier

T Breast, Right
     Mammary duct
     Mammary gland
U Breast, Left
     See T Breast, Right
V Breast, Bilateral
     See T Breast, Right
Y Supernumerary Breast
	Ø Open	Z No Device	Z No Qualifier

Non-OR   All body part, approach, device, and qualifier values

Ø   **Medical and Surgical**
H   **Skin and Breast**
H   **Insertion**   Definition: Putting in a nonbiological appliance that monitors, assists, performs, or prevents a physiological function but does not physically take the place of a body part
                 Explanation: None

Body Part Character 4	Approach Character 5	Device Character 6	Qualifier Character 7
P Skin	**X** External	**Y** Other Device	**Z** No Qualifier

T Breast, Right
   Mammary duct
   Mammary gland
U Breast, Left
   See T Breast, Right
	Ø Open
	3 Percutaneous
	7 Via Natural or Artificial Opening
	8 Via Natural or Artificial Opening Endoscopic
		1 Radioactive Element
		N Tissue Expander
		Y Other Device
			Z No Qualifier

V Breast, Bilateral
   Mammary duct
   Mammary gland
	Ø Open
	3 Percutaneous
	7 Via Natural or Artificial Opening
	8 Via Natural or Artificial Opening Endoscopic
		1 Radioactive Element
		N Tissue Expander
			Z No Qualifier

W Nipple, Right
   Areola
X Nipple, Left
   See W Nipple, Right
	Ø Open
	3 Percutaneous
	7 Via Natural or Artificial Opening
	8 Via Natural or Artificial Opening Endoscopic
		1 Radioactive Element
		N Tissue Expander
			Z No Qualifier

W Nipple, Right
   Areola
X Nipple, Left
   See W Nipple, Right
	X External	**1** Radioactive Element	**Z** No Qualifier

Non-OR   ØHHPXYZ
Non-OR   ØHH[T,U][3,7,8]YZ

Ø   **Medical and Surgical**
H   **Skin and Breast**
J   **Inspection**   Definition: Visually and/or manually exploring a body part
                 Explanation: Visual exploration may be performed with or without optical instrumentation. Manual exploration may be performed directly or through intervening body layers.

Body Part Character 4	Approach Character 5	Device Character 6	Qualifier Character 7

P Skin
   Dermis
   Epidermis
   Sebaceous gland
   Sweat gland
Q Finger Nail
   Nail bed
   Nail plate
R Toe Nail
   See Q Finger Nail
	X External	**Z** No Device	**Z** No Qualifier

T Breast, Right
   Mammary duct
   Mammary gland
U Breast, Left
   See T Breast, Right
	Ø Open
	3 Percutaneous
	7 Via Natural or Artificial Opening
	8 Via Natural or Artificial Opening Endoscopic
		Z No Device	**Z** No Qualifier

Non-OR   All body part, approach, device and qualifier values

NC Noncovered Procedure   **LC** Limited Coverage   **QA** Questionable OB Admit   **NT** New Tech Add-on   ⊞ Combination Member   ♂ Male   ♀ Female

ICD-10-PCS 2022   **435**

ØHH–ØHJ

Ø   **Medical and Surgical**
H   **Skin and Breast**
M   **Reattachment**   Definition: Putting back in or on all or a portion of a separated body part to its normal location or other suitable location
                               Explanation: Vascular circulation and nervous pathways may or may not be reestablished

Body Part Character 4	Approach Character 5	Device Character 6	Qualifier Character 7
Ø Skin, Scalp	**X** External	**Z** No Device	**Z** No Qualifier
1 Skin, Face			
2 Skin, Right Ear			
3 Skin, Left Ear			
4 Skin, Neck			
5 Skin, Chest Breast procedures, skin only			
6 Skin, Back			
7 Skin, Abdomen			
8 Skin, Buttock			
9 Skin, Perineum			
A Skin, Inguinal			
B Skin, Right Upper Arm			
C Skin, Left Upper Arm			
D Skin, Right Lower Arm			
E Skin, Left Lower Arm			
F Skin, Right Hand			
G Skin, Left Hand			
H Skin, Right Upper Leg			
J Skin, Left Upper Leg			
K Skin, Right Lower Leg			
L Skin, Left Lower Leg			
M Skin, Right Foot			
N Skin, Left Foot			

T Breast, Right
    Mammary duct
    Mammary gland			

U Breast, Left *See* T Breast, Right			
V Breast, Bilateral *See* T Breast, Right			
W Nipple, Right Areola			
X Nipple, Left *See* W Nipple, Right			

Non-OR   ØHMØXZZ

Ø   Medical and Surgical
H   Skin and Breast
N   Release   Definition: Freeing a body part from an abnormal physical constraint by cutting or by the use of force
                      Explanation: Some of the restraining tissue may be taken out but none of the body part is taken out

Body Part Character 4	Approach Character 5	Device Character 6	Qualifier Character 7

Ø Skin, Scalp
1 Skin, Face
2 Skin, Right Ear
3 Skin, Left Ear
4 Skin, Neck
5 Skin, Chest
     Breast procedures, skin only
6 Skin, Back
7 Skin, Abdomen
8 Skin, Buttock
9 Skin, Perineum
A Skin, Inguinal
B Skin, Right Upper Arm
C Skin, Left Upper Arm
D Skin, Right Lower Arm
E Skin, Left Lower Arm
F Skin, Right Hand
G Skin, Left Hand
H Skin, Right Upper Leg
J Skin, Left Upper Leg
K Skin, Right Lower Leg
L Skin, Left Lower Leg
M Skin, Right Foot
N Skin, Left Foot
Q Finger Nail
     Nail bed
     Nail plate
R Toe Nail
     See Q Finger Nail
	X External	**Z** No Device	**Z** No Qualifier

T Breast, Right
     Mammary duct
     Mammary gland
U Breast, Left
     See T Breast, Right
V Breast, Bilateral
     See T Breast, Right
	Ø Open
	3 Percutaneous
	7 Via Natural or Artificial Opening
	8 Via Natural or Artificial Opening
	     Endoscopic
		Z No Device	**Z** No Qualifier

W Nipple, Right
     Areola
X Nipple, Left
     See W Nipple, Right
	Ø Open
	3 Percutaneous
	7 Via Natural or Artificial Opening
	8 Via Natural or Artificial Opening
	     Endoscopic
	X External
		Z No Device	**Z** No Qualifier

NC Noncovered Procedure   **LC** Limited Coverage   **QA** Questionable OB Admit   **NT** New Tech Add-on   ⊞ Combination Member   ♂ Male   ♀ Female

ICD-10-PCS 2022   **437**

Ø   Medical and Surgical
H   Skin and Breast
P   Removal   Definition: Taking out or off a device from a body part

Explanation: If a device is taken out and a similar device put in without cutting or puncturing the skin or mucous membrane, the procedure is coded to the root operation CHANGE. Otherwise, the procedure for taking out a device is coded to the root operation REMOVAL.

Body Part Character 4	Approach Character 5	Device Character 6	Qualifier Character 7
P Skin Dermis Epidermis Sebaceous gland Sweat gland	**X** External	**Ø** Drainage Device **7** Autologous Tissue Substitute **J** Synthetic Substitute **K** Nonautologous Tissue Substitute **Y** Other Device	**Z** No Qualifier
Q Finger Nail Nail bed Nail plate **R Toe Nail** *See Q Finger Nail*	**X** External	**Ø** Drainage Device **7** Autologous Tissue Substitute **J** Synthetic Substitute **K** Nonautologous Tissue Substitute	**Z** No Qualifier
S Hair	**X** External	**7** Autologous Tissue Substitute **J** Synthetic Substitute **K** Nonautologous Tissue Substitute	**Z** No Qualifier
T Breast, Right Mammary duct Mammary gland **U Breast, Left** *See T Breast, Right*	**Ø** Open **3** Percutaneous **7** Via Natural or Artificial Opening **8** Via Natural or Artificial Opening Endoscopic	**Ø** Drainage Device **1** Radioactive Element **7** Autologous Tissue Substitute **J** Synthetic Substitute **K** Nonautologous Tissue Substitute **N** Tissue Expander **Y** Other Device	**Z** No Qualifier

Non-OR	ØHPPX[Ø,7,J,K,Y]Z
Non-OR	ØHP[Q,R]X[Ø,7,J,K]Z
Non-OR	ØHPSX[7,J,K]Z
Non-OR	ØHP[T,U]Ø[Ø,1,7,K]Z
Non-OR	ØHP[T,U]3[Ø,1,7,K,Y]Z
Non-OR	ØHP[T,U][7,8][Ø,1,7,J,K,N,Y]Z

Ø   **Medical and Surgical**
H   **Skin and Breast**
Q   **Repair**   Definition: Restoring, to the extent possible, a body part to its normal anatomic structure and function

                                    Explanation: Used only when the method to accomplish the repair is not one of the other root operations

Body Part Character 4	Approach Character 5	Device Character 6	Qualifier Character 7

Ø Skin, Scalp
1 Skin, Face
2 Skin, Right Ear
3 Skin, Left Ear
4 Skin, Neck
5 Skin, Chest
    Breast procedures, skin only
6 Skin, Back
7 Skin, Abdomen
8 Skin, Buttock
9 Skin, Perineum
A Skin, Inguinal
B Skin, Right Upper Arm
C Skin, Left Upper Arm
D Skin, Right Lower Arm
E Skin, Left Lower Arm
F Skin, Right Hand
G Skin, Left Hand
H Skin, Right Upper Leg
J Skin, Left Upper Leg
K Skin, Right Lower Leg
L Skin, Left Lower Leg
M Skin, Right Foot
N Skin, Left Foot
Q Finger Nail
    Nail bed
    Nail plate
R Toe Nail
    See Q Finger Nail
	X External	**Z** No Device	**Z** No Qualifier

T Breast, Right
    Mammary duct
    Mammary gland
U Breast, Left
    See T Breast, Right
V Breast, Bilateral
    See T Breast, Right
Y Supernumerary Breast
	Ø Open
	3 Percutaneous
	7 Via Natural or Artificial Opening
	8 Via Natural or Artificial Opening
	    Endoscopic
		Z No Device	**Z** No Qualifier

W Nipple, Right
    Areola
X Nipple, Left
    See W Nipple, Right
	Ø Open
	3 Percutaneous
	7 Via Natural or Artificial Opening
	8 Via Natural or Artificial Opening
	    Endoscopic
	X External
		Z No Device	**Z** No Qualifier

DRG Non-OR   ØHQ9XZZ
Non-OR   ØHQ[Ø,1,2,3,4,5,6,7,8,A,B,C,D,E,F,G,H,J,K,L,M,N]XZZ

Skin and Breast *(left margin)*

Ø	Medical and Surgical
H	Skin and Breast
R	Replacement

Definition: Putting in or on biological or synthetic material that physically takes the place and/or function of all or a portion of a body part

Explanation: The body part may have been taken out or replaced, or may be taken out, physically eradicated, or rendered nonfunctional during the REPLACEMENT procedure. A REMOVAL procedure is coded for taking out the device used in a previous replacement procedure.

Body Part Character 4		Approach Character 5	Device Character 6	Qualifier Character 7
Ø Skin, Scalp 1 Skin, Face 2 Skin, Right Ear 3 Skin, Left Ear 4 Skin, Neck 5 Skin, Chest Breast procedures, skin only 6 Skin, Back 7 Skin, Abdomen 8 Skin, Buttock 9 Skin, Perineum A Skin, Inguinal	B Skin, Right Upper Arm C Skin, Left Upper Arm D Skin, Right Lower Arm E Skin, Left Lower Arm F Skin, Right Hand G Skin, Left Hand H Skin, Right Upper Leg J Skin, Left Upper Leg K Skin, Right Lower Leg L Skin, Left Lower Leg M Skin, Right Foot N Skin, Left Foot	X External	7 Autologous Tissue Substitute	2 Cell Suspension Technique 3 Full Thickness 4 Partial Thickness
Ø Skin, Scalp 1 Skin, Face 2 Skin, Right Ear 3 Skin, Left Ear 4 Skin, Neck 5 Skin, Chest Breast procedures, skin only 6 Skin, Back 7 Skin, Abdomen 8 Skin, Buttock 9 Skin, Perineum A Skin, Inguinal	B Skin, Right Upper Arm C Skin, Left Upper Arm D Skin, Right Lower Arm E Skin, Left Lower Arm F Skin, Right Hand G Skin, Left Hand H Skin, Right Upper Leg J Skin, Left Upper Leg K Skin, Right Lower Leg L Skin, Left Lower Leg M Skin, Right Foot N Skin, Left Foot	X External	J Synthetic Substitute	3 Full Thickness 4 Partial Thickness Z No Qualifier
Ø Skin, Scalp 1 Skin, Face 2 Skin, Right Ear 3 Skin, Left Ear 4 Skin, Neck 5 Skin, Chest Breast procedures, skin only 6 Skin, Back 7 Skin, Abdomen 8 Skin Buttock 9 Skin, Perineum A Skin, Inguinal	B Skin, Right Upper Arm C Skin, Left Upper Arm D Skin, Right Lower Arm E Skin, Left Lower Arm F Skin, Right Hand G Skin, Left Hand H Skin, Right Upper Leg J Skin, Left Upper Leg K Skin, Right Lower Leg L Skin, Left Lower Leg M Skin, Right Foot N Skin, Left Foot	X External	K Nonautologous Tissue Substitute	3 Full Thickness 4 Partial Thickness

Q Finger Nail
   Nail bed
   Nail plate
	R Toe Nail
	   See Q Finger Nail
	S Hair
		X External	7 Autologous Tissue Substitute
			J Synthetic Substitute
			K Nonautologous Tissue Substitute
				Z No Qualifier

T Breast, Right
   Mammary duct
   Mammary gland
	U Breast, Left
	   See T Breast, Right
	V Breast, Bilateral
	   See T Breast, Right
		Ø Open	7 Autologous Tissue Substitute	5 Latissimus Dorsi Myocutaneous Flap
				6 Transverse Rectus Abdominis Myocutaneous Flap
				7 Deep Inferior Epigastric Artery Perforator Flap
				8 Superficial Inferior Epigastric Artery Flap
				9 Gluteal Artery Perforator Flap
				Z No Qualifier

T Breast, Right
   Mammary duct
   Mammary gland
	U Breast, Left
	   See T Breast, Right
	V Breast, Bilateral
	   See T Breast, Right
		Ø Open	J Synthetic Substitute
			K Nonautologous Tissue Substitute
				Z No Qualifier

T Breast, Right ⊞
   Mammary duct
   Mammary gland
U Breast, Left ⊞
   See T Breast, Right
	V Breast, Bilateral ⊞
	   See T Breast, Right
		3 Percutaneous	7 Autologous Tissue Substitute
			J Synthetic Substitute
			K Nonautologous Tissue Substitute
				Z No Qualifier

W Nipple, Right
   Areola
	X Nipple, Left
	   See W Nipple, Right
		Ø Open
		3 Percutaneous
		X External
			7 Autologous Tissue Substitute
			J Synthetic Substitute
			K Nonautologous Tissue Substitute
				Z No Qualifier

Non-OR   ØHRSX7Z

See Appendix L for Procedure Combinations
  ⊞   ØHR[T,U,V]37Z

Ø Medical and Surgical
H Skin and Breast
S Reposition

Definition: Moving to its normal location, or other suitable location, all or a portion of a body part

Explanation: The body part is moved to a new location from an abnormal location, or from a normal location where it is not functioning correctly. The body part may or may not be cut out or off to be moved to the new location.

Body Part Character 4	Approach Character 5	Device Character 6	Qualifier Character 7

S Hair
W Nipple, Right
   Areola
X Nipple, Left
   See W Nipple, Right
	X External	**Z** No Device	**Z** No Qualifier

T Breast, Right
   Mammary duct
   Mammary gland
U Breast, Left
   See T Breast, Right
V Breast, Bilateral
   See T Breast, Right
	Ø Open	**Z** No Device	**Z** No Qualifier

Non-OR   ØHSSXZZ

Ø Medical and Surgical
H Skin and Breast
T Resection

Definition: Cutting out or off, without replacement, all of a body part

Explanation: None

Body Part Character 4		Approach Character 5	Device Character 6	Qualifier Character 7

Q Finger Nail
   Nail bed
   Nail plate
R Toe Nail
   See Q Finger Nail
W Nipple, Right
   Areola
X Nipple, Left
   See W Nipple, Right
		X External	**Z** No Device	**Z** No Qualifier

T Breast, Right
   Mammary duct
   Mammary gland
U Breast, Left
   See T Breast, Right
V Breast, Bilateral
   See T Breast, Right
Y Supernumerary Breast
	⊞
	
	⊞
	
	⊞
		Ø Open	**Z** No Device	**Z** No Qualifier

Non-OR   ØHT[Q,R]XZZ

See Appendix L for Procedure Combinations
⊞   ØHT[T,U,V]ØZZ

Ø Medical and Surgical
H Skin and Breast
U Supplement

Definition: Putting in or on biological or synthetic material that physically reinforces and/or augments the function of a portion of a body part

Explanation: The biological material is non-living, or is living and from the same individual. The body part may have been previously replaced, and the SUPPLEMENT procedure is performed to physically reinforce and/or augment the function of the replaced body part.

Body Part Character 4	Approach Character 5	Device Character 6	Qualifier Character 7

T Breast, Right
   Mammary duct
   Mammary gland
U Breast, Left
   See T Breast, Right
V Breast, Bilateral
   See T Breast, Right
	Ø Open
	3 Percutaneous
	7 Via Natural or Artificial Opening
	8 Via Natural or Artificial Opening Endoscopic
		7 Autologous Tissue Substitute
		J Synthetic Substitute
		K Nonautologous Tissue Substitute
			Z No Qualifier

W Nipple, Right
   Areola
X Nipple, Left
   See W Nipple, Right
	Ø Open
	3 Percutaneous
	7 Via Natural or Artificial Opening
	8 Via Natural or Artificial Opening Endoscopic
	X External
		7 Autologous Tissue Substitute
		J Synthetic Substitute
		K Nonautologous Tissue Substitute
			Z No Qualifier

Non-OR   ØHU[T,U,V]3JZ

NC Noncovered Procedure   **LC** Limited Coverage   **QA** Questionable OB Admit   **NT** New Tech Add-on   ⊞ Combination Member   ♂ Male   ♀ Female

ICD-10-PCS 2022   **441**

ØHS–ØHU

Ø   Medical and Surgical
H   Skin and Breast
W   Revision

Definition: Correcting, to the extent possible, a portion of a malfunctioning device or the position of a displaced device

Explanation: Revision can include correcting a malfunctioning or displaced device by taking out or putting in components of the device such as a screw or pin

Body Part Character 4	Approach Character 5	Device Character 6	Qualifier Character 7
P Skin Dermis Epidermis Sebaceous gland Sweat gland	X External	Ø Drainage Device 7 Autologous Tissue Substitute J Synthetic Substitute K Nonautologous Tissue Substitute Y Other Device	Z No Qualifier
Q Finger Nail Nail bed Nail plate R Toe Nail See Q Finger Nail	X External	Ø Drainage Device 7 Autologous Tissue Substitute J Synthetic Substitute K Nonautologous Tissue Substitute	Z No Qualifier
S Hair	X External	7 Autologous Tissue Substitute J Synthetic Substitute K Nonautologous Tissue Substitute	Z No Qualifier
T Breast, Right Mammary duct Mammary gland U Breast, Left See T Breast, Right	Ø Open 3 Percutaneous 7 Via Natural or Artificial Opening 8 Via Natural or Artificial Opening Endoscopic	Ø Drainage Device 7 Autologous Tissue Substitute J Synthetic Substitute K Nonautologous Tissue Substitute N Tissue Expander Y Other Device	Z No Qualifier

Non-OR	ØHWPX[Ø,7,J,K,Y]Z
Non-OR	ØHW[Q,R]X[Ø,7,J,K]Z
Non-OR	ØHWSX[7,J,K]Z
Non-OR	ØHW[T,U]Ø[Ø,7,K,N]Z
Non-OR	ØHW[T,U]3[Ø,7,K,N,Y]Z
Non-OR	ØHW[T,U][7,8][Ø,7,J,K,N,Y]Z

Ø   Medical and Surgical
H   Skin and Breast
X   Transfer

Definition: Moving, without taking out, all or a portion of a body part to another location to take over the function of all or a portion of a body part

Explanation: The body part transferred remains connected to its vascular and nervous supply

Body Part Character 4	Approach Character 5	Device Character 6	Qualifier Character 7
Ø Skin, Scalp 1 Skin, Face 2 Skin, Right Ear 3 Skin, Left Ear 4 Skin, Neck 5 Skin, Chest Breast procedures, skin only 6 Skin, Back 7 Skin, Abdomen 8 Skin, Buttock 9 Skin, Perineum A Skin, Inguinal B Skin, Right Upper Arm C Skin, Left Upper Arm D Skin, Right Lower Arm E Skin, Left Lower Arm F Skin, Right Hand G Skin, Left Hand H Skin, Right Upper Leg J Skin, Left Upper Leg K Skin, Right Lower Leg L Skin, Left Lower Leg M Skin, Right Foot N Skin, Left Foot	X External	Z No Device	Z No Qualifier

Subcutaneous Tissue and Fascia ØJØ–ØJX

Character Meanings

This Character Meaning table is provided as a guide to assist the user in the identification of character members that may be found in this section of code tables. It **SHOULD NOT** be used to build a PCS code.

Operation–Character 3	Body Part–Character 4	Approach–Character 5	Device–Character 6	Qualifier–Character 7
Ø Alteration	Ø Subcutaneous Tissue and Fascia, Scalp	Ø Open	Ø Drainage Device OR Monitoring Device, Hemodynamic	B Skin and Subcutaneous Tissue
2 Change	1 Subcutaneous Tissue and Fascia, Face	3 Percutaneous	1 Radioactive Element	C Skin, Subcutaneous Tissue and Fascia
5 Destruction	4 Subcutaneous Tissue and Fascia, Right Neck	X External	2 Monitoring Device	X Diagnostic
8 Division	5 Subcutaneous Tissue and Fascia, Left Neck		3 Infusion Device	Z No Qualifier
9 Drainage	6 Subcutaneous Tissue and Fascia, Chest		4 Pacemaker, Single Chamber	
B Excision	7 Subcutaneous Tissue and Fascia, Back		5 Pacemaker, Single Chamber Rate Responsive	
C Extirpation	8 Subcutaneous Tissue and Fascia, Abdomen		6 Pacemaker, Dual Chamber	
D Extraction	9 Subcutaneous Tissue and Fascia, Buttock		7 Autologous Tissue Substitute OR Cardiac Resynchronization Pacemaker Pulse Generator	
H Insertion	B Subcutaneous Tissue and Fascia, Perineum		8 Defibrillator Generator	
J Inspection	C Subcutaneous Tissue and Fascia, Pelvic Region		9 Cardiac Resynchronization Defibrillator Pulse Generator	
N Release	D Subcutaneous Tissue and Fascia, Right Upper Arm		A Contractility Modulation Device	
P Removal	F Subcutaneous Tissue and Fascia, Left Upper Arm		B Stimulator Generator, Single Array	
Q Repair	G Subcutaneous Tissue and Fascia, Right Lower Arm		C Stimulator Generator, Single Array Rechargeable	
R Replacement	H Subcutaneous Tissue and Fascia, Left Lower Arm		D Stimulator Generator, Multiple Array	
U Supplement	J Subcutaneous Tissue and Fascia, Right Hand		E Stimulator Generator, Multiple Array Rechargeable	
W Revision	K Subcutaneous Tissue and Fascia, Left Hand		F Subcutaneous Defibrillator Lead	
X Transfer	L Subcutaneous Tissue and Fascia, Right Upper Leg		H Contraceptive Device	
	M Subcutaneous Tissue and Fascia, Left Upper Leg		J Synthetic Substitute	
	N Subcutaneous Tissue and Fascia, Right Lower Leg		K Nonautologous Tissue Substitute	
	P Subcutaneous Tissue and Fascia, Left Lower Leg		M Stimulator Generator	
	Q Subcutaneous Tissue and Fascia, Right Foot		N Tissue Expander	
	R Subcutaneous Tissue and Fascia, Left Foot		P Cardiac Rhythm Related Device	
	S Subcutaneous Tissue and Fascia, Head and Neck		V Infusion Device, Pump	
	T Subcutaneous Tissue and Fascia, Trunk		W Vascular Access Device, Totally Implantable	
	V Subcutaneous Tissue and Fascia, Upper Extremity		X Vascular Access Device, Tunneled	
	W Subcutaneous Tissue and Fascia, Lower Extremity		Y Other Device	
			Z No Device	

AHA Coding Clinic for table 0J2

2018, 3Q, 10	Disruption of perma-catheter fibrin sheath via angioplasty of superior vena cava
2017, 2Q, 26	Exchange of tunneled catheter

AHA Coding Clinic for table 0J5

2019, 3Q, 25	Endoscopic removal of pilonidal sinus and cyst

AHA Coding Clinic for table 0J8

2017, 3Q, 11	Bilateral escharotomy of leg, thigh and foot

AHA Coding Clinic for table 0J9

2018, 3Q, 16	Incision and drainage of submandibular space
2018, 3Q, 16	Incision and drainage of neck abscess
2015, 3Q, 23	Incision and drainage of multiple abscess cavities using vessel loop

AHA Coding Clinic for table 0JB

2020, 1Q, 31	Repair of buried penis
2019, 3Q, 25	Endoscopic removal of pilonidal sinus and cyst
2018, 3Q, 17	Excisional debridement of periosteum
2018, 1Q, 7	Placement of fat graft following lumbar decompression surgery
2015, 3Q, 3-8	Excisional and nonexcisional debridement
2015, 2Q, 13	Transfer of free flap to reconstruct orbital defect
2015, 1Q, 29	Fistulectomy with placement of seton
2014, 4Q, 38	Abdominoplasty and abdominal wall plication for hernia repair
2014, 3Q, 22	Transsphenoidal removal of pituitary tumor and fat graft placement

AHA Coding Clinic for table 0JC

2017, 3Q, 22	Replacement of native skull bone flap

AHA Coding Clinic for table 0JD

2016, 3Q, 20	VersaJet™ nonexcisional debridement of leg muscle
2016, 3Q, 21	Nonexcisional debridement of infected lumbar wound
2016, 3Q, 21	Nonexcisional pulsed lavage debridement
2016, 3Q, 22	Debridement of bone and tendon using Tenex ultrasound device
2016, 1Q, 40	Nonexcisional debridement of skin and subcutaneous tissue
2015, 3Q, 3-8	Excisional and nonexcisional debridement
2015, 1Q, 23	Non-Excisional debridement with lavage of wound

AHA Coding Clinic for table 0JH

2020, 4Q, 54	Insertion of other device into subcutaneous tissue and fascia
2020, 4Q, 55	Insertion of subcutaneous pump system for ascites drainage
2020, 2Q, 15	Ommaya Reservoir with Ventricular Catheter Placement
2020, 2Q, 16	Ommaya Reservoir Placement for Cerebrospinal Fluid Infusion Therapy
2019, 4Q, 33	Subcutaneous implantable cardioverter defibrillator lead
2017, 4Q, 63-64	Added and revised device values - Vascular access reservoir
2017, 2Q, 24	Tunneled catheter versus totally implantable catheter
2017, 2Q, 26	Exchange of tunneled catheter
2016, 4Q, 97-98	Phrenic neurostimulator
2016, 2Q, 14	Insertion of peritoneal totally implantable venous access device
2016, 2Q, 15	Removal and replacement of tunneled internal jugular catheter
2015, 4Q, 14	New Section X codes—New Technology procedures
2015, 4Q, 30-31	Vascular access devices
2015, 2Q, 33	Totally implantable central venous access device (Port-a-Cath)
2014, 3Q, 19	End of life replacement of Baclofen pump
2013, 4Q, 116	Device character for Port-A-Cath placement
2012, 4Q, 104	Placement of subcutaneous implantable cardioverter defibrillator

AHA Coding Clinic for table 0JN

2017, 3Q, 11	Bilateral escharotomy of leg, thigh and foot

AHA Coding Clinic for table 0JP

2019, 4Q, 33	Subcutaneous implantable cardioverter defibrillator lead
2018, 4Q, 86	Placement of lumboatrial shunt
2018, 3Q, 29	Decommissioning of left ventricular assist device with exploration of mediastinum
2016, 2Q, 15	Removal and replacement of tunneled internal jugular catheter
2015, 4Q, 31	Vascular access devices
2014, 3Q, 19	End of life replacement of Baclofen pump
2013, 4Q, 109	Separating conjoined twins
2012, 4Q, 104	Placement of subcutaneous implantable cardioverter defibrillator

AHA Coding Clinic for table 0JQ

2017, 3Q, 19	Anterior repair of cystocele
2014, 4Q, 44	Posterior colporrhaphy/rectocele repair

AHA Coding Clinic for table 0JR

2015, 2Q, 13	Transfer of free flap to reconstruct orbital defect

AHA Coding Clinic for table 0JU

2018, 2Q, 20	Prelaminated free flap graft using Alloderm™
2018, 1Q, 7	Placement of fat graft following lumbar decompression surgery

AHA Coding Clinic for table 0JW

2019, 4Q, 33	Subcutaneous implantable cardioverter defibrillator lead
2018, 1Q, 8	Ventricular peritoneal shunt ligation
2015, 4Q, 33	Externalization of peritoneal dialysis catheter
2015, 2Q, 9	Revision of ventriculoperitoneal (VP) shunt
2012, 4Q, 104	Placement of subcutaneous implantable cardioverter defibrillator

AHA Coding Clinic for table 0JX

2021, 2Q, 16	Goldilocks breast reconstruction
2018, 1Q, 10	Complex wound closure using pericranial flap
2014, 3Q, 18	Placement of reverse sural fasciocutaneous pedicle flap
2013, 4Q, 109	Separating conjoined twins

Ø Medical and Surgical
J Subcutaneous Tissue and Fascia
Ø Alteration   Definition: Modifying the anatomic structure of a body part without affecting the function of the body part

                       Explanation: Principal purpose is to improve appearance

Body Part Character 4		Approach Character 5	Device Character 6	Qualifier Character 7
1 Subcutaneous Tissue and Fascia, Face Masseteric fascia Orbital fascia Submandibular space **4 Subcutaneous Tissue and Fascia, Right Neck** Deep cervical fascia Pretracheal fascia Prevertebral fascia **5 Subcutaneous Tissue and Fascia, Left Neck** *See 4 Subcutaneous Tissue and Fascia, Right Neck* **6 Subcutaneous Tissue and Fascia, Chest** Pectoral fascia **7 Subcutaneous Tissue and Fascia, Back** **8 Subcutaneous Tissue and Fascia, Abdomen** **9 Subcutaneous Tissue and Fascia, Buttock** **D Subcutaneous Tissue and Fascia, Right Upper Arm** Axillary fascia Deltoid fascia Infraspinatus fascia Subscapular aponeurosis Supraspinatus fascia	**F Subcutaneous Tissue and Fascia, Left Upper Arm** *See D Subcutaneous Tissue and Fascia, Right Upper Arm* **G Subcutaneous Tissue and Fascia, Right Lower Arm** Antebrachial fascia Bicipital aponeurosis **H Subcutaneous Tissue and Fascia, Left Lower Arm** *See G Subcutaneous Tissue and Fascia, Right Lower Arm* **L Subcutaneous Tissue and Fascia, Right Upper Leg** Crural fascia Fascia lata Iliac fascia Iliotibial tract (band) **M Subcutaneous Tissue and Fascia, Left Upper Leg** *See L Subcutaneous Tissue and Fascia, Right Upper Leg* **N Subcutaneous Tissue and Fascia, Right Lower Leg** **P Subcutaneous Tissue and Fascia, Left Lower Leg**	**Ø Open** **3 Percutaneous**	**Z No Device**	**Z No Qualifier**

Ø Medical and Surgical
J Subcutaneous Tissue and Fascia
2 Change   Definition: Taking out or off a device from a body part and putting back an identical or similar device in or on the same body part without cutting or puncturing the skin or a mucous membrane

                       Explanation: All CHANGE procedures are coded using the approach EXTERNAL

Body Part Character 4	Approach Character 5	Device Character 6	Qualifier Character 7
S Subcutaneous Tissue and Fascia, Head and Neck **T Subcutaneous Tissue and Fascia, Trunk** External oblique aponeurosis Transversalis fascia **V Subcutaneous Tissue and Fascia, Upper Extremity** **W Subcutaneous Tissue and Fascia, Lower Extremity**	**X External**	**Ø Drainage Device** **Y Other Device**	**Z No Qualifier**

Non-OR   All body part, approach, device, and qualifier values

---

NC Noncovered Procedure   LC Limited Coverage   QA Questionable OB Admit   NT New Tech Add-on   ⊞ Combination Member   ♂ Male   ♀ Female

Ø   Medical and Surgical
J   Subcutaneous Tissue and Fascia
5   Destruction   Definition: Physical eradication of all or a portion of a body part by the direct use of energy, force, or a destructive agent
              Explanation: None of the body part is physically taken out

Body Part Character 4		Approach Character 5	Device Character 6	Qualifier Character 7
Ø **Subcutaneous Tissue and Fascia, Scalp** Galea aponeurotica	**G** **Subcutaneous Tissue and Fascia, Right Lower Arm** Antebrachial fascia Bicipital aponeurosis	**Ø** Open **3** Percutaneous	**Z** No Device	**Z** No Qualifier
1 **Subcutaneous Tissue and Fascia, Face** Masseteric fascia Orbital fascia Submandibular space	**H** **Subcutaneous Tissue and Fascia, Left Lower Arm** *See G Subcutaneous Tissue and Fascia, Right Lower Arm*			
4 **Subcutaneous Tissue and Fascia, Right Neck** Deep cervical fascia Pretracheal fascia Prevertebral fascia	**J** **Subcutaneous Tissue and Fascia, Right Hand** Palmar fascia (aponeurosis)			
5 **Subcutaneous Tissue and Fascia, Left Neck** *See 4 Subcutaneous Tissue and Fascia, Right Neck*	**K** **Subcutaneous Tissue and Fascia, Left Hand** *See J Subcutaneous Tissue and Fascia, Right Hand*			
6 **Subcutaneous Tissue and Fascia, Chest** Pectoral fascia	**L** **Subcutaneous Tissue and Fascia, Right Upper Leg** Crural fascia Fascia lata Iliac fascia Iliotibial tract (band)			
7 **Subcutaneous Tissue and Fascia, Back**	**M** **Subcutaneous Tissue and Fascia, Left Upper Leg** *See L Subcutaneous Tissue and Fascia, Right Upper Leg*			
8 **Subcutaneous Tissue and Fascia, Abdomen**	**N** **Subcutaneous Tissue and Fascia, Right Lower Leg**			
9 **Subcutaneous Tissue and Fascia, Buttock**	**P** **Subcutaneous Tissue and Fascia, Left Lower Leg**			
B **Subcutaneous Tissue and Fascia, Perineum**	**Q** **Subcutaneous Tissue and Fascia, Right Foot** Plantar fascia (aponeurosis)			
C **Subcutaneous Tissue and Fascia, Pelvic Region**	**R** **Subcutaneous Tissue and Fascia, Left Foot** *See Q Subcutaneous Tissue and Fascia, Right Foot*			
D **Subcutaneous Tissue and Fascia, Right Upper Arm** Axillary fascia Deltoid fascia Infraspinatus fascia Subscapular aponeurosis Supraspinatus fascia				
F **Subcutaneous Tissue and Fascia, Left Upper Arm** *See D Subcutaneous Tissue and Fascia, Right Upper Arm*				

DRG Non-OR   All body part, approach, device, and qualifier values

Ø　**Medical and Surgical**
J　**Subcutaneous Tissue and Fascia**
8　**Division**　　　Definition: Cutting into a body part, without draining fluids and/or gases from the body part, in order to separate or transect a body part
　　　　　　　　　　　　　Explanation: All or a portion of the body part is separated into two or more portions

Body Part Character 4		Approach Character 5	Device Character 6	Qualifier Character 7
Ø Subcutaneous Tissue and Fascia, Scalp 　Galea aponeurotica **1** Subcutaneous Tissue and Fascia, Face 　Masseteric fascia 　Orbital fascia 　Submandibular space **4** Subcutaneous Tissue and Fascia, Right Neck 　Deep cervical fascia 　Pretracheal fascia 　Prevertebral fascia **5** Subcutaneous Tissue and Fascia, Left Neck 　*See 4 Subcutaneous Tissue and Fascia, Right Neck* **6** Subcutaneous Tissue and Fascia, Chest 　Pectoral fascia **7** Subcutaneous Tissue and Fascia, Back **8** Subcutaneous Tissue and Fascia, Abdomen **9** Subcutaneous Tissue and Fascia, Buttock **B** Subcutaneous Tissue and Fascia, Perineum **C** Subcutaneous Tissue and Fascia, Pelvic Region **D** Subcutaneous Tissue and Fascia, Right Upper Arm 　Axillary fascia 　Deltoid fascia 　Infraspinatus fascia 　Subscapular aponeurosis 　Supraspinatus fascia **F** Subcutaneous Tissue and Fascia, Left Upper Arm 　*See D Subcutaneous Tissue and Fascia, Right Upper Arm* **G** Subcutaneous Tissue and Fascia, Right Lower Arm 　Antebrachial fascia 　Bicipital aponeurosis	**H** Subcutaneous Tissue and Fascia, Left Lower Arm 　*See G Subcutaneous Tissue and Fascia, Right Lower Arm* **J** Subcutaneous Tissue and Fascia, Right Hand 　Palmar fascia (aponeurosis) **K** Subcutaneous Tissue and Fascia, Left Hand 　*See J Subcutaneous Tissue and Fascia, Right Hand* **L** Subcutaneous Tissue and Fascia, Right Upper Leg 　Crural fascia 　Fascia lata 　Iliac fascia 　Iliotibial tract (band) **M** Subcutaneous Tissue and Fascia, Left Upper Leg 　*See L Subcutaneous Tissue and Fascia, Right Upper Leg* **N** Subcutaneous Tissue and Fascia, Right Lower Leg **P** Subcutaneous Tissue and Fascia, Left Lower Leg **Q** Subcutaneous Tissue and Fascia, Right Foot 　Plantar fascia (aponeurosis) **R** Subcutaneous Tissue and Fascia, Left Foot 　*See Q Subcutaneous Tissue and Fascia, Right Foot* **S** Subcutaneous Tissue and Fascia, Head and Neck **T** Subcutaneous Tissue and Fascia, Trunk 　External oblique aponeurosis 　Transversalis fascia **V** Subcutaneous Tissue and Fascia, Upper Extremity **W** Subcutaneous Tissue and Fascia, Lower Extremity	**Ø** Open **3** Percutaneous	**Z** No Device	**Z** No Qualifier

NC Noncovered Procedure　　**LC** Limited Coverage　　**QA** Questionable OB Admit　　**NT** New Tech Add-on　　⊞ Combination Member　　♂ Male　　♀ Female

ICD-10-PCS 2022　　447

ØJ8–ØJ8

Ø   **Medical and Surgical**
J   **Subcutaneous Tissue and Fascia**
9   **Drainage**   Definition: Taking or letting out fluids and/or gases from a body part

                         Explanation: The qualifier DIAGNOSTIC is used to identify drainage procedures that are biopsies

Body Part Character 4		Approach Character 5	Device Character 6	Qualifier Character 7

Ø Subcutaneous Tissue and Fascia, Scalp
    Galea aponeurotica
1 Subcutaneous Tissue and Fascia, Face
    Masseteric fascia
    Orbital fascia
    Submandibular space
4 Subcutaneous Tissue and Fascia, Right Neck
    Deep cervical fascia
    Pretracheal fascia
    Prevertebral fascia
5 Subcutaneous Tissue and Fascia, Left Neck
    See 4 Subcutaneous Tissue and
      Fascia, Right Neck
6 Subcutaneous Tissue and Fascia, Chest
    Pectoral fascia
7 Subcutaneous Tissue and Fascia, Back
8 Subcutaneous Tissue and Fascia, Abdomen
9 Subcutaneous Tissue and Fascia, Buttock
B Subcutaneous Tissue and Fascia, Perineum
C Subcutaneous Tissue and Fascia, Pelvic Region
D Subcutaneous Tissue and Fascia, Right Upper Arm
    Axillary fascia
    Deltoid fascia
    Infraspinatus fascia
    Subscapular aponeurosis
    Supraspinatus fascia
F Subcutaneous Tissue and Fascia, Left Upper Arm
    See D Subcutaneous Tissue and
      Fascia, Right Upper Arm
	G Subcutaneous Tissue and Fascia, Right Lower Arm
	    Antebrachial fascia
	    Bicipital aponeurosis
	H Subcutaneous Tissue and Fascia, Left Lower Arm
	    See G Subcutaneous Tissue and
	      Fascia, Right Lower Arm
	J Subcutaneous Tissue and Fascia, Right Hand
	    Palmar fascia (aponeurosis)
	K Subcutaneous Tissue and Fascia, Left Hand
	    See J Subcutaneous Tissue and
	      Fascia, Right Hand
	L Subcutaneous Tissue and Fascia, Right Upper Leg
	    Crural fascia
	    Fascia lata
	    Iliac fascia
	    Iliotibial tract (band)
	M Subcutaneous Tissue and Fascia, Left Upper Leg
	    See L Subcutaneous Tissue and
	      Fascia, Right Upper Leg
	N Subcutaneous Tissue and Fascia, Right Lower Leg
	P Subcutaneous Tissue and Fascia, Left Lower Leg
	Q Subcutaneous Tissue and Fascia, Right Foot
	    Plantar fascia (aponeurosis)
	R Subcutaneous Tissue and Fascia, Left Foot
	    See Q Subcutaneous Tissue and
	      Fascia, Right Foot
		Ø Open
		3 Percutaneous
			Ø Drainage Device	**Z** No Qualifier

Non-OR   ØJ9[Ø,1,4,5,6,7,8,9,B,C,D,F,G,H,J,K,L,M,N,P,Q,R][Ø,3]ØZ

ØJ9 Continued on next page

ØJ9 Continued

Ø   **Medical and Surgical**
J   **Subcutaneous Tissue and Fascia**
9   **Drainage**   Definition: Taking or letting out fluids and/or gases from a body part
                 Explanation: The qualifier DIAGNOSTIC is used to identify drainage procedures that are biopsies

Body Part Character 4		Approach Character 5	Device Character 6	Qualifier Character 7

Ø **Subcutaneous Tissue and Fascia, Scalp**
  Galea aponeurotica
1 **Subcutaneous Tissue and Fascia, Face**
  Masseteric fascia
  Orbital fascia
  Submandibular space
4 **Subcutaneous Tissue and Fascia, Right Neck**
  Deep cervical fascia
  Pretracheal fascia
  Prevertebral fascia
5 **Subcutaneous Tissue and Fascia, Left Neck**
  See 4 *Subcutaneous Tissue and Fascia, Right Neck*
6 **Subcutaneous Tissue and Fascia, Chest**
  Pectoral fascia
7 **Subcutaneous Tissue and Fascia, Back**
8 **Subcutaneous Tissue and Fascia, Abdomen**
9 **Subcutaneous Tissue and Fascia, Buttock**
B **Subcutaneous Tissue and Fascia, Perineum**
C **Subcutaneous Tissue and Fascia, Pelvic Region**
D **Subcutaneous Tissue and Fascia, Right Upper Arm**
  Axillary fascia
  Deltoid fascia
  Infraspinatus fascia
  Subscapular aponeurosis
  Supraspinatus fascia
F **Subcutaneous Tissue and Fascia, Left Upper Arm**
  See D *Subcutaneous Tissue and Fascia, Right Upper Arm*
	G **Subcutaneous Tissue and Fascia, Right Lower Arm**
	  Antebrachial fascia
	  Bicipital aponeurosis
	H **Subcutaneous Tissue and Fascia, Left Lower Arm**
	  See G *Subcutaneous Tissue and Fascia, Right Lower Arm*
	J **Subcutaneous Tissue and Fascia, Right Hand**
	  Palmar fascia (aponeurosis)
	K **Subcutaenous Tissue and Fascia, Left Hand**
	  See J *Subcutaneous Tissue and Fascia, Right Hand*
	L **Subcutaneous Tissue and Fascia, Right Upper Leg**
	  Crural fascia
	  Fascia lata
	  Iliac fascia
	  Iliotibial tract (band)
	M **Subcutaneous Tissue and Fascia, Left Upper Leg**
	  See L *Subcutaneous Tissue and Fascia, Right Upper Leg*
	N **Subcutaneous Tissue and Fascia, Right Lower Leg**
	P **Subcutaneous Tissue and Fascia, Left Lower Leg**
	Q **Subcutaneous Tissue and Fascia, Right Foot**
	  Plantar fascia (aponeurosis)
	R **Subcutaneous Tissue and Fascia, Left Foot**
	  See Q *Subcutaneous Tissue and Fascia, Right Foot*
		Ø Open
		3 Percutaneous
			Z No Device	X Diagnostic
				Z No Qualifier

Non-OR   ØJ9[Ø,1,4,5,6,7,8,9,B,C,D,F,G,H,J,K,L,M,N,P,Q,R][Ø,3]ZX
Non-OR   ØJ9[Ø,1,4,5,6,7,8,9,B,C,D,F,G,H,J,K,L,M,N,P,Q,R]3ZZ

Ø   Medical and Surgical
J   Subcutaneous Tissue and Fascia
B   Excision   Definition: Cutting out or off, without replacement, a portion of a body part

Explanation: The qualifier DIAGNOSTIC is used to identify excision procedures that are biopsies

Body Part Character 4		Approach Character 5	Device Character 6	Qualifier Character 7
Ø Subcutaneous Tissue and Fascia, Scalp Galea aponeurotica **1 Subcutaneous Tissue and Fascia, Face** Masseteric fascia Orbital fascia Submandibular space **4 Subcutaneous Tissue and Fascia, Right Neck** Deep cervical fascia Pretracheal fascia Prevertebral fascia **5 Subcutaneous Tissue and Fascia, Left Neck** *See 4 Subcutaneous Tissue and Fascia, Right Neck* **6 Subcutaneous Tissue and Fascia, Chest** Pectoral fascia **7 Subcutaneous Tissue and Fascia, Back** **8 Subcutaneous Tissue and Fascia, Abdomen** **9 Subcutaneous Tissue and Fascia, Buttock** **B Subcutaneous Tissue and Fascia, Perineum** **C Subcutaneous Tissue and Fascia, Pelvic Region** **D Subcutaneous Tissue and Fascia, Right Upper Arm** Axillary fascia Deltoid fascia Infraspinatus fascia Subscapular aponeurosis Supraspinatus fascia **F Subcutaneous Tissue and Fascia, Left Upper Arm** *See D Subcutaneous Tissue and Fascia, Right Upper Arm*	**G Subcutaneous Tissue and Fascia, Right Lower Arm** Antebrachial fascia Bicipital aponeurosis **H Subcutaneous Tissue and Fascia, Left Lower Arm** *See G Subcutaneous Tissue and Fascia, Right Lower Arm* **J Subcutaneous Tissue and Fascia, Right Hand** Palmar fascia (aponeurosis) **K Subcutaneous Tissue and Fascia, Left Hand** *See J Subcutaneous Tissue and Fascia, Right Hand* **L Subcutaneous Tissue and Fascia, Right Upper Leg** Crural fascia Fascia lata Iliac fascia Iliotibial tract (band) **M Subcutaneous Tissue and Fascia, Left Upper Leg** *See L Subcutaneous Tissue and Fascia, Right Upper Leg* **N Subcutaneous Tissue and Fascia, Right Lower Leg** **P Subcutaneous Tissue and Fascia, Left Lower Leg** **Q Subcutaneous Tissue and Fascia, Right Foot** Plantar fascia (aponeurosis) **R Subcutaneous Tissue and Fascia, Left Foot** *See Q Subcutaneous Tissue and Fascia, Right Foot*	**Ø Open** **3 Percutaneous**	**Z No Device**	**X Diagnostic** **Z No Qualifier**

DRG Non-OR	ØJB[Ø,4,5,6,7,8,9,B,C,D,F,G,H,L,M,N,P,Q,R]3ZZ
Non-OR	ØJB[Ø,1,4,5,6,7,8,9,B,C,D,F,G,H,J,K,L,M,N,P,Q,R][Ø,3]ZX

Ø   **Medical and Surgical**
J   **Subcutaneous Tissue and Fascia**
C   **Extirpation**   Definition: Taking or cutting out solid matter from a body part

Explanation: The solid matter may be an abnormal byproduct of a biological function or a foreign body; it may be imbedded in a body part or in the lumen of a tubular body part. The solid matter may or may not have been previously broken into pieces.

Body Part Character 4		Approach Character 5	Device Character 6	Qualifier Character 7
Ø **Subcutaneous Tissue and Fascia, Scalp** Galea aponeurotica **1** **Subcutaneous Tissue and Fascia, Face** Masseteric fascia Orbital fascia Submandibular space **4** **Subcutaneous Tissue and Fascia, Right Neck** Deep cervical fascia Pretracheal fascia Prevertebral fascia **5** **Subcutaneous Tissue and Fascia, Left Neck** *See* 4 *Subcutaneous Tissue and Fascia, Right Neck* **6** **Subcutaneous Tissue and Fascia, Chest** Pectoral fascia **7** **Subcutaneous Tissue and Fascia, Back** **8** **Subcutaneous Tissue and Fascia, Abdomen** **9** **Subcutaneous Tissue and Fascia, Buttock** **B** **Subcutaneous Tissue and Fascia, Perineum** **C** **Subcutaneous Tissue and Fascia, Pelvic Region** **D** **Subcutaneous Tissue and Fascia, Right Upper Arm** Axillary fascia Deltoid fascia Infraspinatus fascia Subscapular aponeurosis Supraspinatus fascia **F** **Subcutaneous Tissue and Fascia, Left Upper Arm** *See* D *Subcutaneous Tissue and Fascia, Right Upper Arm*	**G** **Subcutaneous Tissue and Fascia, Right Lower Arm** Antebrachial fascia Bicipital aponeurosis **H** **Subcutaneous Tissue and Fascia, Left Lower Arm** *See* G *Subcutaneous Tissue and Fascia, Right Lower Arm* **J** **Subcutaneous Tissue and Fascia, Right Hand** Palmar fascia (aponeurosis) **K** **Subcutaneous Tissue and Fascia, Left Hand** *See* J *Subcutaneous Tissue and Fascia, Right Hand* **L** **Subcutaneous Tissue and Fascia, Right Upper Leg** Crural fascia Fascia lata Iliac fascia Iliotibial tract (band) **M** **Subcutaneous Tissue and Fascia, Left Upper Leg** *See* L *Subcutaneous Tissue and Fascia, Right Upper Leg* **N** **Subcutaneous Tissue and Fascia, Right Lower Leg** **P** **Subcutaneous Tissue and Fascia, Left Lower Leg** **Q** **Subcutaneous Tissue and Fascia, Right Foot** Plantar fascia (aponeurosis) **R** **Subcutaneous Tissue and Fascia, Left Foot** *See* Q *Subcutaneous Tissue and Fascia, Right Foot*	**Ø** Open **3** Percutaneous	**Z** No Device	**Z** No Qualifier

Non-OR   All body part, approach, device, and qualifier values

NC Noncovered Procedure   **LC** Limited Coverage   **QA** Questionable OB Admit   **NT** New Tech Add-on   ⊞ Combination Member   ♂ Male   ♀ Female

ICD-10-PCS 2022   451

Ø   Medical and Surgical
J   Subcutaneous Tissue and Fascia
D   Extraction   Definition: Pulling or stripping out or off all or a portion of a body part by the use of force
                           Explanation: The qualifier DIAGNOSTIC is used to identify extraction procedures that are biopsies

Body Part Character 4		Approach Character 5	Device Character 6	Qualifier Character 7

Ø Subcutaneous Tissue and Fascia, Scalp
  Galea aponeurotica
	G Subcutaneous Tissue and Fascia, Right Lower Arm
	  Antebrachial fascia
	  Bicipital aponeurosis
		Ø Open
		3 Percutaneous
			Z No Device	**Z** No Qualifier

1 Subcutaneous Tissue and Fascia, Face
  Masseteric fascia
  Orbital fascia
  Submandibular space
	H Subcutaneous Tissue and Fascia, Left Lower Arm
	  See G *Subcutaneous Tissue and Fascia, Right Lower Arm*			

4 Subcutaneous Tissue and Fascia, Right Neck
  Deep cervical fascia
  Pretracheal fascia
  Prevertebral fascia
	J Subcutaneous Tissue and Fascia, Right Hand
	  Palmar fascia (aponeurosis)
	K Subcutaneous Tissue and Fascia, Left Hand			

5 Subcutaneous Tissue and Fascia, Left Neck
  See 4 *Subcutaneous Tissue and Fascia, Right Neck*
	See J *Subcutaneous Tissue and Fascia, Right Hand*
	L Subcutaneous Tissue and Fascia, Right Upper Leg
	  Crural fascia
	  Fascia lata
	  Iliac fascia
	  Iliotibial tract (band)			

6 Subcutaneous Tissue and Fascia, Chest
  Pectoral fascia
	M Subcutaneous Tissue and Fascia, Left Upper Leg
	  See L *Subcutaneous Tissue and Fascia, Right Upper Leg*			

7 Subcutaneous Tissue and Fascia, Back	**N** Subcutaneous Tissue and Fascia, Right Lower Leg			
8 Subcutaneous Tissue and Fascia, Abdomen	**P** Subcutaneous Tissue and Fascia, Left Lower Leg			
9 Subcutaneous Tissue and Fascia, Buttock	**Q** Subcutaneous Tissue and Fascia, Right Foot Plantar fascia (aponeurosis)			
B Subcutaneous Tissue and Fascia, Perineum	**R** Subcutaneous Tissue and Fascia, Left Foot			
C Subcutaneous Tissue and Fascia, Pelvic Region	*See* Q *Subcutaneous Tissue and Fascia, Right Foot*			

D Subcutaneous Tissue and Fascia, Right Upper Arm
  Axillary fascia
  Deltoid fascia
  Infraspinatus fascia
  Subscapular aponeurosis
  Supraspinatus fascia				

F Subcutaneous Tissue and Fascia, Left Upper Arm *See* D *Subcutaneous Tissue and Fascia, Right Upper Arm*				

Non-OR   ØJD[Ø,1,4,5,B,C,D,F,G,H,J,K,N,P,Q,R]3ZZ   **See Appendix L for Procedure Combinations**
                                                         Combo-only   ØJD[6,7,8,9,L,M]3ZZ

Ø   **Medical and Surgical**
J   **Subcutaneous Tissue and Fascia**
H   **Insertion**   Definition: Putting in a nonbiological appliance that monitors, assists, performs, or prevents a physiological function but does not physically take the place of a body part

                  Explanation: None

Body Part Character 4		Approach Character 5	Device Character 6	Qualifier Character 7

Ø Subcutaneous Tissue and Fascia, Scalp
   Galea aponeurotica
1 Subcutaneous Tissue and Fascia, Face
   Masseteric fascia
   Orbital fascia
   Submandibular space
4 Subcutaneous Tissue and Fascia, Right Neck
   Deep cervical fascia
   Pretracheal fascia
   Prevertebral fascia
5 Subcutaneous Tissue and Fascia, Left Neck
   See 4 Subcutaneous Tissue and Fascia, Right Neck
9 Subcutaneous Tissue and Fascia, Buttock
B Subcutaneous Tissue and Fascia, Perineum
	C Subcutaneous Tissue and Fascia, Pelvic Region
	J Subcutaneous Tissue and Fascia, Right Hand
	   Palmar fascia (aponeurosis)
	K Subcutaneous Tissue and Fascia, Left Hand
	   See J Subcutaneous Tissue and Fascia, Right Hand
	Q Subcutaneous Tissue and Fascia, Right Foot
	   Plantar fascia (aponeurosis)
	R Subcutaneous Tissue and Fascia, Left Foot
	   See Q Subcutaneous Tissue and Fascia, Right Foot
		Ø Open
		3 Percutaneous
			N Tissue Expander	**Z** No Qualifier

6 Subcutaneous Tissue and Fascia, Chest ⊞ Pectoral fascia		**Ø** Open **3** Percutaneous	**Ø** Monitoring Device, Hemodynamic **2** Monitoring Device **4** Pacemaker, Single Chamber **5** Pacemaker, Single Chamber Rate Responsive **6** Pacemaker, Dual Chamber **7** Cardiac Resynchronization Pacemaker Pulse Generator **8** Defibrillator Generator **9** Cardiac Resynchronization Defibrillator Pulse Generator **A** Contractility Modulation Device NT **B** Stimulator Generator, Single Array **C** Stimulator Generator, Single Array Rechargeable **D** Stimulator Generator, Multiple Array **E** Stimulator Generator, Multiple Array Rechargeable **F** Subcutaneous Defibrillator Lead **H** Contraceptive Device **M** Stimulator Generator NT **N** Tissue Expander **P** Cardiac Rhythm Related Device **V** Infusion Device, Pump **W** Vascular Access Device, Totally Implantable **X** Vascular Access Device, Tunneled **Y** Other Device	**Z** No Qualifier
7 Subcutaneous Tissue and Fascia, Back NC ⊞		**Ø** Open **3** Percutaneous	**B** Stimulator Generator, Single Array **C** Stimulator Generator, Single Array Rechargeable **D** Stimulator Generator, Multiple Array **E** Stimulator Generator, Multiple Array Rechargeable **M** Stimulator Generator **N** Tissue Expander **V** Infusion Device, Pump **Y** Other Device	**Z** No Qualifier

DRG Non-OR ØJH6[Ø,3][4,5,6,7,H,P,X]Z	NC ØJH7[Ø,3]MZ
DRG Non-OR ØJH63WX	NT ØJH6[Ø,3]AZ
Non-OR ØJH63YZ	*See* Appendix H for applicable device trade name
Non-OR ØJH73YZ	NT ØJH6ØMZ in combination with Ø3HK3MZ or Ø3HL3MZ
HAC ØJH6[Ø,3][4,5,6,7,8,9,P]Z when reported with SDx K68.11 or T81.4Ø-T81.49, T82.6-T82.7 with 7th character A	*See* Appendix H for applicable device trade name
HAC ØJH63XZ when reported with SDx J95.811	**See Appendix L for Procedure Combinations** ⊞ ØJH6[Ø,3][4,5,6,7,8,9,A,B,C,D,E,F,P]Z ⊞ ØJH7[Ø,3][B,C,D,E]Z

ØJH Continued on next page

NC Noncovered Procedure   LC Limited Coverage   QA Questionable OB Admit   NT New Tech Add-on   ⊞ Combination Member   ♂ Male   ♀ Female

Ø   **Medical and Surgical**   *ØJH Continued*
J   **Subcutaneous Tissue and Fascia**
H   **Insertion**   Definition: Putting in a nonbiological appliance that monitors, assists, performs, or prevents a physiological function but does not physically
take the place of a body part
Explanation: None

Body Part Character 4	Approach Character 5	Device Character 6	Qualifier Character 7
8 Subcutaneous Tissue and Fascia, Abdomen NC⊞	**Ø** Open **3** Percutaneous	**Ø** Monitoring Device, Hemodynamic **2** Monitoring Device **4** Pacemaker, Single Chamber **5** Pacemaker, Single Chamber Rate Responsive **6** Pacemaker, Dual Chamber **7** Cardiac Resynchronization Pacemaker Pulse Generator **8** Defibrillator Generator **9** Cardiac Resynchronization Defibrillator Pulse Generator **A** Contractility Modulation Device NT **B** Stimulator Generator, Single Array **C** Stimulator Generator, Single Array Rechargeable **D** Stimulator Generator, Multiple Array **E** Stimulator Generator, Multiple Array Rechargeable **H** Contraceptive Device **M** Stimulator Generator **N** Tissue Expander **P** Cardiac Rhythm Related Device **V** Infusion Device, Pump **W** Vascular Access Device, Totally Implantable **X** Vascular Access Device, Tunneled **Y** Other Device	**Z** No Qualifier
D Subcutaneous Tissue and Fascia, Right Upper Arm Axillary fascia Deltoid fascia Infraspinatus fascia Subscapular aponeurosis Supraspinatus fascia **F** Subcutaneous Tissue and Fascia, Left Upper Arm *See D Subcutaneous Tissue and Fascia, Right Upper Arm* **G** Subcutaneous Tissue and Fascia, Right Lower Arm Antebrachial fascia Bicipital aponeurosis **H** Subcutaneous Tissue and Fascia, Left Lower Arm *See G Subcutaneous Tissue and Fascia, Right Lower Arm* **L** Subcutaneous Tissue and Fascia, Right Upper Leg Crural fascia Fascia lata Iliac fascia Iliotibial tract (band) **M** Subcutaneous Tissue and Fascia, Left Upper Leg *See L Subcutaneous Tissue and Fascia, Right Upper Leg* **N** Subcutaneous Tissue and Fascia, Right Lower Leg **P** Subcutaneous Tissue and Fascia, Left Lower Leg	**Ø** Open **3** Percutaneous	**H** Contraceptive Device **N** Tissue Expander **V** Infusion Device, Pump **W** Vascular Access Device, Totally Implantable **X** Vascular Access Device, Tunneled	**Z** No Qualifier
S Subcutaneous Tissue and Fascia, Head and Neck **V** Subcutaneous Tissue and Fascia, Upper Extremity **W** Subcutaneous Tissue and Fascia, Lower Extremity	**Ø** Open **3** Percutaneous	**1** Radioactive Element **3** Infusion Device **Y** Other Device	**Z** No Qualifier
T Subcutaneous Tissue and Fascia, Trunk External oblique aponeurosis Transversalis fascia	**Ø** Open **3** Percutaneous	**1** Radioactive Element **3** Infusion Device **V** Infusion Device, Pump **Y** Other Device	**Z** No Qualifier

DRG Non-OR   ØJH8[Ø,3][2,4,5,6,7,H,P,X]Z
DRG Non-OR   ØJH83WX
DRG Non-OR   ØJH[D,F,G,H,L,M,N,P]ØXZ
DRG Non-OR   ØJH[D,F,G,H,L,M,N,P]3[W,X]Z
DRG Non-OR   ØJHN3HZ
DRG Non-OR   ØJHP[Ø,3]HZ

Non-OR   ØJH83YZ
Non-OR   ØJH[D,F,G,H,L,M][Ø,3]HZ
Non-OR   ØJHNØHZ
Non-OR   ØJH[S,V,W]Ø3Z
Non-OR   ØJH[S,V,W]3[3,Y]Z
Non-OR   ØJHTØ3Z
Non-OR   ØJHT3[3,Y]Z

HAC   ØJH8[Ø,3][4,5,6,7,8,9,P]Z when reported with SDx K68.11 or T81.4Ø-T81.49, T82.6-T82.7 with 7th character A
NC   ØJH8[Ø,3]MZ
NT   ØJHB[Ø,3]AZ *See Appendix H for applicable device trade name*

See Appendix L for Procedure Combinations
⊞   ØJH8[Ø,3][4,5,6,7,8,9,A,B,C,D,E,P]Z

Ø   **Medical and Surgical**
J   **Subcutaneous Tissue and Fascia**
J   **Inspection**   Definition: Visually and/or manually exploring a body part

Explanation: Visual exploration may be performed with or without optical instrumentation. Manual exploration may be performed directly or through intervening body layers.

Body Part Character 4	Approach Character 5	Device Character 6	Qualifier Character 7
S Subcutaneous Tissue and Fascia, Head and Neck **T** Subcutaneous Tissue and Fascia, Trunk External oblique aponeurosis Transversalis fascia **V** Subcutaneous Tissue and Fascia, Upper Extremity **W** Subcutaneous Tissue and Fascia, Lower Extremity	**Ø** Open **3** Percutaneous **X** External	**Z** No Device	**Z** No Qualifier

Non-OR   All body part, approach, device, and qualifier values

---

Ø   **Medical and Surgical**
J   **Subcutaneous Tissue and Fascia**
N   **Release**   Definition: Freeing a body part from an abnormal physical constraint by cutting or by the use of force

Explanation: Some of the restraining tissue may be taken out but none of the body part is taken out

Body Part Character 4	Approach Character 5	Device Character 6	Qualifier Character 7
Ø Subcutaneous Tissue and Fascia, Scalp Galea aponeurotica **1** Subcutaneous Tissue and Fascia, Face Masseteric fascia Orbital fascia Submandibular space **4** Subcutaneous Tissue and Fascia, Right Neck Deep cervical fascia Pretracheal fascia Prevertebral fascia **5** Subcutaneous Tissue and Fascia, Left Neck *See 4 Subcutaneous Tissue and Fascia, Right Neck* **6** Subcutaneous Tissue and Fascia, Chest Pectoral fascia **7** Subcutaneous Tissue and Fascia, Back **8** Subcutaneous Tissue and Fascia, Abdomen **9** Subcutaneous Tissue and Fascia, Buttock **B** Subcutaneous Tissue and Fascia, Perineum **C** Subcutaneous Tissue and Fascia, Pelvic Region **D** Subcutaneous Tissue and Fascia, Right Upper Arm Axillary fascia Deltoid fascia Infraspinatus fascia Subscapular aponeurosis Supraspinatus fascia **F** Subcutaneous Tissue and Fascia, Left Upper Arm *See D Subcutaneous Tissue and Fascia, Right Upper Arm* **G** Subcutaneous Tissue and Fascia, Right Lower Arm Antebrachial fascia Bicipital aponeurosis **H** Subcutaneous Tissue and Fascia, Left Lower Arm *See G Subcutaneous Tissue and Fascia, Right Lower Arm* **J** Subcutaneous Tissue and Fascia, Right Hand Palmar fascia (aponeurosis) **K** Subcutaneous Tissue and Fascia, Left Hand *See J Subcutaneous Tissue and Fascia, Right Hand* **L** Subcutaneous Tissue and Fascia, Right Upper Leg Crural fascia Fascia lata Iliac fascia Iliotibial tract (band) **M** Subcutaneous Tissue and Fascia, Left Upper Leg *See L Subcutaneous Tissue and Fascia, Right Upper Leg* **N** Subcutaneous Tissue and Fascia, Right Lower Leg **P** Subcutaneous Tissue and Fascia, Left Lower Leg **Q** Subcutaneous Tissue and Fascia, Right Foot Plantar fascia (aponeurosis) **R** Subcutaneous Tissue and Fascia, Left Foot *See Q Subcutaneous Tissue and Fascia, Right Foot*	**Ø** Open **3** Percutaneous **X** External	**Z** No Device	**Z** No Qualifier

Non-OR   ØJN[Ø,1,4,5,6,7,8,9,B,C,D,F,G,H,J,K,L,M,N,P,Q,R]XZZ

NC Noncovered Procedure   **LC** Limited Coverage   **QA** Questionable OB Admit   **NT** New Tech Add-on   ⊞ Combination Member   ♂ Male   ♀ Female

ICD-10-PCS 2022   **455**

Subcutaneous Tissue and Fascia *(left margin)*

Ø   **Medical and Surgical**
J   **Subcutaneous Tissue and Fascia**
P   **Removal**   Definition: Taking out or off a device from a body part

Explanation: If a device is taken out and a similar device put in without cutting or puncturing the skin or mucous membrane, the procedure is coded to the root operation CHANGE. Otherwise, the procedure for taking out a device is coded to the root operation REMOVAL.

Body Part Character 4		Approach Character 5		Device Character 6		Qualifier Character 7
S	Subcutaneous Tissue and Fascia, Head and Neck	Ø Open 3 Percutaneous		Ø Drainage Device 1 Radioactive Element 3 Infusion Device 7 Autologous Tissue Substitute J Synthetic Substitute K Nonautologous Tissue Substitute N Tissue Expander Y Other Device		Z No Qualifier
S	Subcutaneous Tissue and Fascia, Head and Neck	X External		Ø Drainage Device 1 Radioactive Element 3 Infusion Device		Z No Qualifier
T	Subcutaneous Tissue and Fascia, Trunk External oblique aponeurosis Transversalis fascia	Ø Open 3 Percutaneous		Ø Drainage Device 1 Radioactive Element 2 Monitoring Device 3 Infusion Device 7 Autologous Tissue Substitute F Subcutaneous Defibrillator Lead H Contraceptive Device J Synthetic Substitute K Nonautologous Tissue Substitute M Stimulator Generator N Tissue Expander P Cardiac Rhythm Related Device V Infusion Device, Pump W Vascular Access Device, Totally Implantable X Vascular Access Device, Tunneled Y Other Device		Z No Qualifier
T	Subcutaneous Tissue and Fascia, Trunk External oblique aponeurosis Transversalis fascia	X External		Ø Drainage Device 1 Radioactive Element 2 Monitoring Device 3 Infusion Device H Contraceptive Device V Infusion Device, Pump X Vascular Access Device, Tunneled		Z No Qualifier
V	Subcutaneous Tissue and Fascia, Upper Extremity	Ø Open 3 Percutaneous		Ø Drainage Device 1 Radioactive Element 3 Infusion Device 7 Autologous Tissue Substitute H Contraceptive Device J Synthetic Substitute K Nonautologous Tissue Substitute N Tissue Expander V Infusion Device, Pump W Vascular Access Device, Totally Implantable X Vascular Access Device, Tunneled Y Other Device		Z No Qualifier
W	Subcutaneous Tissue and Fascia, Lower Extremity					
V	Subcutaneous Tissue and Fascia, Upper Extremity	X External		Ø Drainage Device 1 Radioactive Element 3 Infusion Device H Contraceptive Device V Infusion Device, Pump X Vascular Access Device, Tunneled		Z No Qualifier
W	Subcutaneous Tissue and Fascia, Lower Extremity					

Non-OR	ØJPS[Ø,3][Ø,1,3,7,J,K,N,Y]Z
Non-OR	ØJPSX[Ø,1,3]Z
Non-OR	ØJPT[Ø,3][Ø,1,2,3,7,H,J,K,M,N,V,W,X,Y]Z
Non-OR	ØJPTX[Ø,1,2,3,H,V,X]Z
Non-OR	ØJP[V,W][Ø,3][Ø,1,3,7,H,J,K,N,V,W,X,Y]Z
Non-OR	ØJP[V,W]X[Ø,1,3,H,V,X]Z
HAC	ØJPT[Ø,3][F,P]Z when reported with SDx K68.11 or T81.4Ø-T81.49, T82.6-T82.7 with 7th character A

Ø   Medical and Surgical
J   Subcutaneous Tissue and Fascia
Q   Repair   Definition: Restoring, to the extent possible, a body part to its normal anatomic structure and function
              Explanation: Used only when the method to accomplish the repair is not one of the other root operations

Body Part Character 4		Approach Character 5	Device Character 6	Qualifier Character 7
Ø Subcutaneous Tissue and Fascia, Scalp Galea aponeurotica **1** Subcutaneous Tissue and Fascia, Face Masseteric fascia Orbital fascia Submandibular space **4** Subcutaneous Tissue and Fascia, Right Neck Deep cervical fascia Pretracheal fascia Prevertebral fascia **5** Subcutaneous Tissue and Fascia, Left Neck *See 4 Subcutaneous Tissue and Fascia, Right Neck* **6** Subcutaneous Tissue and Fascia, Chest Pectoral fascia **7** Subcutaneous Tissue and Fascia, Back **8** Subcutaneous Tissue and Fascia, Abdomen **9** Subcutaneous Tissue and Fascia, Buttock **B** Subcutaneous Tissue and Fascia, Perineum **C** Subcutaneous Tissue and Fascia, Pelvic Region **D** Subcutaneous Tissue and Fascia, Right Upper Arm Axillary fascia Deltoid fascia Infraspinatus fascia Subscapular aponeurosis Supraspinatus fascia **F** Subcutaneous Tissue and Fascia, Left Upper Arm *See D Subcutaneous Tissue and Fascia, Right Upper Arm*	**G** Subcutaneous Tissue and Fascia, Right Lower Arm Antebrachial fascia Bicipital aponeurosis **H** Subcutaneous Tissue and Fascia, Left Lower Arm *See G Subcutaneous Tissue and Fascia, Right Lower Arm* **J** Subcutaneous Tissue and Fascia, Right Hand Palmar fascia (aponeurosis) **K** Subcutaneous Tissue and Fascia, Left Hand *See J Subcutaneous Tissue and Fascia, Right Hand* **L** Subcutaneous Tissue and Fascia, Right Upper Leg Crural fascia Fascia lata Iliac fascia Iliotibial tract (band) **M** Subcutaneous Tissue and Fascia, Left Upper Leg *See L Subcutaneous Tissue and Fascia, Right Upper Leg* **N** Subcutaneous Tissue and Fascia, Right Lower Leg **P** Subcutaneous Tissue and Fascia, Left Lower Leg **Q** Subcutaneous Tissue and Fascia, Right Foot Plantar fascia (aponeurosis) **R** Subcutaneous Tissue and Fascia, Left Foot *See Q Subcutaneous Tissue and Fascia, Right Foot*	**Ø** Open **3** Percutaneous	**Z** No Device	**Z** No Qualifier

Non-OR   ØJQ[Ø,1,4,5,6,7,8,9,B,C,D,F,G,H,J,K,L,M,N,P,Q,R]3ZZ

NC Noncovered Procedure   **LC** Limited Coverage   **QA** Questionable OB Admit   **NT** New Tech Add-on   ⊞ Combination Member   ♂ Male   ♀ Female

ICD-10-PCS 2022   **457**

Ø   Medical and Surgical
J   Subcutaneous Tissue and Fascia
R   Replacement   Definition: Putting in or on biological or synthetic material that physically takes the place and/or function of all or a portion of a body part
Explanation: The body part may have been taken out or replaced, or may be taken out, physically eradicated, or rendered nonfunctional during the REPLACEMENT procedure. A REMOVAL procedure is coded for taking out the device used in a previous replacement procedure.

Body Part Character 4		Approach Character 5	Device Character 6	Qualifier Character 7
Ø **Subcutaneous Tissue and Fascia, Scalp** Galea aponeurotica **1** **Subcutaneous Tissue and Fascia, Face** Masseteric fascia Orbital fascia Submandibular space **4** **Subcutaneous Tissue and Fascia, Right Neck** Deep cervical fascia Pretracheal fascia Prevertebral fascia **5** **Subcutaneous Tissue and Fascia, Left Neck** *See* 4 *Subcutaneous Tissue and Fascia, Right Neck* **6** **Subcutaneous Tissue and Fascia, Chest** Pectoral fascia **7** **Subcutaneous Tissue and Fascia, Back** **8** **Subcutaneous Tissue and Fascia, Abdomen** **9** **Subcutaneous Tissue and Fascia, Buttock** **B** **Subcutaneous Tissue and Fascia, Perineum** **C** **Subcutaneous Tissue and Fascia, Pelvic Region** **D** **Subcutaneous Tissue and Fascia, Right Upper Arm** Axillary fascia Deltoid fascia Infraspinatus fascia Subscapular aponeurosis Supraspinatus fascia **F** **Subcutaneous Tissue and Fascia, Left Upper Arm** *See* D *Subcutaneous Tissue and Fascia, Right Upper Arm*	**G** **Subcutaneous Tissue and Fascia, Right Lower Arm** Antebrachial fascia Bicipital aponeurosis **H** **Subcutaneous Tissue and Fascia, Left Lower Arm** *See* G *Subcutaneous Tissue and Fascia, Right Lower Arm* **J** **Subcutaneous Tissue and Fascia, Right Hand** Palmar fascia (aponeurosis) **K** **Subcutaneous Tissue and Fascia, Left Hand** *See* J *Subcutaneous Tissue and Fascia, Right Hand* **L** **Subcutaneous Tissue and Fascia, Right Upper Leg** Crural fascia Fascia lata Iliac fascia Iliotibial tract (band) **M** **Subcutaneous Tissue and Fascia, Left Upper Leg** *See* L *Subcutaneous Tissue and Fascia, Right Upper Leg* **N** **Subcutaneous Tissue and Fascia, Right Lower Leg** **P** **Subcutaneous Tissue and Fascia, Left Lower Leg** **Q** **Subcutaneous Tissue and Fascia, Right Foot** Plantar fascia (aponeurosis) **R** **Subcutaneous Tissue and Fascia, Left Foot** *See* Q *Subcutaneous Tissue and Fascia, Right Foot*	**Ø** **Open** **3** **Percutaneous**	**7** **Autologous Tissue Substitute** **J** **Synthetic Substitute** **K** **Nonautologous Tissue Substitute**	**Z** **No Qualifier**

Ø   Medical and Surgical
J   Subcutaneous Tissue and Fascia
U   Supplement: Definition: Putting in or on biological or synthetic material that physically reinforces and/or augments the function of a portion of a body part
       Explanation: The biological material is non-living, or is living and from the same individual. The body part may have been previously replaced, and the SUPPLEMENT procedure is performed to physically reinforce and/or augment the function of the replaced body part.

Body Part Character 4		Approach Character 5	Device Character 6	Qualifier Character 7
Ø **Subcutaneous Tissue and Fascia, Scalp** Galea aponeurotica	**G** **Subcutaneous Tissue and Fascia, Right Lower Arm** Antebrachial fascia Bicipital aponeurosis	**Ø** Open **3** Percutaneous	**7** Autologous Tissue Substitute **J** Synthetic Substitute **K** Nonautologous Tissue Substitute	**Z** No Qualifier
1 **Subcutaneous Tissue and Fascia, Face** Masseteric fascia Orbital fascia Submandibular space	**H** **Subcutaneous Tissue and Fascia, Left Lower Arm** *See G Subcutaneous Tissue and Fascia, Right Lower Arm*			
4 **Subcutaneous Tissue and Fascia, Right Neck** Deep cervical fascia Pretracheal fascia Prevertebral fascia	**J** **Subcutaneous Tissue and Fascia, Right Hand** Palmar fascia (aponeurosis)			
5 **Subcutaneous Tissue and Fascia, Left Neck** *See 4 Subcutaneous Tissue and Fascia, Right Neck*	**K** **Subcutaneous Tissue and Fascia, Left Hand** *See J Subcutaneous Tissue and Fascia, Right Hand*			
6 **Subcutaneous Tissue and Fascia, Chest** Pectoral fascia	**L** **Subcutaneous Tissue and Fascia, Right Upper Leg** Crural fascia Fascia lata Iliac fascia Iliotibial tract (band)			
7 **Subcutaneous Tissue and Fascia, Back**	**M** **Subcutaneous Tissue and Fascia, Left Upper Leg** *See L Subcutaneous Tissue and Fascia, Right Upper Leg*			
8 **Subcutaneous Tissue and Fascia, Abdomen**	**N** **Subcutaneous Tissue and Fascia, Right Lower Leg**			
9 **Subcutaneous Tissue and Fascia, Buttock**	**P** **Subcutaneous Tissue and Fascia, Left Lower Leg**			
B **Subcutaneous Tissue and Fascia, Perineum**	**Q** **Subcutaneous Tissue and Fascia, Right Foot** Plantar fascia (aponeurosis)			
C **Subcutaneous Tissue and Fascia, Pelvic Region**	**R** **Subcutaneous Tissue and Fascia, Left Foot** *See Q Subcutaneous Tissue and Fascia, Right Foot*			
D **Subcutaneous Tissue and Fascia, Right Upper Arm** Axillary fascia Deltoid fascia Infraspinatus fascia Subscapular aponeurosis Supraspinatus fascia				
F **Subcutaneous Tissue and Fascia, Left Upper Arm** *See D Subcutaneous Tissue and Fascia, Right Upper Arm*				

NC Noncovered Procedure   **LC** Limited Coverage   **QA** Questionable OB Admit   **NT** New Tech Add-on   ⊞ Combination Member   ♂ Male   ♀ Female

ICD-10-PCS 2022   459

Ø   Medical and Surgical
J   Subcutaneous Tissue and Fascia
W   Revision   Definition: Correcting, to the extent possible, a portion of a malfunctioning device or the position of a displaced device
                       Explanation: Revision can include correcting a malfunctioning or displaced device by taking out or putting in components of the device such as a screw or pin

Body Part Character 4	Approach Character 5	Device Character 6	Qualifier Character 7
S Subcutaneous Tissue and Fascia, Head and Neck	**Ø** Open **3** Percutaneous	**Ø** Drainage Device **3** Infusion Device **7** Autologous Tissue Substitute **J** Synthetic Substitute **K** Nonautologous Tissue Substitute **N** Tissue Expander **Y** Other Device	**Z** No Qualifier
S Subcutaneous Tissue and Fascia, Head and Neck	**X** External	**Ø** Drainage Device **3** Infusion Device **7** Autologous Tissue Substitute **J** Synthetic Substitute **K** Nonautologous Tissue Substitute **N** Tissue Expander	**Z** No Qualifier
T Subcutaneous Tissue and Fascia, Trunk External oblique aponeurosis Transversalis fascia	**Ø** Open **3** Percutaneous	**Ø** Drainage Device **2** Monitoring Device **3** Infusion Device **7** Autologous Tissue Substitute **F** Subcutaneous Defibrillator Lead **H** Contraceptive Device **J** Synthetic Substitute **K** Nonautologous Tissue Substitute **M** Stimulator Generator **N** Tissue Expander **P** Cardiac Rhythm Related Device **V** Infusion Device, Pump **W** Vascular Access Device, Totally Implantable **X** Vascular Access Device, Tunneled **Y** Other Device	**Z** No Qualifier
T Subcutaneous Tissue and Fascia, Trunk External oblique aponeurosis Transversalis fascia	**X** External	**Ø** Drainage Device **2** Monitoring Device **3** Infusion Device **7** Autologous Tissue Substitute **F** Subcutaneous Defibrillator Lead **H** Contraceptive Device **J** Synthetic Substitute **K** Nonautologous Tissue Substitute **M** Stimulator Generator **N** Tissue Expander **P** Cardiac Rhythm Related Device **V** Infusion Device, Pump **W** Vascular Access Device, Totally Implantable **X** Vascular Access Device, Tunneled	**Z** No Qualifier
V Subcutaneous Tissue and Fascia, Upper Extremity **W** Subcutaneous Tissue and Fascia, Lower Extremity	**Ø** Open **3** Percutaneous	**Ø** Drainage Device **3** Infusion Device **7** Autologous Tissue Substitute **H** Contraceptive Device **J** Synthetic Substitute **K** Nonautologous Tissue Substitute **N** Tissue Expander **V** Infusion Device, Pump **W** Vascular Access Device, Totally Implantable **X** Vascular Access Device, Tunneled **Y** Other Device	**Z** No Qualifier
V Subcutaneous Tissue and Fascia, Upper Extremity **W** Subcutaneous Tissue and Fascia, Lower Extremity	**X** External	**Ø** Drainage Device **3** Infusion Device **7** Autologous Tissue Substitute **H** Contraceptive Device **J** Synthetic Substitute **K** Nonautologous Tissue Substitute **N** Tissue Expander **V** Infusion Device, Pump **W** Vascular Access Device, Totally Implantable **X** Vascular Access Device, Tunneled	**Z** No Qualifier

DRG Non-OR	ØJWS[Ø,3][Ø,3,7,J,K,N,Y]Z	**HAC** ØJWT[Ø,3][F,P]Z when reported with SDx K68.11 or T81.4Ø-T81.49, T82.6-T82.7
DRG Non-OR	ØJWT[Ø,3][Ø,3,7,H,J,K,M,N,V,W,X]Z	with 7th character A
DRG Non-OR	ØJWTXMZ	
DRG Non-OR	ØJW[V,W][Ø,3][Ø,3,7,H,J,K,N,V,W,X,Y]Z	
Non-OR	ØJWSX[Ø,3,7,J,K,N]Z	
Non-OR	ØJWT3YZ	
Non-OR	ØJWTX[Ø,2,3,7,F,H,J,K,N,P,V,W,X]Z	
Non-OR	ØJW[V,W]X[Ø,3,7,H,J,K,N,V,W,X]Z	

Ø   Medical and Surgical
J   Subcutaneous Tissue and Fascia
X   Transfer   Definition: Moving, without taking out, all or a portion of a body part to another location to take over the function of all or a portion of a body part
                  Explanation: The body part transferred remains connected to its vascular and nervous supply

Body Part Character 4		Approach Character 5	Device Character 6	Qualifier Character 7

Ø **Subcutaneous Tissue and Fascia, Scalp**
    Galea aponeurotica
	G **Subcutaneous Tissue and Fascia, Right Lower Arm**
	    Antebrachial fascia
	    Bicipital aponeurosis
		Ø Open
		3 Percutaneous
			Z No Device	**B** Skin and Subcutaneous Tissue
				C Skin, Subcutaneous Tissue and Fascia
				Z No Qualifier

1 **Subcutaneous Tissue and Fascia, Face**
    Masseteric fascia
    Orbital fascia
    Submandibular space
	H **Subcutaneous Tissue and Fascia, Left Lower Arm**
	    See G Subcutaneous Tissue and Fascia, Right Lower Arm			

4 **Subcutaneous Tissue and Fascia, Right Neck**
    Deep cervical fascia
    Pretracheal fascia
    Prevertebral fascia
	J **Subcutaneous Tissue and Fascia, Right Hand**
	    Palmar fascia (aponeurosis)			

5 **Subcutaneous Tissue and Fascia, Left Neck**
    See 4 Subcutaneous Tissue and Fascia, Right Neck
	K **Subcutaneous Tissue and Fascia, Left Hand**
	    See J Subcutaneous Tissue and Fascia, Right Hand			

6 **Subcutaneous Tissue and Fascia, Chest**
    Pectoral fascia
	L **Subcutaneous Tissue and Fascia, Right Upper Leg**
	    Crural fascia
	    Fascia lata
	    Iliac fascia
	    Iliotibial tract (band)			

7 **Subcutaneous Tissue and Fascia, Back**	**M** **Subcutaneous Tissue and Fascia, Left Upper Leg** *See L Subcutaneous Tissue and Fascia, Right Upper Leg*			
8 **Subcutaneous Tissue and Fascia, Abdomen**	**N** **Subcutaneous Tissue and Fascia, Right Lower Leg**			
9 **Subcutaneous Tissue and Fascia, Buttock**	**P** **Subcutaneous Tissue and Fascia, Left Lower Leg**			
B **Subcutaneous Tissue and Fascia, Perineum**	**Q** **Subcutaneous Tissue and Fascia, Right Foot** Plantar fascia (aponeurosis)			
C **Subcutaneous Tissue and Fascia, Pelvic Region**	**R** **Subcutaneous Tissue and Fascia, Left Foot** *See Q Subcutaneous Tissue and Fascia, Right Foot*			

D **Subcutaneous Tissue and Fascia, Right Upper Arm**
    Axillary fascia
    Deltoid fascia
    Infraspinatus fascia
    Subscapular aponeurosis
    Supraspinatus fascia				

F **Subcutaneous Tissue and Fascia, Left Upper Arm** *See D Subcutaneous Tissue and Fascia, Right Upper Arm*				

Muscles ØK2–ØKX

Character Meanings

This Character Meaning table is provided as a guide to assist the user in the identification of character members that may be found in this section of code tables. It **SHOULD NOT** be used to build a PCS code.

Operation–Character 3		Body Part–Character 4		Approach–Character 5		Device–Character 6		Qualifier–Character 7	
2	Change	Ø	Head Muscle	Ø	Open	Ø	Drainage Device	Ø	Skin
5	Destruction	1	Facial Muscle	3	Percutaneous	7	Autologous Tissue Substitute	1	Subcutaneous Tissue
8	Division	2	Neck Muscle, Right	4	Percutaneous Endoscopic	J	Synthetic Substitute	2	Skin and Subcutaneous Tissue
9	Drainage	3	Neck Muscle, Left	7	Via Natural or Artificial Opening	K	Nonautologous Tissue Substitute	5	Latissimus Dorsi Myocutaneous Flap
B	Excision	4	Tongue, Palate, Pharynx Muscle	8	Via Natural or Artificial Opening Endoscopic	M	Stimulator Lead	6	Transverse Rectus Abdominis Myocutaneous Flap
C	Extirpation	5	Shoulder Muscle, Right	X	External	Y	Other Device	7	Deep Inferior Epigastric Artery Perforator Flap
D	Extraction	6	Shoulder Muscle, Left			Z	No Device	8	Superficial Inferior Epigastric Artery Flap
H	Insertion	7	Upper Arm Muscle, Right					9	Gluteal Artery Perforator Flap
J	Inspection	8	Upper Arm Muscle, Left					X	Diagnostic
M	Reattachment	9	Lower Arm and Wrist Muscle, Right					Z	No Qualifier
N	Release	B	Lower Arm and Wrist Muscle, Left						
P	Removal	C	Hand Muscle, Right						
Q	Repair	D	Hand Muscle, Left						
R	Replacement	F	Trunk Muscle, Right						
S	Reposition	G	Trunk Muscle, Left						
T	Resection	H	Thorax Muscle, Right						
U	Supplement	J	Thorax Muscle, Left						
W	Revision	K	Abdomen Muscle, Right						
X	Transfer	L	Abdomen Muscle, Left						
		M	Perineum Muscle						
		N	Hip Muscle, Right						
		P	Hip Muscle, Left						
		Q	Upper Leg Muscle, Right						
		R	Upper Leg Muscle, Left						
		S	Lower Leg Muscle, Right						
		T	Lower Leg Muscle, Left						
		V	Foot Muscle, Right						
		W	Foot Muscle, Left						
		X	Upper Muscle						
		Y	Lower Muscle						

AHA Coding Clinic for table ØK8

2020, 2Q, 25   Endoscopic Stapling of Zenker's Diverticulum

AHA Coding Clinic for table ØKB

2020, 1Q, 27   Delayed reconstruction following mastectomy using gracilis musculocutaneous free flap
2016, 3Q, 20   Excisional debridement of sacrum
2015, 3Q, 3-8   Excisional and nonexcisional debridement

AHA Coding Clinic for table ØKD

2017, 4Q, 41-42   Extraction procedures

AHA Coding Clinic for table ØKH

2020, 4Q, 63   Intercompartmental pressure measurement

AHA Coding Clinic for table ØKN

2017, 2Q, 12   Compartment syndrome and fasciotomy of foot
2017, 2Q, 13   Compartment syndrome and fasciotomy of leg
2015, 2Q, 22   Arthroscopic subacromial decompression
2014, 4Q, 39   Abdominal component release with placement of mesh for hernia repair

AHA Coding Clinic for table ØKQ

2018, 2Q, 25   Third and fourth degree obstetric lacerations
2016, 2Q, 34   Assisted vaginal delivery
2016, 1Q, 7   Obstetrical perineal laceration repair
2014, 4Q, 43   Second degree obstetric perineal laceration
2013, 4Q, 120   Repair of second degree perineum obstetric laceration

AHA Coding Clinic for table ØKS

2017, 1Q, 41   Manual reduction of hernia

AHA Coding Clinic for table ØKT

2016, 2Q, 12   Resection of malignant neoplasm of infratemporal fossa
2015, 1Q, 38   Abdominoperineal resection with flap closure of the perineum and colostomy

AHA Coding Clinic for table ØKX

2018, 2Q, 18   Transverse rectus abdominis myocutaneous (TRAM) delay
2017, 4Q, 67   New qualifier values - Pedicle flap procedures
2016, 3Q, 30   Resection of femur with interposition arthroplasty
2015, 3Q, 33   Cleft lip repair using Millard rotation advancement
2015, 2Q, 26   Pharyngeal flap to soft palate
2014, 4Q, 41   Abdominoperineal resection (APR) with flap closure of perineum and colostomy
2014, 2Q, 10   Transverse abdominomyocutaneous (TRAM) breast reconstruction
2014, 2Q, 12   Pedicle latissimus myocutaneous flap with placement of breast tissue expanders

Muscles

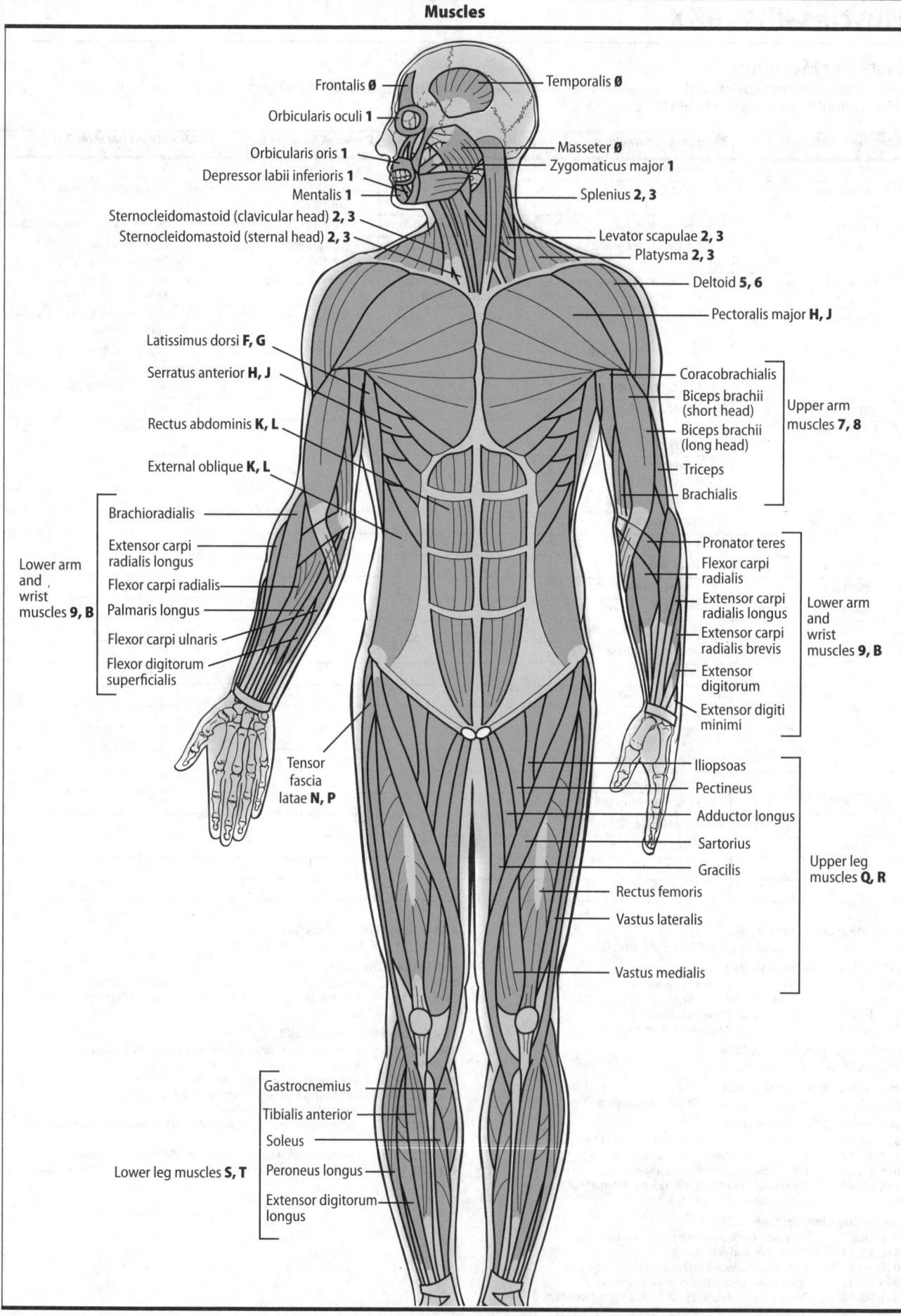

Frontalis **Ø**
Temporalis **Ø**
Orbicularis oculi **1**
Orbicularis oris **1**
Masseter **Ø**
Zygomaticus major **1**
Depressor labii inferioris **1**
Mentalis **1**
Splenius **2, 3**
Sternocleidomastoid (clavicular head) **2, 3**
Sternocleidomastoid (sternal head) **2, 3**
Levator scapulae **2, 3**
Platysma **2, 3**
Deltoid **5, 6**
Pectoralis major **H, J**
Latissimus dorsi **F, G**
Serratus anterior **H, J**
Coracobrachialis
Biceps brachii (short head)
Biceps brachii (long head)
Rectus abdominis **K, L**
Triceps
External oblique **K, L**
Brachialis
Upper arm muscles **7, 8**
Brachioradialis
Pronator teres
Extensor carpi radialis longus
Flexor carpi radialis
Flexor carpi radialis
Extensor carpi radialis longus
Palmaris longus
Extensor carpi radialis brevis
Flexor carpi ulnaris
Extensor digitorum
Flexor digitorum superficialis
Extensor digiti minimi
Lower arm and wrist muscles **9, B**
Lower arm and wrist muscles **9, B**
Tensor fascia latae **N, P**
Iliopsoas
Pectineus
Adductor longus
Sartorius
Gracilis
Rectus femoris
Vastus lateralis
Upper leg muscles **Q, R**
Vastus medialis
Gastrocnemius
Tibialis anterior
Soleus
Peroneus longus
Lower leg muscles **S, T**
Extensor digitorum longus

Ø   Medical and Surgical
K   Muscles
2   Change   Definition: Taking out or off a device from a body part and putting back an identical or similar device in or on the same body part without cutting or puncturing the skin or a mucous membrane

           Explanation: All CHANGE procedures are coded using the approach EXTERNAL

Body Part Character 4	Approach Character 5	Device Character 6	Qualifier Character 7
X Upper Muscle Y Lower Muscle	X External	Ø Drainage Device Y Other Device	Z No Qualifier

Non-OR	All body part, approach, device, and qualifier values

Ø   Medical and Surgical
K   Muscles
5   Destruction   Definition: Physical eradication of all or a portion of a body part by the direct use of energy, force, or a destructive agent

           Explanation: None of the body part is physically taken out

Body Part Character 4			Approach Character 5	Device Character 6	Qualifier Character 7

Ø Head Muscle
Auricularis muscle
Masseter muscle
Pterygoid muscle
Splenius capitis muscle
Temporalis muscle
Temporoparietalis muscle
1 Facial Muscle
Buccinator muscle
Corrugator supercilii muscle
Depressor anguli oris muscle
Depressor labii inferioris muscle
Depressor septi nasi muscle
Depressor supercilii muscle
Levator anguli oris muscle
Levator labii superioris alaeque
    nasi muscle
Levator labii superioris muscle
Mentalis muscle
Nasalis muscle
Occipitofrontalis muscle
Orbicularis oris muscle
Procerus muscle
Risorius muscle
Zygomaticus muscle
2 Neck Muscle, Right
Anterior vertebral muscle
Arytenoid muscle
Cricothyroid muscle
Infrahyoid muscle
Levator scapulae muscle
Platysma muscle
Scalene muscle
Splenius cervicis muscle
Sternocleidomastoid muscle
Suprahyoid muscle
Thyroarytenoid muscle
3 Neck Muscle, Left
See 2 Neck Muscle, Right
4 Tongue, Palate, Pharynx
Muscle
Chondroglossus muscle
Genioglossus muscle
Hyoglossus muscle
Inferior longitudinal muscle
Levator veli palatini muscle
Palatoglossal muscle
Palatopharyngeal muscle
Pharyngeal constrictor muscle
Salpingopharyngeus muscle
Styloglossus muscle
Stylopharyngeus muscle
Superior longitudinal muscle
Tensor veli palatini muscle
5 Shoulder Muscle, Right
Deltoid muscle
Infraspinatus muscle
Subscapularis muscle
Supraspinatus muscle
Teres major muscle
Teres minor muscle
6 Shoulder Muscle, Left
See 5 Shoulder Muscle, Right
	7 Upper Arm Muscle, Right
	Biceps brachii muscle
	Brachialis muscle
	Coracobrachialis muscle
	Triceps brachii muscle
	8 Upper Arm Muscle, Left
	See 7 Upper Arm Muscle, Right
	9 Lower Arm and Wrist Muscle,
	Right
	Anatomical snuffbox
	Brachioradialis muscle
	Extensor carpi radialis muscle
	Extensor carpi ulnaris muscle
	Flexor carpi radialis muscle
	Flexor carpi ulnaris muscle
	Flexor pollicis longus muscle
	Palmaris longus muscle
	Pronator quadratus muscle
	Pronator teres muscle
	B Lower Arm and Wrist Muscle,
	Left
	See 9 Lower Arm and Wrist
	    Muscle, Right
	C Hand Muscle, Right
	Hypothenar muscle
	Palmar interosseous muscle
	Thenar muscle
	D Hand Muscle, Left
	See C Hand Muscle, Right
	F Trunk Muscle, Right
	Coccygeus muscle
	Erector spinae muscle
	Interspinalis muscle
	Intertransversarius muscle
	Latissimus dorsi muscle
	Quadratus lumborum muscle
	Rhomboid major muscle
	Rhomboid minor muscle
	Serratus posterior muscle
	Transversospinalis muscle
	Trapezius muscle
	G Trunk Muscle, Left
	See F Trunk Muscle, Right
	H Thorax Muscle, Right
	Intercostal muscle
	Levatores costarum muscle
	Pectoralis major muscle
	Pectoralis minor muscle
	Serratus anterior muscle
	Subclavius muscle
	Subcostal muscle
	Transverse thoracis muscle
	J Thorax Muscle, Left
	See H Thorax Muscle, Right
	K Abdomen Muscle, Right
	External oblique muscle
	Internal oblique muscle
	Pyramidalis muscle
	Rectus abdominis muscle
	Transversus abdominis muscle
	L Abdomen Muscle, Left
	See K Abdomen Muscle, Right
		M Perineum Muscle
		Bulbospongiosus muscle
		Cremaster muscle
		Deep transverse perineal muscle
		Ischiocavernosus muscle
		Levator ani muscle
		Superficial transverse perineal
		    muscle
		N Hip Muscle, Right
		Gemellus muscle
		Gluteus maximus muscle
		Gluteus medius muscle
		Gluteus minimus muscle
		Iliacus muscle
		Obturator muscle
		Piriformis muscle
		Psoas muscle
		Quadratus femoris muscle
		Tensor fasciae latae muscle
		P Hip Muscle, Left
		See N Hip Muscle, Right
		Q Upper Leg Muscle, Right
		Adductor brevis muscle
		Adductor longus muscle
		Adductor magnus muscle
		Biceps femoris muscle
		Gracilis muscle
		Pectineus muscle
		Quadriceps (femoris)
		Rectus femoris muscle
		Sartorius muscle
		Semimembranosus muscle
		Semitendinosus muscle
		Vastus intermedius muscle
		Vastus lateralis muscle
		Vastus medialis muscle
		R Upper Leg Muscle, Left
		See Q Upper Leg Muscle, Right
		S Lower Leg Muscle, Right
		Extensor digitorum longus muscle
		Extensor hallucis longus muscle
		Fibularis brevis muscle
		Fibularis longus muscle
		Flexor digitorum longus muscle
		Flexor hallucis longus muscle
		Gastrocnemius muscle
		Peroneus brevis muscle
		Peroneus longus muscle
		Popliteus muscle
		Soleus muscle
		Tibialis anterior muscle
		Tibialis posterior muscle
		T Lower Leg Muscle, Left
		See S Lower Leg Muscle, Right
		V Foot Muscle, Right
		Abductor hallucis muscle
		Adductor hallucis muscle
		Extensor digitorum brevis muscle
		Extensor hallucis brevis muscle
		Flexor digitorum brevis muscle
		Flexor hallucis brevis muscle
		Quadratus plantae muscle
		W Foot Muscle, Left
		See V Foot Muscle, Right
			Ø Open
			3 Percutaneous
			4 Percutaneous
			    Endoscopic
				Z No Device	**Z No Qualifier**

NC Noncovered Procedure   **LC** Limited Coverage   **QA** Questionable OB Admit   **NT** New Tech Add-on   ⊞ Combination Member   ♂ Male   ♀ Female

Ø Medical and Surgical
K Muscles
8 Division

Definition: Cutting into a body part, without draining fluids and/or gases from the body part, in order to separate or transect a body part
Explanation: All or a portion of the body part is separated into two or more portions

Body Part Character 4			Approach Character 5	Device Character 6	Qualifier Character 7

Ø Head Muscle
Auricularis muscle
Masseter muscle
Pterygoid muscle
Splenius capitis muscle
Temporalis muscle
Temporoparietalis muscle
1 Facial Muscle
Buccinator muscle
Corrugator supercilii
  muscle
Depressor anguli oris
  muscle
Depressor labii inferioris
  muscle
Depressor septi nasi muscle
Depressor supercilii muscle
Levator anguli oris muscle
Levator labii superioris
  alaeque nasi muscle
Levator labii superioris
  muscle
Mentalis muscle
Nasalis muscle
Occipitofrontalis muscle
Orbicularis oris muscle
Procerus muscle
Risorius muscle
Zygomaticus muscle
2 Neck Muscle, Right
Anterior vertebral muscle
Arytenoid muscle
Cricothyroid muscle
Infrahyoid muscle
Levator scapulae muscle
Platysma muscle
Scalene muscle
Splenius cervicis muscle
Sternocleidomastoid
  muscle
Suprahyoid muscle
Thyroarytenoid muscle
3 Neck Muscle, Left
See 2 Neck Muscle, Right
Tensor veli palatini muscle
5 Shoulder Muscle, Right
Deltoid muscle
Infraspinatus muscle
Subscapularis muscle
Supraspinatus muscle
Teres major muscle
Teres minor muscle
6 Shoulder Muscle, Left
See 5 Shoulder Muscle, Right
7 Upper Arm Muscle, Right
Biceps brachii muscle
Brachialis muscle
Coracobrachialis muscle
Triceps brachii muscle
8 Upper Arm Muscle, Left
See 7 Upper Arm Muscle,
* Right*
	9 Lower Arm and Wrist Muscle,
	Right
	Anatomical snuffbox
	Brachioradialis muscle
	Extensor carpi radialis muscle
	Extensor carpi ulnaris muscle
	Flexor carpi radialis muscle
	Flexor carpi ulnaris muscle
	Flexor pollicis longus muscle
	Palmaris longus muscle
	Pronator quadratus muscle
	Pronator teres muscle
	B Lower Arm and Wrist Muscle,
	Left
	See 9 Lower Arm and Wrist
	* Muscle, Right*
	C Hand Muscle, Right
	Hypothenar muscle
	Palmar interosseous muscle
	Thenar muscle
	D Hand Muscle, Left
	See C Hand Muscle, Right
	F Trunk Muscle, Right
	Coccygeus muscle
	Erector spinae muscle
	Interspinalis muscle
	Intertransversarius muscle
	Latissimus dorsi muscle
	Quadratus lumborum muscle
	Rhomboid major muscle
	Rhomboid minor muscle
	Serratus posterior muscle
	Transversospinalis muscle
	Trapezius muscle
	G Trunk Muscle, Left
	See F Trunk Muscle, Right
	H Thorax Muscle, Right
	Intercostal muscle
	Levatores costarum muscle
	Pectoralis major muscle
	Pectoralis minor muscle
	Serratus anterior muscle
	Subclavius muscle
	Subcostal muscle
	Transverse thoracis muscle
	J Thorax Muscle, Left
	See H Thorax Muscle, Right
	K Abdomen Muscle, Right
	External oblique muscle
	Internal oblique muscle
	Pyramidalis muscle
	Rectus abdominis muscle
	Transversus abdominis muscle
	L Abdomen Muscle, Left
	See K Abdomen Muscle, Right
	M Perineum Muscle
	Bulbospongiosus muscle
	Cremaster muscle
	Deep transverse perineal muscle
	Ischiocavernosus muscle
	Levator ani muscle
	Superficial transverse perineal
	  muscle
		N Hip Muscle, Right
		Gemellus muscle
		Gluteus maximus muscle
		Gluteus medius muscle
		Gluteus minimus muscle
		Iliacus muscle
		Obturator muscle
		Piriformis muscle
		Psoas muscle
		Quadratus femoris muscle
		Tensor fasciae latae muscle
		P Hip Muscle, Left
		See N Hip Muscle, Right
		Q Upper Leg Muscle, Right
		Adductor brevis muscle
		Adductor longus muscle
		Adductor magnus muscle
		Biceps femoris muscle
		Gracilis muscle
		Pectineus muscle
		Quadriceps (femoris)
		Rectus femoris muscle
		Sartorius muscle
		Semimembranosus muscle
		Semitendinosus muscle
		Vastus intermedius muscle
		Vastus lateralis muscle
		Vastus medialis muscle
		R Upper Leg Muscle, Left
		See Q Upper Leg Muscle, Right
		S Lower Leg Muscle, Right
		Extensor digitorum longus
		  muscle
		Extensor hallucis longus
		  muscle
		Fibularis brevis muscle
		Fibularis longus muscle
		Flexor digitorum longus
		  muscle
		Flexor hallucis longus muscle
		Gastrocnemius muscle
		Peroneus brevis muscle
		Peroneus longus muscle
		Popliteus muscle
		Soleus muscle
		Tibialis anterior muscle
		Tibialis posterior muscle
		T Lower Leg Muscle, Left
		See S Lower Leg Muscle, Right
		V Foot Muscle, Right
		Abductor hallucis muscle
		Adductor hallucis muscle
		Extensor digitorum brevis
		  muscle
		Extensor hallucis brevis
		  muscle
		Flexor digitorum brevis
		  muscle
		Flexor hallucis brevis muscle
		Quadratus plantae muscle
		W Foot Muscle, Left
		See V Foot Muscle, Right
			Ø Open
			3 Percutaneous
			4 Percutaneous
			  Endoscopic
				Z No Device	**Z No Qualifier**

4 Tongue, Palate, Pharynx Muscle
Chondroglossus muscle
Genioglossus muscle
Hyoglossus muscle
Inferior longitudinal muscle
Levator veli palatini muscle
Palatoglossal muscle
Palatopharyngeal muscle
Pharyngeal constrictor muscle
Salpingopharyngeus muscle
Styloglossus muscle
Stylopharyngeus muscle
Superior longitudinal muscle
Tensor veli palatini muscle
			Ø Open
			3 Percutaneous
			4 Percutaneous
			  Endoscopic
			7 Via Natural or
			  Artificial Opening
			8 Via Natural or
			  Artificial Opening
			  Endoscopic
				Z No Device	**Z No Qualifier**

0   **Medical and Surgical**
K   **Muscles**
9   **Drainage**   Definition: Taking or letting out fluids and/or gases from a body part
                 Explanation: The qualifier DIAGNOSTIC is used to identify drainage procedures that are biopsies

Body Part Character 4			Approach Character 5	Device Character 6	Qualifier Character 7
0 Head Muscle Auricularis muscle Masseter muscle Pterygoid muscle Splenius capitis muscle Temporalis muscle Temporoparietalis muscle **1 Facial Muscle** Buccinator muscle Corrugator supercilii muscle Depressor anguli oris muscle Depressor labii inferioris muscle Depressor septi nasi muscle Depressor supercilii muscle Levator anguli oris muscle Levator labii superioris alaeque nasi muscle Levator labii superioris muscle Mentalis muscle Nasalis muscle Occipitofrontalis muscle Orbicularis oris muscle Procerus muscle Risorius muscle Zygomaticus muscle **2 Neck Muscle, Right** Anterior vertebral muscle Arytenoid muscle Cricothyroid muscle Infrahyoid muscle Levator scapulae muscle Platysma muscle Scalene muscle Splenius cervicis muscle Sternocleidomastoid muscle Suprahyoid muscle Thyroarytenoid muscle **3 Neck Muscle, Left** *See 2 Neck Muscle, Right* **4 Tongue, Palate, Pharynx Muscle** Chondroglossus muscle Genioglossus muscle Hyoglossus muscle Inferior longitudinal muscle Levator veli palatini muscle Palatoglossal muscle Palatopharyngeal muscle Pharyngeal constrictor muscle Salpingopharyngeus muscle Styloglossus muscle Stylopharyngeus muscle Superior longitudinal muscle Tensor veli palatini muscle **5 Shoulder Muscle, Right** Deltoid muscle Infraspinatus muscle Subscapularis muscle Supraspinatus muscle Teres major muscle Teres minor muscle **6 Shoulder Muscle, Left** *See 5 Shoulder Muscle, Right*	**7 Upper Arm Muscle, Right** Biceps brachii muscle Brachialis muscle Coracobrachialis muscle Triceps brachii muscle **8 Upper Arm Muscle, Left** *See 7 Upper Arm Muscle, Right* **9 Lower Arm and Wrist Muscle, Right** Anatomical snuffbox Brachioradialis muscle Extensor carpi radialis muscle Extensor carpi ulnaris muscle Flexor carpi radialis muscle Flexor carpi ulnaris muscle Flexor pollicis longus muscle Palmaris longus muscle Pronator quadratus muscle Pronator teres muscle **B Lower Arm and Wrist Muscle, Left** *See 9 Lower Arm and Wrist Muscle, Right* **C Hand Muscle, Right** Hypothenar muscle Palmar interosseous muscle Thenar muscle **D Hand Muscle, Left** *See C Hand Muscle, Right* **F Trunk Muscle, Right** Coccygeus muscle Erector spinae muscle Interspinalis muscle Intertransversarius muscle Latissimus dorsi muscle Quadratus lumborum muscle Rhomboid major muscle Rhomboid minor muscle Serratus posterior muscle Transversospinalis muscle Trapezius muscle **G Trunk Muscle, Left** *See F Trunk Muscle, Right* **H Thorax Muscle, Right** Intercostal muscle Levatores costarum muscle Pectoralis major muscle Pectoralis minor muscle Serratus anterior muscle Subclavius muscle Subcostal muscle Transverse thoracis muscle **J Thorax Muscle, Left** *See H Thorax Muscle, Right* **K Abdomen Muscle, Right** External oblique muscle Internal oblique muscle Pyramidalis muscle Rectus abdominis muscle Transversus abdominis muscle **L Abdomen Muscle, Left** *See K Abdomen Muscle, Right*	**M Perineum Muscle** Bulbospongiosus muscle Cremaster muscle Deep transverse perineal muscle Ischiocavernosus muscle Levator ani muscle Superficial transverse perineal muscle **N Hip Muscle, Right** Gemellus muscle Gluteus maximus muscle Gluteus medius muscle Gluteus minimus muscle Iliacus muscle Obturator muscle Piriformis muscle Psoas muscle Quadratus femoris muscle Tensor fasciae latae muscle **P Hip Muscle, Left** *See N Hip Muscle, Right* **Q Upper Leg Muscle, Right** Adductor brevis muscle Adductor longus muscle Adductor magnus muscle Biceps femoris muscle Gracilis muscle Pectineus muscle Quadriceps (femoris) Rectus femoris muscle Sartorius muscle Semimembranosus muscle Semitendinosus muscle Vastus intermedius muscle Vastus lateralis muscle Vastus medialis muscle **R Upper Leg Muscle, Left** *See Q Upper Leg Muscle, Right* **S Lower Leg Muscle, Right** Extensor digitorum longus muscle Extensor hallucis longus muscle Fibularis brevis muscle Fibularis longus muscle Flexor digitorum longus muscle Flexor hallucis longus muscle Gastrocnemius muscle Peroneus brevis muscle Peroneus longus muscle Popliteus muscle Soleus muscle Tibialis anterior muscle Tibialis posterior muscle **T Lower Leg Muscle, Left** *See S Lower Leg Muscle, Right* **V Foot Muscle, Right** Abductor hallucis muscle Adductor hallucis muscle Extensor digitorum brevis muscle Extensor hallucis brevis muscle Flexor digitorum brevis muscle Flexor hallucis brevis muscle Quadratus plantae muscle **W Foot Muscle, Left** *See V Foot Muscle, Right*	**0 Open** **3 Percutaneous** **4 Percutaneous Endoscopic**	**0 Drainage Device**	**Z No Qualifier**

Non-OR   0K9[0,1,2,3,4,5,6,7,8,9,B,C,D,F,G,H,J,K,L,M,N,P,Q,R,S,T,V,W]30Z

0K9 Continued on next page

NC Noncovered Procedure   **LC** Limited Coverage   **QA** Questionable OB Admit   **NT** New Tech Add-on   ⊞ Combination Member   ♂ Male   ♀ Female

ICD-10-PCS 2022   467

0K9–0K9

Muscles

Ø	Medical and Surgical
K	Muscles
9	Drainage

ØK9 Continued

Definition: Taking or letting out fluids and/or gases from a body part
Explanation: The qualifier DIAGNOSTIC is used to identify drainage procedures that are biopsies

Body Part Character 4		Approach Character 5	Device Character 6	Qualifier Character 7

Ø Head Muscle
Auricularis muscle
Masseter muscle
Pterygoid muscle
Splenius capitis muscle
Temporalis muscle
Temporoparietalis muscle
1 Facial Muscle
Buccinator muscle
Corrugator supercilii
  muscle
Depressor anguli oris
  muscle
Depressor labii inferioris
  muscle
Depressor septi nasi
  muscle
Depressor supercilii
  muscle
Levator anguli oris muscle
Levator labii superioris
  alaeque nasi muscle
Levator labii superioris
  muscle
Mentalis muscle
Nasalis muscle
Occipitofrontalis muscle
Orbicularis oris muscle
Procerus muscle
Risorius muscle
Zygomaticus muscle
2 Neck Muscle, Right
Anterior vertebral muscle
Arytenoid muscle
Cricothyroid muscle
Infrahyoid muscle
Levator scapulae muscle
Platysma muscle
Scalene muscle
Splenius cervicis muscle
Sternocleidomastoid
  muscle
Suprahyoid muscle
Thyroarytenoid muscle
3 Neck Muscle, Left
See 2 Neck Muscle, Right
4 Tongue, Palate, Pharynx
Muscle
Chondroglossus muscle
Genioglossus muscle
Hyoglossus muscle
Inferior longitudinal
  muscle
Levator veli palatini
  muscle
Palatoglossal muscle
Palatopharyngeal muscle
Pharyngeal constrictor
  muscle
Salpingopharyngeus
  muscle
Styloglossus muscle
Stylopharyngeus muscle
Superior longitudinal
  muscle
Tensor veli palatini muscle
5 Shoulder Muscle, Right
Deltoid muscle
Infraspinatus muscle
Subscapularis muscle
Supraspinatus muscle
Teres major muscle
Teres minor muscle
6 Shoulder Muscle, Left
See 5 Shoulder Muscle,
Right
	7 Upper Arm Muscle, Right
	Biceps brachii muscle
	Brachialis muscle
	Coracobrachialis muscle
	Triceps brachii muscle
	8 Upper Arm Muscle, Left
	See 7 Upper Arm Muscle,
	Right
	9 Lower Arm and Wrist
	Muscle, Right
	Anatomical snuffbox
	Brachioradialis muscle
	Extensor carpi radialis
	  muscle
	Extensor carpi ulnaris
	  muscle
	Flexor carpi radialis
	  muscle
	Flexor carpi ulnaris muscle
	Flexor pollicis longus
	  muscle
	Palmaris longus muscle
	Pronator quadratus
	  muscle
	Pronator teres muscle
	B Lower Arm and Wrist
	Muscle, Left
	See 9 Lower Arm and Wrist
	Muscle, Right
	C Hand Muscle, Right
	Hypothenar muscle
	Palmar interosseous
	  muscle
	Thenar muscle
	D Hand Muscle, Left
	See C Hand Muscle, Right
	F Trunk Muscle, Right
	Coccygeus muscle
	Erector spinae muscle
	Interspinalis muscle
	Intertransversarius muscle
	Latissimus dorsi muscle
	Quadratus lumborum
	  muscle
	Rhomboid major muscle
	Rhomboid minor muscle
	Serratus posterior muscle
	Transversospinalis muscle
	Trapezius muscle
	G Trunk Muscle, Left
	See F Trunk Muscle, Right
	H Thorax Muscle, Right
	Intercostal muscle
	Levatores costarum
	  muscle
	Pectoralis major muscle
	Pectoralis minor muscle
	Serratus anterior muscle
	Subclavius muscle
	Subcostal muscle
	Transverse thoracis
	  muscle
	J Thorax Muscle, Left
	See H Thorax Muscle, Right
	K Abdomen Muscle, Right
	External oblique muscle
	Internal oblique muscle
	Pyramidalis muscle
	Rectus abdominis muscle
	Transversus abdominis
	  muscle
	L Abdomen Muscle, Left
	See K Abdomen Muscle,
	Right
		M Perineum Muscle
		Bulbospongiosus muscle
		Cremaster muscle
		Deep transverse perineal
		  muscle
		Ischiocavernosus muscle
		Levator ani muscle
		Superficial transverse
		  perineal muscle
		N Hip Muscle, Right
		Gemellus muscle
		Gluteus maximus muscle
		Gluteus medius muscle
		Gluteus minimus muscle
		Iliacus muscle
		Obturator muscle
		Piriformis muscle
		Psoas muscle
		Quadratus femoris muscle
		Tensor fasciae latae
		  muscle
		P Hip Muscle, Left
		See N Hip Muscle, Right
		Q Upper Leg Muscle, Right
		Adductor brevis muscle
		Adductor longus muscle
		Adductor magnus muscle
		Biceps femoris muscle
		Gracilis muscle
		Pectineus muscle
		Quadriceps (femoris)
		Rectus femoris muscle
		Sartorius muscle
		Semimembranosus muscle
		Semitendinosus muscle
		Vastus intermedius muscle
		Vastus lateralis muscle
		Vastus medialis muscle
		R Upper Leg Muscle, Left
		See Q Upper Leg Muscle,
		Right
		S Lower Leg Muscle, Right
		Extensor digitorum longus
		  muscle
		Extensor hallucis longus
		  muscle
		Fibularis brevis muscle
		Fibularis longus muscle
		Flexor digitorum longus
		  muscle
		Flexor hallucis longus
		  muscle
		Gastrocnemius muscle
		Peroneus brevis muscle
		Peroneus longus muscle
		Popliteus muscle
		Soleus muscle
		Tibialis anterior muscle
		Tibialis posterior muscle
		T Lower Leg Muscle, Left
		See S Lower Leg Muscle,
		Right
		V Foot Muscle, Right
		Abductor hallucis muscle
		Adductor hallucis muscle
		Extensor digitorum brevis
		  muscle
		Extensor hallucis brevis
		  muscle
		Flexor digitorum brevis
		  muscle
		Flexor hallucis brevis
		  muscle
		Quadratus plantae muscle
		W Foot Muscle, Left
		See V Foot Muscle, Right
			Ø Open
			3 Percutaneous
			4 Percutaneous
			  Endoscopic
				Z No Device	**X Diagnostic**
					Z No Qualifier

Non-OR	ØK9[Ø,1,2,3,4,5,6,7,8,9,B,F,G,H,J,K,L,M,N,P,Q,R,S,T,V,W]3ZZ
Non-OR	ØK9[C,D][3,4]ZZ

Ø   **Medical and Surgical**
K   **Muscles**
B   **Excision**   Definition: Cutting out or off, without replacement, a portion of a body part
                     Explanation: The qualifier DIAGNOSTIC is used to identify excision procedures that are biopsies

Body Part Character 4			Approach Character 5	Device Character 6	Qualifier Character 7
Ø Head Muscle Auricularis muscle Masseter muscle Pterygoid muscle Splenius capitis muscle Temporalis muscle Temporoparietalis muscle **1 Facial Muscle** Buccinator muscle Corrugator supercilii muscle Depressor anguli oris muscle Depressor labii inferioris muscle Depressor septi nasi muscle Depressor supercilii muscle Levator anguli oris muscle Levator labii superioris alaeque nasi muscle Levator labii superioris muscle Mentalis muscle Nasalis muscle Occipitofrontalis muscle Orbicularis oris muscle Procerus muscle Risorius muscle Zygomaticus muscle **2 Neck Muscle, Right** Anterior vertebral muscle Arytenoid muscle Cricothyroid muscle Infrahyoid muscle Levator scapulae muscle Platysma muscle Scalene muscle Splenius cervicis muscle Sternocleidomastoid muscle Suprahyoid muscle Thyroarytenoid muscle **3 Neck Muscle, Left** *See 2 Neck Muscle, Right* **4 Tongue, Palate, Pharynx Muscle** Chondroglossus muscle Genioglossus muscle Hyoglossus muscle Inferior longitudinal muscle Levator veli palatini muscle Palatoglossal muscle Palatopharyngeal muscle Pharyngeal constrictor muscle Salpingopharyngeus muscle Styloglossus muscle Stylopharyngeus muscle Superior longitudinal muscle Tensor veli palatini muscle **5 Shoulder Muscle, Right** Deltoid muscle Infraspinatus muscle Subscapularis muscle Supraspinatus muscle Teres major muscle Teres minor muscle **6 Shoulder Muscle, Left** *See 5 Shoulder Muscle, Right*	**7 Upper Arm Muscle, Right** Biceps brachii muscle Brachialis muscle Coracobrachialis muscle Triceps brachii muscle **8 Upper Arm Muscle, Left** *See 7 Upper Arm Muscle, Right* **9 Lower Arm and Wrist Muscle, Right** Anatomical snuffbox Brachioradialis muscle Extensor carpi radialis muscle Extensor carpi ulnaris muscle Flexor carpi radialis muscle Flexor carpi ulnaris muscle Flexor pollicis longus muscle Palmaris longus muscle Pronator quadratus muscle Pronator teres muscle **B Lower Arm and Wrist Muscle, Left** *See 9 Lower Arm and Wrist Muscle, Right* **C Hand Muscle, Right** Hypothenar muscle Palmar interosseous muscle Thenar muscle **D Hand Muscle, Left** *See C Hand Muscle, Right* **F Trunk Muscle, Right** Coccygeus muscle Erector spinae muscle Interspinalis muscle Intertransversarius muscle Latissimus dorsi muscle Quadratus lumborum muscle Rhomboid major muscle Rhomboid minor muscle Serratus posterior muscle Transversospinalis muscle Trapezius muscle **G Trunk Muscle, Left** *See F Trunk Muscle, Right* **H Thorax Muscle, Right** Intercostal muscle Levatores costarum muscle Pectoralis major muscle Pectoralis minor muscle Serratus anterior muscle Subclavius muscle Subcostal muscle Transverse thoracis muscle **J Thorax Muscle, Left** *See H Thorax Muscle, Right* **K Abdomen Muscle, Right** External oblique muscle Internal oblique muscle Pyramidalis muscle Rectus abdominis muscle Transversus abdominis muscle **L Abdomen Muscle, Left** *See K Abdomen Muscle, Right*	**M Perineum Muscle** Bulbospongiosus muscle Cremaster muscle Deep transverse perineal muscle Ischiocavernosus muscle Levator ani muscle Superficial transverse perineal muscle **N Hip Muscle, Right** Gemellus muscle Gluteus maximus muscle Gluteus medius muscle Gluteus minimus muscle Iliacus muscle Obturator muscle Piriformis muscle Psoas muscle Quadratus femoris muscle Tensor fasciae latae muscle **P Hip Muscle, Left** *See N Hip Muscle, Right* **Q Upper Leg Muscle, Right** Adductor brevis muscle Adductor longus muscle Adductor magnus muscle Biceps femoris muscle Gracilis muscle Pectineus muscle Quadriceps (femoris) Rectus femoris muscle Sartorius muscle Semimembranosus muscle Semitendinosus muscle Vastus intermedius muscle Vastus lateralis muscle Vastus medialis muscle **R Upper Leg Muscle, Left** *See Q Upper Leg Muscle, Right* **S Lower Leg Muscle, Right** Extensor digitorum longus muscle Extensor hallucis longus muscle Fibularis brevis muscle Fibularis longus muscle Flexor digitorum longus muscle Flexor hallucis longus muscle Gastrocnemius muscle Peroneus brevis muscle Peroneus longus muscle Popliteus muscle Soleus muscle Tibialis anterior muscle Tibialis posterior muscle **T Lower Leg Muscle, Left** *See S Lower Leg Muscle, Right* **V Foot Muscle, Right** Abductor hallucis muscle Adductor hallucis muscle Extensor digitorum brevis muscle Extensor hallucis brevis muscle Flexor digitorum brevis muscle Flexor hallucis brevis muscle Quadratus plantae muscle **W Foot Muscle, Left** *See V Foot Muscle, Right*	**Ø** Open **3** Percutaneous **4** Percutaneous Endoscopic	**Z** No Device	**X** Diagnostic **Z** No Qualifier

NC Noncovered Procedure   **LC** Limited Coverage   **QA** Questionable OB Admit   **NT** New Tech Add-on   ⊞ Combination Member   ♂ Male   ♀ Female

ICD-10-PCS 2022   469

ØKB–ØKB

Muscles

Ø   **Medical and Surgical**
K   **Muscles**
C   **Extirpation**   Definition: Taking or cutting out solid matter from a body part

Explanation: The solid matter may be an abnormal byproduct of a biological function or a foreign body; it may be imbedded in a body part or in the lumen of a tubular body part. The solid matter may or may not have been previously broken into pieces.

Body Part			Approach	Device	Qualifier
Character 4			**Character 5**	**Character 6**	**Character 7**
Ø Head Muscle	**7 Upper Arm Muscle, Right**	**M Perineum Muscle**	**Ø Open**	**Z No Device**	**Z No Qualifier**
Auricularis muscle	Biceps brachii muscle	Bulbospongiosus muscle	**3 Percutaneous**		
Masseter muscle	Brachialis muscle	Cremaster muscle	**4 Percutaneous**		
Pterygoid muscle	Coracobrachialis muscle	Deep transverse perineal	**Endoscopic**		
Splenius capitis muscle	Triceps brachii muscle	muscle			
Temporalis muscle	**8 Upper Arm Muscle, Left**	Ischiocavernosus muscle			
Temporoparietalis muscle	*See 7 Upper Arm Muscle,*	Levator ani muscle			
1 Facial Muscle	*Right*	Superficial transverse			
Buccinator muscle	**9 Lower Arm and Wrist**	perineal muscle			
Corrugator supercilii	**Muscle, Right**	**N Hip Muscle, Right**			
muscle	Anatomical snuffbox	Gemellus muscle			
Depressor anguli oris	Brachioradialis muscle	Gluteus maximus muscle			
muscle	Extensor carpi radialis	Gluteus medius muscle			
Depressor labii inferioris	muscle	Gluteus minimus muscle			
muscle	Extensor carpi ulnaris	Iliacus muscle			
Depressor septi nasi	muscle	Obturator muscle			
muscle	Flexor carpi radialis	Piriformis muscle			
Depressor supercilii	muscle	Psoas muscle			
muscle	Flexor carpi ulnaris muscle	Quadratus femoris muscle			
Levator anguli oris muscle	Flexor pollicis longus	Tensor fasciae latae			
Levator labii superioris	muscle	muscle			
alaeque nasi muscle	Palmaris longus muscle	**P Hip Muscle, Left**			
Levator labii superioris	Pronator quadratus	*See N Hip Muscle, Right*			
muscle	muscle	**Q Upper Leg Muscle, Right**			
Mentalis muscle	Pronator teres muscle	Adductor brevis muscle			
Nasalis muscle	**B Lower Arm and Wrist**	Adductor longus muscle			
Occipitofrontalis muscle	**Muscle, Left**	Adductor magnus muscle			
Orbicularis oris muscle	*See 9 Lower Arm and Wrist*	Biceps femoris muscle			
Procerus muscle	*Muscle, Right*	Gracilis muscle			
Risorius muscle	**C Hand Muscle, Right**	Pectineus muscle			
Zygomaticus muscle	Hypothenar muscle	Quadriceps (femoris)			
2 Neck Muscle, Right	Palmar interosseous	Rectus femoris muscle			
Anterior vertebral muscle	muscle	Sartorius muscle			
Arytenoid muscle	Thenar muscle	Semimembranosus			
Cricothyroid muscle	**D Hand Muscle, Left**	muscle			
Infrahyoid muscle	*See C Hand Muscle, Right*	Semitendinosus muscle			
Levator scapulae muscle	**F Trunk Muscle, Right**	Vastus intermedius muscle			
Platysma muscle	Coccygeus muscle	Vastus lateralis muscle			
Scalene muscle	Erector spinae muscle	Vastus medialis muscle			
Splenius cervicis muscle	Interspinalis muscle	**R Upper Leg Muscle, Left**			
Sternocleidomastoid	Intertransversarius muscle	*See Q Upper Leg Muscle,*			
muscle	Latissimus dorsi muscle	*Right*			
Suprahyoid muscle	Quadratus lumborum	**S Lower Leg Muscle, Right**			
Thyroarytenoid muscle	muscle	Extensor digitorum longus			
3 Neck Muscle, Left	Rhomboid major muscle	muscle			
See 2 Neck Muscle, Right	Rhomboid minor muscle	Extensor hallucis longus			
4 Tongue, Palate, Pharynx	Serratus posterior muscle	muscle			
Muscle	Transversospinalis muscle	Fibularis brevis muscle			
Chondroglossus muscle	Trapezius muscle	Fibularis longus muscle			
Genioglossus muscle	**G Trunk Muscle, Left**	Flexor digitorum longus			
Hyoglossus muscle	*See F Trunk Muscle, Right*	muscle			
Inferior longitudinal	**H Thorax Muscle, Right**	Flexor hallucis longus			
muscle	Intercostal muscle	muscle			
Levator veli palatini	Levatores costarum	Gastrocnemius muscle			
muscle	muscle	Peroneus brevis muscle			
Palatoglossal muscle	Pectoralis major muscle	Peroneus longus muscle			
Palatopharyngeal muscle	Pectoralis minor muscle	Popliteus muscle			
Pharyngeal constrictor	Serratus anterior muscle	Soleus muscle			
muscle	Subclavius muscle	Tibialis anterior muscle			
Salpingopharyngeus	Subcostal muscle	Tibialis posterior muscle			
muscle	Transverse thoracic	**T Lower Leg Muscle, Left**			
Styloglossus muscle	muscle	*See S Lower Leg Muscle,*			
Stylopharyngeus muscle	**J Thorax Muscle, Left**	*Right*			
Superior longitudinal	*See H Thorax Muscle, Right*	**V Foot Muscle, Right**			
muscle	**K Abdomen Muscle, Right**	Abductor hallucis muscle			
Tensor veli palatini muscle	External oblique muscle	Adductor hallucis muscle			
5 Shoulder Muscle, Right	Internal oblique muscle	Extensor digitorum brevis			
Deltoid muscle	Pyramidalis muscle	muscle			
Infraspinatus muscle	Rectus abdominis muscle	Extensor hallucis brevis			
Subscapularis muscle	Transversus abdominis	muscle			
Supraspinatus muscle	muscle	Flexor digitorum brevis			
Teres major muscle	**L Abdomen Muscle, Left**	muscle			
Teres minor muscle	*See K Abdomen Muscle,*	Flexor hallucis brevis			
6 Shoulder Muscle, Left	*Right*	muscle			
See 5 Shoulder Muscle,		Quadratus plantae muscle			
Right		**W Foot Muscle, Left**			
		See V Foot Muscle, Right			

Ø   Medical and Surgical
K   Muscles
D   Extraction   Definition: Pulling or stripping out or off all or a portion of a body part by the use of force
                  Explanation: The qualifier DIAGNOSTIC is used to identify extraction procedures that are biopsies

Body Part Character 4			Approach Character 5	Device Character 6	Qualifier Character 7
Ø Head Muscle Auricularis muscle Masseter muscle Pterygoid muscle Splenius capitis muscle Temporalis muscle Temporoparietalis muscle **1 Facial Muscle** Buccinator muscle Corrugator supercilii muscle Depressor anguli oris muscle Depressor labii inferioris muscle Depressor septi nasi muscle Depressor supercilii muscle Levator anguli oris muscle Levator labii superioris alaeque nasi muscle Levator labii superioris muscle Mentalis muscle Nasalis muscle Occipitofrontalis muscle Orbicularis oris muscle Procerus muscle Risorius muscle Zygomaticus muscle **2 Neck Muscle, Right** Anterior vertebral muscle Arytenoid muscle Cricothyroid muscle Infrahyoid muscle Levator scapulae muscle Platysma muscle Scalene muscle Splenius cervicis muscle Sternocleidomastoid muscle Suprahyoid muscle Thyroarytenoid muscle **3 Neck Muscle, Left** *See 2 Neck Muscle, Right* **4 Tongue, Palate, Pharynx Muscle** Chondroglossus muscle Genioglossus muscle Hyoglossus muscle Inferior longitudinal muscle Levator veli palatini muscle Palatoglossal muscle Palatopharyngeal muscle Pharyngeal constrictor muscle Salpingopharyngeus muscle Styloglossus muscle Stylopharyngeus muscle Superior longitudinal muscle Tensor veli palatini muscle **5 Shoulder Muscle, Right** Deltoid muscle Infraspinatus muscle Subscapularis muscle Supraspinatus muscle Teres major muscle Teres minor muscle **6 Shoulder Muscle, Left** *See 5 Shoulder Muscle, Right*	**7 Upper Arm Muscle, Right** Biceps brachii muscle Brachialis muscle Coracobrachialis muscle Triceps brachii muscle **8 Upper Arm Muscle, Left** *See 7 Upper Arm Muscle, Right* **9 Lower Arm and Wrist Muscle, Right** Anatomical snuffbox Brachioradialis muscle Extensor carpi radialis muscle Extensor carpi ulnaris muscle Flexor carpi radialis muscle Flexor carpi ulnaris muscle Flexor pollicis longus muscle Palmaris longus muscle Pronator quadratus muscle Pronator teres muscle **B Lower Arm and Wrist Muscle, Left** *See 9 Lower Arm and Wrist Muscle, Right* **C Hand Muscle, Right** Hypothenar muscle Palmar interosseous muscle Thenar muscle **D Hand Muscle, Left** *See C Hand Muscle, Right* **F Trunk Muscle, Right** Coccygeus muscle Erector spinae muscle Interspinalis muscle Intertransversarius muscle Latissimus dorsi muscle Quadratus lumborum muscle Rhomboid major muscle Rhomboid minor muscle Serratus posterior muscle Transversospinalis muscle Trapezius muscle **G Trunk Muscle, Left** *See F Trunk Muscle, Right* **H Thorax Muscle, Right** Intercostal muscle Levatores costarum muscle Pectoralis major muscle Pectoralis minor muscle Serratus anterior muscle Subclavius muscle Subcostal muscle Transverse thoracis muscle **J Thorax Muscle, Left** *See H Thorax Muscle, Right* **K Abdomen Muscle, Right** External oblique muscle Internal oblique muscle Pyramidalis muscle Rectus abdominis muscle Transversus abdominis muscle **L Abdomen Muscle, Left** *See K Abdomen Muscle, Right*	**M Perineum Muscle** Bulbospongiosus muscle Cremaster muscle Deep transverse perineal muscle Ischiocavernosus muscle Levator ani muscle Superficial transverse perineal muscle **N Hip Muscle, Right** Gemellus muscle Gluteus maximus muscle Gluteus medius muscle Gluteus minimus muscle Iliacus muscle Obturator muscle Piriformis muscle Psoas muscle Quadratus femoris muscle Tensor fasciae latae muscle **P Hip Muscle, Left** *See N Hip Muscle, Right* **Q Upper Leg Muscle, Right** Adductor brevis muscle Adductor longus muscle Adductor magnus muscle Biceps femoris muscle Gracilis muscle Pectineus muscle Quadriceps (femoris) Rectus femoris muscle Sartorius muscle Semimembranosus muscle Semitendinosus muscle Vastus intermedius muscle Vastus lateralis muscle Vastus medialis muscle **R Upper Leg Muscle, Left** *See Q Upper Leg Muscle, Right* **S Lower Leg Muscle, Right** Extensor digitorum longus muscle Extensor hallucis longus muscle Fibularis brevis muscle Fibularis longus muscle Flexor digitorum longus muscle Flexor hallucis longus muscle Gastrocnemius muscle Peroneus brevis muscle Peroneus longus muscle Popliteus muscle Soleus muscle Tibialis anterior muscle Tibialis posterior muscle **T Lower Leg Muscle, Left** *See S Lower Leg Muscle, Right* **V Foot Muscle, Right** Abductor hallucis muscle Adductor hallucis muscle Extensor digitorum brevis muscle Extensor hallucis brevis muscle Flexor digitorum brevis muscle Flexor hallucis brevis muscle Quadratus plantae muscle **W Foot Muscle, Left** *See V Foot Muscle, Right*	**Ø Open**	**Z No Device**	**Z No Qualifier**

NC Noncovered Procedure   **LC** Limited Coverage   **QA** Questionable OB Admit   **NT** New Tech Add-on   ✚ Combination Member   ♂ Male   ♀ Female

ICD-10-PCS 2022   **471**

Muscles

Ø   **Medical and Surgical**
K   **Muscles**
H   **Insertion**   Definition: Putting in a nonbiological appliance that monitors, assists, performs, or prevents a physiological function but does not physically take the place of a body part
                Explanation: None

Body Part Character 4	Approach Character 5	Device Character 6	Qualifier Character 7
X Upper Muscle Y Lower Muscle	Ø Open 3 Percutaneous 4 Percutaneous Endoscopic	M Stimulator Lead Y Other Device	Z No Qualifier

Non-OR   ØKH[X,Y][3,4]YZ

Ø   **Medical and Surgical**
K   **Muscles**
J   **Inspection**   Definition: Visually and/or manually exploring a body part
                Explanation: Visual exploration may be performed with or without optical instrumentation. Manual exploration may be performed directly or through intervening body layers.

Body Part Character 4	Approach Character 5	Device Character 6	Qualifier Character 7
X Upper Muscle Y Lower Muscle	Ø Open 3 Percutaneous 4 Percutaneous Endoscopic X External	Z No Device	Z No Qualifier

Non-OR   ØKJ[X,Y][3,X]ZZ

Ø   Medical and Surgical
K   Muscles
M   Reattachment   Definition: Putting back in or on all or a portion of a separated body part to its normal location or other suitable location
                           Explanation: Vascular circulation and nervous pathways may or may not be reestablished

Body Part Character 4			Approach Character 5	Device Character 6	Qualifier Character 7

Ø Head Muscle
  Auricularis muscle
  Masseter muscle
  Pterygoid muscle
  Splenius capitis muscle
  Temporalis muscle
  Temporoparietalis muscle
1 Facial Muscle
  Buccinator muscle
  Corrugator supercilii
    muscle
  Depressor anguli oris
    muscle
  Depressor labii inferioris
    muscle
  Depressor septi nasi
    muscle
  Depressor supercilii
    muscle
  Levator anguli oris muscle
  Levator labii superioris
    alaeque nasi muscle
  Levator labii superioris
    muscle
  Mentalis muscle
  Nasalis muscle
  Occipitofrontalis muscle
  Orbicularis oris muscle
  Procerus muscle
  Risorius muscle
  Zygomaticus muscle
2 Neck Muscle, Right
  Anterior vertebral muscle
  Arytenoid muscle
  Cricothyroid muscle
  Infrahyoid muscle
  Levator scapulae muscle
  Platysma muscle
  Scalene muscle
  Splenius cervicis muscle
  Sternocleidomastoid
    muscle
  Suprahyoid muscle
  Thyroarytenoid muscle
3 Neck Muscle, Left
  See 2 Neck Muscle, Right
4 Tongue, Palate, Pharynx
  Muscle
  Chondroglossus muscle
  Genioglossus muscle
  Hyoglossus muscle
  Inferior longitudinal
    muscle
  Levator veli palatini
    muscle
  Palatoglossal muscle
  Palatopharyngeal muscle
  Pharyngeal constrictor
    muscle
  Salpingopharyngeus
    muscle
  Styloglossus muscle
  Stylopharyngeus muscle
  Superior longitudinal
    muscle
  Tensor veli palatini muscle
5 Shoulder Muscle, Right
  Deltoid muscle
  Infraspinatus muscle
  Subscapularis muscle
  Supraspinatus muscle
  Teres major muscle
  Teres minor muscle
6 Shoulder Muscle, Left
  See 5 Shoulder Muscle,
    Right
	7 Upper Arm Muscle, Right
	  Biceps brachii muscle
	  Brachialis muscle
	  Coracobrachialis muscle
	  Triceps brachii muscle
	8 Upper Arm Muscle, Left
	  See 7 Upper Arm Muscle,
	    Right
	9 Lower Arm and Wrist
	  Muscle, Right
	  Anatomical snuffbox
	  Brachioradialis muscle
	  Extensor carpi radialis
	    muscle
	  Extensor carpi ulnaris
	    muscle
	  Flexor carpi radialis
	    muscle
	  Flexor carpi ulnaris muscle
	  Flexor pollicis longus
	    muscle
	  Palmaris longus muscle
	  Pronator quadratus
	    muscle
	  Pronator teres muscle
	B Lower Arm and Wrist
	  Muscle, Left
	  See 9 Lower Arm and Wrist
	    Muscle, Right
	C Hand Muscle, Right
	  Hypothenar muscle
	  Palmar interosseous
	    muscle
	  Thenar muscle
	D Hand Muscle, Left
	  See C Hand Muscle, Right
	F Trunk Muscle, Right
	  Coccygeus muscle
	  Erector spinae muscle
	  Interspinalis muscle
	  Intertransversarius muscle
	  Latissimus dorsi muscle
	  Quadratus lumborum
	    muscle
	  Rhomboid major muscle
	  Rhomboid minor muscle
	  Serratus posterior muscle
	  Transversospinalis muscle
	  Trapezius muscle
	G Trunk Muscle, Left
	  See F Trunk Muscle, Right
	H Thorax Muscle, Right
	  Intercostal muscle
	  Levatores costarum
	    muscle
	  Pectoralis major muscle
	  Pectoralis minor muscle
	  Serratus anterior muscle
	  Subclavius muscle
	  Subcostal muscle
	  Transverse thoracis
	    muscle
	J Thorax Muscle, Left
	  See H Thorax Muscle, Right
	K Abdomen Muscle, Right
	  External oblique muscle
	  Internal oblique muscle
	  Pyramidalis muscle
	  Rectus abdominis muscle
	  Transversus abdominis
	    muscle
	L Abdomen Muscle, Left
	  See K Abdomen Muscle,
	    Right
		M Perineum Muscle
		  Bulbospongiosus muscle
		  Cremaster muscle
		  Deep transverse perineal
		    muscle
		  Ischiocavernosus muscle
		  Levator ani muscle
		  Superficial transverse
		    perineal muscle
		N Hip Muscle, Right
		  Gemellus muscle
		  Gluteus maximus muscle
		  Gluteus medius muscle
		  Gluteus minimus muscle
		  Iliacus muscle
		  Obturator muscle
		  Piriformis muscle
		  Psoas muscle
		  Quadratus femoris muscle
		  Tensor fasciae latae
		    muscle
		P Hip Muscle, Left
		  See N Hip Muscle, Right
		Q Upper Leg Muscle, Right
		  Adductor brevis muscle
		  Adductor longus muscle
		  Adductor magnus muscle
		  Biceps femoris muscle
		  Gracilis muscle
		  Pectineus muscle
		  Quadriceps (femoris)
		  Rectus femoris muscle
		  Sartorius muscle
		  Semimembranosus
		    muscle
		  Semitendinosus muscle
		  Vastus intermedius muscle
		  Vastus lateralis muscle
		  Vastus medialis muscle
		R Upper Leg Muscle, Left
		  See Q Upper Leg Muscle,
		    Right
		S Lower Leg Muscle, Right
		  Extensor digitorum longus
		    muscle
		  Extensor hallucis longus
		    muscle
		  Fibularis brevis muscle
		  Fibularis longus muscle
		  Flexor digitorum longus
		    muscle
		  Flexor hallucis longus
		    muscle
		  Gastrocnemius muscle
		  Peroneus brevis muscle
		  Peroneus longus muscle
		  Popliteus muscle
		  Soleus muscle
		  Tibialis anterior muscle
		  Tibialis posterior muscle
		T Lower Leg Muscle, Left
		  See S Lower Leg Muscle,
		    Right
		V Foot Muscle, Right
		  Abductor hallucis muscle
		  Adductor hallucis muscle
		  Extensor digitorum brevis
		    muscle
		  Extensor hallucis brevis
		    muscle
		  Flexor digitorum brevis
		    muscle
		  Flexor hallucis brevis
		    muscle
		  Quadratus plantae muscle
		W Foot Muscle, Left
		  See V Foot Muscle, Right
			Ø Open
			4 Percutaneous
			  Endoscopic
				Z No Device	**Z No Qualifier**

Ø   **Medical and Surgical**
K   **Muscles**
N   **Release**   Definition: Freeing a body part from an abnormal physical constraint by cutting or by the use of force
                      Explanation: Some of the restraining tissue may be taken out but none of the body part is taken out

Body Part Character 4			Approach Character 5	Device Character 6	Qualifier Character 7
Ø Head Muscle Auricularis muscle Masseter muscle Pterygoid muscle Splenius capitis muscle Temporalis muscle Temporoparietalis muscle **1 Facial Muscle** Buccinator muscle Corrugator supercilii muscle Depressor anguli oris muscle Depressor labii inferioris muscle Depressor septi nasi muscle Depressor supercilii muscle Levator anguli oris muscle Levator labii superioris alaeque nasi muscle Levator labii superioris muscle Mentalis muscle Nasalis muscle Occipitofrontalis muscle Orbicularis oris muscle Procerus muscle Risorius muscle Zygomaticus muscle **2 Neck Muscle, Right** Anterior vertebral muscle Arytenoid muscle Cricothyroid muscle Infrahyoid muscle Levator scapulae muscle Platysma muscle Scalene muscle Splenius cervicis muscle Sternocleidomastoid muscle Suprahyoid muscle Thyroarytenoid muscle **3 Neck Muscle, Left** *See 2 Neck Muscle, Right* **4 Tongue, Palate, Pharynx Muscle** Chondroglossus muscle Genioglossus muscle Hyoglossus muscle Inferior longitudinal muscle Levator veli palatini muscle Palatoglossal muscle Palatopharyngeal muscle Pharyngeal constrictor muscle Salpingopharyngeus muscle Styloglossus muscle Stylopharyngeus muscle Superior longitudinal muscle Tensor veli palatini muscle **5 Shoulder Muscle, Right** Deltoid muscle Infraspinatus muscle Subscapularis muscle Supraspinatus muscle Teres major muscle Teres minor muscle **6 Shoulder Muscle, Left** *See 5 Shoulder Muscle, Right*	**7 Upper Arm Muscle, Right** Biceps brachii muscle Brachialis muscle Coracobrachialis muscle Triceps brachii muscle **8 Upper Arm Muscle, Left** *See 7 Upper Arm Muscle, Right* **9 Lower Arm and Wrist Muscle, Right** Anatomical snuffbox Brachioradialis muscle Extensor carpi radialis muscle Extensor carpi ulnaris muscle Flexor carpi radialis muscle Flexor carpi ulnaris muscle Flexor pollicis longus muscle Palmaris longus muscle Pronator quadratus muscle Pronator teres muscle **B Lower Arm and Wrist Muscle, Left** *See 9 Lower Arm and Wrist Muscle, Right* **C Hand Muscle, Right** Hypothenar muscle Palmar interosseous muscle Thenar muscle **D Hand Muscle, Left** *See C Hand Muscle, Right* **F Trunk Muscle, Right** Coccygeus muscle Erector spinae muscle Interspinalis muscle Intertransversarius muscle Latissimus dorsi muscle Quadratus lumborum muscle Rhomboid major muscle Rhomboid minor muscle Serratus posterior muscle Transversospinalis muscle Trapezius muscle **G Trunk Muscle, Left** *See F Trunk Muscle, Right* **H Thorax Muscle, Right** Intercostal muscle Levatores costarum muscle Pectoralis major muscle Pectoralis minor muscle Serratus anterior muscle Subclavius muscle Subcostal muscle Transverse thoracis muscle **J Thorax Muscle, Left** *See H Thorax Muscle, Right* **K Abdomen Muscle, Right** External oblique muscle Internal oblique muscle Pyramidalis muscle Rectus abdominis muscle Transversus abdominis muscle **L Abdomen Muscle, Left** *See K Abdomen Muscle, Right*	**M Perineum Muscle** Bulbospongiosus muscle Cremaster muscle Deep transverse perineal muscle Ischiocavernosus muscle Levator ani muscle Superficial transverse perineal muscle **N Hip Muscle, Right** Gemellus muscle Gluteus maximus muscle Gluteus medius muscle Gluteus minimus muscle Iliacus muscle Obturator muscle Piriformis muscle Psoas muscle Quadratus femoris muscle Tensor fasciae latae muscle **P Hip Muscle, Left** *See N Hip Muscle, Right* **Q Upper Leg Muscle, Right** Adductor brevis muscle Adductor longus muscle Adductor magnus muscle Biceps femoris muscle Gracilis muscle Pectineus muscle Quadriceps (femoris) Rectus femoris muscle Sartorius muscle Semimembranosus muscle Semitendinosus muscle Vastus intermedius muscle Vastus lateralis muscle Vastus medialis muscle **R Upper Leg Muscle, Left** *See Q Upper Leg Muscle, Right* **S Lower Leg Muscle, Right** Extensor digitorum longus muscle Extensor hallucis longus muscle Fibularis brevis muscle Fibularis longus muscle Flexor digitorum longus muscle Flexor hallucis longus muscle Gastrocnemius muscle Peroneus brevis muscle Peroneus longus muscle Popliteus muscle Soleus muscle Tibialis anterior muscle Tibialis posterior muscle **T Lower Leg Muscle, Left** *See S Lower Leg Muscle, Right* **V Foot Muscle, Right** Abductor hallucis muscle Adductor hallucis muscle Extensor digitorum brevis muscle Extensor hallucis brevis muscle Flexor digitorum brevis muscle Flexor hallucis brevis muscle Quadratus plantae muscle **W Foot Muscle, Left** *See V Foot Muscle, Right*	**Ø Open** **3 Percutaneous** **4 Percutaneous Endoscopic** **X External**	**Z No Device**	**Z No Qualifier**

Non-OR   ØKN[Ø,1,2,3,4,5,6,7,8,9,B,C,D,F,G,H,J,K,L,M,N,P,Q,R,S,T,V,W]XZZ

Ø   **Medical and Surgical**
K   **Muscles**
P   **Removal**   Definition: Taking out or off a device from a body part

                Explanation: If a device is taken out and a similar device put in without cutting or puncturing the skin or mucous membrane, the procedure is coded to the root operation CHANGE. Otherwise, the procedure for taking out a device is coded to the root operation REMOVAL.

Body Part Character 4	Approach Character 5	Device Character 6	Qualifier Character 7
X Upper Muscle Y Lower Muscle	Ø Open 3 Percutaneous 4 Percutaneous Endoscopic	Ø Drainage Device 7 Autologous Tissue Substitute J Synthetic Substitute K Nonautologous Tissue Substitute M Stimulator Lead Y Other Device	Z No Qualifier
X Upper Muscle Y Lower Muscle	X External	Ø Drainage Device M Stimulator Lead	Z No Qualifier

Non-OR	ØKP[X,Y][3,4]YZ
Non-OR	ØKP[X,Y]X[Ø,M]Z

NC Noncovered Procedure   **LC** Limited Coverage   **QA** Questionable OB Admit   **NT** New Tech Add-on   ⊞ Combination Member   ♂ Male   ♀ Female

ICD-10-PCS 2022   **475**

Ø   Medical and Surgical
K   Muscles
Q   Repair   Definition: Restoring, to the extent possible, a body part to its normal anatomic structure and function

Explanation: Used only when the method to accomplish the repair is not one of the other root operations

Body Part Character 4			Approach Character 5	Device Character 6	Qualifier Character 7

Ø Head Muscle	**7 Upper Arm Muscle, Right**	**M Perineum Muscle**	**Ø Open**	**Z No Device**	**Z No Qualifier**
Auricularis muscle	Biceps brachii muscle	Bulbospongiosus muscle	**3 Percutaneous**		
Masseter muscle	Brachialis muscle	Cremaster muscle	**4 Percutaneous**		
Pterygoid muscle	Coracobrachialis muscle	Deep transverse perineal	**Endoscopic**		
Splenius capitis muscle	Triceps brachii muscle	muscle			
Temporalis muscle	**8 Upper Arm Muscle, Left**	Ischiocavernosus muscle			
Temporoparietalis muscle	*See 7 Upper Arm Muscle,*	Levator ani muscle			
1 Facial Muscle	*Right*	Superficial transverse			
Buccinator muscle	**9 Lower Arm and Wrist**	perineal muscle			
Corrugator supercilii	**Muscle, Right**	**N Hip Muscle, Right**			
muscle	Anatomical snuffbox	Gemellus muscle			
Depressor anguli oris	Brachioradialis muscle	Gluteus maximus muscle			
muscle	Extensor carpi radialis	Gluteus medius muscle			
Depressor labii inferioris	muscle	Gluteus minimus muscle			
muscle	Extensor carpi ulnaris	Iliacus muscle			
Depressor septi nasi	muscle	Obturator muscle			
muscle	Flexor carpi radialis	Piriformis muscle			
Depressor supercilii	muscle	Psoas muscle			
muscle	Flexor carpi ulnaris muscle	Quadratus femoris muscle			
Levator anguli oris muscle	Flexor pollicis longus	Tensor fasciae latae			
Levator labii superioris	muscle	muscle			
alaeque nasi muscle	Palmaris longus muscle	**P Hip Muscle, Left**			
Levator labii superioris	Pronator quadratus	*See N Hip Muscle, Right*			
muscle	muscle	**Q Upper Leg Muscle, Right**			
Mentalis muscle	Pronator teres muscle	Adductor brevis muscle			
Nasalis muscle	**B Lower Arm and Wrist**	Adductor longus muscle			
Occipitofrontalis muscle	**Muscle, Left**	Adductor magnus muscle			
Orbicularis oris muscle	*See 9 Lower Arm and Wrist*	Biceps femoris muscle			
Procerus muscle	*Muscle, Right*	Gracilis muscle			
Risorius muscle	**C Hand Muscle, Right**	Pectineus muscle			
Zygomaticus muscle	Hypothenar muscle	Quadriceps (femoris)			
2 Neck Muscle, Right	Palmar interosseous	Rectus femoris muscle			
Anterior vertebral muscle	muscle	Sartorius muscle			
Arytenoid muscle	Thenar muscle	Semimembranosus			
Cricothyroid muscle	**D Hand Muscle, Left**	muscle			
Infrahyoid muscle	*See C Hand Muscle, Right*	Semitendinosus muscle			
Levator scapulae muscle	**F Trunk Muscle, Right**	Vastus intermedius muscle			
Platysma muscle	Coccygeus muscle	Vastus lateralis muscle			
Scalene muscle	Erector spinae muscle	Vastus medialis muscle			
Splenius cervicis muscle	Interspinalis muscle	**R Upper Leg Muscle, Left**			
Sternocleidomastoid	Intertransversarius muscle	*See Q Upper Leg Muscle,*			
muscle	Latissimus dorsi muscle	*Right*			
Suprahyoid muscle	Quadratus lumborum	**S Lower Leg Muscle, Right**			
Thyroarytenoid muscle	muscle	Extensor digitorum longus			
3 Neck Muscle, Left	Rhomboid major muscle	muscle			
See 2 Neck Muscle, Right	Rhomboid minor muscle	Extensor hallucis longus			
4 Tongue, Palate, Pharynx	Serratus posterior muscle	muscle			
Muscle	Transversospinalis muscle	Fibularis brevis muscle			
Chondroglossus muscle	Trapezius muscle	Fibularis longus muscle			
Genioglossus muscle	**G Trunk Muscle, Left**	Flexor digitorum longus			
Hyoglossus muscle	*See F Trunk Muscle, Right*	muscle			
Inferior longitudinal	**H Thorax Muscle, Right**	Flexor hallucis longus			
muscle	Intercostal muscle	muscle			
Levator veli palatini	Levatores costarum	Gastrocnemius muscle			
muscle	muscle	Peroneus brevis muscle			
Palatoglossal muscle	Pectoralis major muscle	Peroneus longus muscle			
Palatopharyngeal muscle	Pectoralis minor muscle	Popliteus muscle			
Pharyngeal constrictor	Serratus anterior muscle	Soleus muscle			
muscle	Subclavius muscle	Tibialis anterior muscle			
Salpingopharyngeus	Subcostal muscle	Tibialis posterior muscle			
muscle	Transverse thoracis	**T Lower Leg Muscle, Left**			
Styloglossus muscle	muscle	*See S Lower Leg Muscle,*			
Stylopharyngeus muscle	**J Thorax Muscle, Left**	*Right*			
Superior longitudinal	*See H Thorax Muscle, Right*	**V Foot Muscle, Right**			
muscle	**K Abdomen Muscle, Right**	Abductor hallucis muscle			
Tensor veli palatini muscle	External oblique muscle	Adductor hallucis muscle			
5 Shoulder Muscle, Right	Internal oblique muscle	Extensor digitorum brevis			
Deltoid muscle	Pyramidalis muscle	muscle			
Infraspinatus muscle	Rectus abdominis muscle	Extensor hallucis brevis			
Subscapularis muscle	Transversus abdominis	muscle			
Supraspinatus muscle	muscle	Flexor digitorum brevis			
Teres major muscle	**L Abdomen Muscle, Left**	muscle			
Teres minor muscle	*See K Abdomen Muscle,*	Flexor hallucis brevis			
6 Shoulder Muscle, Left	*Right*	muscle			
See 5 Shoulder Muscle,		Quadratus plantae muscle			
Right		**W Foot Muscle, Left**			
		See V Foot Muscle, Right			

0   **Medical and Surgical**
K   **Muscles**
R   **Replacement**   Definition: Putting in or on biological or synthetic material that physically takes the place and/or function of all or a portion of a body part
                               Explanation: The body part may have been taken out or replaced, or may be taken out, physically eradicated, or rendered nonfunctional during the REPLACEMENT procedure. A REMOVAL procedure is coded for taking out the device used in a previous replacement procedure.

Body Part Character 4			Approach Character 5	Device Character 6	Qualifier Character 7
0 **Head Muscle** Auricularis muscle Masseter muscle Pterygoid muscle Splenius capitis muscle Temporalis muscle Temporoparietalis muscle **1** **Facial Muscle** Buccinator muscle Corrugator supercilii muscle Depressor anguli oris muscle Depressor labii inferioris muscle Depressor septi nasi muscle Depressor supercilii muscle Levator anguli oris muscle Levator labii superioris alaeque nasi muscle Levator labii superioris muscle Mentalis muscle Nasalis muscle Occipitofrontalis muscle Orbicularis oris muscle Procerus muscle Risorius muscle Zygomaticus muscle **2** **Neck Muscle, Right** Anterior vertebral muscle Arytenoid muscle Cricothyroid muscle Infrahyoid muscle Levator scapulae muscle Platysma muscle Scalene muscle Splenius cervicis muscle Sternocleidomastoid muscle Suprahyoid muscle Thyroarytenoid muscle **3** **Neck Muscle, Left** *See 2 Neck Muscle, Right* **4** **Tongue, Palate, Pharynx Muscle** Chondroglossus muscle Genioglossus muscle Hyoglossus muscle Inferior longitudinal muscle Levator veli palatini muscle Palatoglossal muscle Palatopharyngeal muscle Pharyngeal constrictor muscle Salpingopharyngeus muscle Styloglossus muscle Stylopharyngeus muscle Superior longitudinal muscle Tensor veli palatini muscle **5** **Shoulder Muscle, Right** Deltoid muscle Infraspinatus muscle Subscapularis muscle Supraspinatus muscle Teres major muscle Teres minor muscle **6** **Shoulder Muscle, Left** *See 5 Shoulder Muscle, Right*	**7** **Upper Arm Muscle, Right** Biceps brachii muscle Brachialis muscle Coracobrachialis muscle Triceps brachii muscle **8** **Upper Arm Muscle, Left** *See 7 Upper Arm Muscle, Right* **9** **Lower Arm and Wrist Muscle, Right** Anatomical snuffbox Brachioradialis muscle Extensor carpi radialis muscle Extensor carpi ulnaris muscle Flexor carpi radialis muscle Flexor carpi ulnaris muscle Flexor pollicis longus muscle Palmaris longus muscle Pronator quadratus muscle Pronator teres muscle **B** **Lower Arm and Wrist Muscle, Left** *See 9 Lower Arm and Wrist Muscle, Right* **C** **Hand Muscle, Right** Hypothenar muscle Palmar interosseous muscle Thenar muscle **D** **Hand Muscle, Left** *See C Hand Muscle, Right* **F** **Trunk Muscle, Right** Coccygeus muscle Erector spinae muscle Interspinalis muscle Intertransversarius muscle Latissimus dorsi muscle Quadratus lumborum muscle Rhomboid major muscle Rhomboid minor muscle Serratus posterior muscle Transversospinalis muscle Trapezius muscle **G** **Trunk Muscle, Left** *See F Trunk Muscle, Right* **H** **Thorax Muscle, Right** Intercostal muscle Levatores costarum muscle Pectoralis major muscle Pectoralis minor muscle Serratus anterior muscle Subclavius muscle Subcostal muscle Transverse thoracis muscle **J** **Thorax Muscle, Left** *See H Thorax Muscle, Right* **K** **Abdomen Muscle, Right** External oblique muscle Internal oblique muscle Pyramidalis muscle Rectus abdominis muscle Transversus abdominis muscle **L** **Abdomen Muscle, Left** *See K Abdomen Muscle, Right*	**M** **Perineum Muscle** Bulbospongiosus muscle Cremaster muscle Deep transverse perineal muscle Ischiocavernosus muscle Levator ani muscle Superficial transverse perineal muscle **N** **Hip Muscle, Right** Gemellus muscle Gluteus maximus muscle Gluteus medius muscle Gluteus minimus muscle Iliacus muscle Obturator muscle Piriformis muscle Psoas muscle Quadratus femoris muscle Tensor fasciae latae muscle **P** **Hip Muscle, Left** *See N Hip Muscle, Right* **Q** **Upper Leg Muscle, Right** Adductor brevis muscle Adductor longus muscle Adductor magnus muscle Biceps femoris muscle Gracilis muscle Pectineus muscle Quadriceps (femoris) Rectus femoris muscle Sartorius muscle Semimembranosus muscle Semitendinosus muscle Vastus intermedius muscle Vastus lateralis muscle Vastus medialis muscle **R** **Upper Leg Muscle, Left** *See Q Upper Leg Muscle, Right* **S** **Lower Leg Muscle, Right** Extensor digitorum longus muscle Extensor hallucis longus muscle Fibularis brevis muscle Fibularis longus muscle Flexor digitorum longus muscle Flexor hallucis longus muscle Gastrocnemius muscle Peroneus brevis muscle Peroneus longus muscle Popliteus muscle Soleus muscle Tibialis anterior muscle Tibialis posterior muscle **T** **Lower Leg Muscle, Left** *See S Lower Leg Muscle, Right* **V** **Foot Muscle, Right** Abductor hallucis muscle Adductor hallucis muscle Extensor digitorum brevis muscle Extensor hallucis brevis muscle Flexor digitorum brevis muscle Flexor hallucis brevis muscle Quadratus plantae muscle **W** **Foot Muscle, Left** *See V Foot Muscle, Right*	**0** Open **4** Percutaneous Endoscopic	**7** Autologous Tissue Substitute **J** Synthetic Substitute **K** Nonautologous Tissue Substitute	**Z** No Qualifier

NC Noncovered Procedure   LC Limited Coverage   QA Questionable OB Admit   NT New Tech Add-on   ⊞ Combination Member   ♂ Male   ♀ Female

ICD-10-PCS 2022   477

0KR–0KR

Ø   **Medical and Surgical**
K   **Muscles**
S   **Reposition**   Definition: Moving to its normal location, or other suitable location, all or a portion of a body part
         Explanation: The body part is moved to a new location from an abnormal location, or from a normal location where it is not functioning correctly. The body part may or may not be cut out or off to be moved to the new location.

Body Part Character 4			Approach Character 5	Device Character 6	Qualifier Character 7
Ø **Head Muscle** Auricularis muscle Masseter muscle Pterygoid muscle Splenius capitis muscle Temporalis muscle Temporoparietalis muscle **1** **Facial Muscle** Buccinator muscle Corrugator supercilii muscle Depressor anguli oris muscle Depressor labii inferioris muscle Depressor septi nasi muscle Depressor supercilii muscle Levator anguli oris muscle Levator labii superioris alaeque nasi muscle Levator labii superioris muscle Mentalis muscle Nasalis muscle Occipitofrontalis muscle Orbicularis oris muscle Procerus muscle Risorius muscle Zygomaticus muscle **2** **Neck Muscle, Right** Anterior vertebral muscle Arytenoid muscle Cricothyroid muscle Infrahyoid muscle Levator scapulae muscle Platysma muscle Scalene muscle Splenius cervicis muscle Sternocleidomastoid muscle Suprahyoid muscle Thyroarytenoid muscle **3** **Neck Muscle, Left** *See* 2 Neck Muscle, Right **4** **Tongue, Palate, Pharynx Muscle** Chondroglossus muscle Genioglossus muscle Hyoglossus muscle Inferior longitudinal muscle Levator veli palatini muscle Palatoglossal muscle Palatopharyngeal muscle Pharyngeal constrictor muscle Salpingopharyngeus muscle Styloglossus muscle Stylopharyngeus muscle Superior longitudinal muscle Tensor veli palatini muscle **5** **Shoulder Muscle, Right** Deltoid muscle Infraspinatus muscle Subscapularis muscle Supraspinatus muscle Teres major muscle Teres minor muscle **6** **Shoulder Muscle, Left** *See* 5 Shoulder Muscle, Right	**7** **Upper Arm Muscle, Right** Biceps brachii muscle Brachialis muscle Coracobrachialis muscle Triceps brachii muscle **8** **Upper Arm Muscle, Left** *See* 7 Upper Arm Muscle, Right **9** **Lower Arm and Wrist Muscle, Right** Anatomical snuffbox Brachioradialis muscle Extensor carpi radialis muscle Extensor carpi ulnaris muscle Flexor carpi radialis muscle Flexor carpi ulnaris muscle Flexor pollicis longus muscle Palmaris longus muscle Pronator quadratus muscle Pronator teres muscle **B** **Lower Arm and Wrist Muscle, Left** *See* 9 Lower Arm and Wrist Muscle, Right **C** **Hand Muscle, Right** Hypothenar muscle Palmar interosseous muscle Thenar muscle **D** **Hand Muscle, Left** *See* C Hand Muscle, Right **F** **Trunk Muscle, Right** Coccygeus muscle Erector spinae muscle Interspinalis muscle Intertransversarius muscle Latissimus dorsi muscle Quadratus lumborum muscle Rhomboid major muscle Rhomboid minor muscle Serratus posterior muscle Transversospinalis muscle Trapezius muscle **G** **Trunk Muscle, Left** *See* F Trunk Muscle, Right **H** **Thorax Muscle, Right** Intercostal muscle Levatores costarum muscle Pectoralis major muscle Pectoralis minor muscle Serratus anterior muscle Subclavius muscle Subcostal muscle Transverse thoracis muscle **J** **Thorax Muscle, Left** *See* H Thorax Muscle, Right **K** **Abdomen Muscle, Right** External oblique muscle Internal oblique muscle Pyramidalis muscle Rectus abdominis muscle Transversus abdominis muscle **L** **Abdomen Muscle, Left** *See* K Abdomen Muscle, Right	**M** **Perineum Muscle** Bulbospongiosus muscle Cremaster muscle Deep transverse perineal muscle Ischiocavernosus muscle Levator ani muscle Superficial transverse perineal muscle **N** **Hip Muscle, Right** Gemellus muscle Gluteus maximus muscle Gluteus medius muscle Gluteus minimus muscle Iliacus muscle Obturator muscle Piriformis muscle Psoas muscle Quadratus femoris muscle Tensor fasciae latae muscle **P** **Hip Muscle, Left** *See* N Hip Muscle, Right **Q** **Upper Leg Muscle, Right** Adductor brevis muscle Adductor longus muscle Adductor magnus muscle Biceps femoris muscle Gracilis muscle Pectineus muscle Quadriceps (femoris) Rectus femoris muscle Sartorius muscle Semimembranosus muscle Semitendinosus muscle Vastus intermedius muscle Vastus lateralis muscle Vastus medialis muscle **R** **Upper Leg Muscle, Left** *See* Q Upper Leg Muscle, Right **S** **Lower Leg Muscle, Right** Extensor digitorum longus muscle Extensor hallucis longus muscle Fibularis brevis muscle Fibularis longus muscle Flexor digitorum longus muscle Flexor hallucis longus muscle Gastrocnemius muscle Peroneus brevis muscle Peroneus longus muscle Popliteus muscle Soleus muscle Tibialis anterior muscle Tibialis posterior muscle **T** **Lower Leg Muscle, Left** *See* S Lower Leg Muscle, Right **V** **Foot Muscle, Right** Abductor hallucis muscle Adductor hallucis muscle Extensor digitorum brevis muscle Extensor hallucis brevis muscle Flexor digitorum brevis muscle Flexor hallucis brevis muscle Quadratus plantae muscle **W** **Foot Muscle, Left** *See* V Foot Muscle, Right	**Ø** Open **4** Percutaneous Endoscopic	**Z** No Device	**Z** No Qualifier

Ø　Medical and Surgical
K　Muscles
T　Resection　　Definition: Cutting out or off, without replacement, all of a body part
　　　　　　　　　　　Explanation: None

Body Part Character 4			Approach Character 5	Device Character 6	Qualifier Character 7
Ø　Head Muscle 　　Auricularis muscle 　　Masseter muscle 　　Pterygoid muscle 　　Splenius capitis muscle 　　Temporalis muscle 　　Temporoparietalis muscle **1　Facial Muscle** 　　Buccinator muscle 　　Corrugator supercilii 　　　muscle 　　Depressor anguli oris 　　　muscle 　　Depressor labii inferioris 　　　muscle 　　Depressor septi nasi 　　　muscle 　　Depressor supercilii 　　　muscle 　　Levator anguli oris muscle 　　Levator labii superioris 　　　alaeque nasi muscle 　　Levator labii superioris 　　　muscle 　　Mentalis muscle 　　Nasalis muscle 　　Occipitofrontalis muscle 　　Orbicularis oris muscle 　　Procerus muscle 　　Risorius muscle 　　Zygomaticus muscle **2　Neck Muscle, Right** 　　Anterior vertebral muscle 　　Arytenoid muscle 　　Cricothyroid muscle 　　Infrahyoid muscle 　　Levator scapulae muscle 　　Platysma muscle 　　Scalene muscle 　　Splenius cervicis muscle 　　Sternocleidomastoid 　　　muscle 　　Suprahyoid muscle 　　Thyroarytenoid muscle **3　Neck Muscle, Left** 　　*See 2 Neck Muscle, Right* **4　Tongue, Palate, Pharynx** 　　**Muscle** 　　Chondroglossus muscle 　　Genioglossus muscle 　　Hyoglossus muscle 　　Inferior longitudinal 　　　muscle 　　Levator veli palatini muscle 　　Palatoglossal muscle 　　Palatopharyngeal muscle 　　Pharyngeal constrictor 　　　muscle 　　Salpingopharyngeus 　　　muscle 　　Styloglossus muscle 　　Stylopharyngeus muscle 　　Superior longitudinal 　　　muscle 　　Tensor veli palatini muscle **5　Shoulder Muscle, Right** 　　Deltoid muscle 　　Infraspinatus muscle 　　Subscapularis muscle 　　Supraspinatus muscle 　　Teres major muscle 　　Teres minor muscle **6　Shoulder Muscle, Left** 　　*See 5 Shoulder Muscle,* 　　　*Right*	**7　Upper Arm Muscle, Right** 　　Biceps brachii muscle 　　Brachialis muscle 　　Coracobrachialis muscle 　　Triceps brachii muscle **8　Upper Arm Muscle, Left** 　　*See 7 Upper Arm Muscle,* 　　　*Right* **9　Lower Arm and Wrist** 　　**Muscle, Right** 　　Anatomical snuffbox 　　Brachioradialis muscle 　　Extensor carpi radialis 　　　muscle 　　Extensor carpi ulnaris 　　　muscle 　　Flexor carpi radialis 　　　muscle 　　Flexor carpi ulnaris muscle 　　Flexor pollicis longus 　　　muscle 　　Palmaris longus muscle 　　Pronator quadratus 　　　muscle 　　Pronator teres muscle **B　Lower Arm and Wrist** 　　**Muscle, Left** 　　*See 9 Lower Arm and Wrist* 　　　*Muscle, Right* **C　Hand Muscle, Right** 　　Hypothenar muscle 　　Palmar interosseous 　　　muscle 　　Thenar muscle **D　Hand Muscle, Left** 　　*See C Hand Muscle, Right* **F　Trunk Muscle, Right** 　　Coccygeus muscle 　　Erector spinae muscle 　　Interspinalis muscle 　　Intertransversarius muscle 　　Latissimus dorsi muscle 　　Quadratus lumborum 　　　muscle 　　Rhomboid major muscle 　　Rhomboid minor muscle 　　Serratus posterior muscle 　　Transversospinalis muscle 　　Trapezius muscle **G　Trunk Muscle, Left** 　　*See F Trunk Muscle, Right* **H　Thorax Muscle, Right** ⊞ 　　Intercostal muscle 　　Levatores costarum 　　　muscle 　　Pectoralis major muscle 　　Pectoralis minor muscle 　　Serratus anterior muscle 　　Subclavius muscle 　　Subcostal muscle 　　Transverse thoracis 　　　muscle **J　Thorax Muscle, Left** ⊞ 　　*See H Thorax Muscle, Right* **K　Abdomen Muscle, Right** 　　External oblique muscle 　　Internal oblique muscle 　　Pyramidalis muscle 　　Rectus abdominis muscle 　　Transversus abdominis 　　　muscle **L　Abdomen Muscle, Left** 　　*See K Abdomen Muscle,* 　　　*Right*	**M　Perineum Muscle** 　　Bulbospongiosus muscle 　　Cremaster muscle 　　Deep transverse perineal 　　　muscle 　　Ischiocavernosus muscle 　　Levator ani muscle 　　Superficial transverse 　　　perineal muscle **N　Hip Muscle, Right** 　　Gemellus muscle 　　Gluteus maximus muscle 　　Gluteus medius muscle 　　Gluteus minimus muscle 　　Iliacus muscle 　　Obturator muscle 　　Piriformis muscle 　　Psoas muscle 　　Quadratus femoris muscle 　　Tensor fasciae latae 　　　muscle **P　Hip Muscle, Left** 　　*See N Hip Muscle, Right* **Q　Upper Leg Muscle, Right** 　　Adductor brevis muscle 　　Adductor longus muscle 　　Adductor magnus muscle 　　Biceps femoris muscle 　　Gracilis muscle 　　Pectineus muscle 　　Quadriceps (femoris) 　　Rectus femoris muscle 　　Sartorius muscle 　　Semimembranosus muscle 　　Semitendinosus muscle 　　Vastus intermedius muscle 　　Vastus lateralis muscle 　　Vastus medialis muscle **R　Upper Leg Muscle, Left** 　　*See Q Upper Leg Muscle,* 　　　*Right* **S　Lower Leg Muscle, Right** 　　Extensor digitorum longus 　　　muscle 　　Extensor hallucis longus 　　　muscle 　　Fibularis brevis muscle 　　Fibularis longus muscle 　　Flexor digitorum longus 　　　muscle 　　Flexor hallucis longus 　　　muscle 　　Gastrocnemius muscle 　　Peroneus brevis muscle 　　Peroneus longus muscle 　　Popliteus muscle 　　Soleus muscle 　　Tibialis anterior muscle 　　Tibialis posterior muscle **T　Lower Leg Muscle, Left** 　　*See S Lower Leg Muscle,* 　　　*Right* **V　Foot Muscle, Right** 　　Abductor hallucis muscle 　　Adductor hallucis muscle 　　Extensor digitorum brevis 　　　muscle 　　Extensor hallucis brevis 　　　muscle 　　Flexor digitorum brevis 　　　muscle 　　Flexor hallucis brevis 　　　muscle 　　Quadratus plantae muscle **W　Foot Muscle, Left** 　　*See V Foot Muscle, Right*	**Ø　Open** **4　Percutaneous** 　　**Endoscopic**	**Z　No Device**	**Z　No Qualifier**

See Appendix L for Procedure Combinations
　⊞　　ØKT[H,J]ØZZ

NC Noncovered Procedure　　LC Limited Coverage　　QA Questionable OB Admit　　NT New Tech Add-on　　⊞ Combination Member　　♂ Male　　♀ Female

Muscles

Ø   **Medical and Surgical**
K   **Muscles**
U   **Supplement**   Definition: Putting in or on biological or synthetic material that physically reinforces and/or augments the function of a portion of a body part
                    Explanation: The biological material is non-living, or is living and from the same individual. The body part may have been previously replaced, and the SUPPLEMENT procedure is performed to physically reinforce and/or augment the function of the replaced body part.

Body Part Character 4			Approach Character 5	Device Character 6	Qualifier Character 7
Ø Head Muscle Auricularis muscle Masseter muscle Pterygoid muscle Splenius capitis muscle Temporalis muscle Temporoparietalis muscle **1 Facial Muscle** Buccinator muscle Corrugator supercilii muscle Depressor anguli oris muscle Depressor labii inferioris muscle Depressor septi nasi muscle Depressor supercilii muscle Levator anguli oris muscle Levator labii superioris alaeque nasi muscle Levator labii superioris muscle Mentalis muscle Nasalis muscle Occipitofrontalis muscle Orbicularis oris muscle Procerus muscle Risorius muscle Zygomaticus muscle **2 Neck Muscle, Right** Anterior vertebral muscle Arytenoid muscle Cricothyroid muscle Infrahyoid muscle Levator scapulae muscle Platysma muscle Scalene muscle Splenius cervicis muscle Sternocleidomastoid muscle Suprahyoid muscle Thyroarytenoid muscle **3 Neck Muscle, Left** *See 2 Neck Muscle, Right* **4 Tongue, Palate, Pharynx Muscle** Chondroglossus muscle Genioglossus muscle Hyoglossus muscle Inferior longitudinal muscle Levator veli palatini muscle Palatoglossal muscle Palatopharyngeal muscle Pharyngeal constrictor muscle Salpingopharyngeus muscle Styloglossus muscle Stylopharyngeus muscle Superior longitudinal muscle Tensor veli palatini muscle **5 Shoulder Muscle, Right** Deltoid muscle Infraspinatus muscle Subscapularis muscle Supraspinatus muscle Teres major muscle Teres minor muscle **6 Shoulder Muscle, Left** *See 5 Shoulder Muscle, Right*	**7 Upper Arm Muscle, Right** Biceps brachii muscle Brachialis muscle Coracobrachialis muscle Triceps brachii muscle **8 Upper Arm Muscle, Left** *See 7 Upper Arm Muscle, Right* **9 Lower Arm and Wrist Muscle, Right** Anatomical snuffbox Brachioradialis muscle Extensor carpi radialis muscle Extensor carpi ulnaris muscle Flexor carpi radialis muscle Flexor carpi ulnaris muscle Flexor pollicis longus muscle Palmaris longus muscle Pronator quadratus muscle Pronator teres muscle **B Lower Arm and Wrist Muscle, Left** *See 9 Lower Arm and Wrist Muscle, Right* **C Hand Muscle, Right** Hypothenar muscle Palmar interosseous muscle Thenar muscle **D Hand Muscle, Left** *See C Hand Muscle, Right* **F Trunk Muscle, Right** Coccygeus muscle Erector spinae muscle Interspinalis muscle Intertransversarius muscle Latissimus dorsi muscle Quadratus lumborum muscle Rhomboid major muscle Rhomboid minor muscle Serratus posterior muscle Transversospinalis muscle Trapezius muscle **G Trunk Muscle, Left** *See F Trunk Muscle, Right* **H Thorax Muscle, Right** Intercostal muscle Levatores costarum muscle Pectoralis major muscle Pectoralis minor muscle Serratus anterior muscle Subclavius muscle Subcostal muscle Transverse thoracis muscle **J Thorax Muscle, Left** *See H Thorax Muscle, Right* **K Abdomen Muscle, Right** External oblique muscle Internal oblique muscle Pyramidalis muscle Rectus abdominis muscle Transversus abdominis muscle **L Abdomen Muscle, Left** *See K Abdomen Muscle, Right*	**M Perineum Muscle** Bulbospongiosus muscle Cremaster muscle Deep transverse perineal muscle Ischiocavernosus muscle Levator ani muscle Superficial transverse perineal muscle **N Hip Muscle, Right** Gemellus muscle Gluteus maximus muscle Gluteus medius muscle Gluteus minimus muscle Iliacus muscle Obturator muscle Piriformis muscle Psoas muscle Quadratus femoris muscle Tensor fasciae latae muscle **P Hip Muscle, Left** *See N Hip Muscle, Right* **Q Upper Leg Muscle, Right** Adductor brevis muscle Adductor longus muscle Adductor magnus muscle Biceps femoris muscle Gracilis muscle Pectineus muscle Quadriceps (femoris) Rectus femoris muscle Sartorius muscle Semimembranosus muscle Semitendinosus muscle Vastus intermedius muscle Vastus lateralis muscle Vastus medialis muscle **R Upper Leg Muscle, Left** *See Q Upper Leg Muscle, Right* **S Lower Leg Muscle, Right** Extensor digitorum longus muscle Extensor hallucis longus muscle Fibularis brevis muscle Fibularis longus muscle Flexor digitorum longus muscle Flexor hallucis longus muscle Gastrocnemius muscle Peroneus brevis muscle Peroneus longus muscle Popliteus muscle Soleus muscle Tibialis anterior muscle Tibialis posterior muscle **T Lower Leg Muscle, Left** *See S Lower Leg Muscle, Right* **V Foot Muscle, Right** Abductor hallucis muscle Adductor hallucis muscle Extensor digitorum brevis muscle Extensor hallucis brevis muscle Flexor digitorum brevis muscle Flexor hallucis brevis muscle Quadratus plantae muscle **W Foot Muscle, Left** *See V Foot Muscle, Right*	**Ø Open** **4 Percutaneous Endoscopic**	**7 Autologous Tissue Substitute** **J Synthetic Substitute** **K Nonautologous Tissue Substitute**	**Z No Qualifier**

Non-OR Procedure   DRG Non-OR Procedure   Valid OR Procedure   HAC Associated Procedure   Combination Only   New/Revised GREEN

Ø   Medical and Surgical
K   Muscles
W   Revision   Definition: Correcting, to the extent possible, a portion of a malfunctioning device or the position of a displaced device

Explanation: Revision can include correcting a malfunctioning or displaced device by taking out or putting in components of the device such as a screw or pin

Body Part Character 4	Approach Character 5	Device Character 6	Qualifier Character 7
X Upper Muscle **Y** Lower Muscle	**Ø** Open **3** Percutaneous **4** Percutaneous Endoscopic	**Ø** Drainage Device **7** Autologous Tissue Substitute **J** Synthetic Substitute **K** Nonautologous Tissue Substitute **M** Stimulator Lead **Y** Other Device	**Z** No Qualifier
X Upper Muscle **Y** Lower Muscle	**X** External	**Ø** Drainage Device **7** Autologous Tissue Substitute **J** Synthetic Substitute **K** Nonautologous Tissue Substitute **M** Stimulator Lead	**Z** No Qualifier

Non-OR   ØKW[X,Y][3,4]YZ
Non-OR   ØKW[X,Y]X[Ø,7,J,K,M]Z

Muscles

Ø Medical and Surgical
K Muscles
X Transfer Definition: Moving, without taking out, all or a portion of a body part to another location to take over the function of all or a portion of a body part
Explanation: The body part transferred remains connected to its vascular and nervous supply

Body Part Character 4			Approach Character 5	Device Character 6	Qualifier Character 7

Ø Head Muscle
Auricularis muscle
Masseter muscle
Pterygoid muscle
Splenius capitis muscle
Temporalis muscle
Temporoparietalis muscle

1 Facial Muscle
Buccinator muscle
Corrugator supercilii muscle
Depressor anguli oris muscle
Depressor labii inferioris muscle
Depressor septi nasi muscle
Depressor supercilii muscle
Levator anguli oris muscle
Levator labii superioris alaeque nasi muscle
Levator labii superioris muscle
Mentalis muscle
Nasalis muscle
Occipitofrontalis muscle
Orbicularis oris muscle
Procerus muscle
Risorius muscle
Zygomaticus muscle

2 Neck Muscle, Right
Anterior vertebral muscle
Arytenoid muscle
Cricothyroid muscle
Infrahyoid muscle
Levator scapulae muscle
Platysma muscle
Scalene muscle
Splenius cervicis muscle
Sternocleidomastoid muscle
Suprahyoid muscle
Thyroarytenoid muscle

3 Neck Muscle, Left
See 2 Neck Muscle, Right

4 Tongue, Palate, Pharynx Muscle
Chondroglossus muscle
Genioglossus muscle
Hyoglossus muscle
Inferior longitudinal muscle
Levator veli palatini muscle
Palatoglossal muscle
Palatopharyngeal muscle
Pharyngeal constrictor muscle
Salpingopharyngeus muscle
Styloglossus muscle
Stylopharyngeus muscle
Superior longitudinal muscle
Tensor veli palatini muscle

5 Shoulder Muscle, Right
Deltoid muscle
Infraspinatus muscle
Subscapularis muscle
Supraspinatus muscle
Teres major muscle
Teres minor muscle

6 Shoulder Muscle, Left
See 5 Shoulder Muscle, Right

7 Upper Arm Muscle, Right
Biceps brachii muscle
Brachialis muscle
Coracobrachialis muscle
Triceps brachii muscle

8 Upper Arm Muscle, Left
See 7 Upper Arm Muscle, Right

9 Lower Arm and Wrist Muscle, Right
Anatomical snuffbox
Brachioradialis muscle
Extensor carpi radialis muscle
Extensor carpi ulnaris muscle
Flexor carpi radialis muscle
Flexor carpi ulnaris muscle
Flexor pollicis longus muscle
Palmaris longus muscle
Pronator quadratus muscle
Pronator teres muscle

B Lower Arm and Wrist Muscle, Left
See 9 Lower Arm and Wrist Muscle, Right

C Hand Muscle, Right
Hypothenar muscle
Palmar interosseous muscle
Thenar muscle

D Hand Muscle, Left
See C Hand Muscle, Right

H Thorax Muscle, Right
Intercostal muscle
Levatores costarum muscle
Pectoralis major muscle
Pectoralis minor muscle
Serratus anterior muscle
Subclavius muscle
Subcostal muscle
Transverse thoracis muscle

J Thorax Muscle, Left
See H Thorax Muscle, Right

M Perineum Muscle
Bulbospongiosus muscle
Cremaster muscle
Deep transverse perineal muscle
Ischiocavernosus muscle
Levator ani muscle
Superficial transverse perineal muscle

N Hip Muscle, Right
Gemellus muscle
Gluteus maximus muscle
Gluteus medius muscle
Gluteus minimus muscle
Iliacus muscle
Obturator muscle
Piriformis muscle
Psoas muscle
Quadratus femoris muscle
Tensor fasciae latae muscle

P Hip Muscle, Left
See N Hip Muscle, Right

Q Upper Leg Muscle, Right
Adductor brevis muscle
Adductor longus muscle
Adductor magnus muscle
Biceps femoris muscle
Gracilis muscle
Pectineus muscle
Quadriceps (femoris)
Rectus femoris muscle
Sartorius muscle
Semimembranosus muscle
Semitendinosus muscle
Vastus intermedius muscle
Vastus lateralis muscle
Vastus medialis muscle

R Upper Leg Muscle, Left
See Q Upper Leg Muscle, Right

S Lower Leg Muscle, Right
Extensor digitorum longus muscle
Extensor hallucis longus muscle
Fibularis brevis muscle
Fibularis longus muscle
Flexor digitorum longus muscle
Flexor hallucis longus muscle
Gastrocnemius muscle
Peroneus brevis muscle
Peroneus longus muscle
Popliteus muscle
Soleus muscle
Tibialis anterior muscle
Tibialis posterior muscle

T Lower Leg Muscle, Left
See S Lower Leg Muscle, Right

V Foot Muscle, Right
Abductor hallucis muscle
Adductor hallucis muscle
Extensor digitorum brevis muscle
Extensor hallucis brevis muscle
Flexor digitorum brevis muscle
Flexor hallucis brevis muscle
Quadratus plantae muscle

W Foot Muscle, Left
See V Foot Muscle, Right

Ø Open
4 Percutaneous Endoscopic

Z No Device

Ø Skin
1 Subcutaneous Tissue
2 Skin and Subcutaneous Tissue
Z No Qualifier

ØKX Continued on next page

Ø Medical and Surgical
K Muscles
X Transfer

ØKX Continued

Definition: Moving, without taking out, all or a portion of a body part to another location to take over the function of all or a portion of a body part
Explanation: The body part transferred remains connected to its vascular and nervous supply

Body Part Character 4	Approach Character 5	Device Character 6	Qualifier Character 7
F Trunk Muscle, Right Coccygeus muscle Erector spinae muscle Interspinalis muscle Intertransversarius muscle Latissimus dorsi muscle Quadratus lumborum muscle Rhomboid major muscle Rhomboid minor muscle Serratus posterior muscle Transversospinalis muscle Trapezius muscle **G Trunk Muscle, Left** *See F Trunk Muscle, Right*	**Ø Open** **4 Percutaneous Endoscopic**	**Z No Device**	**Ø Skin** **1 Subcutaneous Tissue** **2 Skin and Subcutaneous Tissue** **5 Latissimus Dorsi Myocutaneous Flap** **7 Deep Inferior Epigastric Artery Perforator Flap** **8 Superficial Inferior Epigastric Artery Flap** **9 Gluteal Artery Perforator Flap** **Z No Qualifier**
K Abdomen Muscle, Right External oblique muscle Internal oblique muscle Pyramidalis muscle Rectus abdominis muscle Transversus abdominis muscle **L Abdomen Muscle, Left** *See K Abdomen Muscle, Right*	**Ø Open** **4 Percutaneous Endoscopic**	**Z No Device**	**Ø Skin** **1 Subcutaneous Tissue** **2 Skin and Subcutaneous Tissue** **6 Transverse Rectus Abdominis Myocutaneous Flap** **Z No Qualifier**

NC Noncovered Procedure   LC Limited Coverage   QA Questionable OB Admit   NT New Tech Add-on   ⊞ Combination Member   ♂ Male   ♀ Female

ICD-10-PCS 2022   **483**

ØKX–ØKX

Tendons ØL2–ØLX

Character Meanings*

This Character Meaning table is provided as a guide to assist the user in the identification of character members that may be found in this section of code tables. It **SHOULD NOT** be used to build a PCS code.

Operation–Character 3	Body Part–Character 4	Approach–Character 5	Device–Character 6	Qualifier–Character 7
2 Change	Ø Head and Neck Tendon	Ø Open	Ø Drainage Device	X Diagnostic
5 Destruction	1 Shoulder Tendon, Right	3 Percutaneous	7 Autologous Tissue Substitute	Z No Qualifier
8 Division	2 Shoulder Tendon, Left	4 Percutaneous Endoscopic	J Synthetic Substitute	
9 Drainage	3 Upper Arm Tendon, Right	X External	K Nonautologous Tissue Substitute	
B Excision	4 Upper Arm Tendon, Left		Y Other Device	
C Extirpation	5 Lower Arm and Wrist Tendon, Right		Z No Device	
D Extraction	6 Lower Arm and Wrist Tendon, Left			
H Insertion	7 Hand Tendon, Right			
J Inspection	8 Hand Tendon, Left			
M Reattachment	9 Trunk Tendon, Right			
N Release	B Trunk Tendon, Left			
P Removal	C Thorax Tendon, Right			
Q Repair	D Thorax Tendon, Left			
R Replacement	F Abdomen Tendon, Right			
S Reposition	G Abdomen Tendon, Left			
T Resection	H Perineum Tendon			
U Supplement	J Hip Tendon, Right			
W Revision	K Hip Tendon, Left			
X Transfer	L Upper Leg Tendon, Right			
	M Upper Leg Tendon, Left			
	N Lower Leg Tendon, Right			
	P Lower Leg Tendon, Left			
	Q Knee Tendon, Right			
	R Knee Tendon, Left			
	S Ankle Tendon, Right			
	T Ankle Tendon, Left			
	V Foot Tendon, Right			
	W Foot Tendon, Left			
	X Upper Tendon			
	Y Lower Tendon			

* Includes synovial membrane.

AHA Coding Clinic for table ØL8
2016, 3Q, 30   Resection of femur with interposition arthroplasty

AHA Coding Clinic for table ØLB
2017, 2Q, 21   Arthroscopic anterior cruciate ligament revision using autograft with anterolateral ligament reconstruction
2015, 3Q, 26   Thumb arthroplasty with resection of trapezium
2014, 3Q, 14   Application of TheraSkin® and excisional debridement
2014, 3Q, 18   Placement of reverse sural fasciocutaneous pedicle flap

AHA Coding Clinic for table ØLD
2017, 4Q, 41   Extraction procedures

AHA Coding Clinic for table ØLQ
2016, 3Q, 32   Rotator cuff repair, tenodesis, decompression, acromioplasty and coracoplasty
2015, 2Q, 11   Repair of patellar and quadriceps tendons with allograft
2013, 3Q, 20   Superior labrum anterior posterior (SLAP) repair and subacromial decompression

AHA Coding Clinic for table ØLS
2016, 3Q, 32   Rotator cuff repair, tenodesis, decompression, acromioplasty and coracoplasty
2015, 3Q, 14   Endoprosthetic replacement of humerus and tendon reattachment

AHA Coding Clinic for table ØLU
2015, 2Q, 11   Repair of patellar and quadriceps tendons with allograft

Foot Tendons

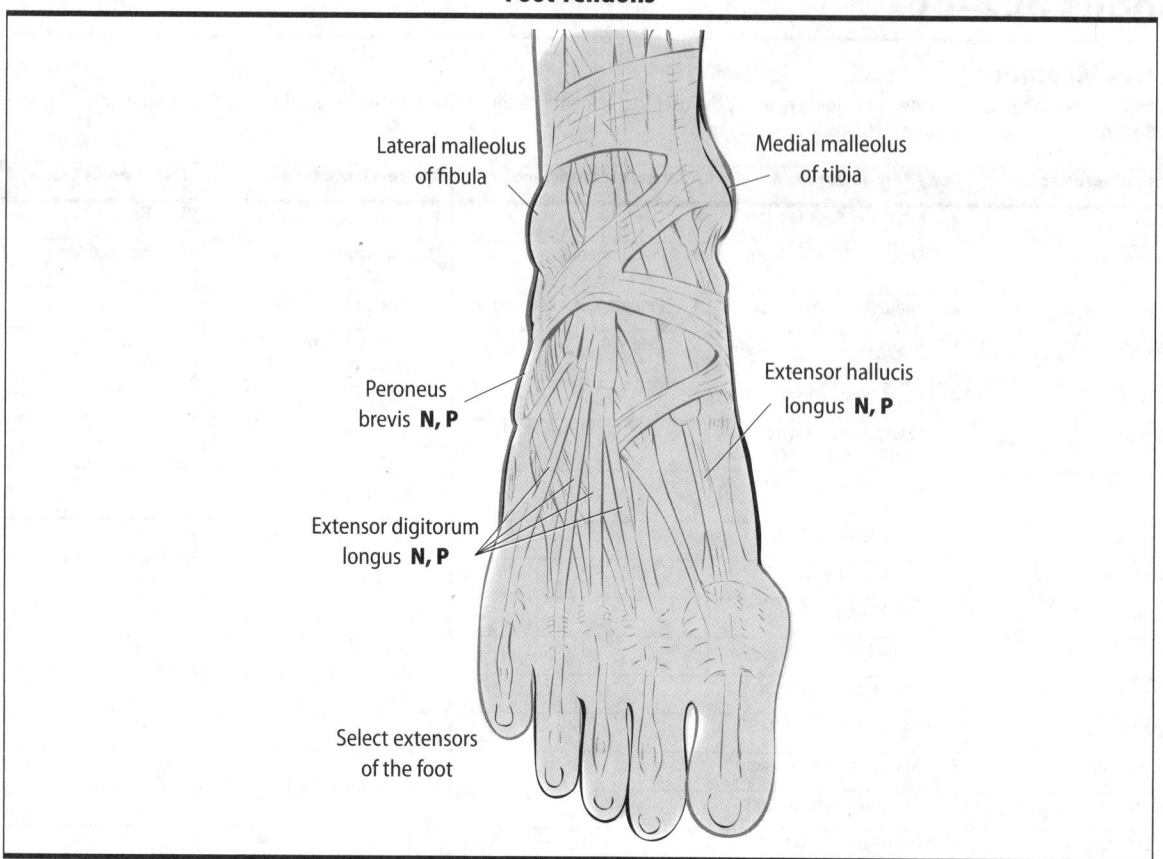

Lateral malleolus
of fibula

Medial malleolus
of tibia

Peroneus
brevis **N, P**

Extensor hallucis
longus **N, P**

Extensor digitorum
longus **N, P**

Select extensors
of the foot

Shoulder Tendons

Posterior view

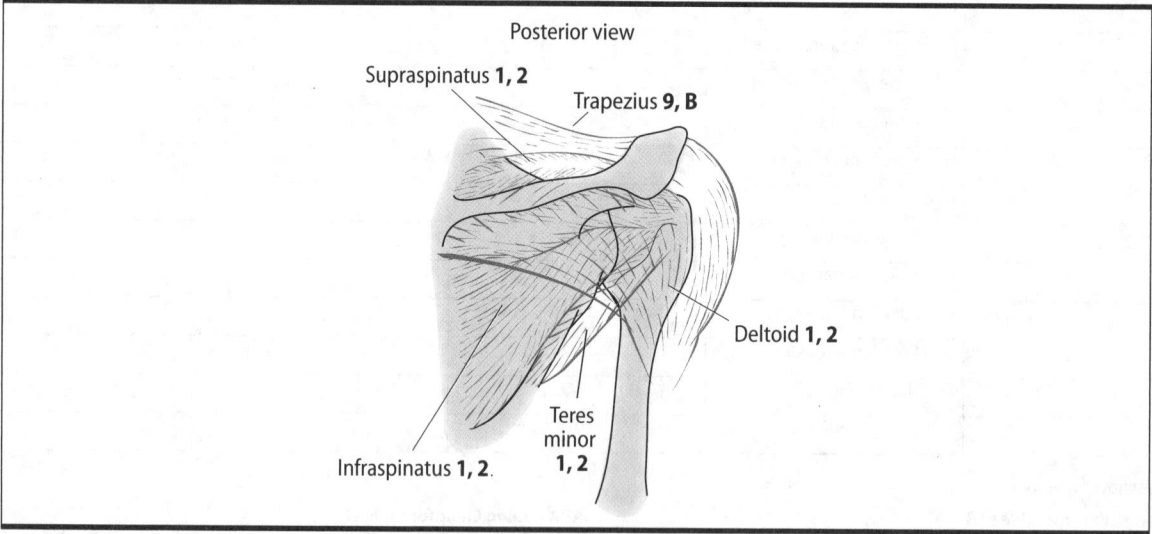

Supraspinatus **1, 2**

Trapezius **9, B**

Deltoid **1, 2**

Infraspinatus **1, 2**

Teres
minor
1, 2

Tendons of Wrist and Hand

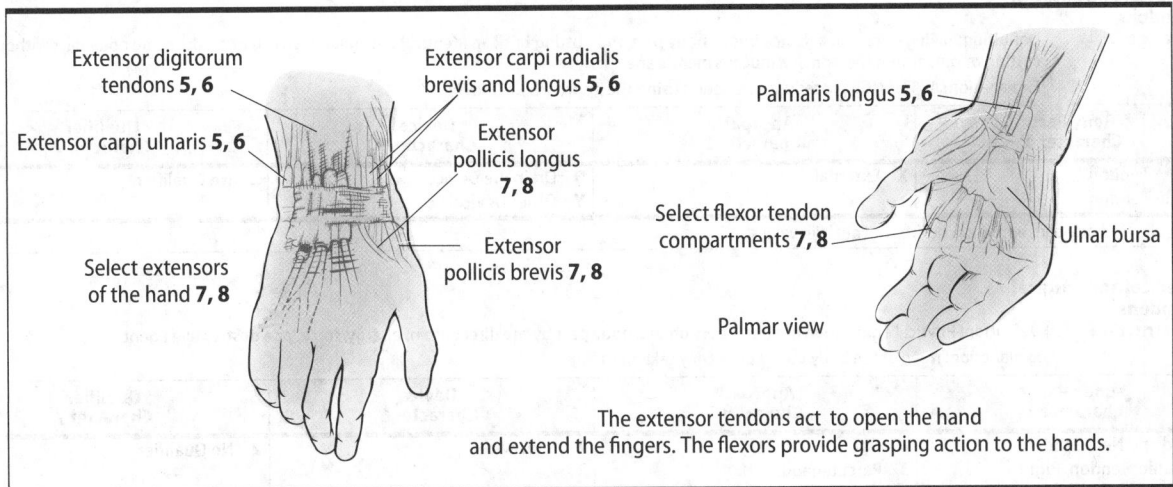

Extensor digitorum tendons **5, 6**

Extensor carpi ulnaris **5, 6**

Select extensors of the hand **7, 8**

Extensor carpi radialis brevis and longus **5, 6**

Extensor pollicis longus **7, 8**

Extensor pollicis brevis **7, 8**

Palmaris longus **5, 6**

Select flexor tendon compartments **7, 8**

Ulnar bursa

Palmar view

The extensor tendons act to open the hand and extend the fingers. The flexors provide grasping action to the hands.

Leg Muscles and Tendons

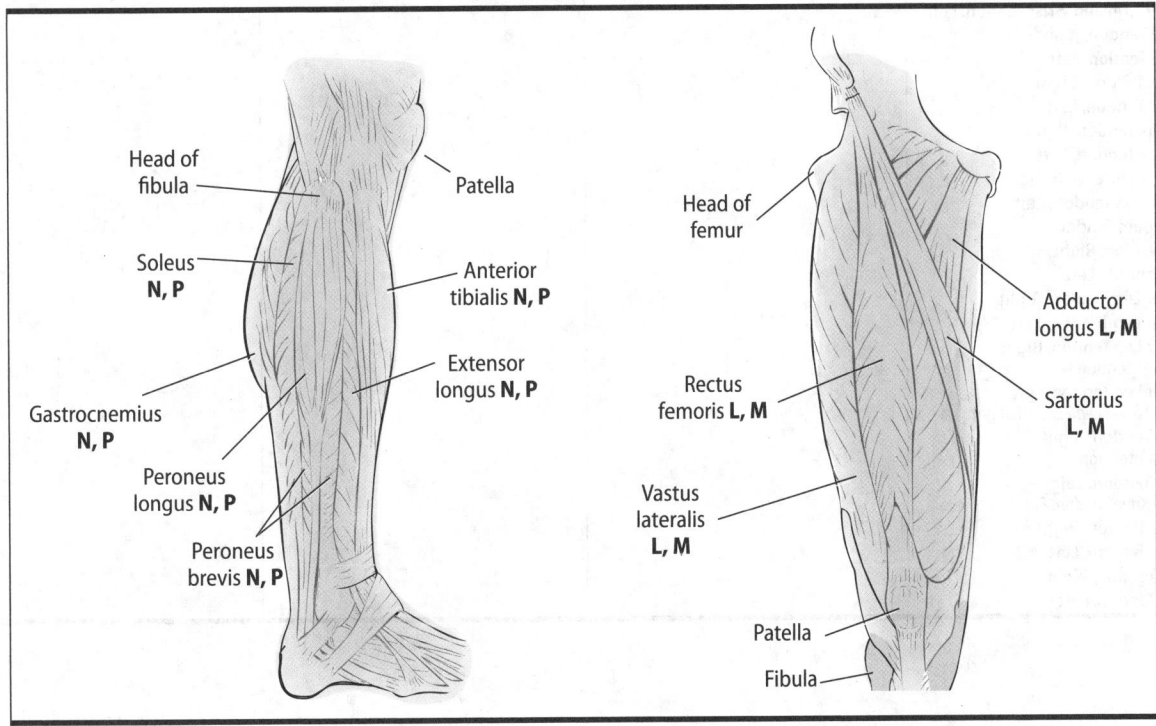

Head of fibula

Soleus **N, P**

Gastrocnemius **N, P**

Peroneus longus **N, P**

Peroneus brevis **N, P**

Patella

Anterior tibialis **N, P**

Extensor longus **N, P**

Head of femur

Rectus femoris **L, M**

Vastus lateralis **L, M**

Patella

Fibula

Adductor longus **L, M**

Sartorius **L, M**

Ø   Medical and Surgical
L   Tendons
2   Change   Definition: Taking out or off a device from a body part and putting back an identical or similar device in or on the same body part without
                         cutting or puncturing the skin or a mucous membrane
                         Explanation: All CHANGE procedures are coded using the approach EXTERNAL

Body Part Character 4	Approach Character 5	Device Character 6	Qualifier Character 7
X Upper Tendon Y Lower Tendon	X External	Ø Drainage Device Y Other Device	Z No Qualifier

Non-OR	All body part, approach, device, and qualifier values

Ø   Medical and Surgical
L   Tendons
5   Destruction   Definition: Physical eradication of all or a portion of a body part by the direct use of energy, force, or a destructive agent
                        Explanation: None of the body part is physically taken out

Body Part Character 4	Approach Character 5	Device Character 6	Qualifier Character 7

Ø Head and Neck Tendon
1 Shoulder Tendon, Right
2 Shoulder Tendon, Left
3 Upper Arm Tendon, Right
4 Upper Arm Tendon, Left
5 Lower Arm and Wrist Tendon, Right
6 Lower Arm and Wrist Tendon, Left
7 Hand Tendon, Right
8 Hand Tendon, Left
9 Trunk Tendon, Right
B Trunk Tendon, Left
C Thorax Tendon, Right
D Thorax Tendon, Left
F Abdomen Tendon, Right
G Abdomen Tendon, Left
H Perineum Tendon
J Hip Tendon, Right
K Hip Tendon, Left
L Upper Leg Tendon, Right
M Upper Leg Tendon, Left
N Lower Leg Tendon, Right
   Achilles tendon
P Lower Leg Tendon, Left
   See N Lower Leg Tendon, Right
Q Knee Tendon, Right
   Patellar tendon
R Knee Tendon, Left
   See Q Knee Tendon, Right
S Ankle Tendon, Right
T Ankle Tendon, Left
V Foot Tendon, Right
W Foot Tendon, Left
	Ø Open
	3 Percutaneous
	4 Percutaneous Endoscopic
		Z No Device	Z No Qualifier

Ø   **Medical and Surgical**
L   **Tendons**
8   **Division**   Definition: Cutting into a body part, without draining fluids and/or gases from the body part, in order to separate or transect a body part
                 Explanation: All or a portion of the body part is separated into two or more portions

Body Part Character 4	Approach Character 5	Device Character 6	Qualifier Character 7
Ø Head and Neck Tendon	**Ø** Open	**Z** No Device	**Z** No Qualifier
1 Shoulder Tendon, Right	**3** Percutaneous		
2 Shoulder Tendon, Left	**4** Percutaneous Endoscopic		
3 Upper Arm Tendon, Right			
4 Upper Arm Tendon, Left			
5 Lower Arm and Wrist Tendon, Right			
6 Lower Arm and Wrist Tendon, Left			
7 Hand Tendon, Right			
8 Hand Tendon, Left			
9 Trunk Tendon, Right			
B Trunk Tendon, Left			
C Thorax Tendon, Right			
D Thorax Tendon, Left			
F Abdomen Tendon, Right			
G Abdomen Tendon, Left			
H Perineum Tendon			
J Hip Tendon, Right			
K Hip Tendon, Left			
L Upper Leg Tendon, Right			
M Upper Leg Tendon, Left			
N Lower Leg Tendon, Right Achilles tendon			
P Lower Leg Tendon, Left *See N Lower Leg Tendon, Right*			
Q Knee Tendon, Right Patellar tendon			
R Knee Tendon, Left *See Q Knee Tendon, Right*			
S Ankle Tendon, Right			
T Ankle Tendon, Left			
V Foot Tendon, Right			
W Foot Tendon, Left			

NC Noncovered Procedure   LC Limited Coverage   QA Questionable OB Admit   NT New Tech Add-on   ✛ Combination Member   ♂ Male   ♀ Female

ICD-10-PCS 2022   **489**

ØL8–ØL8

Ø   Medical and Surgical
L   Tendons
9   Drainage   Definition: Taking or letting out fluids and/or gases from a body part

Explanation: The qualifier DIAGNOSTIC is used to identify drainage procedures that are biopsies

Body Part Character 4	Approach Character 5	Device Character 6	Qualifier Character 7

Ø Head and Neck Tendon
1 Shoulder Tendon, Right
2 Shoulder Tendon, Left
3 Upper Arm Tendon, Right
4 Upper Arm Tendon, Left
5 Lower Arm and Wrist Tendon, Right
6 Lower Arm and Wrist Tendon, Left
7 Hand Tendon, Right
8 Hand Tendon, Left
9 Trunk Tendon, Right
B Trunk Tendon, Left
C Thorax Tendon, Right
D Thorax Tendon, Left
F Abdomen Tendon, Right
G Abdomen Tendon, Left
H Perineum Tendon
J Hip Tendon, Right
K Hip Tendon, Left
L Upper Leg Tendon, Right
M Upper Leg Tendon, Left
N Lower Leg Tendon, Right
    Achilles tendon
P Lower Leg Tendon, Left
    See N Lower Leg Tendon, Right
Q Knee Tendon, Right
    Patellar tendon
R Knee Tendon, Left
    See Q Knee Tendon, Right
S Ankle Tendon, Right
T Ankle Tendon, Left
V Foot Tendon, Right
W Foot Tendon, Left
	Ø Open
	3 Percutaneous
	4 Percutaneous Endoscopic
		Ø Drainage Device	**Z** No Qualifier

Ø Head and Neck Tendon
1 Shoulder Tendon, Right
2 Shoulder Tendon, Left
3 Upper Arm Tendon, Right
4 Upper Arm Tendon, Left
5 Lower Arm and Wrist Tendon, Right
6 Lower Arm and Wrist Tendon, Left
7 Hand Tendon, Right
8 Hand Tendon, Left
9 Trunk Tendon, Right
B Trunk Tendon, Left
C Thorax Tendon, Right
D Thorax Tendon, Left
F Abdomen Tendon, Right
G Abdomen Tendon, Left
H Perineum Tendon
J Hip Tendon, Right
K Hip Tendon, Left
L Upper Leg Tendon, Right
M Upper Leg Tendon, Left
N Lower Leg Tendon, Right
    Achilles tendon
P Lower Leg Tendon, Left
    See N Lower Leg Tendon, Right
Q Knee Tendon, Right
    Patellar tendon
R Knee Tendon, Left
    See Q Knee Tendon, Right
S Ankle Tendon, Right
T Ankle Tendon, Left
V Foot Tendon, Right
W Foot Tendon, Left
	Ø Open
	3 Percutaneous
	4 Percutaneous Endoscopic
		Z No Device	**X** Diagnostic
			Z No Qualifier

Non-OR   ØL9[Ø,1,2,3,4,5,6,7,8,9,B,C,D,F,G,H,J,K,L,M,N,P,Q,R,S,T,V,W]3ØZ
Non-OR   ØL9[Ø,1,2,3,4,5,6,7,8,9,B,C,D,F,G,H,J,K,L,M,N,P,Q,R,S,T,V,W]3ZZ
Non-OR   ØL9[7,8]4ZZ

Ø   **Medical and Surgical**
L   **Tendons**
B   **Excision**   Definition: Cutting out or off, without replacement, a portion of a body part

                       Explanation: The qualifier DIAGNOSTIC is used to identify excision procedures that are biopsies

Body Part Character 4	Approach Character 5	Device Character 6	Qualifier Character 7

Ø   Head and Neck Tendon
1   Shoulder Tendon, Right
2   Shoulder Tendon, Left
3   Upper Arm Tendon, Right
4   Upper Arm Tendon, Left
5   Lower Arm and Wrist Tendon, Right
6   Lower Arm and Wrist Tendon, Left
7   Hand Tendon, Right
8   Hand Tendon, Left
9   Trunk Tendon, Right
B   Trunk Tendon, Left
C   Thorax Tendon, Right
D   Thorax Tendon, Left
F   Abdomen Tendon, Right
G   Abdomen Tendon, Left
H   Perineum Tendon
J   Hip Tendon, Right
K   Hip Tendon, Left
L   Upper Leg Tendon, Right
M   Upper Leg Tendon, Left
N   Lower Leg Tendon, Right
     Achilles tendon
P   Lower Leg Tendon, Left
     See N Lower Leg Tendon, Right
Q   Knee Tendon, Right
     Patellar tendon
R   Knee Tendon, Left
     See Q Knee Tendon, Right
S   Ankle Tendon, Right
T   Ankle Tendon, Left
V   Foot Tendon, Right
W   Foot Tendon, Left
	Ø Open
	3 Percutaneous
	4 Percutaneous Endoscopic
		Z No Device	**X** Diagnostic
			Z No Qualifier

NC Noncovered Procedure   LC Limited Coverage   QA Questionable OB Admit   NT New Tech Add-on   ⊞ Combination Member   ♂ Male   ♀ Female

ICD-10-PCS 2022   **491**

Ø   Medical and Surgical
L   Tendons
C   Extirpation

Definition: Taking or cutting out solid matter from a body part

Explanation: The solid matter may be an abnormal byproduct of a biological function or a foreign body; it may be imbedded in a body part or in the lumen of a tubular body part. The solid matter may or may not have been previously broken into pieces.

Body Part Character 4	Approach Character 5	Device Character 6	Qualifier Character 7

Ø   Head and Neck Tendon
1   Shoulder Tendon, Right
2   Shoulder Tendon, Left
3   Upper Arm Tendon, Right
4   Upper Arm Tendon, Left
5   Lower Arm and Wrist Tendon, Right
6   Lower Arm and Wrist Tendon, Left
7   Hand Tendon, Right
8   Hand Tendon, Left
9   Trunk Tendon, Right
B   Trunk Tendon, Left
C   Thorax Tendon, Right
D   Thorax Tendon, Left
F   Abdomen Tendon, Right
G   Abdomen Tendon, Left
H   Perineum Tendon
J   Hip Tendon, Right
K   Hip Tendon, Left
L   Upper Leg Tendon, Right
M   Upper Leg Tendon, Left
N   Lower Leg Tendon, Right
     Achilles tendon
P   Lower Leg Tendon, Left
     See N Lower Leg Tendon, Right
Q   Knee Tendon, Right
     Patellar tendon
R   Knee Tendon, Left
     See Q Knee Tendon, Right
S   Ankle Tendon, Right
T   Ankle Tendon, Left
V   Foot Tendon, Right
W   Foot Tendon, Left
	Ø Open
	3 Percutaneous
	4 Percutaneous Endoscopic
		Z No Device	Z No Qualifier

Ø Medical and Surgical
L Tendons
D Extraction   Definition: Pulling or stripping out or off all or a portion of a body part by the use of force

Explanation: The qualifier DIAGNOSTIC is used to identify extraction procedures that are biopsies

Body Part Character 4	Approach Character 5	Device Character 6	Qualifier Character 7
Ø Head and Neck Tendon	Ø Open	Z No Device	Z No Qualifier
1 Shoulder Tendon, Right			
2 Shoulder Tendon, Left			
3 Upper Arm Tendon, Right			
4 Upper Arm Tendon, Left			
5 Lower Arm and Wrist Tendon, Right			
6 Lower Arm and Wrist Tendon, Left			
7 Hand Tendon, Right			
8 Hand Tendon, Left			
9 Trunk Tendon, Right			
B Trunk Tendon, Left			
C Thorax Tendon, Right			
D Thorax Tendon, Left			
F Abdomen Tendon, Right			
G Abdomen Tendon, Left			
H Perineum Tendon			
J Hip Tendon, Right			
K Hip Tendon, Left			
L Upper Leg Tendon, Right			
M Upper Leg Tendon, Left			
N Lower Leg Tendon, Right Achilles tendon			
P Lower Leg Tendon, Left See N Lower Leg Tendon, Right			
Q Knee Tendon, Right Patellar tendon			
R Knee Tendon, Left See Q Knee Tendon, Right			
S Ankle Tendon, Right			
T Ankle Tendon, Left			
V Foot Tendon, Right			
W Foot Tendon, Left			

Ø Medical and Surgical
L Tendons
H Insertion   Definition: Putting in a nonbiological appliance that monitors, assists, performs, or prevents a physiological function but does not physically take the place of a body part

Explanation: None

Body Part Character 4	Approach Character 5	Device Character 6	Qualifier Character 7
X Upper Tendon Y Lower Tendon	Ø Open 3 Percutaneous 4 Percutaneous Endoscopic	Y Other Device	Z No Qualifier

Non-OR   ØLH[X,Y][3,4]YZ

Ø Medical and Surgical
L Tendons
J Inspection   Definition: Visually and/or manually exploring a body part

Explanation: Visual exploration may be performed with or without optical instrumentation. Manual exploration may be performed directly or through intervening body layers.

Body Part Character 4	Approach Character 5	Device Character 6	Qualifier Character 7
X Upper Tendon Y Lower Tendon	Ø Open 3 Percutaneous 4 Percutaneous Endoscopic X External	Z No Device	Z No Qualifier

Non-OR   ØLJ[X,Y][3,X]ZZ

NC Noncovered Procedure   LC Limited Coverage   QA Questionable OB Admit   NT New Tech Add-on   ⊞ Combination Member   ♂ Male   ♀ Female

ICD-10-PCS 2022   493   ØLD–ØLJ

Ø   Medical and Surgical
L   Tendons
M   Reattachment   Definition: Putting back in or on all or a portion of a separated body part to its normal location or other suitable location

Explanation: Vascular circulation and nervous pathways may or may not be reestablished

Body Part Character 4	Approach Character 5	Device Character 6	Qualifier Character 7

Ø   Head and Neck Tendon
1   Shoulder Tendon, Right
2   Shoulder Tendon, Left
3   Upper Arm Tendon, Right
4   Upper Arm Tendon, Left
5   Lower Arm and Wrist Tendon, Right
6   Lower Arm and Wrist Tendon, Left
7   Hand Tendon, Right
8   Hand Tendon, Left
9   Trunk Tendon, Right
B   Trunk Tendon, Left
C   Thorax Tendon, Right
D   Thorax Tendon, Left
F   Abdomen Tendon, Right
G   Abdomen Tendon, Left
H   Perineum Tendon
J   Hip Tendon, Right
K   Hip Tendon, Left
L   Upper Leg Tendon, Right
M   Upper Leg Tendon, Left
N   Lower Leg Tendon, Right
    Achilles tendon
P   Lower Leg Tendon, Left
    See N Lower Leg Tendon, Right
Q   Knee Tendon, Right
    Patellar tendon
R   Knee Tendon, Left
    See Q Knee Tendon, Right
S   Ankle Tendon, Right
T   Ankle Tendon, Left
V   Foot Tendon, Right
W   Foot Tendon, Left
	Ø Open
	4 Percutaneous Endoscopic
		Z No Device	Z No Qualifier

Ø   Medical and Surgical
L   Tendons
N   Release   Definition: Freeing a body part from an abnormal physical constraint by cutting or by the use of force

Explanation: Some of the restraining tissue may be taken out but none of the body part is taken out

Body Part Character 4	Approach Character 5	Device Character 6	Qualifier Character 7

Ø   Head and Neck Tendon
1   Shoulder Tendon, Right
2   Shoulder Tendon, Left
3   Upper Arm Tendon, Right
4   Upper Arm Tendon, Left
5   Lower Arm and Wrist Tendon, Right
6   Lower Arm and Wrist Tendon, Left
7   Hand Tendon, Right
8   Hand Tendon, Left
9   Trunk Tendon, Right
B   Trunk Tendon, Left
C   Thorax Tendon, Right
D   Thorax Tendon, Left
F   Abdomen Tendon, Right
G   Abdomen Tendon, Left
H   Perineum Tendon
J   Hip Tendon, Right
K   Hip Tendon, Left
L   Upper Leg Tendon, Right
M   Upper Leg Tendon, Left
N   Lower Leg Tendon, Right
    Achilles tendon
P   Lower Leg Tendon, Left
    See N Lower Leg Tendon, Right
Q   Knee Tendon, Right
    Patellar tendon
R   Knee Tendon, Left
    See Q Knee Tendon, Right
S   Ankle Tendon, Right
T   Ankle Tendon, Left
V   Foot Tendon, Right
W   Foot Tendon, Left
	Ø Open
	3 Percutaneous
	4 Percutaneous Endoscopic
	X External
		Z No Device	Z No Qualifier

Non-OR   ØLN[Ø,1,2,3,4,5,6,7,8,9,B,C,D,F,G,H,J,K,L,M,N,P,Q,R,S,T,V,W]XZZ

Non-OR Procedure   DRG Non-OR Procedure   Valid OR Procedure   HAC Associated Procedure   Combination Only   New/Revised GREEN

Ø   Medical and Surgical
L   Tendons
P   Removal   Definition: Taking out or off a device from a body part

           Explanation: If a device is taken out and a similar device put in without cutting or puncturing the skin or mucous membrane, the procedure is coded to the root operation CHANGE. Otherwise, the procedure for taking out a device is coded to the root operation REMOVAL.

Body Part Character 4	Approach Character 5	Device Character 6	Qualifier Character 7
X Upper Tendon Y Lower Tendon	Ø Open 3 Percutaneous 4 Percutaneous Endoscopic	Ø Drainage Device 7 Autologous Tissue Substitute J Synthetic Substitute K Nonautologous Tissue Substitute Y Other Device	Z No Qualifier
X Upper Tendon Y Lower Tendon	X External	Ø Drainage Device	Z No Qualifier

Non-OR   ØLP[X,Y]3ØZ
Non-OR   ØLP[X,Y][3,4]YZ
Non-OR   ØLP[X,Y]XØZ

Ø   Medical and Surgical
L   Tendons
Q   Repair   Definition: Restoring, to the extent possible, a body part to its normal anatomic structure and function

           Explanation: Used only when the method to accomplish the repair is not one of the other root operations

Body Part Character 4	Approach Character 5	Device Character 6	Qualifier Character 7

Ø   Head and Neck Tendon
1   Shoulder Tendon, Right
2   Shoulder Tendon, Left
3   Upper Arm Tendon, Right
4   Upper Arm Tendon, Left
5   Lower Arm and Wrist Tendon, Right
6   Lower Arm and Wrist Tendon, Left
7   Hand Tendon, Right
8   Hand Tendon, Left
9   Trunk Tendon, Right
B   Trunk Tendon, Left
C   Thorax Tendon, Right
D   Thorax Tendon, Left
F   Abdomen Tendon, Right
G   Abdomen Tendon, Left
H   Perineum Tendon
J   Hip Tendon, Right
K   Hip Tendon, Left
L   Upper Leg Tendon, Right
M   Upper Leg Tendon, Left
N   Lower Leg Tendon, Right
     Achilles tendon
P   Lower Leg Tendon, Left
     See N Lower Leg Tendon, Right
Q   Knee Tendon, Right
     Patellar tendon
R   Knee Tendon, Left
     See Q Knee Tendon, Right
S   Ankle Tendon, Right
T   Ankle Tendon, Left
V   Foot Tendon, Right
W   Foot Tendon, Left
	Ø Open
	3 Percutaneous
	4 Percutaneous Endoscopic
		Z No Device	Z No Qualifier

NC Noncovered Procedure   LC Limited Coverage   QA Questionable OB Admit   NT New Tech Add-on   ⊞ Combination Member   ♂ Male   ♀ Female

ICD-10-PCS 2022   495

Ø Medical and Surgical
L Tendons
R Replacement

Definition: Putting in or on biological or synthetic material that physically takes the place and/or function of all or a portion of a body part

Explanation: The body part may have been taken out or replaced, or may be taken out, physically eradicated, or rendered nonfunctional during the REPLACEMENT procedure. A REMOVAL procedure is coded for taking out the device used in a previous replacement procedure.

Body Part Character 4	Approach Character 5	Device Character 6	Qualifier Character 7

Ø Head and Neck Tendon
1 Shoulder Tendon, Right
2 Shoulder Tendon, Left
3 Upper Arm Tendon, Right
4 Upper Arm Tendon, Left
5 Lower Arm and Wrist Tendon, Right
6 Lower Arm and Wrist Tendon, Left
7 Hand Tendon, Right
8 Hand Tendon, Left
9 Trunk Tendon, Right
B Trunk Tendon, Left
C Thorax Tendon, Right
D Thorax Tendon, Left
F Abdomen Tendon, Right
G Abdomen Tendon, Left
H Perineum Tendon
J Hip Tendon, Right
K Hip Tendon, Left
L Upper Leg Tendon, Right
M Upper Leg Tendon, Left
N Lower Leg Tendon, Right
   Achilles tendon
P Lower Leg Tendon, Left
   See N Lower Leg Tendon, Right
Q Knee Tendon, Right
   Patellar tendon
R Knee Tendon, Left
   See Q Knee Tendon, Right
S Ankle Tendon, Right
T Ankle Tendon, Left
V Foot Tendon, Right
W Foot Tendon, Left
	Ø Open
	4 Percutaneous Endoscopic
		7 Autologous Tissue Substitute
		J Synthetic Substitute
		K Nonautologous Tissue Substitute
			Z No Qualifier

Ø Medical and Surgical
L Tendons
S Reposition

Definition: Moving to its normal location, or other suitable location, all or a portion of a body part

Explanation: The body part is moved to a new location from an abnormal location, or from a normal location where it is not functioning correctly. The body part may or may not be cut out or off to be moved to the new location.

Body Part Character 4	Approach Character 5	Device Character 6	Qualifier Character 7

Ø Head and Neck Tendon
1 Shoulder Tendon, Right
2 Shoulder Tendon, Left
3 Upper Arm Tendon, Right
4 Upper Arm Tendon, Left
5 Lower Arm and Wrist Tendon, Right
6 Lower Arm and Wrist Tendon, Left
7 Hand Tendon, Right
8 Hand Tendon, Left
9 Trunk Tendon, Right
B Trunk Tendon, Left
C Thorax Tendon, Right
D Thorax Tendon, Left
F Abdomen Tendon, Right
G Abdomen Tendon, Left
H Perineum Tendon
J Hip Tendon, Right
K Hip Tendon, Left
L Upper Leg Tendon, Right
M Upper Leg Tendon, Left
N Lower Leg Tendon, Right
   Achilles tendon
P Lower Leg Tendon, Left
   See N Lower Leg Tendon, Right
Q Knee Tendon, Right
   Patellar tendon
R Knee Tendon, Left
   See Q Knee Tendon, Right
S Ankle Tendon, Right
T Ankle Tendon, Left
V Foot Tendon, Right
W Foot Tendon, Left
	Ø Open
	4 Percutaneous Endoscopic
		Z No Device	Z No Qualifier

Ø   **Medical and Surgical**
L   **Tendons**
T   **Resection**   Definition: Cutting out or off, without replacement, all of a body part
                         Explanation: None

Body Part Character 4	Approach Character 5	Device Character 6	Qualifier Character 7

Ø Head and Neck Tendon
1 Shoulder Tendon, Right
2 Shoulder Tendon, Left
3 Upper Arm Tendon, Right
4 Upper Arm Tendon, Left
5 Lower Arm and Wrist Tendon, Right
6 Lower Arm and Wrist Tendon, Left
7 Hand Tendon, Right
8 Hand Tendon, Left
9 Trunk Tendon, Right
B Trunk Tendon, Left
C Thorax Tendon, Right
D Thorax Tendon, Left
F Abdomen Tendon, Right
G Abdomen Tendon, Left
H Perineum Tendon
J Hip Tendon, Right
K Hip Tendon, Left
L Upper Leg Tendon, Right
M Upper Leg Tendon, Left
N Lower Leg Tendon, Right
    Achilles tendon
P Lower Leg Tendon, Left
    See N Lower Leg Tendon, Right
Q Knee Tendon, Right
    Patellar tendon
R Knee Tendon, Left
    See Q Knee Tendon, Right
S Ankle Tendon, Right
T Ankle Tendon, Left
V Foot Tendon, Right
W Foot Tendon, Left
	Ø Open
	4 Percutaneous Endoscopic
		Z No Device	**Z** No Qualifier

Ø   **Medical and Surgical**
L   **Tendons**
U   **Supplement**   Definition: Putting in or on biological or synthetic material that physically reinforces and/or augments the function of a portion of a body part
                         Explanation: The biological material is non-living, or is living and from the same individual. The body part may have been previously replaced, and the SUPPLEMENT procedure is performed to physically reinforce and/or augment the function of the replaced body part.

Body Part Character 4	Approach Character 5	Device Character 6	Qualifier Character 7

Ø Head and Neck Tendon
1 Shoulder Tendon, Right
2 Shoulder Tendon, Left
3 Upper Arm Tendon, Right
4 Upper Arm Tendon, Left
5 Lower Arm and Wrist Tendon, Right
6 Lower Arm and Wrist Tendon, Left
7 Hand Tendon, Right
8 Hand Tendon, Left
9 Trunk Tendon, Right
B Trunk Tendon, Left
C Thorax Tendon, Right
D Thorax Tendon, Left
F Abdomen Tendon, Right
G Abdomen Tendon, Left
H Perineum Tendon
J Hip Tendon, Right
K Hip Tendon, Left
L Upper Leg Tendon, Right
M Upper Leg Tendon, Left
N Lower Leg Tendon, Right
    Achilles tendon
P Lower Leg Tendon, Left
    See N Lower Leg Tendon, Right
Q Knee Tendon, Right
    Patellar tendon
R Knee Tendon, Left
    See Q Knee Tendon, Right
S Ankle Tendon, Right
T Ankle Tendon, Left
V Foot Tendon, Right
W Foot Tendon, Left
	Ø Open
	4 Percutaneous Endoscopic
		7 Autologous Tissue Substitute
		J Synthetic Substitute
		K Nonautologous Tissue Substitute
			Z No Qualifier

NC Noncovered Procedure   **LC** Limited Coverage   **QA** Questionable OB Admit   **NT** New Tech Add-on   ⊞ Combination Member   ♂ Male   ♀ Female

Ø   Medical and Surgical
L   Tendons
W   Revision   Definition: Correcting, to the extent possible, a portion of a malfunctioning device or the position of a displaced device

Explanation: Revision can include correcting a malfunctioning or displaced device by taking out or putting in components of the device such as a screw or pin

Body Part Character 4	Approach Character 5	Device Character 6	Qualifier Character 7
X Upper Tendon Y Lower Tendon	Ø Open 3 Percutaneous 4 Percutaneous Endoscopic	Ø Drainage Device 7 Autologous Tissue Substitute J Synthetic Substitute K Nonautologous Tissue Substitute Y Other Device	Z No Qualifier
X Upper Tendon Y Lower Tendon	X External	Ø Drainage Device 7 Autologous Tissue Substitute J Synthetic Substitute K Nonautologous Tissue Substitute	Z No Qualifier

Non-OR	ØLW[X,Y][3,4]YZ
Non-OR	ØLW[X,Y]X[Ø,7,J,K]Z

Ø   Medical and Surgical
L   Tendons
X   Transfer   Definition: Moving, without taking out, all or a portion of a body part to another location to take over the function of all or a portion of a body part

Explanation: The body part transferred remains connected to its vascular and nervous supply

Body Part Character 4	Approach Character 5	Device Character 6	Qualifier Character 7

Ø   Head and Neck Tendon
1   Shoulder Tendon, Right
2   Shoulder Tendon, Left
3   Upper Arm Tendon, Right
4   Upper Arm Tendon, Left
5   Lower Arm and Wrist Tendon, Right
6   Lower Arm and Wrist Tendon, Left
7   Hand Tendon, Right
8   Hand Tendon, Left
9   Trunk Tendon, Right
B   Trunk Tendon, Left
C   Thorax Tendon, Right
D   Thorax Tendon, Left
F   Abdomen Tendon, Right
G   Abdomen Tendon, Left
H   Perineum Tendon
J   Hip Tendon, Right
K   Hip Tendon, Left
L   Upper Leg Tendon, Right
M   Upper Leg Tendon, Left
N   Lower Leg Tendon, Right
     Achilles tendon
P   Lower Leg Tendon, Left
     See N Lower Leg Tendon, Right
Q   Knee Tendon, Right
     Patellar tendon
R   Knee Tendon, Left
     See Q Knee Tendon, Right
S   Ankle Tendon, Right
T   Ankle Tendon, Left
V   Foot Tendon, Right
W   Foot Tendon, Left
	Ø Open
	4 Percutaneous Endoscopic
		Z No Device	Z No Qualifier

Bursae and Ligaments ØM2–ØMX

Character Meanings*

This Character Meaning table is provided as a guide to assist the user in the identification of character members that may be found in this section of code tables. It **SHOULD NOT** be used to build a PCS code.

Operation–Character 3	Body Part–Character 4	Approach–Character 5	Device–Character 6	Qualifier–Character 7
2 Change	Ø Head and Neck Bursa and Ligament	Ø Open	Ø Drainage Device	X Diagnostic
5 Destruction	1 Shoulder Bursa and Ligament, Right	3 Percutaneous	7 Autologous Tissue Substitute	Z No Qualifier
8 Division	2 Shoulder Bursa and Ligament, Left	4 Percutaneous Endoscopic	J Synthetic Substitute	
9 Drainage	3 Elbow Bursa and Ligament, Right	X External	K Nonautologous Tissue Substitute	
B Excision	4 Elbow Bursa and Ligament, Left		Y Other Device	
C Extirpation	5 Wrist Bursa and Ligament, Right		Z No Device	
D Extraction	6 Wrist Bursa and Ligament, Left			
H Insertion	7 Hand Bursa and Ligament, Right			
J Inspection	8 Hand Bursa and Ligament, Left			
M Reattachment	9 Upper Extremity Bursa and Ligament, Right			
N Release	B Upper Extremity Bursa and Ligament, Left			
P Removal	C Upper Spine Bursa and Ligament			
Q Repair	D Lower Spine Bursa and Ligament			
R Replacement	F Sternum Bursa and Ligament			
S Reposition	G Rib(s) Bursa and Ligament			
T Resection	H Abdomen Bursa and Ligament, Right			
U Supplement	J Abdomen Bursa and Ligament, Left			
W Revision	K Perineum Bursa and Ligament			
X Transfer	L Hip Bursa and Ligament, Right			
	M Hip Bursa and Ligament, Left			
	N Knee Bursa and Ligament, Right			
	P Knee Bursa and Ligament, Left			
	Q Ankle Bursa and Ligament, Right			
	R Ankle Bursa and Ligament, Left			
	S Foot Bursa and Ligament, Right			
	T Foot Bursa and Ligament, Left			
	V Lower Extremity Bursa and Ligament, Right			
	W Lower Extremity Bursa and Ligament, Left			
	X Upper Bursa and Ligament			
	Y Lower Bursa and Ligament			

* Includes synovial membrane.

AHA Coding Clinic for table ØMB
2018, 3Q, 17   Excisional debridement of periosteum

AHA Coding Clinic for table ØMM
2013, 3Q, 20   Superior labrum anterior posterior (SLAP) repair and subacromial decompression

AHA Coding Clinic for table ØMQ
2014, 3Q, 9   Interspinous ligamentoplasty

AHA Coding Clinic for table ØMT
2017, 2Q, 21   Arthroscopic anterior cruciate ligament revision using autograft with anterolateral ligament reconstruction

AHA Coding Clinic for table ØMU
2017, 2Q, 21   Arthroscopic anterior cruciate ligament revision using autograft with anterolateral ligament reconstruction

Shoulder Ligaments

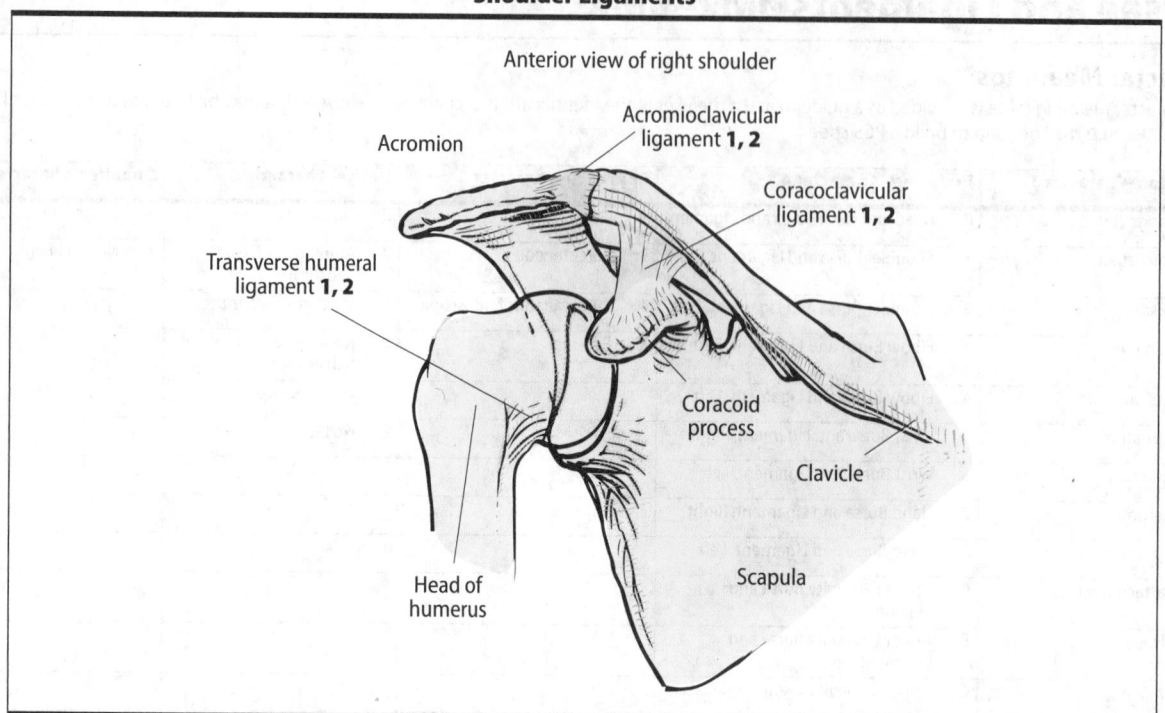

Anterior view of right shoulder

Acromion

Acromioclavicular ligament **1, 2**

Coracoclavicular ligament **1, 2**

Transverse humeral ligament **1, 2**

Coracoid process

Clavicle

Head of humerus

Scapula

Knee Bursae

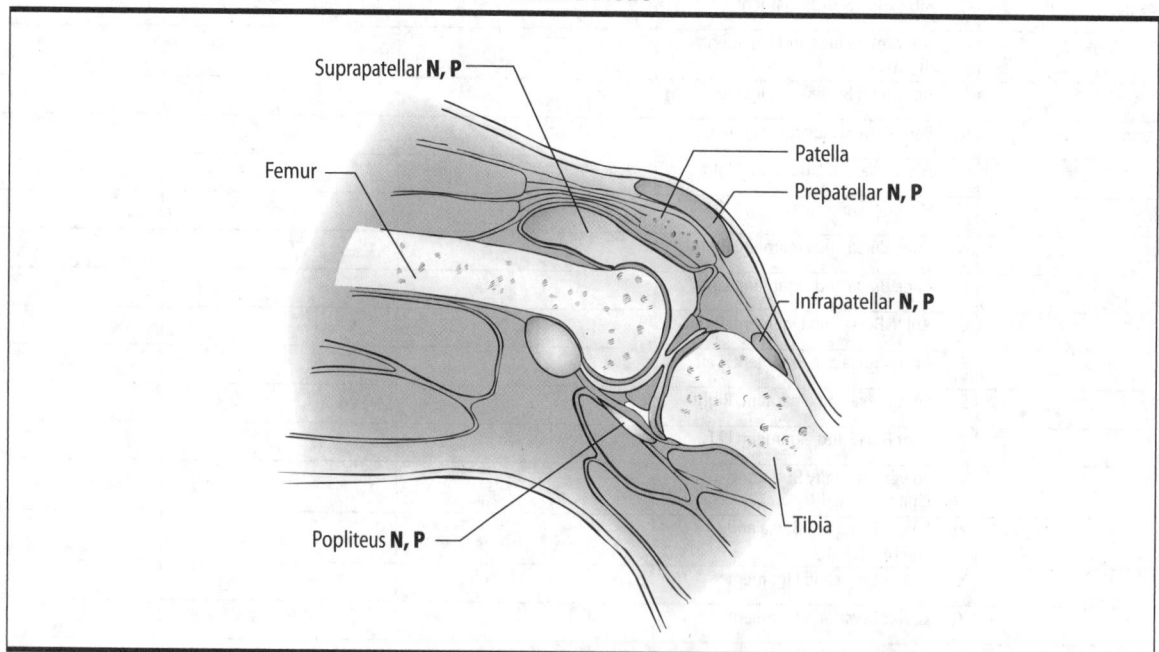

Suprapatellar **N, P**

Femur

Patella

Prepatellar **N, P**

Infrapatellar **N, P**

Popliteus **N, P**

Tibia

Knee Ligaments

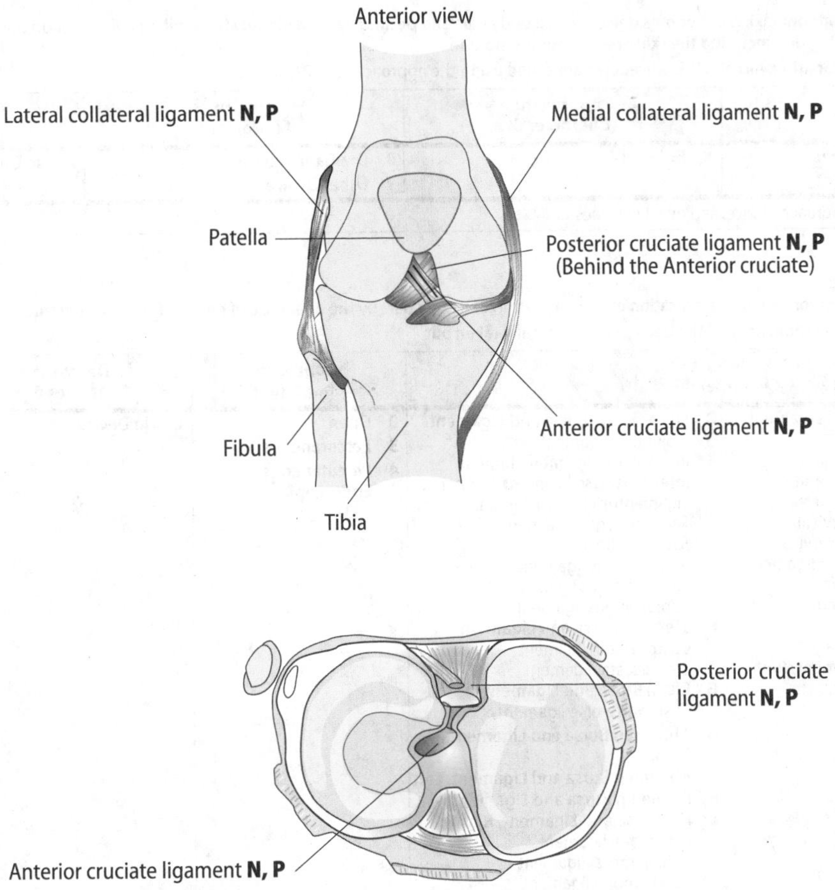

Anterior view

Lateral collateral ligament **N, P**

Medial collateral ligament **N, P**

Patella

Posterior cruciate ligament **N, P**
(Behind the Anterior cruciate)

Anterior cruciate ligament **N, P**

Fibula

Tibia

Posterior cruciate
ligament **N, P**

Anterior cruciate ligament **N, P**

Wrist Ligaments

Palmar view

Flexor carpi
ulnaris **5, 6**

Radial collateral
carpal **5, 6**

Ulnar collateral
carpal **5, 6**

Palmar radiocarpal **5, 6**

Dorsal view

Radial collateral
carpal **5, 6**

Ulnar collateral
carpal **5, 6**

Dorsal
radiocarpal **5, 6**

Ulnocarpal **5, 6**

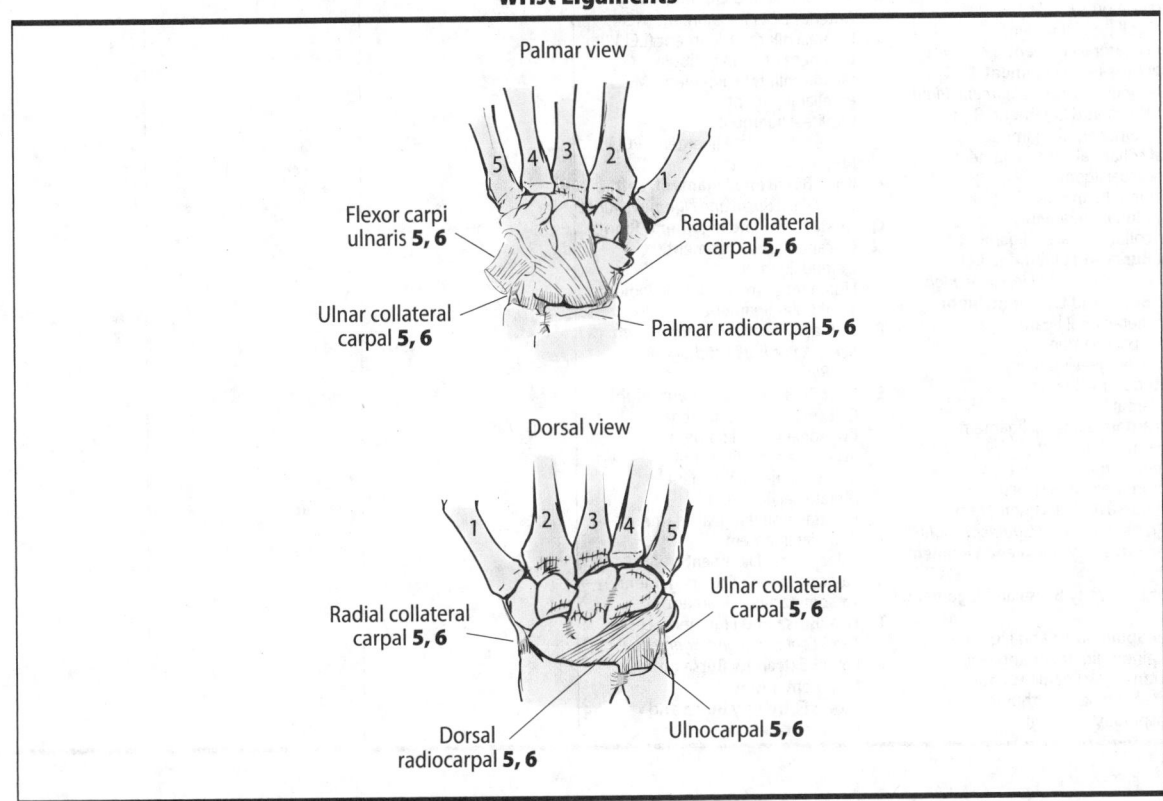

Ø   **Medical and Surgical**
M   **Bursae and Ligaments**
2   **Change**   Definition: Taking out or off a device from a body part and putting back an identical or similar device in or on the same body part without cutting or puncturing the skin or a mucous membrane
                   Explanation: All CHANGE procedures are coded using the approach EXTERNAL

Body Part Character 4	Approach Character 5	Device Character 6	Qualifier Character 7
X Upper Bursa and Ligament Y Lower Bursa and Ligament	X External	Ø Drainage Device Y Other Device	Z No Qualifier

Non-OR   All body part, approach, device, and qualifier values

Ø   **Medical and Surgical**
M   **Bursae and Ligaments**
5   **Destruction**   Definition: Physical eradication of all or a portion of a body part by the direct use of energy, force, or a destructive agent
                       Explanation: None of the body part is physically taken out

Body Part Character 4		Approach Character 5	Device Character 6	Qualifier Character 7

Ø   **Head and Neck Bursa and Ligament**
     Alar ligament of axis
     Cervical interspinous ligament
     Cervical intertransverse ligament
     Cervical ligamentum flavum
     Interspinous ligament, cervical
     Intertransverse ligament, cervical
     Lateral temporomandibular ligament
     Ligamentum flavum, cervical
     Sphenomandibular ligament
     Stylomandibular ligament
     Transverse ligament of atlas
1   **Shoulder Bursa and Ligament, Right**
     Acromioclavicular ligament
     Coracoacromial ligament
     Coracoclavicular ligament
     Coracohumeral ligament
     Costoclavicular ligament
     Glenohumeral ligament
     Interclavicular ligament
     Sternoclavicular ligament
     Subacromial bursa
     Transverse humeral ligament
     Transverse scapular ligament
2   **Shoulder Bursa and Ligament, Left**
     See 1 Shoulder Bursa and Ligament, Right
3   **Elbow Bursa and Ligfament, Right**
     Annular ligament
     Olecranon bursa
     Radial collateral ligament
     Ulnar collateral ligament
4   **Elbow Bursa and Ligament, Left**
     See 3 Elbow Bursa and Ligament, Right
5   **Wrist Bursa and Ligament, Right**
     Palmar ulnocarpal ligament
     Radial collateral carpal ligament
     Radiocarpal ligament
     Radioulnar ligament
     Scapholunate ligament
     Ulnar collateral carpal ligament
6   **Wrist Bursa and Ligament, Left**
     See 5 Wrist Bursa and Ligament, Right
7   **Hand Bursa and Ligament, Right**
     Carpometacarpal ligament
     Intercarpal ligament
     Interphalangeal ligament
     Lunotriquetral ligament
     Metacarpal ligament
     Metacarpophalangeal ligament
     Pisohamate ligament
     Pisometacarpal ligament
     Scaphotrapezium ligament
8   **Hand Bursa and Ligament, Left**
     See 7 Hand Bursa and Ligament, Right
9   **Upper Extremity Bursa and Ligament, Right**
B   **Upper Extremity Bursa and Ligament, Left**
C   **Upper Spine Bursa and Ligament**
     Interspinous ligament, thoracic
     Intertransverse ligament, thoracic
     Ligamentum flavum, thoracic
     Supraspinous ligament
	D **Lower Spine Bursa and Ligament**
	     Iliolumbar ligament
	     Interspinous ligament, lumbar
	     Intertransverse ligament, lumbar
	     Ligamentum flavum, lumbar
	     Sacrococcygeal ligament
	     Sacroiliac ligament
	     Sacrospinous ligament
	     Sacrotuberous ligament
	     Supraspinous ligament
	F **Sternum Bursa and Ligament**
	     Costoxiphoid ligament
	     Sternocostal ligament
	G **Rib(s) Bursa and Ligament**
	     Costotransverse ligament
	H **Abdomen Bursa and Ligament, Right**
	J **Abdomen Bursa and Ligament, Left**
	K **Perineum Bursa and Ligament**
	L **Hip Bursa and Ligament, Right**
	     Iliofemoral ligament
	     Ischiofemoral ligament
	     Pubofemoral ligament
	     Transverse acetabular ligament
	     Trochanteric bursa
	M **Hip Bursa and Ligament, Left**
	     See L Hip Bursa and Ligament, Right
	N **Knee Bursa and Ligament, Right**
	     Anterior cruciate ligament (ACL)
	     Lateral collateral ligament (LCL)
	     Ligament of head of fibula
	     Medial collateral ligament (MCL)
	     Patellar ligament
	     Popliteal ligament
	     Posterior cruciate ligament (PCL)
	     Prepatellar bursa
	P **Knee Bursa and Ligament, Left**
	     See N Knee Bursa and Ligament, Right
	Q **Ankle Bursa and Ligament, Right**
	     Calcaneofibular ligament
	     Deltoid ligament
	     Ligament of the lateral malleolus
	     Talofibular ligament
	R **Ankle Bursa and Ligament, Left**
	     See Q Ankle Bursa and Ligament, Right
	S **Foot Bursa and Ligament, Right**
	     Calcaneocuboid ligament
	     Cuneonavicular ligament
	     Intercuneiform ligament
	     Interphalangeal ligament
	     Metatarsal ligament
	     Metatarsophalangeal ligament
	     Subtalar ligament
	     Talocalcaneal ligament
	     Talocalcaneonavicular ligament
	     Tarsometatarsal ligament
	T **Foot Bursa and Ligament, Left**
	     See S Foot Bursa and Ligament, Right
	V **Lower Extremity Bursa and Ligament, Right**
	W **Lower Extremity Bursa and Ligament, Left**
		Ø Open
		3 Percutaneous
		4 Percutaneous Endoscopic
			Z No Device	Z No Qualifier

Non-OR Procedure   DRG Non-OR Procedure   Valid OR Procedure   HAC Associated Procedure   Combination Only   New/Revised GREEN

Ø   **Medical and Surgical**
M   **Bursae and Ligaments**
8   **Division**   Definition: Cutting into a body part, without draining fluids and/or gases from the body part, in order to separate or transect a body part
                   Explanation: All or a portion of the body part is separated into two or more portions

Body Part Character 4		Approach Character 5	Device Character 6	Qualifier Character 7
Ø Head and Neck Bursa and Ligament	**D Lower Spine Bursa and Ligament**	**Ø Open**	**Z No Device**	**Z No Qualifier**
Alar ligament of axis	Iliolumbar ligament	**3 Percutaneous**		
Cervical interspinous ligament	Interspinous ligament, lumbar	**4 Percutaneous Endoscopic**		
Cervical intertransverse ligament	Intertransverse ligament, lumbar			
Cervical ligamentum flavum	Ligamentum flavum, lumbar			
Interspinous ligament, cervical	Sacrococcygeal ligament			
Intertransverse ligament, cervical	Sacroiliac ligament			
Lateral temporomandibular ligament	Sacrospinous ligament			
Ligamentum flavum, cervical	Sacrotuberous ligament			
Sphenomandibular ligament	Supraspinous ligament			
Stylomandibular ligament	**F Sternum Bursa and Ligament**			
Transverse ligament of atlas	Costoxiphoid ligament			
1 Shoulder Bursa and Ligament, Right	Sternocostal ligament			
Acromioclavicular ligament	**G Rib(s) Bursa and Ligament**			
Coracoacromial ligament	Costotransverse ligament			
Coracoclavicular ligament	**H Abdomen Bursa and Ligament, Right**			
Coracohumeral ligament	**J Abdomen Bursa and Ligament, Left**			
Costoclavicular ligament	**K Perineum Bursa and Ligament**			
Glenohumeral ligament	**L Hip Bursa and Ligament, Right**			
Interclavicular ligament	Iliofemoral ligament			
Sternoclavicular ligament	Ischiofemoral ligament			
Subacromial bursa	Pubofemoral ligament			
Transverse humeral ligament	Transverse acetabular ligament			
Transverse scapular ligament	Trochanteric bursa			
2 Shoulder Bursa and Ligament, Left	**M Hip Bursa and Ligament, Left**			
See 1 Shoulder Bursa and Ligament, Right	**See** L Hip Bursa and Ligament, Right			
3 Elbow Bursa and Ligament, Right	**N Knee Bursa and Ligament, Right**			
Annular ligament	Anterior cruciate ligament (ACL)			
Olecranon bursa	Lateral collateral ligament (LCL)			
Radial collateral ligament	Ligament of head of fibula			
Ulnar collateral ligament	Medial collateral ligament (MCL)			
4 Elbow Bursa and Ligament, Left	Patellar ligament			
See 3 Elbow Bursa and Ligament, Right	Popliteal ligament			
5 Wrist Bursa and Ligament, Right	Posterior cruciate ligament (PCL)			
Palmar ulnocarpal ligament	Prepatellar bursa			
Radial collateral carpal ligament	**P Knee Bursa and Ligament, Left**			
Radiocarpal ligament	**See** N Knee Bursa and Ligament, Right			
Radioulnar ligament	**Q Ankle Bursa and Ligament, Right**			
Scapholunate ligament	Calcaneofibular ligament			
Ulnar collateral carpal ligament	Deltoid ligament			
6 Wrist Bursa and Ligament, Left	Ligament of the lateral malleolus			
See 5 Wrist Bursa and Ligament, Right	Talofibular ligament			
7 Hand Bursa and Ligament, Right	**R Ankle Bursa and Ligament, Left**			
Carpometacarpal ligament	**See** Q Ankle Bursa and Ligament, Right			
Intercarpal ligament	**S Foot Bursa and Ligament, Right**			
Interphalangeal ligament	Calcaneocuboid ligament			
Lunotriquetral ligament	Cuneonavicular ligament			
Metacarpal ligament	Intercuneiform ligament			
Metacarpophalangeal ligament	Interphalangeal ligament			
Pisohamate ligament	Metatarsal ligament			
Pisometacarpal ligament	Metatarsophalangeal ligament			
Scaphotrapezium ligament	Subtalar ligament			
8 Hand Bursa and Ligament, Left	Talocalcaneal ligament			
See 7 Hand Bursa and Ligament, Right	Talocalcaneonavicular ligament			
9 Upper Extremity Bursa and Ligament, Right	Tarsometatarsal ligament			
B Upper Extremity Bursa and Ligament, Left	**T Foot Bursa and Ligament, Left**			
C Upper Spine Bursa and Ligament	**See** S Foot Bursa and Ligament, Right			
Interspinous ligament, thoracic	**V Lower Extremity Bursa and Ligament, Right**			
Intertransverse ligament, thoracic	**W Lower Extremity Bursa and Ligament, Left**			
Ligamentum flavum, thoracic				
Supraspinous ligament				

NC Noncovered Procedure   **LC** Limited Coverage   **QA** Questionable OB Admit   **NT** New Tech Add-on   ⊞ Combination Member   ♂ Male   ♀ Female

ICD-10-PCS 2022   503

ØM8–ØM8

Bursae and Ligaments

Ø   **Medical and Surgical**
M   **Bursae and Ligaments**
9   **Drainage**   Definition: Taking or letting out fluids and/or gases from a body part
                     Explanation: The qualifier DIAGNOSTIC is used to identify drainage procedures that are biopsies

Body Part Character 4		Approach Character 5	Device Character 6	Qualifier Character 7
Ø **Head and Neck Bursa and Ligament** Alar ligament of axis Cervical interspinous ligament Cervical intertransverse ligament Cervical ligamentum flavum Interspinous ligament, cervical Intertransverse ligament, cervical Lateral temporomandibular ligament Ligamentum flavum, cervical Sphenomandibular ligament Stylomandibular ligament Transverse ligament of atlas **1** **Shoulder Bursa and Ligament, Right** Acromioclavicular ligament Coracoacromial ligament Coracoclavicular ligament Coracohumeral ligament Costoclavicular ligament Glenohumeral ligament Interclavicular ligament Sternoclavicular ligament Subacromial bursa Transverse humeral ligament Transverse scapular ligament **2** **Shoulder Bursa and Ligament, Left** See 1 Shoulder Bursa and Ligament, Right **3** **Elbow Bursa and Ligament, Right** Annular ligament Olecranon bursa Radial collateral ligament Ulnar collateral ligament **4** **Elbow Bursa and Ligament, Left** See 3 Elbow Bursa and Ligament, Right **5** **Wrist Bursa and Ligament, Right** Palmar ulnocarpal ligament Radial collateral carpal ligament Radiocarpal ligament Radioulnar ligament Scapholunate ligament Ulnar collateral carpal ligament **6** **Wrist Bursa and Ligament, Left** See 5 Wrist Bursa and Ligament, Right **7** **Hand Bursa and Ligament, Right** Carpometacarpal ligament Intercarpal ligament Interphalangeal ligament Lunotriquetral ligament Metacarpal ligament Metacarpophalangeal ligament Pisohamate ligament Pisometacarpal ligament Scaphotrapezium ligament **8** **Hand Bursa and Ligament, Left** See 7 Hand Bursa and Ligament, Right **9** **Upper Extremity Bursa and Ligament, Right** **B** **Upper Extremity Bursa and Ligament, Left** **C** **Upper Spine Bursa and Ligament** Interspinous ligament, thoracic Intertransverse ligament, thoracic Ligamentum flavum, thoracic Supraspinous ligament	**D** **Lower Spine Bursa and Ligament** Iliolumbar ligament Interspinous ligament, lumbar Intertransverse ligament, lumbar Ligamentum flavum, lumbar Sacrococcygeal ligament Sacroiliac ligament Sacrospinous ligament Sacrotuberous ligament Supraspinous ligament **F** **Sternum Bursa and Ligament** Costoxiphoid ligament Sternocostal ligament **G** **Rib(s) Bursa and Ligament** Costotransverse ligament **H** **Abdomen Bursa and Ligament, Right** **J** **Abdomen Bursa and Ligament, Left** **K** **Perineum Bursa and Ligament** **L** **Hip Bursa and Ligament, Right** Iliofemoral ligament Ischiofemoral ligament Pubofemoral ligament Transverse acetabular ligament Trochanteric bursa **M** **Hip Bursa and Ligament, Left** See L Hip Bursa and Ligament, Right **N** **Knee Bursa and Ligament, Right** Anterior cruciate ligament (ACL) Lateral collateral ligament (LCL) Ligament of head of fibula Medial collateral ligament (MCL) Patellar ligament Popliteal ligament Posterior cruciate ligament (PCL) Prepatellar bursa **P** **Knee Bursa and Ligament, Left** See N Knee Bursa and Ligament, Right **Q** **Ankle Bursa and Ligament, Right** Calcaneofibular ligament Deltoid ligament Ligament of the lateral malleolus Talofibular ligament **R** **Ankle Bursa and Ligament, Left** See Q Ankle Bursa and Ligament, Right **S** **Foot Bursa and Ligament, Right** Calcaneocuboid ligament Cuneonavicular ligament Intercuneiform ligament Interphalangeal ligament Metatarsal ligament Metatarsophalangeal ligament Subtalar ligament Talocalcaneal ligament Talocalcaneonavicular ligament Tarsometatarsal ligament **T** **Foot Bursa and Ligament, Left** See S Foot Bursa and Ligament, Right **V** **Lower Extremity Bursa and Ligament, Right** **W** **Lower Extremity Bursa and Ligament, Left**	**Ø** Open **3** Percutaneous **4** Percutaneous Endoscopic	**Ø** Drainage Device	**Z** No Qualifier

Non-OR	ØM9[Ø,1,2,3,4,5,6,7,8,9,B,C,D,F,G,H,J,K,L,M,N,P,Q,R,S,T,V,W]3ØZ
Non-OR	ØM9[1,2,3,4,7,8,9,B,C,D,F,G,H,J,K,L,M,V,W]4ØZ

ØM9 Continued on next page

Ø   **Medical and Surgical**
M   **Bursae and Ligaments**
9   **Drainage**   Definition: Taking or letting out fluids and/or gases from a body part

ØM9 Continued

                      Explanation: The qualifier DIAGNOSTIC is used to identify drainage procedures that are biopsies

Body Part Character 4		Approach Character 5	Device Character 6	Qualifier Character 7
Ø **Head and Neck Bursa and Ligament** Alar ligament of axis Cervical interspinous ligament Cervical intertransverse ligament Cervical ligamentum flavum Interspinous ligament, cervical Intertransverse ligament, cervical Lateral temporomandibular ligament Ligamentum flavum, cervical Sphenomandibular ligament Stylomandibular ligament Transverse ligament of atlas	**D** **Lower Spine Bursa and Ligament** Iliolumbar ligament Interspinous ligament, lumbar Intertransverse ligament, lumbar Ligamentum flavum, lumbar Sacrococcygeal ligament Sacroiliac ligament Sacrospinous ligament Sacrotuberous ligament Supraspinous ligament	**Ø** Open **3** Percutaneous **4** Percutaneous Endoscopic	**Z** No Device	**X** Diagnostic **Z** No Qualifier
1 **Shoulder Bursa and Ligament, Right** Acromioclavicular ligament Coracoacromial ligament Coracoclavicular ligament Coracohumeral ligament Costoclavicular ligament Glenohumeral ligament Interclavicular ligament Sternoclavicular ligament Subacromial bursa Transverse humeral ligament Transverse scapular ligament	**F** **Sternum Bursa and Ligament** Costoxiphoid ligament Sternocostal ligament **G** **Rib(s) Bursa and Ligament** Costotransverse ligament **H** **Abdomen Bursa and Ligament, Right** **J** **Abdomen Bursa and Ligament, Left** **K** **Perineum Bursa and Ligament**			
2 **Shoulder Bursa and Ligament, Left** *See* 1 Shoulder Bursa and Ligament, Right	**L** **Hip Bursa and Ligament, Right** Iliofemoral ligament Ischiofemoral ligament Pubofemoral ligament Transverse acetabular ligament Trochanteric bursa			
3 **Elbow Bursa and Ligament, Right** Annular ligament Olecranon bursa Radial collateral ligament Ulnar collateral ligament	**M** **Hip Bursa and Ligament, Left** *See* L Hip Bursa and Ligament, Right			
4 **Elbow Bursa and Ligament, Left** *See* 3 Elbow Bursa and Ligament, Right	**N** **Knee Bursa and Ligament, Right** Anterior cruciate ligament (ACL) Lateral collateral ligament (LCL) Ligament of head of fibula Medial collateral ligament (MCL) Patellar ligament Popliteal ligament Posterior cruciate ligament (PCL) Prepatellar bursa			
5 **Wrist Bursa and Ligament, Right** Palmar ulnocarpal ligament Radial collateral carpal ligament Radiocarpal ligament Radioulnar ligament Scapholunate ligament Ulnar collateral carpal ligament	**P** **Knee Bursa and Ligament, Left** *See* N Knee Bursa and Ligament, Right			
6 **Wrist Bursa and Ligament, Left** *See* 5 Wrist Bursa and Ligament, Right	**Q** **Ankle Bursa and Ligament, Right** Calcaneofibular ligament Deltoid ligament Ligament of the lateral malleolus Talofibular ligament			
7 **Hand Bursa and Ligament, Right** Carpometacarpal ligament Intercarpal ligament Interphalangeal ligament Lunotriquetral ligament Metacarpal ligament Metacarpophalangeal ligament Pisohamate ligament Pisometacarpal ligament Scaphotrapezium ligament	**R** **Ankle Bursa and Ligament, Left** *See* Q Ankle Bursa and Ligament, Right **S** **Foot Bursa and Ligament, Right** Calcaneocuboid ligament Cuneonavicular ligament Intercuneiform ligament Interphalangeal ligament Metatarsal ligament Metatarsophalangeal ligament Subtalar ligament Talocalcaneal ligament Talocalcaneonavicular ligament Tarsometatarsal ligament			
8 **Hand Bursa and Ligament, Left** *See* 7 Hand Bursa and Ligament, Right	**T** **Foot Bursa and Ligament, Left** *See* S Foot Bursa and Ligament, Right			
9 **Upper Extremity Bursa and Ligament, Right** **B** **Upper Extremity Bursa and Ligament, Left** **C** **Upper Spine Bursa and Ligament** Interspinous ligament, thoracic Intertransverse ligament, thoracic Ligamentum flavum, thoracic Supraspinous ligament	**V** **Lower Extremity Bursa and Ligament, Right** **W** **Lower Extremity Bursa and Ligament, Left**			

Non-OR   ØM9[Ø,1,2,3,4,5,6,7,8,C,D,F,G,L,M,N,P,Q,R,S,T][Ø,3,4]ZX
Non-OR   ØM9[Ø,1,2,3,4,5,6,7,8,9,B,C,D,F,G,H,J,K,L,M,N,P,Q,R,S,T,V,W]3ZZ
Non-OR   ØM9[Ø,5,6,7,8,9,B,C,D,F,G,H,J,K,N,P,Q,R,S,T,V,W]4ZZ

NC Noncovered Procedure   **LC** Limited Coverage   **QA** Questionable OB Admit   **NT** New Tech Add-on   ⊞ Combination Member   ♂ Male   ♀ Female

ICD-10-PCS 2022   **505**

ØM9–ØM9

Ø   **Medical and Surgical**
M   **Bursae and Ligaments**
B   **Excision**   Definition: Cutting out or off, without replacement, a portion of a body part
                  Explanation: The qualifier DIAGNOSTIC is used to identify excision procedures that are biopsies

Body Part Character 4		Approach Character 5	Device Character 6	Qualifier Character 7

Ø **Head and Neck Bursa and Ligament**
  Alar ligament of axis
  Cervical interspinous ligament
  Cervical intertransverse ligament
  Cervical ligamentum flavum
  Interspinous ligament, cervical
  Intertransverse ligament, cervical
  Lateral temporomandibular
    ligament
  Ligamentum flavum, cervical
  Sphenomandibular ligament
  Stylomandibular ligament
  Transverse ligament of atlas
1 **Shoulder Bursa and Ligament, Right**
  Acromioclavicular ligament
  Coracoacromial ligament
  Coracoclavicular ligament
  Coracohumeral ligament
  Costoclavicular ligament
  Glenohumeral ligament
  Interclavicular ligament
  Sternoclavicular ligament
  Subacromial bursa
  Transverse humeral ligament
  Transverse scapular ligament
2 **Shoulder Bursa and Ligament, Left**
  See *1 Shoulder Bursa and Ligament, Right*
3 **Elbow Bursa and Ligament, Right**
  Annular ligament
  Olecranon bursa
  Radial collateral ligament
  Ulnar collateral ligament
4 **Elbow Bursa and Ligament, Left**
  See *3 Elbow Bursa and Ligament, Right*
5 **Wrist Bursa and Ligament, Right**
  Palmar ulnocarpal ligament
  Radial collateral carpal ligament
  Radiocarpal ligament
  Radioulnar ligament
  Scapholunate ligament
  Ulnar collateral carpal ligament
6 **Wrist Bursa and Ligament, Left**
  See *5 Wrist Bursa and Ligament, Right*
7 **Hand Bursa and Ligament, Right**
  Carpometacarpal ligament
  Intercarpal ligament
  Interphalangeal ligament
  Lunotriquetral ligament
  Metacarpal ligament
  Metacarpophalangeal ligament
  Pisohamate ligament
  Pisometacarpal ligament
  Scaphotrapezium ligament
8 **Hand Bursa and Ligament, Left**
  See *7 Hand Bursa and Ligament, Right*
9 **Upper Extremity Bursa and Ligament, Right**
B **Upper Extremity Bursa and Ligament, Left**
C **Upper Spine Bursa and Ligament**
  Interspinous ligament, thoracic
  Intertransverse ligament, thoracic
  Ligamentum flavum, thoracic
  Supraspinous ligament
	D **Lower Spine Bursa and Ligament**
	  Iliolumbar ligament
	  Interspinous ligament, lumbar
	  Intertransverse ligament, lumbar
	  Ligamentum flavum, lumbar
	  Sacrococcygeal ligament
	  Sacroiliac ligament
	  Sacrospinous ligament
	  Sacrotuberous ligament
	  Supraspinous ligament
	F **Sternum Bursa and Ligament**
	  Costoxiphoid ligament
	  Sternocostal ligament
	G **Rib(s) Bursa and Ligament**
	  Costotransverse ligament
	H **Abdomen Bursa and Ligament, Right**
	J **Abdomen Bursa and Ligament, Left**
	K **Perineum Bursa and Ligament**
	L **Hip Bursa and Ligament, Right**
	  Iliofemoral ligament
	  Ischiofemoral ligament
	  Pubofemoral ligament
	  Transverse acetabular ligament
	  Trochanteric bursa
	M **Hip Bursa and Ligament, Left**
	  See *L Hip Bursa and Ligament, Right*
	N **Knee Bursa and Ligament, Right**
	  Anterior cruciate ligament (ACL)
	  Lateral collateral ligament (LCL)
	  Ligament of head of fibula
	  Medial collateral ligament (MCL)
	  Patellar ligament
	  Popliteal ligament
	  Posterior cruciate ligament (PCL)
	  Prepatellar bursa
	P **Knee Bursa and Ligament, Left**
	  See *N Knee Bursa and Ligament, Right*
	Q **Ankle Bursa and Ligament, Right**
	  Calcaneofibular ligament
	  Deltoid ligament
	  Ligament of the lateral malleolus
	  Talofibular ligament
	R **Ankle Bursa and Ligament, Left**
	  See *Q Ankle Bursa and Ligament, Right*
	S **Foot Bursa and Ligament, Right**
	  Calcaneocuboid ligament
	  Cuneonavicular ligament
	  Intercuneiform ligament
	  Interphalangeal ligament
	  Metatarsal ligament
	  Metatarsophalangeal ligament
	  Subtalar ligament
	  Talocalcaneal ligament
	  Talocalcaneonavicular ligament
	  Tarsometatarsal ligament
	T **Foot Bursa and Ligament, Left**
	  See *S Foot Bursa and Ligament, Right*
	V **Lower Extremity Bursa and Ligament, Right**
	W **Lower Extremity Bursa and Ligament, Left**
		Ø Open
		3 Percutaneous
		4 Percutaneous
		   Endoscopic
			Z No Device	X Diagnostic
				Z No Qualifier

Non-OR	ØMB[Ø,1,2,3,4,5,6,7,8,B,C,D,F,G,L,M,N,P,Q,R,S,T][Ø,3,4]ZX
Non-OR	ØMB94ZX

Ø   **Medical and Surgical**
M   **Bursae and Ligaments**
C   **Extirpation**   Definition: Taking or cutting out solid matter from a body part

Explanation: The solid matter may be an abnormal byproduct of a biological function or a foreign body; it may be imbedded in a body part or in the lumen of a tubular body part. The solid matter may or may not have been previously broken into pieces.

Body Part Character 4		Approach Character 5	Device Character 6	Qualifier Character 7
Ø **Head and Neck Bursa and Ligament** Alar ligament of axis Cervical interspinous ligament Cervical intertransverse ligament Cervical ligamentum flavum Interspinous ligament, cervical Intertransverse ligament, cervical Lateral temporomandibular ligament Ligamentum flavum, cervical Sphenomandibular ligament Stylomandibular ligament Transverse ligament of atlas **1** **Shoulder Bursa and Ligament, Right** Acromioclavicular ligament Coracoacromial ligament Coracoclavicular ligament Coracohumeral ligament Costoclavicular ligament Glenohumeral ligament Interclavicular ligament Sternoclavicular ligament Subacromial bursa Transverse humeral ligament Transverse scapular ligament **2** **Shoulder Bursa and Ligament, Left** *See 1 Shoulder Bursa and Ligament, Right* **3** **Elbow Bursa and Ligament, Right** Annular ligament Olecranon bursa Radial collateral ligament Ulnar collateral ligament **4** **Elbow Bursa and Ligament, Left** *See 3 Elbow Bursa and Ligament, Right* **5** **Wrist Bursa and Ligament, Right** Palmar ulnocarpal ligament Radial collateral carpal ligament Radiocarpal ligament Radioulnar ligament Scapholunate ligament Ulnar collateral carpal ligament **6** **Wrist Bursa and Ligament, Left** *See 5 Wrist Bursa and Ligament, Right* **7** **Hand Bursa and Ligament, Right** Carpometacarpal ligament Intercarpal ligament Interphalangeal ligament Lunotriquetral ligament Metacarpal ligament Metacarpophalangeal ligament Pisohamate ligament Pisometacarpal ligament Scaphotrapezium ligament **8** **Hand Bursa and Ligament, Left** *See 7 Hand Bursa and Ligament, Right* **9** **Upper Extremity Bursa and Ligament, Right** **B** **Upper Extremity Bursa and Ligament, Left** **C** **Upper Spine Bursa and Ligament** Interspinous ligament, thoracic Intertransverse ligament, thoracic Ligamentum flavum, thoracic Supraspinous ligament	**D** **Lower Spine Bursa and Ligament** Iliolumbar ligament Interspinous ligament, lumbar Intertransverse ligament, lumbar Ligamentum flavum, lumbar Sacrococcygeal ligament Sacroiliac ligament Sacrospinous ligament Sacrotuberous ligament Supraspinous ligament **F** **Sternum Bursa and Ligament** Costoxiphoid ligament Sternocostal ligament **G** **Rib(s) Bursa and Ligament** Costotransverse ligament **H** **Abdomen Bursa and Ligament, Right** **J** **Abdomen Bursa and Ligament, Left** **K** **Perineum Bursa and Ligament** **L** **Hip Bursa and Ligament, Right** Iliofemoral ligament Ischiofemoral ligament Pubofemoral ligament Transverse acetabular ligament Trochanteric bursa **M** **Hip Bursa and Ligament, Left** *See L Hip Bursa and Ligament, Right* **N** **Knee Bursa and Ligament, Right** Anterior cruciate ligament (ACL) Lateral collateral ligament (LCL) Ligament of head of fibula Medial collateral ligament (MCL) Patellar ligament Popliteal ligament Posterior cruciate ligament (PCL) Prepatellar bursa **P** **Knee Bursa and Ligament, Left** *See N Knee Bursa and Ligament, Right* **Q** **Ankle Bursa and Ligament, Right** Calcaneofibular ligament Deltoid ligament Ligament of the lateral malleolus Talofibular ligament **R** **Ankle Bursa and Ligament, Left** *See Q Ankle Bursa and Ligament, Right* **S** **Foot Bursa and Ligament, Right** Calcaneocuboid ligament Cuneonavicular ligament Intercuneiform ligament Interphalangeal ligament Metatarsal ligament Metatarsophalangeal ligament Subtalar ligament Talocalcaneal ligament Talocalcaneonavicular ligament Tarsometatarsal ligament **T** **Foot Bursa and Ligament, Left** *See S Foot Bursa and Ligament, Right* **V** **Lower Extremity Bursa and Ligament, Right** **W** **Lower Extremity Bursa and Ligament, Left**	**Ø** Open **3** Percutaneous **4** Percutaneous Endoscopic	**Z** No Device	**Z** No Qualifier

NC Noncovered Procedure   **LC** Limited Coverage   **QA** Questionable OB Admit   **NT** New Tech Add-on   ⊞ Combination Member   ♂ Male   ♀ Female

ICD-10-PCS 2022   **507**

Ø Medical and Surgical
M Bursae and Ligaments
D Extraction Definition: Pulling or stripping out or off all or a portion of a body part by the use of force
Explanation: The qualifier DIAGNOSTIC is used to identify extraction procedures that are biopsies

Body Part Character 4		Approach Character 5	Device Character 6	Qualifier Character 7
Ø Head and Neck Bursa and Ligament Alar ligament of axis Cervical interspinous ligament Cervical intertransverse ligament Cervical ligamentum flavum Interspinous ligament, cervical Intertransverse ligament, cervical Lateral temporomandibular ligament Ligamentum flavum, cervical Sphenomandibular ligament Stylomandibular ligament Transverse ligament of atlas **1 Shoulder Bursa and Ligament, Right** Acromioclavicular ligament Coracoacromial ligament Coracoclavicular ligament Coracohumeral ligament Costoclavicular ligament Glenohumeral ligament Interclavicular ligament Sternoclavicular ligament Subacromial bursa Transverse humeral ligament Transverse scapular ligament **2 Shoulder Bursa and Ligament, Left** *See 1 Shoulder Bursa and Ligament, Right* **3 Elbow Bursa and Ligament, Right** Annular ligament Olecranon bursa Radial collateral ligament Ulnar collateral ligament **4 Elbow Bursa and Ligament, Left** *See 3 Elbow Bursa and Ligament, Right* **5 Wrist Bursa and Ligament, Right** Palmar ulnocarpal ligament Radial collateral carpal ligament Radiocarpal ligament Radioulnar ligament Scapholunate ligament Ulnar collateral carpal ligament **6 Wrist Bursa and Ligament, Left** *See 5 Wrist Bursa and Ligament, Right* **7 Hand Bursa and Ligament, Right** Carpometacarpal ligament Intercarpal ligament Interphalangeal ligament Lunotriquetral ligament Metacarpal ligament Metacarpophalangeal ligament Pisohamate ligament Pisometacarpal ligament Scaphotrapezium ligament **8 Hand Bursa and Ligament, Left** *See 7 Hand Bursa and Ligament, Right* **9 Upper Extremity Bursa and Ligament, Right** **B Upper Extremity Bursa and Ligament, Left** **C Upper Spine Bursa and Ligament** Interspinous ligament, thoracic Intertransverse ligament, thoracic Ligamentum flavum, thoracic Supraspinous ligament	**D Lower Spine Bursa and Ligament** Iliolumbar ligament Interspinous ligament, lumbar Intertransverse ligament, lumbar Ligamentum flavum, lumbar Sacrococcygeal ligament Sacroiliac ligament Sacrospinous ligament Sacrotuberous ligament Supraspinous ligament **F Sternum Bursa and Ligament** Costoxiphoid ligament Sternocostal ligament **G Rib(s) Bursa and Ligament** Costotransverse ligament **H Abdomen Bursa and Ligament, Right** **J Abdomen Bursa and Ligament, Left** **K Perineum Bursa and Ligament** **L Hip Bursa and Ligament, Right** Iliofemoral ligament Ischiofemoral ligament Pubofemoral ligament Transverse acetabular ligament Trochanteric bursa **M Hip Bursa and Ligament, Left** *See L Hip Bursa and Ligament, Right* **N Knee Bursa and Ligament, Right** Anterior cruciate ligament (ACL) Lateral collateral ligament (LCL) Ligament of head of fibula Medial collateral ligament (MCL) Patellar ligament Popliteal ligament Posterior cruciate ligament (PCL) Prepatellar bursa **P Knee Bursa and Ligament, Left** *See N Knee Bursa and Ligament, Right* **Q Ankle Bursa and Ligament, Right** Calcaneofibular ligament Deltoid ligament Ligament of the lateral malleolus Talofibular ligament **R Ankle Bursa and Ligament, Left** *See Q Ankle Bursa and Ligament, Right* **S Foot Bursa and Ligament, Right** Calcaneocuboid ligament Cuneonavicular ligament Intercuneiform ligament Interphalangeal ligament Metatarsal ligament Metatarsophalangeal ligament Subtalar ligament Talocalcaneal ligament Talocalcaneonavicular ligament Tarsometatarsal ligament **T Foot Bursa and Ligament, Left** *See S Foot Bursa and Ligament, Right* **V Lower Extremity Bursa and Ligament, Right** **W Lower Extremity Bursa and Ligament, Left**	**Ø Open** **3 Percutaneous** **4 Percutaneous Endoscopic**	**Z No Device**	**Z No Qualifier**

Non-OR Procedure   DRG Non-OR Procedure   Valid OR Procedure   HAC Associated Procedure   Combination Only   New/Revised GREEN

Ø   Medical and Surgical
M   Bursae and Ligaments
H   Insertion   Definition: Putting in a nonbiological appliance that monitors, assists, performs, or prevents a physiological function but does not physically take the place of a body part

                         Explanation: None

Body Part Character 4	Approach Character 5	Device Character 6	Qualifier Character 7
X Upper Bursa and Ligament **Y** Lower Bursa and Ligament	**Ø** Open **3** Percutaneous **4** Percutaneous Endoscopic	**Y** Other Device	**Z** No Qualifier

Non-OR   ØMH[X,Y][3,4]YZ

Ø   Medical and Surgical
M   Bursae and Ligaments
J   Inspection   Definition: Visually and/or manually exploring a body part

                         Explanation: Visual exploration may be performed with or without optical instrumentation. Manual exploration may be performed directly or through intervening body layers.

Body Part Character 4	Approach Character 5	Device Character 6	Qualifier Character 7
X Upper Bursa and Ligament **Y** Lower Bursa and Ligament	**Ø** Open **3** Percutaneous **4** Percutaneous Endoscopic **X** External	**Z** No Device	**Z** No Qualifier

Non-OR   ØMJ[X,Y][3,X]ZZ

Ø Medical and Surgical
M Bursae and Ligaments
M Reattachment   Definition: Putting back in or on all or a portion of a separated body part to its normal location or other suitable location
                         Explanation: Vascular circulation and nervous pathways may or may not be reestablished

Body Part Character 4		Approach Character 5	Device Character 6	Qualifier Character 7
Ø Head and Neck Bursa and Ligament Alar ligament of axis Cervical interspinous ligament Cervical intertransverse ligament Cervical ligamentum flavum Interspinous ligament, cervical Intertransverse ligament, cervical Lateral temporomandibular ligament Ligamentum flavum, cervical Sphenomandibular ligament Stylomandibular ligament Transverse ligament of atlas **1 Shoulder Bursa and Ligament, Right** Acromioclavicular ligament Coracoacromial ligament Coracoclavicular ligament Coracohumeral ligament Costoclavicular ligament Glenohumeral ligament Interclavicular ligament Sternoclavicular ligament Subacromial bursa Transverse humeral ligament Transverse scapular ligament **2 Shoulder Bursa and Ligament, Left** *See 1 Shoulder Bursa and Ligament, Right* **3 Elbow Bursa and Ligament, Right** Annular ligament Olecranon bursa Radial collateral ligament Ulnar collateral ligament **4 Elbow Bursa and Ligament, Left** *See 3 Elbow Bursa and Ligament, Right* **5 Wrist Bursa and Ligament, Right** Palmar ulnocarpal ligament Radial collateral carpal ligament Radiocarpal ligament Radioulnar ligament Scapholunate ligament Ulnar collateral carpal ligament **6 Wrist Bursa and Ligament, Left** *See 5 Wrist Bursa and Ligament, Right* **7 Hand Bursa and Ligament, Right** Carpometacarpal ligament Intercarpal ligament Interphalangeal ligament Lunotriquetral ligament Metacarpal ligament Metacarpophalangeal ligament Pisohamate ligament Pisometacarpal ligament Scaphotrapezium ligament **8 Hand Bursa and Ligament, Left** *See 7 Hand Bursa and Ligament, Right* **9 Upper Extremity Bursa and Ligament, Right** **B Upper Extremity Bursa and Ligament, Left** **C Upper Spine Bursa and Ligament** Interspinous ligament, thoracic Intertransverse ligament, thoracic Ligamentum flavum, thoracic Supraspinous ligament	**D Lower Spine Bursa and Ligament** Iliolumbar ligament Interspinous ligament, lumbar Intertransverse ligament, lumbar Ligamentum flavum, lumbar Sacrococcygeal ligament Sacroiliac ligament Sacrospinous ligament Sacrotuberous ligament Supraspinous ligament **F Sternum Bursa and Ligament** Costoxiphoid ligament Sternocostal ligament **G Rib(s) Bursa and Ligament** Costotransverse ligament **H Abdomen Bursa and Ligament, Right** **J Abdomen Bursa and Ligament, Left** **K Perineum Bursa and Ligament** **L Hip Bursa and Ligament, Right** Iliofemoral ligament Ischiofemoral ligament Pubofemoral ligament Transverse acetabular ligament Trochanteric bursa **M Hip Bursa and Ligament, Left** *See L Hip Bursa and Ligament, Right* **N Knee Bursa and Ligament, Right** Anterior cruciate ligament (ACL) Lateral collateral ligament (LCL) Ligament of head of fibula Medial collateral ligament (MCL) Patellar ligament Popliteal ligament Posterior cruciate ligament (PCL) Prepatellar bursa **P Knee Bursa and Ligament, Left** *See N Knee Bursa and Ligament, Right* **Q Ankle Bursa and Ligament, Right** Calcaneofibular ligament Deltoid ligament Ligament of the lateral malleolus Talofibular ligament **R Ankle Bursa and Ligament, Left** *See Q Ankle Bursa and Ligament, Right* **S Foot Bursa and Ligament, Right** Calcaneocuboid ligament Cuneonavicular ligament Intercuneiform ligament Interphalangeal ligament Metatarsal ligament Metatarsophalangeal ligament Subtalar ligament Talocalcaneal ligament Talocalcaneonavicular ligament Tarsometatarsal ligament **T Foot Bursa and Ligament, Left** *See S Foot Bursa and Ligament, Right* **V Lower Extremity Bursa and Ligament, Right** **W Lower Extremity Bursa and Ligament, Left**	**Ø Open** **4 Percutaneous Endoscopic**	**Z No Device**	**Z No Qualifier**

Ø　**Medical and Surgical**
M　**Bursae and Ligaments**
N　**Release**　　Definition: Freeing a body part from an abnormal physical constraint by cutting or by the use of force
　　　　　　　　Explanation: Some of the restraining tissue may be taken out but none of the body part is taken out

Body Part Character 4		Approach Character 5	Device Character 6	Qualifier Character 7
Ø **Head and Neck Bursa and Ligament** Alar ligament of axis Cervical interspinous ligament Cervical intertransverse ligament Cervical ligamentum flavum Interspinous ligament, cervical Intertransverse ligament, cervical Lateral temporomandibular ligament Ligamentum flavum, cervical Sphenomandibular ligament Stylomandibular ligament Transverse ligament of atlas	D **Lower Spine Bursa and Ligament** Iliolumbar ligament Interspinous ligament, lumbar Intertransverse ligament, lumbar Ligamentum flavum, lumbar Sacrococcygeal ligament Sacroiliac ligament Sacrospinous ligament Sacrotuberous ligament Supraspinous ligament	Ø Open 3 Percutaneous 4 Percutaneous Endoscopic X External	Z No Device	Z No Qualifier
1 **Shoulder Bursa and Ligament, Right** Acromioclavicular ligament Coracoacromial ligament Coracoclavicular ligament Coracohumeral ligament Costoclavicular ligament Glenohumeral ligament Interclavicular ligament Sternoclavicular ligament Subacromial bursa Transverse humeral ligament Transverse scapular ligament	F **Sternum Bursa and Ligament** Costoxiphoid ligament Sternocostal ligament G **Rib(s) Bursa and Ligament** Costotransverse ligament H **Abdomen Bursa and Ligament, Right** J **Abdomen Bursa and Ligament, Left** K **Perineum Bursa and Ligament** L **Hip Bursa and Ligament, Right** Iliofemoral ligament Ischiofemoral ligament Pubofemoral ligament Transverse acetabular ligament Trochanteric bursa			
2 **Shoulder Bursa and Ligament, Left** *See 1 Shoulder Bursa and Ligament, Right*	M **Hip Bursa and Ligament, Left** *See L Hip Bursa and Ligament, Right*			
3 **Elbow Bursa and Ligament, Right** Annular ligament Olecranon bursa Radial collateral ligament Ulnar collateral ligament	N **Knee Bursa and Ligament, Right** Anterior cruciate ligament (ACL) Lateral collateral ligament (LCL) Ligament of head of fibula Medial collateral ligament (MCL) Patellar ligament Popliteal ligament Posterior cruciate ligament (PCL) Prepatellar bursa			
4 **Elbow Bursa and Ligament, Left** *See 3 Elbow Bursa and Ligament, Right*	P **Knee Bursa and Ligament, Left** *See N Knee Bursa and Ligament, Right*			
5 **Wrist Bursa and Ligament, Right** Palmar ulnocarpal ligament Radial collateral carpal ligament Radiocarpal ligament Radioulnar ligament Scapholunate ligament Ulnar collateral carpal ligament	Q **Ankle Bursa and Ligament, Right** Calcaneofibular ligament Deltoid ligament Ligament of the lateral malleolus Talofibular ligament			
6 **Wrist Bursa and Ligament, Left** *See 5 Wrist Bursa and Ligament, Right*	R **Ankle Bursa and Ligament, Left** *See Q Ankle Bursa and Ligament, Right*			
7 **Hand Bursa and Ligament, Right** Carpometacarpal ligament Intercarpal ligament Interphalangeal ligament Lunotriquetral ligament Metacarpal ligament Metacarpophalangeal ligament Pisohamate ligament Pisometacarpal ligament Scaphotrapezium ligament	S **Foot Bursa and Ligament, Right** Calcaneocuboid ligament Cuneonavicular ligament Intercuneiform ligament Interphalangeal ligament Metatarsal ligament Metatarsophalangeal ligament Subtalar ligament Talocalcaneal ligament Talocalcaneonavicular ligament Tarsometatarsal ligament			
8 **Hand Bursa and Ligament, Left** *See 7 Hand Bursa and Ligament, Right*	T **Foot Bursa and Ligament, Left** *See S Foot Bursa and Ligament, Right*			
9 **Upper Extremity Bursa and Ligament, Right** B **Upper Extremity Bursa and Ligament, Left** C **Upper Spine Bursa and Ligament** Interspinous ligament, thoracic Intertransverse ligament, thoracic Ligamentum flavum, thoracic Supraspinous ligament	V **Lower Extremity Bursa and Ligament, Right** W **Lower Extremity Bursa and Ligament, Left**			

Non-OR　ØMN[Ø,1,2,3,4,5,6,7,8,9,B,C,D,F,G,H,J,K,L,M,N,P,Q,R,S,T,V,W]XZZ

🆖 Noncovered Procedure　　🆛 Limited Coverage　　🆀🅰 Questionable OB Admit　　🆕🆃 New Tech Add-on　　➕ Combination Member　　♂ Male　　♀ Female

ICD-10-PCS 2022　　　　　　　　　　　　　　　　　　　　　　　　　　　　　　　　　　　511

Bursae and Ligaments

Ø   **Medical and Surgical**
M   **Bursae and Ligaments**
P   **Removal**   Definition: Taking out or off a device from a body part

Explanation: If a device is taken out and a similar device put in without cutting or puncturing the skin or mucous membrane, the procedure is coded to the root operation CHANGE. Otherwise, the procedure for taking out a device is coded to the root operation REMOVAL.

Body Part Character 4	Approach Character 5	Device Character 6	Qualifier Character 7
X Upper Bursa and Ligament Y Lower Bursa and Ligament	Ø Open 3 Percutaneous 4 Percutaneous Endoscopic	Ø Drainage Device 7 Autologous Tissue Substitute J Synthetic Substitute K Nonautologous Tissue Substitute Y Other Device	Z No Qualifier
X Upper Bursa and Ligament Y Lower Bursa and Ligament	X External	Ø Drainage Device	Z No Qualifier

Non-OR   ØMP[X,Y]3ØZ
Non-OR   ØMP[X,Y][3,4]YZ
Non-OR   ØMP[X,Y]XØZ

Ø   **Medical and Surgical**
M   **Bursae and Ligaments**
Q   **Repair**   Definition: Restoring, to the extent possible, a body part to its normal anatomic structure and function

Explanation: Used only when the method to accomplish the repair is not one of the other root operations

Body Part Character 4		Approach Character 5	Device Character 6	Qualifier Character 7
Ø Head and Neck Bursa and Ligament Alar ligament of axis Cervical interspinous ligament Cervical intertransverse ligament Cervical ligamentum flavum Interspinous ligament, cervical Intertransverse ligament, cervical Lateral temporomandibular ligament Ligamentum flavum, cervical Sphenomandibular ligament Stylomandibular ligament Transverse ligament of atlas **1** Shoulder Bursa and Ligament, Right Acromioclavicular ligament Coracoacromial ligament Coracoclavicular ligament Coracohumeral ligament Costoclavicular ligament Glenohumeral ligament Interclavicular ligament Sternoclavicular ligament Subacromial bursa Transverse humeral ligament Transverse scapular ligament **2** Shoulder Bursa and Ligament, Left *See 1 Shoulder Bursa and Ligament, Right* **3** Elbow Bursa and Ligament, Right Annular ligament Olecranon bursa Radial collateral ligament Ulnar collateral ligament **4** Elbow Bursa and Ligament, Left *See 3 Elbow Bursa and Ligament, Right* **5** Wrist Bursa and Ligament, Right Palmar ulnocarpal ligament Radial collateral carpal ligament Radiocarpal ligament Radioulnar ligament Scapholunate ligament Ulnar collateral carpal ligament **6** Wrist Bursa and Ligament, Left *See 5 Wrist Bursa and Ligament, Right* **7** Hand Bursa and Ligament, Right Carpometacarpal ligament Intercarpal ligament Interphalangeal ligament Lunotriquetral ligament Metacarpal ligament Metacarpophalangeal ligament Pisohamate ligament Pisometacarpal ligament Scaphotrapezium ligament **8** Hand Bursa and Ligament, Left *See 7 Hand Bursa and Ligament, Right* **9** Upper Extremity Bursa and Ligament, Right **B** Upper Extremity Bursa and Ligament, Left **C** Upper Spine Bursa and Ligament Interspinous ligament, thoracic Intertransverse ligament, thoracic Ligamentum flavum, thoracic Supraspinous ligament	**D** Lower Spine Bursa and Ligament Iliolumbar ligament Interspinous ligament, lumbar Intertransverse ligament, lumbar Ligamentum flavum, lumbar Sacrococcygeal ligament Sacroiliac ligament Sacrospinous ligament Sacrotuberous ligament Supraspinous ligament **F** Sternum Bursa and Ligament Costoxiphoid ligament Sternocostal ligament **G** Rib(s) Bursa and Ligament Costotransverse ligament **H** Abdomen Bursa and Ligament, Right **J** Abdomen Bursa and Ligament, Left **K** Perineum Bursa and Ligament **L** Hip Bursa and Ligament, Right Iliofemoral ligament Ischiofemoral ligament Pubofemoral ligament Transverse acetabular ligament Trochanteric bursa **M** Hip Bursa and Ligament, Left *See L Hip Bursa and Ligament, Right* **N** Knee Bursa and Ligament, Right Anterior cruciate ligament (ACL) Lateral collateral ligament (LCL) Ligament of head of fibula Medial collateral ligament (MCL) Patellar ligament Popliteal ligament Posterior cruciate ligament (PCL) Prepatellar bursa **P** Knee Bursa and Ligament, Left *See N Knee Bursa and Ligament, Right* **Q** Ankle Bursa and Ligament, Right Calcaneofibular ligament Deltoid ligament Ligament of the lateral malleolus Talofibular ligament **R** Ankle Bursa and Ligament, Left *See Q Ankle Bursa and Ligament, Right* **S** Foot Bursa and Ligament, Right Calcaneocuboid ligament Cuneonavicular ligament Intercuneiform ligament Interphalangeal ligament Metatarsal ligament Metatarsophalangeal ligament Subtalar ligament Talocalcaneal ligament Talocalcaneonavicular ligament Tarsometatarsal ligament **T** Foot Bursa and Ligament, Left *See S Foot Bursa and Ligament, Right* **V** Lower Extremity Bursa and Ligament, Right **W** Lower Extremity Bursa and Ligament, Left	**Ø** Open **3** Percutaneous **4** Percutaneous Endoscopic	**Z** No Device	**Z** No Qualifier

NC Noncovered Procedure   **LC** Limited Coverage   **QA** Questionable OB Admit   **NT** New Tech Add-on   ⊞ Combination Member   ♂ Male   ♀ Female

ICD-10-PCS 2022   513

ØMQ–ØMQ

Bursae and Ligaments

Ø   **Medical and Surgical**
M   **Bursae and Ligaments**
R   **Replacement**   Definition: Putting in or on biological or synthetic material that physically takes the place and/or function of all or a portion of a body part
                         Explanation: The body part may have been taken out or replaced, or may be taken out, physically eradicated, or rendered nonfunctional during the REPLACEMENT procedure. A REMOVAL procedure is coded for taking out the device used in a previous replacement procedure.

Body Part Character 4		Approach Character 5	Device Character 6	Qualifier Character 7
Ø Head and Neck Bursa and Ligament Alar ligament of axis Cervical interspinous ligament Cervical intertransverse ligament Cervical ligamentum flavum Interspinous ligament, cervical Intertransverse ligament, cervical Lateral temporomandibular ligament Ligamentum flavum, cervical Sphenomandibular ligament Stylomandibular ligament Transverse ligament of atlas **1 Shoulder Bursa and Ligament, Right** Acromioclavicular ligament Coracoacromial ligament Coracoclavicular ligament Coracohumeral ligament Costoclavicular ligament Glenohumeral ligament Interclavicular ligament Sternoclavicular ligament Subacromial bursa Transverse humeral ligament Transverse scapular ligament **2 Shoulder Bursa and Ligament, Left** *See 1 Shoulder Bursa and Ligament, Right* **3 Elbow Bursa and Ligament, Right** Annular ligament Olecranon bursa Radial collateral ligament Ulnar collateral ligament **4 Elbow Bursa and Ligament, Left** *See 3 Elbow Bursa and Ligament, Right* **5 Wrist Bursa and Ligament, Right** Palmar ulnocarpal ligament Radial collateral carpal ligament Radiocarpal ligament Radioulnar ligament Scapholunate ligament Ulnar collateral carpal ligament **6 Wrist Bursa and Ligament, Left** *See 5 Wrist Bursa and Ligament, Right* **7 Hand Bursa and Ligament, Right** Carpometacarpal ligament Intercarpal ligament Interphalangeal ligament Lunotriquetral ligament Metacarpal ligament Metacarpophalangeal ligament Pisohamate ligament Pisometacarpal ligament Scaphotrapezium ligament **8 Hand Bursa and Ligament, Left** *See 7 Hand Bursa and Ligament, Right* **9 Upper Extremity Bursa and Ligament, Right** **B Upper Extremity Bursa and Ligament, Left** **C Upper Spine Bursa and Ligament** Interspinous ligament, thoracic Intertransverse ligament, thoracic Ligamentum flavum, thoracic Supraspinous ligament	**D Lower Spine Bursa and Ligament** Iliolumbar ligament Interspinous ligament, lumbar Intertransverse ligament, lumbar Ligamentum flavum, lumbar Sacrococcygeal ligament Sacroiliac ligament Sacrospinous ligament Sacrotuberous ligament Supraspinous ligament **F Sternum Bursa and Ligament** Costoxiphoid ligament Sternocostal ligament **G Rib(s) Bursa and Ligament** Costotransverse ligament **H Abdomen Bursa and Ligament, Right** **J Abdomen Bursa and Ligament, Left** **K Perineum Bursa and Ligament** **L Hip Bursa and Ligament, Right** Iliofemoral ligament Ischiofemoral ligament Pubofemoral ligament Transverse acetabular ligament Trochanteric bursa **M Hip Bursa and Ligament, Left** *See L Hip Bursa and Ligament, Right* **N Knee Bursa and Ligament, Right** Anterior cruciate ligament (ACL) Lateral collateral ligament (LCL) Ligament of head of fibula Medial collateral ligament (MCL) Patellar ligament Popliteal ligament Posterior cruciate ligament (PCL) Prepatellar bursa **P Knee Bursa and Ligament, Left** *See N Knee Bursa and Ligament, Right* **Q Ankle Bursa and Ligament, Right** Calcaneofibular ligament Deltoid ligament Ligament of the lateral malleolus Talofibular ligament **R Ankle Bursa and Ligament, Left** *See Q Ankle Bursa and Ligament, Right* **S Foot Bursa and Ligament, Right** Calcaneocuboid ligament Cuneonavicular ligament Intercuneiform ligament Interphalangeal ligament Metatarsal ligament Metatarsophalangeal ligament Subtalar ligament Talocalcaneal ligament Talocalcaneonavicular ligament Tarsometatarsal ligament **T Foot Bursa and Ligament, Left** *See S Foot Bursa and Ligament, Right* **V Lower Extremity Bursa and Ligament, Right** **W Lower Extremity Bursa and Ligament, Left**	**Ø Open** **4 Percutaneous Endoscopic**	**7 Autologous Tissue Substitute** **J Synthetic Substitute** **K Nonautologous Tissue Substitute**	**Z No Qualifier**

Ø   **Medical and Surgical**
M   **Bursae and Ligaments**
S   **Reposition**   Definition: Moving to its normal location, or other suitable location, all or a portion of a body part

Explanation: The body part is moved to a new location from an abnormal location, or from a normal location where it is not functioning correctly. The body part may or may not be cut out or off to be moved to the new location.

Body Part Character 4		Approach Character 5	Device Character 6	Qualifier Character 7
Ø Head and Neck Bursa and Ligament Alar ligament of axis Cervical interspinous ligament Cervical intertransverse ligament Cervical ligamentum flavum Interspinous ligament, cervical Intertransverse ligament, cervical Lateral temporomandibular ligament Ligamentum flavum, cervical Sphenomandibular ligament Stylomandibular ligament Transverse ligament of atlas **1 Shoulder Bursa and Ligament, Right** Acromioclavicular ligament Coracoacromial ligament Coracoclavicular ligament Coracohumeral ligament Costoclavicular ligament Glenohumeral ligament Interclavicular ligament Sternoclavicular ligament Subacromial bursa Transverse humeral ligament Transverse scapular ligament **2 Shoulder Bursa and Ligament, Left** *See 1 Shoulder Bursa and Ligament, Right* **3 Elbow Bursa and Ligament, Right** Annular ligament Olecranon bursa Radial collateral ligament Ulnar collateral ligament **4 Elbow Bursa and Ligament, Left** *See 3 Elbow Bursa and Ligament, Right* **5 Wrist Bursa and Ligament, Right** Palmar ulnocarpal ligament Radial collateral carpal ligament Radiocarpal ligament Radioulnar ligament Scapholunate ligament Ulnar collateral carpal ligament **6 Wrist Bursa and Ligament, Left** *See 5 Wrist Bursa and Ligament, Right* **7 Hand Bursa and Ligament, Right** Carpometacarpal ligament Intercarpal ligament Interphalangeal ligament Lunotriquetral ligament Metacarpal ligament Metacarpophalangeal ligament Pisohamate ligament Pisometacarpal ligament Scaphotrapezium ligament **8 Hand Bursa and Ligament, Left** *See 7 Hand Bursa and Ligament, Right* **9 Upper Extremity Bursa and Ligament, Right** **B Upper Extremity Bursa and Ligament, Left** **C Upper Spine Bursa and Ligament** Interspinous ligament, thoracic Intertransverse ligament, thoracic Ligamentum flavum, thoracic Supraspinous ligament	**D Lower Spine Bursa and Ligament** Iliolumbar ligament Interspinous ligament, lumbar Intertransverse ligament, lumbar Ligamentum flavum, lumbar Sacrococcygeal ligament Sacroiliac ligament Sacrospinous ligament Sacrotuberous ligament Supraspinous ligament **F Sternum Bursa and Ligament** Costoxiphoid ligament Sternocostal ligament **G Rib(s) Bursa and Ligament** Costotransverse ligament **H Abdomen Bursa and Ligament, Right** **J Abdomen Bursa and Ligament, Left** **K Perineum Bursa and Ligament** **L Hip Bursa and Ligament, Right** Iliofemoral ligament Ischiofemoral ligament Pubofemoral ligament Transverse acetabular ligament Trochanteric bursa **M Hip Bursa and Ligament, Left** *See L Hip Bursa and Ligament, Right* **N Knee Bursa and Ligament, Right** Anterior cruciate ligament (ACL) Lateral collateral ligament (LCL) Ligament of head of fibula Medial collateral ligament (MCL) Patellar ligament Popliteal ligament Posterior cruciate ligament (PCL) Prepatellar bursa **P Knee Bursa and Ligament, Left** *See N Knee Bursa and Ligament, Right* **Q Ankle Bursa and Ligament, Right** Calcaneofibular ligament Deltoid ligament Ligament of the lateral malleolus Talofibular ligament **R Ankle Bursa and Ligament, Left** *See Q Ankle Bursa and Ligament, Right* **S Foot Bursa and Ligament, Right** Calcaneocuboid ligament Cuneonavicular ligament Intercuneiform ligament Interphalangeal ligament Metatarsal ligament Metatarsophalangeal ligament Subtalar ligament Talocalcaneal ligament Talocalcaneonavicular ligament Tarsometatarsal ligament **T Foot Bursa and Ligament, Left** *See S Foot Bursa and Ligament, Right* **V Lower Extremity Bursa and Ligament, Right** **W Lower Extremity Bursa and Ligament, Left**	**Ø** Open **4** Percutaneous Endoscopic	**Z** No Device	**Z** No Qualifier

Ø Medical and Surgical
M Bursae and Ligaments
T Resection   Definition: Cutting out or off, without replacement, all of a body part
           Explanation: None

Body Part Character 4		Approach Character 5	Device Character 6	Qualifier Character 7

Ø Head and Neck Bursa and Ligament
  Alar ligament of axis
  Cervical interspinous ligament
  Cervical intertransverse ligament
  Cervical ligamentum flavum
  Interspinous ligament, cervical
  Intertransverse ligament, cervical
  Lateral temporomandibular
    ligament
  Ligamentum flavum, cervical
  Sphenomandibular ligament
  Stylomandibular ligament
  Transverse ligament of atlas
1 Shoulder Bursa and Ligament, Right
  Acromioclavicular ligament
  Coracoacromial ligament
  Coracoclavicular ligament
  Coracohumeral ligament
  Costoclavicular ligament
  Glenohumeral ligament
  Interclavicular ligament
  Sternoclavicular ligament
  Subacromial bursa
  Transverse humeral ligament
  Transverse scapular ligament
2 Shoulder Bursa and Ligament, Left
  See 1 Shoulder Bursa and Ligament, Right
3 Elbow Bursa and Ligament, Right
  Annular ligament
  Olecranon bursa
  Radial collateral ligament
  Ulnar collateral ligament
4 Elbow Bursa and Ligament, Left
  See 3 Elbow Bursa and Ligament, Right
5 Wrist Bursa and Ligament, Right
  Palmar ulnocarpal ligament
  Radial collateral carpal ligament
  Radiocarpal ligament
  Radioulnar ligament
  Scapholunate ligament
  Ulnar collateral carpal ligament
6 Wrist Bursa and Ligament, Left
  See 5 Wrist Bursa and Ligament, Right
7 Hand Bursa and Ligament, Right
  Carpometacarpal ligament
  Intercarpal ligament
  Interphalangeal ligament
  Lunotriquetral ligament
  Metacarpal ligament
  Metacarpophalangeal ligament
  Pisohamate ligament
  Pisometacarpal ligament
  Scaphotrapezium ligament
8 Hand Bursa and Ligament, Left
  See 7 Hand Bursa and Ligament, Right
9 Upper Extremity Bursa and Ligament, Right
B Upper Extremity Bursa and Ligament, Left
C Upper Spine Bursa and Ligament
  Interspinous ligament, thoracic
  Intertransverse ligament, thoracic
  Ligamentum flavum, thoracic
  Supraspinous ligament
	D Lower Spine Bursa and Ligament
	  Iliolumbar ligament
	  Interspinous ligament, lumbar
	  Intertransverse ligament, lumbar
	  Ligamentum flavum, lumbar
	  Sacrococcygeal ligament
	  Sacroiliac ligament
	  Sacrospinous ligament
	  Sacrotuberous ligament
	  Supraspinous ligament
	F Sternum Bursa and Ligament
	  Costoxiphoid ligament
	  Sternocostal ligament
	G Rib(s) Bursa and Ligament
	  Costotransverse ligament
	H Abdomen Bursa and Ligament, Right
	J Abdomen Bursa and Ligament, Left
	K Perineum Bursa and Ligament
	L Hip Bursa and Ligament, Right
	  Iliofemoral ligament
	  Ischiofemoral ligament
	  Pubofemoral ligament
	  Transverse acetabular ligament
	  Trochanteric bursa
	M Hip Bursa and Ligament, Left
	  See L Hip Bursa and Ligament, Right
	N Knee Bursa and Ligament, Right
	  Anterior cruciate ligament (ACL)
	  Lateral collateral ligament (LCL)
	  Ligament of head of fibula
	  Medial collateral ligament (MCL)
	  Patellar ligament
	  Popliteal ligament
	  Posterior cruciate ligament (PCL)
	  Prepatellar bursa
	P Knee Bursa and Ligament, Left
	  See N Knee Bursa and Ligament, Right
	Q Ankle Bursa and Ligament, Right
	  Calcaneofibular ligament
	  Deltoid ligament
	  Ligament of the lateral malleolus
	  Talofibular ligament
	R Ankle Bursa and Ligament, Left
	  See Q Ankle Bursa and Ligament, Right
	S Foot Bursa and Ligament, Right
	  Calcaneocuboid ligament
	  Cuneonavicular ligament
	  Intercuneiform ligament
	  Interphalangeal ligament
	  Metatarsal ligament
	  Metatarsophalangeal ligament
	  Subtalar ligament
	  Talocalcaneal ligament
	  Talocalcaneonavicular ligament
	  Tarsometatarsal ligament
	T Foot Bursa and Ligament, Left
	  See S Foot Bursa and Ligament, Right
	V Lower Extremity Bursa and Ligament, Right
	W Lower Extremity Bursa and Ligament, Left
		Ø Open
		4 Percutaneous Endoscopic
			Z No Device	**Z No Qualifier**

Ø   **Medical and Surgical**
M   **Bursae and Ligaments**
U   **Supplement**   Definition: Putting in or on biological or synthetic material that physically reinforces and/or augments the function of a portion of a body part
                      Explanation: The biological material is non-living, or is living and from the same individual. The body part may have been previously replaced, and the SUPPLEMENT procedure is performed to physically reinforce and/or augment the function of the replaced body part.

Body Part Character 4		Approach Character 5	Device Character 6	Qualifier Character 7
Ø **Head and Neck Bursa and Ligament** Alar ligament of axis Cervical interspinous ligament Cervical intertransverse ligament Cervical ligamentum flavum Interspinous ligament, cervical Intertransverse ligament, cervical Lateral temporomandibular ligament Ligamentum flavum, cervical Sphenomandibular ligament Stylomandibular ligament Transverse ligament of atlas **1** **Shoulder Bursa and Ligament, Right** Acromioclavicular ligament Coracoacromial ligament Coracoclavicular ligament Coracohumeral ligament Costoclavicular ligament Glenohumeral ligament Interclavicular ligament Sternoclavicular ligament Subacromial bursa Transverse humeral ligament Transverse scapular ligament **2** **Shoulder Bursa and Ligament, Left** *See 1 Shoulder Bursa and Ligament, Right* **3** **Elbow Bursa and Ligament, Right** Annular ligament Olecranon bursa Radial collateral ligament Ulnar collateral ligament **4** **Elbow Bursa and Ligament, Left** *See 3 Elbow Bursa and Ligament, Right* **5** **Wrist Bursa and Ligament, Right** Palmar ulnocarpal ligament Radial collateral carpal ligament Radiocarpal ligament Radioulnar ligament Scapholunate ligament Ulnar collateral carpal ligament **6** **Wrist Bursa and Ligament, Left** *See 5 Wrist Bursa and Ligament, Right* **7** **Hand Bursa and Ligament, Right** Carpometacarpal ligament Intercarpal ligament Interphalangeal ligament Lunotriquetral ligament Metacarpal ligament Metacarpophalangeal ligament Pisohamate ligament Pisometacarpal ligament Scaphotrapezium ligament **8** **Hand Bursa and Ligament, Left** *See 7 Hand Bursa and Ligament, Right* **9** **Upper Extremity Bursa and Ligament, Right** **B** **Upper Extremity Bursa and Ligament, Left** **C** **Upper Spine Bursa and Ligament** Interspinous ligament, thoracic Intertransverse ligament, thoracic Ligamentum flavum, thoracic Supraspinous ligament	**D** **Lower Spine Bursa and Ligament** Iliolumbar ligament Interspinous ligament, lumbar Intertransverse ligament, lumbar Ligamentum flavum, lumbar Sacrococcygeal ligament Sacroiliac ligament Sacrospinous ligament Sacrotuberous ligament Supraspinous ligament **F** **Sternum Bursa and Ligament** Costoxiphoid ligament Sternocostal ligament **G** **Rib(s) Bursa and Ligament** Costotransverse ligament **H** **Abdomen Bursa and Ligament, Right** **J** **Abdomen Bursa and Ligament, Left** **K** **Perineum Bursa and Ligament** **L** **Hip Bursa and Ligament, Right** Iliofemoral ligament Ischiofemoral ligament Pubofemoral ligament Transverse acetabular ligament Trochanteric bursa **M** **Hip Bursa and Ligament, Left** *See L Hip Bursa and Ligament, Right* **N** **Knee Bursa and Ligament, Right** Anterior cruciate ligament (ACL) Lateral collateral ligament (LCL) Ligament of head of fibula Medial collateral ligament (MCL) Patellar ligament Popliteal ligament Posterior cruciate ligament (PCL) Prepatellar bursa **P** **Knee Bursa and Ligament, Left** *See N Knee Bursa and Ligament, Right* **Q** **Ankle Bursa and Ligament, Right** Calcaneofibular ligament Deltoid ligament Ligament of the lateral malleolus Talofibular ligament **R** **Ankle Bursa and Ligament, Left** *See Q Ankle Bursa and Ligament, Right* **S** **Foot Bursa and Ligament, Right** Calcaneocuboid ligament Cuneonavicular ligament Intercuneiform ligament Interphalangeal ligament Metatarsal ligament Metatarsophalangeal ligament Subtalar ligament Talocalcaneal ligament Talocalcaneonavicular ligament Tarsometatarsal ligament **T** **Foot Bursa and Ligament, Left** *See S Foot Bursa and Ligament, Right* **V** **Lower Extremity Bursa and Ligament, Right** **W** **Lower Extremity Bursa and Ligament, Left**	**Ø** Open **4** Percutaneous Endoscopic	**7** Autologous Tissue Substitute **J** Synthetic Substitute **K** Nonautologous Tissue Substitute	**Z** No Qualifier

Ø Medical and Surgical
M Bursae and Ligaments
W Revision — Definition: Correcting, to the extent possible, a portion of a malfunctioning device or the position of a displaced device

Explanation: Revision can include correcting a malfunctioning or displaced device by taking out or putting in components of the device such as a screw or pin

Body Part Character 4	Approach Character 5	Device Character 6	Qualifier Character 7
X Upper Bursa and Ligament **Y** Lower Bursa and Ligament	**Ø** Open **3** Percutaneous **4** Percutaneous Endoscopic	**Ø** Drainage Device **7** Autologous Tissue Substitute **J** Synthetic Substitute **K** Nonautologous Tissue Substitute **Y** Other Device	**Z** No Qualifier
X Upper Bursa and Ligament **Y** Lower Bursa and Ligament	**X** External	**Ø** Drainage Device **7** Autologous Tissue Substitute **J** Synthetic Substitute **K** Nonautologous Tissue Substitute	**Z** No Qualifier

Non-OR ØMW[X,Y][3,4]YZ
Non-OR ØMW[X,Y]X[Ø,7,J,K]Z

Ø Medical and Surgical
M Bursae and Ligaments
X Transfer — Definition: Moving, without taking out, all or a portion of a body part to another location to take over the function of all or a portion of a body part
Explanation: The body part transferred remains connected to its vascular and nervous supply

Body Part — Character 4	Approach — Character 5	Device — Character 6	Qualifier — Character 7
Ø Head and Neck Bursa and Ligament Alar ligament of axis Cervical interspinous ligament Cervical intertransverse ligament Cervical ligamentum flavum Interspinous ligament, cervical Intertransverse ligament, cervical Lateral temporomandibular ligament Ligamentum flavum, cervical Sphenomandibular ligament Stylomandibular ligament Transverse ligament of atlas **1** Shoulder Bursa and Ligament, Right Acromioclavicular ligament Coracoacromial ligament Coracoclavicular ligament Coracohumeral ligament Costoclavicular ligament Glenohumeral ligament Interclavicular ligament Sternoclavicular ligament Subacromial bursa Transverse humeral ligament Transverse scapular ligament **2** Shoulder Bursa and Ligament, Left *See 1 Shoulder Bursa and Ligament, Right* **3** Elbow Bursa and Ligament, Right Annular ligament Olecranon bursa Radial collateral ligament Ulnar collateral ligament **4** Elbow Bursa and Ligament, Left *See 3 Elbow Bursa and Ligament, Right* **5** Wrist Bursa and Ligament, Right Palmar ulnocarpal ligament Radial collateral carpal ligament Radiocarpal ligament Radioulnar ligament Scapholunate ligament Ulnar collateral carpal ligament **6** Wrist Bursa and Ligament, Left *See 5 Wrist Bursa and Ligament, Right* **7** Hand Bursa and Ligament, Right Carpometacarpal ligament Intercarpal ligament Interphalangeal ligament Lunotriquetral ligament Metacarpal ligament Metacarpophalangeal ligament Pisohamate ligament Pisometacarpal ligament Scaphotrapezium ligament **8** Hand Bursa and Ligament, Left *See 7 Hand Bursa and Ligament, Right* **9** Upper Extremity Bursa and Ligament, Right **B** Upper Extremity Bursa and Ligament, Left **C** Upper Spine Bursa and Ligament Interspinous ligament, thoracic Intertransverse ligament, thoracic Ligamentum flavum, thoracic Supraspinous ligament **D** Lower Spine Bursa and Ligament Iliolumbar ligament Interspinous ligament, lumbar Intertransverse ligament, lumbar Ligamentum flavum, lumbar Sacrococcygeal ligament Sacroiliac ligament Sacrospinous ligament Sacrotuberous ligament Supraspinous ligament **F** Sternum Bursa and Ligament Costoxiphoid ligament Sternocostal ligament **G** Rib(s) Bursa and Ligament Costotransverse ligament **H** Abdomen Bursa and Ligament, Right **J** Abdomen Bursa and Ligament, Left **K** Perineum Bursa and Ligament **L** Hip Bursa and Ligament, Right Iliofemoral ligament Ischiofemoral ligament Pubofemoral ligament Transverse acetabular ligament Trochanteric bursa **M** Hip Bursa and Ligament, Left *See L Hip Bursa and Ligament, Right* **N** Knee Bursa and Ligament, Right Anterior cruciate ligament (ACL) Lateral collateral ligament (LCL) Ligament of head of fibula Medial collateral ligament (MCL) Patellar ligament Popliteal ligament Posterior cruciate ligament (PCL) Prepatellar bursa **P** Knee Bursa and Ligament, Left *See N Knee Bursa and Ligament, Right* **Q** Ankle Bursa and Ligament, Right Calcaneofibular ligament Deltoid ligament Ligament of the lateral malleolus Talofibular ligament **R** Ankle Bursa and Ligament, Left *See Q Ankle Bursa and Ligament, Right* **S** Foot Bursa and Ligament, Right Calcaneocuboid ligament Cuneonavicular ligament Intercuneiform ligament Interphalangeal ligament Metatarsal ligament Metatarsophalangeal ligament Subtalar ligament Talocalcaneal ligament Talocalcaneonavicular ligament Tarsometatarsal ligament **T** Foot Bursa and Ligament, Left *See S Foot Bursa and Ligament, Right* **V** Lower Extremity Bursa and Ligament, Right **W** Lower Extremity Bursa and Ligament, Left	**Ø** Open **4** Percutaneous Endoscopic	**Z** No Device	**Z** No Qualifier

NC Noncovered Procedure   **LC** Limited Coverage   **QA** Questionable OB Admit   **NT** New Tech Add-on   ⊞ Combination Member   ♂ Male   ♀ Female

ICD-10-PCS 2022

519

ØMX–ØMX

Head and Facial Bones ØN2–ØNW

Character Meanings

This Character Meaning table is provided as a guide to assist the user in the identification of character members that may be found in this section of code tables. It **SHOULD NOT** be used to build a PCS code.

Operation–Character 3	Body Part–Character 4	Approach–Character 5	Device–Character 6	Qualifier–Character 7
2 Change	Ø Skull	Ø Open	Ø Drainage Device	X Diagnostic
5 Destruction	1 Frontal Bone	3 Percutaneous	3 Infusion Device	Z No Qualifier
8 Division	3 Parietal Bone, Right	4 Percutaneous Endoscopic	4 Internal Fixation Device	
9 Drainage	4 Parietal Bone, Left	X External	5 External Fixation Device	
B Excision	5 Temporal Bone, Right		7 Autologous Tissue Substitute	
C Extirpation	6 Temporal Bone, Left		J Synthetic Substitute	
D Extraction	7 Occipital Bone		K Nonautologous Tissue Substitute	
H Insertion	B Nasal Bone		M Bone Growth Stimulator	
J Inspection	C Sphenoid Bone		N Neurostimulator Generator	
N Release	F Ethmoid Bone, Right		S Hearing Device	
P Removal	G Ethmoid Bone, Left		Y Other Device	
Q Repair	H Lacrimal Bone, Right		Z No Device	
R Replacement	J Lacrimal Bone, Left			
S Reposition	K Palatine Bone, Right			
T Resection	L Palatine Bone, Left			
U Supplement	M Zygomatic Bone, Right			
W Revision	N Zygomatic Bone, Left			
	P Orbit, Right			
	Q Orbit, Left			
	R Maxilla			
	T Mandible, Right			
	V Mandible, Left			
	W Facial Bone			
	X Hyoid Bone			

AHA Coding Clinic for table ØNB
2021, 1Q, 21   Maxillectomy with reconstruction of maxilla
2017, 1Q, 20   Preparatory nasal adhesion repair before definitive cleft palate repair
2015, 3Q, 3-8   Excisional and nonexcisional debridement
2015, 2Q, 12   Orbital exenteration

AHA Coding Clinic for table ØND
2017, 4Q, 41   Extraction procedures

AHA Coding Clinic for table ØNH
2015, 3Q, 13   Nonexcisional debridement of cranial wound with removal and replacement of hardware

AHA Coding Clinic for table ØNP
2015, 3Q, 13   Nonexcisional debridement of cranial wound with removal and replacement of hardware

AHA Coding Clinic for table ØNQ
2016, 3Q, 29   Closure of bilateral alveolar clefts

AHA Coding Clinic for table ØNR
2021, 1Q, 21   Maxillectomy with reconstruction of maxilla
2017, 3Q, 17   Resection of schwannoma and placement of DuraGen and Lorenz cranial plating system
2017, 3Q, 22   Replacement of native skull bone flap
2017, 1Q, 23   Reconstruction of mandible using titanium and bone
2014, 3Q, 7   Hemi-cranioplasty for repair of cranial defect

AHA Coding Clinic for table ØNS
2017, 3Q, 22   Replacement of native skull bone flap
2017, 1Q, 20   Preparatory nasal adhesion repair before definitive cleft palate repair
2016, 2Q, 30   Clipping (occlusion) of cerebral artery, decompressive craniectomy and storage of bone flap in abdominal wall
2015, 3Q, 17   Craniosynostosis with cranial vault reconstruction
2015, 3Q, 27   Moyamoya disease and hemispheric pial synagiosis with craniotomy
2014, 3Q, 23   Le Fort I osteotomy
2013, 3Q, 24   Distraction osteogenesis
2013, 3Q, 25   Fracture of frontal bone with repair and coagulation for hemostasis

AHA Coding Clinic for table ØNU
2016, 3Q, 29   Closure of bilateral alveolar clefts
2013, 3Q, 24   Distraction osteogenesis

Head and Facial Bones

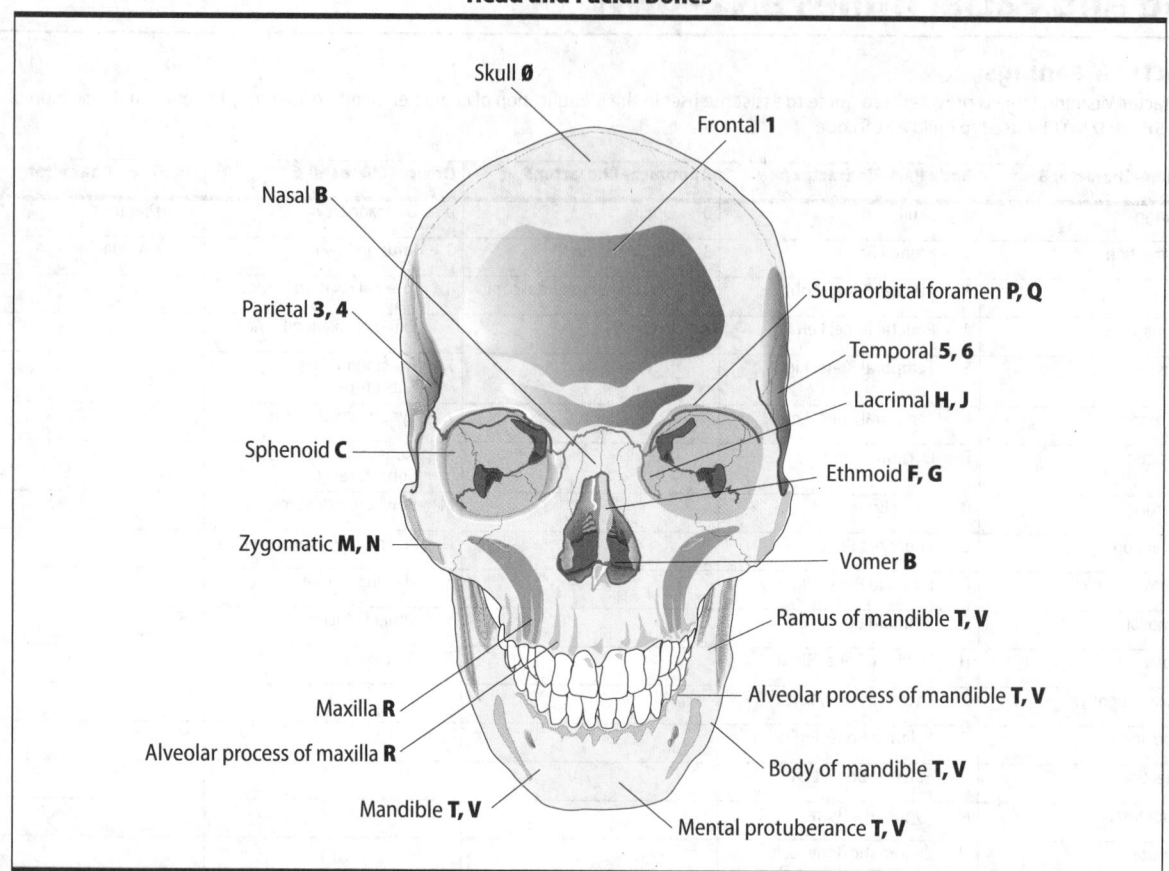

Skull **Ø**

Frontal **1**

Nasal **B**

Supraorbital foramen **P, Q**

Parietal **3, 4**

Temporal **5, 6**

Lacrimal **H, J**

Sphenoid **C**

Ethmoid **F, G**

Zygomatic **M, N**

Vomer **B**

Ramus of mandible **T, V**

Alveolar process of mandible **T, V**

Maxilla **R**

Alveolar process of maxilla **R**

Body of mandible **T, V**

Mandible **T, V**

Mental protuberance **T, V**

Skull Bones

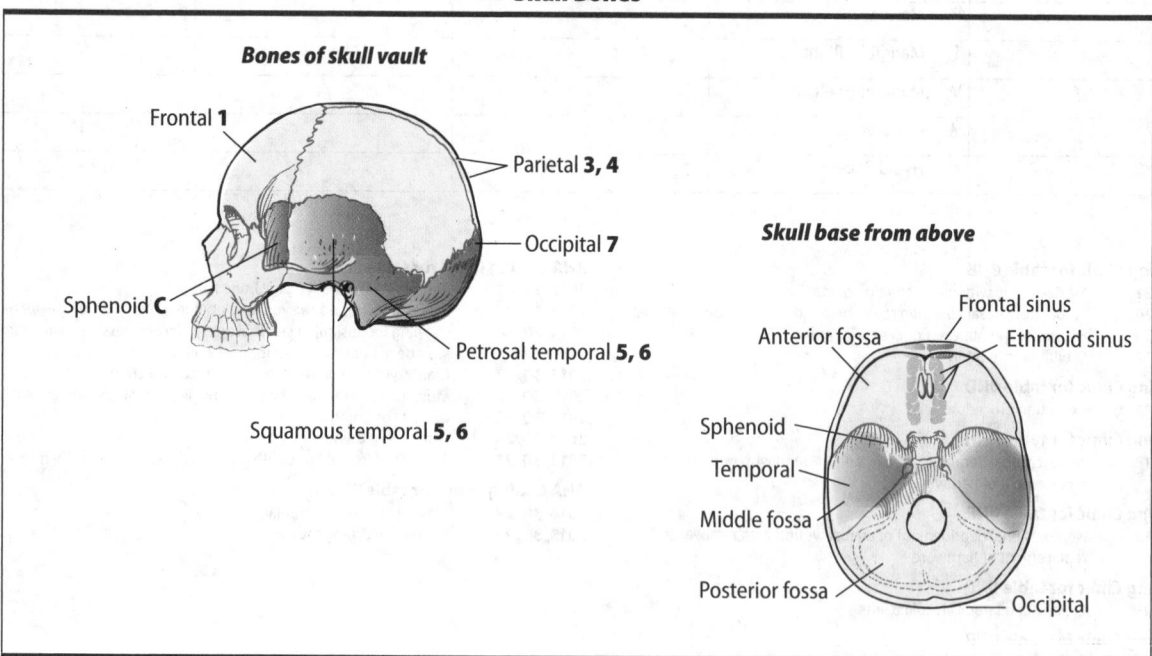

Bones of skull vault

Frontal **1**

Parietal **3, 4**

Occipital **7**

Sphenoid **C**

Petrosal temporal **5, 6**

Squamous temporal **5, 6**

Skull base from above

Frontal sinus

Anterior fossa

Ethmoid sinus

Sphenoid

Temporal

Middle fossa

Posterior fossa

Occipital

Ø   Medical and Surgical
N   Head and Facial Bones
2   Change   Definition: Taking out or off a device from a body part and putting back an identical or similar device in or on the same body part without cutting or puncturing the skin or a mucous membrane

Explanation: ALL CHANGE procedures are coded using the approach EXTERNAL

Body Part Character 4	Approach Character 5	Device Character 6	Qualifier Character 7
Ø Skull **B Nasal Bone** Vomer of nasal septum **W Facial Bone**	**X External**	**Ø Drainage Device** **Y Other Device**	**Z No Qualifier**

Non-OR   All body part, approach, device, and qualifier values

Ø   Medical and Surgical
N   Head and Facial Bones
5   Destruction   Definition: Physical eradication of all or a portion of a body part by the direct use of energy, force, or a destructive agent

Explanation: None of the body part is physically taken out

Body Part Character 4	Approach Character 5	Device Character 6	Qualifier Character 7

Ø Skull
1 Frontal Bone
  Zygomatic process of frontal bone
3 Parietal Bone, Right
4 Parietal Bone, Left
5 Temporal Bone, Right
  Mastoid process
  Petrous part of temporal bone
  Tympanic part of temporal bone
  Zygomatic process of temporal bone
6 Temporal Bone, Left
  See 5 Temporal Bone, Right
7 Occipital Bone
  Foramen magnum
B Nasal Bone
  Vomer of nasal septum
C Sphenoid Bone
  Greater wing
  Lesser wing
  Optic foramen
  Pterygoid process
  Sella turcica
F Ethmoid Bone, Right
  Cribriform plate
G Ethmoid Bone, Left
  See F Ethmoid Bone, Right
H Lacrimal Bone, Right
J Lacrimal Bone, Left
K Palatine Bone, Right
L Palatine Bone, Left
M Zygomatic Bone, Right
N Zygomatic Bone, Left
P Orbit, Right
  Bony orbit
  Orbital portion of ethmoid bone
  Orbital portion of frontal bone
  Orbital portion of lacrimal bone
  Orbital portion of maxilla
  Orbital portion of palatine bone
  Orbital portion of sphenoid bone
  Orbital portion of zygomatic bone
Q Orbit, Left
  See P Orbit, Right
R Maxilla
  Alveolar process of maxilla
T Mandible, Right
  Alveolar process of mandible
  Condyloid process
  Mandibular notch
  Mental foramen
V Mandible, Left
  See T Mandible, Right
X Hyoid Bone
	Ø Open
	3 Percutaneous
	4 Percutaneous Endoscopic
		Z No Device	**Z No Qualifier**

NC Noncovered Procedure   **LC** Limited Coverage   **QA** Questionable OB Admit   **NT** New Tech Add-on   ⊞ Combination Member   ♂ Male   ♀ Female

ICD-10-PCS 2022   **523**

Ø **Medical and Surgical**
N **Head and Facial Bones**
8 **Division**   Definition: Cutting into a body part, without draining fluids and/or gases from the body part, in order to separate or transect a body part
                           Explanation: All or a portion of the body part is separated into two or more portions

Body Part Character 4	Approach Character 5	Device Character 6	Qualifier Character 7
Ø **Skull**	**Ø** **Open**	**Z** **No Device**	**Z** **No Qualifier**
1 **Frontal Bone**	**3** **Percutaneous**		
Zygomatic process of frontal bone	**4** **Percutaneous Endoscopic**		
3 **Parietal Bone, Right**			
4 **Parietal Bone, Left**			
5 **Temporal Bone, Right**			
Mastoid process			
Petrous part of temporal bone			
Tympanic part of temporal bone			
Zygomatic process of temporal bone			
6 **Temporal Bone, Left**			
See 5 Temporal Bone, Right			
7 **Occipital Bone**			
Foramen magnum			
B **Nasal Bone**			
Vomer of nasal septum			
C **Sphenoid Bone**			
Greater wing			
Lesser wing			
Optic foramen			
Pterygoid process			
Sella turcica			
F **Ethmoid Bone, Right**			
Cribriform plate			
G **Ethmoid Bone, Left**			
See F Ethmoid Bone, Right			
H **Lacrimal Bone, Right**			
J **Lacrimal Bone, Left**			
K **Palatine Bone, Right**			
L **Palatine Bone, Left**			
M **Zygomatic Bone, Right**			
N **Zygomatic Bone, Left**			
P **Orbit, Right**			
Bony orbit			
Orbital portion of ethmoid bone			
Orbital portion of frontal bone			
Orbital portion of lacrimal bone			
Orbital portion of maxilla			
Orbital portion of palatine bone			
Orbital portion of sphenoid bone			
Orbital portion of zygomatic bone			
Q **Orbit, Left**			
See P Orbit, Right			
R **Maxilla**			
Alveolar process of maxilla			
T **Mandible, Right**			
Alveolar process of mandible			
Condyloid process			
Mandibular notch			
Mental foramen			
V **Mandible, Left**			
See T Mandible, Right			
X **Hyoid Bone**			

Non-OR   ØN8B[Ø,3,4]ZZ

Ø   Medical and Surgical
N   Head and Facial Bones
9   Drainage   Definition: Taking or letting out fluids and/or gases from a body part

                        Explanation: The qualifier DIAGNOSTIC is used to identify drainage procedures that are biopsies

Body Part Character 4	Approach Character 5	Device Character 6	Qualifier Character 7

Ø   Skull
1   Frontal Bone
     Zygomatic process of frontal bone
3   Parietal Bone, Right
4   Parietal Bone, Left
5   Temporal Bone, Right
     Mastoid process
     Petrous part of temporal bone
     Tympanic part of temporal bone
     Zygomatic process of temporal bone
6   Temporal Bone, Left
     See 5 Temporal Bone, Right
7   Occipital Bone
     Foramen magnum
B   Nasal Bone
     Vomer of nasal septum
C   Sphenoid Bone
     Greater wing
     Lesser wing
     Optic foramen
     Pterygoid process
     Sella turcica
F   Ethmoid Bone, Right
     Cribriform plate
G   Ethmoid Bone, Left
     See F Ethmoid Bone, Right
H   Lacrimal Bone, Right
J   Lacrimal Bone, Left
K   Palatine Bone, Right
L   Palatine Bone, Left
M   Zygomatic Bone, Right
N   Zygomatic Bone, Left
P   Orbit, Right
     Bony orbit
     Orbital portion of ethmoid bone
     Orbital portion of frontal bone
     Orbital portion of lacrimal bone
     Orbital portion of maxilla
     Orbital portion of palatine bone
     Orbital portion of sphenoid bone
     Orbital portion of zygomatic bone
Q   Orbit, Left
     See P Orbit, Right
R   Maxilla
     Alveolar process of maxilla
T   Mandible, Right
     Alveolar process of mandible
     Condyloid process
     Mandibular notch
     Mental foramen
V   Mandible, Left
     See T Mandible, Right
X   Hyoid Bone
	Ø Open
	3 Percutaneous
	4 Percutaneous Endoscopic
		Ø Drainage Device	**Z** No Qualifier

Non-OR   ØN9[Ø,1,3,4,5,6,7,C,F,G,H,J,K,L,M,N,P,Q,X]3ØZ
Non-OR   ØN9[B,R,T,V][Ø,3,4]ØZ

ØN9 Continued on next page

Head and Facial Bones

Ø   **Medical and Surgical**
N   **Head and Facial Bones**
9   **Drainage**   Definition: Taking or letting out fluids and/or gases from a body part

ØN9 Continued

                    Explanation: The qualifier DIAGNOSTIC is used to identify drainage procedures that are biopsies

Body Part Character 4	Approach Character 5	Device Character 6	Qualifier Character 7
Ø **Skull**	**Ø** Open	**Z** No Device	**X** Diagnostic
1 **Frontal Bone**	**3** Percutaneous		**Z** No Qualifier
Zygomatic process of frontal bone	**4** Percutaneous Endoscopic		
3 **Parietal Bone, Right**			
4 **Parietal Bone, Left**			
5 **Temporal Bone, Right**			
Mastoid process			
Petrous part of temporal bone			
Tympanic part of temporal bone			
Zygomatic process of temporal bone			
6 **Temporal Bone, Left**			
See 5 Temporal Bone, Right			
7 **Occipital Bone**			
Foramen magnum			
B **Nasal Bone**			
Vomer of nasal septum			
C **Sphenoid Bone**			
Greater wing			
Lesser wing			
Optic foramen			
Pterygoid process			
Sella turcica			
F **Ethmoid Bone, Right**			
Cribriform plate			
G **Ethmoid Bone, Left**			
See F Ethmoid Bone, Right			
H **Lacrimal Bone, Right**			
J **Lacrimal Bone, Left**			
K **Palatine Bone, Right**			
L **Palatine Bone, Left**			
M **Zygomatic Bone, Right**			
N **Zygomatic Bone, Left**			
P **Orbit, Right**			
Bony orbit			
Orbital portion of ethmoid bone			
Orbital portion of frontal bone			
Orbital portion of lacrimal bone			
Orbital portion of maxilla			
Orbital portion of palatine bone			
Orbital portion of sphenoid bone			
Orbital portion of zygomatic bone			
Q **Orbit, Left**			
See P Orbit, Right			
R **Maxilla**			
Alveolar process of maxilla			
T **Mandible, Right**			
Alveolar process of mandible			
Condyloid process			
Mandibular notch			
Mental foramen			
V **Mandible, Left**			
See T Mandible, Right			
X **Hyoid Bone**			

Non-OR   ØN9[Ø,1,3,4,5,6,7,C,F,G,H,J,K,L,M,N,P,Q,X]3ZZ
Non-OR   ØN9B[Ø,3,4]Z[X,Z]
Non-OR   ØN9[R,T,V][Ø,3,4]ZZ

Ø   **Medical and Surgical**
N   **Head and Facial Bones**
B   **Excision**   Definition: Cutting out or off, without replacement, a portion of a body part
                  Explanation: The qualifier DIAGNOSTIC is used to identify excision procedures that are biopsies

Body Part Character 4	Approach Character 5	Device Character 6	Qualifier Character 7
Ø **Skull**	**Ø** **Open**	**Z** **No Device**	**X** **Diagnostic**
1 **Frontal Bone**	**3** **Percutaneous**		**Z** **No Qualifier**
Zygomatic process of frontal bone	**4** **Percutaneous Endoscopic**		
3 **Parietal Bone, Right**			
4 **Parietal Bone, Left**			
5 **Temporal Bone, Right**			
Mastoid process			
Petrous part of temporal bone			
Tympanic part of temporal bone			
Zygomatic process of temporal bone			
6 **Temporal Bone, Left**			
See 5 Temporal Bone, Right			
7 **Occipital Bone**			
Foramen magnum			
B Nasal Bone			
Vomer of nasal septum			
C **Sphenoid Bone**			
Greater wing			
Lesser wing			
Optic foramen			
Pterygoid process			
Sella turcica			
F **Ethmoid Bone, Right**			
Cribriform plate			
G **Ethmoid Bone, Left**			
See F Ethmoid Bone, Right			
H **Lacrimal Bone, Right**			
J **Lacrimal Bone, Left**			
K **Palatine Bone, Right**			
L **Palatine Bone, Left**			
M **Zygomatic Bone, Right**			
N **Zygomatic Bone, Left**			
P **Orbit, Right**			
Bony orbit			
Orbital portion of ethmoid bone			
Orbital portion of frontal bone			
Orbital portion of lacrimal bone			
Orbital portion of maxilla			
Orbital portion of palatine bone			
Orbital portion of sphenoid bone			
Orbital portion of zygomatic bone			
Q **Orbit, Left**			
See P Orbit, Right			
R Maxilla			
Alveolar process of maxilla			
T Mandible, Right			
Alveolar process of mandible			
Condyloid process			
Mandibular notch			
Mental foramen			
V Mandible, Left			
See T Mandible, Right			
X **Hyoid Bone**			

Non-OR   ØNB[B,R,T,V][Ø,3,4]ZX

Head and Facial Bones

Ø   **Medical and Surgical**
N   **Head and Facial Bones**
C   **Extirpation**   Definition: Taking or cutting out solid matter from a body part

                     Explanation: The solid matter may be an abnormal byproduct of a biological function or a foreign body; it may be imbedded in a body part or in the lumen of a tubular body part. The solid matter may or may not have been previously broken into pieces.

Body Part Character 4	Approach Character 5	Device Character 6	Qualifier Character 7

1   **Frontal Bone**
     Zygomatic process of frontal bone
3   **Parietal Bone, Right**
4   **Parietal Bone, Left**
5   **Temporal Bone, Right**
     Mastoid process
     Petrous part of temporal bone
     Tympanic part of temporal bone
     Zygomatic process of temporal bone
6   **Temporal Bone, Left**
     See 5 Temporal Bone, Right
7   **Occipital Bone**
     Foramen magnum
B   Nasal Bone
     Vomer of nasal septum
C   **Sphenoid Bone**
     Greater wing
     Lesser wing
     Optic foramen
     Pterygoid process
     Sella turcica
F   **Ethmoid Bone, Right**
     Cribriform plate
G   **Ethmoid Bone, Left**
     See F Ethmoid Bone, Right
H   **Lacrimal Bone, Right**
J   **Lacrimal Bone, Left**
K   **Palatine Bone, Right**
L   **Palatine Bone, Left**
M   **Zygomatic Bone, Right**
N   **Zygomatic Bone, Left**
P   **Orbit, Right**
     Bony orbit
     Orbital portion of ethmoid bone
     Orbital portion of frontal bone
     Orbital portion of lacrimal bone
     Orbital portion of maxilla
     Orbital portion of palatine bone
     Orbital portion of sphenoid bone
     Orbital portion of zygomatic bone
Q   **Orbit, Left**
     See P Orbit, Right
R   Maxilla
     Alveolar process of maxilla
T   Mandible, Right
     Alveolar process of mandible
     Condyloid process
     Mandibular notch
     Mental foramen
V   Mandible, Left
     See T Mandible, Right
X   **Hyoid Bone**
	Ø Open
	3 Percutaneous
	4 Percutaneous Endoscopic
		Z No Device	**Z** No Qualifier

Non-OR	ØNC[B,R,T,V][Ø,3,4]ZZ

Ø   **Medical and Surgical**
N   **Head and Facial Bones**
D   **Extraction**   Definition: Pulling or stripping out or off all or a portion of a body part by the use of force
                        Explanation: The qualifier DIAGNOSTIC is used to identify extraction procedures that are biopsies

Body Part Character 4	Approach Character 5	Device Character 6	Qualifier Character 7
Ø Skull	**Ø Open**	**Z No Device**	**Z No Qualifier**
1 Frontal Bone Zygomatic process of frontal bone			
3 Parietal Bone, Right			
4 Parietal Bone, Left			
5 Temporal Bone, Right Mastoid process Petrous part of temporal bone Tympanic part of temporal bone Zygomatic process of temporal bone			
6 Temporal Bone, Left *See 5 Temporal Bone, Right*			
7 Occipital Bone Foramen magnum			
B Nasal Bone Vomer of nasal septum			
C Sphenoid Bone Greater wing Lesser wing Optic foramen Pterygoid process Sella turcica			
F Ethmoid Bone, Right Cribriform plate			
G Ethmoid Bone, Left *See F Ethmoid Bone, Right*			
H Lacrimal Bone, Right			
J Lacrimal Bone, Left			
K Palatine Bone, Right			
L Palatine Bone, Left			
M Zygomatic Bone, Right			
N Zygomatic Bone, Left			
P Orbit, Right Bony orbit Orbital portion of ethmoid bone Orbital portion of frontal bone Orbital portion of lacrimal bone Orbital portion of maxilla Orbital portion of palatine bone Orbital portion of sphenoid bone Orbital portion of zygomatic bone			
Q Orbit, Left *See P Orbit, Right*			
R Maxilla Alveolar process of maxilla			
T Mandible, Right Alveolar process of mandible Condyloid process Mandibular notch Mental foramen			
V Mandible, Left *See T Mandible, Right*			
X Hyoid Bone			

Head and Facial Bones

Ø   **Medical and Surgical**
N   **Head and Facial Bones**
H   **Insertion**   Definition: Putting in a nonbiological appliance that monitors, assists, performs, or prevents a physiological function but does not physically take the place of a body part
                     Explanation: None

Body Part Character 4	Approach Character 5	Device Character 6	Qualifier Character 7
Ø Skull ⊞	Ø Open	3 Infusion Device 4 Internal Fixation Device 5 External Fixation Device M Bone Growth Stimulator N Neurostimulator Generator	Z No Qualifier
Ø Skull	3 Percutaneous 4 Percutaneous Endoscopic	3 Infusion Device 4 Internal Fixation Device 5 External Fixation Device M Bone Growth Stimulator	Z No Qualifier

1   **Frontal Bone**
     Zygomatic process of frontal bone
3   **Parietal Bone, Right**
4   **Parietal Bone, Left**
7   **Occipital Bone**
     Foramen magnum
C   **Sphenoid Bone**
     Greater wing
     Lesser wing
     Optic foramen
     Pterygoid process
     Sella turcica
F   **Ethmoid Bone, Right**
     Cribriform plate
G   **Ethmoid Bone, Left**
     See F Ethmoid Bone, Right
H   **Lacrimal Bone, Right**
J   **Lacrimal Bone, Left**
K   **Palatine Bone, Right**
L   **Palatine Bone, Left**
M   **Zygomatic Bone, Right**
N   **Zygomatic Bone, Left**
P   **Orbit, Right**
     Bony orbit
     Orbital portion of ethmoid bone
     Orbital portion of frontal bone
     Orbital portion of lacrimal bone
     Orbital portion of maxilla
     Orbital portion of palatine bone
     Orbital portion of sphenoid bone
     Orbital portion of zygomatic bone
Q   **Orbit, Left**
     See P Orbit, Right
X   **Hyoid Bone**
	Ø Open
	3 Percutaneous
	4 Percutaneous Endoscopic
		4 Internal Fixation Device	Z No Qualifier

5   **Temporal Bone, Right**
     Mastoid process
     Petrous part of temporal bone
     Tympanic part of temporal bone
     Zygomatic process of temporal bone
6   **Temporal Bone, Left**
     See 5 Temporal Bone, Right
	Ø Open
	3 Percutaneous
	4 Percutaneous Endoscopic
		4 Internal Fixation Device
		S Hearing Device
			Z No Qualifier

B Nasal Bone Vomer of nasal septum	Ø Open 3 Percutaneous 4 Percutaneous Endoscopic	4 Internal Fixation Device M Bone Growth Stimulator	Z No Qualifier

R   **Maxilla**
     Alveolar process of maxilla
T   **Mandible, Right**
     Alveolar process of mandible
     Condyloid process
     Mandibular notch
     Mental foramen
V   **Mandible, Left**
     See T Mandible, Right
	Ø Open
	3 Percutaneous
	4 Percutaneous Endoscopic
		4 Internal Fixation Device
		5 External Fixation Device
			Z No Qualifier

W **Facial Bone**	Ø Open 3 Percutaneous 4 Percutaneous Endoscopic	M Bone Growth Stimulator	Z No Qualifier

Non-OR ØNHØØ5Z **Non-OR** ØNHØ[3,4]5Z **Non-OR** ØNHB[Ø,3,4][4,M]Z	**See Appendix L for Procedure Combinations** ⊞ ØNHØØNZ	

Ø   Medical and Surgical
N   Head and Facial Bones
J   Inspection   Definition: Visually and/or manually exploring a body part

Explanation: Visual exploration may be performed with or without optical instrumentation. Manual exploration may be performed directly or through intervening body layers.

Body Part Character 4	Approach Character 5	Device Character 6	Qualifier Character 7
Ø Skull B Nasal Bone Vomer of nasal septum W Facial Bone	Ø Open 3 Percutaneous 4 Percutaneous Endoscopic X External	Z No Device	Z No Qualifier

Non-OR   ØNJ[Ø,B,W][3,X]ZZ

Ø   Medical and Surgical
N   Head and Facial Bones
N   Release   Definition: Freeing a body part from an abnormal physical constraint by cutting or by the use of force

Explanation: Some of the restraining tissue may be taken out but none of the body part is taken out

Body Part Character 4	Approach Character 5	Device Character 6	Qualifier Character 7

1 Frontal Bone
    Zygomatic process of frontal bone
3 Parietal Bone, Right
4 Parietal Bone, Left
5 Temporal Bone, Right
    Mastoid process
    Petrous part of temporal bone
    Tympanic part of temporal bone
    Zygomatic process of temporal bone
6 Temporal Bone, Left
    See 5 Temporal Bone, Right
7 Occipital Bone
    Foramen magnum
B Nasal Bone
    Vomer of nasal septum
C Sphenoid Bone
    Greater wing
    Lesser wing
    Optic foramen
    Pterygoid process
    Sella turcica
F Ethmoid Bone, Right
    Cribriform plate
G Ethmoid Bone, Left
    See F Ethmoid Bone, Right
H Lacrimal Bone, Right
J Lacrimal Bone, Left
K Palatine Bone, Right
L Palatine Bone, Left
M Zygomatic Bone, Right
N Zygomatic Bone, Left
P Orbit, Right
    Bony orbit
    Orbital portion of ethmoid bone
    Orbital portion of frontal bone
    Orbital portion of lacrimal bone
    Orbital portion of maxilla
    Orbital portion of palatine bone
    Orbital portion of sphenoid bone
    Orbital portion of zygomatic bone
Q Orbit, Left
    See P Orbit, Right
R Maxilla
    Alveolar process of maxilla
T Mandible, Right
    Alveolar process of mandible
    Condyloid process
    Mandibular notch
    Mental foramen
V Mandible, Left
    See T Mandible, Right
X Hyoid Bone
	Ø Open
	3 Percutaneous
	4 Percutaneous Endoscopic
		Z No Device	Z No Qualifier

Non-OR   ØNNB[Ø,3,4]ZZ

NC Noncovered Procedure   **LC** Limited Coverage   **DA** Questionable OB Admit   **NT** New Tech Add-on   ⊕ Combination Member   ♂ Male   ♀ Female

ICD-10-PCS 2022   531

ØNJ–ØNN

Ø   Medical and Surgical
N   Head and Facial Bones
P   Removal   Definition: Taking out or off a device from a body part

Explanation: If a device is taken out and a similar device put in without cutting or puncturing the skin or mucous membrane, the procedure is coded to the root operation CHANGE. Otherwise, the procedure for taking out a device is coded to the root operation REMOVAL.

Body Part Character 4	Approach Character 5	Device Character 6	Qualifier Character 7
Ø Skull	Ø Open	Ø Drainage Device 4 Internal Fixation Device 5 External Fixation Device 7 Autologous Tissue Substitute J Synthetic Substitute K Nonautologous Tissue Substitute M Bone Growth Stimulator N Neurostimulator Generator S Hearing Device	Z No Qualifier
Ø Skull	3 Percutaneous 4 Percutaneous Endoscopic	Ø Drainage Device 4 Internal Fixation Device 5 External Fixation Device 7 Autologous Tissue Substitute J Synthetic Substitute K Nonautologous Tissue Substitute M Bone Growth Stimulator S Hearing Device	Z No Qualifier
Ø Skull	X External	Ø Drainage Device 4 Internal Fixation Device 5 External Fixation Device M Bone Growth Stimulator S Hearing Device	Z No Qualifier
B Nasal Bone Vomer of nasal septum W Facial Bone	Ø Open 3 Percutaneous 4 Percutaneous Endoscopic	Ø Drainage Device 4 Internal Fixation Device 7 Autologous Tissue Substitute J Synthetic Substitute K Nonautologous Tissue Substitute M Bone Growth Stimulator	Z No Qualifier
B Nasal Bone Vomer of nasal septum W Facial Bone	X External	Ø Drainage Device 4 Internal Fixation Device M Bone Growth Stimulator	Z No Qualifier

Non-OR   ØNPØ[3,4]5Z
Non-OR   ØNPØX[Ø,5]Z
Non-OR   ØNPB[Ø,3,4][Ø,4,7,J,K,M]Z
Non-OR   ØNPBX[Ø,4,M]Z
Non-OR   ØNPWX[Ø,M]Z

Ø **Medical and Surgical**
N **Head and Facial Bones**
Q **Repair**   Definition: Restoring, to the extent possible, a body part to its normal anatomic structure and function

                       Explanation: Used only when the method to accomplish the repair is not one of the other root operations

Body Part Character 4	Approach Character 5	Device Character 6	Qualifier Character 7
Ø **Skull**	Ø **Open**	Z **No Device**	Z **No Qualifier**
1 **Frontal Bone** Zygomatic process of frontal bone	3 **Percutaneous**		
3 **Parietal Bone, Right**	4 **Percutaneous Endoscopic**		
4 **Parietal Bone, Left**	X **External**		

5 **Temporal Bone, Right**
   Mastoid process
   Petrous part of temporal bone
   Tympanic part of temporal bone
   Zygomatic process of temporal bone			

6 **Temporal Bone, Left** *See 5 Temporal Bone, Right*			
7 **Occipital Bone** Foramen magnum			
B **Nasal Bone** Vomer of nasal septum			

C **Sphenoid Bone**
   Greater wing
   Lesser wing
   Optic foramen
   Pterygoid process
   Sella turcica			

F **Ethmoid Bone, Right** Cribriform plate			
G **Ethmoid Bone, Left** *See F Ethmoid Bone, Right*			
H **Lacrimal Bone, Right**			
J **Lacrimal Bone, Left**			
K **Palatine Bone, Right**			
L **Palatine Bone, Left**			
M **Zygomatic Bone, Right**			
N **Zygomatic Bone, Left**			

P **Orbit, Right**
   Bony orbit
   Orbital portion of ethmoid bone
   Orbital portion of frontal bone
   Orbital portion of lacrimal bone
   Orbital portion of maxilla
   Orbital portion of palatine bone
   Orbital portion of sphenoid bone
   Orbital portion of zygomatic bone			

Q **Orbit, Left** *See P Orbit, Right*			
R **Maxilla** Alveolar process of maxilla			

T **Mandible, Right**
   Alveolar process of mandible
   Condyloid process
   Mandibular notch
   Mental foramen			

V **Mandible, Left** *See T Mandible, Right*			
X **Hyoid Bone**			

Non-OR   ØNQ[Ø,1,3,4,5,6,7,B,C,F,G,H,J,K,L,M,N,P,Q,R,T,V,X]XZZ

NC Noncovered Procedure   LC Limited Coverage   QA Questionable OB Admit   NT New Tech Add-on   ⊞ Combination Member   ♂ Male   ♀ Female

ICD-10-PCS 2022   533

ØNQ–ØNQ

Ø   Medical and Surgical
N   Head and Facial Bones
R   Replacement   Definition: Putting in or on biological or synthetic material that physically takes the place and/or function of all or a portion of a body part

Explanation: The body part may have been taken out or replaced, or may be taken out, physically eradicated, or rendered nonfunctional during the REPLACEMENT procedure. A REMOVAL procedure is coded for taking out the device used in a previous replacement procedure.

Body Part Character 4	Approach Character 5	Device Character 6	Qualifier Character 7
Ø Skull	**Ø Open**	**7 Autologous Tissue Substitute**	**Z No Qualifier**
1 Frontal Bone Zygomatic process of frontal bone	**3 Percutaneous**	**J Synthetic Substitute**	
3 Parietal Bone, Right	**4 Percutaneous Endoscopic**	**K Nonautologous Tissue Substitute**	
4 Parietal Bone, Left			
5 Temporal Bone, Right Mastoid process Petrous part of temporal bone Tympanic part of temporal bone Zygomatic process of temporal bone			
6 Temporal Bone, Left *See 5 Temporal Bone, Right*			
7 Occipital Bone Foramen magnum			
B Nasal Bone Vomer of nasal septum			
C Sphenoid Bone Greater wing Lesser wing Optic foramen Pterygoid process Sella turcica			
F Ethmoid Bone, Right Cribriform plate			
G Ethmoid Bone, Left *See F Ethmoid Bone, Right*			
H Lacrimal Bone, Right			
J Lacrimal Bone, Left			
K Palatine Bone, Right			
L Palatine Bone, Left			
M Zygomatic Bone, Right			
N Zygomatic Bone, Left			
P Orbit, Right Bony orbit Orbital portion of ethmoid bone Orbital portion of frontal bone Orbital portion of lacrimal bone Orbital portion of maxilla Orbital portion of palatine bone Orbital portion of sphenoid bone Orbital portion of zygomatic bone			
Q Orbit, Left *See P Orbit, Right*			
R Maxilla Alveolar process of maxilla			
T Mandible, Right Alveolar process of mandible Condyloid process Mandibular notch Mental foramen			
V Mandible, Left *See T Mandible, Right*			
X Hyoid Bone			

Ø   Medical and Surgical
N   Head and Facial Bones
S   Reposition   Definition: Moving to its normal location, or other suitable location, all or a portion of a body part

Explanation: The body part is moved to a new location from an abnormal location, or from a normal location where it is not functioning correctly. The body part may or may not be cut out or off to be moved to the new location.

Body Part Character 4	Approach Character 5	Device Character 6	Qualifier Character 7

Ø Skull
R Maxilla
    Alveolar process of maxilla
T Mandible, Right
    Alveolar process of mandible
    Condyloid process
    Mandibular notch
    Mental foramen
V Mandible, Left
    See T Mandible, Right
	Ø Open
	3 Percutaneous
	4 Percutaneous Endoscopic
		4 Internal Fixation Device
		5 External Fixation Device
		Z No Device
			Z No Qualifier

Ø Skull
R Maxilla
    Alveolar process of maxilla
T Mandible, Right
    Alveolar process of mandible
    Condyloid process
    Mandibular notch
    Mental foramen
V Mandible, Left
    See T Mandible, Right
	X External	**Z No Device**	**Z No Qualifier**

1 Frontal Bone
    Zygomatic process of frontal bone
3 Parietal Bone, Right
4 Parietal Bone, Left
5 Temporal Bone, Right
    Mastoid process
    Petrous part of temporal bone
    Tympanic part of temporal bone
    Zygomatic process of temporal bone
6 Temporal Bone, Left
    See 5 Temporal Bone, Right
7 Occipital Bone
    Foramen magnum
B Nasal Bone
    Vomer of nasal septum
C Sphenoid Bone
    Greater wing
    Lesser wing
    Optic foramen
    Pterygoid process
    Sella turcica
F Ethmoid Bone, Right
    Cribriform plate
G Ethmoid Bone, Left
    See F Ethmoid Bone, Right
H Lacrimal Bone, Right
J Lacrimal Bone, Left
K Palatine Bone, Right
L Palatine Bone, Left
M Zygomatic Bone, Right
N Zygomatic Bone, Left
P Orbit, Right
    Bony orbit
    Orbital portion of ethmoid bone
    Orbital portion of frontal bone
    Orbital portion of lacrimal bone
    Orbital portion of maxilla
    Orbital portion of palatine bone
    Orbital portion of sphenoid bone
    Orbital portion of zygomatic bone
Q Orbit, Left
    See P Orbit, Right
X Hyoid Bone
	Ø Open
	3 Percutaneous
	4 Percutaneous Endoscopic
		4 Internal Fixation Device
		Z No Device
			Z No Qualifier

Non-OR	ØNS[R,T,V][3,4][4,5,Z]Z
Non-OR	ØNS[Ø,R,T,V]XZZ
Non-OR	ØNS[B,C,F,G,H,J,K,L,M,N,P,Q,X][3,4][4,Z]Z

ØNS Continued on next page

NC Noncovered Procedure   **LC** Limited Coverage   **QA** Questionable OB Admit   **NT** New Tech Add-on   **➕** Combination Member   ♂ Male   ♀ Female

ICD-10-PCS 2022   **535**

Head and Facial Bones

Ø Medical and Surgical
N Head and Facial Bones
S Reposition   Definition: Moving to its normal location, or other suitable location, all or a portion of a body part

Explanation: The body part is moved to a new location from an abnormal location, or from a normal location where it is not functioning correctly. The body part may or may not be cut out or off to be moved to the new location.

Body Part Character 4	Approach Character 5	Device Character 6	Qualifier Character 7
1 Frontal Bone Zygomatic process of frontal bone	**X External**	**Z No Device**	**Z No Qualifier**
3 Parietal Bone, Right			
4 Parietal Bone, Left			
5 Temporal Bone, Right Mastoid process Petrous part of temporal bone Tympanic part of temporal bone Zygomatic process of temporal bone			
6 Temporal Bone, Left *See 5 Temporal Bone, Right*			
7 Occipital Bone Foramen magnum			
B Nasal Bone Vomer of nasal septum			
C Sphenoid Bone Greater wing Lesser wing Optic foramen Pterygoid process Sella turcica			
F Ethmoid Bone, Right Cribriform plate			
G Ethmoid Bone, Left *See F Ethmoid Bone, Right*			
H Lacrimal Bone, Right			
J Lacrimal Bone, Left			
K Palatine Bone, Right			
L Palatine Bone, Left			
M Zygomatic Bone, Right			
N Zygomatic Bone, Left			
P Orbit, Right Bony orbit Orbital portion of ethmoid bone Orbital portion of frontal bone Orbital portion of lacrimal bone Orbital portion of maxilla Orbital portion of palatine bone Orbital portion of sphenoid bone Orbital portion of zygomatic bone			
Q Orbit, Left *See P Orbit, Right*			
X Hyoid Bone			

Non-OR   ØNS[1,3,4,5,6,7,B,C,F,G,H,J,K,L,M,N,P,Q,X]XZZ

Ø   Medical and Surgical
N   Head and Facial Bones
T   Resection   Definition: Cutting out or off, without replacement, all of a body part
                     Explanation: None

Body Part Character 4	Approach Character 5	Device Character 6	Qualifier Character 7

1   Frontal Bone
   Zygomatic process of frontal bone
3   Parietal Bone, Right
4   Parietal Bone, Left
5   Temporal Bone, Right
   Mastoid process
   Petrous part of temporal bone
   Tympanic part of temporal bone
   Zygomatic process of temporal bone
6   Temporal Bone, Left
   See 5 Temporal Bone, Right
7   Occipital Bone
   Foramen magnum
B   Nasal Bone
   Vomer of nasal septum
C   Sphenoid Bone
   Greater wing
   Lesser wing
   Optic foramen
   Pterygoid process
   Sella turcica
F   Ethmoid Bone, Right
   Cribriform plate
G   Ethmoid Bone, Left
   See F Ethmoid Bone, Right
H   Lacrimal Bone, Right
J   Lacrimal Bone, Left
K   Palatine Bone, Right
L   Palatine Bone, Left
M   Zygomatic Bone, Right
N   Zygomatic Bone, Left
P   Orbit, Right
   Bony orbit
   Orbital portion of ethmoid bone
   Orbital portion of frontal bone
   Orbital portion of lacrimal bone
   Orbital portion of maxilla
   Orbital portion of palatine bone
   Orbital portion of sphenoid bone
   Orbital portion of zygomatic bone
Q   Orbit, Left
   See P Orbit, Right
R   Maxilla
   Alveolar process of maxilla
T   Mandible, Right
   Alveolar process of mandible
   Condyloid process
   Mandibular notch
   Mental foramen
V   Mandible, Left
   See T Mandible, Right
X   Hyoid Bone
	Ø Open	**Z No Device**	**Z No Qualifier**

NC Noncovered Procedure   **LC** Limited Coverage   **QA** Questionable OB Admit   **NT** New Tech Add-on   ⊞ Combination Member   ♂ Male   ♀ Female

ICD-10-PCS 2022   537

Head and Facial Bones

Ø   **Medical and Surgical**
N   **Head and Facial Bones**
U   **Supplement**   Definition: Putting in or on biological or synthetic material that physically reinforces and/or augments the function of a portion of a body part

                             Explanation: The biological material is non-living, or is living and from the same individual. The body part may have been previously replaced, and the SUPPLEMENT procedure is performed to physically reinforce and/or augment the function of the replaced body part.

Body Part Character 4	Approach Character 5	Device Character 6	Qualifier Character 7

Ø   Skull
1   **Frontal Bone**
     Zygomatic process of frontal bone
3   **Parietal Bone, Right**
4   **Parietal Bone, Left**
5   **Temporal Bone, Right**
     Mastoid process
     Petrous part of temporal bone
     Tympanic part of temporal bone
     Zygomatic process of temporal bone
6   **Temporal Bone, Left**
     See 5 Temporal Bone, Right
7   **Occipital Bone**
     Foramen magnum
B   **Nasal Bone**
     Vomer of nasal septum
C   **Sphenoid Bone**
     Greater wing
     Lesser wing
     Optic foramen
     Pterygoid process
     Sella turcica
F   **Ethmoid Bone, Right**
     Cribriform plate
G   **Ethmoid Bone, Left**
     See F Ethmoid Bone, Right
H   **Lacrimal Bone, Right**
J   **Lacrimal Bone, Left**
K   **Palatine Bone, Right**
L   **Palatine Bone, Left**
M   **Zygomatic Bone, Right**
N   **Zygomatic Bone, Left**
P   **Orbit, Right**
     Bony orbit
     Orbital portion of ethmoid bone
     Orbital portion of frontal bone
     Orbital portion of lacrimal bone
     Orbital portion of maxilla
     Orbital portion of palatine bone
     Orbital portion of sphenoid bone
     Orbital portion of zygomatic bone
Q   **Orbit, Left**
     See P Orbit, Right
R   **Maxilla**
     Alveolar process of maxilla
T   **Mandible, Right**
     Alveolar process of mandible
     Condyloid process
     Mandibular notch
     Mental foramen
V   **Mandible, Left**
     See T Mandible, Right
X   **Hyoid Bone**
	Ø Open
	3 Percutaneous
	4 Percutaneous Endoscopic
		7 Autologous Tissue Substitute
		J Synthetic Substitute
		K Nonautologous Tissue Substitute
			Z No Qualifier

Ø   **Medical and Surgical**
N   **Head and Facial Bones**
W   **Revision**   Definition: Correcting, to the extent possible, a portion of a malfunctioning device or the position of a displaced device

                  Explanation: Revision can include correcting a malfunctioning or displaced device by taking out or putting in components of the device such as a screw or pin

Body Part Character 4	Approach Character 5	Device Character 6	Qualifier Character 7
Ø Skull	**Ø** Open	**Ø** Drainage Device **4** Internal Fixation Device **5** External Fixation Device **7** Autologous Tissue Substitute **J** Synthetic Substitute **K** Nonautologous Tissue Substitute **M** Bone Growth Stimulator **N** Neurostimulator Generator **S** Hearing Device	**Z** No Qualifier
Ø Skull	**3** Percutaneous **4** Percutaneous Endoscopic **X** External	**Ø** Drainage Device **4** Internal Fixation Device **5** External Fixation Device **7** Autologous Tissue Substitute **J** Synthetic Substitute **K** Nonautologous Tissue Substitute **M** Bone Growth Stimulator **S** Hearing Device	**Z** No Qualifier
B Nasal Bone Vomer of nasal septum **W** Facial Bone	**Ø** Open **3** Percutaneous **4** Percutaneous Endoscopic **X** External	**Ø** Drainage Device **4** Internal Fixation Device **7** Autologous Tissue Substitute **J** Synthetic Substitute **K** Nonautologous Tissue Substitute **M** Bone Growth Stimulator	**Z** No Qualifier

Non-OR   ØNWØX[Ø,4,5,7,J,K,M,S]Z
Non-OR   ØNWB[Ø,3,4,X][Ø,4,7,J,K,M]Z
Non-OR   ØNWWX[Ø,4,7,J,K,M]Z

NC Noncovered Procedure   **LC** Limited Coverage   **QA** Questionable OB Admit   **NT** New Tech Add-on   ⊞ Combination Member   ♂ Male   ♀ Female

ICD-10-PCS 2022   **539**

Upper Bones ØP2–ØPW

Character Meanings

This Character Meaning table is provided as a guide to assist the user in the identification of character members that may be found in this section of code tables. It **SHOULD NOT** be used to build a PCS code.

Operation–Character 3	Body Part–Character 4	Approach–Character 5	Device–Character 6	Qualifier–Character 7
2 Change	Ø Sternum	Ø Open	Ø Drainage Device OR Internal Fixation Device, Rigid Plate	X Diagnostic
5 Destruction	1 Ribs, 1 to 2	3 Percutaneous	3 Spinal Stabilization Device, Vertebral Body Tether	Z No Qualifier
8 Division	2 Ribs, 3 or more	4 Percutaneous Endoscopic	4 Internal Fixation Device	
9 Drainage	3 Cervical Vertebra	X External	5 External Fixation Device	
B Excision	4 Thoracic Vertebra		6 Internal Fixation Device, Intramedullary	
C Extirpation	5 Scapula, Right		7 Autologous Tissue Substitute OR Internal Fixation Device, Intramedullary Limb Lengthening	
D Extraction	6 Scapula, Left		8 External Fixation Device, Limb Lengthening	
H Insertion	7 Glenoid Cavity, Right		B External Fixation Device, Monoplanar	
J Inspection	8 Glenoid Cavity, Left		C External Fixation Device, Ring	
N Release	9 Clavicle, Right		D External Fixation Device, Hybrid	
P Removal	B Clavicle, Left		J Synthetic Substitute	
Q Repair	C Humeral Head, Right		K Nonautologous Tissue Substitute	
R Replacement	D Humeral Head, Left		M Bone Growth Stimulator	
S Reposition	F Humeral Shaft, Right		Y Other Device	
T Resection	G Humeral Shaft, Left		Z No Device	
U Supplement	H Radius, Right			
W Revision	J Radius, Left			
	K Ulna, Right			
	L Ulna, Left			
	M Carpal, Right			
	N Carpal, Left			
	P Metacarpal, Right			
	Q Metacarpal, Left			
	R Thumb Phalanx, Right			
	S Thumb Phalanx, Left			
	T Finger Phalanx, Right			
	V Finger Phalanx, Left			
	Y Upper Bone			

AHA Coding Clinic for table ØPB
2015, 3Q, 3-8 Excisional and nonexcisional debridement
2015, 2Q, 34 Decompressive laminectomy
2013, 4Q, 109 Separating conjoined twins
2013, 4Q, 116 Spinal decompression
2013, 3Q, 20 Superior labrum anterior posterior (SLAP) repair and subacromial decompression
2012, 4Q, 101 Rib resection with reconstruction of anterior chest wall
2012, 2Q, 19 Multiple decompressive cervical laminectomies

AHA Coding Clinic for table ØPC
2019, 3Q, 19 Removal of sternal wire

AHA Coding Clinic for table ØPD
2017, 4Q, 41 Extraction procedures

AHA Coding Clinic for table ØPH
2020, 1Q, 29 Repair of sternal dehiscence using Sternal Talon® device
2019, 4Q, 34 Intramedullary limb lengthening internal fixation device
2019, 2Q, 40 Decompression of spinal cord and placement of instrumentation
2018, 3Q, 26 Anterior vertebral tethering using Dynesys Tethering System
2017, 2Q, 20 Exchange of intramedullary antibiotic impregnated spacer
2016, 4Q, 117 Placement of magnetic growth rods
2014, 4Q, 28 Removal and replacement of displaced growing rods

AHA Coding Clinic for table ØPP
2019, 3Q, 19 Removal of sternal wire
2017, 2Q, 20 Exchange of intramedullary antibiotic impregnated spacer
2016, 4Q, 117 Placement of magnetic growth rods
2014, 4Q, 28 Removal and replacement of displaced growing rods

AHA Coding Clinic for table ØPR
2018, 4Q, 92 Radial head arthroplasty

AHA Coding Clinic for table ØPS
2020, 1Q, 33 Spinal fusion without use of bone graft
2018, 3Q, 26 Anterior vertebral tethering using Dynesys Tethering System
2017, 4Q, 53 New and revised body part values - Ribs
2016, 1Q, 21 Elongation derotation flexion casting
2015, 4Q, 33 Ravitch operation
2015, 2Q, 35 Application of tongs to reduce and stabilize cervical fracture
2014, 4Q, 26 Placement of vertical expandable prosthetic titanium rib (VEPTR)
2014, 4Q, 32 Open reduction internal fixation of fracture with debridement
2014, 3Q, 33 Radial fracture treatment with open reduction internal fixation, and release of carpal ligament

AHA Coding Clinic for table ØPT
2015, 3Q, 26 Thumb arthroplasty with resection of trapezium

AHA Coding Clinic for table ØPU
2015, 2Q, 20 Cervical laminoplasty
2013, 4Q, 109 Separating conjoined twins

AHA Coding Clinic for table ØPW
2014, 4Q, 26 Adjustment of VEPTR lengthening mechanism
2014, 4Q, 27 Bilateral lengthening of growing rods

Upper Bones

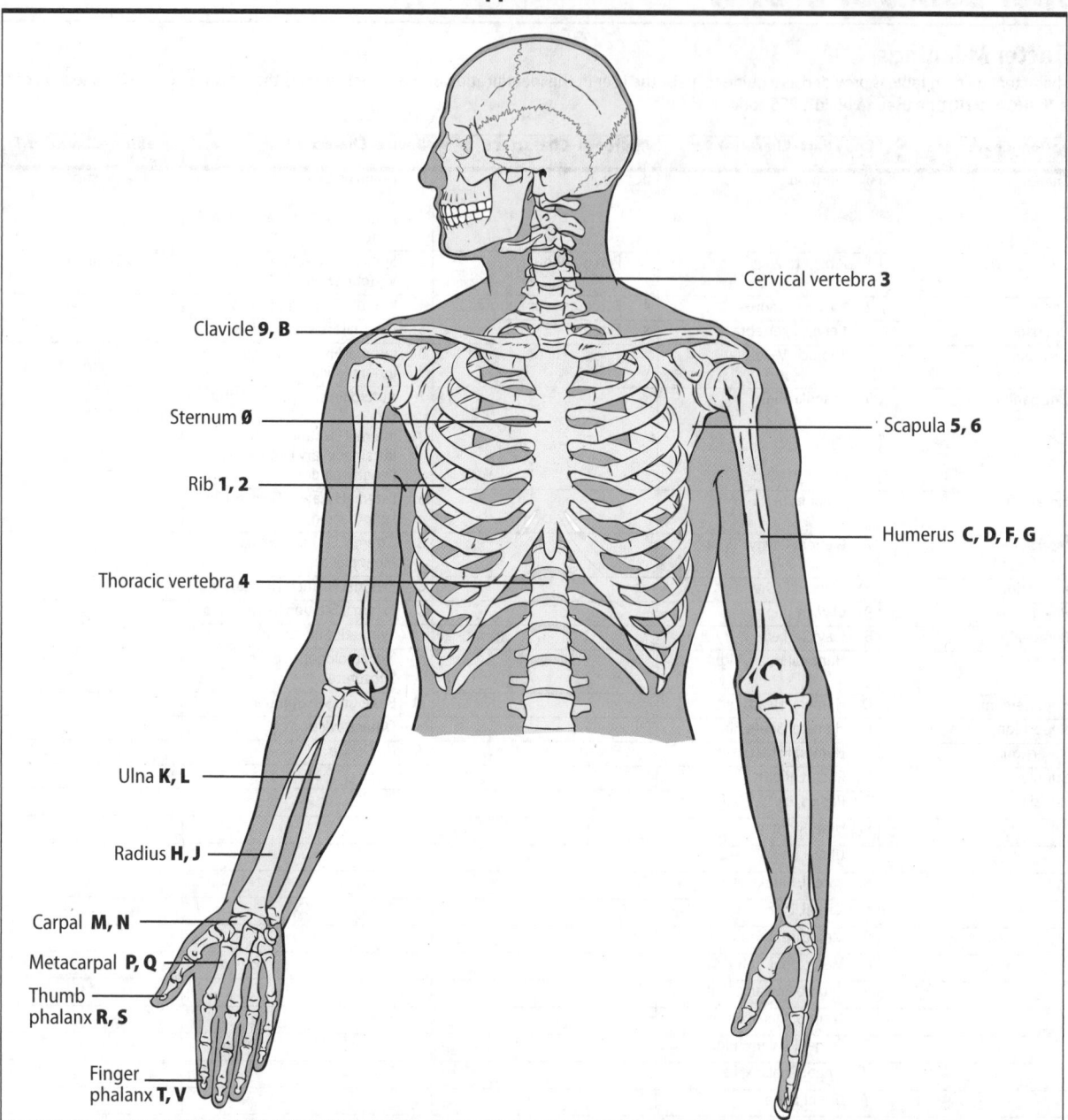

Cervical vertebra **3**

Clavicle **9, B**

Sternum **Ø**

Scapula **5, 6**

Rib **1, 2**

Humerus **C, D, F, G**

Thoracic vertebra **4**

Ulna **K, L**

Radius **H, J**

Carpal **M, N**

Metacarpal **P, Q**

Thumb phalanx **R, S**

Finger phalanx **T, V**

Humerus and Scapula

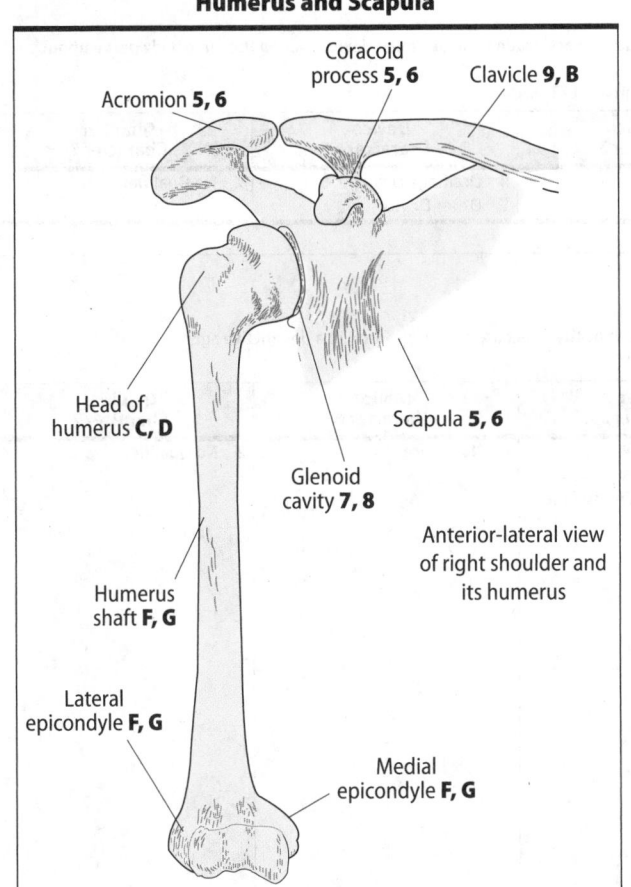

Coracoid process **5, 6**

Acromion **5, 6**

Clavicle **9, B**

Head of humerus **C, D**

Scapula **5, 6**

Glenoid cavity **7, 8**

Anterior-lateral view of right shoulder and its humerus

Humerus shaft **F, G**

Lateral epicondyle **F, G**

Medial epicondyle **F, G**

Radius and Ulna

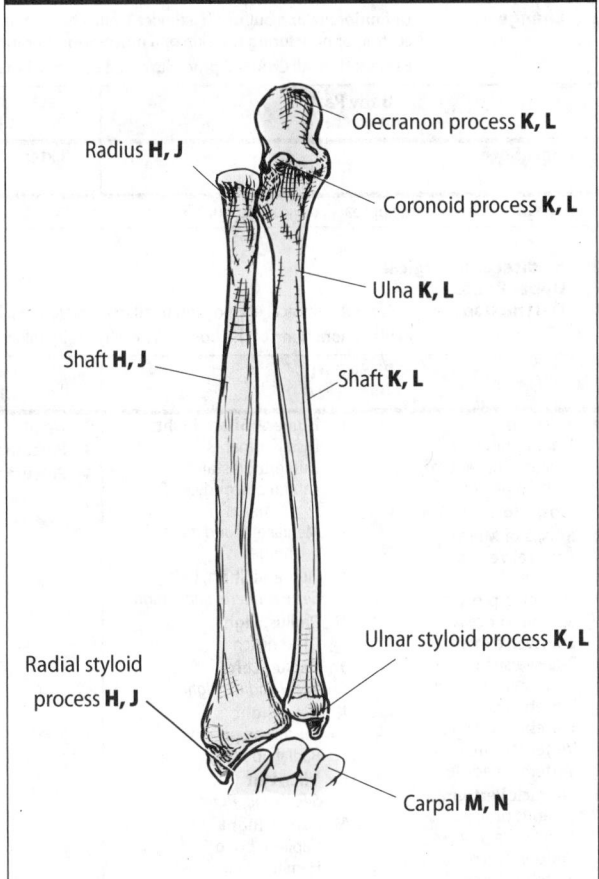

Olecranon process **K, L**

Radius **H, J**

Coronoid process **K, L**

Ulna **K, L**

Shaft **H, J**

Shaft **K, L**

Ulnar styloid process **K, L**

Radial styloid process **H, J**

Carpal **M, N**

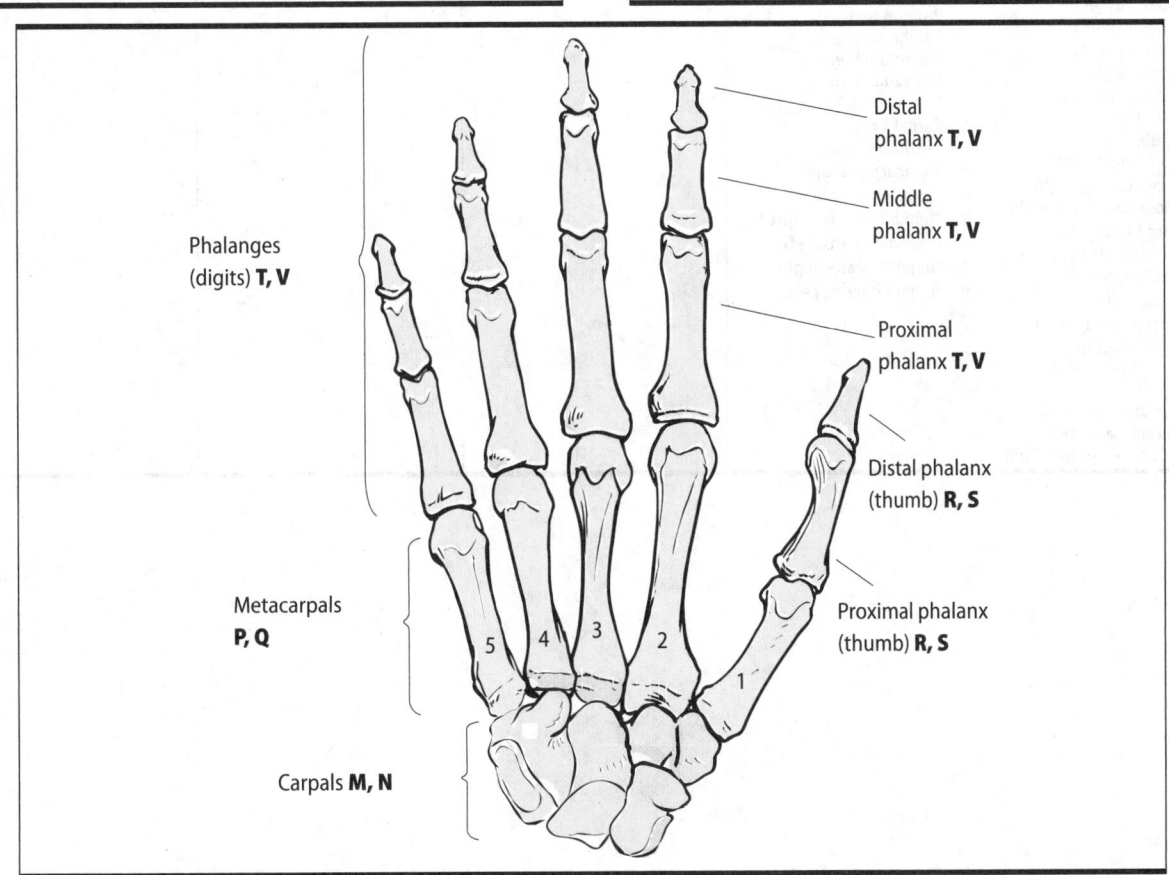

Phalanges (digits) **T, V**

Distal phalanx **T, V**

Middle phalanx **T, V**

Proximal phalanx **T, V**

Distal phalanx (thumb) **R, S**

Metacarpals **P, Q**

Proximal phalanx (thumb) **R, S**

Carpals **M, N**

Ø Medical and Surgical
P Upper Bones
2 Change

Definition: Taking out or off a device from a body part and putting back an identical or similar device in or on the same body part without cutting or puncturing the skin or a mucous membrane

Explanation: All CHANGE procedures are coded using the approach EXTERNAL

Body Part Character 4	Approach Character 5	Device Character 6	Qualifier Character 7
Y Upper Bone	X External	Ø Drainage Device Y Other Device	Z No Qualifier

Non-OR   All body part, approach, device, and qualifier values

Ø Medical and Surgical
P Upper Bones
5 Destruction

Definition: Physical eradication of all or a portion of a body part by the direct use of energy, force, or a destructive agent

Explanation: None of the body part is physically taken out

Body Part Character 4	Approach Character 5	Device Character 6	Qualifier Character 7

Ø   Sternum
    Manubrium
    Suprasternal notch
    Xiphoid process
1   Ribs, 1 to 2
2   Ribs, 3 or More
3   Cervical Vertebra
    Dens
    Odontoid process
    Spinous process
    Transverse foramen
    Transverse process
    Vertebral arch
    Vertebral body
    Vertebral foramen
    Vertebral lamina
    Vertebral pedicle
4   Thoracic Vertebra
    Spinous process
    Transverse process
    Vertebral arch
    Vertebral body
    Vertebral foramen
    Vertebral lamina
    Vertebral pedicle
5   Scapula, Right
    Acromion (process)
    Coracoid process
6   Scapula, Left
    See 5 Scapula, Right
7   Glenoid Cavity, Right
    Glenoid fossa (of scapula)
8   Glenoid Cavity, Left
    See 7 Glenoid Cavity, Right
9   Clavicle, Right
B   Clavicle, Left
C   Humeral Head, Right
    Greater tuberosity
    Lesser tuberosity
    Neck of humerus
      (anatomical)(surgical)
D   Humeral Head, Left
    See C Humeral Head, Right
	F Humeral Shaft, Right
	    Distal humerus
	    Humerus, distal
	    Lateral epicondyle of
	      humerus
	    Medial epicondyle of
	      humerus
	G Humeral Shaft, Left
	    See F Humeral Shaft, Right
	H Radius, Right
	    Ulnar notch
	J Radius, Left
	    See H Radius, Right
	K Ulna, Right
	    Olecranon process
	    Radial notch
	L Ulna, Left
	    See K Ulna, Right
	M Carpal, Right
	    Capitate bone
	    Hamate bone
	    Lunate bone
	    Pisiform bone
	    Scaphoid bone
	    Trapezium bone
	    Trapezoid bone
	    Triquetral bone
	N Carpal, Left
	    See M Carpal, Right
	P Metacarpal, Right
	Q Metacarpal, Left
	R Thumb Phalanx, Right
	S Thumb Phalanx, Left
	T Finger Phalanx, Right
	V Finger Phalanx, Left
		Ø Open
		3 Percutaneous
		4 Percutaneous Endoscopic
			Z No Device	Z No Qualifier

0   **Medical and Surgical**
P   **Upper Bones**
8   **Division**   Definition: Cutting into a body part, without draining fluids and/or gases from the body part, in order to separate or transect a body part
                             Explanation: All or a portion of the body part is separated into two or more portions

Body Part Character 4	Approach Character 5	Device Character 6	Qualifier Character 7

0   **Sternum**
    Manubrium
    Suprasternal notch
    Xiphoid process
1   **Ribs, 1 to 2**
2   **Ribs, 3 or More**
3   **Cervical Vertebra**
    Dens
    Odontoid process
    Spinous process
    Transverse foramen
    Transverse process
    Vertebral arch
    Vertebral body
    Vertebral foramen
    Vertebral lamina
    Vertebral pedicle
4   **Thoracic Vertebra**
    Spinous process
    Transverse process
    Vertebral arch
    Vertebral body
    Vertebral foramen
    Vertebral lamina
    Vertebral pedicle
5   **Scapula, Right**
    Acromion (process)
    Coracoid process
6   **Scapula, Left**
    See 5 Scapula, Right
7   **Glenoid Cavity, Right**
    Glenoid fossa (of scapula)
8   **Glenoid Cavity, Left**
    See 7 Glenoid Cavity, Right
9   **Clavicle, Right**
B   **Clavicle, Left**
C   **Humeral Head, Right**
    Greater tuberosity
    Lesser tuberosity
    Neck of humerus (anatomical)(surgical)
D   **Humeral Head, Left**
    See C Humeral Head, Right
F   **Humeral Shaft, Right**
    Distal humerus
    Humerus, distal
    Lateral epicondyle of humerus
    Medial epicondyle of humerus
G   **Humeral Shaft, Left**
    See F Humeral Shaft, Right
H   **Radius, Right**
    Ulnar notch
J   **Radius, Left**
    See H Radius, Right
K   **Ulna, Right**
    Olecranon process
    Radial notch
L   **Ulna, Left**
    See K Ulna, Right
M   **Carpal, Right**
    Capitate bone
    Hamate bone
    Lunate bone
    Pisiform bone
    Scaphoid bone
    Trapezium bone
    Trapezoid bone
    Triquetral bone
N   **Carpal, Left**
    See M Carpal, Right
P   **Metacarpal, Right**
Q   **Metacarpal, Left**
R   **Thumb Phalanx, Right**
S   **Thumb Phalanx, Left**
T   **Finger Phalanx, Right**
V   **Finger Phalanx, Left**
	0 Open
	3 Percutaneous
	4 Percutaneous Endoscopic
		Z No Device	**Z** No Qualifier

NC Noncovered Procedure   **LC** Limited Coverage   **QA** Questionable OB Admit   **NT** New Tech Add-on   ⊞ Combination Member   ♂ Male   ♀ Female

ICD-10-PCS 2022   **545**

Upper Bones

Ø   **Medical and Surgical**
P   **Upper Bones**
9   **Drainage**   Definition: Taking or letting out fluids and/or gases from a body part

                               Explanation: The qualifier DIAGNOSTIC is used to identify drainage procedures that are biopsies

Body Part Character 4		Approach Character 5	Device Character 6	Qualifier Character 7

Ø   **Sternum**
    Manubrium
    Suprasternal notch
    Xiphoid process
1   **Ribs, 1 to 2**
2   **Ribs, 3 or More**
3   **Cervical Vertebra**
    Dens
    Odontoid process
    Spinous process
    Transverse foramen
    Transverse process
    Vertebral arch
    Vertebral body
    Vertebral foramen
    Vertebral lamina
    Vertebral pedicle
4   **Thoracic Vertebra**
    Spinous process
    Transverse process
    Vertebral arch
    Vertebral body
    Vertebral foramen
    Vertebral lamina
    Vertebral pedicle
5   **Scapula, Right**
    Acromion (process)
    Coracoid process
6   **Scapula, Left**
    See 5 Scapula, Right
7   **Glenoid Cavity, Right**
    Glenoid fossa (of scapula)
8   **Glenoid Cavity, Left**
    See 7 Glenoid Cavity, Right
9   **Clavicle, Right**
B   **Clavicle, Left**
C   **Humeral Head, Right**
    Greater tuberosity
    Lesser tuberosity
    Neck of humerus
      (anatomical)(surgical)
	D **Humeral Head, Left**
	    See C Humeral Head, Right
	F **Humeral Shaft, Right**
	    Distal humerus
	    Humerus, distal
	    Lateral epicondyle of
	      humerus
	    Medial epicondyle of
	      humerus
	G **Humeral Shaft, Left**
	    See F Humeral Shaft, Right
	H **Radius, Right**
	    Ulnar notch
	J **Radius, Left**
	    See H Radius, Right
	K **Ulna, Right**
	    Olecranon process
	    Radial notch
	L **Ulna, Left**
	    See K Ulna, Right
	M **Carpal, Right**
	    Capitate bone
	    Hamate bone
	    Lunate bone
	    Pisiform bone
	    Scaphoid bone
	    Trapezium bone
	    Trapezoid bone
	    Triquetral bone
	N **Carpal, Left**
	    See M Carpal, Right
	P **Metacarpal, Right**
	Q **Metacarpal, Left**
	R **Thumb Phalanx, Right**
	S **Thumb Phalanx, Left**
	T **Finger Phalanx, Right**
	V **Finger Phalanx, Left**
		Ø Open
		3 Percutaneous
		4 Percutaneous Endoscopic
			Ø Drainage Device	**Z** No Qualifier

Non-OR   ØP9[Ø,1,2,3,4,5,6,7,8,9,B,C,D,F,G,H,J,K,L,M,N,P,Q,R,S,T,V]3ØZ

ØP9 Continued on next page

Ø   **Medical and Surgical**
P   **Upper Bones**
9   **Drainage**   Definition: Taking or letting out fluids and/or gases from a body part

ØP9 Continued

Explanation: The qualifier DIAGNOSTIC is used to identify drainage procedures that are biopsies

Body Part — Character 4		Approach — Character 5	Device — Character 6	Qualifier — Character 7

Ø **Sternum**
 Manubrium
 Suprasternal notch
 Xiphoid process
 1 **Ribs, 1 to 2**
 2 **Ribs, 3 or More**
 3 **Cervical Vertebra**
 Dens
 Odontoid process
 Spinous process
 Transverse foramen
 Transverse process
 Vertebral arch
 Vertebral body
 Vertebral foramen
 Vertebral lamina
 Vertebral pedicle
 4 **Thoracic Vertebra**
 Spinous process
 Transverse process
 Vertebral arch
 Vertebral body
 Vertebral foramen
 Vertebral lamina
 Vertebral pedicle
 5 **Scapula, Right**
 Acromion (process)
 Coracoid process
 6 **Scapula, Left**
 See 5 Scapula, Right
 7 **Glenoid Cavity, Right**
 Glenoid fossa (of scapula)
 8 **Glenoid Cavity, Left**
 See 7 Glenoid Cavity, Right
 9 **Clavicle, Right**
 B **Clavicle, Left**
 C **Humeral Head, Right**
 Greater tuberosity
 Lesser tuberosity
 Neck of humerus
   (anatomical)(surgical)
	D **Humeral Head, Left**
	 See C Humeral Head, Right
	 F **Humeral Shaft, Right**
	 Distal humerus
	 Humerus, distal
	 Lateral epicondyle of
	   humerus
	 Medial epicondyle of
	   humerus
	 G **Humeral Shaft, Left**
	 See F Humeral Shaft, Right
	 H **Radius, Right**
	 Ulnar notch
	 J **Radius, Left**
	 See H Radius, Right
	 K **Ulna, Right**
	 Olecranon process
	 Radial notch
	 L **Ulna, Left**
	 See K Ulna, Right
	 M **Carpal, Right**
	 Capitate bone
	 Hamate bone
	 Lunate bone
	 Pisiform bone
	 Scaphoid bone
	 Trapezium bone
	 Trapezoid bone
	 Triquetral bone
	 N **Carpal, Left**
	 See M Carpal, Right
	 P **Metacarpal, Right**
	 Q **Metacarpal, Left**
	 R **Thumb Phalanx, Right**
	 S **Thumb Phalanx, Left**
	 T **Finger Phalanx, Right**
	 V **Finger Phalanx, Left**
		Ø Open
		 3 Percutaneous
		 4 Percutaneous Endoscopic
			Z No Device	**X** Diagnostic
				 Z No Qualifier

Non-OR   ØP9[Ø,1,2,3,4,5,6,7,8,9,B,C,D,F,G,H,J,K,L,M,N,P,Q,R,S,T,V]3ZZ

NC Noncovered Procedure   **LC** Limited Coverage   **QA** Questionable OB Admit   **NT** New Tech Add-on   ⊞ Combination Member   ♂ Male   ♀ Female

ICD-10-PCS 2022   547

Ø   Medical and Surgical
P   Upper Bones
B   Excision   Definition: Cutting out or off, without replacement, a portion of a body part

Explanation: The qualifier DIAGNOSTIC is used to identify excision procedures that are biopsies

Body Part Character 4	Approach Character 5	Device Character 6	Qualifier Character 7

Ø   **Sternum**
   Manubrium
   Suprasternal notch
   Xiphoid process
	Ø Open
	3 Percutaneous
	4 Percutaneous Endoscopic
		Z No Device	**X** Diagnostic
			Z No Qualifier

1 **Ribs, 1 to 2**			
2 **Ribs, 3 or More**			

3   **Cervical Vertebra**
   Dens
   Odontoid process
   Spinous process
   Transverse foramen
   Transverse process
   Vertebral arch
   Vertebral body
   Vertebral foramen
   Vertebral lamina
   Vertebral pedicle			

4   **Thoracic Vertebra**
   Spinous process
   Transverse process
   Vertebral arch
   Vertebral body
   Vertebral foramen
   Vertebral lamina
   Vertebral pedicle			

5   **Scapula, Right**
   Acromion (process)
   Coracoid process			

6 **Scapula, Left** *See 5 Scapula, Right*			
7 **Glenoid Cavity, Right** Glenoid fossa (of scapula)			
8 **Glenoid Cavity, Left** *See 7 Glenoid Cavity, Right*			
9 **Clavicle, Right**			
B **Clavicle, Left**			

C   **Humeral Head, Right**
   Greater tuberosity
   Lesser tuberosity
   Neck of humerus (anatomical)(surgical)			

D **Humeral Head, Left** *See C Humeral Head, Right*			

F   **Humeral Shaft, Right**
   Distal humerus
   Humerus, distal
   Lateral epicondyle of humerus
   Medial epicondyle of humerus			

G **Humeral Shaft, Left** *See F Humeral Shaft, Right*			
H **Radius, Right** Ulnar notch			
J **Radius, Left** *See H Radius, Right*			

K   **Ulna, Right**
   Olecranon process
   Radial notch			

L **Ulna, Left** *See K Ulna, Right*			

M   **Carpal, Right**
   Capitate bone
   Hamate bone
   Lunate bone
   Pisiform bone
   Scaphoid bone
   Trapezium bone
   Trapezoid bone
   Triquetral bone			

N **Carpal, Left** *See M Carpal, Right*			
P **Metacarpal, Right**			
Q **Metacarpal, Left**			
R **Thumb Phalanx, Right**			
S **Thumb Phalanx, Left**			
T **Finger Phalanx, Right**			
V **Finger Phalanx, Left**			

Ø   Medical and Surgical
P   Upper Bones
C   Extirpation   Definition: Taking or cutting out solid matter from a body part

                       Explanation: The solid matter may be an abnormal byproduct of a biological function or a foreign body; it may be imbedded in a body part or in the lumen of a tubular body part. The solid matter may or may not have been previously broken into pieces.

Body Part Character 4	Approach Character 5	Device Character 6	Qualifier Character 7

Ø Sternum
   Manubrium
   Suprasternal notch
   Xiphoid process
1 Ribs, 1 to 2
2 Ribs, 3 or More
3 Cervical Vertebra
   Dens
   Odontoid process
   Spinous process
   Transverse foramen
   Transverse process
   Vertebral arch
   Vertebral body
   Vertebral foramen
   Vertebral lamina
   Vertebral pedicle
4 Thoracic Vertebra
   Spinous process
   Transverse process
   Vertebral arch
   Vertebral body
   Vertebral foramen
   Vertebral lamina
   Vertebral pedicle
5 Scapula, Right
   Acromion (process)
   Coracoid process
6 Scapula, Left
   See 5 Scapula, Right
7 Glenoid Cavity, Right
   Glenoid fossa (of scapula)
8 Glenoid Cavity, Left
   See 7 Glenoid Cavity, Right
9 Clavicle, Right
B Clavicle, Left
C Humeral Head, Right
   Greater tuberosity
   Lesser tuberosity
   Neck of humerus (anatomical)(surgical)
D Humeral Head, Left
   See C Humeral Head, Right
F Humeral Shaft, Right
   Distal humerus
   Humerus, distal
   Lateral epicondyle of humerus
   Medial epicondyle of humerus
G Humeral Shaft, Left
   See F Humeral Shaft, Right
H Radius, Right
   Ulnar notch
J Radius, Left
   See H Radius, Right
K Ulna, Right
   Olecranon process
   Radial notch
L Ulna, Left
   See K Ulna, Right
M Carpal, Right
   Capitate bone
   Hamate bone
   Lunate bone
   Pisiform bone
   Scaphoid bone
   Trapezium bone
   Trapezoid bone
   Triquetral bone
N Carpal, Left
   See M Carpal, Right
P Metacarpal, Right
Q Metacarpal, Left
R Thumb Phalanx, Right
S Thumb Phalanx, Left
T Finger Phalanx, Right
V Finger Phalanx, Left
	Ø Open
	3 Percutaneous
	4 Percutaneous Endoscopic
		Z No Device	**Z No Qualifier**

Upper Bones

Ø   **Medical and Surgical**
P   **Upper Bones**
D   **Extraction**   Definition: Pulling or stripping out or off all or a portion of a body part by the use of force
                      Explanation: The qualifier DIAGNOSTIC is used to identify extraction procedures that are biopsies

Body Part Character 4	Approach Character 5	Device Character 6	Qualifier Character 7
Ø Sternum Manubrium Suprasternal notch Xiphoid process	**Ø Open**	**Z No Device**	**Z No Qualifier**
1 Ribs, 1 to 2			
2 Ribs, 3 or More			
3 Cervical Vertebra Dens Odontoid process Spinous process Transverse foramen Transverse process Vertebral arch Vertebral body Vertebral foramen Vertebral lamina Vertebral pedicle			
4 Thoracic Vertebra Spinous process Transverse process Vertebral arch Vertebral body Vertebral foramen Vertebral lamina Vertebral pedicle			
5 Scapula, Right Acromion (process) Coracoid process			
6 Scapula, Left *See 5 Scapula, Right*			
7 Glenoid Cavity, Right Glenoid fossa (of scapula)			
8 Glenoid Cavity, Left *See 7 Glenoid Cavity, Right*			
9 Clavicle, Right			
B Clavicle, Left			
C Humeral Head, Right Greater tuberosity Lesser tuberosity Neck of humerus (anatomical)(surgical)			
D Humeral Head, Left *See C Humeral Head, Right*			
F Humeral Shaft, Right Distal humerus Humerus, distal Lateral epicondyle of humerus Medial epicondyle of humerus			
G Humeral Shaft, Left *See F Humeral Shaft, Right*			
H Radius, Right Ulnar notch			
J Radius, Left *See H Radius, Right*			
K Ulna, Right Olecranon process Radial notch			
L Ulna, Left *See K Ulna, Right*			
M Carpal, Right Capitate bone Hamate bone Lunate bone Pisiform bone Scaphoid bone Trapezium bone Trapezoid bone Triquetral bone			
N Carpal, Left *See M Carpal, Right*			
P Metacarpal, Right			
Q Metacarpal, Left			
R Thumb Phalanx, Right			
S Thumb Phalanx, Left			
T Finger Phalanx, Right			
V Finger Phalanx, Left			

Non-OR Procedure   DRG Non-OR Procedure   Valid OR Procedure   HAC Associated Procedure   Combination Only   New/Revised GREEN

Ø   Medical and Surgical
P   Upper Bones
H   Insertion   Definition: Putting in a nonbiological appliance that monitors, assists, performs, or prevents a physiological function but does not physically take the place of a body part
                Explanation: None

Body Part Character 4		Approach Character 5	Device Character 6	Qualifier Character 7
Ø Sternum Manubrium Suprasternal notch Xiphoid process		**Ø** Open **3** Percutaneous **4** Percutaneous Endoscopic	**Ø** Internal Fixation Device, Rigid Plate **4** Internal Fixation Device	**Z** No Qualifier
1 Ribs, 1 to 2 **2** Ribs, 3 or More **3** Cervical Vertebra Dens Odontoid process Spinous process Transverse foramen Transverse process Vertebral arch Vertebral body Vertebral foramen Vertebral lamina Vertebral pedicle **4** Thoracic Vertebra Spinous process Transverse process Vertebral arch Vertebral body Vertebral foramen Vertebral lamina Vertebral pedicle	**5** Scapula, Right Acromion (process) Coracoid process **6** Scapula, Left *See 5 Scapula, Right* **7** Glenoid Cavity, Right Glenoid fossa (of scapula) **8** Glenoid Cavity, Left *See 7 Glenoid Cavity, Right* **9** Clavicle, Right **B** Clavicle, Left	**Ø** Open **3** Percutaneous **4** Percutaneous Endoscopic	**4** Internal Fixation Device	**Z** No Qualifier
C Humeral Head, Right Greater tuberosity Lesser tuberosity Neck of humerus (anatomical)(surgical) **D** Humeral Head, Left *See C Humeral Head, Right*	**H** Radius, Right Ulnar notch **J** Radius, Left *See H Radius, Right* **K** Ulna, Right Olecranon process Radial notch **L** Ulna, Left *See K Ulna, Right*	**Ø** Open **3** Percutaneous **4** Percutaneous Endoscopic	**4** Internal Fixation Device **5** External Fixation Device **6** Internal Fixation Device, Intramedullary **8** External Fixation Device, Limb Lengthening **B** External Fixation Device, Monoplanar **C** External Fixation Device, Ring **D** External Fixation Device, Hybrid	**Z** No Qualifier
F Humeral Shaft, Right Distal humerus Humerus, distal Lateral epicondyle of humerus Medial epicondyle of humerus	**G** Humeral Shaft, Left *See F Humeral Shaft, Right*	**Ø** Open **3** Percutaneous **4** Percutaneous Endoscopic	**4** Internal Fixation Device **5** External Fixation Device **6** Internal Fixation Device, Intramedullary **7** Internal Fixation Device, Intramedullary Limb Lengthening **8** External Fixation Device, Limb Lengthening **B** External Fixation Device, Monoplanar **C** External Fixation Device, Ring **D** External Fixation Device, Hybrid	**Z** No Qualifier
M Carpal, Right Capitate bone Hamate bone Lunate bone Pisiform bone Scaphoid bone Trapezium bone Trapezoid bone Triquetral bone **N** Carpal, Left *See M Carpal, Right*	**P** Metacarpal, Right **Q** Metacarpal, Left **R** Thumb Phalanx, Right **S** Thumb Phalanx, Left **T** Finger Phalanx, Right **V** Finger Phalanx, Left	**Ø** Open **3** Percutaneous **4** Percutaneous Endoscopic	**4** Internal Fixation Device **5** External Fixation Device	**Z** No Qualifier
Y Upper Bone		**Ø** Open **3** Percutaneous **4** Percutaneous Endoscopic	**M** Bone Growth Stimulator	**Z** No Qualifier

Non-OR   ØPH[C,D,H,J,K,L][Ø,3,4]8Z
Non-OR   ØPH[F,G][Ø,3,4]8Z

NC Noncovered Procedure   LC Limited Coverage   QA Questionable OB Admit   NT New Tech Add-on   ⊞ Combination Member   ♂ Male   ♀ Female

Ø   Medical and Surgical
P   Upper Bones
J   Inspection   Definition: Visually and/or manually exploring a body part

Explanation: Visual exploration may be performed with or without optical instrumentation. Manual exploration may be performed directly or through intervening body layers.

Body Part Character 4	Approach Character 5	Device Character 6	Qualifier Character 7
Y Upper Bone	Ø Open 3 Percutaneous 4 Percutaneous Endoscopic X External	Z No Device	Z No Qualifier

Non-OR   ØPJY[3,X]ZZ

Ø   Medical and Surgical
P   Upper Bones
N   Release   Definition: Freeing a body part from an abnormal physical constraint by cutting or by the use of force

Explanation: Some of the restraining tissue may be taken out but none of the body part is taken out

Body Part Character 4	Approach Character 5	Device Character 6	Qualifier Character 7

Ø   Sternum
    Manubrium
    Suprasternal notch
    Xiphoid process
1   Ribs, 1 to 2
2   Ribs, 3 or More
3   Cervical Vertebra
    Dens
    Odontoid process
    Spinous process
    Transverse foramen
    Transverse process
    Vertebral arch
    Vertebral body
    Vertebral foramen
    Vertebral lamina
    Vertebral pedicle
4   Thoracic Vertebra
    Spinous process
    Transverse process
    Vertebral arch
    Vertebral body
    Vertebral foramen
    Vertebral lamina
    Vertebral pedicle
5   Scapula, Right
    Acromion (process)
    Coracoid process
6   Scapula, Left
    See 5 Scapula, Right
7   Glenoid Cavity, Right
    Glenoid fossa (of scapula)
8   Glenoid Cavity, Left
    See 7 Glenoid Cavity, Right
9   Clavicle, Right
B   Clavicle, Left
C   Humeral Head, Right
    Greater tuberosity
    Lesser tuberosity
    Neck of humerus
      (anatomical) (surgical)
D   Humeral Head, Left
    See C Humeral Head, Right
	F Humeral Shaft, Right
	    Distal humerus
	    Humerus, distal
	    Lateral epicondyle of
	      humerus
	    Medial epicondyle of
	      humerus
	G Humeral Shaft, Left
	    See F Humeral Shaft, Right
	H Radius, Right
	    Ulnar notch
	J Radius, Left
	    See H Radius, Right
	K Ulna, Right
	    Olecranon process
	    Radial notch
	L Ulna, Left
	    See K Ulna, Right
	M Carpal, Right
	    Capitate bone
	    Hamate bone
	    Lunate bone
	    Pisiform bone
	    Scaphoid bone
	    Trapezium bone
	    Trapezoid bone
	    Triquetral bone
	N Carpal, Left
	    See M Carpal, Right
	P Metacarpal, Right
	Q Metacarpal, Left
	R Thumb Phalanx, Right
	S Thumb Phalanx, Left
	T Finger Phalanx, Right
	V Finger Phalanx, Left
		Ø Open
		3 Percutaneous
		4 Percutaneous Endoscopic
			Z No Device	Z No Qualifier

Ø   Medical and Surgical
P   Upper Bones
P   Removal   Definition: Taking out or off a device from a body part

Explanation: If a device is taken out and a similar device put in without cutting or puncturing the skin or mucous membrane, the procedure is coded to the root operation CHANGE. Otherwise, the procedure for taking out a device is coded to the root operation REMOVAL.

Body Part Character 4		Approach Character 5	Device Character 6	Qualifier Character 7
Ø Sternum Manubrium Suprasternal notch Xiphoid process **1 Ribs, 1 to 2** **2 Ribs, 3 or More** **3 Cervical Vertebra** Dens Odontoid process Spinous process Transverse foramen Transverse process Vertebral arch Vertebral body Vertebral foramen Vertebral lamina Vertebral pedicle	**4 Thoracic Vertebra** Spinous process Transverse process Vertebral arch Vertebral body Vertebral foramen Vertebral lamina Vertebral pedicle **5 Scapula, Right** Acromion (process) Coracoid process **6 Scapula, Left** *See 5 Scapula, Right* **7 Glenoid Cavity, Right** Glenoid fossa (of scapula) **8 Glenoid Cavity, Left** *See 7 Glenoid Cavity, Right* **9 Clavicle, Right** **B Clavicle, Left**	**Ø Open** **3 Percutaneous** **4 Percutaneous Endoscopic**	**4 Internal Fixation Device** **7 Autologous Tissue Substitute** **J Synthetic Substitute** **K Nonautologous Tissue Substitute**	**Z No Qualifier**
Ø Sternum Manubrium Suprasternal notch Xiphoid process **1 Ribs, 1 to 2** **2 Ribs, 3 or More** **3 Cervical Vertebra** Dens Odontoid process Spinous process Transverse foramen Transverse process Vertebral arch Vertebral body Vertebral foramen Vertebral lamina Vertebral pedicle	**4 Thoracic Vertebra** Spinous process Transverse process Vertebral arch Vertebral body Vertebral foramen Vertebral lamina Vertebral pedicle **5 Scapula, Right** Acromion (process) Coracoid process **6 Scapula, Left** *See 5 Scapula, Right* **7 Glenoid Cavity, Right** Glenoid fossa (of scapula) **8 Glenoid Cavity, Left** *See 7 Glenoid Cavity, Right* **9 Clavicle, Right** **B Clavicle, Left**	**X External**	**4 Internal Fixation Device**	**Z No Qualifier**

C Humeral Head, Right
Greater tuberosity
Lesser tuberosity
Neck of humerus
  (anatomical) (surgical)
D Humeral Head, Left
See C Humeral Head, Right
F Humeral Shaft, Right
Distal humerus
Humerus, distal
Lateral epicondyle of
  humerus
Medial epicondyle of
  humerus
G Humeral Shaft, Left
See F Humeral Shaft, Right
H Radius, Right
Ulnar notch
J Radius, Left
See H Radius, Right
K Ulna, Right
Olecranon process
Radial notch
	L Ulna, Left
	See K Ulna, Right
	M Carpal, Right
	Capitate bone
	Hamate bone
	Lunate bone
	Pisiform bone
	Scaphoid bone
	Trapezium bone
	Trapezoid bone
	Triquetral bone
	N Carpal, Left
	See M Carpal, Right
	P Metacarpal, Right
	Q Metacarpal, Left
	R Thumb Phalanx, Right
	S Thumb Phalanx, Left
	T Finger Phalanx, Right
	V Finger Phalanx, Left
		Ø Open
		3 Percutaneous
		4 Percutaneous Endoscopic
			4 Internal Fixation Device
			5 External Fixation Device
			7 Autologous Tissue Substitute
			J Synthetic Substitute
			K Nonautologous Tissue Substitute
				Z No Qualifier

Non-OR   ØPP[Ø,1,2,3,4,5,6,7,8,9,B]X4Z

ØPP Continued on next page

NC Noncovered Procedure   **LC** Limited Coverage   **QA** Questionable OB Admit   **NT** New Tech Add-on   ⊞ Combination Member   ♂ Male   ♀ Female

ICD-10-PCS 2022   553

Ø   Medical and Surgical
P   Upper Bones   *ØPP Continued*
P   Removal   Definition: Taking out or off a device from a body part

Explanation: If a device is taken out and a similar device put in without cutting or puncturing the skin or mucous membrane, the procedure is coded to the root operation CHANGE. Otherwise, the procedure for taking out a device is coded to the root operation REMOVAL.

Body Part Character 4		Approach Character 5	Device Character 6	Qualifier Character 7

C Humeral Head, Right
  Greater tuberosity
  Lesser tuberosity
  Neck of humerus
    (anatomical) (surgical)
D Humeral Head, Left
  See C Humeral Head, Right
F Humeral Shaft, Right
  Distal humerus
  Humerus, distal
  Lateral epicondyle of
    humerus
  Medial epicondyle of
    humerus
G Humeral Shaft, Left
  See F Humeral Shaft, Right
H Radius, Right
  Ulnar notch
J Radius, Left
  See H Radius, Right
K Ulna, Right
  Olecranon process
Radial notch
	L Ulna, Left
	  See K Ulna, Right
	M Carpal, Right
	  Capitate bone
	  Hamate bone
	  Lunate bone
	  Pisiform bone
	  Scaphoid bone
	  Trapezium bone
	  Trapezoid bone
	  Triquetral bone
	N Carpal, Left
	  See M Carpal, Right
	P Metacarpal, Right
	Q Metacarpal, Left
	R Thumb Phalanx, Right
	S Thumb Phalanx, Left
	T Finger Phalanx, Right
	V Finger Phalanx, Left
		X External	**4** Internal Fixation Device
			5 External Fixation Device
				Z No Qualifier

Y Upper Bone		**Ø** Open **3** Percutaneous **4** Percutaneous Endoscopic **X** External	**Ø** Drainage Device **M** Bone Growth Stimulator	**Z** No Qualifier

Non-OR	ØPP[C,D,F,G,H,J,K,L,M,N,P,Q,R,S,T,V]X[4,5]Z
Non-OR	ØPPY3ØZ
Non-OR	ØPPYX[Ø,M]Z

Ø   Medical and Surgical
P   Upper Bones
Q   Repair   Definition: Restoring, to the extent possible, a body part to its normal anatomic structure and function
                   Explanation: Used only when the method to accomplish the repair is not one of the other root operations

Body Part Character 4		Approach Character 5	Device Character 6	Qualifier Character 7

Ø Sternum
  Manubrium
  Suprasternal notch
  Xiphoid process
1 Ribs, 1 to 2
2 Ribs, 3 or More
3 Cervical Vertebra
  Dens
  Odontoid process
  Spinous process
  Transverse foramen
  Transverse process
  Vertebral arch
  Vertebral body
  Vertebral foramen
  Vertebral lamina
  Vertebral pedicle
4 Thoracic Vertebra
  Spinous process
  Transverse process
  Vertebral arch
  Vertebral body
  Vertebral foramen
  Vertebral lamina
  Vertebral pedicle
5 Scapula, Right
  Acromion (process)
  Coracoid process
6 Scapula, Left
  See 5 Scapula, Right
7 Glenoid Cavity, Right
  Glenoid fossa (of scapula)
8 Glenoid Cavity, Left
  See 7 Glenoid Cavity, Right
9 Clavicle, Right
B Clavicle, Left
C Humeral Head, Right
  Greater tuberosity
  Lesser tuberosity
  Neck of humerus
    (anatomical)(surgical)
D Humeral Head, Left
  See C Humeral Head, Right
	F Humeral Shaft, Right
	  Distal humerus
	  Humerus, distal
	  Lateral epicondyle of
	    humerus
	  Medial epicondyle of
	    humerus
	G Humeral Shaft, Left
	  See F Humeral Shaft, Right
	H Radius, Right
	  Ulnar notch
	J Radius, Left
	  See H Radius, Right
	K Ulna, Right
	  Olecranon process
	  Radial notch
	L Ulna, Left
	  See K Ulna, Right
	M Carpal, Right
	  Capitate bone
	  Hamate bone
	  Lunate bone
	  Pisiform bone
	  Scaphoid bone
	  Trapezium bone
	  Trapezoid bone
	  Triquetral bone
	N Carpal, Left
	  See M Carpal, Right
	P Metacarpal, Right
	Q Metacarpal, Left
	R Thumb Phalanx, Right
	S Thumb Phalanx, Left
	T Finger Phalanx, Right
	V Finger Phalanx, Left
		Ø Open
		3 Percutaneous
		4 Percutaneous Endoscopic
		X External
			Z No Device	**Z No Qualifier**

Non-OR   ØPQ[Ø,1,2,3,4,5,6,7,8,9,B,C,D,F,G,H,J,K,L,M,N,P,Q,R,S,T,V]XZZ

Ø   **Medical and Surgical**
P   **Upper Bones**
R   **Replacement**

Definition: Putting in or on biological or synthetic material that physically takes the place and/or function of all or a portion of a body part

Explanation: The body part may have been taken out or replaced, or may be taken out, physically eradicated, or rendered nonfunctional during the REPLACEMENT procedure. A REMOVAL procedure is coded for taking out the device used in a previous replacement procedure.

Body Part Character 4		Approach Character 5	Device Character 6	Qualifier Character 7

Ø Sternum
   Manubrium
   Suprasternal notch
   Xiphoid process
1 Ribs, 1 to 2
2 Ribs, 3 or More
3 Cervical Vertebra
   Dens
   Odontoid process
   Spinous process
   Transverse foramen
   Transverse process
   Vertebral arch
   Vertebral body
   Vertebral foramen
   Vertebral lamina
   Vertebral pedicle
4 Thoracic Vertebra
   Spinous process
   Transverse process
   Vertebral arch
   Vertebral body
   Vertebral foramen
   Vertebral lamina
   Vertebral pedicle
5 Scapula, Right
   Acromion (process)
   Coracoid process
6 Scapula, Left
   See 5 Scapula, Right
7 Glenoid Cavity, Right
   Glenoid fossa (of scapula)
8 Glenoid Cavity, Left
   See 7 Glenoid Cavity, Right
9 Clavicle, Right
B Clavicle, Left
C Humeral Head, Right
   Greater tuberosity
   Lesser tuberosity
   Neck of humerus
     (anatomical)(surgical)
D Humeral Head, Left
   See C Humeral Head, Right
	F Humeral Shaft, Right
	   Distal humerus
	   Humerus, distal
	   Lateral epicondyle of
	     humerus
	   Medial epicondyle of
	     humerus
	G Humeral Shaft, Left
	   See F Humeral Shaft, Right
	H Radius, Right
	   Ulnar notch
	J Radius, Left
	   See H Radius, Right
	K Ulna, Right
	   Olecranon process
	   Radial notch
	L Ulna, Left
	   See K Ulna, Right
	M Carpal, Right
	   Capitate bone
	   Hamate bone
	   Lunate bone
	   Pisiform bone
	   Scaphoid bone
	   Trapezium bone
	   Trapezoid bone
	   Triquetral bone
	N Carpal, Left
	   See M Carpal, Right
	P Metacarpal, Right
	Q Metacarpal, Left
	R Thumb Phalanx, Right
	S Thumb Phalanx, Left
	T Finger Phalanx, Right
	V Finger Phalanx, Left
		Ø Open
		3 Percutaneous
		4 Percutaneous Endoscopic
			7 Autologous Tissue
			   Substitute
			J Synthetic Substitute
			K Nonautologous Tissue
			   Substitute
				Z No Qualifier

Ø   Medical and Surgical
P   Upper Bones
S   Reposition   Definition: Moving to its normal location, or other suitable location, all or a portion of a body part

Explanation: The body part is moved to a new location from an abnormal location, or from a normal location where it is not functioning correctly. The body part may or may not be cut out or off to be moved to the new location.

Body Part Character 4		Approach Character 5	Device Character 6	Qualifier Character 7
Ø Sternum Manubrium Suprasternal notch Xiphoid process		**Ø Open** **3 Percutaneous** **4 Percutaneous Endoscopic**	**Ø Internal Fixation Device, Rigid Plate** **4 Internal Fixation Device** **Z No Device**	**Z No Qualifier**
Ø Sternum Manubrium Suprasternal notch Xiphoid process		**X External**	**Z No Device**	**Z No Qualifier**
1 Ribs, 1 to 2 **2 Ribs, 3 or More** **3 Cervical Vertebra** ⊞ Dens Odontoid process Spinous process Transverse foramen Transverse process Vertebral arch Vertebral body Vertebral foramen Vertebral lamina Vertebral pedicle	**5 Scapula, Right** Acromion (process) Coracoid process **6 Scapula, Left** *See 5 Scapula, Right* **7 Glenoid Cavity, Right** Glenoid fossa (of scapula) **8 Glenoid Cavity, Left** *See 7 Glenoid Cavity, Right* **9 Clavicle, Right** **B Clavicle, Left**	**Ø Open** **3 Percutaneous** **4 Percutaneous Endoscopic**	**4 Internal Fixation Device** **Z No Device**	**Z No Qualifier**
1 Ribs, 1 to 2 **2 Ribs, 3 or More** **3 Cervical Vertebra** Dens Odontoid process Spinous process Transverse foramen Transverse process Vertebral arch Vertebral body Vertebral foramen Vertebral lamina Vertebral pedicle	**5 Scapula, Right** Acromion (process) Coracoid process **6 Scapula, Left** *See 5 Scapula, Right* **7 Glenoid Cavity, Right** Glenoid fossa (of scapula) **8 Glenoid Cavity, Left** *See 7 Glenoid Cavity, Right* **9 Clavicle, Right** **B Clavicle, Left**	**X External**	**Z No Device**	**Z No Qualifier**
4 Thoracic Vertebra ⊞ Spinous process Transverse process Vertebral arch Vertebral body Vertebral foramen Vertebral lamina Vertebral pedicle		**Ø Open** **4 Percutaneous Endoscopic**	**3 Spinal Stabilization Device, Vertebral Body Tether** **4 Internal Fixation Device** **Z No Device**	**Z No Qualifier**
4 Thoracic Vertebra Spinous process Transverse process Vertebral arch Vertebral body Vertebral foramen Vertebral lamina Vertebral pedicle		**3 Percutaneous**	**4 Internal Fixation Device** **Z No Device**	**Z No Qualifier**
4 Thoracic Vertebra Spinous process Transverse process Vertebral arch Vertebral body Vertebral foramen Vertebral lamina Vertebral pedicle		**X External**	**Z No Device**	**Z No Qualifier**
C Humeral Head, Right Greater tuberosity Lesser tuberosity Neck of humerus (anatomical)(surgical) **D Humeral Head, Left** *See C Humeral Head, Right* **F Humeral Shaft, Right** Distal humerus Humerus, distal Lateral epicondyle of humerus Medial epicondyle of humerus	**G Humeral Shaft, Left** *See F Humeral Shaft, Right* **H Radius, Right** Ulnar notch **J Radius, Left** *See H Radius, Right* **K Ulna, Right** Olecranon process Radial notch **L Ulna, Left** *See K Ulna, Right*	**Ø Open** **3 Percutaneous** **4 Percutaneous Endoscopic**	**4 Internal Fixation Device** **5 External Fixation Device** **6 Internal Fixation Device, Intramedullary** **B External Fixation Device, Monoplanar** **C External Fixation Device, Ring** **D External Fixation Device, Hybrid** **Z No Device**	**Z No Qualifier**

Non-OR ØPSØ[3,4]ZZ	**Non-OR** ØPS[1,2,3,5,6,7,8,9,B]XZZ	**See Appendix L for Procedure Combinations**
Non-OR ØPSØXZZ	**Non-OR** ØPS4XZZ	⊞ ØPS[3,4]3ZZ
Non-OR ØPS[1,2,5,6,7,8,9,B][3,4]ZZ	**Non-OR** ØPS[C,D,F,G,H,J,K,L][3,4]ZZ	

ØPS Continued on next page

ØPS–ØPS

[NC] Noncovered Procedure   [LC] Limited Coverage   [QA] Questionable OB Admit   [NT] New Tech Add-on   ⊞ Combination Member   ♂ Male   ♀ Female

Ø   Medical and Surgical
P   Upper Bones
S   Reposition

ØPS Continued

Definition: Moving to its normal location, or other suitable location, all or a portion of a body part

Explanation: The body part is moved to a new location from an abnormal location, or from a normal location where it is not functioning correctly. The body part may or may not be cut out or off to be moved to the new location.

Body Part Character 4		Approach Character 5	Device Character 6	Qualifier Character 7
C Humeral Head, Right	**G Humeral Shaft, Left**	**X External**	**Z No Device**	**Z No Qualifier**
Greater tuberosity	*See F Humeral Shaft, Right*			
Lesser tuberosity	**H Radius, Right**			
Neck of humerus	Ulnar notch			
(anatomical)(surgical)	**J Radius, Left**			
D Humeral Head, Left	*See H Radius, Right*			
See C Humeral Head, Right	**K Ulna, Right**			
F Humeral Shaft, Right	Olecranon process			
Distal humerus	Radial notch			
Humerus, distal	**L Ulna, Left**			
Lateral epicondyle of humerus	*See K Ulna, Right*			
Medial epicondyle of humerus				
M Carpal, Right	**N Carpal, Left**	**Ø Open**	**4 Internal Fixation Device**	**Z No Qualifier**
Capitate bone	*See M Carpal, Right*	**3 Percutaneous**	**5 External Fixation Device**	
Hamate bone	**P Metacarpal, Right**	**4 Percutaneous Endoscopic**	**Z No Device**	
Lunate bone	**Q Metacarpal, Left**			
Pisiform bone	**R Thumb Phalanx, Right**			
Scaphoid bone	**S Thumb Phalanx, Left**			
Trapezium bone	**T Finger Phalanx, Right**			
Trapezoid bone	**V Finger Phalanx, Left**			
Triquetral bone				
M Carpal, Right	**N Carpal, Left**	**X External**	**Z No Device**	**Z No Qualifier**
Capitate bone	*See M Carpal, Right*			
Hamate bone	**P Metacarpal, Right**			
Lunate bone	**Q Metacarpal, Left**			
Pisiform bone	**R Thumb Phalanx, Right**			
Scaphoid bone	**S Thumb Phalanx, Left**			
Trapezium bone	**T Finger Phalanx, Right**			
Trapezoid bone	**V Finger Phalanx, Left**			
Triquetral bone				

Non-OR	ØPS[C,D,F,G,H,J,K,L]XZZ
Non-OR	ØPS[M,N,P,Q,R,S,T,V][3,4]ZZ
Non-OR	ØPS[M,N,P,Q,R,S,T,V]XZZ

Ø   Medical and Surgical
P   Upper Bones
T   Resection

Definition: Cutting out or off, without replacement, all of a body part

Explanation: None

Body Part Character 4		Approach Character 5	Device Character 6	Qualifier Character 7
Ø Sternum	**G Humeral Shaft, Left**	**Ø Open**	**Z No Device**	**Z No Qualifier**
Manubrium	*See F Humeral Shaft, Right*			
Suprasternal notch	**H Radius, Right**			
Xiphoid process	Ulnar notch			
1 Ribs, 1 to 2	**J Radius, Left**			
2 Ribs, 3 or More	*See H Radius, Right*			
5 Scapula, Right	**K Ulna, Right**			
Acromion (process)	Olecranon process			
Coracoid process	Radial notch			
6 Scapula, Left	**L Ulna, Left**			
See 5 Scapula, Right	*See K Ulna, Right*			
7 Glenoid Cavity, Right	**M Carpal, Right**			
Glenoid fossa (of scapula)	Capitate bone			
8 Glenoid Cavity, Left	Hamate bone			
See 7 Glenoid Cavity, Right	Lunate bone			
9 Clavicle, Right	Pisiform bone			
B Clavicle, Left	Scaphoid bone			
C Humeral Head, Right	Trapezium bone			
Greater tuberosity	Trapezoid bone			
Lesser tuberosity	Triquetral bone			
Neck of humerus	**N Carpal, Left**			
(anatomical) (surgical)	*See M Carpal, Right*			
D Humeral Head, Left	**P Metacarpal, Right**			
See C Humeral Head, Right	**Q Metacarpal, Left**			
F Humeral Shaft, Right	**R Thumb Phalanx, Right**			
Distal humerus	**S Thumb Phalanx, Left**			
Humerus, distal	**T Finger Phalanx, Right**			
Lateral epicondyle of humerus	**V Finger Phalanx, Left**			
Medial epicondyle of humerus				

Ø   Medical and Surgical
P   Upper Bones
U   Supplement   Definition: Putting in or on biological or synthetic material that physically reinforces and/or augments the function of a portion of a body part
                         Explanation: The biological material is non-living, or is living and from the same individual. The body part may have been previously replaced, and the SUPPLEMENT procedure is performed to physically reinforce and/or augment the function of the replaced body part.

Body Part Character 4		Approach Character 5	Device Character 6	Qualifier Character 7

Ø Sternum
   Manubrium
   Suprasternal notch
   Xiphoid process
1 Ribs, 1 to 2
2 Ribs, 3 or More
3 Cervical Vertebra ⊞
   Dens
   Odontoid process
   Spinous process
   Transverse foramen
   Transverse process
   Vertebral arch
   Vertebral body
   Vertebral foramen
   Vertebral lamina
   Vertebral pedicle
4 Thoracic Vertebra ⊞
   Spinous process
   Transverse process
   Vertebral arch
   Vertebral body
   Vertebral foramen
   Vertebral lamina
   Vertebral pedicle
5 Scapula, Right
   Acromion (process)
   Coracoid process
6 Scapula, Left
   See 5 Scapula, Right
7 Glenoid Cavity, Right
   Glenoid fossa (of scapula)
8 Glenoid Cavity, Left
   See 7 Glenoid Cavity, Right
9 Clavicle, Right
B Clavicle, Left
C Humeral Head, Right
   Greater tuberosity
   Lesser tuberosity
   Neck of humerus
     (anatomical) (surgical)
	D Humeral Head, Left
	   See C Humeral Head, Right
	F Humeral Shaft, Right
	   Distal humerus
	   Humerus, distal
	   Lateral epicondyle of humerus
	   Medial epicondyle of humerus
	G Humeral Shaft, Left
	   See F Humeral Shaft, Right
	H Radius, Right
	   Ulnar notch
	J Radius, Left
	   See H Radius, Right
	K Ulna, Right
	   Olecranon process
	   Radial notch
	L Ulna, Left
	   See K Ulna, Right
	M Carpal, Right
	   Capitate bone
	   Hamate bone
	   Lunate bone
	   Pisiform bone
	   Scaphoid bone
	   Trapezium bone
	   Trapezoid bone
	   Triquetral bone
	N Carpal, Left
	   See M Carpal, Right
	P Metacarpal, Right
	Q Metacarpal, Left
	R Thumb Phalanx, Right
	S Thumb Phalanx, Left
	T Finger Phalanx, Right
	V Finger Phalanx, Left
		Ø Open
		3 Percutaneous
		4 Percutaneous Endoscopic
			7 Autologous Tissue Substitute
			J Synthetic Substitute
			K Nonautologous Tissue Substitute
				Z No Qualifier

See Appendix L for Procedure Combinations
⊞   ØPU[3,4]3JZ

NC Noncovered Procedure   LC Limited Coverage   QA Questionable OB Admit   NT New Tech Add-on   ⊞ Combination Member   ♂ Male   ♀ Female

ICD-10-PCS 2022   559

ØPU–ØPU

Upper Bones

Ø   Medical and Surgical
P   Upper Bones
W   Revision   Definition: Correcting, to the extent possible, a portion of a malfunctioning device or the position of a displaced device

Explanation: Revision can include correcting a malfunctioning or displaced device by taking out or putting in components of the device such as a screw or pin

Body Part Character 4		Approach Character 5	Device Character 6	Qualifier Character 7
Ø **Sternum** Manubrium Suprasternal notch Xiphoid process **1** **Ribs, 1 to 2** **2** **Ribs, 3 or More** **3** **Cervical Vertebra** Dens Odontoid process Spinous process Transverse foramen Transverse process Vertebral arch Vertebral body Vertebral foramen Vertebral lamina Vertebral pedicle **4** **Thoracic Vertebra** Spinous process Transverse process Vertebral arch Vertebral body Vertebral foramen Vertebral lamina Vertebral pedicle	**5** **Scapula, Right** Acromion (process) Coracoid process **6** **Scapula, Left** *See 5 Scapula, Right* **7** **Glenoid Cavity, Right** Glenoid fossa (of scapula) **8** **Glenoid Cavity, Left** *See 7 Glenoid Cavity, Right* **9** **Clavicle, Right** **B** **Clavicle, Left**	**Ø** Open **3** Percutaneous **4** Percutaneous Endoscopic **X** External	**4** Internal Fixation Device **7** Autologous Tissue Substitute **J** Synthetic Substitute **K** Nonautologous Tissue Substitute	**Z** No Qualifier
C **Humeral Head, Right** Greater tuberosity Lesser tuberosity Neck of humerus (anatomical)(surgical) **D** **Humeral Head, Left** *See C Humeral Head, Right* **F** **Humeral Shaft, Right** Distal humerus Humerus, distal Lateral epicondyle of humerus Medial epicondyle of humerus **G** **Humeral Shaft, Left** *See F Humeral Shaft, Right* **H** **Radius, Right** Ulnar notch **J** **Radius, Left** *See H Radius, Right* **K** **Ulna, Right** Olecranon process Radial notch	**L** **Ulna, Left** *See K Ulna, Right* **M** **Carpal, Right** Capitate bone Hamate bone Lunate bone Pisiform bone Scaphoid bone Trapezium bone Trapezoid bone Triquetral bone **N** **Carpal, Left** *See M Carpal, Right* **P** **Metacarpal, Right** **Q** **Metacarpal, Left** **R** **Thumb Phalanx, Right** **S** **Thumb Phalanx, Left** **T** **Finger Phalanx, Right** **V** **Finger Phalanx, Left**	**Ø** Open **3** Percutaneous **4** Percutaneous Endoscopic **X** External	**4** Internal Fixation Device **5** External Fixation Device **7** Autologous Tissue Substitute **J** Synthetic Substitute **K** Nonautologous Tissue Substitute	**Z** No Qualifier
Y **Upper Bone**		**Ø** Open **3** Percutaneous **4** Percutaneous Endoscopic **X** External	**Ø** Drainage Device **M** Bone Growth Stimulator	**Z** No Qualifier

Non-OR   ØPW[Ø,1,2,3,4,5,6,7,8,9,B]X[4,7,J,K]Z
Non-OR   ØPW[C,D,F,G,H,J,K,L,M,N,P,Q,R,S,T,V]X[4,5,7,J,K]Z
Non-OR   ØPWYX[Ø,M]Z

Lower Bones 0Q2–0QW

Character Meanings

This Character Meaning table is provided as a guide to assist the user in the identification of character members that may be found in this section of code tables. It **SHOULD NOT** be used to build a PCS code.

Operation–Character 3	Body Part–Character 4	Approach–Character 5	Device–Character 6	Qualifier–Character 7
2 Change	0 Lumbar Vertebra	0 Open	0 Drainage Device	2 Sesamoid Bone(s) 1st Toe
5 Destruction	1 Sacrum	3 Percutaneous	3 Spinal Stabilization Device, Vertebral Body Tether	X Diagnostic
8 Division	2 Pelvic Bone, Right	4 Percutaneous Endoscopic	4 Internal Fixation Device	Z No Qualifier
9 Drainage	3 Pelvic Bone, Left	X External	5 External Fixation Device	
B Excision	4 Acetabulum, Right		6 Internal Fixation Device, Intramedullary	
C Extirpation	5 Acetabulum, Left		7 Autologous Tissue Substitute OR Internal Fixation Device, Intramedullary Limb Lengthening	
D Extraction	6 Upper Femur, Right		8 External Fixation Device, Limb Lengthening	
H Insertion	7 Upper Femur, Left		B External Fixation Device, Monoplanar	
J Inspection	8 Femoral Shaft, Right		C External Fixation Device, Ring	
N Release	9 Femoral Shaft, Left		D External Fixation Device, Hybrid	
P Removal	B Lower Femur, Right		J Synthetic Substitute	
Q Repair	C Lower Femur, Left		K Nonautologous Tissue Substitute	
R Replacement	D Patella, Right		M Bone Growth Stimulator	
S Reposition	F Patella, Left		Y Other Device	
T Resection	G Tibia, Right		Z No Device	
U Supplement	H Tibia, Left			
W Revision	J Fibula, Right			
	K Fibula, Left			
	L Tarsal, Right			
	M Tarsal, Left			
	N Metatarsal, Right			
	P Metatarsal, Left			
	Q Toe Phalanx, Right			
	R Toe Phalanx, Left			
	S Coccyx			
	Y Lower Bone			

AHA Coding Clinic for table 0Q8
| 2018, 1Q, 25 | Periacetabular osteotomy for repair of congenital hip dysplasia |
| 2016, 2Q, 31 | Periacetabular osteotomy for repair of congenital hip dysplasia |

AHA Coding Clinic for table 0QB
2021, 2Q, 18	Excision of tibial sesamoid
2020, 2Q, 26	Sacral Pressure Ulcer with Excisional and Nonexcisional Debridement of Same Site
2019, 2Q, 19	Cervical spinal fusion, decompression and placement of interfacet stabilization device
2018, 3Q, 17	Excisional debridement of periosteum
2017, 1Q, 23	Reconstruction of mandible using titanium and bone
2016, 3Q, 30	Resection of femur with interposition arthroplasty
2015, 3Q, 3-8	Excisional and nonexcisional debridement
2015, 3Q, 26	Femoral head resection
2015, 2Q, 34	Decompressive laminectomy
2014, 4Q, 25	Femoroacetabular impingement and labral tear with repair
2014, 2Q, 6	Posterior lumbar fusion with discectomy
2013, 4Q, 116	Spinal decompression
2013, 2Q, 39	Ankle fusion, osteotomy, and removal of hardware
2012, 2Q, 19	Multiple decompressive cervical laminectomies

AHA Coding Clinic for table 0QD
| 2017, 4Q, 41 | Extraction procedures |

AHA Coding Clinic for table 0QH
2019, 4Q, 34	Intramedullary limb lengthening internal fixation device
2017, 1Q, 21	Staged scoliosis surgery with iliac fixation and spinal fusion
2016, 3Q, 34	Tibial/fibula epiphysiodesis

AHA Coding Clinic for table 0QP
2020, 4Q, 56	Removal of external fixation device
2017, 4Q, 74-75	Magnetic growth rods
2015, 2Q, 6	Planned implant break

AHA Coding Clinic for table 0QQ
| 2018, 1Q, 15 | Pubic symphysis fusion |
| 2014, 3Q, 24 | Repair of lipomyelomeningocele and tethered cord |

AHA Coding Clinic for table 0QR
| 2017, 1Q, 22 | Total knee replacement and patellar component |
| 2016, 3Q, 30 | Resection of femur with interposition arthroplasty |

AHA Coding Clinic for table 0QS
2020, 1Q, 33	Spinal fusion without use of bone graft
2019, 3Q, 26	Open reduction with internal fixation and placement of strut allograft
2018, 1Q, 13	Bilateral cuboid osteotomy for repair of congenital talipes equinovarus
2018, 1Q, 25	Periacetabular osteotomy for repair of congenital hip dysplasia
2016, 3Q, 34	Tibial/fibula epiphysiodesis
2014, 4Q, 29	Rotational osteosynthesis
2014, 4Q, 31	Reposition of femur for correction of valgus and recurvatum deformities

AHA Coding Clinic for table 0QT
2017, 1Q, 22	Chopart amputation of foot
2016, 3Q, 30	Resection of femur with interposition arthroplasty
2015, 3Q, 26	Femoral head resection
2014, 4Q, 29	Rotational osteosynthesis

AHA Coding Clinic for table 0QU
2019, 3Q, 26	Open reduction with internal fixation and placement of strut allograft
2019, 2Q, 35	Kiva® kyphoplasty
2015, 3Q, 18	Total hip replacement with acetabular reconstruction
2014, 4Q, 29	Reposition of femur for correction of valgus and recurvatum deformities
2014, 2Q, 12	Percutaneous vertebroplasty using cement
2013, 2Q, 35	Use of bone void filler in grafting

AHA Coding Clinic for table 0QW
| 2017, 4Q, 74-75 | Magnetic growth rods |

Lower Bones

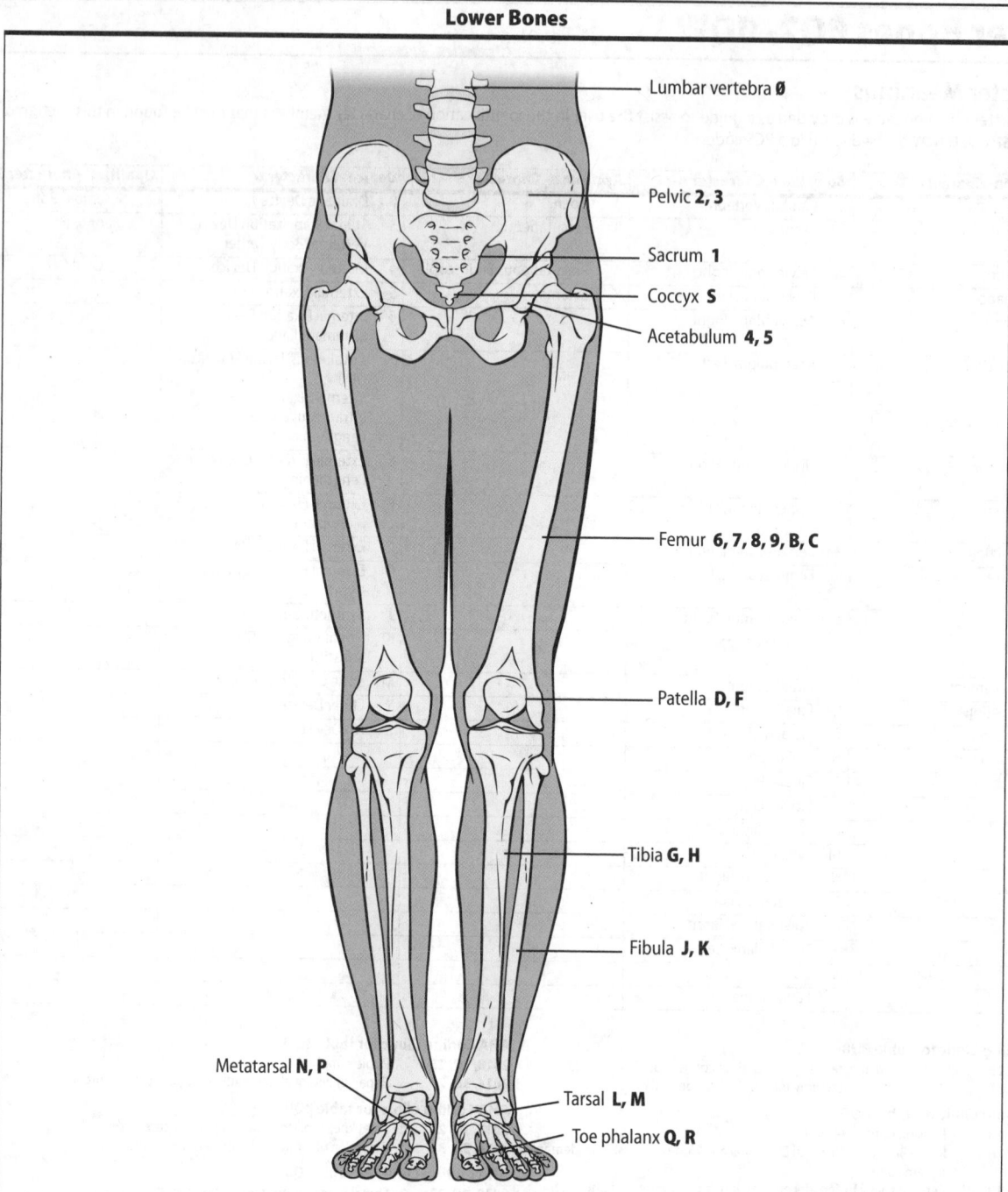

Lumbar vertebra **Ø**

Pelvic **2, 3**

Sacrum **1**

Coccyx **S**

Acetabulum **4, 5**

Femur **6, 7, 8, 9, B, C**

Patella **D, F**

Tibia **G, H**

Fibula **J, K**

Metatarsal **N, P**

Tarsal **L, M**

Toe phalanx **Q, R**

Hip Bone Anatomy

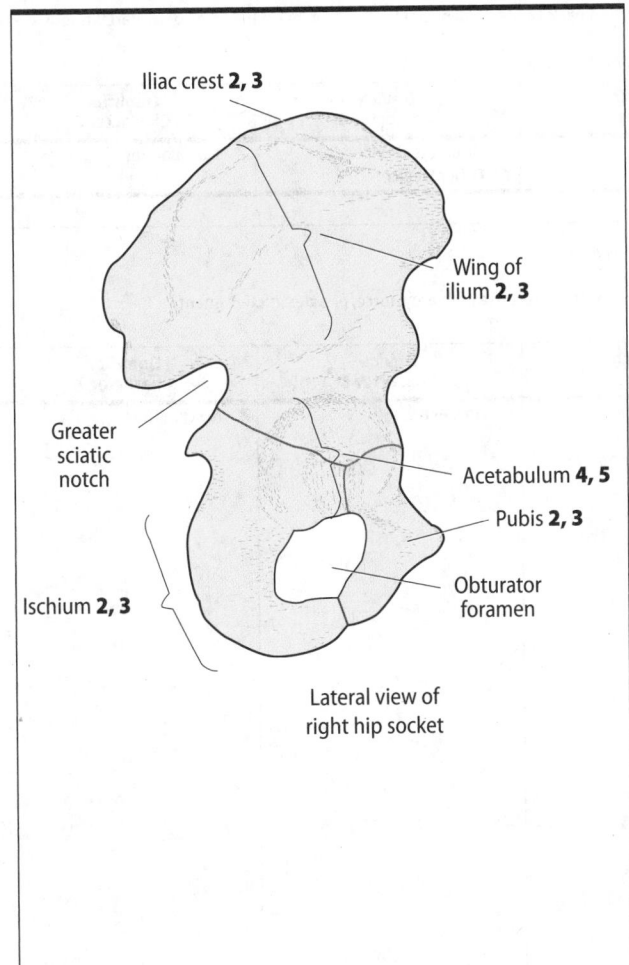

Iliac crest **2, 3**

Wing of ilium **2, 3**

Greater sciatic notch

Acetabulum **4, 5**

Pubis **2, 3**

Obturator foramen

Ischium **2, 3**

Lateral view of right hip socket

Pelvic and Lower Extremity Bones

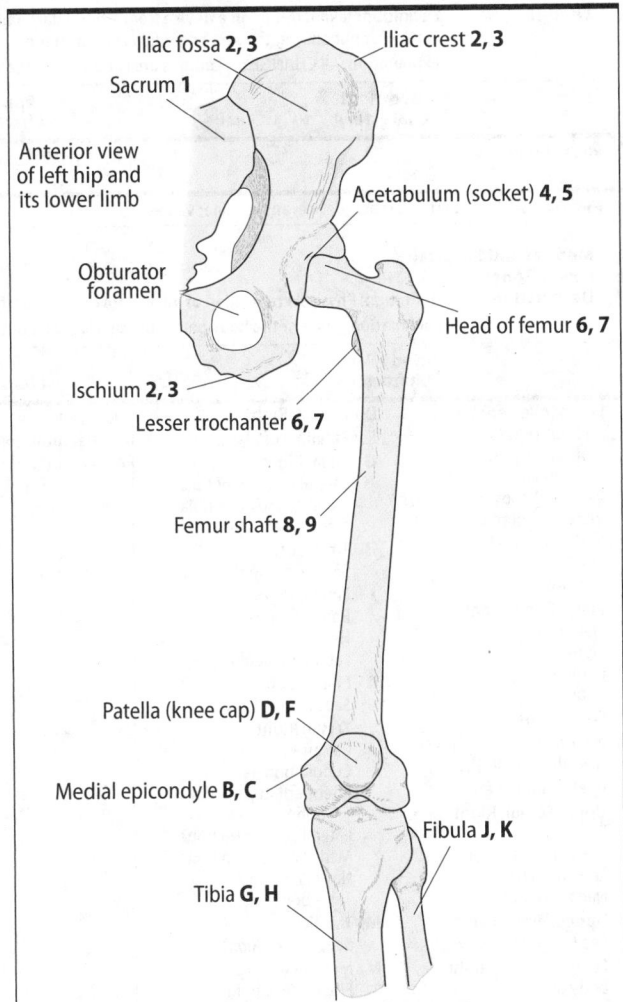

Iliac fossa **2, 3**

Iliac crest **2, 3**

Sacrum **1**

Anterior view of left hip and its lower limb

Acetabulum (socket) **4, 5**

Obturator foramen

Head of femur **6, 7**

Ischium **2, 3**

Lesser trochanter **6, 7**

Femur shaft **8, 9**

Patella (knee cap) **D, F**

Medial epicondyle **B, C**

Fibula **J, K**

Tibia **G, H**

Foot Bones

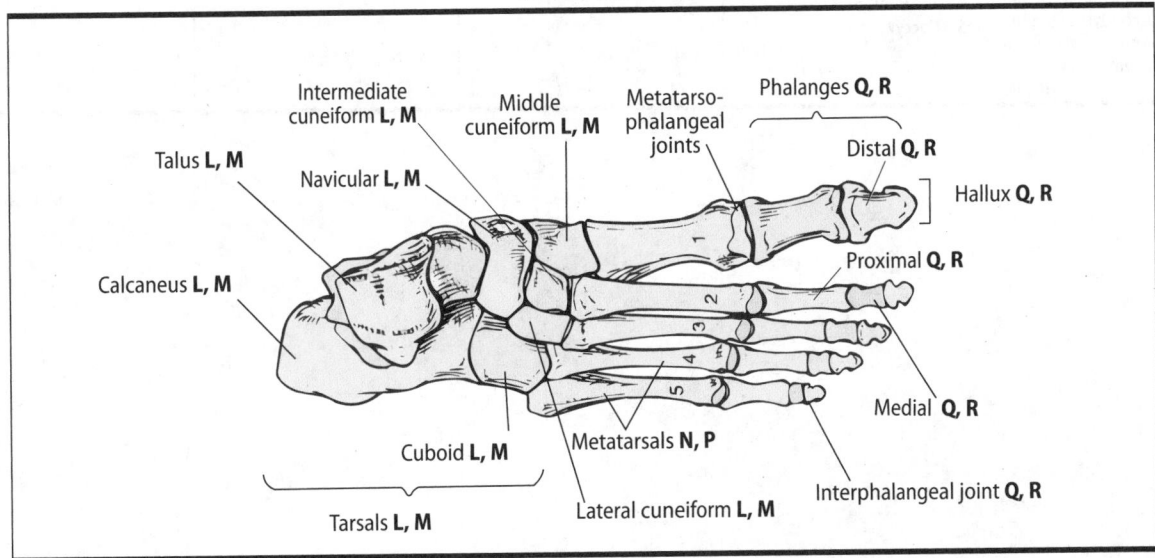

Intermediate cuneiform **L, M**

Middle cuneiform **L, M**

Metatarso-phalangeal joints

Phalanges **Q, R**

Talus **L, M**

Navicular **L, M**

Distal **Q, R**

Hallux **Q, R**

Calcaneus **L, M**

Proximal **Q, R**

Medial **Q, R**

Cuboid **L, M**

Metatarsals **N, P**

Interphalangeal joint **Q, R**

Tarsals **L, M**

Lateral cuneiform **L, M**

0 **Medical and Surgical**
Q **Lower Bones**
2 **Change**　　　Definition: Taking out or off a device from a body part and putting back an identical or similar device in or on the same body part without cutting or puncturing the skin or a mucous membrane

Explanation: All CHANGE procedures are coded using the approach EXTERNAL

Body Part Character 4	Approach Character 5	Device Character 6	Qualifier Character 7
Y　Lower Bone	X　External	0　Drainage Device Y　Other Device	Z　No Qualifier

Non-OR　All body part, approach, device, and qualifier values

0 **Medical and Surgical**
Q **Lower Bones**
5 **Destruction**　　　Definition: Physical eradication of all or a portion of a body part by the direct use of energy, force, or a destructive agent

Explanation: None of the body part is physically taken out

Body Part Character 4		Approach Character 5	Device Character 6	Qualifier Character 7
0　Lumbar Vertebra 　　Spinous process 　　Transverse process 　　Vertebral arch 　　Vertebral body 　　Vertebral foramen 　　Vertebral lamina 　　Vertebral pedicle 1　Sacrum 2　Pelvic Bone, Right 　　Iliac crest 　　Ilium 　　Ischium 　　Pubis 3　Pelvic Bone, Left 　　*See 2 Pelvic Bone, Right* 4　Acetabulum, Right 5　Acetabulum, Left 6　Upper Femur, Right 　　Femoral head 　　Greater trochanter 　　Lesser trochanter 　　Neck of femur 7　Upper Femur, Left 　　*See 6 Upper Femur, Right* 8　Femoral Shaft, Right 　　Body of femur 9　Femoral Shaft, Left 　　*See 8 Femoral Shaft, Right* B　Lower Femur, Right 　　Lateral condyle of femur 　　Lateral epicondyle of femur 　　Medial condyle of femur 　　Medial epicondyle of femur C　Lower Femur, Left 　　*See B Lower Femur, Right*	D　Patella, Right F　Patella, Left G　Tibia, Right 　　Lateral condyle of tibia 　　Medial condyle of tibia 　　Medial malleolus H　Tibia, Left 　　*See G Tibia, Right* J　Fibula, Right 　　Body of fibula 　　Head of fibula 　　Lateral malleolus K　Fibula, Left 　　*See J Fibula, Right* L　Tarsal, Right 　　Calcaneus 　　Cuboid bone 　　Intermediate cuneiform 　　　bone 　　Lateral cuneiform bone 　　Medial cuneiform bone 　　Navicular bone 　　Talus bone M　Tarsal, Left 　　*See L Tarsal, Right* N　Metatarsal, Right 　　Fibular sesamoid 　　Tibial sesamoid P　Metatarsal, Left 　　*See N Metatarsal, Right* Q　Toe Phalanx, Right R　Toe Phalanx, Left S　Coccyx	0　Open 3　Percutaneous 4　Percutaneous Endoscopic	Z　No Device	Z　No Qualifier

0   **Medical and Surgical**
Q   **Lower Bones**
8   **Division**   Definition: Cutting into a body part, without draining fluids and/or gases from the body part, in order to separate or transect a body part
                              Explanation: All or a portion of the body part is separated into two or more portions

Body Part Character 4	Approach Character 5	Device Character 6	Qualifier Character 7

0   **Lumbar Vertebra**
    Spinous process
    Transverse process
    Vertebral arch
    Vertebral body
    Vertebral foramen
    Vertebral lamina
    Vertebral pedicle
	0 Open
	3 Percutaneous
	4 Percutaneous Endoscopic
		Z No Device	**Z** No Qualifier

1 **Sacrum**			

2   **Pelvic Bone, Right**
    Iliac crest
    Ilium
    Ischium
    Pubis			

3 **Pelvic Bone, Left** *See 2 Pelvic Bone, Right*			
4 **Acetabulum, Right**			
5 **Acetabulum, Left**			

6   **Upper Femur, Right**
    Femoral head
    Greater trochanter
    Lesser trochanter
    Neck of femur			

7 **Upper Femur, Left** *See 6 Upper Femur, Right*			
8 **Femoral Shaft, Right** Body of femur			
9 **Femoral Shaft, Left** *See 8 Femoral Shaft, Right*			

B   **Lower Femur, Right**
    Lateral condyle of femur
    Lateral epicondyle of femur
    Medial condyle of femur
    Medial epicondyle of femur			

C **Lower Femur, Left** *See B Lower Femur, Right*			
D **Patella, Right**			
F **Patella, Left**			

G   **Tibia, Right**
    Lateral condyle of tibia
    Medial condyle of tibia
    Medial malleolus			

H **Tibia, Left** *See G Tibia, Right*			

J   **Fibula, Right**
    Body of fibula
    Head of fibula
    Lateral malleolus			

K **Fibula, Left** *See J Fibula, Right*			

L   **Tarsal, Right**
    Calcaneus
    Cuboid bone
    Intermediate cuneiform bone
    Lateral cuneiform bone
    Medial cuneiform bone
    Navicular bone
    Talus bone			

M **Tarsal, Left** *See L Tarsal, Right*			

N   **Metatarsal, Right**
    Fibular sesamoid
    Tibial sesamoid			

P **Metatarsal, Left** *See N Metatarsal, Right*			
Q **Toe Phalanx, Right**			
R **Toe Phalanx, Left**			
S **Coccyx**			

NC Noncovered Procedure   **LC** Limited Coverage   **QA** Questionable OB Admit   **NT** New Tech Add-on   ⊞ Combination Member   ♂ Male   ♀ Female

ICD-10-PCS 2022   **565**

0Q8–0Q8

Lower Bones

0   **Medical and Surgical**
Q   **Lower Bones**
9   **Drainage**   Definition: Taking or letting out fluids and/or gases from a body part
                     Explanation: The qualifier DIAGNOSTIC is used to identify drainage procedures that are biopsies

Body Part Character 4		Approach Character 5	Device Character 6	Qualifier Character 7

0 Lumbar Vertebra
  Spinous process
  Transverse process
  Vertebral arch
  Vertebral body
  Vertebral foramen
  Vertebral lamina
  Vertebral pedicle
1 Sacrum
2 Pelvic Bone, Right
  Iliac crest
  Ilium
  Ischium
  Pubis
3 Pelvic Bone, Left
  See 2 Pelvic Bone, Right
4 Acetabulum, Right
5 Acetabulum, Left
6 Upper Femur, Right
  Femoral head
  Greater trochanter
  Lesser trochanter
  Neck of femur
7 Upper Femur, Left
  See 6 Upper Femur, Right
8 Femoral Shaft, Right
  Body of femur
9 Femoral Shaft, Left
  See 8 Femoral Shaft, Right
B Lower Femur, Right
  Lateral condyle of femur
  Lateral epicondyle of femur
  Medial condyle of femur
  Medial epicondyle of femur
	C Lower Femur, Left
	  See B Lower Femur, Right
	D Patella, Right
	F Patella, Left
	G Tibia, Right
	  Lateral condyle of tibia
	  Medial condyle of tibia
	  Medial malleolus
	H Tibia, Left
	  See G Tibia, Right
	J Fibula, Right
	  Body of fibula
	  Head of fibula
	  Lateral malleolus
	K Fibula, Left
	  See J Fibula, Right
	L Tarsal, Right
	  Calcaneus
	  Cuboid bone
	  Intermediate cuneiform bone
	  Lateral cuneiform bone
	  Medial cuneiform bone
	  Navicular bone
	  Talus bone
	M Tarsal, Left
	  See L Tarsal, Right
	N Metatarsal, Right
	  Fibular sesamoid
	  Tibial sesamoid
	P Metatarsal, Left
	  See N Metatarsal, Right
	Q Toe Phalanx, Right
	R Toe Phalanx, Left
	S Coccyx
		0 Open
		3 Percutaneous
		4 Percutaneous Endoscopic
			0 Drainage Device	**Z** No Qualifier

0 Lumbar Vertebra
  Spinous process
  Transverse process
  Vertebral arch
  Vertebral body
  Vertebral foramen
  Vertebral lamina
  Vertebral pedicle
1 Sacrum
2 Pelvic Bone, Right
  Iliac crest
  Ilium
  Ischium
  Pubis
3 Pelvic Bone, Left
  See 2 Pelvic Bone, Right
4 Acetabulum, Right
5 Acetabulum, Left
6 Upper Femur, Right
  Femoral head
  Greater trochanter
  Lesser trochanter
  Neck of femur
7 Upper Femur, Left
  See 6 Upper Femur, Right
8 Femoral Shaft, Right
  Body of femur
9 Femoral Shaft, Left
  See 8 Femoral Shaft, Right
B Lower Femur, Right
  Lateral condyle of femur
  Lateral epicondyle of femur
  Medial condyle of femur
  Medial epicondyle of femur
	C Lower Femur, Left
	  See B Lower Femur, Right
	D Patella, Right
	F Patella, Left
	G Tibia, Right
	  Lateral condyle of tibia
	  Medial condyle of tibia
	  Medial malleolus
	H Tibia, Left
	  See G Tibia, Right
	J Fibula, Right
	  Body of fibula
	  Head of fibula
	  Lateral malleolus
	K Fibula, Left
	  See J Fibula, Right
	L Tarsal, Right
	  Calcaneus
	  Cuboid bone
	  Intermediate cuneiform bone
	  Lateral cuneiform bone
	  Medial cuneiform bone
	  Navicular bone
	  Talus bone
	M Tarsal, Left
	  See L Tarsal, Right
	N Metatarsal, Right
	  Fibular sesamoid
	  Tibial sesamoid
	P Metatarsal, Left
	  See N Metatarsal, Right
	Q Toe Phalanx, Right
	R Toe Phalanx, Left
	S Coccyx
		0 Open
		3 Percutaneous
		4 Percutaneous Endoscopic
			Z No Device	**X** Diagnostic
				Z No Qualifier

Non-OR   0Q9[0,1,2,3,4,5,6,7,8,9,B,C,D,F,G,H,J,K,L,M,P,Q,R,S]30Z
Non-OR   0Q9[0,1,2,3,4,5,6,7,8,9,B,C,D,F,G,H,J,K,L,M,P,Q,R,S]3ZZ

Lower Bones

Ø   Medical and Surgical
Q   Lower Bones
B   Excision   Definition: Cutting out or off, without replacement, a portion of a body part
                       Explanation: The qualifier DIAGNOSTIC is used to identify excision procedures that are biopsies

Body Part Character 4	Approach Character 5	Device Character 6	Qualifier Character 7

Ø   Lumbar Vertebra
    Spinous process
    Transverse process
    Vertebral arch
    Vertebral body
    Vertebral foramen
    Vertebral lamina
    Vertebral pedicle
1   Sacrum
2   Pelvic Bone, Right
    Iliac crest
    Ilium
    Ischium
    Pubis
3   Pelvic Bone, Left
    See 2 Pelvic Bone, Right
4   Acetabulum, Right
5   Acetabulum, Left
6   Upper Femur, Right
    Femoral head
    Greater trochanter
    Lesser trochanter
    Neck of femur
7   Upper Femur, Left
    See 6 Upper Femur, Right
8   Femoral Shaft, Right
    Body of femur
9   Femoral Shaft, Left
    See 8 Femoral Shaft, Right
B   Lower Femur, Right
    Lateral condyle of femur
    Lateral epicondyle of femur
    Medial condyle of femur
    Medial epicondyle of femur
C   Lower Femur, Left
    See B Lower Femur, Right
D   Patella, Right
F   Patella, Left
G   Tibia, Right
    Lateral condyle of tibia
    Medial condyle of tibia
    Medial malleolus
H   Tibia, Left
    See G Tibia, Right
J   Fibula, Right
    Body of fibula
    Head of fibula
    Lateral malleolus
K   Fibula, Left
    See J Fibula, Right
L   Tarsal, Right
    Calcaneus
    Cuboid bone
    Intermediate cuneiform bone
    Lateral cuneiform bone
    Medial cuneiform bone
    Navicular bone
    Talus bone
M   Tarsal, Left
    See L Tarsal, Right
Q   Toe Phalanx, Right
R   Toe Phalanx, Left
S   Coccyx
	Ø Open
	3 Percutaneous
	4 Percutaneous Endoscopic
		Z No Device	**X Diagnostic**
			Z No Qualifier

N   Metatarsal, Right
    Fibular sesamoid
    Tibial sesamoid
P   Metatarsal, Left
    See N Metatarsal, Right
	Ø Open
	3 Percutaneous
	4 Percutaneous Endoscopic
		Z No Device	**2 Sesamoid Bone(s) 1st Toe**
			X Diagnostic
			Z No Qualifier

NC Noncovered Procedure   **LC** Limited Coverage   **OA** Questionable OB Admit   **NT** New Tech Add-on   ⊞ Combination Member   ♂ Male   ♀ Female

ICD-10-PCS 2022   **567**

Lower Bones

Ø   **Medical and Surgical**
Q   **Lower Bones**
C   **Extirpation**   Definition: Taking or cutting out solid matter from a body part

Explanation: The solid matter may be an abnormal byproduct of a biological function or a foreign body; it may be imbedded in a body part or in the lumen of a tubular body part. The solid matter may or may not have been previously broken into pieces.

Body Part Character 4	Approach Character 5	Device Character 6	Qualifier Character 7
Ø Lumbar Vertebra Spinous process Transverse process Vertebral arch Vertebral body Vertebral foramen Vertebral lamina Vertebral pedicle **1** Sacrum **2** Pelvic Bone, Right Iliac crest Ilium Ischium Pubis **3** Pelvic Bone, Left *See 2 Pelvic Bone, Right* **4** Acetabulum, Right **5** Acetabulum, Left **6** Upper Femur, Right Femoral head Greater trochanter Lesser trochanter Neck of femur **7** Upper Femur, Left *See 6 Upper Femur, Right* **8** Femoral Shaft, Right Body of femur **9** Femoral Shaft, Left *See 8 Femoral Shaft, Right* **B** Lower Femur, Right Lateral condyle of femur Lateral epicondyle of femur Medial condyle of femur Medial epicondyle of femur **C** Lower Femur, Left *See B Lower Femur, Right* **D** Patella, Right **F** Patella, Left **G** Tibia, Right Lateral condyle of tibia Medial condyle of tibia Medial malleolus **H** Tibia, Left *See G Tibia, Right* **J** Fibula, Right Body of fibula Head of fibula Lateral malleolus **K** Fibula, Left *See J Fibula, Right* **L** Tarsal, Right Calcaneus Cuboid bone Intermediate cuneiform bone Lateral cuneiform bone Medial cuneiform bone Navicular bone Talus bone **M** Tarsal, Left *See L Tarsal, Right* **N** Metatarsal, Right Fibular sesamoid Tibial sesamoid **P** Metatarsal, Left *See N Metatarsal, Right* **Q** Toe Phalanx, Right **R** Toe Phalanx, Left **S** Coccyx	**Ø** Open **3** Percutaneous **4** Percutaneous Endoscopic	**Z** No Device	**Z** No Qualifier

Ø   **Medical and Surgical**
Q   **Lower Bones**
D   **Extraction**   Definition: Pulling or stripping out or off all or a portion of a body part by the use of force
                            Explanation: The qualifier DIAGNOSTIC is used to identify extraction procedures that are biopsies

Body Part Character 4	Approach Character 5	Device Character 6	Qualifier Character 7

Ø   **Lumbar Vertebra**
    Spinous process
    Transverse process
    Vertebral arch
    Vertebral body
    Vertebral foramen
    Vertebral lamina
    Vertebral pedicle
	Ø Open	**Z** No Device	**Z** No Qualifier

1 **Sacrum**			

2   **Pelvic Bone, Right**
    Iliac crest
    Ilium
    Ischium
    Pubis			

3 **Pelvic Bone, Left** *See 2 Pelvic Bone, Right*			
4 **Acetabulum, Right**			
5 **Acetabulum, Left**			

6   **Upper Femur, Right**
    Femoral head
    Greater trochanter
    Lesser trochanter
    Neck of femur			

7 **Upper Femur, Left** *See 6 Upper Femur, Right*			
8 **Femoral Shaft, Right** Body of femur			
9 **Femoral Shaft, Left** *See 8 Femoral Shaft, Right*			

B   **Lower Femur, Right**
    Lateral condyle of femur
    Lateral epicondyle of femur
    Medial condyle of femur
    Medial epicondyle of femur			

C **Lower Femur, Left** *See B Lower Femur, Right*			
D **Patella, Right**			
F **Patella, Left**			

G   **Tibia, Right**
    Lateral condyle of tibia
    Medial condyle of tibia
    Medial malleolus			

H **Tibia, Left** *See G Tibia, Right*			

J   **Fibula, Right**
    Body of fibula
    Head of fibula
    Lateral malleolus			

K **Fibula, Left** *See J Fibula, Right*			

L   **Tarsal, Right**
    Calcaneus
    Cuboid bone
    Intermediate cuneiform bone
    Lateral cuneiform bone
    Medial cuneiform bone
    Navicular bone
    Talus bone			

M **Tarsal, Left** *See L Tarsal, Right*			

N   **Metatarsal, Right**
    Fibular sesamoid
    Tibial sesamoid			

P **Metatarsal, Left** *See N Metatarsal, Right*			
Q **Toe Phalanx, Right**			
R **Toe Phalanx, Left**			
S **Coccyx**			

NC Noncovered Procedure   **LC** Limited Coverage   **QA** Questionable OB Admit   **NT** New Tech Add-on   ⊞ Combination Member   ♂ Male   ♀ Female

ICD-10-PCS 2022   **569**

ØQD–ØQD

Ø   **Medical and Surgical**
Q   **Lower Bones**
H   **Insertion**

Definition: Putting in a nonbiological appliance that monitors, assists, performs, or prevents a physiological function but does not physically take the place of a body part

Explanation: None

Body Part Character 4		Approach Character 5	Device Character 6	Qualifier Character 7
Ø Lumbar Vertebra Spinous process Transverse process Vertebral arch Vertebral body Vertebral foramen Vertebral lamina Vertebral pedicle **1 Sacrum** **2 Pelvic Bone, Right** Iliac crest Ilium Ischium Pubis **3 Pelvic Bone, Left** *See 2 Pelvic Bone, Right* **4 Acetabulum, Right** **5 Acetabulum, Left**	**D Patella, Right** **F Patella, Left** **L Tarsal, Right** Calcaneus Cuboid bone Intermediate cuneiform bone Lateral cuneiform bone Medial cuneiform bone Navicular bone Talus bone **M Tarsal, Left** *See L Tarsal, Right* **N Metatarsal, Right** Fibular sesamoid Tibial sesamoid **P Metatarsal, Left** *See N Metatarsal, Right* **Q Toe Phalanx, Right** **R Toe Phalanx, Left** **S Coccyx**	**Ø Open** **3 Percutaneous** **4 Percutaneous Endoscopic**	**4 Internal Fixation Device** **5 External Fixation Device**	**Z No Qualifier**
6 Upper Femur, Right Femoral head Greater trochanter Lesser trochanter Neck of femur **7 Upper Femur, Left** *See 6 Upper Femur, Right* **B Lower Femur, Right** Lateral condyle of femur Lateral epicondyle of femur Medial condyle of femur Medial epicondyle of femur	**C Lower Femur, Left** *See B Lower Femur, Right* **J Fibula, Right** Body of fibula Head of fibula Lateral malleolus **K Fibula, Left** *See J Fibula, Right*	**Ø Open** **3 Percutaneous** **4 Percutaneous Endoscopic**	**4 Internal Fixation Device** **5 External Fixation Device** **6 Internal Fixation Device, Intramedullary** **8 External Fixation Device, Limb Lengthening** **B External Fixation Device, Monoplanar** **C External Fixation Device, Ring** **D External Fixation Device, Hybrid**	**Z No Qualifier**
8 Femoral Shaft, Right Body of femur **9 Femoral Shaft, Left** *See 8 Femoral Shaft, Right*	**G Tibia, Right** Lateral condyle of tibia Medial condyle of tibia Medial malleolus **H Tibia, Left** *See G Tibia, Right*	**Ø Open** **3 Percutaneous** **4 Percutaneous Endoscopic**	**4 Internal Fixation Device** **5 External Fixation Device** **6 Internal Fixation Device, Intramedullary** **7 Internal Fixation Device, Intramedullary Limb Lengthening** **8 External Fixation Device, Limb Lengthening** **B External Fixation Device, Monoplanar** **C External Fixation Device, Ring** **D External Fixation Device, Hybrid**	**Z No Qualifier**
Y Lower Bone		**Ø Open** **3 Percutaneous** **4 Percutaneous Endoscopic**	**M Bone Growth Stimulator**	**Z No Qualifier**

Non-OR   ØQH[6,7,B,C,J,K][Ø,3,4]8Z
Non-OR   ØQH[8,9,G,H][Ø,3,4]8Z

Ø   **Medical and Surgical**
Q   **Lower Bones**
J   **Inspection**

Definition: Visually and/or manually exploring a body part

Explanation: Visual exploration may be performed with or without optical instrumentation. Manual exploration may be performed directly or through intervening body layers.

Body Part Character 4	Approach Character 5	Device Character 6	Qualifier Character 7
Y Lower Bone	**Ø Open** **3 Percutaneous** **4 Percutaneous Endoscopic** **X External**	**Z No Device**	**Z No Qualifier**

Non-OR   ØQJY[3,X]ZZ

Ø   Medical and Surgical
Q   Lower Bones
N   Release   Definition: Freeing a body part from an abnormal physical constraint by cutting or by the use of force

Explanation: Some of the restraining tissue may be taken out but none of the body part is taken out

Body Part Character 4	Approach Character 5	Device Character 6	Qualifier Character 7
Ø Lumbar Vertebra Spinous process Transverse process Vertebral arch Vertebral body Vertebral foramen Vertebral lamina Vertebral pedicle **1 Sacrum** **2 Pelvic Bone, Right** Iliac crest Ilium Ischium Pubis **3 Pelvic Bone, Left** *See 2 Pelvic Bone, Right* **4 Acetabulum, Right** **5 Acetabulum, Left** **6 Upper Femur, Right** Femoral head Greater trochanter Lesser trochanter Neck of femur **7 Upper Femur, Left** *See 6 Upper Femur, Right* **8 Femoral Shaft, Right** Body of femur **9 Femoral Shaft, Left** *See 8 Femoral Shaft, Right* **B Lower Femur, Right** Lateral condyle of femur Lateral epicondyle of femur Medial condyle of femur Medial epicondyle of femur **C Lower Femur, Left** *See B Lower Femur, Right* **D Patella, Right** **F Patella, Left** **G Tibia, Right** Lateral condyle of tibia Medial condyle of tibia Medial malleolus **H Tibia, Left** *See G Tibia, Right* **J Fibula, Right** Body of fibula Head of fibula Lateral malleolus **K Fibula, Left** *See J Fibula, Right* **L Tarsal, Right** Calcaneus Cuboid bone Intermediate cuneiform bone Lateral cuneiform bone Medial cuneiform bone Navicular bone Talus bone **M Tarsal, Left** *See L Tarsal, Right* **N Metatarsal, Right** Fibular sesamoid Tibial sesamoid **P Metatarsal, Left** *See N Metatarsal, Right* **Q Toe Phalanx, Right** **R Toe Phalanx, Left** **S Coccyx**	**Ø Open** **3 Percutaneous** **4 Percutaneous Endoscopic**	**Z No Device**	**Z No Qualifier**

NC Noncovered Procedure   **LC** Limited Coverage   **QA** Questionable OB Admit   **NT** New Tech Add-on   ⊞ Combination Member   ♂ Male   ♀ Female

ICD-10-PCS 2022   571

ØQN–ØQN

Lower Bones

Ø   **Medical and Surgical**
Q   **Lower Bones**
P   **Removal**   Definition: Taking out or off a device from a body part

Explanation: If a device is taken out and a similar device put in without cutting or puncturing the skin or mucous membrane, the procedure is coded to the root operation CHANGE. Otherwise, the procedure for taking out a device is coded to the root operation REMOVAL.

Body Part Character 4		Approach Character 5	Device Character 6	Qualifier Character 7

Ø Lumbar Vertebra
  Spinous process
  Transverse process
  Vertebral arch
  Vertebral body
  Vertebral foramen
  Vertebral lamina
  Vertebral pedicle
1 Sacrum
2 Pelvic Bone, Right
  Iliac crest
  Ilium
  Ischium
  Pubis
3 Pelvic Bone, Left
  See 2 Pelvic Bone, Right
4 Acetabulum, Right
5 Acetabulum, Left
6 Upper Femur, Right
  Femoral head
  Greater trochanter
  Lesser trochanter
  Neck of femur
7 Upper Femur, Left
  See 6 Upper Femur, Right
8 Femoral Shaft, Right
  Body of femur
9 Femoral Shaft, Left
  See 8 Femoral Shaft, Right
B Lower Femur, Right
  Lateral condyle of femur
  Lateral epicondyle of femur
  Medial condyle of femur
  Medial epicondyle of femur
	C Lower Femur, Left
	  See B Lower Femur, Right
	D Patella, Right
	F Patella, Left
	G Tibia, Right
	  Lateral condyle of tibia
	  Medial condyle of tibia
	  Medial malleolus
	H Tibia, Left
	  See G Tibia, Right
	J Fibula, Right
	  Body of fibula
	  Head of fibula
	  Lateral malleolus
	K Fibula, Left
	  See J Fibula, Right
	L Tarsal, Right
	  Calcaneus
	  Cuboid bone
	  Intermediate cuneiform bone
	  Lateral cuneiform bone
	  Medial cuneiform bone
	  Navicular bone
	  Talus bone
	M Tarsal, Left
	  See L Tarsal, Right
	N Metatarsal, Right
	  Fibular sesamoid
	  Tibial sesamoid
	P Metatarsal, Left
	  See N Metatarsal, Right
	Q Toe Phalanx, Right
	R Toe Phalanx, Left
	S Coccyx
		Ø Open
		3 Percutaneous
		4 Percutaneous Endoscopic
			4 Internal Fixation Device
			5 External Fixation Device
			7 Autologous Tissue Substitute
			J Synthetic Substitute
			K Nonautologous Tissue Substitute
				Z No Qualifier

Ø Lumbar Vertebra
  Spinous process
  Transverse process
  Vertebral arch
  Vertebral body
  Vertebral foramen
  Vertebral lamina
  Vertebral pedicle
1 Sacrum
2 Pelvic Bone, Right
  Iliac crest
  Ilium
  Ischium
  Pubis
3 Pelvic Bone, Left
  See 2 Pelvic Bone, Right
4 Acetabulum, Right
5 Acetabulum, Left
6 Upper Femur, Right
  Femoral head
  Greater trochanter
  Lesser trochanter
  Neck of femur
7 Upper Femur, Left
  See 6 Upper Femur, Right
8 Femoral Shaft, Right
  Body of femur
9 Femoral Shaft, Left
  See 8 Femoral Shaft, Right
B Lower Femur, Right
  Lateral condyle of femur
  Lateral epicondyle of femur
  Medial condyle of femur
  Medial epicondyle of femur
	C Lower Femur, Left
	  See B Lower Femur, Right
	D Patella, Right
	F Patella, Left
	G Tibia, Right
	  Lateral condyle of tibia
	  Medial condyle of tibia
	  Medial malleolus
	H Tibia, Left
	  See G Tibia, Right
	J Fibula, Right
	  Body of fibula
	  Head of fibula
	  Lateral malleolus
	K Fibula, Left
	  See J Fibula, Right
	L Tarsal, Right
	  Calcaneus
	  Cuboid bone
	  Intermediate cuneiform bone
	  Lateral cuneiform bone
	  Medial cuneiform bone
	  Navicular bone
	  Talus bone
	M Tarsal, Left
	  See L Tarsal, Right
	N Metatarsal, Right
	  Fibular sesamoid
	  Tibial sesamoid
	P Metatarsal, Left
	  See N Metatarsal, Right
	Q Toe Phalanx, Right
	R Toe Phalanx, Left
	S Coccyx
		X External	4 Internal Fixation Device
			5 External Fixation Device
				Z No Qualifier

Y Lower Bone		Ø Open 3 Percutaneous 4 Percutaneous Endoscopic X External	Ø Drainage Device M Bone Growth Stimulator	Z No Qualifier

Non-OR	ØQPYX[Ø,M]Z	Non-OR	ØQPY3ØZ	Non-OR	ØQP[Ø,1,2,3,4,5,6,7,8,9,B,C,D,F,G,H,J,K,L,M,N,P,Q,R,S]X[4,5]Z

Non-OR Procedure   DRG Non-OR Procedure   Valid OR Procedure   HAC Associated Procedure   Combination Only   New/Revised GREEN

Ø   **Medical and Surgical**
Q   **Lower Bones**
Q   **Repair**   Definition: Restoring, to the extent possible, a body part to its normal anatomic structure and function

                     Explanation: Used only when the method to accomplish the repair is not one of the other root operations

Body Part Character 4	Approach Character 5	Device Character 6	Qualifier Character 7

Ø   **Lumbar Vertebra**
    Spinous process
    Transverse process
    Vertebral arch
    Vertebral body
    Vertebral foramen
    Vertebral lamina
    Vertebral pedicle
	Ø Open
	3 Percutaneous
	4 Percutaneous Endoscopic
	X External
		Z No Device	Z No Qualifier

1 **Sacrum**			

2   **Pelvic Bone, Right**
    Iliac crest
    Ilium
    Ischium
    Pubis			

3 **Pelvic Bone, Left** *See 2 Pelvic Bone, Right*			
4 **Acetabulum, Right**			
5 **Acetabulum, Left**			

6   **Upper Femur, Right**
    Femoral head
    Greater trochanter
    Lesser trochanter
    Neck of femur			

7 **Upper Femur, Left** *See 6 Upper Femur, Right*			
8 **Femoral Shaft, Right** Body of femur			
9 **Femoral Shaft, Left** *See 8 Femoral Shaft, Right*			

B   **Lower Femur, Right**
    Lateral condyle of femur
    Lateral epicondyle of femur
    Medial condyle of femur
    Medial epicondyle of femur			

C **Lower Femur, Left** *See B Lower Femur, Right*			
D **Patella, Right**			
F **Patella, Left**			

G   **Tibia, Right**
    Lateral condyle of tibia
    Medial condyle of tibia
    Medial malleolus			

H **Tibia, Left** *See G Tibia, Right*			

J   **Fibula, Right**
    Body of fibula
    Head of fibula
    Lateral malleolus			

K **Fibula, Left** *See J Fibula, Right*			

L   **Tarsal, Right**
    Calcaneus
    Cuboid bone
    Intermediate cuneiform bone
    Lateral cuneiform bone
    Medial cuneiform bone
    Navicular bone
    Talus bone			

M **Tarsal, Left** *See L Tarsal, Right*			

N   **Metatarsal, Right**
    Fibular sesamoid
    Tibial sesamoid			

P **Metatarsal, Left** *See N Metatarsal, Right*			
Q **Toe Phalanx, Right**			
R **Toe Phalanx, Left**			
S **Coccyx**			

Non-OR   ØQQ[Ø,1,2,3,4,5,6,7,8,9,B,C,D,F,G,H,J,K,L,M,N,P,Q,R,S]XZZ

NC Noncovered Procedure   LC Limited Coverage   QA Questionable OB Admit   NT New Tech Add-on   ⊞ Combination Member   ♂Male   ♀Female

ICD-10-PCS 2022   **573**

ØQQ–ØQQ

Ø Medical and Surgical
Q Lower Bones
R Replacement

Definition: Putting in or on biological or synthetic material that physically takes the place and/or function of all or a portion of a body part
Explanation: The body part may have been taken out or replaced, or may be taken out, physically eradicated, or rendered nonfunctional during the REPLACEMENT procedure. A REMOVAL procedure is coded for taking out the device used in a previous replacement procedure.

Body Part Character 4	Approach Character 5	Device Character 6	Qualifier Character 7
Ø Lumbar Vertebra Spinous process Transverse process Vertebral arch Vertebral body Vertebral foramen Vertebral lamina Vertebral pedicle **1 Sacrum** **2 Pelvic Bone, Right** Iliac crest Ilium Ischium Pubis **3 Pelvic Bone, Left** *See 2 Pelvic Bone, Right* **4 Acetabulum, Right** **5 Acetabulum, Left** **6 Upper Femur, Right** Femoral head Greater trochanter Lesser trochanter Neck of femur **7 Upper Femur, Left** *See 6 Upper Femur, Right* **8 Femoral Shaft, Right** Body of femur **9 Femoral Shaft, Left** *See 8 Femoral Shaft, Right* **B Lower Femur, Right** Lateral condyle of femur Lateral epicondyle of femur Medial condyle of femur Medial epicondyle of femur **C Lower Femur, Left** *See B Lower Femur, Right* **D Patella, Right** **F Patella, Left** **G Tibia, Right** Lateral condyle of tibia Medial condyle of tibia Medial malleolus **H Tibia, Left** *See G Tibia, Right* **J Fibula, Right** Body of fibula Head of fibula Lateral malleolus **K Fibula, Left** *See J Fibula, Right* **L Tarsal, Right** Calcaneus Cuboid bone Intermediate cuneiform bone Lateral cuneiform bone Medial cuneiform bone Navicular bone Talus bone **M Tarsal, Left** *See L Tarsal, Right* **N Metatarsal, Right** Fibular sesamoid Tibial sesamoid **P Metatarsal, Left** *See N Metatarsal, Right* **Q Toe Phalanx, Right** **R Toe Phalanx, Left** **S Coccyx**	**Ø Open** **3 Percutaneous** **4 Percutaneous Endoscopic**	**7 Autologous Tissue Substitute** **J Synthetic Substitute** **K Nonautologous Tissue Substitute**	**Z No Qualifier**

0   **Medical and Surgical**
Q   **Lower Bones**
S   **Reposition**   Definition: Moving to its normal location, or other suitable location, all or a portion of a body part

Explanation: The body part is moved to a new location from an abnormal location, or from a normal location where it is not functioning correctly. The body part may or may not be cut out or off to be moved to the new location.

Body Part Character 4		Approach Character 5	Device Character 6	Qualifier Character 7
0 **Lumbar Vertebra** Spinous process Transverse process Vertebral arch Vertebral body Vertebral foramen Vertebral lamina Vertebral pedicle		**0** Open **4** Percutaneous Endoscopic	**3** Spinal Stabilization Device, Vertebral Body Tether **4** Internal Fixation Device **Z** No Device	**Z** No Qualifier
0 **Lumbar Vertebra** ⊞ Spinous process Transverse process Vertebral arch Vertebral body Vertebral foramen Vertebral lamina Vertebral pedicle		**3** Percutaneous	**4** Internal Fixation Device **Z** No Device	**Z** No Qualifier
0 **Lumbar Vertebra** Spinous process Transverse process Vertebral arch Vertebral body Vertebral foramen Vertebral lamina Vertebral pedicle		**X** External	**Z** No Device	**Z** No Qualifier
1 **Sacrum** ⊞ **4** **Acetabulum, Right** **5** **Acetabulum, Left** **S** **Coccyx** ⊞		**0** Open **3** Percutaneous **4** Percutaneous Endoscopic	**4** Internal Fixation Device **Z** No Device	**Z** No Qualifier
1 **Sacrum** **4** **Acetabulum, Right** **5** **Acetabulum, Left** **S** **Coccyx**		**X** External	**Z** No Device	**Z** No Qualifier

2   **Pelvic Bone, Right**
Iliac crest
Ilium
Ischium
Pubis
3   **Pelvic Bone, Left**
See 2 Pelvic Bone, Right
D   **Patella, Right**
F   **Patella, Left**
L   **Tarsal, Right**
Calcaneus
Cuboid bone
Intermediate cuneiform
    bone
Lateral cuneiform bone
Medial cuneiform bone
Navicular bone
Talus bone
	M **Tarsal, Left**
	     See L Tarsal, Right
	Q **Toe Phalanx, Right**
	R **Toe Phalanx, Left**
		0 Open
		3 Percutaneous
		4 Percutaneous Endoscopic
			4 Internal Fixation Device
			5 External Fixation Device
			Z No Device
				Z No Qualifier

2   **Pelvic Bone, Right**
Iliac crest
Ilium
Ischium
Pubis
3   **Pelvic Bone, Left**
See 2 Pelvic Bone, Right
D   **Patella, Right**
F   **Patella, Left**
L   **Tarsal, Right**
Calcaneus
Cuboid bone
Intermediate cuneiform
    bone
Lateral cuneiform bone
Medial cuneiform bone
Navicular bone
Talus bone
	M **Tarsal, Left**
	     See L Tarsal, Right
	Q **Toe Phalanx, Right**
	R **Toe Phalanx, Left**
		X External	**Z** No Device	**Z** No Qualifier

Non-OR	0QS0XZZ
Non-OR	0QS[4,5][3,4]ZZ
Non-OR	0QS[1,4,5,S]XZZ
Non-OR	0QS[2,3,D,F,L,M,Q,R][3,4]ZZ
Non-OR	0QS[2,3,D,F,L,M,Q,R]XZZ

See Appendix L for Procedure Combinations
⊞   0QS03ZZ
⊞   0QS[1,S]3ZZ

0QS Continued on next page

NC Noncovered Procedure   **LC** Limited Coverage   **QA** Questionable OB Admit   **NT** New Tech Add-on   ⊞ Combination Member   ♂ Male   ♀ Female

ICD-10-PCS 2022   **575**

0QS–0QS

Lower Bones

Ø Medical and Surgical
Q Lower Bones
S Reposition

ØQS Continued

Definition: Moving to its normal location, or other suitable location, all or a portion of a body part

Explanation: The body part is moved to a new location from an abnormal location, or from a normal location where it is not functioning correctly. The body part may or may not be cut out or off to be moved to the new location.

Body Part Character 4	Approach Character 5	Device Character 6	Qualifier Character 7
6 Upper Femur, Right 　Femoral head 　Greater trochanter 　Lesser trochanter 　Neck of femur 7 Upper Femur, Left 　*See 6 Upper Femur, Right* 8 Femoral Shaft, Right 　Body of femur 9 Femoral Shaft, Left 　*See 8 Femoral Shaft, Right* B Lower Femur, Right 　Lateral condyle of femur 　Lateral epicondyle of femur 　Medial condyle of femur 　Medial epicondyle of femur C Lower Femur, Left 　*See B Lower Femur, Right* G Tibia, Right 　Lateral condyle of tibia 　Medial condyle of tibia 　Medial malleolus H Tibia, Left 　*See G Tibia, Right* J Fibula, Right 　Body of fibula 　Head of fibula 　Lateral malleolus K Fibula, Left 　*See J Fibula, Right*	Ø Open 3 Percutaneous 4 Percutaneous Endoscopic	4 Internal Fixation Device 5 External Fixation Device 6 Internal Fixation Device, 　Intramedullary B External Fixation Device, 　Monoplanar C External Fixation Device, Ring D External Fixation Device, Hybrid Z No Device	Z No Qualifier
6 Upper Femur, Right 　Femoral head 　Greater trochanter 　Lesser trochanter 　Neck of femur 7 Upper Femur, Left 　*See 6 Upper Femur, Right* 8 Femoral Shaft, Right 　Body of femur 9 Femoral Shaft, Left 　*See 8 Femoral Shaft, Right* B Lower Femur, Right 　Lateral condyle of femur 　Lateral epicondyle of femur 　Medial condyle of femur 　Medial epicondyle of femur C Lower Femur, Left 　*See B Lower Femur, Right* G Tibia, Right 　Lateral condyle of tibia 　Medial condyle of tibia 　Medial malleolus H Tibia, Left 　*See G Tibia, Right* J Fibula, Right 　Body of fibula 　Head of fibula 　Lateral malleolus K Fibula, Left 　*See J Fibula, Right*	X External	Z No Device	Z No Qualifier
N Metatarsal, Right 　Fibular sesamoid 　Tibial sesamoid P Metatarsal, Left 　*See N Metatarsal, Right*	Ø Open 3 Percutaneous 4 Percutaneous Endoscopic	4 Internal Fixation Device 5 External Fixation Device Z No Device	2 Sesamoid Bone(s) 1st Toe Z No Qualifier
N Metatarsal, Right 　Fibular sesamoid 　Tibial sesamoid P Metatarsal, Left 　*See N Metatarsal, Right*	X External	Z No Device	2 Sesamoid Bone(s) 1st Toe Z No Qualifier

Non-OR　ØQS[6,7,8,9,B,C,G,H,J,K][3,4]ZZ
Non-OR　ØQS[6,7,8,9,B,C,G,H,J,K]XZZ
Non-OR　ØQS[N,P][3,4]Z[2,Z]
Non-OR　ØQS[N,P]XZ[2,Z]

Non-OR Procedure　　DRG Non-OR Procedure　　Valid OR Procedure　　HAC Associated Procedure　　Combination Only　　New/Revised GREEN

0   **Medical and Surgical**
Q   **Lower Bones**
T   **Resection**   Definition: Cutting out or off, without replacement, all of a body part

Explanation: None

Body Part Character 4		Approach Character 5	Device Character 6	Qualifier Character 7

2 Pelvic Bone, Right
  Iliac crest
  Ilium
  Ischium
  Pubis
3 Pelvic Bone, Left
  See 2 Pelvic Bone, Right
4 Acetabulum, Right
5 Acetabulum, Left
6 Upper Femur, Right
  Femoral head
  Greater trochanter
  Lesser trochanter
  Neck of femur
7 Upper Femur, Left
  See 6 Upper Femur, Right
8 Femoral Shaft, Right
  Body of femur
9 Femoral Shaft, Left
  See 8 Femoral Shaft, Right
B Lower Femur, Right
  Lateral condyle of femur
  Lateral epicondyle of femur
  Medial condyle of femur
  Medial epicondyle of femur
C Lower Femur, Left
  See B Lower Femur, Right
D Patella, Right
	F Patella, Left
	G Tibia, Right
	  Lateral condyle of tibia
	  Medial condyle of tibia
	  Medial malleolus
	H Tibia, Left
	  See G Tibia, Right
	J Fibula, Right
	  Body of fibula
	  Head of fibula
	  Lateral malleolus
	K Fibula, Left
	  See J Fibula, Right
	L Tarsal, Right
	  Calcaneus
	  Cuboid bone
	  Intermediate cuneiform bone
	  Lateral cuneiform bone
	  Medial cuneiform bone
	  Navicular bone
	  Talus bone
	M Tarsal, Left
	  See L Tarsal, Right
	N Metatarsal, Right
	  Fibular sesamoid
	  Tibial sesamoid
	P Metatarsal, Left
	  See N Metatarsal, Right
	Q Toe Phalanx, Right
	R Toe Phalanx, Left
	S Coccyx
		0 Open	**Z No Device**	**Z No Qualifier**

0   **Medical and Surgical**
Q   **Lower Bones**
U   **Supplement**   Definition: Putting in or on biological or synthetic material that physically reinforces and/or augments the function of a portion of a body part

Explanation: The biological material is non-living, or is living and from the same individual. The body part may have been previously replaced, and the SUPPLEMENT procedure is performed to physically reinforce and/or augment the function of the replaced body part.

Body Part Character 4		Approach Character 5	Device Character 6	Qualifier Character 7

0 Lumbar Vertebra ⊞
  Spinous process
  Transverse process
  Vertebral arch
  Vertebral body
  Vertebral foramen
  Vertebral lamina
  Vertebral pedicle
1 Sacrum ⊞
2 Pelvic Bone, Right
  Iliac crest
  Ilium
  Ischium
  Pubis
3 Pelvic Bone, Left
  See 2 Pelvic Bone, Right
4 Acetabulum, Right
5 Acetabulum, Left
6 Upper Femur, Right
  Femoral head
  Greater trochanter
  Lesser trochanter
  Neck of femur
7 Upper Femur, Left
  See 6 Upper Femur, Right
8 Femoral Shaft, Right
  Body of femur
9 Femoral Shaft, Left
  See 8 Femoral Shaft, Right
B Lower Femur, Right
  Lateral condyle of femur
  Lateral epicondyle of femur
  Medial condyle of femur
  Medial epicondyle of femur
	C Lower Femur, Left
	  See B Lower Femur, Right
	D Patella, Right
	F Patella, Left
	G Tibia, Right
	  Lateral condyle of tibia
	  Medial condyle of tibia
	  Medial malleolus
	H Tibia, Left
	  See G Tibia, Right
	J Fibula, Right
	  Body of fibula
	  Head of fibula
	  Lateral malleolus
	K Fibula, Left
	  See J Fibula, Right
	L Tarsal, Right
	  Calcaneus
	  Cuboid bone
	  Intermediate cuneiform bone
	  Lateral cuneiform bone
	  Medial cuneiform bone
	  Navicular bone
	  Talus bone
	M Tarsal, Left
	  See L Tarsal, Right
	N Metatarsal, Right
	  Fibular sesamoid
	  Tibial sesamoid
	P Metatarsal, Left
	  See N Metatarsal, Right
	Q Toe Phalanx, Right
	R Toe Phalanx, Left
	S Coccyx ⊞
		0 Open
		3 Percutaneous
		4 Percutaneous Endoscopic
			7 Autologous Tissue
			  Substitute
			J Synthetic Substitute
			K Nonautologous Tissue
			  Substitute
				Z No Qualifier

See Appendix L for Procedure Combinations
⊞   0QU[0,1,S]3JZ

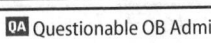 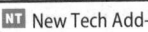

NC Noncovered Procedure   **LC** Limited Coverage   **QA** Questionable OB Admit   **NT** New Tech Add-on   ⊞ Combination Member   ♂ Male   ♀ Female

ICD-10-PCS 2022   577

Ø **Medical and Surgical**
Q **Lower Bones**
W **Revision**

Definition: Correcting, to the extent possible, a portion of a malfunctioning device or the position of a displaced device

Explanation: Revision can include correcting a malfunctioning or displaced device by taking out or putting in components of the device such as a screw or pin

Body Part Character 4	Approach Character 5	Device Character 6	Qualifier Character 7
Ø **Lumbar Vertebra** Spinous process Transverse process Vertebral arch Vertebral body Vertebral foramen Vertebral lamina Vertebral pedicle **1** **Sacrum** **4** **Acetabulum, Right** **5** **Acetabulum, Left** **S** **Coccyx**	**Ø** Open **3** Percutaneous **4** Percutaneous Endoscopic **X** External	**4** Internal Fixation Device **7** Autologous Tissue Substitute **J** Synthetic Substitute **K** Nonautologous Tissue Substitute	**Z** No Qualifier
2 **Pelvic Bone, Right** Iliac crest Ilium Ischium Pubis **3** **Pelvic Bone, Left** See 2 Pelvic Bone, Right **6** **Upper Femur, Right** Femoral head Greater trochanter Lesser trochanter Neck of femur **7** **Upper Femur, Left** See 6 Upper Femur, Right **8** **Femoral Shaft, Right** Body of femur **9** **Femoral Shaft, Left** See 8 Femoral Shaft, Right **B** **Lower Femur, Right** Lateral condyle of femur Lateral epicondyle of femur Medial condyle of femur Medial epicondyle of femur **C** **Lower Femur, Left** See B Lower Femur, Right **D** **Patella, Right** **F** **Patella, Left** **G** **Tibia, Right** Lateral condyle of tibia Medial condyle of tibia Medial malleolus **H** **Tibia, Left** See G Tibia, Right **J** **Fibula, Right** Body of fibula Head of fibula Lateral malleolus **K** **Fibula, Left** See J Fibula, Right **L** **Tarsal, Right** Calcaneus Cuboid bone Intermediate cuneiform bone Lateral cuneiform bone Medial cuneiform bone Navicular bone Talus bone **M** **Tarsal, Left** See L Tarsal, Right **N** **Metatarsal, Right** Fibular sesamoid Tibial sesamoid **P** **Metatarsal, Left** See N Metatarsal, Right **Q** **Toe Phalanx, Right** **R** **Toe Phalanx, Left**	**Ø** Open **3** Percutaneous **4** Percutaneous Endoscopic **X** External	**4** Internal Fixation Device **5** External Fixation Device **7** Autologous Tissue Substitute **J** Synthetic Substitute **K** Nonautologous Tissue Substitute	**Z** No Qualifier
Y **Lower Bone**	**Ø** Open **3** Percutaneous **4** Percutaneous Endoscopic **X** External	**Ø** Drainage Device **M** Bone Growth Stimulator	**Z** No Qualifier

Non-OR ØQW[Ø,1,4,5,S]X[4,7,J,K]Z
Non-OR ØQW[2,3,6,7,8,9,B,C,D,F,G,H,J,K,L,M,N,P,Q,R]X[4,5,7,J,K]Z

Non-OR ØQWYX[Ø,M]Z

Non-OR Procedure   DRG Non-OR Procedure   Valid OR Procedure   HAC Associated Procedure   Combination Only   New/Revised GREEN

Upper Joints ØR2–ØRW

Character Meanings*

This Character Meaning table is provided as a guide to assist the user in the identification of character members that may be found in this section of code tables. It **SHOULD NOT** be used to build a PCS code.

Operation–Character 3	Body Part–Character 4	Approach–Character 5	Device–Character 6	Qualifier–Character 7
2 Change	Ø Occipital-cervical Joint	Ø Open	Ø Drainage Device OR Synthetic Substitute, Reverse Ball and Socket	Ø Anterior Approach, Anterior Column
5 Destruction	1 Cervical Vertebral Joint	3 Percutaneous	3 Infusion Device OR Internal Fixation Device, Sustained Compression	1 Posterior Approach, Posterior Column
9 Drainage	2 Cervical Vertebral Joint, 2 or more	4 Percutaneous Endoscopic	4 Internal Fixation Device	6 Humeral Surface
B Excision	3 Cervical Vertebral Disc	X External	5 External Fixation Device	7 Glenoid Surface
C Extirpation	4 Cervicothoracic Vertebral Joint		7 Autologous Tissue Substitute	J Posterior Approach, Anterior Column
G Fusion	5 Cervicothoracic Vertebral Disc		8 Spacer	X Diagnostic
H Insertion	6 Thoracic Vertebral Joint		A Interbody Fusion Device	Z No Qualifier
J Inspection	7 Thoracic Vertebral Joint, 2 to 7		B Spinal Stabilization Device, Interspinous Process	
N Release	8 Thoracic Vertebral Joint, 8 or more		C Spinal Stabilization Device, Pedicle-Based	
P Removal	9 Thoracic Vertebral Disc		D Spinal Stabilization Device, Facet Replacement	
Q Repair	A Thoracolumbar Vertebral Joint		J Synthetic Substitute	
R Replacement	B Thoracolumbar Vertebral Disc		K Nonautologous Tissue Substitute	
S Reposition	C Temporomandibular Joint, Right		Y Other Device	
T Resection	D Temporomandibular Joint, Left		Z No Device	
U Supplement	E Sternoclavicular Joint, Right			
W Revision	F Sternoclavicular Joint, Left			
	G Acromioclavicular Joint, Right			
	H Acromioclavicular Joint, Left			
	J Shoulder Joint, Right			
	K Shoulder Joint, Left			
	L Elbow Joint, Right			
	M Elbow Joint, Left			
	N Wrist Joint, Right			
	P Wrist Joint, Left			
	Q Carpal Joint, Right			
	R Carpal Joint, Left			
	S Carpometacarpal Joint, Right			
	T Carpometacarpal Joint, Left			
	U Metacarpophalangeal Joint, Right			
	V Metacarpophalangeal Joint, Left			
	W Finger Phalangeal Joint, Right			
	X Finger Phalangeal Joint, Left			
	Y Upper Joint			

* Includes synovial membrane.

AHA Coding Clinic for table ØRB

2019, 3Q, 26	Acromioclavicular joint reconstruction using allograft

AHA Coding Clinic for table ØRG

2021, 1Q, 18	Placement of interspinous distraction device (spacer) for decompression
2021, 1Q, 53	Official guidelines for coding and reporting for interbody fusion device B3.10c
2020, 4Q, 56-58	Intramedullary sustained compression joint fusion
2020, 2Q, 27	Spinal Fusion with NuVasive® VersaTie®
2020, 1Q, 33	Spinal fusion without use of bone graft
2019, 3Q, 28	Use of VERTE-STACK™ implant with fusion
2019, 3Q, 35	Fusion procedures of the spine (guideline B3.10c)
2019, 2Q, 19	Cervical spinal fusion, decompression and placement of interfacet stabilization device
2019, 1Q, 30	Spinal fusion performed at same level as decompressive laminectomy
2018, 4Q, 43	Joint fusion device value
2018, 1Q, 22	Spinal fusion procedures without bone graft
2017, 4Q, 62	Added and revised device values - Nerve substitutes
2017, 4Q, 76	Radiolucent porous interbody fusion device
2017, 2Q, 23	Decompression of spinal cord and placement of instrumentation
2014, 3Q, 30	Spinal fusion and fixation instrumentation
2014, 2Q, 7	Anterior cervical thoracic fusion with total discectomy
2013, 1Q, 21-23	Spinal fusion of thoracic and lumbar vertebrae
2013, 1Q, 29	Cervical and thoracic spinal fusion

AHA Coding Clinic for table ØRH

2021, 1Q, 18	Placement of interspinous distraction device (spacer) for decompression
2019, 2Q, 40	Decompression of spinal cord and placement of instrumentation
2018, 3Q, 26	Anterior vertebral tethering using Dynesys Tethering System
2017, 2Q, 23	Decompression of spinal cord and placement of instrumentation
2016, 3Q, 32	Rotator cuff repair, tenodesis, decompression, acromioplasty and coracoplasty

AHA Coding Clinic for table ØRN

2019, 1Q, 30	Spinal fusion performed at same level as decompressive laminectomy
2016, 3Q, 32	Rotator cuff repair, tenodesis, decompression, acromioplasty and coracoplasty
2015, 2Q, 22	Arthroscopic subacromial decompression
2015, 2Q, 23	Arthroscopic release of shoulder joint

AHA Coding Clinic for table ØRP

2017, 4Q, 107	Total ankle replacement versus revision

AHA Coding Clinic for table ØRQ

2016, 1Q, 30	Thermal capsulorrhapy of shoulder

AHA Coding Clinic for table ØRR

2018, 4Q, 92	Radial head arthroplasty
2017, 4Q, 107	Total ankle replacement versus revision
2015, 3Q, 14	Endoprosthetic replacement of humerus and tendon reattachment
2015, 1Q, 27	Reverse total shoulder arthroplasty

AHA Coding Clinic for table ØRS

2019, 3Q, 26	Acromioclavicular joint reconstruction using allograft
2018, 3Q, 26	Anterior vertebral tethering using Dynesys Tethering System
2015, 2Q, 35	Application of tongs to reduce and stabilize cervical fracture
2014, 4Q, 32	Open reduction internal fixation of fracture with debridement
2014, 3Q, 33	Radial fracture treatment with open reduction internal fixation, and release of carpal ligament
2013, 2Q, 39	Application of cervical tongs for reduction of cervical fracture

AHA Coding Clinic for table ØRT

2019, 3Q, 26	Acromioclavicular joint reconstruction using allograft
2014, 2Q, 7	Anterior cervical thoracic fusion with total discectomy

AHA Coding Clinic for table ØRU

2019, 3Q, 26	Acromioclavicular joint reconstruction using allograft
2015, 3Q, 26	Thumb arthroplasty with resection of trapezium

AHA Coding Clinic for table ØRW

2017, 4Q, 107	Total ankle replacement versus revision

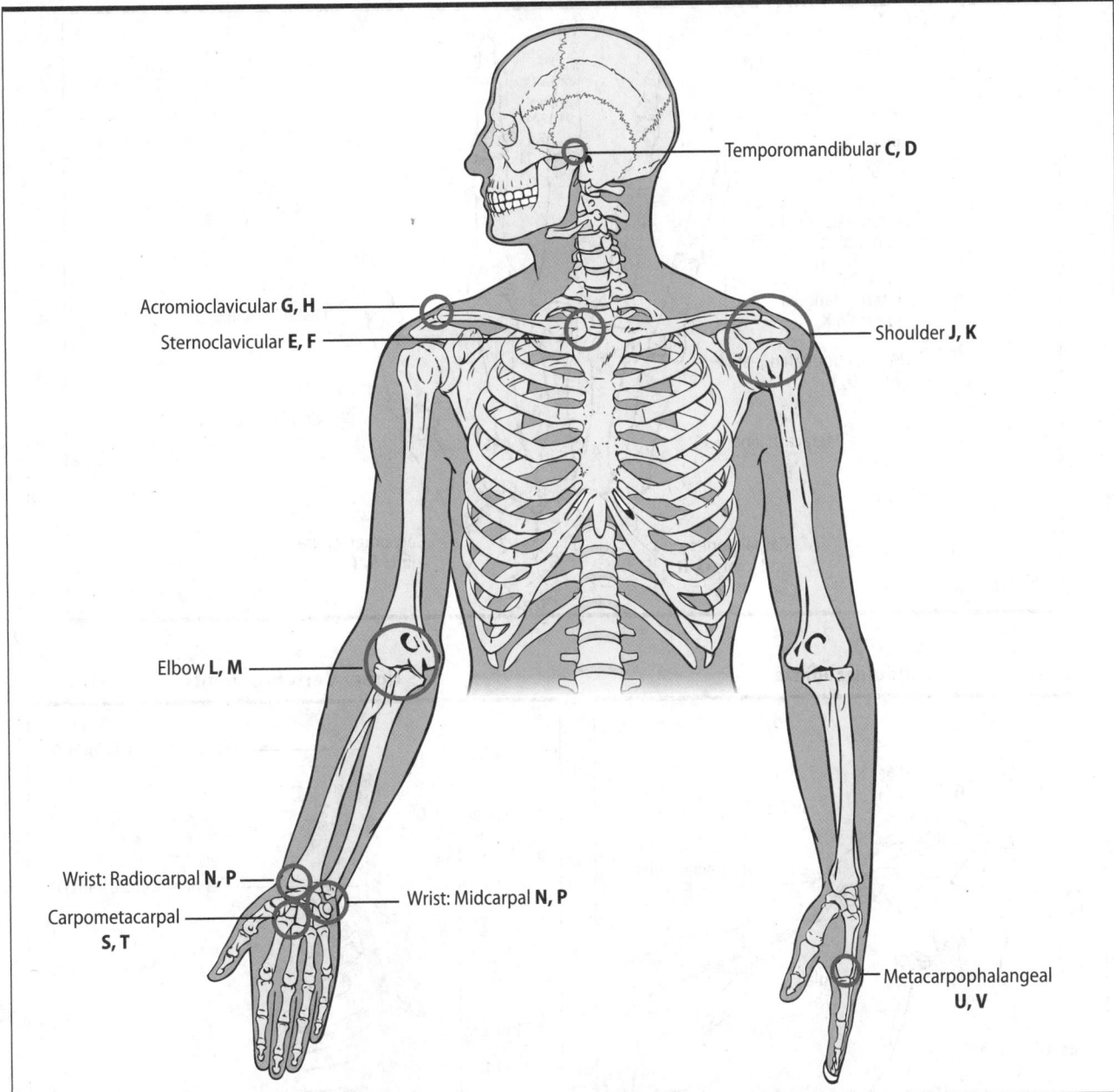

Temporomandibular **C, D**

Acromioclavicular **G, H**

Sternoclavicular **E, F**

Shoulder **J, K**

Elbow **L, M**

Wrist: Radiocarpal **N, P**

Wrist: Midcarpal **N, P**

Carpometacarpal **S, T**

Metacarpophalangeal **U, V**

Hand Joints

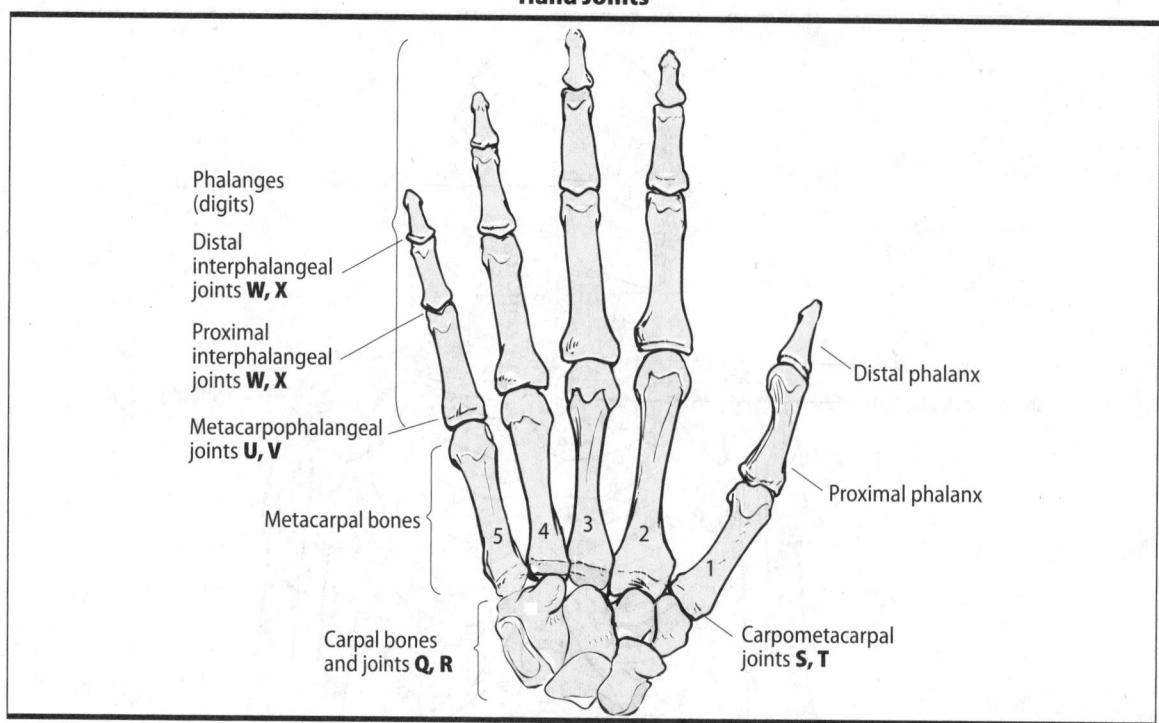

Phalanges
(digits)

Distal
interphalangeal
joints **W, X**

Proximal
interphalangeal
joints **W, X**

Metacarpophalangeal
joints **U, V**

Metacarpal bones

Carpal bones
and joints **Q, R**

Distal phalanx

Proximal phalanx

Carpometacarpal
joints **S, T**

5 4 3 2 1

Shoulder Joints

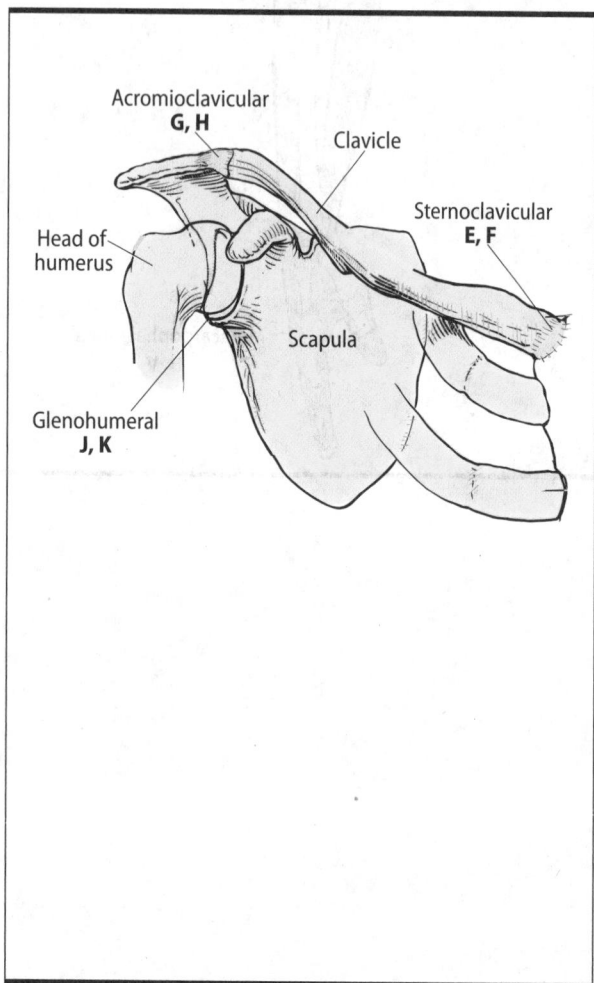

Acromioclavicular
G, H

Clavicle

Sternoclavicular
E, F

Head of
humerus

Glenohumeral
J, K

Scapula

Upper Vertebral Joints

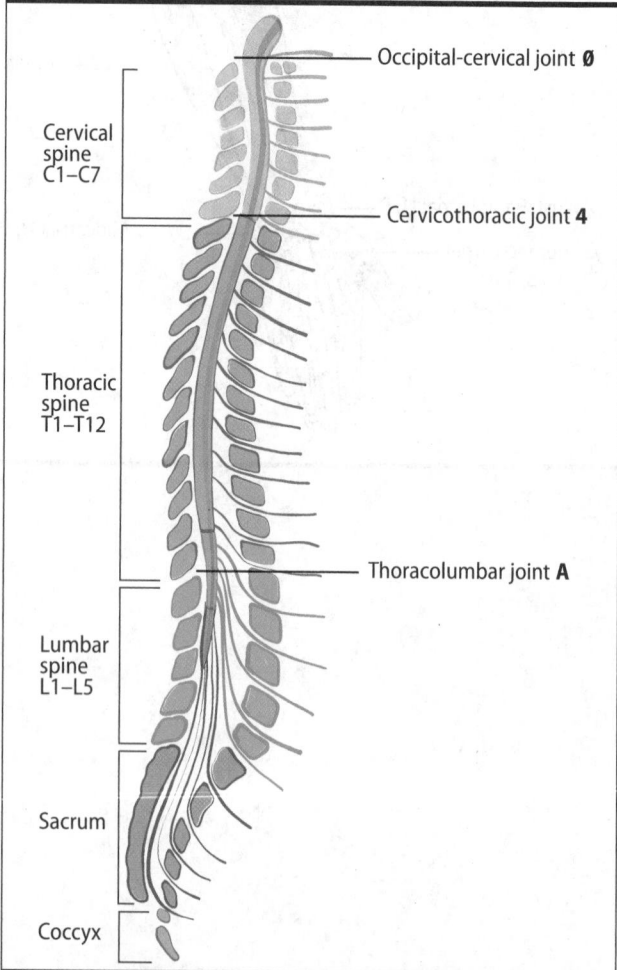

Occipital-cervical joint **Ø**

Cervicothoracic joint **4**

Cervical
spine
C1–C7

Thoracic
spine
T1–T12

Thoracolumbar joint **A**

Lumbar
spine
L1–L5

Sacrum

Coccyx

0   **Medical and Surgical**
R   **Upper Joints**
2   **Change**   Definition: Taking out or off a device from a body part and putting back an identical or similar device in or on the same body part without cutting or puncturing the skin or a mucous membrane

                 Explanation: All CHANGE procedures are coded using the approach EXTERNAL

Body Part Character 4	Approach Character 5	Device Character 6	Qualifier Character 7
Y Upper Joint	X External	0 Drainage Device Y Other Device	Z No Qualifier

Non-OR   All body part, approach, device, and qualifier values

---

0   **Medical and Surgical**
R   **Upper Joints**
5   **Destruction**   Definition: Physical eradication of all or a portion of a body part by the direct use of energy, force, or a destructive agent

                     Explanation: None of the body part is physically taken out

Body Part Character 4	Approach Character 5	Device Character 6	Qualifier Character 7

0   Occipital-cervical Joint
1   Cervical Vertebral Joint
     Atlantoaxial joint
     Cervical facet joint
3   Cervical Vertebral Disc
4   Cervicothoracic Vertebral Joint
     Cervicothoracic facet joint
5   Cervicothoracic Vertebral Disc
6   Thoracic Vertebral Joint
     Costotransverse joint
     Costovertebral joint
     Thoracic facet joint
9   Thoracic Vertebral Disc
A   Thoracolumbar Vertebral Joint
     Thoracolumbar facet joint
B   Thoracolumbar Vertebral Disc
C   Temporomandibular Joint, Right
D   Temporomandibular Joint, Left
E   Sternoclavicular Joint, Right
F   Sternoclavicular Joint, Left
G   Acromioclavicular Joint, Right
H   Acromioclavicular Joint, Left
J   Shoulder Joint, Right
     Glenohumeral joint
     Glenoid ligament (labrum)
K   Shoulder Joint, Left
     See J Shoulder Joint, Right
L   Elbow Joint, Right
     Distal humerus, involving joint
     Humeroradial joint
     Humeroulnar joint
     Proximal radioulnar joint
M   Elbow Joint, Left
     See L Elbow Joint, Right
N   Wrist Joint, Right
     Distal radioulnar joint
     Radiocarpal joint
P   Wrist Joint, Left
     See N Wrist Joint, Right
Q   Carpal Joint, Right
     Intercarpal joint
     Midcarpal joint
R   Carpal Joint, Left
     See Q Carpal Joint, Right
S   Carpometacarpal Joint, Right
T   Carpometacarpal Joint, Left
U   Metacarpophalangeal Joint, Right
V   Metacarpophalangeal Joint, Left
W   Finger Phalangeal Joint, Right
     Interphalangeal (IP) joint
X   Finger Phalangeal Joint, Left
     See W Finger Phalangeal Joint, Right
	0 Open
	3 Percutaneous
	4 Percutaneous Endoscopic
		Z No Device	Z No Qualifier

Non-OR   0R5[3,5,9,B][3,4]ZZ

NC Noncovered Procedure   LC Limited Coverage   QA Questionable OB Admit   NT New Tech Add-on   ⊞ Combination Member   ♂ Male   ♀ Female

Upper Joints

Ø   **Medical and Surgical**
R   **Upper Joints**
9   **Drainage**   Definition: Taking or letting out fluids and/or gases from a body part
                          Explanation: The qualifier DIAGNOSTIC is used to identify drainage procedures that are biopsies

Body Part Character 4		Approach Character 5	Device Character 6	Qualifier Character 7

Ø Occipital-cervical Joint
1 Cervical Vertebral Joint
  Atlantoaxial joint
  Cervical facet joint
3 Cervical Vertebral Disc
4 Cervicothoracic Vertebral Joint
  Cervicothoracic facet joint
5 Cervicothoracic Vertebral Disc
6 Thoracic Vertebral Joint
  Costotransverse joint
  Costovertebral joint
  Thoracic facet joint
9 Thoracic Vertebral Disc
A Thoracolumbar Vertebral Joint
  Thoracolumbar facet joint
B Thoracolumbar Vertebral Disc
C Temporomandibular Joint, Right
D Temporomandibular Joint, Left
E Sternoclavicular Joint, Right
F Sternoclavicular Joint, Left
G Acromioclavicular Joint, Right
H Acromioclavicular Joint, Left
J Shoulder Joint, Right
  Glenohumeral joint
  Glenoid ligament (labrum)
K Shoulder Joint, Left
  See J Shoulder Joint, Right
	L Elbow Joint, Right
	  Distal humerus, involving joint
	  Humeroradial joint
	  Humeroulnar joint
	  Proximal radioulnar joint
	M Elbow Joint, Left
	  See L Elbow Joint, Right
	N Wrist Joint, Right
	  Distal radioulnar joint
	  Radiocarpal joint
	P Wrist Joint, Left
	  See N Wrist Joint, Right
	Q Carpal Joint, Right
	  Intercarpal joint
	  Midcarpal joint
	R Carpal Joint, Left
	  See Q Carpal Joint, Right
	S Carpometacarpal Joint, Right
	T Carpometacarpal Joint, Left
	U Metacarpophalangeal Joint, Right
	V Metacarpophalangeal Joint, Left
	W Finger Phalangeal Joint, Right
	  Interphalangeal (IP) joint
	X Finger Phalangeal Joint, Left
	  See W Finger Phalangeal Joint, Right
		Ø Open
		3 Percutaneous
		4 Percutaneous Endoscopic
			Ø Drainage Device	Z No Qualifier

Ø Occipital-cervical Joint
1 Cervical Vertebral Joint
  Atlantoaxial joint
  Cervical facet joint
3 Cervical Vertebral Disc
4 Cervicothoracic Vertebral Joint
  Cervicothoracic facet joint
5 Cervicothoracic Vertebral Disc
6 Thoracic Vertebral Joint
  Costotransverse joint
  Costovertebral joint
  Thoracic facet joint
9 Thoracic Vertebral Disc
A Thoracolumbar Vertebral Joint
  Thoracolumbar facet joint
B Thoracolumbar Vertebral Disc
C Temporomandibular Joint, Right
D Temporomandibular Joint, Left
E Sternoclavicular Joint, Right
F Sternoclavicular Joint, Left
G Acromioclavicular Joint, Right
H Acromioclavicular Joint, Left
J Shoulder Joint, Right
  Glenohumeral joint
  Glenoid ligament (labrum)
K Shoulder Joint, Left
  See J Shoulder Joint, Right
	L Elbow Joint, Right
	  Distal humerus, involving joint
	  Humeroradial joint
	  Humeroulnar joint
	  Proximal radioulnar joint
	M Elbow Joint, Left
	  See L Elbow Joint, Right
	N Wrist Joint, Right
	  Distal radioulnar joint
	  Radiocarpal joint
	P Wrist Joint, Left
	  See N Wrist Joint, Right
	Q Carpal Joint, Right
	  Intercarpal joint
	  Midcarpal joint
	R Carpal Joint, Left
	  See Q Carpal Joint, Right
	S Carpometacarpal Joint, Right
	T Carpometacarpal Joint, Left
	U Metacarpophalangeal Joint, Right
	V Metacarpophalangeal Joint, Left
	W Finger Phalangeal Joint, Right
	  Interphalangeal (IP) joint
	X Finger Phalangeal Joint, Left
	  See W Finger Phalangeal Joint, Right
		Ø Open
		3 Percutaneous
		4 Percutaneous Endoscopic
			Z No Device	X Diagnostic
				Z No Qualifier

Non-OR   ØR9[Ø,1,3,4,5,6,9,A,B,E,F,G,H,J,K,L,M,N,P,Q,R,S,T,U,V,W,X][3,4]ØZ
Non-OR   ØR9[C,D]3ØZ
Non-OR   ØR9[Ø,1,3,4,5,6,9,A,B,E,F,G,H,J,K,L,M,N,P,Q,R,S,T,U,V,W,X][Ø,3,4]ZX
Non-OR   ØR9[Ø,1,3,4,5,6,9,A,B,E,F,G,H,J,K,L,M,N,P,Q,R,S,T,U,V,W,X][3,4]ZZ
Non-OR   ØR9[C,D]3ZZ

Ø   Medical and Surgical
R   Upper Joints
B   Excision   Definition: Cutting out or off, without replacement, a portion of a body part
                  Explanation: The qualifier DIAGNOSTIC is used to identify excision procedures that are biopsies

Body Part Character 4	Approach Character 5	Device Character 6	Qualifier Character 7
Ø **Occipital-cervical Joint**	**Ø** Open	**Z** No Device	**X** Diagnostic
1 **Cervical Vertebral Joint**	**3** Percutaneous		**Z** No Qualifier
Atlantoaxial joint	**4** Percutaneous Endoscopic		
Cervical facet joint			
3 **Cervical Vertebral Disc**			
4 **Cervicothoracic Vertebral Joint**			
Cervicothoracic facet joint			
5 **Cervicothoracic Vertebral Disc**			
6 **Thoracic Vertebral Joint**			
Costotransverse joint			
Costovertebral joint			
Thoracic facet joint			
9 **Thoracic Vertebral Disc**			
A **Thoracolumbar Vertebral Joint**			
Thoracolumbar facet joint			
B **Thoracolumbar Vertebral Disc**			
C **Temporomandibular Joint, Right**			
D **Temporomandibular Joint, Left**			
E **Sternoclavicular Joint, Right**			
F **Sternoclavicular Joint, Left**			
G **Acromioclavicular Joint, Right**			
H **Acromioclavicular Joint, Left**			
J **Shoulder Joint, Right**			
Glenohumeral joint			
Glenoid ligament (labrum)			
K **Shoulder Joint, Left**			
See J Shoulder Joint, Right			
L **Elbow Joint, Right**			
Distal humerus, involving joint			
Humeroradial joint			
Humeroulnar joint			
Proximal radioulnar joint			
M **Elbow Joint, Left**			
See L Elbow Joint, Right			
N **Wrist Joint, Right**			
Distal radioulnar joint			
Radiocarpal joint			
P **Wrist Joint, Left**			
See N Wrist Joint, Right			
Q **Carpal Joint, Right**			
Intercarpal joint			
Midcarpal joint			
R **Carpal Joint, Left**			
See Q Carpal Joint, Right			
S **Carpometacarpal Joint, Right**			
T **Carpometacarpal Joint, Left**			
U **Metacarpophalangeal Joint, Right**			
V **Metacarpophalangeal Joint, Left**			
W **Finger Phalangeal Joint, Right**			
Interphalangeal (IP) joint			
X **Finger Phalangeal Joint, Left**			
See W Finger Phalangeal Joint, Right			

Non-OR   ØRB[Ø,1,3,4,5,6,9,A,B,E,F,G,H,J,K,L,M,N,P,Q,R,S,T,U,V,W,X][Ø,3,4]ZX

Ø   Medical and Surgical
R   Upper Joints
C   Extirpation   Definition: Taking or cutting out solid matter from a body part

Explanation: The solid matter may be an abnormal byproduct of a biological function or a foreign body; it may be imbedded in a body part or in the lumen of a tubular body part. The solid matter may or may not have been previously broken into pieces.

Body Part Character 4	Approach Character 5	Device Character 6	Qualifier Character 7
Ø **Occipital-cervical Joint**	**Ø** Open	**Z** No Device	**Z** No Qualifier
1 **Cervical Vertebral Joint**	**3** Percutaneous		
Atlantoaxial joint	**4** Percutaneous Endoscopic		
Cervical facet joint			
3 **Cervical Vertebral Disc**			
4 **Cervicothoracic Vertebral Joint**			
Cervicothoracic facet joint			
5 **Cervicothoracic Vertebral Disc**			
6 **Thoracic Vertebral Joint**			
Costotransverse joint			
Costovertebral joint			
Thoracic facet joint			
9 **Thoracic Vertebral Disc**			
A **Thoracolumbar Vertebral Joint**			
Thoracolumbar facet joint			
B **Thoracolumbar Vertebral Disc**			
C **Temporomandibular Joint, Right**			
D **Temporomandibular Joint, Left**			
E **Sternoclavicular Joint, Right**			
F **Sternoclavicular Joint, Left**			
G **Acromioclavicular Joint, Right**			
H **Acromioclavicular Joint, Left**			
J **Shoulder Joint, Right**			
Glenohumeral joint			
Glenoid ligament (labrum)			
K **Shoulder Joint, Left**			
See J Shoulder Joint, Right			
L **Elbow Joint, Right**			
Distal humerus, involving joint			
Humeroradial joint			
Humeroulnar joint			
Proximal radioulnar joint			
M **Elbow Joint, Left**			
See L Elbow Joint, Right			
N **Wrist Joint, Right**			
Distal radioulnar joint			
Radiocarpal joint			
P **Wrist Joint, Left**			
See N Wrist Joint, Right			
Q **Carpal Joint, Right**			
Intercarpal joint			
Midcarpal joint			
R **Carpal Joint, Left**			
See Q Carpal Joint, Right			
S **Carpometacarpal Joint, Right**			
T **Carpometacarpal Joint, Left**			
U **Metacarpophalangeal Joint, Right**			
V **Metacarpophalangeal Joint, Left**			
W **Finger Phalangeal Joint, Right**			
Interphalangeal (IP) joint			
X **Finger Phalangeal Joint, Left**			
See W Finger Phalangeal Joint, Right			

Non-OR Procedure   DRG Non-OR Procedure   Valid OR Procedure   HAC Associated Procedure   Combination Only   New/Revised GREEN

Ø   **Medical and Surgical**
R   **Upper Joints**
G   **Fusion**   Definition: Joining together portions of an articular body part rendering the articular body part immobile

                       Explanation: The body part is joined together by fixation device, bone graft, or other means

Body Part Character 4	Approach Character 5	Device Character 6	Qualifier Character 7

Ø **Occipital-cervical Joint**
1 **Cervical Vertebral Joint**
   Atlantoaxial joint
   Cervical facet joint
2 **Cervical Vertebral Joints, 2 or more**
   Cervical facet joint
4 **Cervicothoracic Vertebral Joint**
   Cervicothoracic facet joint
6 **Thoracic Vertebral Joint**
   Costotransverse joint
   Costovertebral joint
   Thoracic facet joint
7 **Thoracic Vertebral Joints, 2 to 7** ⊞
8 **Thoracic Vertebral Joints, 8 or more**
A **Thoracolumbar Vertebral Joint**
   Thoracolumbar facet joint
	Ø Open
	3 Percutaneous
	4 Percutaneous Endoscopic
		7 Autologous Tissue Substitute
		J Synthetic Substitute
		K Nonautologous Tissue Substitute
			Ø Anterior Approach, Anterior Column
			1 Posterior Approach, Posterior Column
			J Posterior Approach, Anterior Column

Ø **Occipital-cervical Joint**
1 **Cervical Vertebral Joint**
   Atlantoaxial joint
   Cervical facet joint
2 **Cervical Vertebral Joints, 2 or more**
   Cervical facet joint
4 **Cervicothoracic Vertebral Joint**
   Cervicothoracic facet joint
6 **Thoracic Vertebral Joint**
   Costotransverse joint
   Costovertebral joint
   Thoracic facet joint
7 **Thoracic Vertebral Joints, 2 to 7** ⊞
8 **Thoracic Vertebral Joints, 8 or more**
A **Thoracolumbar Vertebral Joint**
   Thoracolumbar facet joint
	Ø Open
	3 Percutaneous
	4 Percutaneous Endoscopic
		A Interbody Fusion Device	**Ø** Anterior Approach, Anterior Column
			J Posterior Approach, Anterior Column

C **Temporomandibular Joint, Right**
D **Temporomandibular Joint, Left**
E **Sternoclavicular Joint, Right**
F **Sternoclavicular Joint, Left**
G **Acromioclavicular Joint, Right**
H **Acromioclavicular Joint, Left**
J **Shoulder Joint, Right**
   Glenohumeral joint
   Glenoid ligament (labrum)
K **Shoulder Joint, Left**
   See J Shoulder Joint, Right
	Ø Open
	3 Percutaneous
	4 Percutaneous Endoscopic
		4 Internal Fixation Device
		7 Autologous Tissue Substitute
		J Synthetic Substitute
		K Nonautologous Tissue Substitute
			Z No Qualifier

L **Elbow Joint, Right**
   Distal humerus, involving joint
   Humeroradial joint
   Humeroulnar joint
   Proximal radioulnar joint
M **Elbow Joint, Left**
   See L Elbow Joint, Right
N **Wrist Joint, Right**
   Distal radioulnar joint
   Radiocarpal joint
P **Wrist Joint, Left**
   See N Wrist Joint, Right
Q **Carpal Joint, Right**
   Intercarpal joint
   Midcarpal joint
 	
R **Carpal Joint, Left**
   See Q Carpal Joint, Right
S **Carpometacarpal Joint, Right**
T **Carpometacarpal Joint, Left**
U **Metacarpophalangeal Joint, Right**
V **Metacarpophalangeal Joint, Left**
W **Finger Phalangeal Joint, Right**
   Interphalangeal (IP) joint
X **Finger Phalangeal Joint, Left**
   See W Finger Phalangeal Joint, Right
	Ø Open
	3 Percutaneous
	4 Percutaneous Endoscopic
		3 Internal Fixation Device, Sustained Compression
		4 Internal Fixation Device
		5 External Fixation Device
		7 Autologous Tissue Substitute
		J Synthetic Substitute
		K Nonautologous Tissue Substitute
			Z No Qualifier

HAC ØRG[Ø,1,2,4,6,7,8,A][Ø,3,4][7,J,K][Ø,1,J] when reported with SDx K68.11 or T81.4Ø–T81.49, T84.6Ø-T84.619, T84.63-T84.7 with 7th character A	**See Appendix L for Procedure Combinations** ⊞ ØRG7[Ø,3,4][7,J,K][Ø,1,J]
HAC ØRG[Ø,1,2,4,6,7,8,A][Ø,3,4]A[Ø,J] when reported with SDx K68.11 or T81.4Ø–T81.49, T84.6Ø-T84.619, T84.63-T84.7 with 7th character A	⊞ ØRG7[Ø,3,4]A[Ø,J]
HAC ØRG[E,F,G,H,J,K][Ø,3,4][4,7,J,K]Z when reported with SDx K68.11 or T81.4Ø–T81.49, T84.6Ø-T84.619, T84.63-T84.7 with 7th character A	
HAC ØRG[L,M][Ø,3,4][3,4,5,7,J,K]Z when reported with SDx K68.11 or T81.4Ø–T81.49, T84.6Ø-T84.619, T84.63-T84.7 with 7th character A	

NC Noncovered Procedure   **LC** Limited Coverage   **UA** Questionable OB Admit   **NT** New Tech Add-on   ⊞ Combination Member   ♂Male   ♀Female

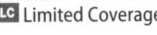

ICD-10-PCS 2022   587

ØRG–ØRG

Ø　Medical and Surgical
R　Upper Joints
H　Insertion　　　Definition: Putting in a nonbiological appliance that monitors, assists, performs, or prevents a physiological function but does not physically take the place of a body part
　　　　　　　　　　　Explanation: None

Body Part Character 4	Approach Character 5	Device Character 6	Qualifier Character 7
Ø Occipital-cervical Joint 1 Cervical Vertebral Joint 　Atlantoaxial joint 　Cervical facet joint 4 Cervicothoracic Vertebral Joint 　Cervicothoracic facet joint 6 Thoracic Vertebral Joint 　Costotransverse joint 　Costovertebral joint 　Thoracic facet joint A Thoracolumbar Vertebral Joint 　Thoracolumbar facet joint	Ø Open 3 Percutaneous 4 Percutaneous Endoscopic	3 Infusion Device 4 Internal Fixation Device 8 Spacer B Spinal Stabilization Device, 　Interspinous Process C Spinal Stabilization Device, 　Pedicle-Based D Spinal Stabilization Device, 　Facet Replacement	Z No Qualifier
3 Cervical Vertebral Disc 5 Cervicothoracic Vertebral Disc 9 Thoracic Vertebral Disc B Thoracolumbar Vertebral Disc	Ø Open 3 Percutaneous 4 Percutaneous Endoscopic	3 Infusion Device	Z No Qualifier
C Temporomandibular Joint, Right D Temporomandibular Joint, Left E Sternoclavicular Joint, Right F Sternoclavicular Joint, Left G Acromioclavicular Joint, Right H Acromioclavicular Joint, Left J Shoulder Joint, Right 　Glenohumeral joint 　Glenoid ligament (labrum) K Shoulder Joint, Left 　See J Shoulder Joint, Right	Ø Open 3 Percutaneous 4 Percutaneous Endoscopic	3 Infusion Device 4 Internal Fixation Device 8 Spacer	Z No Qualifier
L Elbow Joint, Right 　Distal humerus, involving joint 　Humeroradial joint 　Humeroulnar joint 　Proximal radioulnar joint M Elbow Joint, Left 　See L Elbow Joint, Right N Wrist Joint, Right 　Distal radioulnar joint 　Radiocarpal joint P Wrist Joint, Left 　See N Wrist Joint, Right Q Carpal Joint, Right 　Intercarpal joint 　Midcarpal joint R Carpal Joint, Left 　See Q Carpal Joint, Right S Carpometacarpal Joint, Right T Carpometacarpal Joint, Left U Metacarpophalangeal Joint, Right V Metacarpophalangeal Joint, Left W Finger Phalangeal Joint, Right 　Interphalangeal (IP) joint X Finger Phalangeal Joint, Left 　See W Finger Phalangeal Joint, Right	Ø Open 3 Percutaneous 4 Percutaneous Endoscopic	3 Infusion Device 4 Internal Fixation Device 5 External Fixation Device 8 Spacer	Z No Qualifier

Non-OR	ØRH[Ø,1,4,6,A][Ø,3,4][3,8]Z
Non-OR	ØRH[3,5,9,B][Ø,3,4]3Z
Non-OR	ØRH[C,D][Ø,4]8Z
Non-OR	ØRH[C,D]3[3,8]Z
Non-OR	ØRH[E,F,G,H,J,K][Ø,3,4][3,8]Z
Non-OR	ØRH[L,M,N,P,Q,R,S,T,U,V,W,X][Ø,3,4][3,8]Z

Ø   **Medical and Surgical**
R   **Upper Joints**
J   **Inspection**   Definition: Visually and/or manually exploring a body part

                     Explanation: Visual exploration may be performed with or without optical instrumentation. Manual exploration may be performed directly or through intervening body layers.

Body Part Character 4	Approach Character 5	Device Character 6	Qualifier Character 7
Ø **Occipital-cervical Joint**	**Ø** Open	**Z** No Device	**Z** No Qualifier
1 **Cervical Vertebral Joint**	**3** Percutaneous		
Atlantoaxial joint	**4** Percutaneous Endoscopic		
Cervical facet joint	**X** External		
3 **Cervical Vertebral Disc**			
4 **Cervicothoracic Vertebral Joint**			
Cervicothoracic facet joint			
5 **Cervicothoracic Vertebral Disc**			
6 **Thoracic Vertebral Joint**			
Costotransverse joint			
Costovertebral joint			
Thoracic facet joint			
9 **Thoracic Vertebral Disc**			
A **Thoracolumbar Vertebral Joint**			
Thoracolumbar facet joint			
B **Thoracolumbar Vertebral Disc**			
C **Temporomandibular Joint, Right**			
D **Temporomandibular Joint, Left**			
E **Sternoclavicular Joint, Right**			
F **Sternoclavicular Joint, Left**			
G **Acromioclavicular Joint, Right**			
H **Acromioclavicular Joint, Left**			
J **Shoulder Joint, Right**			
Glenohumeral joint			
Glenoid ligament (labrum)			
K **Shoulder Joint, Left**			
See J Shoulder Joint, Right			
L **Elbow Joint, Right**			
Distal humerus, involving joint			
Humeroradial joint			
Humeroulnar joint			
Proximal radioulnar joint			
M **Elbow Joint, Left**			
See L Elbow Joint, Right			
N **Wrist Joint, Right**			
Distal radioulnar joint			
Radiocarpal joint			
P **Wrist Joint, Left**			
See N Wrist Joint, Right			
Q **Carpal Joint, Right**			
Intercarpal joint			
Midcarpal joint			
R **Carpal Joint, Left**			
See Q Carpal Joint, Right			
S **Carpometacarpal Joint, Right**			
T **Carpometacarpal Joint, Left**			
U **Metacarpophalangeal Joint, Right**			
V **Metacarpophalangeal Joint, Left**			
W **Finger Phalangeal Joint, Right**			
Interphalangeal (IP) joint			
X **Finger Phalangeal Joint, Left**			
See W Finger Phalangeal Joint, Right			

Non-OR   ØRJ[Ø,1,3,4,5,6,9,A,B,C,D,E,F,G,H,J,K,L,M,N,P,Q,R,S,T,U,V,W,X][3,X]ZZ

NC Noncovered Procedure   **LC** Limited Coverage   **QA** Questionable OB Admit   **NT** New Tech Add-on   ⊞ Combination Member   ♂ Male   ♀ Female

ICD-10-PCS 2022   589

Ø   Medical and Surgical
R   Upper Joints
N   Release   Definition: Freeing a body part from an abnormal physical constraint by cutting or by the use of force
                       Explanation: Some of the restraining tissue may be taken out but none of the body part is taken out

Body Part Character 4	Approach Character 5	Device Character 6	Qualifier Character 7
Ø **Occipital-cervical Joint**	**Ø** Open	**Z** No Device	**Z** No Qualifier
1 **Cervical Vertebral Joint**	**3** Percutaneous		
Atlantoaxial joint	**4** Percutaneous Endoscopic		
Cervical facet joint	**X** External		
3 **Cervical Vertebral Disc**			
4 **Cervicothoracic Vertebral Joint**			
Cervicothoracic facet joint			
5 **Cervicothoracic Vertebral Disc**			
6 **Thoracic Vertebral Joint**			
Costotransverse joint			
Costovertebral joint			
Thoracic facet joint			
9 **Thoracic Vertebral Disc**			
A **Thoracolumbar Vertebral Joint**			
Thoracolumbar facet joint			
B **Thoracolumbar Vertebral Disc**			
C **Temporomandibular Joint, Right**			
D **Temporomandibular Joint, Left**			
E **Sternoclavicular Joint, Right**			
F **Sternoclavicular Joint, Left**			
G **Acromioclavicular Joint, Right**			
H **Acromioclavicular Joint, Left**			
J **Shoulder Joint, Right**			
Glenohumeral joint			
Glenoid ligament (labrum)			
K **Shoulder Joint, Left**			
See J Shoulder Joint, Right			
L **Elbow Joint, Right**			
Distal humerus, involving joint			
Humeroradial joint			
Humeroulnar joint			
Proximal radioulnar joint			
M **Elbow Joint, Left**			
See L Elbow Joint, Right			
N **Wrist Joint, Right**			
Distal radioulnar joint			
Radiocarpal joint			
P **Wrist Joint, Left**			
See N Wrist Joint, Right			
Q **Carpal Joint, Right**			
Intercarpal joint			
Midcarpal joint			
R **Carpal Joint, Left**			
See Q Carpal Joint, Right			
S **Carpometacarpal Joint, Right**			
T **Carpometacarpal Joint, Left**			
U **Metacarpophalangeal Joint, Right**			
V **Metacarpophalangeal Joint, Left**			
W **Finger Phalangeal Joint, Right**			
Interphalangeal (IP) joint			
X **Finger Phalangeal Joint, Left**			
See W Finger Phalangeal Joint, Right			

Non-OR   ØRN[Ø,1,3,4,5,6,9,A,B,C,D,E,F,G,H,J,K,L,M,N,P,Q,R,S,T,U,V,W,X]XZZ

Non-OR Procedure   DRG Non-OR Procedure   Valid OR Procedure   HAC Associated Procedure   Combination Only   New/Revised GREEN
590   ICD-10-PCS 2022

ØRN–ØRN

Ø　**Medical and Surgical**
R　**Upper Joints**
P　**Removal**　　Definition: Taking out or off a device from a body part

Explanation: If a device is taken out and a similar device put in without cutting or puncturing the skin or mucous membrane, the procedure is coded to the root operation CHANGE. Otherwise, the procedure for taking out the device is coded to the root operation REMOVAL.

Body Part Character 4	Approach Character 5	Device Character 6	Qualifier Character 7
Ø　Occipital-cervical Joint 1　Cervical Vertebral Joint 　　Atlantoaxial joint 　　Cervical facet joint 4　Cervicothoracic Vertebral Joint 　　Cervicothoracic facet joint 6　Thoracic Vertebral Joint 　　Costotransverse joint 　　Costovertebral joint 　　Thoracic facet joint A　Thoracolumbar Vertebral Joint 　　Thoracolumbar facet joint	Ø　Open 3　Percutaneous 4　Percutaneous Endoscopic	Ø　Drainage Device 3　Infusion Device 4　Internal Fixation Device 7　Autologous Tissue Substitute 8　Spacer A　Interbody Fusion Device J　Synthetic Substitute K　Nonautologous Tissue Substitute	Z　No Qualifier
Ø　Occipital-cervical Joint 1　Cervical Vertebral Joint 　　Atlantoaxial joint 　　Cervical facet joint 4　Cervicothoracic Vertebral Joint 　　Cervicothoracic facet joint 6　Thoracic Vertebral Joint 　　Costotransverse joint 　　Costovertebral joint 　　Thoracic facet joint A　Thoracolumbar Vertebral Joint 　　Thoracolumbar facet joint	X　External	Ø　Drainage Device 3　Infusion Device 4　Internal Fixation Device	Z　No Qualifier
3　Cervical Vertebral Disc 5　Cervicothoracic Vertebral Disc 9　Thoracic Vertebral Disc B　Thoracolumbar Vertebral Disc	Ø　Open 3　Percutaneous 4　Percutaneous Endoscopic	Ø　Drainage Device 3　Infusion Device 7　Autologous Tissue Substitute J　Synthetic Substitute K　Nonautologous Tissue Substitute	Z　No Qualifier
3　Cervical Vertebral Disc 5　Cervicothoracic Vertebral Disc 9　Thoracic Vertebral Disc B　Thoracolumbar Vertebral Disc	X　External	Ø　Drainage Device 3　Infusion Device	Z　No Qualifier
C　Temporomandibular Joint, Right D　Temporomandibular Joint, Left E　Sternoclavicular Joint, Right F　Sternoclavicular Joint, Left G　Acromioclavicular Joint, Right H　Acromioclavicular Joint, Left	Ø　Open 3　Percutaneous 4　Percutaneous Endoscopic	Ø　Drainage Device 3　Infusion Device 4　Internal Fixation Device 7　Autologous Tissue Substitute 8　Spacer J　Synthetic Substitute K　Nonautologous Tissue Substitute	Z　No Qualifier
C　Temporomandibular Joint, Right D　Temporomandibular Joint, Left E　Sternoclavicular Joint, Right F　Sternoclavicular Joint, Left G　Acromioclavicular Joint, Right H　Acromioclavicular Joint, Left	X　External	Ø　Drainage Device 3　Infusion Device 4　Internal Fixation Device	Z　No Qualifier
J　Shoulder Joint, Right 　　Glenohumeral joint 　　Glenoid ligament (labrum) K　Shoulder Joint, Left 　　*See J Shoulder Joint, Right*	Ø　Open 3　Percutaneous 4　Percutaneous Endoscopic	Ø　Drainage Device 3　Infusion Device 4　Internal Fixation Device 7　Autologous Tissue Substitute 8　Spacer K　Nonautologous Tissue Substitute	Z　No Qualifier
J　Shoulder Joint, Right 　　Glenohumeral joint 　　Glenoid ligament (labrum) K　Shoulder Joint, Left 　　*See J Shoulder Joint, Right*	Ø　Open 3　Percutaneous 4　Percutaneous Endoscopic	J　Synthetic Substitute	6　Humeral Surface 7　Glenoid Surface Z　No Qualifier
J　Shoulder Joint, Right 　　Glenohumeral joint 　　Glenoid ligament (labrum) K　Shoulder Joint, Left 　　*See J Shoulder Joint, Right*	X　External	Ø　Drainage Device 3　Infusion Device 4　Internal Fixation Device	Z　No Qualifier

Non-OR　ØRP[Ø,1,4,6,A]3[Ø,3,8]Z	**Non-OR**　ØRP[C,D,E,F,G,H][Ø,4]8Z
Non-OR　ØRP[Ø,1,4,6,A][Ø,4]8Z	**Non-OR**　ØRP[C,D]X[Ø,3]Z
Non-OR　ØRP[Ø,1,4,6,A]X[Ø,3,4]Z	**Non-OR**　ØRP[E,F,G,H,J,K]X[Ø,3,4]Z
Non-OR　ØRP[3,5,9,B]3[Ø,3]Z	**Non-OR**　ØRP[J,K]3[Ø,3,8]Z
Non-OR　ØRP[3,5,9,B]X[Ø,3]Z	**Non-OR**　ØRP[J,K][Ø,4]8Z
Non-OR　ØRP[C,D,E,F,G,H]3[Ø,3,8]Z	**Non-OR**　ØRP[J,K]X[Ø,3,4]Z

ØRP Continued on next page

NC Noncovered Procedure　　LC Limited Coverage　　QA Questionable OB Admit　　NT New Tech Add-on　　⊞ Combination Member　　♂ Male　　♀ Female

Ø   **Medical and Surgical**   *ØRP Continued*
R   **Upper Joints**
P   **Removal**   Definition: Taking out or off a device from a body part

Explanation: If a device is taken out and a similar device put in without cutting or puncturing the skin or mucous membrane, the procedure is coded to the root operation CHANGE. Otherwise, the procedure for taking out the device is coded to the root operation REMOVAL.

Body Part Character 4	Approach Character 5	Device Character 6	Qualifier Character 7
L **Elbow Joint, Right** Distal humerus, involving joint Humeroradial joint Humeroulnar joint Proximal radioulnar joint **M** **Elbow Joint, Left** *See L Elbow Joint, Right* **N** **Wrist Joint, Right** Distal radioulnar joint Radiocarpal joint **P** **Wrist Joint, Left** *See N Wrist Joint, Right* **Q** **Carpal Joint, Right** Intercarpal joint Midcarpal joint **R** **Carpal Joint, Left** *See Q Carpal Joint, Right* **S** **Carpometacarpal Joint, Right** **T** **Carpometacarpal Joint, Left** **U** **Metacarpophalangeal Joint, Right** **V** **Metacarpophalangeal Joint, Left** **W** **Finger Phalangeal Joint, Right** Interphalangeal (IP) joint **X** **Finger Phalangeal Joint, Left** *See W Finger Phalangeal Joint, Right*	**Ø** Open **3** Percutaneous **4** Percutaneous Endoscopic	**Ø** Drainage Device **3** Infusion Device **4** Internal Fixation Device **5** External Fixation Device **7** Autologous Tissue Substitute **8** Spacer **J** Synthetic Substitute **K** Nonautologous Tissue Substitute	**Z** No Qualifier
L **Elbow Joint, Right** Distal humerus, involving joint Humeroradial joint Humeroulnar joint Proximal radioulnar joint **M** **Elbow Joint, Left** *See L Elbow Joint, Right* **N** **Wrist Joint, Right** Distal radioulnar joint Radiocarpal joint **P** **Wrist Joint, Left** *See N Wrist Joint, Right* **Q** **Carpal Joint, Right** Intercarpal joint Midcarpal joint **R** **Carpal Joint, Left** *See Q Carpal Joint, Right* **S** **Carpometacarpal Joint, Right** **T** **Carpometacarpal Joint, Left** **U** **Metacarpophalangeal Joint, Right** **V** **Metacarpophalangeal Joint, Left** **W** **Finger Phalangeal Joint, Right** Interphalangeal (IP) joint **X** **Finger Phalangeal Joint, Left** *See W Finger Phalangeal Joint, Right*	**X** External	**Ø** Drainage Device **3** Infusion Device **4** Internal Fixation Device **5** External Fixation Device	**Z** No Qualifier

Non-OR	ØRP[L,M,N,P,Q,R,S,T,U,V,W,X]3[Ø,3,8]Z
Non-OR	ØRP[L,M,N,P,Q,R,S,T,U,V,W,X][Ø,4]8Z
Non-OR	ØRP[L,M,N,P,Q,R,S,T,U,V,W,X]X[Ø,3,4,5]Z

Ø　Medical and Surgical
R　Upper Joints
Q　Repair　　Definition: Restoring, to the extent possible, a body part to its normal anatomic structure and function
　　　　　　　　　Explanation: Used only when the method to accomplish the repair is not one of the other root operations

Body Part Character 4	Approach Character 5	Device Character 6	Qualifier Character 7
Ø Occipital-cervical Joint	**Ø** Open	**Z** No Device	**Z** No Qualifier
1 Cervical Vertebral Joint	**3** Percutaneous		
Atlantoaxial joint	**4** Percutaneous Endoscopic		
Cervical facet joint	**X** External		
3 Cervical Vertebral Disc			
4 Cervicothoracic Vertebral Joint			
Cervicothoracic facet joint			
5 Cervicothoracic Vertebral Disc			
6 Thoracic Vertebral Joint			
Costotransverse joint			
Costovertebral joint			
Thoracic facet joint			
9 Thoracic Vertebral Disc			
A Thoracolumbar Vertebral Joint			
Thoracolumbar facet joint			
B Thoracolumbar Vertebral Disc			
C Temporomandibular Joint, Right			
D Temporomandibular Joint, Left			
E Sternoclavicular Joint, Right			
F Sternoclavicular Joint, Left			
G Acromioclavicular Joint, Right			
H Acromioclavicular Joint, Left			
J Shoulder Joint, Right			
Glenohumeral joint			
Glenoid ligament (labrum)			
K Shoulder Joint, Left			
See J Shoulder Joint, Right			
L Elbow Joint, Right			
Distal humerus, involving joint			
Humeroradial joint			
Humeroulnar joint			
Proximal radioulnar joint			
M Elbow Joint, Left			
See L Elbow Joint, Right			
N Wrist Joint, Right			
Distal radioulnar joint			
Radiocarpal joint			
P Wrist Joint, Left			
See N Wrist Joint, Right			
Q Carpal Joint, Right			
Intercarpal joint			
Midcarpal joint			
R Carpal Joint, Left			
See Q Carpal Joint, Right			
S Carpometacarpal Joint, Right			
T Carpometacarpal Joint, Left			
U Metacarpophalangeal Joint, Right			
V Metacarpophalangeal Joint, Left			
W Finger Phalangeal Joint, Right			
Interphalangeal (IP) joint			
X Finger Phalangeal Joint, Left			
See W Finger Phalangeal Joint, Right			

Non-OR　ØRQ[Ø,1,3,4,5,6,9,A,B,C,D,E,F,G,H,J,K,L,M,N,P,Q,R,S,T,U,V,W,X]XZZ
HAC　　ØRQ[E,F,G,H,J,K,L,M][Ø,3,4]ZZ when reported with SDx K68.11 or T81.4Ø–T81.49, T84.6Ø-T84.619, T84.63-T84.7 with 7th character A

NC Noncovered Procedure　　**LC** Limited Coverage　　**QA** Questionable OB Admit　　**NT** New Tech Add-on　　⊞ Combination Member　　♂ Male　　♀ Female

ICD-10-PCS 2022　　593

ØRQ–ØRQ

Ø Medical and Surgical
R Upper Joints
R Replacement

Definition: Putting in or on biological or synthetic material that physically takes the place and/or function of all or a portion of a body part

Explanation: The body part may have been taken out or replaced, or may be taken out, physically eradicated, or rendered nonfunctional during the REPLACEMENT procedure. A REMOVAL procedure is coded for taking out the device used in a previous replacement procedure.

Body Part Character 4	Approach Character 5	Device Character 6	Qualifier Character 7

Ø Occipital-cervical Joint
1 Cervical Vertebral Joint
  Atlantoaxial joint
  Cervical facet joint
3 Cervical Vertebral Disc
4 Cervicothoracic Vertebral Joint
  Cervicothoracic facet joint
5 Cervicothoracic Vertebral Disc
6 Thoracic Vertebral Joint
  Costotransverse joint
  Costovertebral joint
  Thoracic facet joint
9 Thoracic Vertebral Disc
A Thoracolumbar Vertebral Joint
  Thoracolumbar facet joint
B Thoracolumbar Vertebral Disc
C Temporomandibular Joint, Right
D Temporomandibular Joint, Left
E Sternoclavicular Joint, Right
F Sternoclavicular Joint, Left
G Acromioclavicular Joint, Right
H Acromioclavicular Joint, Left
L Elbow Joint, Right
  Distal humerus, involving joint
  Humeroradial joint
  Humeroulnar joint
  Proximal radioulnar joint
M Elbow Joint, Left
  See L Elbow Joint, Right
N Wrist Joint, Right
  Distal radioulnar joint
  Radiocarpal joint
P Wrist Joint, Left
  See N Wrist Joint, Right
Q Carpal Joint, Right
  Intercarpal joint
  Midcarpal joint
R Carpal Joint, Left
  See Q Carpal Joint, Right
S Carpometacarpal Joint, Right
T Carpometacarpal Joint, Left
U Metacarpophalangeal Joint, Right
V Metacarpophalangeal Joint, Left
W Finger Phalangeal Joint, Right
  Interphalangeal (IP) joint
X Finger Phalangeal Joint, Left
  See W Finger Phalangeal Joint, Right
	Ø Open	**7** Autologous Tissue
		  Substitute
		J Synthetic Substitute
		K Nonautologous Tissue
		  Substitute
			Z No Qualifier

J Shoulder Joint, Right
  Glenohumeral joint
  Glenoid ligament (labrum)
K Shoulder Joint, Left
  See J Shoulder Joint, Right
	Ø Open	**Ø** Synthetic Substitute,
		  Reverse Ball and Socket
		7 Autologous Tissue
		  Substitute
		K Nonautologous Tissue
		  Substitute
			Z No Qualifier

J Shoulder Joint, Right
  Glenohumeral joint
  Glenoid ligament (labrum)
K Shoulder Joint, Left
  See J Shoulder Joint, Right
	Ø Open	**J** Synthetic Substitute	**6** Humeral Surface
			7 Glenoid Surface
			Z No Qualifier

Ø   **Medical and Surgical**
R   **Upper Joints**
S   **Reposition**   Definition: Moving to its normal location, or other suitable location, all or a portion of a body part

                         Explanation: The body part is moved to a new location from an abnormal location, or from a normal location where it is not functioning correctly. The body part may or may not be cut out or off to be moved to the new location.

Body Part Character 4	Approach Character 5	Device Character 6	Qualifier Character 7

Ø   **Occipital-cervical Joint**
1   **Cervical Vertebral Joint**
     Atlantoaxial joint
     Cervical facet joint
4   **Cervicothoracic Vertebral Joint**
     Cervicothoracic facet joint
6   **Thoracic Vertebral Joint**
     Costotransverse joint
     Costovertebral joint
     Thoracic facet joint
A   **Thoracolumbar Vertebral Joint**
     Thoracolumbar facet joint
C   **Temporomandibular Joint, Right**
D   **Temporomandibular Joint, Left**
E   **Sternoclavicular Joint, Right**
F   **Sternoclavicular Joint, Left**
G   **Acromioclavicular Joint, Right**
H   **Acromioclavicular Joint, Left**
J   **Shoulder Joint, Right**
     Glenohumeral joint
     Glenoid ligament (labrum)
K   **Shoulder Joint, Left**
     See J Shoulder Joint, Right
	Ø Open
	3 Percutaneous
	4 Percutaneous Endoscopic
	X External
		4 Internal Fixation Device
		Z No Device
			Z No Qualifier

L   **Elbow Joint, Right**
     Distal humerus, involving joint
     Humeroradial joint
     Humeroulnar joint
     Proximal radioulnar joint
M   **Elbow Joint, Left**
     See L Elbow Joint, Right
N   **Wrist Joint, Right**
     Distal radioulnar joint
     Radiocarpal joint
P   **Wrist Joint, Left**
     See N Wrist Joint, Right
Q   **Carpal Joint, Right**
     Intercarpal joint
     Midcarpal joint
R   **Carpal Joint, Left**
     See Q Carpal Joint, Right
S   **Carpometacarpal Joint, Right**
T   **Carpometacarpal Joint, Left**
U   **Metacarpophalangeal Joint, Right**
V   **Metacarpophalangeal Joint, Left**
W   **Finger Phalangeal Joint, Right**
     Interphalangeal (IP) joint
X   **Finger Phalangeal Joint, Left**
     See W Finger Phalangeal Joint, Right
	Ø Open
	3 Percutaneous
	4 Percutaneous Endoscopic
	X External
		4 Internal Fixation Device
		5 External Fixation Device
		Z No Device
			Z No Qualifier

Non-OR   ØRS[Ø,1,4,6,A,C,D,E,F,G,H,J,K][3,4,X][4,Z]Z
Non-OR   ØRS[L,M,N,P,Q,R,S,T,U,V,W,X][3,4,X][4,5,Z]Z

Ø   Medical and Surgical
R   Upper Joints
T   Resection   Definition: Cutting out or off, without replacement, all of a body part
                      Explanation: None

Body Part Character 4	Approach Character 5	Device Character 6	Qualifier Character 7
3 Cervical Vertebral Disc	**Ø** Open	**Z** No Device	**Z** No Qualifier
4 Cervicothoracic Vertebral Joint Cervicothoracic facet joint			
5 Cervicothoracic Vertebral Disc			
9 Thoracic Vertebral Disc			
B Thoracolumbar Vertebral Disc			
C Temporomandibular Joint, Right			
D Temporomandibular Joint, Left			
E Sternoclavicular Joint, Right			
F Sternoclavicular Joint, Left			
G Acromioclavicular Joint, Right			
H Acromioclavicular Joint, Left			

J   Shoulder Joint, Right
      Glenohumeral joint
      Glenoid ligament (labrum)			

K Shoulder Joint, Left *See J Shoulder Joint, Right*			

L   Elbow Joint, Right
      Distal humerus, involving joint
      Humeroradial joint
      Humeroulnar joint
      Proximal radioulnar joint			

M Elbow Joint, Left *See L Elbow Joint, Right*			

N   Wrist Joint, Right
      Distal radioulnar joint
      Radiocarpal joint			

P Wrist Joint, Left *See N Wrist Joint, Right*			

Q   Carpal Joint, Right
      Intercarpal joint
      Midcarpal joint			

R Carpal Joint, Left *See Q Carpal Joint, Right*			
S Carpometacarpal Joint, Right			
T Carpometacarpal Joint, Left			
U Metacarpophalangeal Joint, Right			
V Metacarpophalangeal Joint, Left			
W Finger Phalangeal Joint, Right Interphalangeal (IP) joint			
X Finger Phalangeal Joint, Left *See W Finger Phalangeal Joint, Right*			

Ø   **Medical and Surgical**
R   **Upper Joints**
U   **Supplement**   Definition: Putting in or on biological or synthetic material that physically reinforces and/or augments the function of a portion of a body part
                              Explanation: The biological material is non-living, or is living and from the same individual. The body part may have been previously replaced, and the SUPPLEMENT procedure is performed to physically reinforce and/or augment the function of the replaced body part.

Body Part Character 4	Approach Character 5	Device Character 6	Qualifier Character 7

Ø Occipital-cervical Joint
1 Cervical Vertebral Joint
   Atlantoaxial joint
   Cervical facet joint
3 Cervical Vertebral Disc
4 Cervicothoracic Vertebral Joint
   Cervicothoracic facet joint
5 Cervicothoracic Vertebral Disc
6 Thoracic Vertebral Joint
   Costotransverse joint
   Costovertebral joint
   Thoracic facet joint
9 Thoracic Vertebral Disc
A Thoracolumbar Vertebral Joint
   Thoracolumbar facet joint
B Thoracolumbar Vertebral Disc
C Temporomandibular Joint, Right
D Temporomandibular Joint, Left
E Sternoclavicular Joint, Right
F Sternoclavicular Joint, Left
G Acromioclavicular Joint, Right
H Acromioclavicular Joint, Left
J Shoulder Joint, Right
   Glenohumeral joint
   Glenoid ligament (labrum)
K Shoulder Joint, Left
   See J Shoulder Joint, Right
L Elbow Joint, Right
   Distal humerus, involving joint
   Humeroradial joint
   Humeroulnar joint
   Proximal radioulnar joint
M Elbow Joint, Left
   See L Elbow Joint, Right
N Wrist Joint, Right
   Distal radioulnar joint
   Radiocarpal joint
P Wrist Joint, Left
   See N Wrist Joint, Right
Q Carpal Joint, Right
   Intercarpal joint
   Midcarpal joint
R Carpal Joint, Left
   See Q Carpal Joint, Right
S Carpometacarpal Joint, Right
T Carpometacarpal Joint, Left
U Metacarpophalangeal Joint, Right
V Metacarpophalangeal Joint, Left
W Finger Phalangeal Joint, Right
   Interphalangeal (IP) joint
X Finger Phalangeal Joint, Left
   See W Finger Phalangeal Joint, Right
	Ø Open
	3 Percutaneous
	4 Percutaneous Endoscopic
		7 Autologous Tissue
		   Substitute
		J Synthetic Substitute
		K Nonautologous Tissue
		   Substitute
			Z No Qualifier

HAC   ØRU[E,F,G,H,J,K,L,M][Ø,3,4][7,J,K]Z when reported with SDx K68.11 or T81.4Ø–T81.49, T84.6Ø-T84.619, T84.63-T84.7 with 7th character A

NC Noncovered Procedure   LC Limited Coverage   QA Questionable OB Admit   NT New Tech Add-on   ✛ Combination Member   ♂ Male   ♀ Female

Upper Joints

Ø   **Medical and Surgical**
R   **Upper Joints**
W   **Revision**   Definition: Correcting, to the extent possible, a portion of a malfunctioning device or the position of a displaced device

Explanation: Revision can include correcting a malfunctioning or displaced device by taking out or putting in components of the device such as a screw or pin

Body Part Character 4	Approach Character 5	Device Character 6	Qualifier Character 7

Ø Occipital-cervical Joint
1 Cervical Vertebral Joint
   Atlantoaxial joint
   Cervical facet joint
4 Cervicothoracic Vertebral Joint
   Cervicothoracic facet joint
6 Thoracic Vertebral Joint
   Costotransverse joint
   Costovertebral joint
   Thoracic facet joint
A Thoracolumbar Vertebral Joint
   Thoracolumbar facet joint
	Ø Open
	3 Percutaneous
	4 Percutaneous Endoscopic
	X External
		Ø Drainage Device
		3 Infusion Device
		4 Internal Fixation Device
		7 Autologous Tissue Substitute
		8 Spacer
		A Interbody Fusion Device
		J Synthetic Substitute
		K Nonautologous Tissue Substitute
			Z No Qualifier

3 Cervical Vertebral Disc 5 Cervicothoracic Vertebral Disc 9 Thoracic Vertebral Disc B Thoracolumbar Vertebral Disc	Ø Open 3 Percutaneous 4 Percutaneous Endoscopic X External	Ø Drainage Device 3 Infusion Device 7 Autologous Tissue Substitute J Synthetic Substitute K Nonautologous Tissue Substitute	Z No Qualifier
C Temporomandibular Joint, Right D Temporomandibular Joint, Left E Sternoclavicular Joint, Right F Sternoclavicular Joint, Left G Acromioclavicular Joint, Right H Acromioclavicular Joint, Left	Ø Open 3 Percutaneous 4 Percutaneous Endoscopic X External	Ø Drainage Device 3 Infusion Device 4 Internal Fixation Device 7 Autologous Tissue Substitute 8 Spacer J Synthetic Substitute K Nonautologous Tissue Substitute	Z No Qualifier

J Shoulder Joint, Right
   Glenohumeral joint
   Glenoid ligament (labrum)
K Shoulder Joint, Left
   See J Shoulder Joint, Right
	Ø Open
	3 Percutaneous
	4 Percutaneous Endoscopic
	X External
		Ø Drainage Device
		3 Infusion Device
		4 Internal Fixation Device
		7 Autologous Tissue Substitute
		8 Spacer
		J Synthetic Substitute
		K Nonautologous Tissue Substitute
			Z No Qualifier

J Shoulder Joint, Right
   Glenohumeral joint
   Glenoid ligament (labrum)
K Shoulder Joint, Left
   See J Shoulder Joint, Right
	Ø Open
	3 Percutaneous
	4 Percutaneous Endoscopic
	X External
		J Synthetic Substitute	6 Humeral Surgace
			7 Glenoid Surface
			Z No Qualifier

L Elbow Joint, Right
   Distal humerus, involving joint
   Humeroradial joint
   Humeroulnar joint
   Proximal radioulnar joint
M Elbow Joint, Left
   See L Elbow Joint, Right
N Wrist Joint, Right
   Distal radioulnar joint
   Radiocarpal joint
P Wrist Joint, Left
   See N Wrist Joint, Right
Q Carpal Joint, Right
   Intercarpal joint
   Midcarpal joint
R Carpal Joint, Left
   See Q Carpal Joint, Right
S Carpometacarpal Joint, Right
T Carpometacarpal Joint, Left
U Metacarpophalangeal Joint, Right
V Metacarpophalangeal Joint, Left
W Finger Phalangeal Joint, Right
   Interphalangeal (IP) joint
X Finger Phalangeal Joint, Left
   See W Finger Phalangeal Joint, Right
	Ø Open
	3 Percutaneous
	4 Percutaneous Endoscopic
	X External
		Ø Drainage Device
		3 Infusion Device
		4 Internal Fixation Device
		5 External Fixation Device
		7 Autologous Tissue Substitute
		8 Spacer
		J Synthetic Substitute
		K Nonautologous Tissue Substitute
			Z No Qualifier

Non-OR   ØRW[Ø,1,4,6,A]X[Ø,3,4,7,8,A,J,K]Z
Non-OR   ØRW[3,5,9,B]X[Ø,3,7,J,K]Z
Non-OR   ØRW[C,D,E,F,G,H]X[Ø,3,4,7,8,J,K]Z
Non-OR   ØRW[J,K]X[Ø,3,4,7,8,J,K]Z
Non-OR   ØRW[J,K]XJ[6,7]
Non-OR   ØRW[L,M,N,P,Q,R,S,T,U,V,W,X]X[Ø,3,4,5,7,8,J,K]Z

Lower Joints ØS2–ØSW

Character Meanings*

This Character Meaning table is provided as a guide to assist the user in the identification of character members that may be found in this section of code tables. It **SHOULD NOT** be used to build a PCS code.

Operation–Character 3	Body Part–Character 4	Approach–Character 5	Device–Character 6	Qualifier–Character 7
2 Change	Ø Lumbar Vertebral Joint	Ø Open	Ø Drainage Device OR Synthetic Substitute, Polyethylene	Ø Anterior Approach, Anterior Column
5 Destruction	1 Lumbar Vertebral Joint, 2 or more	3 Percutaneous	1 Synthetic Substitute, Metal	1 Posterior Approach, Posterior Column
9 Drainage	2 Lumbar Vertebral Disc	4 Percutaneous Endoscopic	2 Synthetic Substitute, Metal on Polyethylene	9 Cemented
B Excision	3 Lumbosacral Joint	X External	3 Infusion Device OR Internal Fixation Device, Sustained Compression OR Synthetic Substitute, Ceramic	A Uncemented
C Extirpation	4 Lumbosacral Disc		4 Internal Fixation Device OR Synthetic Substitute, Ceramic on Polyethylene	C Patellar Surface
G Fusion	5 Sacrococcygeal Joint		5 External Fixation Device	J Posterior Approach, Anterior Column
H Insertion	6 Coccygeal Joint		6 Synthetic Substitute, Oxidized Zirconium on Polyethylene	X Diagnostic
J Inspection	7 Sacroiliac Joint, Right		7 Autologous Tissue Substitute	Z No Qualifier
N Release	8 Sacroiliac Joint, Left		8 Spacer	
P Removal	9 Hip Joint, Right		9 Liner	
Q Repair	A Hip Joint, Acetabular Surface, Right		A Interbody Fusion Device	
R Replacement	B Hip Joint, Left		B Resurfacing Device OR Spinal Stabilization Device, Interspinous Process	
S Reposition	C Knee Joint, Right		C Spinal Stabilization Device, Pedicle-Based	
T Resection	D Knee Joint, Left		D Spinal Stabilization Device, Facet Replacement	
U Supplement	E Hip Joint, Acetabular Surface, Left		E Articulating Spacer	
W Revision	F Ankle Joint, Right		J Synthetic Substitute	
	G Ankle Joint, Left		K Nonautologous Tissue Substitute	
	H Tarsal Joint, Right		L Synthetic Substitute, Unicondylar Medial	
	J Tarsal Joint, Left		M Synthetic Substitute, Unicondylar Lateral	
	K Tarsometatarsal Joint, Right		N Synthetic Substitute, Patellofemoral	
	L Tarsometatarsal Joint, Left		Y Other Device	
	M Metatarsal-Phalangeal Joint, Right		Z No Device	
	N Metatarsal-Phalangeal Joint, Left			
	P Toe Phalangeal Joint, Right			
	Q Toe Phalangeal Joint, Left			
	R Hip Joint, Femoral Surface, Right			
	S Hip Joint, Femoral Surface, Left			
	T Knee Joint, Femoral Surface, Right			
	U Knee Joint, Femoral Surface, Left			
	V Knee Joint, Tibial Surface, Right			
	W Knee Joint, Tibial Surface, Left			
	Y Lower Joint			

* Includes synovial membrane.

AHA Coding Clinic for table ØS9

2018, 2Q, 17	Arthroscopic drainage of knee and nonexcisional debridement
2017, 1Q, 50	Dry aspiration of ankle joint

AHA Coding Clinic for table ØSB

2017, 4Q, 76	Radiolucent porous interbody fusion device
2016, 2Q, 16	Decompressive laminectomy/foraminotomy and lumbar discectomy
2016, 1Q, 20	Metatarsophalangeal joint resection arthroplasty
2015, 1Q, 34	Arthroscopic meniscectomy with debridement and abrasion chondroplasty
2014, 2Q, 6	Posterior lumbar fusion with discectomy

AHA Coding Clinic for table ØSG

2021, 1Q, 18	Placement of interspinous distraction device (spacer) for decompression
2021, 1Q, 53	Official guidelines for coding and reporting for interbody fusion device B3.10c
2020, 4Q, 56-58	Intramedullary sustained compression joint fusion
2020, 2Q, 27	Spinal Fusion with NuVasive® VersaTie®
2020, 1Q, 33	Spinal fusion without use of bone graft
2019, 3Q, 35	Fusion procedures of the spine (guideline B3.10c)
2019, 1Q, 30	Spinal fusion performed at same level as decompressive laminectomy
2018, 4Q, 43	Joint fusion device value
2018, 1Q, 22	Spinal fusion procedures without bone graft
2017, 4Q, 76	Radiolucent porous interbody fusion device
2017, 2Q, 23	Decompression of spinal cord and placement of instrumentation
2014, 3Q, 30	Spinal fusion and fixation instrumentation
2014, 3Q, 36	Lumbar interbody fusion of two vertebral levels
2014, 2Q, 6	Posterior lumbar fusion with discectomy
2013, 3Q, 25	360-degree spinal fusion
2013, 2Q, 39	Ankle fusion, osteotomy, and removal of hardware
2013, 1Q, 21-23	Spinal fusion of thoracic and lumbar vertebrae

AHA Coding Clinic for table ØSH

2021, 1Q, 18	Placement of interspinous distraction device (spacer) for decompression
2017, 2Q, 23	Decompression of spinal cord and placement of instrumentation

AHA Coding Clinic for table ØSJ

2017, 1Q, 50	Dry aspiration of ankle joint

AHA Coding Clinic for table ØSN

2020, 2Q, 26	Arthroscopic Manipulation and Nonexcisional Debridement of Knee Joint
2019, 1Q, 30	Spinal fusion performed at same level as decompressive laminectomy

AHA Coding Clinic for table ØSP

2021, 1Q, 17	Revision of ankle arthroplasty with placement of tibial insert
2018, 4Q, 43	Articulating spacer for hip and knee joint
2018, 2Q, 16	Exchange of tibial polyethylene component with stabilizing insert (tibial tray)
2017, 4Q, 107	Total ankle replacement versus revision
2016, 4Q, 110-112	Removal and revision of hip and knee devices
2015, 2Q, 18	Total knee revision
2015, 2Q, 19	Revision of femoral head and acetabular liner
2013, 2Q, 39	Ankle fusion, osteotomy, and removal of hardware

AHA Coding Clinic for table ØSQ

2014, 4Q, 25	Femoroacetabular impingement and labral tear with repair

AHA Coding Clinic for table ØSR

2021, 1Q, 17	Revision of ankle arthroplasty with placement of tibial insert
2020, 3Q, 33	Total hip arthroplasty using dual mobility components
2018, 4Q, 43	Articulating spacer for hip and knee joint
2018, 2Q, 16	Exchange of tibial polyethylene component with stabilizing insert (tibial tray)
2017, 4Q, 38-39	Oxidized zirconium on polyethylene bearing surface
2017, 4Q, 107	Total ankle replacement versus revision
2017, 1Q, 22	Total knee replacement and patellar component
2016, 4Q, 110-111	Partial (unicondylar) knee replacement
2016, 4Q, 111-112	Removal and revision of hip and knee devices
2016, 3Q, 35	Use of cemented versus uncemented qualifier for joint replacement
2015, 3Q, 18	Total hip replacement with acetabular reconstruction
2015, 2Q, 18	Total knee revision
2015, 2Q, 19	Revision of femoral head and acetabular liner

AHA Coding Clinic for table ØSS

2016, 2Q, 31	Periacetabular ostectomy for repair of congenital hip dysplasia

AHA Coding Clinic for table ØST

2016, 1Q, 20	Metatarsophalangeal joint resection arthroplasty
2014, 4Q, 29	Rotational osteosynthesis

AHA Coding Clinic for table ØSU

2021, 1Q, 17	Revision of ankle arthroplasty with placement of tibial insert
2018, 2Q, 16	Exchange of tibial polyethylene component with stabilizing insert (tibial tray)
2016, 4Q, 111	Removal and revision of hip and knee devices
2015, 2Q, 19	Revision of femoral head and acetabular liner

AHA Coding Clinic for table ØSW

2017, 4Q, 107	Total ankle replacement versus revision
2016, 4Q, 110-112	Removal and revision of hip and knee devices
2015, 2Q, 18	Total knee revision
2015, 2Q, 19	Revision of femoral head and acetabular liner

Lower Joints

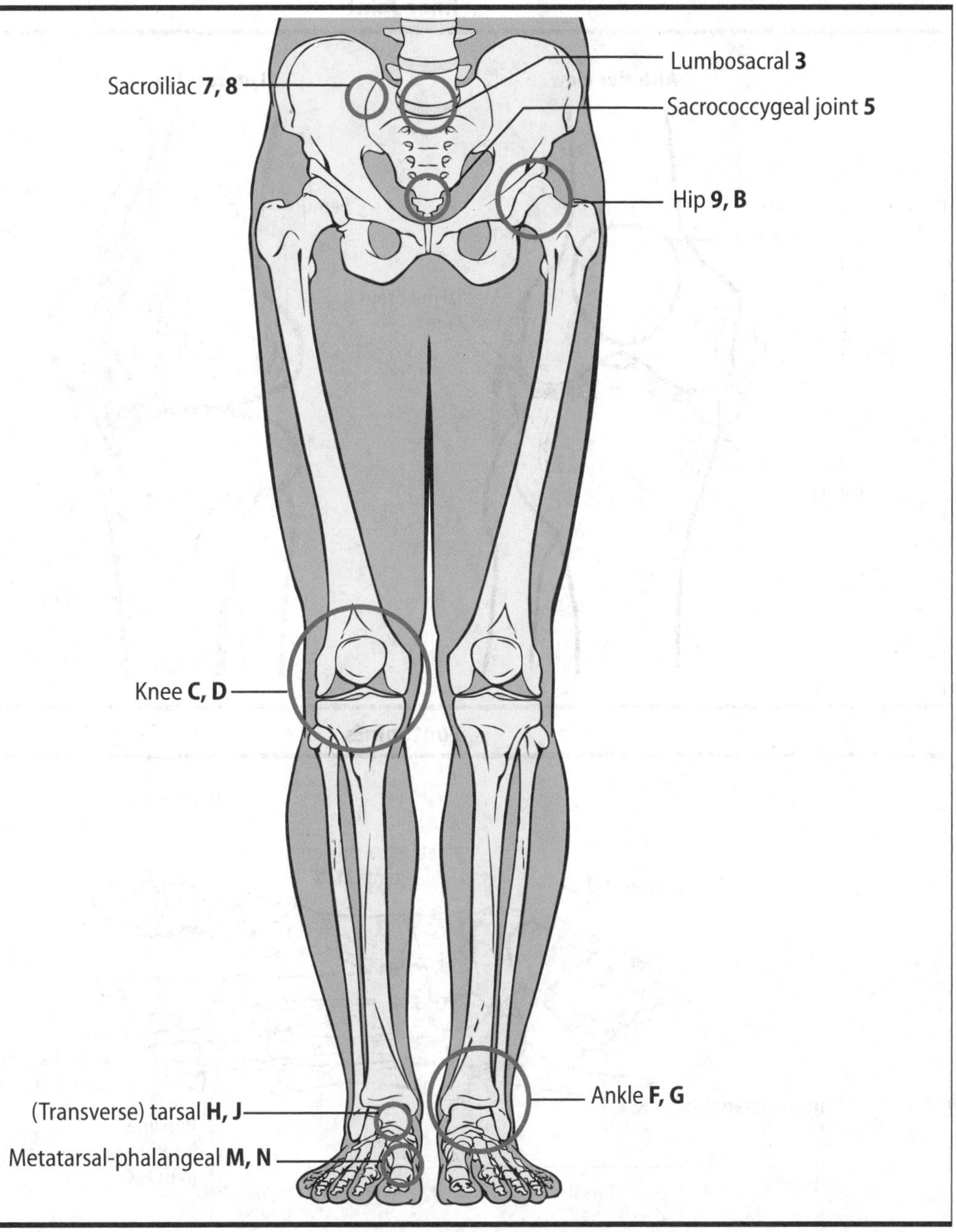

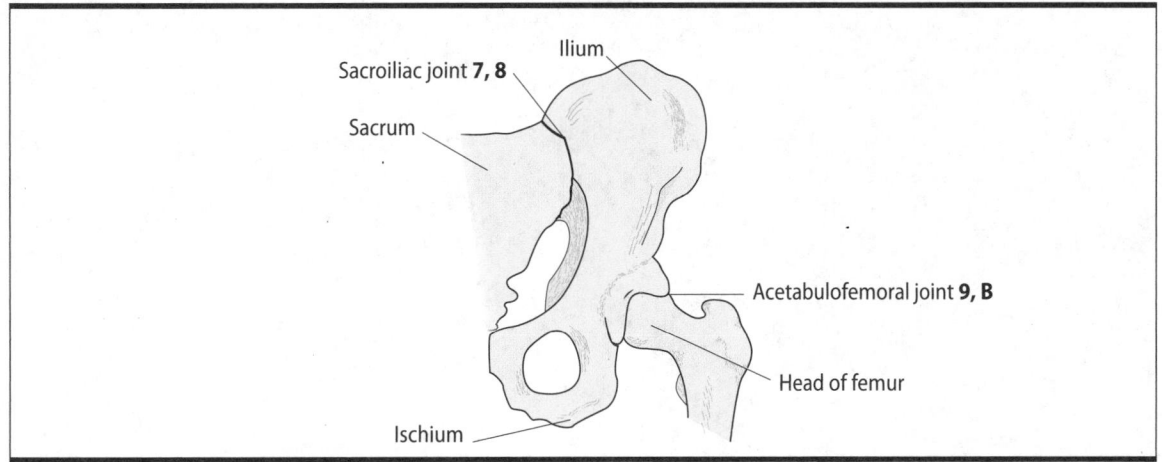

Sacroiliac **7, 8**

Lumbosacral **3**

Sacrococcygeal joint **5**

Hip **9, B**

Knee **C, D**

(Transverse) tarsal **H, J**

Metatarsal-phalangeal **M, N**

Ankle **F, G**

Hip Joint

Sacroiliac joint **7, 8**

Ilium

Sacrum

Acetabulofemoral joint **9, B**

Head of femur

Ischium

Knee Joint

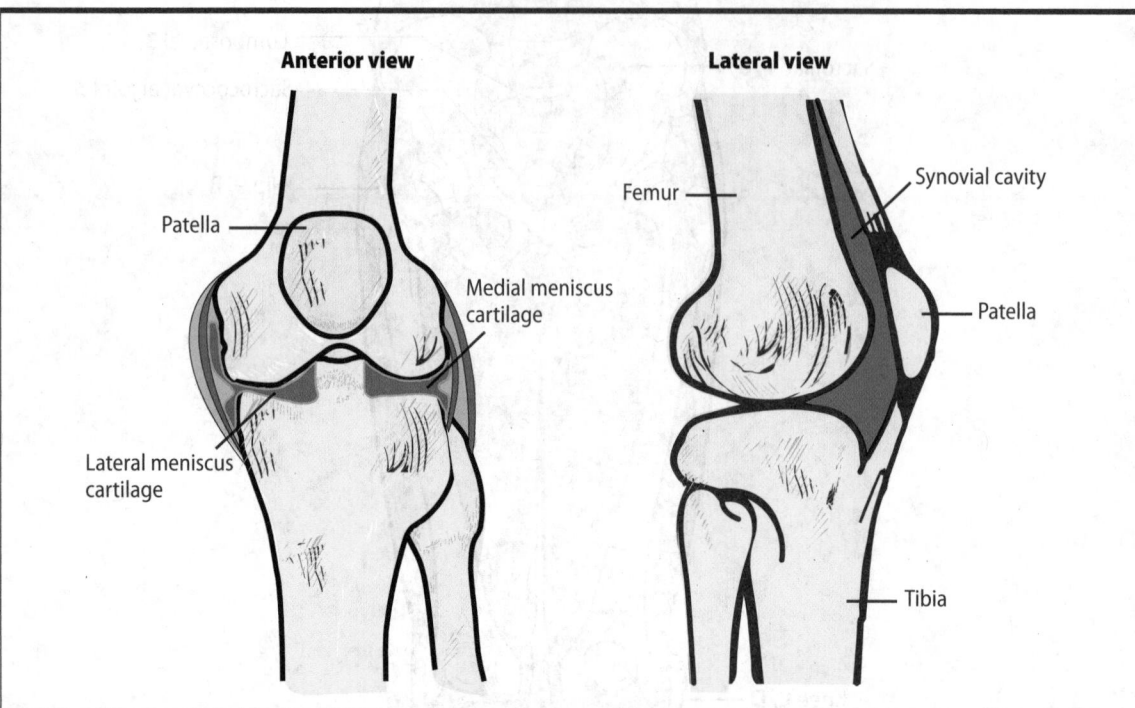

Anterior view

Patella

Medial meniscus cartilage

Lateral meniscus cartilage

Lateral view

Femur

Synovial cavity

Patella

Tibia

Foot Joints

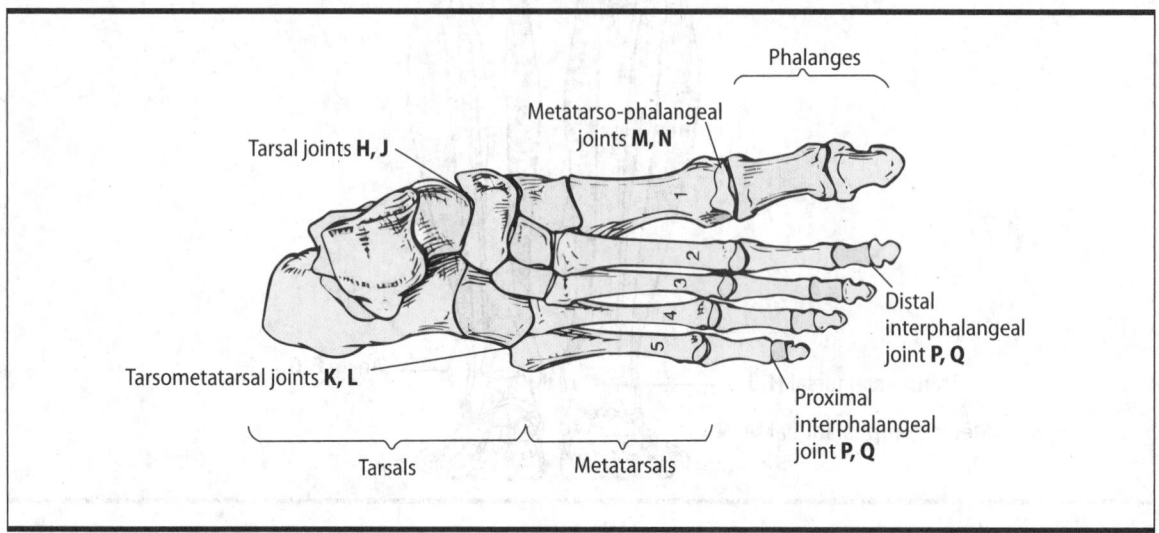

Phalanges

Metatarso-phalangeal joints **M, N**

Tarsal joints **H, J**

Tarsometatarsal joints **K, L**

Distal interphalangeal joint **P, Q**

Proximal interphalangeal joint **P, Q**

Tarsals

Metatarsals

Ø   Medical and Surgical
S   Lower Joints
2   Change   Definition: Taking out or off a device from a body part and putting back an identical or similar device in or on the same body part without cutting or puncturing the skin or a mucous membrane

                   Explanation: All CHANGE procedures are coded using the approach EXTERNAL

Body Part Character 4	Approach Character 5	Device Character 6	Qualifier Character 7
Y Lower Joint	X External	Ø Drainage Device Y Other Device	Z No Qualifier

Non-OR	All body part, approach, device, and qualifier values

Ø   Medical and Surgical
S   Lower Joints
5   Destruction   Definition: Physical eradication of all or a portion of a body part by the direct use of energy, force, or a destructive agent

                   Explanation: None of the body part is physically taken out

Body Part Character 4	Approach Character 5	Device Character 6	Qualifier Character 7

Ø   **Lumbar Vertebral Joint**
    Lumbar facet joint
2   **Lumbar Vertebral Disc**
3   **Lumbosacral Joint**
    Lumbosacral facet joint
4   **Lumbosacral Disc**
5   **Sacrococcygeal Joint**
    Sacrococcygeal symphysis
6   **Coccygeal Joint**
7   **Sacroiliac Joint, Right**
8   **Sacroiliac Joint, Left**
9   **Hip Joint, Right**
    Acetabulofemoral joint
B   **Hip Joint, Left**
    See 9 Hip Joint, Right
C   **Knee Joint, Right**
    Femoropatellar joint
    Femorotibial joint
    Lateral meniscus
    Medial meniscus
    Patellofemoral joint
    Tibiofemoral joint
D   **Knee Joint, Left**
    See C Knee Joint, Right
F   **Ankle Joint, Right**
    Inferior tibiofibular joint
    Talocrural joint
G   **Ankle Joint, Left**
    See F Ankle Joint, Right
H   **Tarsal Joint, Right**
    Calcaneocuboid joint
    Cuboideonavicular joint
    Cuneonavicular joint
    Intercuneiform joint
    Subtalar (talocalcaneal) joint
    Talocalcaneal (subtalar) joint
    Talocalcaneonavicular joint
J   **Tarsal Joint, Left**
    See H Tarsal Joint, Right
K   **Tarsometatarsal Joint, Right**
L   **Tarsometatarsal Joint, Left**
M   **Metatarsal-Phalangeal Joint, Right**
    Metatarsophalangeal (MTP) joint
N   **Metatarsal-Phalangeal Joint, Left**
    See M Metatarsal-Phalangeal Joint, Right
P   **Toe Phalangeal Joint, Right**
    Interphalangeal (IP) joint
Q   **Toe Phalangeal Joint, Left**
    See P Toe Phalangeal Joint, Right
	Ø Open
	3 Percutaneous
	4 Percutaneous Endoscopic
		Z No Device	Z No Qualifier

NC Noncovered Procedure   LC Limited Coverage   QA Questionable OB Admit   NT New Tech Add-on   ⊞ Combination Member   ♂ Male   ♀ Female

ICD-10-PCS 2022   603

ØS2–ØS5

Ø **Medical and Surgical**
S **Lower Joints**
9 **Drainage**　　Definition: Taking or letting out fluids and/or gases from a body part
　　　　　　　　　　Explanation: The qualifier DIAGNOSTIC is used to identify drainage procedures that are biopsies

Body Part — Character 4		Approach — Character 5	Device — Character 6	Qualifier — Character 7
Ø **Lumbar Vertebral Joint** Lumbar facet joint **2** **Lumbar Vertebral Disc** **3** **Lumbosacral Joint** Lumbosacral facet joint **4** **Lumbosacral Disc** **5** **Sacrococcygeal Joint** Sacrococcygeal symphysis **6** **Coccygeal Joint** **7** **Sacroiliac Joint, Right** **8** **Sacroiliac Joint, Left** **9** **Hip Joint, Right** Acetabulofemoral joint **B** **Hip Joint, Left** *See 9 Hip Joint, Right* **C** **Knee Joint, Right** Femoropatellar joint Femorotibial joint Lateral meniscus Medial meniscus Patellofemoral joint Tibiofemoral joint **D** **Knee Joint, Left** *See C Knee Joint, Right* **F** **Ankle Joint, Right** Inferior tibiofibular joint Talocrural joint **G** **Ankle Joint, Left** *See F Ankle Joint, Right*	**H** **Tarsal Joint, Right** Calcaneocuboid joint Cuboideonavicular joint Cuneonavicular joint Intercuneiform joint Subtalar (talocalcaneal) joint Talocalcaneal (subtalar) joint Talocalcaneonavicular joint **J** **Tarsal Joint, Left** *See H Tarsal Joint, Right* **K** **Tarsometatarsal Joint, Right** **L** **Tarsometatarsal Joint, Left** **M** **Metatarsal-Phalangeal Joint, Right** Metatarsophalangeal (MTP) joint **N** **Metatarsal-Phalangeal Joint, Left** *See M Metatarsal-Phalangeal Joint, Right* **P** **Toe Phalangeal Joint, Right** Interphalangeal (IP) joint **Q** **Toe Phalangeal Joint, Left** *See P Toe Phalangeal Joint, Right*	**Ø** Open **3** Percutaneous **4** Percutaneous Endoscopic	**Ø** Drainage Device	**Z** No Qualifier
Ø **Lumbar Vertebral Joint** Lumbar facet joint **2** **Lumbar Vertebral Disc** **3** **Lumbosacral Joint** Lumbosacral facet joint **4** **Lumbosacral Disc** **5** **Sacrococcygeal Joint** Sacrococcygeal symphysis **6** **Coccygeal Joint** **7** **Sacroiliac Joint, Right** **8** **Sacroiliac Joint, Left** **9** **Hip Joint, Right** Acetabulofemoral joint **B** **Hip Joint, Left** *See 9 Hip Joint, Right* **C** **Knee Joint, Right** Femoropatellar joint Femorotibial joint Lateral meniscus Medial meniscus Patellofemoral joint Tibiofemoral joint **D** **Knee Joint, Left** *See C Knee Joint, Right* **F** **Ankle Joint, Right** Inferior tibiofibular joint Talocrural joint **G** **Ankle Joint, Left** *See F Ankle Joint, Right*	**H** **Tarsal Joint, Right** Calcaneocuboid joint Cuboideonavicular joint Cuneonavicular joint Intercuneiform joint Subtalar (talocalcaneal) joint Talocalcaneal (subtalar) joint Talocalcaneonavicular joint **J** **Tarsal Joint, Left** *See H Tarsal Joint, Right* **K** **Tarsometatarsal Joint, Right** **L** **Tarsometatarsal Joint, Left** **M** **Metatarsal-Phalangeal Joint, Right** Metatarsophalangeal (MTP) joint **N** **Metatarsal-Phalangeal Joint, Left** *See M Metatarsal-Phalangeal Joint, Right* **P** **Toe Phalangeal Joint, Right** Interphalangeal (IP) joint **Q** **Toe Phalangeal Joint, Left** *See P Toe Phalangeal Joint, Right*	**Ø** Open **3** Percutaneous **4** Percutaneous Endoscopic	**Z** No Device	**X** Diagnostic **Z** No Qualifier

Non-OR　　ØS9[Ø,2,3,4,5,6,7,8,9,B,C,D,F,G,H,J,K,L,M,N,P,Q][3,4]ØZ
Non-OR　　ØS9[Ø,2,3,4,5,6,7,8,9,B,C,D,F,G,H,J,K,L,M,N,P,Q][Ø,3,4]ZX
Non-OR　　ØS9[Ø,2,3,4,5,6,7,8,9,B,C,D,F,G,H,J,K,L,M,N,P,Q][3,4]ZZ

Ø　**Medical and Surgical**
S　**Lower Joints**
B　**Excision**　　　Definition: Cutting out or off, without replacement, a portion of a body part
　　　　　　　　　　　Explanation: The qualifier DIAGNOSTIC is used to identify excision procedures that are biopsies

Body Part Character 4	Approach Character 5	Device Character 6	Qualifier Character 7
Ø **Lumbar Vertebral Joint** Lumbar facet joint **2** **Lumbar Vertebral Disc** **3** **Lumbosacral Joint** Lumbosacral facet joint **4** **Lumbosacral Disc** **5** **Sacrococcygeal Joint** Sacrococcygeal symphysis **6** **Coccygeal Joint** **7** **Sacroiliac Joint, Right** **8** **Sacroiliac Joint, Left** **9** **Hip Joint, Right** Acetabulofemoral joint **B** **Hip Joint, Left** *See 9 Hip Joint, Right* **C** **Knee Joint, Right** Femoropatellar joint Femorotibial joint Lateral meniscus Medial meniscus Patellofemoral joint Tibiofemoral joint **D** **Knee Joint, Left** *See C Knee Joint, Right* **F** **Ankle Joint, Right** Inferior tibiofibular joint Talocrural joint **G** **Ankle Joint, Left** *See F Ankle Joint, Right* **H** **Tarsal Joint, Right** Calcaneocuboid joint Cuboideonavicular joint Cuneonavicular joint Intercuneiform joint Subtalar (talocalcaneal) joint Talocalcaneal (subtalar) joint Talocalcaneonavicular joint **J** **Tarsal Joint, Left** *See H Tarsal Joint, Right* **K** **Tarsometatarsal Joint, Right** **L** **Tarsometatarsal Joint, Left** **M** **Metatarsal-Phalangeal Joint, Right** Metatarsophalangeal (MTP) joint **N** **Metatarsal-Phalangeal Joint, Left** *See M Metatarsal-Phalangeal Joint, Right* **P** **Toe Phalangeal Joint, Right** Interphalangeal (IP) joint **Q** **Toe Phalangeal Joint, Left** *See P Toe Phalangeal Joint, Right*	**Ø** Open **3** Percutaneous **4** Percutaneous Endoscopic	**Z** No Device	**X** Diagnostic **Z** No Qualifier

Non-OR　ØSB[Ø,2,3,4,5,6,7,8,9,B,C,D,F,G,H,J,K,L,M,N,P,Q][Ø,3,4]ZX

NC Noncovered Procedure　　LC Limited Coverage　　QA Questionable OB Admit　　NT New Tech Add-on　　⊞ Combination Member　　♂ Male　　♀ Female

ICD-10-PCS 2022　　　605

Ø   **Medical and Surgical**
S   **Lower Joints**
C   **Extirpation**   Definition: Taking or cutting out solid matter from a body part

                              Explanation: The solid matter may be an abnormal byproduct of a biological function or a foreign body; it may be imbedded in a body part or in the lumen of a tubular body part. The solid matter may or may not have been previously broken into pieces.

Body Part Character 4	Approach Character 5	Device Character 6	Qualifier Character 7

Ø **Lumbar Vertebral Joint**
    Lumbar facet joint
2 **Lumbar Vertebral Disc**
3 **Lumbosacral Joint**
    Lumbosacral facet joint
4 **Lumbosacral Disc**
5 **Sacrococcygeal Joint**
    Sacrococcygeal symphysis
6 **Coccygeal Joint**
7 **Sacroiliac Joint, Right**
8 **Sacroiliac Joint, Left**
9 **Hip Joint, Right**
    Acetabulofemoral joint
B **Hip Joint, Left**
    See 9 Hip Joint, Right
C **Knee Joint, Right**
    Femoropatellar joint
    Femorotibial joint
    Lateral meniscus
    Medial meniscus
    Patellofemoral joint
    Tibiofemoral joint
D **Knee Joint, Left**
    See C Knee Joint, Right
F **Ankle Joint, Right**
    Inferior tibiofibular joint
    Talocrural joint
G **Ankle Joint, Left**
    See F Ankle Joint, Right
H **Tarsal Joint, Right**
    Calcaneocuboid joint
    Cuboideonavicular joint
    Cuneonavicular joint
    Intercuneiform joint
    Subtalar (talocalcaneal) joint
    Talocalcaneal (subtalar) joint
    Talocalcaneonavicular joint
J **Tarsal Joint, Left**
    See H Tarsal Joint, Right
K **Tarsometatarsal Joint, Right**
L **Tarsometatarsal Joint, Left**
M **Metatarsal-Phalangeal Joint, Right**
    Metatarsophalangeal (MTP) joint
N **Metatarsal-Phalangeal Joint, Left**
    See M Metatarsal-Phalangeal Joint, Right
P **Toe Phalangeal Joint, Right**
    Interphalangeal (IP) joint
Q **Toe Phalangeal Joint, Left**
    See P Toe Phalangeal Joint, Right
	Ø Open
	3 Percutaneous
	4 Percutaneous Endoscopic
		Z No Device	**Z** No Qualifier

Ø   Medical and Surgical
S   Lower Joints
G   Fusion   Definition: Joining together portions of an articular body part rendering the articular body part immobile
               Explanation: The body part is joined together by fixation device, bone graft, or other means

Body Part Character 4	Approach Character 5	Device Character 6	Qualifier Character 7

Ø Lumbar Vertebral Joint
   Lumbar facet joint
1 Lumbar Vertebral Joints, 2 or more ⊞
3 Lumbosacral Joint
   Lumbosacral facet joint
	Ø Open
	3 Percutaneous
	4 Percutaneous Endoscopic
		7 Autologous Tissue Substitute
		J Synthetic Substitute
		K Nonautologous Tissue Substitute
			Ø Anterior Approach, Anterior
			   Column
			1 Posterior Approach, Posterior
			   Column
			J Posterior Approach, Anterior
			   Column

Ø Lumbar Vertebral Joint
   Lumbar facet joint
1 Lumbar Vertebral Joints, 2 or more ⊞
3 Lumbosacral Joint
   Lumbosacral facet joint
	Ø Open
	3 Percutaneous
	4 Percutaneous Endoscopic
		A Interbody Fusion Device	**Ø** Anterior Approach, Anterior
			   Column
			J Posterior Approach, Anterior
			   Column

5 Sacrococcygeal Joint Sacrococcygeal symphysis **6** Coccygeal Joint **7** Sacroiliac Joint, Right **8** Sacroiliac Joint, Left	**Ø** Open **3** Percutaneous **4** Percutaneous Endoscopic	**4** Internal Fixation Device **7** Autologous Tissue Substitute **J** Synthetic Substitute **K** Nonautologous Tissue Substitute	**Z** No Qualifier

9 Hip Joint, Right
   Acetabulofemoral joint
B Hip Joint, Left
   See 9 Hip Joint, Right
C Knee Joint, Right
   Femoropatellar joint
   Femorotibial joint
   Lateral meniscus
   Medial meniscus
   Patellofemoral joint
   Tibiofemoral joint
D Knee Joint, Left
   See C Knee Joint, Right
F Ankle Joint, Right
   Inferior tibiofibular joint
   Talocrural joint
G Ankle Joint, Left
   See F Ankle Joint, Right
H Tarsal Joint, Right
   Calcaneocuboid joint
   Cuboideonavicular joint
   Cuneonavicular joint
   Intercuneiform joint
   Subtalar (talocalcaneal) joint
   Talocalcaneal (subtalar) joint
   Talocalcaneonavicular joint
J Tarsal Joint, Left
   See H Tarsal Joint, Right
K Tarsometatarsal Joint, Right
L Tarsometatarsal Joint, Left
M Metatarsal-Phalangeal Joint, Right
   Metatarsophalangeal (MTP) joint
N Metatarsal-Phalangeal Joint, Left
   See M Metatarsal-Phalangeal Joint, Right
P Toe Phalangeal Joint, Right
   Interphalangeal (IP) joint
Q Toe Phalangeal Joint, Left
   See P Toe Phalangeal Joint, Right
	Ø Open
	3 Percutaneous
	4 Percutaneous Endoscopic
		3 Internal Fixation Device,
		   Sustained Compression
		4 Internal Fixation Device
		5 External Fixation Device
		7 Autologous Tissue Substitute
		J Synthetic Substitute
		K Nonautologous Tissue Substitute
			Z No Qualifier

HAC   ØSG[Ø,1,3][Ø,3,4][7,J,K][Ø,1,J] when reported with SDx K68.11 or T81.4Ø–
       T81.49, T84.6Ø-T84.619, T84.63-T84.7 with 7th character A
HAC   ØSG[Ø,1,3][Ø,3,4]A[Ø,J] when reported with SDx K68.11 or T81.4Ø–T81.49,
       T84.6Ø-T84.619, T84.63-T84.7 with 7th character A
HAC   ØSG[7,8][Ø,3,4][4,7,J,K]Z when reported with SDx K68.11 or T81.4Ø–T81.49,
       T84.6Ø-T84.619, T84.63-T84.7 with 7th character A

See Appendix L for Procedure Combinations
⊞   ØSG1[Ø,3,4][7,J,K][Ø,1,J]
⊞   ØSG1[Ø,3,4]A[Ø,J]

NC Noncovered Procedure   **LC** Limited Coverage   **QA** Questionable OB Admit   **NT** New Tech Add-on   ⊞ Combination Member   ♂ Male   ♀ Female

ICD-10-PCS 2022   607

ØSG–ØSG

Ø   Medical and Surgical
S   Lower Joints
H   Insertion   Definition: Putting in a nonbiological appliance that monitors, assists, performs, or prevents a physiological function but does not physically take the place of a body part
                     Explanation: None

Body Part Character 4	Approach Character 5	Device Character 6	Qualifier Character 7
Ø Lumbar Vertebral Joint Lumbar facet joint **3 Lumbosacral Joint** Lumbosacral facet joint	**Ø** Open **3** Percutaneous **4** Percutaneous Endoscopic	**3** Infusion Device **4** Internal Fixation Device **8** Spacer **B** Spinal Stabilization Device, Interspinous Process **C** Spinal Stabilization Device, Pedicle-Based **D** Spinal Stabilization Device, Facet Replacement	**Z** No Qualifier
2 Lumbar Vertebral Disc **4 Lumbosacral Disc**	**Ø** Open **3** Percutaneous **4** Percutaneous Endoscopic	**3** Infusion Device **8** Spacer	**Z** No Qualifier
5 Sacrococcygeal Joint Sacrococcygeal symphysis **6 Coccygeal Joint** **7 Sacroiliac Joint, Right** **8 Sacroiliac Joint, Left**	**Ø** Open **3** Percutaneous **4** Percutaneous Endoscopic	**3** Infusion Device **4** Internal Fixation Device **8** Spacer	**Z** No Qualifier
9 Hip Joint, Right Acetabulofemoral joint **B Hip Joint, Left** *See 9 Hip Joint, Right* **C Knee Joint, Right** Femoropatellar joint Femorotibial joint Lateral meniscus Medial meniscus Patellofemoral joint Tibiofemoral joint **D Knee Joint, Left** *See C Knee Joint, Right* **F Ankle Joint, Right** Inferior tibiofibular joint Talocrural joint **G Ankle Joint, Left** *See F Ankle Joint, Right* **H Tarsal Joint, Right** Calcaneocuboid joint Cuboideonavicular joint Cuneonavicular joint Intercuneiform joint Subtalar (talocalcaneal) joint Talocalcaneal (subtalar) joint Talocalcaneonavicular joint **J Tarsal Joint, Left** *See H Tarsal Joint, Right* **K Tarsometatarsal Joint, Right** **L Tarsometatarsal Joint, Left** **M Metatarsal-Phalangeal Joint, Right** Metatarsophalangeal (MTP) joint **N Metatarsal-Phalangeal Joint, Left** *See M Metatarsal-Phalangeal Joint, Right* **P Toe Phalangeal Joint, Right** Interphalangeal (IP) joint **Q Toe Phalangeal Joint, Left** *See P Toe Phalangeal Joint, Right*	**Ø** Open **3** Percutaneous **4** Percutaneous Endoscopic	**3** Infusion Device **4** Internal Fixation Device **5** External Fixation Device **8** Spacer	**Z** No Qualifier

Non-OR	ØSH[Ø,3][Ø,3,4][3,8]Z
Non-OR	ØSH[2,4][Ø,3,4][3,8]Z
Non-OR	ØSH[5,6,7,8][Ø,3,4][3,8]Z
Non-OR	ØSH[9,B,C,D][Ø,3,4]3Z
Non-OR	ØSH[9,B,C,D][3,4]8Z
Non-OR	ØSH[F,G,H,J,K,L,M,N,P,Q][Ø,3,4][3,8]Z

Ø   Medical and Surgical
S   Lower Joints
J   Inspection   Definition: Visually and/or manually exploring a body part

Explanation: Visual exploration may be performed with or without optical instrumentation. Manual exploration may be performed directly or through intervening body layers.

Body Part Character 4		Approach Character 5	Device Character 6	Qualifier Character 7

Ø Lumbar Vertebral Joint
Lumbar facet joint
2 Lumbar Vertebral Disc
3 Lumbosacral Joint
Lumbosacral facet joint
4 Lumbosacral Disc
5 Sacrococcygeal Joint
Sacrococcygeal symphysis
6 Coccygeal Joint
7 Sacroiliac Joint, Right
8 Sacroiliac Joint, Left
9 Hip Joint, Right
Acetabulofemoral joint
B Hip Joint, Left
See 9 Hip Joint, Right
C Knee Joint, Right
Femoropatellar joint
Femorotibial joint
Lateral meniscus
Medial meniscus
Patellofemoral joint
Tibiofemoral joint
D Knee Joint, Left
See C Knee Joint, Right
F Ankle Joint, Right
Inferior tibiofibular joint
Talocrural joint
G Ankle Joint, Left
See F Ankle Joint, Right
	H Tarsal Joint, Right
	Calcaneocuboid joint
	Cuboideonavicular joint
	Cuneonavicular joint
	Intercuneiform joint
	Subtalar (talocalcaneal) joint
	Talocalcaneal (subtalar)
	  joint
	Talocalcaneonavicular joint
	J Tarsal Joint, Left
	See H Tarsal Joint, Right
	K Tarsometatarsal Joint, Right
	L Tarsometatarsal Joint, Left
	M Metatarsal-Phalangeal Joint, Right
	Metatarsophalangeal (MTP)
	  joint
	N Metatarsal-Phalangeal Joint, Left
	See M Metatarsal-Phalangeal Joint, Right
	P Toe Phalangeal Joint, Right
	Interphalangeal (IP) joint
	Q Toe Phalangeal Joint, Left
	See P Toe Phalangeal Joint, Right
		Ø Open
		3 Percutaneous
		4 Percutaneous Endoscopic
		X External
			Z No Device	**Z** No Qualifier

Non-OR   ØSJ[Ø,2,3,4,5,6,7,8,9,B,C,D,F,G,H,J,K,L,M,N,P,Q][3,X]ZZ

Ø   Medical and Surgical
S   Lower Joints
N   Release   Definition: Freeing a body part from an abnormal physical constraint by cutting or by the use of force

Explanation: Some of the restraining tissue may be taken out but none of the body part is taken out

Body Part Character 4		Approach Character 5	Device Character 6	Qualifier Character 7

Ø Lumbar Vertebral Joint
Lumbar facet joint
2 Lumbar Vertebral Disc
3 Lumbosacral Joint
Lumbosacral facet joint
4 Lumbosacral Disc
5 Sacrococcygeal Joint
Sacrococcygeal symphysis
6 Coccygeal Joint
7 Sacroiliac Joint, Right
8 Sacroiliac Joint, Left
9 Hip Joint, Right
Acetabulofemoral joint
B Hip Joint, Left
See 9 Hip Joint, Right
C Knee Joint, Right
Femoropatellar joint
Femorotibial joint
Lateral meniscus
Medial meniscus
Patellofemoral joint
Tibiofemoral joint
D Knee Joint, Left
See C Knee Joint, Right
F Ankle Joint, Right
Inferior tibiofibular joint
Talocrural joint
G Ankle Joint, Left
See F Ankle Joint, Right
	H Tarsal Joint, Right
	Calcaneocuboid joint
	Cuboideonavicular joint
	Cuneonavicular joint
	Intercuneiform joint
	Subtalar (talocalcaneal) joint
	Talocalcaneal (subtalar)
	  joint
	Talocalcaneonavicular joint
	J Tarsal Joint, Left
	See H Tarsal Joint, Right
	K Tarsometatarsal Joint, Right
	L Tarsometatarsal Joint, Left
	M Metatarsal-Phalangeal Joint, Right
	Metatarsophalangeal (MTP)
	  joint
	N Metatarsal-Phalangeal Joint, Left
	See M Metatarsal-Phalangeal Joint, Right
	P Toe Phalangeal Joint, Right
	Interphalangeal (IP) joint
	Q Toe Phalangeal Joint, Left
	See P Toe Phalangeal Joint, Right
		Ø Open
		3 Percutaneous
		4 Percutaneous Endoscopic
		X External
			Z No Device	**Z** No Qualifier

Non-OR   ØSN[Ø,2,3,4,5,6,7,8,9,B,C,D,F,G,H,J,K,L,M,N,P,Q]XZZ

NC Noncovered Procedure   LC Limited Coverage   QA Questionable OB Admit   NT New Tech Add-on   ⊞ Combination Member   ♂ Male   ♀ Female

ICD-10-PCS 2022   609

ØSJ–ØSN

Ø   Medical and Surgical
S   Lower Joints
P   Removal   Definition: Taking out or off a device from a body part

Explanation: If a device is taken out and a similar device put in without cutting or puncturing the skin or mucous membrane, the procedure is coded to the root operation CHANGE. Otherwise, the procedure for taking out the device is coded to the root operation REMOVAL.

Body Part Character 4	Approach Character 5	Device Character 6	Qualifier Character 7

Ø   Lumbar Vertebral Joint
     Lumbar facet joint
3   Lumbosacral Joint
     Lumbosacral facet joint
	Ø Open
	3 Percutaneous
	4 Percutaneous Endoscopic
		Ø Drainage Device
		3 Infusion Device
		4 Internal Fixation Device
		7 Autologous Tissue Substitute
		8 Spacer
		A Interbody Fusion Device
		J Synthetic Substitute
		K Nonautologous Tissue Substitute
			Z No Qualifier

Ø   Lumbar Vertebral Joint
     Lumbar facet joint
3   Lumbosacral Joint
     Lumbosacral facet joint
	X External	Ø Drainage Device
		3 Infusion Device
		4 Internal Fixation Device
			Z No Qualifier

2 Lumbar Vertebral Disc 4 Lumbosacral Disc	Ø Open 3 Percutaneous 4 Percutaneous Endoscopic	Ø Drainage Device 3 Infusion Device 7 Autologous Tissue Substitute J Synthetic Substitute K Nonautologous Tissue Substitute	Z No Qualifier
2 Lumbar Vertebral Disc 4 Lumbosacral Disc	X External	Ø Drainage Device 3 Infusion Device	Z No Qualifier
5 Sacrococcygeal Joint Sacrococcygeal symphysis 6 Coccygeal Joint 7 Sacroiliac Joint, Right 8 Sacroiliac Joint, Left	Ø Open 3 Percutaneous 4 Percutaneous Endoscopic	Ø Drainage Device 3 Infusion Device 4 Internal Fixation Device 7 Autologous Tissue Substitute 8 Spacer J Synthetic Substitute K Nonautologous Tissue Substitute	Z No Qualifier
5 Sacrococcygeal Joint Sacrococcygeal symphysis 6 Coccygeal Joint 7 Sacroiliac Joint, Right 8 Sacroiliac Joint, Left	X External	Ø Drainage Device 3 Infusion Device 4 Internal Fixation Device	Z No Qualifier

9   Hip Joint, Right ⊞
     Acetabulofemoral joint
B   Hip Joint, Left ⊞
     See 9 Hip Joint, Right
	Ø Open	Ø Drainage Device
		3 Infusion Device
		4 Internal Fixation Device
		5 External Fixation Device
		7 Autologous Tissue Substitute
		8 Spacer
		9 Liner
		B Resurfacing Device
		E Articulating Spacer
		J Synthetic Substitute
		K Nonautologous Tissue Substitute
			Z No Qualifier

9   Hip Joint, Right ⊞
     Acetabulofemoral joint
B   Hip Joint, Left ⊞
     See 9 Hip Joint, Right
	3 Percutaneous
	4 Percutaneous Endoscopic
		Ø Drainage Device
		3 Infusion Device
		4 Internal Fixation Device
		5 External Fixation Device
		7 Autologous Tissue Substitute
		8 Spacer
		J Synthetic Substitute
		K Nonautologous Tissue Substitute
			Z No Qualifier

9   Hip Joint, Right ⊞
     Acetabulofemoral joint
B   Hip Joint, Left ⊞
     See 9 Hip Joint, Right
	X External	Ø Drainage Device
		3 Infusion Device
		4 Internal Fixation Device
		5 External Fixation Device
			Z No Qualifier

Non-OR ØSP[Ø,3][Ø,3,4]8Z		
Non-OR ØSP[Ø,3]3[Ø,3]Z	**See Appendix L for Procedure Combinations**	
Non-OR ØSP[Ø,3]X[Ø,3,4]Z	**Combo-only** ØSP[9,B]48Z	
Non-OR ØSP[2,4]3[Ø,3]Z	⊞ ØSP[9,B]Ø[8,9,B,E,J]Z	
Non-OR ØSP[2,4]X[Ø,3]Z	⊞ ØSP[9,B]4JZ	
Non-OR ØSP[5,6,7,8][Ø,3,4]8Z		
Non-OR ØSP[5,6,7,8]3[Ø,3]Z		
Non-OR ØSP[5,6,7,8]X[Ø,3,4]Z		
Non-OR ØSP[9,B]3[Ø,3,8]Z		
Non-OR ØSP[9,B]X[Ø,3,4,5]Z		

ØSP Continued on next page

Lower Joints

ØSP Continued

Ø   **Medical and Surgical**
S   **Lower Joints**
P   **Removal**   Definition: Taking out or off a device from a body part

Explanation: If a device is taken out and a similar device put in without cutting or puncturing the skin or mucous membrane, the procedure is coded to the root operation CHANGE. Otherwise, the procedure for taking out the device is coded to the root operation REMOVAL.

Body Part Character 4	Approach Character 5	Device Character 6	Qualifier Character 7

A Hip Joint, Acetabular Surface, Right ⊞
E Hip Joint, Acetabular Surface, Left ⊞
R Hip Joint, Femoral Surface, Right ⊞
S Hip Joint, Femoral Surface, Left ⊞
T Knee Joint, Femoral Surface, Right ⊞
   Femoropatellar joint
   Patellofemoral joint
U Knee Joint, Femoral Surface, Left ⊞
   See T Knee Joint, Femoral Surface, Right
V Knee Joint, Tibial Surface, Right ⊞
   Femorotibial joint
   Tibiofemoral joint
W Knee Joint, Tibial Surface, Left ⊞
   See V Knee Joint, Tibial Surface, Right
	Ø Open
	3 Percutaneous
	4 Percutaneous Endoscopic
		J Synthetic Substitute	**Z** No Qualifier

C Knee Joint, Right ⊞
   Femoropatellar joint
   Femorotibial joint
   Lateral meniscus
   Medial meniscus
   Patellofemoral joint
   Tibiofemoral joint
D Knee Joint, Left ⊞
   See C Knee Joint, Right
	Ø Open	**Ø** Drainage Device
		3 Infusion Device
		4 Internal Fixation Device
		5 External Fixation Device
		7 Autologous Tissue Substitute
		8 Spacer
		9 Liner
		E Articulating Spacer
		K Nonautologous Tissue Substitute
		L Synthetic Substitute, Unicondylar Medial
		M Synthetic Substitute, Unicondylar Lateral
		N Synthetic Substitute, Patellofemoral
			Z No Qualifier

C Knee Joint, Right ⊞
   Femoropatellar joint
   Femorotibial joint
   Lateral meniscus
   Medial meniscus
   Patellofemoral joint
   Tibiofemoral joint
D Knee Joint, Left ⊞
   See C Knee Joint, Right
	Ø Open	**J** Synthetic Substitute	**C** Patellar Surface
			Z No Qualifier

C Knee Joint, Right ⊞
   Femoropatellar joint
   Femorotibial joint
   Lateral meniscus
   Medial meniscus
   Patellofemoral joint
   Tibiofemoral joint
D Knee Joint, Left ⊞
   See C Knee Joint, Right
	3 Percutaneous
	4 Percutaneous Endoscopic
		Ø Drainage Device
		3 Infusion Device
		4 Internal Fixation Device
		5 External Fixation Device
		7 Autologous Tissue Substitute
		8 Spacer
		K Nonautologous Tissue Substitute
		L Synthetic Substitute, Unicondylar Medial
		M Synthetic Substitute, Unicondylar Lateral
		N Synthetic Substitute, Patellofemoral
			Z No Qualifier

C Knee Joint, Right ⊞
   Femoropatellar joint
   Femorotibial joint
   Lateral meniscus
   Medial meniscus
   Patellofemoral joint
   Tibiofemoral joint
D Knee Joint, Left ⊞
   See C Knee Joint, Right
	3 Percutaneous
	4 Percutaneous Endoscopic
		J Synthetic Substitute	**C** Patellar Surface
			Z No Qualifier

Non-OR   ØSP[C,D]3[Ø,3]Z

See Appendix L for Procedure Combinations
Combo-only   ØSP[C,D][3,4]8Z   ⊞   ØSP[C,D]ØJ[C,Z]
⊞   ØSP[A,E,R,S,T,U,V,W][Ø,4]JZ   ⊞   ØSP[C,D]4[L,M,N]Z
⊞   ØSP[C,D]Ø[8,9,E,L,M,N]Z   ⊞   ØSP[C,D]4J[C,Z]

ØSP Continued on next page

NC Noncovered Procedure   **LC** Limited Coverage   **QA** Questionable OB Admit   **NT** New Tech Add-on   ⊞ Combination Member   ♂ Male   ♀ Female

ICD-10-PCS 2022   611

ØSP–ØSP

0   Medical and Surgical
S   Lower Joints
P   Removal   Definition: Taking out or off a device from a body part

ØSP Continued

Explanation: If a device is taken out and a similar device put in without cutting or puncturing the skin or mucous membrane, the procedure is coded to the root operation CHANGE. Otherwise, the procedure for taking out the device is coded to the root operation REMOVAL.

Body Part Character 4	Approach Character 5	Device Character 6	Qualifier Character 7
C Knee Joint, Right Femoropatellar joint Femorotibial joint Lateral meniscus Medial meniscus Patellofemoral joint Tibiofemoral joint **D Knee Joint, Left** *See C Knee Joint, Right*	**X** External	**Ø** Drainage Device **3** Infusion Device **4** Internal Fixation Device **5** External Fixation Device	**Z** No Qualifier
F Ankle Joint, Right Inferior tibiofibular joint Talocrural joint **G Ankle Joint, Left** *See F Ankle Joint, Right* **H Tarsal Joint, Right** Calcaneocuboid joint Cuboideonavicular joint Cuneonavicular joint Intercuneiform joint Subtalar (talocalcaneal) joint Talocalcaneal (subtalar) joint Talocalcaneonavicular joint **J Tarsal Joint, Left** *See H Tarsal Joint, Right* **K Tarsometatarsal Joint, Right** **L Tarsometatarsal Joint, Left** **M Metatarsal-Phalangeal Joint, Right** Metatarsophalangeal (MTP) joint **N Metatarsal-Phalangeal Joint, Left** *See M Metatarsal-Phalangeal Joint, Right* **P Toe Phalangeal Joint, Right** Interphalangeal (IP) joint **Q Toe Phalangeal Joint, Left** *See P Toe Phalangeal Joint, Right*	**Ø** Open **3** Percutaneous **4** Percutaneous Endoscopic	**Ø** Drainage Device **3** Infusion Device **4** Internal Fixation Device **5** External Fixation Device **7** Autologous Tissue Substitute **8** Spacer **J** Synthetic Substitute **K** Nonautologous Tissue Substitute	**Z** No Qualifier
F Ankle Joint, Right Inferior tibiofibular joint Talocrural joint **G Ankle Joint, Left** *See F Ankle Joint, Right* **H Tarsal Joint, Right** Calcaneocuboid joint Cuboideonavicular joint Cuneonavicular joint Intercuneiform joint Subtalar (talocalcaneal) joint Talocalcaneal (subtalar) joint Talocalcaneonavicular joint **J Tarsal Joint, Left** *See H Tarsal Joint, Right* **K Tarsometatarsal Joint, Right** **L Tarsometatarsal Joint, Left** **M Metatarsal-Phalangeal Joint, Right** Metatarsophalangeal (MTP) joint **N Metatarsal-Phalangeal Joint, Left** *See M Metatarsal-Phalangeal Joint, Right* **P Toe Phalangeal Joint, Right** Interphalangeal (IP) joint **Q Toe Phalangeal Joint, Left** *See P Toe Phalangeal Joint, Right*	**X** External	**Ø** Drainage Device **3** Infusion Device **4** Internal Fixation Device **5** External Fixation Device	**Z** No Qualifier

Non-OR	ØSP[C,D]X[Ø,3,4,5]Z
Non-OR	ØSP[F,G,H,J,K,L,M,N,P,Q]3[Ø,3,8]Z
Non-OR	ØSP[F,G,H,J,K,L,M,N,P,Q][Ø,4]8Z
Non-OR	ØSP[F,G,H,J,K,L,M,N,P,Q]X[Ø,3,4,5]Z

0 **Medical and Surgical**
S **Lower Joints**
Q **Repair**　　　Definition: Restoring, to the extent possible, a body part to its normal anatomic structure and function
　　　　　　　　　　Explanation: Used only when the method to accomplish the repair is not one of the other root operations

Body Part Character 4	Approach Character 5	Device Character 6	Qualifier Character 7
0 **Lumbar Vertebral Joint** 　Lumbar facet joint **2** **Lumbar Vertebral Disc** **3** **Lumbosacral Joint** 　Lumbosacral facet joint **4** **Lumbosacral Disc** **5** **Sacrococcygeal Joint** 　Sacrococcygeal symphysis **6** **Coccygeal Joint** **7** **Sacroiliac Joint, Right** **8** **Sacroiliac Joint, Left** **9** **Hip Joint, Right** 　Acetabulofemoral joint **B** **Hip Joint, Left** 　*See 9 Hip Joint, Right* **C** **Knee Joint, Right** 　Femoropatellar joint 　Femorotibial joint 　Lateral meniscus 　Medial meniscus 　Patellofemoral joint 　Tibiofemoral joint **D** **Knee Joint, Left** 　*See C Knee Joint, Right* **F** **Ankle Joint, Right** 　Inferior tibiofibular joint 　Talocrural joint **G** **Ankle Joint, Left** 　*See F Ankle Joint, Right* **H** **Tarsal Joint, Right** 　Calcaneocuboid joint 　Cuboideonavicular joint 　Cuneonavicular joint 　Intercuneiform joint 　Subtalar (talocalcaneal) joint 　Talocalcaneal (subtalar) joint 　Talocalcaneonavicular joint **J** **Tarsal Joint, Left** 　*See H Tarsal Joint, Right* **K** **Tarsometatarsal Joint, Right** **L** **Tarsometatarsal Joint, Left** **M** **Metatarsal-Phalangeal Joint, Right** 　Metatarsophalangeal (MTP) joint **N** **Metatarsal-Phalangeal Joint, Left** 　*See M Metatarsal-Phalangeal Joint, Right* **P** **Toe Phalangeal Joint, Right** 　Interphalangeal (IP) joint **Q** **Toe Phalangeal Joint, Left** 　*See P Toe Phalangeal Joint, Right*	**0** Open **3** Percutaneous **4** Percutaneous Endoscopic **X** External	**Z** No Device	**Z** No Qualifier

Non-OR　0SQ[0,2,3,4,5,6,7,8,9,B,C,D,F,G,H,J,K,L,M,N,P,Q]XZZ

NC Noncovered Procedure　　**LC** Limited Coverage　　**OA** Questionable OB Admit　　**NT** New Tech Add-on　　⊞ Combination Member　　♂ Male　　♀ Female

ICD-10-PCS 2022　　**613**

0SQ–0SQ

Ø Medical and Surgical
S Lower Joints
R Replacement   Definition: Putting in or on biological or synthetic material that physically takes the place and/or function of all or a portion of a body part

Explanation: The body part may have been taken out or replaced, or may be taken out, physically eradicated, or rendered nonfunctional during the REPLACEMENT procedure. A REMOVAL procedure is coded for taking out the device used in a previous replacement procedure.

Body Part Character 4	Approach Character 5	Device Character 6	Qualifier Character 7

Ø Lumbar Vertebral Joint
  Lumbar facet joint
2 Lumbar Vertebral Disc NC
3 Lumbosacral Joint
  Lumbosacral facet joint
4 Lumbosacral Disc NC
5 Sacrococcygeal Joint
  Sacrococcygeal symphysis
6 Coccygeal Joint
7 Sacroiliac Joint, Right
8 Sacroiliac Joint, Left
H Tarsal Joint, Right
  Calcaneocuboid joint
  Cuboideonavicular joint
  Cuneonavicular joint
  Intercuneiform joint
  Subtalar (talocalcaneal) joint
  Talocalcaneal (subtalar) joint
  Talocalcaneonavicular joint
J Tarsal Joint, Left
  See H Tarsal Joint, Right
K Tarsometatarsal Joint, Right
L Tarsometatarsal Joint, Left
M Metatarsal-Phalangeal Joint, Right
  Metatarsophalangeal (MTP) joint
N Metatarsal-Phalangeal Joint, Left
  See M Metatarsal-Phalangeal Joint, Right
P Toe Phalangeal Joint, Right
  Interphalangeal (IP) joint
Q Toe Phalangeal Joint, Left
  See P Toe Phalangeal Joint, Right
	Ø Open	7 Autologous Tissue Substitute
		J Synthetic Substitute
		K Nonautologous Tissue Substitute
			Z No Qualifier

9 Hip Joint, Right ⊞
  Acetabulofemoral joint
B Hip Joint, Left ⊞
  See 9 Hip Joint, Right
	Ø Open	1 Synthetic Substitute, Metal
		2 Synthetic Substitute, Metal on
		  Polyethylene
		3 Synthetic Substitute, Ceramic
		4 Synthetic Substitute, Ceramic on
		  Polyethylene
		6 Synthetic Substitute, Oxidized
		  Zirconium on Polyethylene
		J Synthetic Substitute
			9 Cemented
			A Uncemented
			Z No Qualifier

9 Hip Joint, Right ⊞
  Acetabulofemoral joint
B Hip Joint, Left ⊞
  See 9 Hip Joint, Right
	Ø Open	7 Autologous Tissue Substitute
		E Articulating Spacer
		K Nonautologous Tissue Substitute
			Z No Qualifier

A Hip Joint, Acetabular Surface, ⊞
  Right
E Hip Joint, Acetabular Surface, ⊞
  Left
	Ø Open	Ø Synthetic Substitute, Polyethylene
		1 Synthetic Substitute, Metal
		3 Synthetic Substitute, Ceramic
		J Synthetic Substitute
			9 Cemented
			A Uncemented
			Z No Qualifier

A Hip Joint, Acetabular Surface, Right E Hip Joint, Acetabular Surface, Left	Ø Open	7 Autologous Tissue Substitute K Nonautologous Tissue Substitute	Z No Qualifier

HAC	ØSR[9,B]Ø[1,2,3,4,6,J][9,A,Z] when reported with SDx of I26.Ø2-I26.Ø9, I26.92-I26.99, or I82.4Ø1-I82.4Z9
HAC	ØSR[9,B]Ø[7,E,K]Z when reported with SDx of I26.Ø2-I26.Ø9, I26.92-I26.99, or I82.4Ø1-I82.4Z9
HAC	ØSR[A,E]Ø[Ø,1,3,J][9,A,Z] when reported with SDx of I26.Ø2-I26.Ø9, I26.92-I26.99, or I82.4Ø1-I82.4Z9
HAC	ØSR[A,E]Ø[7,K]Z when reported with SDx of I26.Ø2-I26.Ø9, I26.92-I26.99, or I82.4Ø1-I82.4Z9
NC	ØSR[2,4]ØJZ when beneficiary age is over 6Ø

See Appendix L for Procedure Combinations
⊞ ØSR[9,B]Ø[1,2,3,4,6,J][9,A,Z]
⊞ ØSR[9,B]ØEZ
⊞ ØSR[A,E]Ø[Ø,1,3,J][9,A,Z]

ØSR Continued on next page

ØSR Continued

Ø **Medical and Surgical**
S **Lower Joints**
R **Replacement**

Definition: Putting in or on biological or synthetic material that physically takes the place and/or function of all or a portion of a body part

Explanation: The body part may have been taken out or replaced, or may be taken out, physically eradicated, or rendered nonfunctional during the REPLACEMENT procedure. A REMOVAL procedure is coded for taking out the device used in a previous replacement procedure.

Body Part Character 4	Approach Character 5	Device Character 6	Qualifier Character 7
C **Knee Joint, Right** Femoropatellar joint Femorotibial joint Lateral meniscus Medial meniscus Patellofemoral joint Tibiofemoral joint D **Knee Joint, Left** ⊞ *See C Knee Joint, Right*	Ø Open	6 Synthetic Substitute, Oxidized Zirconium on Polyethylene J Synthetic Substitute L Synthetic Substitute, Unicondylar Medial M Synthetic Substitute, Unicondylar Lateral N Synthetic Substitute, Patellofemoral	9 Cemented A Uncemented Z No Qualifier
C **Knee Joint, Right** Femoropatellar joint Femorotibial joint Lateral meniscus Medial meniscus Patellofemoral joint Tibiofemoral joint D **Knee Joint, Left** ⊞ *See C Knee Joint, Right*	Ø Open	7 Autologous Tissue Substitute E Articulating Spacer K Nonautologous Tissue Substitute	Z No Qualifier
F **Ankle Joint, Right** Inferior tibiofibular joint Talocrural joint G **Ankle Joint, Left** *See F Ankle Joint, Right* T **Knee Joint, Femoral Surface, Right** Femoropatellar joint Patellofemoral joint U **Knee Joint, Femoral Surface, Left** *See T Knee Joint, Femoral Surface, Right* V **Knee Joint, Tibial Surface, Right** Femorotibial joint Tibiofemoral joint W **Knee Joint, Tibial Surface, Left** *See V Knee Joint, Tibial Surface, Right*	Ø Open	7 Autologous Tissue Substitute K Nonautologous Tissue Substitute	Z No Qualifier
F **Ankle Joint, Right** Inferior tibiofibular joint Talocrural joint G **Ankle Joint, Left** *See F Ankle Joint, Right* T **Knee Joint, Femoral Surface, Right** ⊞ Femoropatellar joint Patellofemoral joint U **Knee Joint, Femoral Surface, Left** ⊞ *See T Knee Joint, Femoral Surface, Right* V **Knee Joint, Tibial Surface, Right** ⊞ Femorotibial joint Tibiofemoral joint W **Knee Joint, Tibial Surface, Left** ⊞ *See V Knee Joint, Tibial Surface, Right*	Ø Open	J Synthetic Substitute	9 Cemented A Uncemented Z No Qualifier
R **Hip Joint, Femoral Surface, Right** ⊞ S **Hip Joint, Femoral Surface, Left** ⊞	Ø Open	1 Synthetic Substitute, Metal 3 Synthetic Substitute, Ceramic J Synthetic Substitute	9 Cemented A Uncemented Z No Qualifier
R **Hip Joint, Femoral Surface, Right** S **Hip Joint, Femoral Surface, Left**	Ø Open	7 Autologous Tissue Substitute K Nonautologous Tissue Substitute	Z No Qualifier

HAC ØSR[C,D]Ø[6,J,L,M,N][9,A,Z] when reported with SDx of I26.Ø2-I26.Ø9, I26.92-I26.99 or I82.4Ø1-I82.4Z9

HAC ØSR[C,D]Ø[7,E,K]Z when reported with SDx of I26.Ø2-I26.Ø9, I26.92-I26.99 or I82.4Ø1-I82.4Z9

HAC ØSR[T,U,V,W]Ø[7,K]Z when reported with SDx of I26.Ø2-I26.Ø9, I26.92-I26.99 or I82.4Ø1-I82.4Z9

HAC ØSR[T,U,V,W]ØJ[9,A,Z] when reported with SDx of I26.Ø2-I26.Ø9, I26.92-I26.99 or I82.4Ø1-I82.4Z9

HAC ØSR[R,S]Ø[1,3,J][9,A,Z] when reported with SDx of I26.Ø2-I26.Ø9, I26.92-I26.99, or I82.4Ø1-I82.4Z9

HAC ØSR[R,S]Ø[7,K]Z when reported with SDx of I26.Ø2-I26.Ø9, I26.92-I26.99, or I82.4Ø1-I82.4Z9

See Appendix L for Procedure Combinations
⊞ ØSR[C,D]Ø[6,J,L,M,N][9,A,Z]
⊞ ØSR[C,D]ØEZ
⊞ ØSR[T,U,V,W]ØJ[9,A,Z]
⊞ ØSR[R,S]Ø[1,3,J][9,A,Z]

NC Noncovered Procedure   **LC** Limited Coverage   **QA** Questionable OB Admit   **NT** New Tech Add-on   ⊞ Combination Member   ♂Male   ♀Female

ICD-10-PCS 2022   **615**

ØSR–ØSR

Ø   **Medical and Surgical**
S   **Lower Joints**
S   **Reposition**   Definition: Moving to its normal location, or other suitable location, all or a portion of a body part

Explanation: The body part is moved to a new location from an abnormal location, or from a normal location where it is not functioning correctly. The body part may or may not be cut out or off to be moved to the new location.

Body Part Character 4		Approach Character 5	Device Character 6	Qualifier Character 7

Ø **Lumbar Vertebral Joint**
   Lumbar facet joint
3 **Lumbosacral Joint**
   Lumbosacral facet joint
5 **Sacrococcygeal Joint**
   Sacrococcygeal symphysis
6 **Coccygeal Joint**
7 **Sacroiliac Joint, Right**
8 **Sacroiliac Joint, Left**
		Ø Open
		3 Percutaneous
		4 Percutaneous Endoscopic
		X External
			4 Internal Fixation Device
			Z No Device
				Z No Qualifier

9 **Hip Joint, Right**
   Acetabulofemoral joint
B **Hip Joint, Left**
   See 9 Hip Joint, Right
C **Knee Joint, Right**
   Femoropatellar joint
   Femorotibial joint
   Lateral meniscus
   Medial meniscus
   Patellofemoral joint
   Tibiofemoral joint
D **Knee Joint, Left**
   See C Knee Joint, Right
F **Ankle Joint, Right**
   Inferior tibiofibular joint
   Talocrural joint
G **Ankle Joint, Left**
   See F Ankle Joint, Right
H **Tarsal Joint, Right**
   Calcaneocuboid joint
   Cuboideonavicular joint
   Cuneonavicular joint
   Intercuneiform joint
   Subtalar (talocalcaneal) joint
   Talocalcaneal (subtalar)
      joint
   Talocalcaneonavicular joint
	J **Tarsal Joint, Left**
	   See H Tarsal Joint, Right
	K **Tarsometatarsal Joint,
	   Right**
	L **Tarsometatarsal Joint, Left**
	M **Metatarsal-Phalangeal
	   Joint, Right**
	   Metatarsophalangeal (MTP)
	      joint
	N **Metatarsal-Phalangeal
	   Joint, Left**
	   *See M Metatarsal-Phalangeal
	      Joint, Right*
	P **Toe Phalangeal Joint, Right**
	   Interphalangeal (IP) joint
	Q **Toe Phalangeal Joint, Left**
	   *See P Toe Phalangeal Joint,
	      Right*
		Ø Open
		3 Percutaneous
		4 Percutaneous Endoscopic
		X External
			4 Internal Fixation Device
			5 External Fixation Device
			Z No Device
				Z No Qualifier

Non-OR	ØSS[Ø,3,5,6,7,8][3,4,X][4,Z]Z
Non-OR	ØSS[9,B,C,D,F,G,H,J,K,L,M,N,P,Q][3,4,X][4,5,Z]Z

Ø   **Medical and Surgical**
S   **Lower Joints**
T   **Resection**   Definition: Cutting out or off, without replacement, all of a body part

Explanation: None

Body Part Character 4		Approach Character 5	Device Character 6	Qualifier Character 7

2 **Lumbar Vertebral Disc**
4 **Lumbosacral Disc**
5 **Sacrococcygeal Joint**
   Sacrococcygeal symphysis
6 **Coccygeal Joint**
7 **Sacroiliac Joint, Right**
8 **Sacroiliac Joint, Left**
9 **Hip Joint, Right**
   Acetabulofemoral joint
B **Hip Joint, Left**
   See 9 Hip Joint, Right
C **Knee Joint, Right**
   Femoropatellar joint
   Femorotibial joint
   Lateral meniscus
   Medial meniscus
   Patellofemoral joint
   Tibiofemoral joint
D **Knee Joint, Left**
   See C Knee Joint, Right
F **Ankle Joint, Right**
   Inferior tibiofibular joint
   Talocrural joint
G **Ankle Joint, Left**
   See F Ankle Joint, Right
	H **Tarsal Joint, Right**
	   Calcaneocuboid joint
	   Cuboideonavicular joint
	   Cuneonavicular joint
	   Intercuneiform joint
	   Subtalar (talocalcaneal) joint
	   Talocalcaneal (subtalar) joint
	   Talocalcaneonavicular joint
	J **Tarsal Joint, Left**
	   See H Tarsal Joint, Right
	K **Tarsometatarsal Joint,
	   Right**
	L **Tarsometatarsal Joint, Left**
	M **Metatarsal-Phalangeal
	   Joint, Right**
	   Metatarsophalangeal (MTP)
	      joint
	N **Metatarsal-Phalangeal
	   Joint, Left**
	   *See M Metatarsal-Phalangeal
	      Joint, Right*
	P **Toe Phalangeal Joint, Right**
	   Interphalangeal (IP) joint
	Q **Toe Phalangeal Joint, Left**
	   *See P Toe Phalangeal Joint,
	      Right*
		Ø Open	**Z** No Device	**Z** No Qualifier

Non-OR Procedure   DRG Non-OR Procedure   Valid OR Procedure   HAC Associated Procedure   Combination Only   New/Revised GREEN

Ø   Medical and Surgical
S   Lower Joints
U   Supplement   Definition: Putting in or on biological or synthetic material that physically reinforces and/or augments the function of a portion of a body part
               Explanation: The biological material is non-living, or is living and from the same individual. The body part may have been previously replaced, and the SUPPLEMENT procedure is performed to physically reinforce and/or augment the function of the replaced body part.

Body Part Character 4	Approach Character 5	Device Character 6	Qualifier Character 7

Ø Lumbar Vertebral Joint
   Lumbar facet joint
2 Lumbar Vertebral Disc
3 Lumbosacral Joint
   Lumbosacral facet joint
4 Lumbosacral Disc
5 Sacrococcygeal Joint
   Sacrococcygeal symphysis
6 Coccygeal Joint
7 Sacroiliac Joint, Right
8 Sacroiliac Joint, Left
F Ankle Joint, Right
   Inferior tibiofibular joint
   Talocrural joint
G Ankle Joint, Left
   See F Ankle Joint, Right
H Tarsal Joint, Right
   Calcaneocuboid joint
   Cuboideonavicular joint
   Cuneonavicular joint
   Intercuneiform joint
   Subtalar (talocalcaneal) joint
   Talocalcaneal (subtalar) joint
   Talocalcaneonavicular joint
J Tarsal Joint, Left
   See H Tarsal Joint, Right
K Tarsometatarsal Joint, Right
L Tarsometatarsal Joint, Left
M Metatarsal-Phalangeal Joint, Right
   Metatarsophalangeal (MTP) joint
N Metatarsal-Phalangeal Joint, Left
   See M Metatarsal-Phalangeal Joint, Right
P Toe Phalangeal Joint, Right
   Interphalangeal (IP) joint
Q Toe Phalangeal Joint, Left
   See P Toe Phalangeal Joint, Right
	Ø Open
	3 Percutaneous
	4 Percutaneous Endoscopic
		7 Autologous Tissue Substitute
		J Synthetic Substitute
		K Nonautologous Tissue Substitute
			Z No Qualifier

9 Hip Joint, Right ⊞
   Acetabulofemoral joint
B Hip Joint, Left ⊞
   See 9 Hip Joint, Right
	Ø Open	**7** Autologous Tissue Substitute
		9 Liner
		B Resurfacing Device
		J Synthetic Substitute
		K Nonautologous Tissue Substitute
			Z No Qualifier

9 Hip Joint, Right
   Acetabulofemoral joint
B Hip Joint, Left
   See 9 Hip Joint, Right
	3 Percutaneous
	4 Percutaneous Endoscopic
		7 Autologous Tissue Substitute
		J Synthetic Substitute
		K Nonautologous Tissue Substitute
			Z No Qualifier

A Hip Joint, Acetabular Surface, Right ⊞ **E** Hip Joint, Acetabular Surface, Left ⊞ **R** Hip Joint, Femoral Surface, Right ⊞ **S** Hip Joint, Femoral Surface, Left ⊞	**Ø** Open	**9** Liner **B** Resurfacing Device	**Z** No Qualifier

C Knee Joint, Right
   Femoropatellar joint
   Femorotibial joint
   Lateral meniscus
   Medial meniscus
   Patellofemoral joint
   Tibiofemoral joint
D Knee Joint, Left
   See C Knee Joint, Right
	Ø Open	**7** Autologous Tissue Substitute
		J Synthetic Substitute
		K Nonautologous Tissue Substitute
			Z No Qualifier

C Knee Joint, Right
   Femoropatellar joint
   Femorotibial joint
   Lateral meniscus
   Medial meniscus
   Patellofemoral joint
   Tibiofemoral joint
D Knee Joint, Left
   See C Knee Joint, Right
	Ø Open	**9** Liner	**C** Patellar Surface
			Z No Qualifier

HAC   ØSU[9,B]ØBZ when reported with SDx of I26.Ø2-I26.Ø9,
          I26.92-I26.99, or I82.4Ø1-I82.4Z9
HAC   ØSU[A,E,R,S]ØBZ when reported with SDx of I26.Ø2-I26.Ø9,
          I26.92-I26.99, or I82.4Ø1-I82.4Z9

See Appendix L for Procedure Combinations
⊞   ØSU[9,B]Ø9Z
⊞   ØSU[A,E,R,S]Ø9Z

ØSU Continued on next page

NC Noncovered Procedure   **LC** Limited Coverage   **QA** Questionable OB Admit   **NT** New Tech Add-on   ⊞ Combination Member   ♂ Male   ♀ Female

Lower Joints

Ø Medical and Surgical
S Lower Joints
U Supplement

ØSU Continued

Definition: Putting in or on biological or synthetic material that physically reinforces and/or augments the function of a portion of a body part

Explanation: The biological material is non-living, or is living and from the same individual. The body part may have been previously replaced, and the SUPPLEMENT procedure is performed to physically reinforce and/or augment the function of the replaced body part.

Body Part Character 4	Approach Character 5	Device Character 6	Qualifier Character 7
C Knee Joint, Right Femoropatellar joint Femorotibial joint Lateral meniscus Medial meniscus Patellofemoral joint Tibiofemoral joint **D Knee Joint, Left** *See C Knee Joint, Right*	**3** Percutaneous **4** Percutaneous Endoscopic	**7** Autologous Tissue Substitute **J** Synthetic Substitute **K** Nonautologous Tissue Substitute	**Z** No Qualifier
T Knee Joint, Femoral Surface, Right Femoropatellar joint Patellofemoral joint **U Knee Joint, Femoral Surface, Left** *See T Knee Joint, Femoral Surface, Right* **V Knee Joint, Tibial Surface, Right** ⊞ Femorotibial joint Tibiofemoral joint **W Knee Joint, Tibial Surface, Left** ⊞ *See V Knee Joint, Tibial Surface, Right*	**Ø** Open	**9** Liner	**Z** No Qualifier

See Appendix L for Procedure Combinations
⊞   ØSU[V,W]Ø9Z

Ø   Medical and Surgical
S   Lower Joints
W   Revision   Definition: Correcting, to the extent possible, a portion of a malfunctioning device or the position of a displaced device

Explanation: Revision can include correcting a malfunctioning or displaced device by taking out or putting in components of the device such as a screw or pin

Body Part Character 4	Approach Character 5	Device Character 6	Qualifier Character 7

Ø Lumbar Vertebral Joint
   Lumbar facet joint
3 Lumbosacral Joint
   Lumbosacral facet joint
	Ø Open
	3 Percutaneous
	4 Percutaneous Endoscopic
	X External
		Ø Drainage Device
		3 Infusion Device
		4 Internal Fixation Device
		7 Autologous Tissue Substitute
		8 Spacer
		A Interbody Fusion Device
		J Synthetic Substitute
		K Nonautologous Tissue Substitute
			Z No Qualifier

2 Lumbar Vertebral Disc 4 Lumbosacral Disc	Ø Open 3 Percutaneous 4 Percutaneous Endoscopic X External	Ø Drainage Device 3 Infusion Device 7 Autologous Tissue Substitute J Synthetic Substitute K Nonautologous Tissue Substitute	Z No Qualifier
5 Sacrococcygeal Joint Sacrococcygeal symphysis 6 Coccygeal Joint 7 Sacroiliac Joint, Right 8 Sacroiliac Joint, Left	Ø Open 3 Percutaneous 4 Percutaneous Endoscopic X External	Ø Drainage Device 3 Infusion Device 4 Internal Fixation Device 7 Autologous Tissue Substitute 8 Spacer J Synthetic Substitute K Nonautologous Tissue Substitute	Z No Qualifier

9 Hip Joint, Right
   Acetabulofemoral joint
B Hip Joint, Left
   See 9 Hip Joint, Right
	Ø Open	Ø Drainage Device
		3 Infusion Device
		4 Internal Fixation Device
		5 External Fixation Device
		7 Autologous Tissue Substitute
		8 Spacer
		9 Liner
		B Resurfacing Device
		J Synthetic Substitute
		K Nonautologous Tissue Substitute
			Z No Qualifier

9 Hip Joint, Right
   Acetabulofemoral joint
B Hip Joint, Left
   See 9 Hip Joint, Right
	3 Percutaneous
	4 Percutaneous Endoscopic
	X External
		Ø Drainage Device
		3 Infusion Device
		4 Internal Fixation Device
		5 External Fixation Device
		7 Autologous Tissue Substitute
		8 Spacer
		J Synthetic Substitute
		K Nonautologous Tissue Substitute
			Z No Qualifier

A Hip Joint, Acetabular Surface, Right
E Hip Joint, Acetabular Surface, Left
R Hip Joint, Femoral Surface, Right
S Hip Joint, Femoral Surface, Left
T Knee Joint, Femoral Surface, Right
   Femoropatellar joint
   Patellofemoral joint
U Knee Joint, Femoral Surface, Left
   See T Knee Joint, Femoral Surface, Right
V Knee Joint, Tibial Surface, Right
   Femorotibial joint
   Tibiofemoral joint
W Knee Joint, Tibial Surface, Left
   See V Knee Joint, Tibial Surface, Right
	Ø Open
	3 Percutaneous
	4 Percutaneous Endoscopic
	X External
		J Synthetic Substitute	Z No Qualifier

C Knee Joint, Right
   Femoropatellar joint
   Femorotibial joint
   Lateral meniscus
   Medial meniscus
   Patellofemoral joint
   Tibiofemoral joint
D Knee Joint, Left
   See C Knee Joint, Right
	Ø Open	Ø Drainage Device
		3 Infusion Device
		4 Internal Fixation Device
		5 External Fixation Device
		7 Autologous Tissue Substitute
		8 Spacer
		9 Liner
		K Nonautologous Tissue Substitute
			Z No Qualifier

Non-OR   ØSW[Ø,3]X[Ø,3,4,7,8,A,J,K]Z
Non-OR   ØSW[2,4]X[Ø,3,7,J,K]Z
Non-OR   ØSW[5,6,7,8]X[Ø,3,4,7,8,J,K]Z
Non-OR   ØSW[9,B]X[Ø,3,4,5,7,8,J,K]Z
Non-OR   ØSW[A,E,R,S,T,U,V,W]XJZ

ØSW Continued on next page

NC Noncovered Procedure   LC Limited Coverage   QA Questionable OB Admit   NT New Tech Add-on   ⊞ Combination Member   ♂ Male   ♀ Female

Ø Medical and Surgical
S Lower Joints
W Revision

ØSW Continued

Definition: Correcting, to the extent possible, a portion of a malfunctioning device or the position of a displaced device

Explanation: Revision can include correcting a malfunctioning or displaced device by taking out or putting in components of the device such as a screw or pin

Body Part Character 4	Approach Character 5	Device Character 6	Qualifier Character 7
C Knee Joint, Right Femoropatellar joint Femorotibial joint Lateral meniscus Medial meniscus Patellofemoral joint Tibiofemoral joint **D Knee Joint, Left** *See C Knee Joint, Right*	**Ø Open**	**J Synthetic Substitute**	**C Patellar Surface** **Z No Qualifier**
C Knee Joint, Right Femoropatellar joint Femorotibial joint Lateral meniscus Medial meniscus Patellofemoral joint Tibiofemoral joint **D Knee Joint, Left** *See C Knee Joint, Right*	**3 Percutaneous** **4 Percutaneous Endoscopic** **X External**	**Ø Drainage Device** **3 Infusion Device** **4 Internal Fixation Device** **5 External Fixation Device** **7 Autologous Tissue Substitute** **8 Spacer** **K Nonautologous Tissue Substitute**	**Z No Qualifier**
C Knee Joint, Right Femoropatellar joint Femorotibial joint Lateral meniscus Medial meniscus Patellofemoral joint Tibiofemoral joint **D Knee Joint, Left** *See C Knee Joint, Right*	**3 Percutaneous** **4 Percutaneous Endoscopic** **X External**	**J Synthetic Substitute**	**C Patellar Surface** **Z No Qualifier**
F Ankle Joint, Right Inferior tibiofibular joint Talocrural joint **G Ankle Joint, Left** *See F Ankle Joint, Right* **H Tarsal Joint, Right** Calcaneocuboid joint Cuboideonavicular joint Cuneonavicular joint Intercuneiform joint Subtalar (talocalcaneal) joint Talocalcaneal (subtalar) joint Talocalcaneonavicular joint **J Tarsal Joint, Left** *See H Tarsal Joint, Right* **K Tarsometatarsal Joint, Right** **L Tarsometatarsal Joint, Left** **M Metatarsal-Phalangeal Joint, Right** Metatarsophalangeal (MTP) joint **N Metatarsal-Phalangeal Joint, Left** *See M Metatarsal-Phalangeal Joint, Right* **P Toe Phalangeal Joint, Right** Interphalangeal (IP) joint **Q Toe Phalangeal Joint, Left** *See P Toe Phalangeal Joint, Right*	**Ø Open** **3 Percutaneous** **4 Percutaneous Endoscopic** **X External**	**Ø Drainage Device** **3 Infusion Device** **4 Internal Fixation Device** **5 External Fixation Device** **7 Autologous Tissue Substitute** **8 Spacer** **J Synthetic Substitute** **K Nonautologous Tissue Substitute**	**Z No Qualifier**

Non-OR ØSW[C,D]X[Ø,3,4,5,7,8,K]Z
Non-OR ØSW[C,D]XJ[C,Z]
Non-OR ØSW[F,G,H,J,K,L,M,N,P,Q]X[Ø,3,4,5,7,8,J,K]Z

Urinary System ØT1–ØTY

Character Meanings

This Character Meaning table is provided as a guide to assist the user in the identification of character members that may be found in this section of code tables. It **SHOULD NOT** be used to build a PCS code.

Operation–Character 3	Body Part–Character 4	Approach–Character 5	Device–Character 6	Qualifier–Character 7
1　Bypass	Ø　Kidney, Right	Ø　Open	Ø　Drainage Device	Ø　Allogeneic
2　Change	1　Kidney, Left	3　Percutaneous	1　Radioactive Element	1　Syngeneic
5　Destruction	2　Kidneys, Bilateral	4　Percutaneous Endoscopic	2　Monitoring Device	2　Zooplastic
7　Dilation	3　Kidney Pelvis, Right	7　Via Natural or Artificial Opening	3　Infusion Device	3　Kidney Pelvis, Right
8　Division	4　Kidney Pelvis, Left	8　Via Natural or Artificial Opening Endoscopic	7　Autologous Tissue Substitute	4　Kidney Pelvis, Left
9　Drainage	5　Kidney	X　External	C　Extraluminal Device	6　Ureter, Right
B　Excision	6　Ureter, Right		D　Intraluminal Device	7　Ureter, Left
C　Extirpation	7　Ureter, Left		J　Synthetic Substitute	8　Colon
D　Extraction	8　Ureters, Bilateral		K　Nonautologous Tissue Substitute	9　Colocutaneous
F　Fragmentation	9　Ureter		L　Artificial Sphincter	A　Ileum
H　Insertion	B　Bladder		M　Stimulator Lead	B　Bladder
J　Inspection	C　Bladder Neck		Y　Other Device	C　Ileocutaneous
L　Occlusion	D　Urethra		Z　No Device	D　Cutaneous
M　Reattachment				X　Diagnostic
N　Release				Z　No Qualifier
P　Removal				
Q　Repair				
R　Replacement				
S　Reposition				
T　Resection				
U　Supplement				
V　Restriction				
W　Revision				
Y　Transplantation				

AHA Coding Clinic for table ØT1
2017, 3Q, 20　　Creation of Indiana pouch
2017, 3Q, 21　　Augmentation cystoplasty with Indiana pouch and continent urinary diversion
2017, 1Q, 37　　Perineal urethrostomy
2015, 3Q, 34　　Redo urinary diversion surgery via left ureteral reimplantation

AHA Coding Clinic for table ØT7
2019, 2Q, 16　　Reimplantation of ureters with insertion of tubes
2017, 4Q, 111　　Exchange of ureteral stent
2016, 2Q, 27　　Exchange of ureteral stents
2015, 2Q, 8　　Urinary calculi fragmentation and evacuation
2013, 4Q, 123　　Urolift® procedure

AHA Coding Clinic for table ØT9
2017, 3Q, 19　　Ureteral stent placement for urinary leakage
2017, 3Q, 20　　Creation of Indiana pouch
2017, 3Q, 21　　Augmentation cystoplasty with Indiana pouch and continent urinary diversion

AHA Coding Clinic for table ØTB
2016, 1Q, 19　　Biopsy of neobladder malignancy
2015, 3Q, 34　　Excision of Mitrofanoff polyp
2014, 2Q, 8　　Ileoscopy with excision of polyp of Ileal loop urinary diversion

AHA Coding Clinic for table ØTC
2019, 3Q, 4　　Evacuation of clots from bladder dome
2016, 3Q, 23　　Ureteral stone migrating into bladder
2015, 2Q, 7　　Urinary calculi fragmentation and evacuation
2015, 2Q, 8　　Urinary calculi fragmentation and evacuation
2013, 4Q, 122　　Laser lithotripsy with removal of fragments

AHA Coding Clinic for table ØTF
2015, 2Q, 7　　Urinary calculi fragmentation and evacuation
2013, 4Q, 122　　Extracorporeal shock wave lithotripsy
2013, 4Q, 122　　Laser lithotripsy with removal of fragments

AHA Coding Clinic for table ØTH
2020, 4Q, 43-44　　Insertion of radioactive element
2019, 2Q, 16　　Reimplantation of ureters with insertion of tubes

AHA Coding Clinic for table ØTP
2017, 4Q, 111　　Exchange of ureteral stent
2016, 2Q, 27　　Exchange of ureteral stents

AHA Coding Clinic for table ØTQ
2018, 2Q, 27　　Dismembered pyeloplasty
2017, 1Q, 37　　Perineal urethrostomy

AHA Coding Clinic for table ØTR
2017, 3Q, 20　　Creation of Indiana pouch

AHA Coding Clinic for table ØTS
2019, 1Q, 29　　Young-Dees-Leadbetter bladder neck reconstruction
2018, 2Q, 27　　Dismembered pyeloplasty
2017, 1Q, 36　　Dismembered pyeloplasty
2016, 1Q, 15　　Pubovaginal sling placement

AHA Coding Clinic for table ØTT
2014, 3Q, 16　　Hand-assisted laparoscopy nephroureterectomy

AHA Coding Clinic for table ØTU
2019, 1Q, 29　　Young-Dees-Leadbetter bladder neck reconstruction
2017, 3Q, 21　　Augmentation cystoplasty with Indiana pouch and continent urinary diversion

AHA Coding Clinic for table ØTV
2015, 2Q, 11　　Cystourethroscopic Deflux® injection

Urinary System

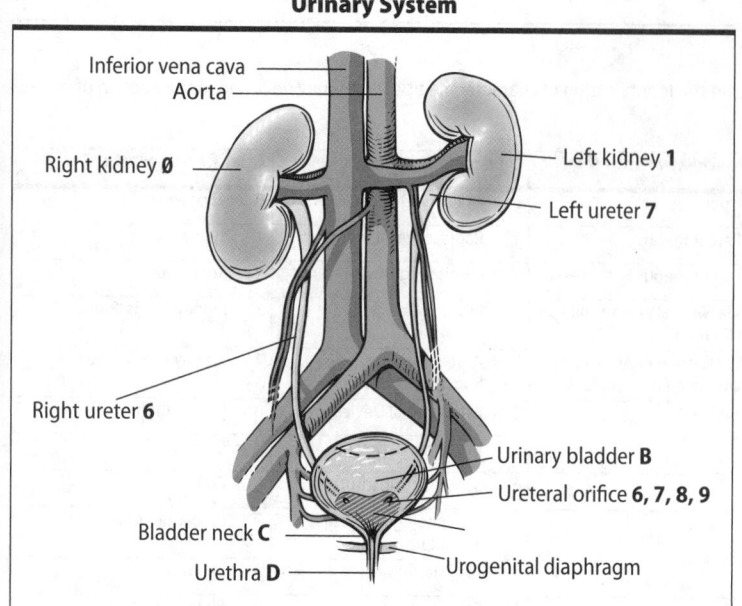

- Inferior vena cava
- Aorta
- Right kidney Ø
- Left kidney **1**
- Left ureter **7**
- Right ureter **6**
- Urinary bladder **B**
- Ureteral orifice **6, 7, 8, 9**
- Bladder neck **C**
- Urethra **D**
- Urogenital diaphragm

Kidney

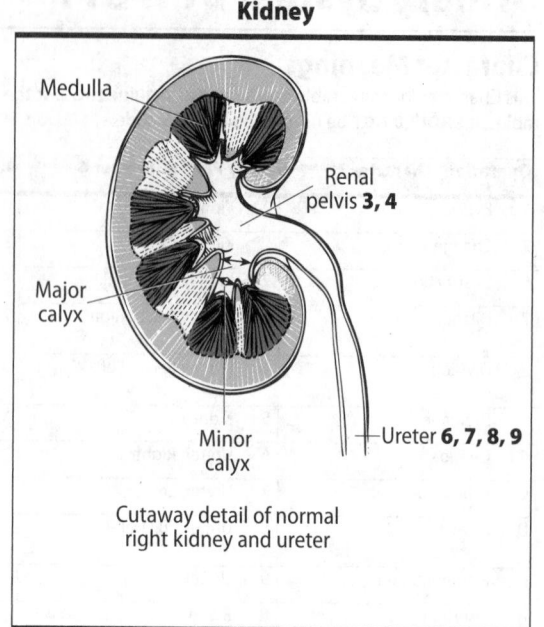

- Medulla
- Renal pelvis **3, 4**
- Major calyx
- Minor calyx
- Ureter **6, 7, 8, 9**

Cutaway detail of normal right kidney and ureter

Bladder

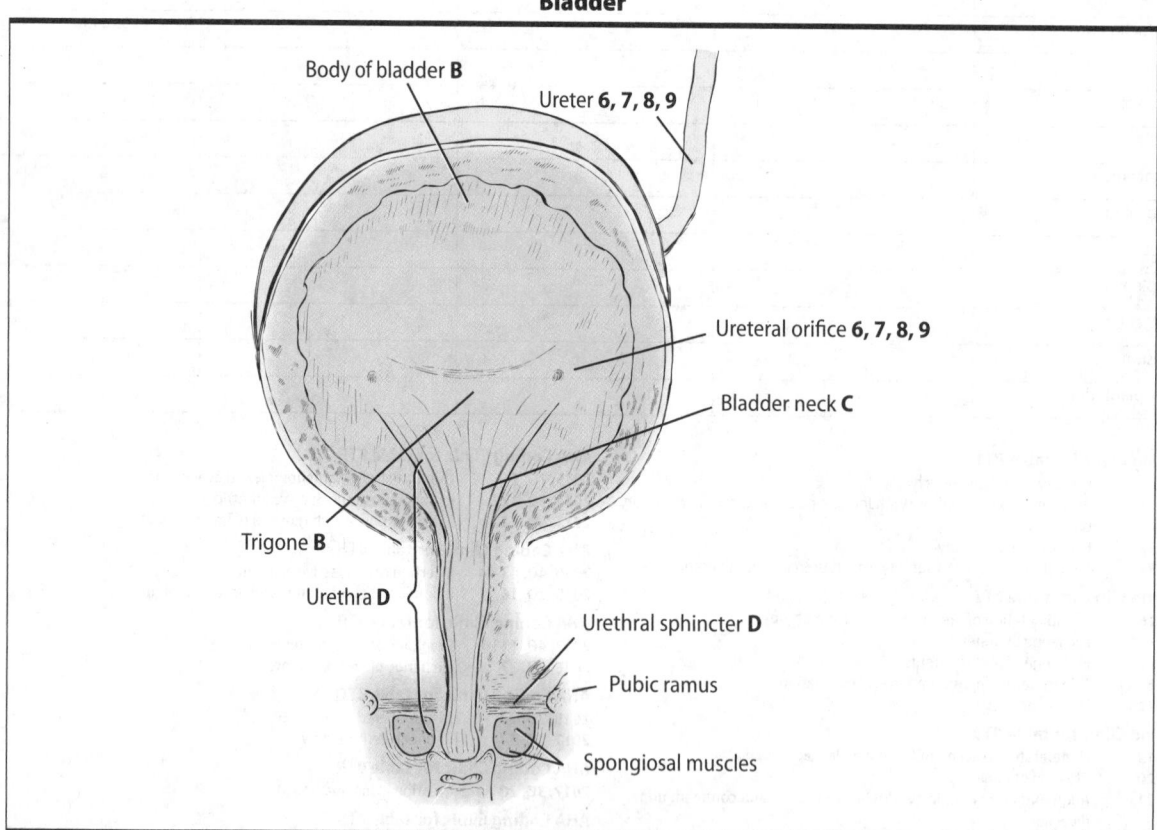

- Body of bladder **B**
- Ureter **6, 7, 8, 9**
- Ureteral orifice **6, 7, 8, 9**
- Bladder neck **C**
- Trigone **B**
- Urethra **D**
- Urethral sphincter **D**
- Pubic ramus
- Spongiosal muscles

Ø Medical and Surgical
T Urinary System
1 Bypass   Definition: Altering the route of passage of the contents of a tubular body part

Explanation: Rerouting contents of a body part to a downstream area of the normal route, to a similar route and body part, or to an abnormal route and dissimilar body part. Includes one or more anastomoses, with or without the use of a device.

Body Part Character 4	Approach Character 5	Device Character 6	Qualifier Character 7
3 Kidney Pelvis, Right Ureteropelvic junction (UPJ) **4 Kidney Pelvis, Left** *See 3 Kidney Pelvis, Right*	**Ø** Open **4** Percutaneous Endoscopic	**7** Autologous Tissue Substitute **J** Synthetic Substitute **K** Nonautologous Tissue Substitute **Z** No Device	**3** Kidney Pelvis, Right **4** Kidney Pelvis, Left **6** Ureter, Right **7** Ureter, Left **8** Colon **9** Colocutaneous **A** Ileum **B** Bladder **C** Ileocutaneous **D** Cutaneous
3 Kidney Pelvis, Right Ureteropelvic junction (UPJ) **4 Kidney Pelvis, Left** *See 3 Kidney Pelvis, Right*	**3** Percutaneous	**J** Synthetic Substitute	**D** Cutaneous
6 Ureter, Right Ureteral orifice Ureterovesical orifice **7 Ureter, Left** *See 6 Ureter, Right* **8 Ureters, Bilateral** *See 6 Ureter, Right*	**Ø** Open **4** Percutaneous Endoscopic	**7** Autologous Tissue Substitute **J** Synthetic Substitute **K** Nonautologous Tissue Substitute **Z** No Device	**6** Ureter, Right **7** Ureter, Left **8** Colon **9** Colocutaneous **A** Ileum **B** Bladder **C** Ileocutaneous **D** Cutaneous
6 Ureter, Right Ureteral orifice Ureterovesical orifice **7 Ureter, Left** *See 6 Ureter, Right* **8 Ureters, Bilateral** *See 6 Ureter, Right*	**3** Percutaneous	**J** Synthetic Substitute	**D** Cutaneous
B Bladder Trigone of bladder	**Ø** Open **4** Percutaneous Endoscopic	**7** Autologous Tissue Substitute **J** Synthetic Substitute **K** Nonautologous Tissue Substitute **Z** No Device	**9** Colocutaneous **C** Ileocutaneous **D** Cutaneous
B Bladder Trigone of bladder	**3** Percutaneous	**J** Synthetic Substitute	**D** Cutaneous

Ø Medical and Surgical
T Urinary System
2 Change   Definition: Taking out or off a device from a body part and putting back an identical or similar device in or on the same body part without cutting or puncturing the skin or a mucous membrane

Explanation: All CHANGE procedures are coded using the approach EXTERNAL

Body Part Character 4	Approach Character 5	Device Character 6	Qualifier Character 7
5 Kidney Renal calyx Renal capsule Renal cortex Renal segment **9 Ureter** Ureteral orifice Ureterovesical orifice **B Bladder** Trigone of bladder **D Urethra** Bulbourethral (Cowper's) gland Cowper's (bulbourethral) gland External urethral sphincter Internal urethral sphincter Membranous urethra Penile urethra Prostatic urethra	**X** External	**Ø** Drainage Device **Y** Other Device	**Z** No Qualifier

Non-OR   All body part, approach, device, and qualifier values

NC Noncovered Procedure   **LC** Limited Coverage   **QA** Questionable OB Admit   **NT** New Tech Add-on   ⊞ Combination Member   ♂ Male   ♀ Female

ICD-10-PCS 2022   **623**

ØT1–ØT2

Urinary System

Ø Medical and Surgical
T Urinary System
5 Destruction   Definition: Physical eradication of all or a portion of a body part by the direct use of energy, force, or a destructive agent
                     Explanation: None of the body part is physically taken out

Body Part Character 4	Approach Character 5	Device Character 6	Qualifier Character 7
Ø Kidney, Right Renal calyx Renal capsule Renal cortex Renal segment **1 Kidney, Left** *See Ø Kidney, Right* **3 Kidney Pelvis, Right** Ureteropelvic junction (UPJ) **4 Kidney Pelvis, Left** *See 3 Kidney Pelvis, Right* **6 Ureter, Right** Ureteral orifice Ureterovesical orifice **7 Ureter, Left** *See 6 Ureter, Right* **B Bladder** Trigone of bladder **C Bladder Neck**	**Ø** Open **3** Percutaneous **4** Percutaneous Endoscopic **7** Via Natural or Artificial Opening **8** Via Natural or Artificial Opening Endoscopic	**Z** No Device	**Z** No Qualifier
D Urethra Bulbourethral (Cowper's) gland Cowper's (bulbourethral) gland External urethral sphincter Internal urethral sphincter Membranous urethra Penile urethra Prostatic urethra	**Ø** Open **3** Percutaneous **4** Percutaneous Endoscopic **7** Via Natural or Artificial Opening **8** Via Natural or Artificial Opening Endoscopic **X** External	**Z** No Device	**Z** No Qualifier

Non-OR   ØT5D[Ø,3,4,7,8,X]ZZ

Ø Medical and Surgical
T Urinary System
7 Dilation   Definition: Expanding an orifice or the lumen of a tubular body part
                 Explanation: The orifice can be a natural orifice or an artificially created orifice. Accomplished by stretching a tubular body part using intraluminal pressure or by cutting part of the orifice or wall of the tubular body part.

Body Part Character 4	Approach Character 5	Device Character 6	Qualifier Character 7
3 Kidney Pelvis, Right Ureteropelvic junction (UPJ) **4 Kidney Pelvis, Left** *See 3 Kidney Pelvis, Right* **6 Ureter, Right** Ureteral orifice Ureterovesical orifice **7 Ureter, Left** *See 6 Ureter, Right* **8 Ureters, Bilateral** *See 6 Ureter, Right* **B Bladder** Trigone of bladder **C Bladder Neck** **D Urethra** Bulbourethral (Cowper's) gland Cowper's (bulbourethral) gland External urethral sphincter Internal urethral sphincter Membranous urethra Penile urethra Prostatic urethra	**Ø** Open **3** Percutaneous **4** Percutaneous Endoscopic **7** Via Natural or Artificial Opening **8** Via Natural or Artificial Opening Endoscopic	**D** Intraluminal Device **Z** No Device	**Z** No Qualifier

Non-OR   ØT7[6,7,8][Ø,3,4,7]DZ   **Non-OR**   ØT7B7[D,Z]Z   **Non-OR**   ØT7[C,D][7,8][D,Z]Z
Non-OR   ØT7[6,7,8]7ZZ   **Non-OR**   ØT7C[Ø,3,4]ZZ
Non-OR   ØT788ZZ   **Non-OR**   ØT7[C,D][Ø,3,4]DZ

Ø Medical and Surgical
T Urinary System
8 Division   Definition: Cutting into a body part, without draining fluids and/or gases from the body part, in order to separate or transect a body part
                 Explanation: All or a portion of the body part is separated into two or more portions

Body Part Character 4	Approach Character 5	Device Character 6	Qualifier Character 7
2 Kidneys, Bilateral Renal calyx Renal capsule Renal cortex Renal segment **C Bladder Neck**	**Ø** Open **3** Percutaneous **4** Percutaneous Endoscopic	**Z** No Device	**Z** No Qualifier

Ø   Medical and Surgical
T   Urinary System
9   Drainage   Definition: Taking or letting out fluids and/or gases from a body part
                        Explanation: The qualifier DIAGNOSTIC is used to identify drainage procedures that are biopsies

Body Part Character 4	Approach Character 5	Device Character 6	Qualifier Character 7
Ø Kidney, Right Renal calyx Renal capsule Renal cortex Renal segment **1 Kidney, Left** *See Ø Kidney, Right* **3 Kidney Pelvis, Right** Ureteropelvic junction (UPJ) **4 Kidney Pelvis, Left** *See 3 Kidney Pelvis, Right* **6 Ureter, Right** Ureteral orifice Ureterovesical orifice **7 Ureter, Left** *See 6 Ureter, Right* **8 Ureters, Bilateral** *See 6 Ureter, Right* **B Bladder** Trigone of bladder **C Bladder Neck**	**Ø** Open **3** Percutaneous **4** Percutaneous Endoscopic **7** Via Natural or Artificial Opening **8** Via Natural or Artificial Opening Endoscopic	**Ø** Drainage Device	**Z** No Qualifier
Ø Kidney, Right Renal calyx Renal capsule Renal cortex Renal segment **1 Kidney, Left** *See Ø Kidney, Right* **3 Kidney Pelvis, Right** Ureteropelvic junction (UPJ) **4 Kidney Pelvis, Left** *See 3 Kidney Pelvis, Right* **6 Ureter, Right** Ureteral orifice Ureterovesical orifice **7 Ureter, Left** *See 6 Ureter, Right* **8 Ureters, Bilateral** *See 6 Ureter, Right* **B Bladder** Trigone of bladder **C Bladder Neck**	**Ø** Open **3** Percutaneous **4** Percutaneous Endoscopic **7** Via Natural or Artificial Opening **8** Via Natural or Artificial Opening Endoscopic	**Z** No Device	**X** Diagnostic **Z** No Qualifier
D Urethra Bulbourethral (Cowper's) gland Cowper's (bulbourethral) gland External urethral sphincter Internal urethral sphincter Membranous urethra Penile urethra Prostatic urethra	**Ø** Open **3** Percutaneous **4** Percutaneous Endoscopic **7** Via Natural or Artificial Opening **8** Via Natural or Artificial Opening Endoscopic **X** External	**Ø** Drainage Device	**Z** No Qualifier
D Urethra Bulbourethral (Cowper's) gland Cowper's (bulbourethral) gland External urethral sphincter Internal urethral sphincter Membranous urethra Penile urethra Prostatic urethra	**Ø** Open **3** Percutaneous **4** Percutaneous Endoscopic **7** Via Natural or Artificial Opening **8** Via Natural or Artificial Opening Endoscopic **X** External	**Z** No Device	**X** Diagnostic **Z** No Qualifier

Non-OR	ØT9[Ø,1,3,4]3ØZ
Non-OR	ØT9[6,7,8][Ø,3,4,7,8]ØZ
Non-OR	ØT9[B,C][3,4,7,8]ØZ
Non-OR	ØT9[Ø,1,3,4,6,7,8][3,4,7,8]ZX
Non-OR	ØT9[Ø,1,3,4][3,4]ZZ
Non-OR	ØT9[6,7,8]3ZZ
Non-OR	ØT9[B,C][3,4,7,8]ZZ
Non-OR	ØT9D3ØZ
Non-OR	ØT9D[Ø,3,4,7,8,X]ZX
Non-OR	ØT9D3ZZ

NC Noncovered Procedure   **LC** Limited Coverage   **QA** Questionable OB Admit   **NT** New Tech Add-on   ⊞ Combination Member   ♂ Male   ♀ Female

ICD-10-PCS 2022   **625**

ØT9–ØT9

Ø   Medical and Surgical
T   Urinary System
B   Excision   Definition: Cutting out or off, without replacement, a portion of a body part

Explanation: The qualifier DIAGNOSTIC is used to identify excision procedures that are biopsies

Body Part Character 4	Approach Character 5	Device Character 6	Qualifier Character 7

Ø **Kidney, Right**
  Renal calyx
  Renal capsule
  Renal cortex
  Renal segment
1 **Kidney, Left**
  See Ø Kidney, Right
3 **Kidney Pelvis, Right**
  Ureteropelvic junction (UPJ)
4 **Kidney Pelvis, Left**
  See 3 Kidney Pelvis, Right
6 **Ureter, Right**
  Ureteral orifice
  Ureterovesical orifice
7 **Ureter, Left**
  See 6 Ureter, Right
B **Bladder**
  Trigone of bladder
C **Bladder Neck**
	Ø Open
	3 Percutaneous
	4 Percutaneous Endoscopic
	7 Via Natural or Artificial Opening
	8 Via Natural or Artificial Opening
	  Endoscopic
		Z No Device	**X** Diagnostic
			Z No Qualifier

D **Urethra**
  Bulbourethral (Cowper's) gland
  Cowper's (bulbourethral) gland
  External urethral sphincter
  Internal urethral sphincter
  Membranous urethra
  Penile urethra
  Prostatic urethra
	Ø Open
	3 Percutaneous
	4 Percutaneous Endoscopic
	7 Via Natural or Artificial Opening
	8 Via Natural or Artificial Opening
	  Endoscopic
	X External
		Z No Device	**X** Diagnostic
			Z No Qualifier

Non-OR	ØTB[Ø,1,3,4,6,7][3,4,7,8]ZX
Non-OR	ØTBD[Ø,3,4,7,8,X]ZX

Ø   Medical and Surgical
T   Urinary System
C   Extirpation   Definition: Taking or cutting out solid matter from a body part

Explanation: The solid matter may be an abnormal byproduct of a biological function or a foreign body; it may be imbedded in a body part or in the lumen of a tubular body part. The solid matter may or may not have been previously broken into pieces.

Body Part Character 4	Approach Character 5	Device Character 6	Qualifier Character 7

Ø **Kidney, Right**
  Renal calyx
  Renal capsule
  Renal cortex
  Renal segment
1 **Kidney, Left**
  See Ø Kidney, Right
3 **Kidney Pelvis, Right**
  Ureteropelvic junction (UPJ)
4 **Kidney Pelvis, Left**
  See 3 Kidney Pelvis, Right
6 **Ureter, Right**
  Ureteral orifice
  Ureterovesical orifice
7 **Ureter, Left**
  See 6 Ureter, Right
B **Bladder**
  Trigone of bladder
C **Bladder Neck**
	Ø Open
	3 Percutaneous
	4 Percutaneous Endoscopic
	7 Via Natural or Artificial Opening
	8 Via Natural or Artificial Opening
	  Endoscopic
		Z No Device	**Z** No Qualifier

D **Urethra**
  Bulbourethral (Cowper's) gland
  Cowper's (bulbourethral) gland
  External urethral sphincter
  Internal urethral sphincter
  Membranous urethra
  Penile urethra
  Prostatic urethra
	Ø Open
	3 Percutaneous
	4 Percutaneous Endoscopic
	7 Via Natural or Artificial Opening
	8 Via Natural or Artificial Opening
	  Endoscopic
	X External
		Z No Device	**Z** No Qualifier

Non-OR	ØTC[B,C][7,8]ZZ
Non-OR	ØTCD[7,8,X]ZZ

Ø   Medical and Surgical
T   Urinary System
D   Extraction   Definition: Pulling or stripping out or off all or a portion of a body part by the use of force

                         Explanation: The qualifier DIAGNOSTIC is used to identify extraction procedures that are biopsies

Body Part Character 4	Approach Character 5	Device Character 6	Qualifier Character 7

Ø   Kidney, Right
    Renal calyx
    Renal capsule
    Renal cortex
    Renal segment
1   Kidney, Left
    See Ø Kidney, Right
	Ø Open
	3 Percutaneous
	4 Percutaneous Endoscopic
		Z No Device	**Z No Qualifier**

Ø   Medical and Surgical
T   Urinary System
F   Fragmentation   Definition: Breaking solid matter in a body part into pieces

                         Explanation: Physical force (e.g., manual, ultrasonic) applied directly or indirectly is used to break the solid matter into pieces. The solid matter may be an abnormal byproduct of a biological function or a foreign body. The pieces of solid matter are not taken out.

Body Part Character 4	Approach Character 5	Device Character 6	Qualifier Character 7

3   Kidney Pelvis, Right
    Ureteropelvic junction (UPJ)
4   Kidney Pelvis, Left
    See 3 Kidney Pelvis, Right
6   Ureter, Right
    Ureteral orifice
    Ureterovesical orifice
7   Ureter, Left
    See 6 Ureter, Right
B   Bladder
    Trigone of bladder
C   Bladder Neck
D   Urethra   `NC`
    Bulbourethral (Cowper's) gland
    Cowper's (bulbourethral) gland
    External urethral sphincter
    Internal urethral sphincter
    Membranous urethra
    Penile urethra
    Prostatic urethra
	Ø Open
	3 Percutaneous
	4 Percutaneous Endoscopic
	7 Via Natural or Artificial Opening
	**8 Via Natural or Artificial Opening
	    Endoscopic**
	X External
		Z No Device	**Z No Qualifier**

    Non-OR   ØTF[3,4][Ø,7,8]ZZ
    Non-OR   ØTF[6,7,B,C,D][Ø,3,4,7,8]ZZ
    Non-OR   ØTF[3,4,6,7,B,C,D]XZZ
    `NC`   ØTFDXZZ

`NC` Noncovered Procedure   `LC` Limited Coverage   `QA` Questionable OB Admit   `NT` New Tech Add-on   ⊞ Combination Member   ♂ Male   ♀ Female

ICD-10-PCS 2022   627

Urinary System

Ø Medical and Surgical
T Urinary System
H Insertion

Definition: Putting in a nonbiological appliance that monitors, assists, performs, or prevents a physiological function but does not physically take the place of a body part

Explanation: None

Body Part Character 4	Approach Character 5	Device Character 6	Qualifier Character 7
5 Kidney Renal calyx Renal capsule Renal cortex Renal segment	Ø Open 3 Percutaneous 4 Percutaneous Endoscopic 7 Via Natural or Artificial Opening 8 Via Natural or Artificial Opening Endoscopic	1 Radioactive Element 2 Monitoring Device 3 Infusion Device Y Other Device	Z No Qualifier
9 Ureter Ureteral orifice Ureterovesical orifice	Ø Open 3 Percutaneous 4 Percutaneous Endoscopic 7 Via Natural or Artificial Opening 8 Via Natural or Artificial Opening Endoscopic	1 Radioactive Element 2 Monitoring Device 3 Infusion Device M Stimulator Lead Y Other Device	Z No Qualifier
B Bladder NC Trigone of bladder	Ø Open 3 Percutaneous 4 Percutaneous Endoscopic 7 Via Natural or Artificial Opening 8 Via Natural or Artificial Opening Endoscopic	1 Radioactive Element 2 Monitoring Device 3 Infusion Device L Artificial Sphincter M Stimulator Lead Y Other Device	Z No Qualifier
C Bladder Neck	Ø Open 3 Percutaneous 4 Percutaneous Endoscopic 7 Via Natural or Artificial Opening 8 Via Natural or Artificial Opening Endoscopic	L Artificial Sphincter	Z No Qualifier
D Urethra Bulbourethral (Cowper's) gland Cowper's (bulbourethral) gland External urethral sphincter Internal urethral sphincter Membranous urethra Penile urethra Prostatic urethra	Ø Open 3 Percutaneous 4 Percutaneous Endoscopic 7 Via Natural or Artificial Opening 8 Via Natural or Artificial Opening Endoscopic	1 Radioactive Element 2 Monitoring Device 3 Infusion Device L Artificial Sphincter Y Other Device	Z No Qualifier
D Urethra Bulbourethral (Cowper's) gland Cowper's (bulbourethral) gland External urethral sphincter Internal urethral sphincter Membranous urethra Penile urethra Prostatic urethra	X External	2 Monitoring Device 3 Infusion Device L Artificial Sphincter	Z No Qualifier

Non-OR	ØTH5Ø3Z	Non-OR	ØTHB3[1,3,Y]Z
Non-OR	ØTH53[1,3,Y]Z	Non-OR	ØTHB4[3,Y]Z
Non-OR	ØTH54[3,Y]Z	Non-OR	ØTHB7[1,2,3,Y]Z
Non-OR	ØTH57[1,2,3,Y]Z	Non-OR	ØTHB8[2,3]Z
Non-OR	ØTH58[2,3]Z	Non-OR	ØTHDØ3Z
Non-OR	ØTH9Ø3Z	Non-OR	ØTHD3[1,3,Y]Z
Non-OR	ØTH93[1,3,Y]Z	Non-OR	ØTHD4[3,Y]Z
Non-OR	ØTH94[3,Y]Z	Non-OR	ØTHD7[1,2,3,Y]Z
Non-OR	ØTH97[1,2,3,Y]Z	Non-OR	ØTHD8[2,3,Y]Z
Non-OR	ØTH98[2,3]Z	Non-OR	ØTHDX3Z
Non-OR	ØTHBØ3Z	NC	ØTHB[Ø,3,4,7,8]MZ

Ø   Medical and Surgical
T   Urinary System
J   Inspection   Definition: Visually and/or manually exploring a body part

Explanation: Visual exploration may be performed with or without optical instrumentation. Manual exploration may be performed directly or through intervening body layers.

Body Part Character 4	Approach Character 5	Device Character 6	Qualifier Character 7

5   **Kidney**
    Renal calyx
    Renal capsule
    Renal cortex
    Renal segment
9   **Ureter**
    Ureteral orifice
    Ureterovesical orifice
B   **Bladder**
    Trigone of bladder
D   **Urethra**
    Bulbourethral (Cowper's) gland
    Cowper's (bulbourethral) gland
    External urethral sphincter
    Internal urethral sphincter
    Membranous urethra
    Penile urethra
    Prostatic urethra
	Ø Open
	3 Percutaneous
	4 Percutaneous Endoscopic
	7 Via Natural or Artificial Opening
	8 Via Natural or Artificial Opening
	    Endoscopic
	X External
		Z No Device	Z No Qualifier

Non-OR	ØTJ[5,9,D][3,4,7,8,X]ZZ
Non-OR	ØTJB[3,7,8,X]ZZ

Ø   Medical and Surgical
T   Urinary System
L   Occlusion   Definition: Completely closing an orifice or the lumen of a tubular body part

Explanation: The orifice can be a natural orifice or an artificially created orifice

Body Part Character 4	Approach Character 5	Device Character 6	Qualifier Character 7

3   **Kidney Pelvis, Right**
    Ureteropelvic junction (UPJ)
4   **Kidney Pelvis, Left**
    See 3 Kidney Pelvis, Right
6   **Ureter, Right**
    Ureteral orifice
    Ureterovesical orifice
7   **Ureter, Left**
    See 6 Ureter, Right
B   **Bladder**
    Trigone of bladder
C   **Bladder Neck**
	Ø Open
	3 Percutaneous
	4 Percutaneous Endoscopic
		C Extraluminal Device
		D Intraluminal Device
		Z No Device
			Z No Qualifier

3   **Kidney Pelvis, Right**
    Ureteropelvic junction (UPJ)
4   **Kidney Pelvis, Left**
    See 3 Kidney Pelvis, Right
6   **Ureter, Right**
    Ureteral orifice
    Ureterovesical orifice
7   **Ureter, Left**
    See 6 Ureter, Right
B   **Bladder**
    Trigone of bladder
C   **Bladder Neck**
	7 Via Natural or Artificial Opening
	8 Via Natural or Artificial Opening
	    Endoscopic
		D Intraluminal Device
		Z No Device
			Z No Qualifier

D   **Urethra**
    Bulbourethral (Cowper's) gland
    Cowper's (bulbourethral) gland
    External urethral sphincter
    Internal urethral sphincter
    Membranous urethra
    Penile urethra
    Prostatic urethra
	Ø Open
	3 Percutaneous
	4 Percutaneous Endoscopic
	X External
		C Extraluminal Device
		D Intraluminal Device
		Z No Device
			Z No Qualifier

D   **Urethra**
    Bulbourethral (Cowper's) gland
    Cowper's (bulbourethral) gland
    External urethral sphincter
    Internal urethral sphincter
    Membranous urethra
    Penile urethra
    Prostatic urethra
	7 Via Natural or Artificial Opening
	8 Via Natural or Artificial Opening
	    Endoscopic
		D Intraluminal Device
		Z No Device
			Z No Qualifier

NC Noncovered Procedure   **LC** Limited Coverage   **QA** Questionable OB Admit   **NT** New Tech Add-on   ⊞ Combination Member   ♂ Male   ♀ Female

ICD-10-PCS 2022   629

Ø   Medical and Surgical
T   Urinary System
M   Reattachment   Definition: Putting back in or on all or a portion of a separated body part to its normal location or other suitable location
Explanation: Vascular circulation and nervous pathways may or may not be reestablished

Body Part Character 4	Approach Character 5	Device Character 6	Qualifier Character 7
Ø **Kidney, Right** Renal calyx Renal capsule Renal cortex Renal segment 1 **Kidney, Left** *See Ø Kidney, Right* 2 **Kidneys, Bilateral** *See Ø Kidney, Right* 3 **Kidney Pelvis, Right** Ureteropelvic junction (UPJ) 4 **Kidney Pelvis, Left** *See 3 Kidney Pelvis, Right* 6 **Ureter, Right** Ureteral orifice Ureterovesical orifice 7 **Ureter, Left** *See 6 Ureter, Right* 8 **Ureters, Bilateral** *See 6 Ureter, Right* B **Bladder** Trigone of bladder C **Bladder Neck** D **Urethra** Bulbourethral (Cowper's) gland Cowper's (bulbourethral) gland External urethral sphincter Internal urethral sphincter Membranous urethra Penile urethra Prostatic urethra	Ø **Open** 4 **Percutaneous Endoscopic**	Z **No Device**	Z **No Qualifier**

Ø   Medical and Surgical
T   Urinary System
N   Release   Definition: Freeing a body part from an abnormal physical constraint by cutting or by the use of force
Explanation: Some of the restraining tissue may be taken out but none of the body part is taken out

Body Part Character 4	Approach Character 5	Device Character 6	Qualifier Character 7
Ø **Kidney, Right** Renal calyx Renal capsule Renal cortex Renal segment 1 **Kidney, Left** *See Ø Kidney, Right* 3 **Kidney Pelvis, Right** Ureteropelvic junction (UPJ) 4 **Kidney Pelvis, Left** *See 3 Kidney Pelvis, Right* 6 **Ureter, Right** Ureteral orifice Ureterovesical orifice 7 **Ureter, Left** *See 6 Ureter, Right* B **Bladder** Trigone of bladder C **Bladder Neck**	Ø **Open** 3 **Percutaneous** 4 **Percutaneous Endoscopic** 7 **Via Natural or Artificial Opening** 8 **Via Natural or Artificial Opening Endoscopic**	Z **No Device**	Z **No Qualifier**
D **Urethra** Bulbourethral (Cowper's) gland Cowper's (bulbourethral) gland External urethral sphincter Internal urethral sphincter Membranous urethra Penile urethra Prostatic urethra	Ø **Open** 3 **Percutaneous** 4 **Percutaneous Endoscopic** 7 **Via Natural or Artificial Opening** 8 **Via Natural or Artificial Opening Endoscopic** X **External**	Z **No Device**	Z **No Qualifier**

Urinary System

Ø   **Medical and Surgical**
T   **Urinary System**
P   **Removal**   Definition: Taking out or off a device from a body part

Explanation: If a device is taken out and a similar device put in without cutting or puncturing the skin or mucous membrane, the procedure is coded to the root operation CHANGE. Otherwise, the procedure for taking out the device is coded to the root operation REMOVAL.

Body Part Character 4	Approach Character 5	Device Character 6	Qualifier Character 7
5 Kidney Renal calyx Renal capsule Renal cortex Renal segment	Ø Open 3 Percutaneous 4 Percutaneous Endoscopic 7 Via Natural or Artificial Opening 8 Via Natural or Artificial Opening Endoscopic	Ø Drainage Device 2 Monitoring Device 3 Infusion Device 7 Autologous Tissue Substitute C Extraluminal Device D Intraluminal Device J Synthetic Substitute K Nonautologous Tissue Substitute Y Other Device	Z No Qualifier
5 Kidney Renal calyx Renal capsule Renal cortex Renal segment	X External	Ø Drainage Device 2 Monitoring Device 3 Infusion Device D Intraluminal Device	Z No Qualifier
9 Ureter Ureteral orifice Ureterovesical orifice	Ø Open 3 Percutaneous 4 Percutaneous Endoscopic 7 Via Natural or Artificial Opening 8 Via Natural or Artificial Opening Endoscopic	Ø Drainage Device 2 Monitoring Device 3 Infusion Device 7 Autologous Tissue Substitute C Extraluminal Device D Intraluminal Device J Synthetic Substitute K Nonautologous Tissue Substitute M Stimulator Lead Y Other Device	Z No Qualifier
9 Ureter Ureteral orifice Ureterovesical orifice	X External	Ø Drainage Device 2 Monitoring Device 3 Infusion Device D Intraluminal Device M Stimulator Lead	Z No Qualifier
B Bladder `NC` Trigone of bladder	Ø Open 3 Percutaneous 4 Percutaneous Endoscopic 7 Via Natural or Artificial Opening 8 Via Natural or Artificial Opening Endoscopic	Ø Drainage Device 2 Monitoring Device 3 Infusion Device 7 Autologous Tissue Substitute C Extraluminal Device D Intraluminal Device J Synthetic Substitute K Nonautologous Tissue Substitute L Artificial Sphincter M Stimulator Lead Y Other Device	Z No Qualifier
B Bladder Trigone of bladder	X External	Ø Drainage Device 2 Monitoring Device 3 Infusion Device D Intraluminal Device L Artificial Sphincter M Stimulator Lead	Z No Qualifier
D Urethra Bulbourethral (Cowper's) gland Cowper's (bulbourethral) gland External urethral sphincter Internal urethral sphincter Membranous urethra Penile urethra Prostatic urethra	Ø Open 3 Percutaneous 4 Percutaneous Endoscopic 7 Via Natural or Artificial Opening 8 Via Natural or Artificial Opening Endoscopic	Ø Drainage Device 2 Monitoring Device 3 Infusion Device 7 Autologous Tissue Substitute C Extraluminal Device D Intraluminal Device J Synthetic Substitute K Nonautologous Tissue Substitute L Artificial Sphincter Y Other Device	Z No Qualifier
D Urethra Bulbourethral (Cowper's) gland Cowper's (bulbourethral) gland External urethral sphincter Internal urethral sphincter Membranous urethra Penile urethra Prostatic urethra	X External	Ø Drainage Device 2 Monitoring Device 3 Infusion Device D Intraluminal Device L Artificial Sphincter	Z No Qualifier

Non-OR   ØTP5[3,4,7]YZ
Non-OR   ØTP5[7,8][Ø,2,3,D]Z
Non-OR   ØTP5X[Ø,2,3,D]Z
Non-OR   ØTP9[3,4,7]YZ

Non-OR   ØTP9[7,8][Ø,2,3,D]Z
Non-OR   ØTP9X[Ø,2,3,D]Z
Non-OR   ØTPB[3,4,7]YZ

Non-OR   ØTPB[7,8][Ø,2,3,D]Z
Non-OR   ØTPBX[Ø,2,3,D,L]Z
Non-OR   ØTPD[3,4]YZ

Non-OR   ØTPD[7,8][Ø,2,3,D,Y]Z
Non-OR   ØTPDX[Ø,2,3,D]Z
`NC`   ØTPB[Ø,3,4,7,8]MZ

`NC` Noncovered Procedure   `LC` Limited Coverage   `QA` Questionable OB Admit   `NT` New Tech Add-on   ⊞ Combination Member   ♂ Male   ♀ Female

Ø   **Medical and Surgical**
T   **Urinary System**
Q   **Repair**   Definition: Restoring, to the extent possible, a body part to its normal anatomic structure and function
                  Explanation: Used only when the method to accomplish the repair is not one of the other root operations

Body Part Character 4	Approach Character 5	Device Character 6	Qualifier Character 7

Ø **Kidney, Right**
   Renal calyx
   Renal capsule
   Renal cortex
   Renal segment
1 **Kidney, Left**
   See Ø Kidney, Right
3 **Kidney Pelvis, Right**
   Ureteropelvic junction (UPJ)
4 **Kidney Pelvis, Left**
   See 3 Kidney Pelvis, Right
6 **Ureter, Right**
   Ureteral orifice
   Ureterovesical orifice
7 **Ureter, Left**
   See 6 Ureter, Right
B **Bladder**   ⊞
   Trigone of bladder
C **Bladder Neck**
	Ø Open
	3 Percutaneous
	4 Percutaneous Endoscopic
	7 Via Natural or Artificial Opening
	8 Via Natural or Artificial Opening
	   Endoscopic
		Z No Device	**Z** No Qualifier

D **Urethra**
   Bulbourethral (Cowper's) gland
   Cowper's (bulbourethral) gland
   External urethral sphincter
   Internal urethral sphincter
   Membranous urethra
   Penile urethra
   Prostatic urethra
	Ø Open
	3 Percutaneous
	4 Percutaneous Endoscopic
	7 Via Natural or Artificial Opening
	8 Via Natural or Artificial Opening
	   Endoscopic
	X External
		Z No Device	**Z** No Qualifier

See Appendix L for Procedure Combinations
  ⊞   ØTQB[Ø,3,4]ZZ

Ø   **Medical and Surgical**
T   **Urinary System**
R   **Replacement**   Definition: Putting in or on biological or synthetic material that physically takes the place and/or function of all or a portion of a body part
                      Explanation: The body part may have been taken out or replaced, or may be taken out, physically eradicated, or rendered nonfunctional during
                      the REPLACEMENT procedure. A REMOVAL procedure is coded for taking out the device used in a previous replacement procedure.

Body Part Character 4	Approach Character 5	Device Character 6	Qualifier Character 7

3 **Kidney Pelvis, Right**
   Ureteropelvic junction (UPJ)
4 **Kidney Pelvis, Left**
   See 3 Kidney Pelvis, Right
6 **Ureter, Right**
   Ureteral orifice
   Ureterovesical orifice
7 **Ureter, Left**
   See 6 Ureter, Right
B **Bladder**
   Trigone of bladder
C **Bladder Neck**
	Ø Open
	4 Percutaneous Endoscopic
	7 Via Natural or Artificial Opening
	8 Via Natural or Artificial Opening
	   Endoscopic
		7 Autologous Tissue Substitute
		J Synthetic Substitute
		K Nonautologous Tissue Substitute
			Z No Qualifier

D **Urethra**
   Bulbourethral (Cowper's) gland
   Cowper's (bulbourethral) gland
   External urethral sphincter
   Internal urethral sphincter
   Membranous urethra
   Penile urethra
   Prostatic urethra
	Ø Open
	4 Percutaneous Endoscopic
	7 Via Natural or Artificial Opening
	8 Via Natural or Artificial Opening
	   Endoscopic
	X External
		7 Autologous Tissue Substitute
		J Synthetic Substitute
		K Nonautologous Tissue Substitute
			Z No Qualifier

0   **Medical and Surgical**
T   **Urinary System**
S   **Reposition**   Definition: Moving to its normal location, or other suitable location, all or a portion of a body part

Explanation: The body part is moved to a new location from an abnormal location, or from a normal location where it is not functioning correctly. The body part may or may not be cut out or off to be moved to the new location.

Body Part Character 4	Approach Character 5	Device Character 6	Qualifier Character 7

0   **Kidney, Right**
   Renal calyx
   Renal capsule
   Renal cortex
   Renal segment
1   **Kidney, Left**
   See 0 Kidney, Right
2   **Kidneys, Bilateral**
   See 0 Kidney, Right
3   **Kidney Pelvis, Right**
   Ureteropelvic junction (UPJ)
4   **Kidney Pelvis, Left**
   See 3 Kidney Pelvis, Right
6   **Ureter, Right**
   Ureteral orifice
   Ureterovesical orifice
7   **Ureter, Left**
   See 6 Ureter, Right
8   **Ureters, Bilateral**
   See 6 Ureter, Right
B   **Bladder**
   Trigone of bladder
C   **Bladder Neck**
D   **Urethra**
   Bulbourethral (Cowper's) gland
   Cowper's (bulbourethral) gland
   External urethral sphincter
   Internal urethral sphincter
   Membranous urethra
   Penile urethra
   Prostatic urethra
	0 Open
	4 Percutaneous Endoscopic
		Z No Device	**Z** No Qualifier

0   **Medical and Surgical**
T   **Urinary System**
T   **Resection**   Definition: Cutting out or off, without replacement, all of a body part

Explanation: None

Body Part Character 4	Approach Character 5	Device Character 6	Qualifier Character 7

0   **Kidney, Right**
   Renal calyx
   Renal capsule
   Renal cortex
   Renal segment
1   **Kidney, Left**
   See 0 Kidney, Right
2   **Kidneys, Bilateral**
   See 0 Kidney, Right
	0 Open
	4 Percutaneous Endoscopic
		Z No Device	**Z** No Qualifier

3   **Kidney Pelvis, Right**
   Ureteropelvic junction (UPJ)
4   **Kidney Pelvis, Left**
   See 3 Kidney Pelvis, Right
6   **Ureter, Right**
   Ureteral orifice
   Ureterovesical orifice
7   **Ureter, Left**
   See 6 Ureter, Right
B   **Bladder**   ⊞
   Trigone of bladder
C   **Bladder Neck**
D   Urethra
   Bulbourethral (Cowper's) gland
   Cowper's (bulbourethral) gland
   External urethral sphincter
   Internal urethral sphincter
   Membranous urethra
   Penile urethra
   Prostatic urethra
	0 Open
	4 Percutaneous Endoscopic
	7 Via Natural or Artificial Opening
	8 Via Natural or Artificial Opening Endoscopic
		Z No Device	**Z** No Qualifier

Non-OR   0TTD[4,7,8]ZZ

See Appendix L for Procedure Combinations
   Combo-only   0TTD0ZZ
   ⊞   0TTB0ZZ

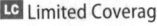 Noncovered Procedure   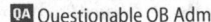 Limited Coverage   **QA** Questionable OB Admit   **NT** New Tech Add-on   ⊞ Combination Member   ♂ Male   ♀ Female

Urinary System

Ø   Medical and Surgical
T   Urinary System
U   Supplement   Definition: Putting in or on biological or synthetic material that physically reinforces and/or augments the function of a portion of a body part

Explanation: The biological material is non-living, or is living and from the same individual. The body part may have been previously replaced, and the SUPPLEMENT procedure is performed to physically reinforce and/or augment the function of the replaced body part.

Body Part Character 4	Approach Character 5	Device Character 6	Qualifier Character 7
3 Kidney Pelvis, Right Ureteropelvic junction (UPJ) **4 Kidney Pelvis, Left** *See 3 Kidney Pelvis, Right* **6 Ureter, Right** Ureteral orifice Ureterovesical orifice **7 Ureter, Left** *See 6 Ureter, Right* **B Bladder** Trigone of bladder **C Bladder Neck**	**Ø** Open **4** Percutaneous Endoscopic **7** Via Natural or Artificial Opening **8** Via Natural or Artificial Opening Endoscopic	**7** Autologous Tissue Substitute **J** Synthetic Substitute **K** Nonautologous Tissue Substitute	**Z** No Qualifier
D Urethra Bulbourethral (Cowper's) gland Cowper's (bulbourethral) gland External urethral sphincter Internal urethral sphincter Membranous urethra Penile urethra Prostatic urethra	**Ø** Open **4** Percutaneous Endoscopic **7** Via Natural or Artificial Opening **8** Via Natural or Artificial Opening Endoscopic **X** External	**7** Autologous Tissue Substitute **J** Synthetic Substitute **K** Nonautologous Tissue Substitute	**Z** No Qualifier

Ø   Medical and Surgical
T   Urinary System
V   Restriction   Definition: Partially closing an orifice or the lumen of a tubular body part

Explanation: The orifice can be a natural orifice or an artificially created orifice

Body Part Character 4	Approach Character 5	Device Character 6	Qualifier Character 7
3 Kidney Pelvis, Right Ureteropelvic junction (UPJ) **4 Kidney Pelvis, Left** *See 3 Kidney Pelvis, Right* **6 Ureter, Right** Ureteral orifice Ureterovesical orifice **7 Ureter, Left** *See 6 Ureter, Right* **B Bladder** Trigone of bladder **C Bladder Neck**	**Ø** Open **3** Percutaneous **4** Percutaneous Endoscopic	**C** Extraluminal Device **D** Intraluminal Device **Z** No Device	**Z** No Qualifier
3 Kidney Pelvis, Right Ureteropelvic junction (UPJ) **4 Kidney Pelvis, Left** *See 3 Kidney Pelvis, Right* **6 Ureter, Right** Ureteral orifice Ureterovesical orifice **7 Ureter, Left** *See 6 Ureter, Right* **B Bladder** Trigone of bladder **C Bladder Neck**	**7** Via Natural or Artificial Opening **8** Via Natural or Artificial Opening Endoscopic	**D** Intraluminal Device **Z** No Device	**Z** No Qualifier
D Urethra Bulbourethral (Cowper's) gland Cowper's (bulbourethral) gland External urethral sphincter Internal urethral sphincter Membranous urethra Penile urethra Prostatic urethra	**Ø** Open **3** Percutaneous **4** Percutaneous Endoscopic	**C** Extraluminal Device **D** Intraluminal Device **Z** No Device	**Z** No Qualifier
D Urethra Bulbourethral (Cowper's) gland Cowper's (bulbourethral) gland External urethral sphincter Internal urethral sphincter Membranous urethra Penile urethra Prostatic urethra	**7** Via Natural or Artificial Opening **8** Via Natural or Artificial Opening Endoscopic	**D** Intraluminal Device **Z** No Device	**Z** No Qualifier
D Urethra Bulbourethral (Cowper's) gland Cowper's (bulbourethral) gland External urethral sphincter Internal urethral sphincter Membranous urethra Penile urethra Prostatic urethra	**X** External	**Z** No Device	**Z** No Qualifier

Ø   **Medical and Surgical**
T   **Urinary System**
W   **Revision**   Definition: Correcting, to the extent possible, a portion of a malfunctioning device or the position of a displaced device
                 Explanation: Revision can include correcting a malfunctioning or displaced device by taking out or putting in components of the device such as a screw or pin

Body Part Character 4	Approach Character 5	Device Character 6	Qualifier Character 7

5   Kidney
    Renal calyx
    Renal capsule
    Renal cortex
    Renal segment
	Ø Open
	3 Percutaneous
	4 Percutaneous Endoscopic
	7 Via Natural or Artificial Opening
	8 Via Natural or Artificial Opening Endoscopic
		Ø Drainage Device
		2 Monitoring Device
		3 Infusion Device
		7 Autologous Tissue Substitute
		C Extraluminal Device
		D Intraluminal Device
		J Synthetic Substitute
		K Nonautologous Tissue Substitute
		Y Other Device
			Z No Qualifier

5   Kidney
    Renal calyx
    Renal capsule
    Renal cortex
    Renal segment
	X External	**Ø** Drainage Device
		2 Monitoring Device
		3 Infusion Device
		7 Autologous Tissue Substitute
		C Extraluminal Device
		D Intraluminal Device
		J Synthetic Substitute
		K Nonautologous Tissue Substitute
			Z No Qualifier

9   Ureter
    Ureteral orifice
    Ureterovesical orifice
	Ø Open
	3 Percutaneous
	4 Percutaneous Endoscopic
	7 Via Natural or Artificial Opening
	8 Via Natural or Artificial Opening Endoscopic
		Ø Drainage Device
		2 Monitoring Device
		3 Infusion Device
		7 Autologous Tissue Substitute
		C Extraluminal Device
		D Intraluminal Device
		J Synthetic Substitute
		K Nonautologous Tissue Substitute
		M Stimulator Lead
		Y Other Device
			Z No Qualifier

9   Ureter
    Ureteral orifice
    Ureterovesical orifice
	X External	**Ø** Drainage Device
		2 Monitoring Device
		3 Infusion Device
		7 Autologous Tissue Substitute
		C Extraluminal Device
		D Intraluminal Device
		J Synthetic Substitute
		K Nonautologous Tissue Substitute
		M Stimulator Lead
			Z No Qualifier

B Bladder Trigone of bladder	**Ø** Open **3** Percutaneous **4** Percutaneous Endoscopic **7** Via Natural or Artificial Opening **8** Via Natural or Artificial Opening Endoscopic	**Ø** Drainage Device **2** Monitoring Device **3** Infusion Device **7** Autologous Tissue Substitute **C** Extraluminal Device **D** Intraluminal Device **J** Synthetic Substitute **K** Nonautologous Tissue Substitute **L** Artificial Sphincter **M** Stimulator Lead **Y** Other Device	**Z** No Qualifier
B Bladder Trigone of bladder	**X** External	**Ø** Drainage Device **2** Monitoring Device **3** Infusion Device **7** Autologous Tissue Substitute **C** Extraluminal Device **D** Intraluminal Device **J** Synthetic Substitute **K** Nonautologous Tissue Substitute **L** Artificial Sphincter **M** Stimulator Lead	**Z** No Qualifier

Non-OR ØTW5[3,4,7]YZ	**Non-OR** ØTW9X[Ø,2,3,7,C,D,J,K,M]Z	
Non-OR ØTW5X[Ø,2,3,7,C,D,J,K]Z	**Non-OR** ØTWB[3,4,7]YZ	
Non-OR ØTW9[3,4,7]YZ	**Non-OR** ØTWBX[Ø,2,3,7,C,D,J,K,L,M]Z	

ØTW Continued on next page

NC Noncovered Procedure   **LC** Limited Coverage   **QA** Questionable OB Admit   **NT** New Tech Add-on   ✛ Combination Member   ♂ Male   ♀ Female

Ø   **Medical and Surgical**
T   **Urinary System**
W   **Revision**   *ØTW Continued*

Definition: Correcting, to the extent possible, a portion of a malfunctioning device or the position of a displaced device

Explanation: Revision can include correcting a malfunctioning or displaced device by taking out or putting in components of the device such as a screw or pin

Body Part Character 4	Approach Character 5	Device Character 6	Qualifier Character 7

D Urethra
   Bulbourethral (Cowper's) gland
   Cowper's (bulbourethral) gland
   External urethral sphincter
   Internal urethral sphincter
   Membranous urethra
   Penile urethra
   Prostatic urethra
	Ø Open
	3 Percutaneous
	4 Percutaneous Endoscopic
	7 Via Natural or Artificial Opening
	8 Via Natural or Artificial Opening
	    Endoscopic
		Ø Drainage Device
		2 Monitoring Device
		3 Infusion Device
		7 Autologous Tissue Substitute
		C Extraluminal Device
		D Intraluminal Device
		J Synthetic Substitute
		K Nonautologous Tissue Substitute
		L Artificial Sphincter
		Y Other Device
			Z No Qualifier

D Urethra
   Bulbourethral (Cowper's) gland
   Cowper's (bulbourethral) gland
   External urethral sphincter
   Internal urethral sphincter
   Membranous urethra
   Penile urethra
   Prostatic urethra
	X External	**Ø** Drainage Device
		2 Monitoring Device
		3 Infusion Device
		7 Autologous Tissue Substitute
		C Extraluminal Device
		D Intraluminal Device
		J Synthetic Substitute
		K Nonautologous Tissue Substitute
		L Artificial Sphincter
			Z No Qualifier

Non-OR   ØTWD[3,4,7,8]YZ
Non-OR   ØTWDX[Ø,2,3,7,C,D,J,K,L]Z

Ø   **Medical and Surgical**
T   **Urinary System**
Y   **Transplantation**   Definition: Putting in or on all or a portion of a living body part taken from another individual or animal to physically take the place and/or function of all or a portion of a similar body part

Explanation: The native body part may or may not be taken out, and the transplanted body part may take over all or a portion of its function

Body Part Character 4	Approach Character 5	Device Character 6	Qualifier Character 7

Ø Kidney, Right   LC ⊞
   Renal calyx
   Renal capsule
   Renal cortex
   Renal segment
1 Kidney, Left   LC ⊞
   See Ø Kidney, Right
	Ø Open	**Z** No Device	**Ø** Allogeneic
			1 Syngeneic
			2 Zooplastic

LC   ØTY[Ø,1]ØZ[Ø,1,2]

See Appendix L for Procedure Combinations
⊞   ØTY[Ø,1]ØZ[Ø,1,2]

Female Reproductive System ØU1–ØUY

Character Meanings

This Character Meaning table is provided as a guide to assist the user in the identification of character members that may be found in this section of code tables. It **SHOULD NOT** be used to build a PCS code.

Operation–Character 3	Body Part–Character 4	Approach–Character 5	Device–Character 6	Qualifier–Character 7
1 Bypass	Ø Ovary, Right	Ø Open	Ø Drainage Device	Ø Allogeneic
2 Change	1 Ovary, Left	3 Percutaneous	1 Radioactive Element	1 Syngeneic
5 Destruction	2 Ovaries, Bilateral	4 Percutaneous Endoscopic	3 Infusion Device	2 Zooplastic
7 Dilation	3 Ovary	7 Via Natural or Artificial Opening	7 Autologous Tissue Substitute	5 Fallopian Tube, Right
8 Division	4 Uterine Supporting Structure	8 Via Natural or Artificial Opening Endoscopic	C Extraluminal Device	6 Fallopian Tube, Left
9 Drainage	5 Fallopian Tube, Right	F Via Natural or Artificial Opening With Percutaneous Endoscopic Assistance	D Intraluminal Device	9 Uterus
B Excision	6 Fallopian Tube, Left	X External	G Intraluminal Device, Pessary	L Supracervical
C Extirpation	7 Fallopian Tubes, Bilateral		H Contraceptive Device	X Diagnostic
D Extraction	8 Fallopian Tube		J Synthetic Substitute	Z No Qualifier
F Fragmentation	9 Uterus		K Nonautologous Tissue Substitute	
H Insertion	B Endometrium		Y Other Device	
J Inspection	C Cervix		Z No Device	
L Occlusion	D Uterus and Cervix			
M Reattachment	F Cul-de-sac			
N Release	G Vagina			
P Removal	H Vagina and Cul-de-sac			
Q Repair	J Clitoris			
S Reposition	K Hymen			
T Resection	L Vestibular Gland			
U Supplement	M Vulva			
V Restriction	N Ova			
W Revision				
Y Transplantation				

AHA Coding Clinic for table ØU5
2015, 3Q, 31   Tubal ligation for sterilization

AHA Coding Clinic for table ØU7
2020, 2Q, 30   Duhrssen Cervical Incision

AHA Coding Clinic for table ØU9
2016, 4Q, 58   Longitudinal vaginal septum

AHA Coding Clinic for table ØUB
2018, 1Q, 23   Tubal ligation procedure
2015, 3Q, 31   Laparoscopic partial salpingectomy for ectopic pregnancy
2015, 3Q, 31   Tubal ligation for sterilization
2014, 4Q, 16   Excision of multiple uterine fibroids
2014, 3Q, 12   Excision of skin tag from labia majora

AHA Coding Clinic for table ØUC
2015, 3Q, 30   Removal of cervical cerclage
2013, 2Q, 38   Evacuation of clot post-partum

AHA Coding Clinic for table ØUH
2020, 4Q, 43-44   Insertion of radioactive element
2018, 1Q, 25   Intrauterine brachytherapy & placement of tandems & ovoids
2013, 2Q, 34   Placement of intrauterine device via open approach

AHA Coding Clinic for table ØUJ
2015, 1Q, 33   Robotic-assisted laparoscopic hysterectomy converted to open procedure

AHA Coding Clinic for table ØUL
2018, 1Q, 23   Tubal ligation procedure
2015, 3Q, 31   Tubal ligation for sterilization

AHA Coding Clinic for table ØUQ
2020, 4Q, 59-60   Extraction of ectopic products of conception
2014, 4Q, 18   Obstetrical periurethral laceration
2013, 4Q, 120   Repair of clitoral obstetric laceration

AHA Coding Clinic for table ØUS
2016, 1Q, 9   Anteversion of retroverted pregnant uterus

AHA Coding Clinic for table ØUT
2017, 4Q, 68   New qualifier values - Supracervical hysterectomy
2015, 1Q, 33   Robotic-assisted laparoscopic hysterectomy converted to open procedure
2013, 3Q, 28   Total hysterectomy
2013, 1Q, 24   Excision versus Resection of remaining ovarian remnant following previous excision

AHA Coding Clinic for table ØUV
2015, 3Q, 30   Insertion of cervical cerclage

AHA Coding Clinic for table ØUY
2018, 4Q, 40   Uterus transplant

Female Reproductive System

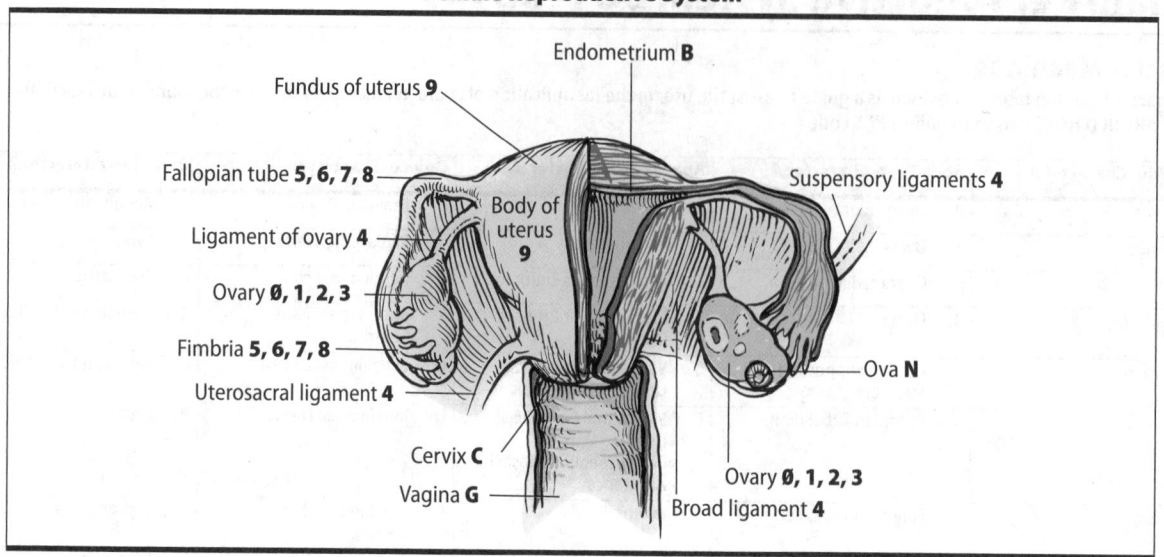

Endometrium **B**

Fundus of uterus **9**

Fallopian tube **5, 6, 7, 8**

Ligament of ovary **4**

Body of uterus **9**

Ovary **Ø, 1, 2, 3**

Fimbria **5, 6, 7, 8**

Uterosacral ligament **4**

Cervix **C**

Vagina **G**

Suspensory ligaments **4**

Ova **N**

Ovary **Ø, 1, 2, 3**

Broad ligament **4**

Female Internal/External Structures

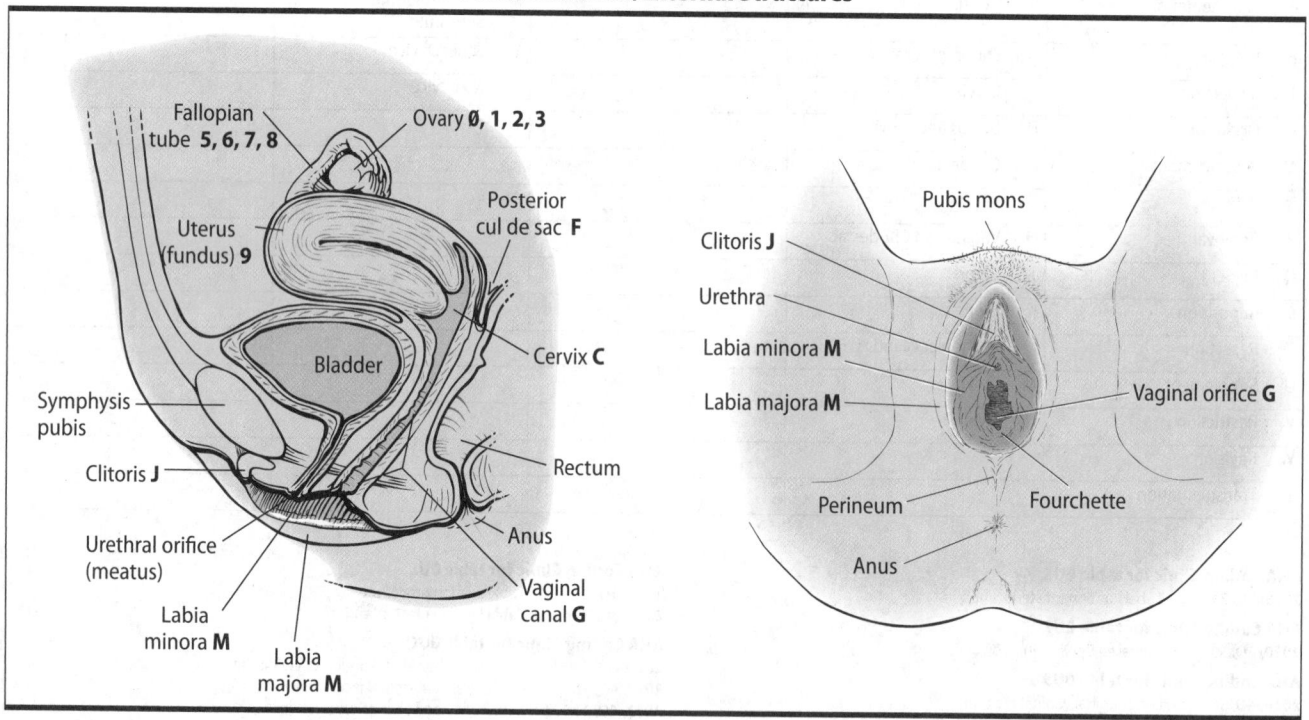

Fallopian tube **5, 6, 7, 8**

Ovary **Ø, 1, 2, 3**

Uterus (fundus) **9**

Posterior cul de sac **F**

Bladder

Cervix **C**

Symphysis pubis

Clitoris **J**

Rectum

Urethral orifice (meatus)

Anus

Labia minora **M**

Vaginal canal **G**

Labia majora **M**

Pubis mons

Clitoris **J**

Urethra

Labia minora **M**

Labia majora **M**

Vaginal orifice **G**

Perineum

Fourchette

Anus

Ø   Medical and Surgical
U   Female Reproductive System
1   Bypass   Definition: Altering the route of passage of the contents of a tubular body part

Explanation: Rerouting contents of a body part to a downstream area of the normal route, to a similar route and body part, or to an abnormal route and dissimilar body part. Includes one or more anastomoses, with or without the use of a device.

Body Part Character 4		Approach Character 5	Device Character 6	Qualifier Character 7
5 Fallopian Tube, Right ♀ Oviduct Salpinx Uterine tube 6 Fallopian Tube, Left ♀ *See 5 Fallopian Tube, Right*		Ø Open 4 Percutaneous Endoscopic	7 Autologous Tissue Substitute J Synthetic Substitute K Nonautologous Tissue Substitute Z No Device	5 Fallopian Tube, Right 6 Fallopian Tube, Left 9 Uterus

♀   All body part, approach, device, and qualifier values

Ø   Medical and Surgical
U   Female Reproductive System
2   Change   Definition: Taking out or off a device from a body part and putting back an identical or similar device in or on the same body part without cutting or puncturing the skin or a mucous membrane

Explanation: All CHANGE procedures are coded using the approach EXTERNAL

Body Part Character 4		Approach Character 5	Device Character 6	Qualifier Character 7
3 Ovary ♀ 8 Fallopian Tube ♀ M Vulva ♀ Labia majora Labia minora		X External	Ø Drainage Device Y Other Device	Z No Qualifier
D Uterus and Cervix ♀		X External	Ø Drainage Device H Contraceptive Device Y Other Device	Z No Qualifier
H Vagina and Cul-de-sac ♀		X External	Ø Drainage Device G Intraluminal Device, Pessary Y Other Device	Z No Qualifier

Non-OR   All body part, approach, device, and qualifier values   ♀   All body part, approach, device, and qualifier values

NC Noncovered Procedure   LC Limited Coverage   QA Questionable OB Admit   NT New Tech Add-on   ⊞ Combination Member   ♂ Male   ♀ Female

ICD-10-PCS 2022   639

Female Reproductive System

Ø   **Medical and Surgical**
U   **Female Reproductive System**
5   **Destruction**   Definition: Physical eradication of all or a portion of a body part by the direct use of energy, force, or a destructive agent
                         Explanation: None of the body part is physically taken out

Body Part Character 4	Approach Character 5	Device Character 6	Qualifier Character 7

Ø Ovary, Right ♀
1 Ovary, Left ♀
2 Ovaries, Bilateral ♀
4 Uterine Supporting Structure ♀
    Broad ligament
    Infundibulopelvic ligament
    Ovarian ligament
    Round ligament of uterus
	Ø Open
	3 Percutaneous
	4 Percutaneous Endoscopic
	8 Via Natural or Artificial Opening
	    Endoscopic
		Z No Device	**Z** No Qualifier

5 Fallopian Tube, Right ♀
    Oviduct
    Salpinx
    Uterine tube
6 Fallopian Tube, Left ♀
    See 5 Fallopian Tube, Right
7 Fallopian Tubes, Bilateral NC ♀
9 Uterus ♀
    Fundus uteri
    Myometrium
    Perimetrium
    Uterine cornu
B Endometrium ♀
C Cervix ♀
F Cul-de-sac ♀
	Ø Open
	3 Percutaneous
	4 Percutaneous Endoscopic
	7 Via Natural or Artificial Opening
	8 Via Natural or Artificial Opening
	    Endoscopic
		Z No Device	**Z** No Qualifier

G Vagina ♀ **K** Hymen ♀	**Ø** Open **3** Percutaneous **4** Percutaneous Endoscopic **7** Via Natural or Artificial Opening **8** Via Natural or Artificial Opening Endoscopic **X** External	**Z** No Device	**Z** No Qualifier

J Clitoris ♀
L Vestibular Gland ♀
    Bartholin's (greater vestibular) gland
    Greater vestibular (Bartholin's) gland
    Paraurethral (Skene's) gland
    Skene's (paraurethral) gland
M Vulva ♀
    Labia majora
    Labia minora
	Ø Open
	X External
		Z No Device	**Z** No Qualifier

NC   ØU57[Ø,3,4,7,8]ZZ with principal or secondary diagnosis of Z3Ø.2   ♀   All body part, approach, device, and qualifier values

Non-OR Procedure   DRG Non-OR Procedure   Valid OR Procedure   HAC Associated Procedure   Combination Only   New/Revised GREEN

Ø   **Medical and Surgical**
U   **Female Reproductive System**
7   **Dilation**   Definition: Expanding an orifice or the lumen of a tubular body part

                    Explanation: The orifice can be a natural orifice or an artificially created orifice. Accomplished by stretching a tubular body part using intraluminal pressure or by cutting part of the orifice or wall of the tubular body part.

Body Part Character 4	Approach Character 5	Device Character 6	Qualifier Character 7

5 Fallopian Tube, Right ♀
   Oviduct
   Salpinx
   Uterine tube
6 Fallopian Tube, Left ♀
   See 5 Fallopian Tube, Right
7 Fallopian Tubes, Bilateral ♀
9 Uterus ♀
   Fundus uteri
   Myometrium
   Perimetrium
   Uterine cornu
C Cervix ♀
G Vagina ♀
	Ø Open
	3 Percutaneous
	4 Percutaneous Endoscopic
	7 Via Natural or Artificial Opening
	8 Via Natural or Artificial Opening
	   Endoscopic
		D Intraluminal Device
		Z No Device
			Z No Qualifier

K Hymen ♀	Ø Open 3 Percutaneous 4 Percutaneous Endoscopic 7 Via Natural or Artificial Opening 8 Via Natural or Artificial Opening Endoscopic X External	D Intraluminal Device Z No Device	Z No Qualifier

Non-OR   ØU7C[Ø,3,4,7,8][D,Z]Z   ♀   All body part, approach, device, and qualifier values
Non-OR   ØU7G[7,8][D,Z]Z

Ø   **Medical and Surgical**
U   **Female Reproductive System**
8   **Division**   Definition: Cutting into a body part, without draining fluids and/or gases from the body part, in order to separate or transect a body part

                    Explanation: All or a portion of the body part is separated into two or more portions

Body Part Character 4	Approach Character 5	Device Character 6	Qualifier Character 7

Ø Ovary, Right ♀
1 Ovary, Left ♀
2 Ovaries, Bilateral ♀
4 Uterine Supporting Structure ♀
   Broad ligament
   Infundibulopelvic ligament
   Ovarian ligament
   Round ligament of uterus
	Ø Open
	3 Percutaneous
	4 Percutaneous Endoscopic
		Z No Device	Z No Qualifier

K Hymen ♀	7 Via Natural or Artificial Opening 8 Via Natural or Artificial Opening Endoscopic X External	Z No Device	Z No Qualifier

Non-OR   ØU8K[7,8,X]ZZ   ♀   All body part, approach, device, and qualifier values

NC Noncovered Procedure   LC Limited Coverage   QA Questionable OB Admit   NT New Tech Add-on   ⊞ Combination Member   ♂ Male   ♀ Female

ICD-10-PCS 2022   641

Female Reproductive System

Ø   Medical and Surgical
U   Female Reproductive System
9   Drainage   Definition: Taking or letting out fluids and/or gases from a body part
                     Explanation: The qualifier DIAGNOSTIC is used to identify drainage procedures that are biopsies

Body Part Character 4	Approach Character 5	Device Character 6	Qualifier Character 7
Ø Ovary, Right ♀ **1** Ovary, Left ♀ **2** Ovaries, Bilateral ♀	**Ø** Open **3** Percutaneous **4** Percutaneous Endoscopic **8** Via Natural or Artificial Opening Endoscopic	**Ø** Drainage Device	**Z** No Qualifier
Ø Ovary, Right ♀ **1** Ovary, Left ♀ **2** Ovaries, Bilateral ♀	**Ø** Open **3** Percutaneous **4** Percutaneous Endoscopic **8** Via Natural or Artificial Opening Endoscopic	**Z** No Device	**X** Diagnostic **Z** No Qualifier
Ø Ovary, Right ♀ **1** Ovary, Left ♀ **2** Ovaries, Bilateral ♀	**X** External	**Z** No Device	**Z** No Qualifier

4 Uterine Supporting Structure ♀
   Broad ligament
   Infundibulopelvic ligament
   Ovarian ligament
   Round ligament of uterus
	Ø Open
	3 Percutaneous
	4 Percutaneous Endoscopic
	8 Via Natural or Artificial Opening
	    Endoscopic
		Ø Drainage Device	**Z** No Qualifier

4 Uterine Supporting Structure ♀
   Broad ligament
   Infundibulopelvic ligament
   Ovarian ligament
   Round ligament of uterus
	Ø Open
	3 Percutaneous
	4 Percutaneous Endoscopic
	8 Via Natural or Artificial Opening
	    Endoscopic
		Z No Device	**X** Diagnostic
			Z No Qualifier

5 Fallopian Tube, Right ♀
   Oviduct
   Salpinx
   Uterine tube
6 Fallopian Tube, Left ♀
   See 5 Fallopian Tube, Right
7 Fallopian Tubes, Bilateral ♀
9 Uterus ♀
   Fundus uteri
   Myometrium
   Perimetrium
   Uterine cornu
C Cervix ♀
F Cul-de-sac ♀
	Ø Open
	3 Percutaneous
	4 Percutaneous Endoscopic
	7 Via Natural or Artificial Opening
	8 Via Natural or Artificial Opening
	    Endoscopic
		Ø Drainage Device	**Z** No Qualifier

5 Fallopian Tube, Right ♀
   Oviduct
   Salpinx
   Uterine tube
6 Fallopian Tube, Left ♀
   See 5 Fallopian Tube, Right
7 Fallopian Tubes, Bilateral ♀
9 Uterus ♀
   Fundus uteri
   Myometrium
   Perimetrium
   Uterine cornu
C Cervix ♀
F Cul-de-sac ♀
	Ø Open
	3 Percutaneous
	4 Percutaneous Endoscopic
	7 Via Natural or Artificial Opening
	8 Via Natural or Artificial Opening
	    Endoscopic
		Z No Device	**X** Diagnostic
			Z No Qualifier

Non-OR ØU9[Ø,1,2][3,8]ØZ		**Non-OR** ØU9[5,6,7,9,C]3ØZ	
Non-OR ØU9[Ø,1,2][3,8]ZZ		**Non-OR** ØU9F[3,4]ØZ	
Non-OR ØU9[Ø,1,2]8ZX		**Non-OR** ØU9[5,6,7][3,4,7,8]ZZ	
Non-OR ØU94[3,8]ØZ		**Non-OR** ØU9[9,C]3ZZ	
Non-OR ØU94[3,8]ZZ		**Non-OR** ØU9F[3,4]ZZ	
Non-OR ØU948ZX		♀ All body part, approach, device, and qualifier values	

ØU9 Continued on next page

0U9 Continued

0 **Medical and Surgical**
U **Female Reproductive System**
9 **Drainage**   Definition: Taking or letting out fluids and/or gases from a body part
      Explanation: The qualifier DIAGNOSTIC is used to identify drainage procedures that are biopsies

Body Part Character 4	Approach Character 5	Device Character 6	Qualifier Character 7
G Vagina ♀ K Hymen ♀	0 Open 3 Percutaneous 4 Percutaneous Endoscopic 7 Via Natural or Artificial Opening 8 Via Natural or Artificial Opening Endoscopic X External	0 Drainage Device	Z No Qualifier
G Vagina ♀ K Hymen ♀	0 Open 3 Percutaneous 4 Percutaneous Endoscopic 7 Via Natural or Artificial Opening 8 Via Natural or Artificial Opening Endoscopic X External	Z No Device	X Diagnostic Z No Qualifier

J Clitoris ♀
L Vestibular Gland ♀
  Bartholin's (greater vestibular) gland
  Greater vestibular (Bartholin's) gland
  Paraurethral (Skene's) gland
  Skene's (paraurethral) gland
M Vulva ♀
  Labia majora
  Labia minora
	0 Open
	X External
		0 Drainage Device	Z No Qualifier

J Clitoris ♀
L Vestibular Gland ♀
  Bartholin's (greater vestibular) gland
  Greater vestibular (Bartholin's) gland
  Paraurethral (Skene's) gland
  Skene's (paraurethral) gland
M Vulva ♀
  Labia majora
  Labia minora
	0 Open
	X External
		Z No Device	X Diagnostic
			Z No Qualifier

Non-OR   0U9G30Z
Non-OR   0U9K[0,3,4,7,8,X]0Z
Non-OR   0U9G3ZZ
Non-OR   0U9K[0,3,4,7,8,X]ZZ

Non-OR   0U9L[0,X]0Z
Non-OR   0U9L[0,X]ZZ
♀   All body part, approach, device, and qualifier values

Female Reproductive System *(left margin)*

Ø **Medical and Surgical**
U **Female Reproductive System**
B **Excision**   Definition: Cutting out or off, without replacement, a portion of a body part
                    Explanation: The qualifier DIAGNOSTIC is used to identify excision procedures that are biopsies

Body Part Character 4	Approach Character 5	Device Character 6	Qualifier Character 7

Ø Ovary, Right ♀
1 Ovary, Left ♀
2 Ovaries, Bilateral ♀
4 Uterine Supporting Structure ♀
  Broad ligament
  Infundibulopelvic ligament
  Ovarian ligament
  Round ligament of uterus
5 Fallopian Tube, Right ♀
  Oviduct
  Salpinx
  Uterine tube
6 Fallopian Tube, Left ♀
  See 5 Fallopian Tube, Right
7 Fallopian Tubes, Bilateral ♀
9 Uterus ♀
  Fundus uteri
  Myometrium
  Perimetrium
  Uterine cornu
C Cervix ♀
F Cul-de-sac ♀
	Ø Open
	3 Percutaneous
	4 Percutaneous Endoscopic
	7 Via Natural or Artificial Opening
	8 Via Natural or Artificial Opening
	  Endoscopic
		Z No Device	X Diagnostic
			Z No Qualifier

G Vagina ♀ K Hymen ♀	Ø Open 3 Percutaneous 4 Percutaneous Endoscopic 7 Via Natural or Artificial Opening 8 Via Natural or Artificial Opening Endoscopic X External	Z No Device	X Diagnostic Z No Qualifier

J Clitoris ♀
L Vestibular Gland ♀
  Bartholin's (greater vestibular) gland
  Greater vestibular (Bartholin's) gland
  Paraurethral (Skene's) gland
  Skene's (paraurethral) gland
M Vulva ♀
  Labia majora
  Labia minora
	Ø Open
	X External
		Z No Device	X Diagnostic
			Z No Qualifier

♀   All body part, approach, device, and qualifier values

Ø   Medical and Surgical
U   Female Reproductive System
C   Extirpation   Definition: Taking or cutting out solid matter from a body part

                 Explanation: The solid matter may be an abnormal byproduct of a biological function or a foreign body; it may be imbedded in a body part or in the lumen of a tubular body part. The solid matter may or may not have been previously broken into pieces.

Body Part Character 4	Approach Character 5	Device Character 6	Qualifier Character 7

Ø Ovary, Right ♀
1 Ovary, Left ♀
2 Ovaries, Bilateral ♀
4 Uterine Supporting Structure ♀
   Broad ligament
   Infundibulopelvic ligament
   Ovarian ligament
   Round ligament of uterus
	Ø Open
	3 Percutaneous
	4 Percutaneous Endoscopic
	8 Via Natural or Artificial Opening
	   Endoscopic
		Z No Device	Z No Qualifier

5 Fallopian Tube, Right ♀
   Oviduct
   Salpinx
   Uterine tube
6 Fallopian Tube, Left ♀
   See 5 Fallopian Tube, Right
7 Fallopian Tubes, Bilateral ♀
9 Uterus ♀
   Fundus uteri
   Myometrium
   Perimetrium
   Uterine cornu
B Endometrium ♀
C Cervix ♀
F Cul-de-sac ♀
	Ø Open
	3 Percutaneous
	4 Percutaneous Endoscopic
	7 Via Natural or Artificial Opening
	8 Via Natural or Artificial Opening
	   Endoscopic
		Z No Device	Z No Qualifier

G Vagina ♀ K Hymen ♀	Ø Open 3 Percutaneous 4 Percutaneous Endoscopic 7 Via Natural or Artificial Opening 8 Via Natural or Artificial Opening Endoscopic X External	Z No Device	Z No Qualifier

J Clitoris ♀
L Vestibular Gland ♀
   Bartholin's (greater vestibular) gland
   Greater vestibular (Bartholin's) gland
   Paraurethral (Skene's) gland
   Skene's (paraurethral) gland
M Vulva ♀
   Labia majora
   Labia minora
	Ø Open
	X External
		Z No Device	Z No Qualifier

Non-OR   ØUC9[7,8]ZZ
Non-OR   ØUCG[7,8,X]ZZ
Non-OR   ØUCK[Ø,3,4,7,8,X]ZZ

Non-OR   ØUCMXZZ
♀   All body part, approach, device, and qualifier values

Ø   Medical and Surgical
U   Female Reproductive System
D   Extraction   Definition: Pulling or stripping out or off all or a portion of a body part by the use of force

                 Explanation: The qualifier DIAGNOSTIC is used to identify extraction procedures that are biopsies

Body Part Character 4	Approach Character 5	Device Character 6	Qualifier Character 7
B Endometrium ♀	7 Via Natural or Artificial Opening 8 Via Natural or Artificial Opening Endoscopic	Z No Device	X Diagnostic Z No Qualifier
N Ova ♀	Ø Open 3 Percutaneous 4 Percutaneous Endoscopic	Z No Device	Z No Qualifier

♀   All body part, approach, device, and qualifier values

Female Reproductive System

Ø   **Medical and Surgical**
U   **Female Reproductive System**
F   **Fragmentation**   Definition: Breaking solid matter in a body part into pieces

               Explanation: Physical force (e.g., manual, ultrasonic) applied directly or indirectly is used to break the solid matter into pieces. The solid matter may be an abnormal byproduct of a biological function or a foreign body. The pieces of solid matter are not taken out.

Body Part Character 4	Approach Character 5	Device Character 6	Qualifier Character 7

5 Fallopian Tube, Right   NC ♀
   Oviduct
   Salpinx
   Uterine tube
6 Fallopian Tube, Left   NC ♀
   See 5 Fallopian Tube, Right
7 Fallopian Tubes, Bilateral   NC ♀
9 Uterus   NC ♀
   Fundus uteri
   Myometrium
   Perimetrium
   Uterine cornu
	Ø Open
	3 Percutaneous
	4 Percutaneous Endoscopic
	7 Via Natural or Artificial Opening
	8 Via Natural or Artificial Opening Endoscopic
	X External
		Z No Device	**Z** No Qualifier

Non-OR ØUF[5,6,7,9]XZZ		
NC ØUF[5,6,7,9]XZZ	♀ All body part, approach, device, and qualifier values	

Ø   **Medical and Surgical**
U   **Female Reproductive System**
H   **Insertion**   Definition: Putting in a nonbiological appliance that monitors, assists, performs, or prevents a physiological function but does not physically take the place of a body part

               Explanation: None

Body Part Character 4	Approach Character 5	Device Character 6	Qualifier Character 7
3 Ovary ♀	**Ø** Open **3** Percutaneous **4** Percutaneous Endoscopic	**1** Radioactive Element **3** Infusion Device **Y** Other Device	**Z** No Qualifier
3 Ovary ♀	**7** Via Natural or Artificial Opening **8** Via Natural or Artificial Opening Endoscopic	**1** Radioactive Element **Y** Other Device	**Z** No Qualifier
8 Fallopian Tube ♀ **D** Uterus and Cervix ♀ **H** Vagina and Cul-de-sac ♀	**Ø** Open **3** Percutaneous **4** Percutaneous Endoscopic **7** Via Natural or Artificial Opening **8** Via Natural or Artificial Opening Endoscopic	**3** Infusion Device **Y** Other Device	**Z** No Qualifier

9 Uterus   ♀
   Fundus uteri
   Myometrium
   Perimetrium
   Uterine cornu
	Ø Open
	7 Via Natural or Artificial Opening
	8 Via Natural or Artificial Opening Endoscopic
		1 Radioactive Element
		H Contraceptive Device
			Z No Qualifier

C Cervix ♀	**Ø** Open **3** Percutaneous **4** Percutaneous Endoscopic	**1** Radioactive Element	**Z** No Qualifier
C Cervix ♀	**7** Via Natural or Artificial Opening **8** Via Natural or Artificial Opening Endoscopic	**1** Radioactive Element **H** Contraceptive Device	**Z** No Qualifier
F Cul-de-sac ♀	**7** Via Natural or Artificial Opening **8** Via Natural or Artificial Opening Endoscopic	**G** Intraluminal Device, Pessary	**Z** No Qualifier
G Vagina ♀	**Ø** Open **3** Percutaneous **4** Percutaneous Endoscopic **X** External	**1** Radioactive Element	**Z** No Qualifier
G Vagina ♀	**7** Via Natural or Artificial Opening **8** Via Natural or Artificial Opening Endoscopic	**1** Radioactive Element **G** Intraluminal Device, Pessary	**Z** No Qualifier

Non-OR ØUH3[Ø,4][3,Y]Z	**Non-OR** ØUH9[Ø,7,8][1,H]Z
Non-OR ØUH33[1,3,Y]Z	**Non-OR** ØUHC[7,8]HZ
Non-OR ØUH3[7,8][1,Y]Z	**Non-OR** ØÜHF[7,8]HZ
Non-OR ØUH[8,D][Ø,3,4,7,8][3,Y]Z	**Non-OR** ØUHG[7,8]HZ
Non-OR ØUHH[3,4]YZ	♀ All body part, approach, device, and qualifier values
Non-OR ØUHH[7,8][3,Y]Z	

Ø   **Medical and Surgical**
U   **Female Reproductive System**
J   **Inspection**   Definition: Visually and/or manually exploring a body part

         Explanation: Visual exploration may be performed with or without optical instrumentation. Manual exploration may be performed directly or through intervening body layers.

Body Part Character 4	Approach Character 5	Device Character 6	Qualifier Character 7
3 Ovary ♀	**Ø** Open **3** Percutaneous **4** Percutaneous Endoscopic **8** Via Natural or Artificial Opening Endoscopic **X** External	**Z** No Device	**Z** No Qualifier
8 Fallopian Tube ♀ **D** Uterus and Cervix ♀ **H** Vagina and Cul-de-sac ♀	**Ø** Open **3** Percutaneous **4** Percutaneous Endoscopic **7** Via Natural or Artificial Opening **8** Via Natural or Artificial Opening Endoscopic **X** External	**Z** No Device	**Z** No Qualifier
M Vulva ♀ Labia majora Labia minora	**Ø** Open **X** External	**Z** No Device	**Z** No Qualifier

Non-OR ØUJ3[3,8,X]ZZ	**Non-OR** ØUJMXZZ	
Non-OR ØUJ[8,D,H][3,7,8,X]ZZ	♀ All body part, approach, device, and qualifier values	

Ø   **Medical and Surgical**
U   **Female Reproductive System**
L   **Occlusion**   Definition: Completely closing an orifice or the lumen of a tubular body part

         Explanation: The orifice can be a natural orifice or an artificially created orifice

Body Part Character 4	Approach Character 5	Device Character 6	Qualifier Character 7
5 Fallopian Tube, Right ♀ Oviduct Salpinx Uterine tube **6** Fallopian Tube, Left ♀ *See 5 Fallopian Tube, Right* **7** Fallopian Tubes, Bilateral NC♀	**Ø** Open **3** Percutaneous **4** Percutaneous Endoscopic	**C** Extraluminal Device **D** Intraluminal Device **Z** No Device	**Z** No Qualifier
5 Fallopian Tube, Right ♀ Oviduct Salpinx Uterine tube **6** Fallopian Tube, Left ♀ *See 5 Fallopian Tube, Right* **7** Fallopian Tubes, Bilateral NC♀	**7** Via Natural or Artificial Opening **8** Via Natural or Artificial Opening Endoscopic	**D** Intraluminal Device **Z** No Device	**Z** No Qualifier
F Cul-de-sac ♀ **G** Vagina ♀	**7** Via Natural or Artificial Opening **8** Via Natural or Artificial Opening Endoscopic	**D** Intraluminal Device **Z** No Device	**Z** No Qualifier

NC ØUL7[Ø,3,4][C,D,Z]Z with principal or secondary diagnosis of Z3Ø.2	♀ All body part, approach, device, and qualifier values
NC ØUL7[7,8][D,Z]Z with principal or secondary diagnosis of Z3Ø.2	

Female Reproductive System *(left margin)*

Ø **Medical and Surgical**
U **Female Reproductive System**
M **Reattachment**   Definition: Putting back in or on all or a portion of a separated body part to its normal location or other suitable location
                       Explanation: Vascular circulation and nervous pathways may or may not be reestablished

Body Part Character 4	Approach Character 5	Device Character 6	Qualifier Character 7

Ø **Ovary, Right** ♀
1 **Ovary, Left** ♀
2 **Ovaries, Bilateral** ♀
4 **Uterine Supporting Structure** ♀
   Broad ligament
   Infundibulopelvic ligament
   Ovarian ligament
   Round ligament of uterus
5 **Fallopian Tube, Right** ♀
   Oviduct
   Salpinx
   Uterine tube
6 **Fallopian Tube, Left** ♀
   See 5 Fallopian Tube, Right
7 **Fallopian Tubes, Bilateral** ♀
9 **Uterus** ♀
   Fundus uteri
   Myometrium
   Perimetrium
   Uterine cornu
C **Cervix** ♀
F **Cul-de-sac** ♀
G **Vagina** ♀
	Ø **Open**
	4 **Percutaneous Endoscopic**
		Z **No Device**	Z **No Qualifier**

J **Clitoris** ♀
M **Vulva** ♀
   Labia majora
   Labia minora
	X **External**	Z **No Device**	Z **No Qualifier**

K **Hymen** ♀	Ø **Open** 4 **Percutaneous Endoscopic** X **External**	Z **No Device**	Z **No Qualifier**

♀   All body part, approach, device, and qualifier values

Ø　Medical and Surgical
U　Female Reproductive System
N　Release　　Definition: Freeing a body part from an abnormal physical constraint by cutting or by the use of force
　　　　　　　　　Explanation: Some of the restraining tissue may be taken out but none of the body part is taken out

Body Part Character 4	Approach Character 5	Device Character 6	Qualifier Character 7
Ø Ovary, Right ♀ **1** Ovary, Left ♀ **2** Ovaries, Bilateral ♀ **4** Uterine Supporting Structure ♀ 　Broad ligament 　Infundibulopelvic ligament 　Ovarian ligament 　Round ligament of uterus	**Ø** Open **3** Percutaneous **4** Percutaneous Endoscopic **8** Via Natural or Artificial Opening 　Endoscopic	**Z** No Device	**Z** No Qualifier
5 Fallopian Tube, Right ♀ 　Oviduct 　Salpinx 　Uterine tube **6** Fallopian Tube, Left ♀ 　*See 5 Fallopian Tube, Right* **7** Fallopian Tubes, Bilateral ♀ **9** Uterus ♀ 　Fundus uteri 　Myometrium 　Perimetrium 　Uterine cornu **C** Cervix ♀ **F** Cul-de-sac ♀	**Ø** Open **3** Percutaneous **4** Percutaneous Endoscopic **7** Via Natural or Artificial Opening **8** Via Natural or Artificial Opening 　Endoscopic	**Z** No Device	**Z** No Qualifier
G Vagina ♀ **K** Hymen ♀	**Ø** Open **3** Percutaneous **4** Percutaneous Endoscopic **7** Via Natural or Artificial Opening **8** Via Natural or Artificial Opening 　Endoscopic **X** External	**Z** No Device	**Z** No Qualifier
J Clitoris ♀ **L** Vestibular Gland ♀ 　Bartholin's (greater vestibular) gland 　Greater vestibular (Bartholin's) gland 　Paraurethral (Skene's) gland 　Skene's (paraurethral) gland **M** Vulva ♀ 　Labia majora 　Labia minora	**Ø** Open **X** External	**Z** No Device	**Z** No Qualifier

　♀　　All body part, approach, device, and qualifier values

NC Noncovered Procedure　**LC** Limited Coverage　**QA** Questionable OB Admit　**NT** New Tech Add-on　⊞ Combination Member　♂ Male　♀ Female

ICD-10-PCS 2022
649

Female Reproductive System *(left margin)*

Ø   **Medical and Surgical**
U   **Female Reproductive System**
P   **Removal**   Definition: Taking out or off a device from a body part

Explanation: If a device is taken out and a similar device put in without cutting or puncturing the skin or mucous membrane, the procedure is coded to the root operation CHANGE. Otherwise, the procedure for taking out the device is coded to the root operation REMOVAL.

Body Part Character 4	Approach Character 5	Device Character 6	Qualifier Character 7
3 Ovary ♀	Ø Open 3 Percutaneous 4 Percutaneous Endoscopic	Ø Drainage Device 3 Infusion Device Y Other Device	Z No Qualifier
3 Ovary ♀	7 Via Natural or Artificial Opening 8 Via Natural or Artificial Opening Endoscopic	Y Other Device	Z No Qualifier
3 Ovary ♀	X External	Ø Drainage Device 3 Infusion Device	Z No Qualifier
8 Fallopian Tube ♀	Ø Open 3 Percutaneous 4 Percutaneous Endoscopic 7 Via Natural or Artificial Opening 8 Via Natural or Artificial Opening Endoscopic	Ø Drainage Device 3 Infusion Device 7 Autologous Tissue Substitute C Extraluminal Device D Intraluminal Device J Synthetic Substitute K Nonautologous Tissue Substitute Y Other Device	Z No Qualifier
8 Fallopian Tube ♀	X External	Ø Drainage Device 3 Infusion Device D Intraluminal Device	Z No Qualifier
D Uterus and Cervix ♀	Ø Open 3 Percutaneous 4 Percutaneous Endoscopic 7 Via Natural or Artificial Opening 8 Via Natural or Artificial Opening Endoscopic	Ø Drainage Device 1 Radioactive Element 3 Infusion Device 7 Autologous Tissue Substitute C Extraluminal Device D Intraluminal Device H Contraceptive Device J Synthetic Substitute K Nonautologous Tissue Substitute Y Other Device	Z No Qualifier
D Uterus and Cervix ♀	X External	Ø Drainage Device 3 Infusion Device D Intraluminal Device H Contraceptive Device	Z No Qualifier
H Vagina and Cul-de-sac ♀	Ø Open 3 Percutaneous 4 Percutaneous Endoscopic 7 Via Natural or Artificial Opening 8 Via Natural or Artificial Opening Endoscopic	Ø Drainage Device 1 Radioactive Element 3 Infusion Device 7 Autologous Tissue Substitute D Intraluminal Device J Synthetic Substitute K Nonautologous Tissue Substitute Y Other Device	Z No Qualifier
H Vagina and Cul-de-sac ♀	X External	Ø Drainage Device 1 Radioactive Element 3 Infusion Device D Intraluminal Device	Z No Qualifier
M Vulva ♀ Labia majora Labia minora	Ø Open	Ø Drainage Device 7 Autologous Tissue Substitute J Synthetic Substitute K Nonautologous Tissue Substitute	Z No Qualifier
M Vulva ♀ Labia majora Labia minora	X External	Ø Drainage Device	Z No Qualifier

Non-OR	ØUP3[3,4]YZ	**Non-OR**	ØUPD[7,8][Ø,3,C,D,H,Y]Z
Non-OR	ØUP3[7,8]YZ	**Non-OR**	ØUPDX[Ø,3,D,H]Z
Non-OR	ØUP3X[Ø,3]Z	**Non-OR**	ØUPH[3,4]YZ
Non-OR	ØUP8[3,4]YZ	**Non-OR**	ØUPH[7,8][Ø,3,D,Y]Z
Non-OR	ØUP8[7,8][Ø,3,D,Y]Z	**Non-OR**	ØUPHX[Ø,1,3,D]Z
Non-OR	ØUP8X[Ø,3,D]Z	**Non-OR**	ØUPMXØZ
Non-OR	ØUPD[3,4][C,Y]Z	♀	All body part, approach, device, and qualifier values

0   **Medical and Surgical**
U   **Female Reproductive System**
Q   **Repair**   Definition: Restoring, to the extent possible, a body part to its normal anatomic structure and function
                       Explanation: Used only when the method to accomplish the repair is not one of the other root operations

Body Part Character 4	Approach Character 5	Device Character 6	Qualifier Character 7

0 Ovary, Right ♀
1 Ovary, Left ♀
2 Ovaries, Bilateral ♀
4 Uterine Supporting Structure ♀
    Broad ligament
    Infundibulopelvic ligament
    Ovarian ligament
    Round ligament of uterus
	0 Open
	3 Percutaneous
	4 Percutaneous Endoscopic
	8 Via Natural or Artificial Opening
	    Endoscopic
		Z No Device	**Z** No Qualifier

5 Fallopian Tube, Right ♀
    Oviduct
    Salpinx
    Uterine tube
6 Fallopian Tube, Left ♀
    See 5 Fallopian Tube, Right
7 Fallopian Tubes, Bilateral ♀
9 Uterus ♀
    Fundus uteri
    Myometrium
    Perimetrium
    Uterine cornu
C Cervix ♀
F Cul-de-sac ♀
	0 Open
	3 Percutaneous
	4 Percutaneous Endoscopic
	7 Via Natural or Artificial Opening
	8 Via Natural or Artificial Opening
	    Endoscopic
		Z No Device	**Z** No Qualifier

G Vagina ♀ **K** Hymen ♀	**0** Open **3** Percutaneous **4** Percutaneous Endoscopic **7** Via Natural or Artificial Opening **8** Via Natural or Artificial Opening Endoscopic **X** External	**Z** No Device	**Z** No Qualifier

J Clitoris ♀
L Vestibular Gland ♀
    Bartholin's (greater vestibular) gland
    Greater vestibular (Bartholin's) gland
    Paraurethral (Skene's) gland
    Skene's (paraurethral) gland
M Vulva ♀
    Labia majora
    Labia minora
	0 Open
	X External
		Z No Device	**Z** No Qualifier

Non-OR   0UQG[7,X]ZZ
Non-OR   0UQKXZZ
Non-OR   0UQMXZZ
♀   All body part, approach, device, and qualifier values

0   **Medical and Surgical**
U   **Female Reproductive System**
S   **Reposition**   Definition: Moving to its normal location, or other suitable location, all or a portion of a body part
                       Explanation: The body part is moved to a new location from an abnormal location, or from a normal location where it is not functioning
                       correctly. The body part may or may not be cut out or off to be moved to the new location.

Body Part Character 4	Approach Character 5	Device Character 6	Qualifier Character 7

0 Ovary, Right ♀
1 Ovary, Left ♀
2 Ovaries, Bilateral ♀
4 Uterine Supporting Structure ♀
    Broad ligament
    Infundibulopelvic ligament
    Ovarian ligament
    Round ligament of uterus
5 Fallopian Tube, Right ♀
    Oviduct
    Salpinx
    Uterine tube
6 Fallopian Tube, Left ♀
    See 5 Fallopian Tube, Right
7 Fallopian Tubes, Bilateral ♀
C Cervix ♀
F Cul-de-sac ♀
	0 Open
	4 Percutaneous Endoscopic
	8 Via Natural or Artificial Opening
	    Endoscopic
		Z No Device	**Z** No Qualifier

9 Uterus ♀
    Fundus uteri
    Myometrium
    Perimetrium
    Uterine cornu
G Vagina ♀
	0 Open
	4 Percutaneous Endoscopic
	7 Via Natural or Artificial Opening
	8 Via Natural or Artificial Opening
	    Endoscopic
	X External
		Z No Device	**Z** No Qualifier

Non-OR   0US9XZZ
♀   All body part, approach, device, and qualifier values

NC Noncovered Procedure   **LC** Limited Coverage   **QA** Questionable OB Admit   **NT** New Tech Add-on   ⊞ Combination Member   ♂ Male   ♀ Female

Ø   Medical and Surgical
U   Female Reproductive System
T   Resection   Definition: Cutting out or off, without replacement, all of a body part
                            Explanation: None

Body Part Character 4	Approach Character 5	Device Character 6	Qualifier Character 7
Ø Ovary, Right ♀ **1** Ovary, Left ♀ **2** Ovaries, Bilateral ⊞♀ **5** Fallopian Tube, Right ♀ 　Oviduct 　Salpinx 　Uterine tube **6** Fallopian Tube, Left ♀ 　*See 5 Fallopian Tube, Right* **7** Fallopian Tubes, Bilateral ⊞♀	**Ø** Open **4** Percutaneous Endoscopic **7** Via Natural or Artificial Opening **8** Via Natural or Artificial Opening 　Endoscopic **F** Via Natural or Artificial Opening 　With Percutaneous Endoscopic 　Assistance	**Z** No Device	**Z** No Qualifier
4 Uterine Supporting Structure ⊞♀ 　Broad ligament 　Infundibulopelvic ligament 　Ovarian ligament 　Round ligament of uterus **C** Cervix ⊞♀ **F** Cul-de-sac ♀ **G** Vagina ⊞♀	**Ø** Open **4** Percutaneous Endoscopic **7** Via Natural or Artificial Opening **8** Via Natural or Artificial Opening 　Endoscopic	**Z** No Device	**Z** No Qualifier
9 Uterus ⊞♀ 　Fundus uteri 　Myometrium 　Perimetrium 　Uterine cornu	**Ø** Open **4** Percutaneous Endoscopic **7** Via Natural or Artificial Opening **8** Via Natural or Artificial Opening 　Endoscopic **F** Via Natural or Artificial Opening 　With Percutaneous Endoscopic 　Assistance	**Z** No Device	**L** Supracervical **Z** No Qualifier
J Clitoris ♀ **L** Vestibular Gland ♀ 　Bartholin's (greater vestibular) 　　gland 　Greater vestibular (Bartholin's) 　　gland 　Paraurethral (Skene's) gland 　Skene's (paraurethral) gland **M** Vulva ⊞♀ 　Labia majora 　Labia minora	**Ø** Open **X** External	**Z** No Device	**Z** No Qualifier
K Hymen ♀	**Ø** Open **4** Percutaneous Endoscopic **7** Via Natural or Artificial Opening **8** Via Natural or Artificial Opening 　Endoscopic **X** External	**Z** No Device	**Z** No Device

♀　　All body part, approach, device, and qualifier values

See Appendix L for Procedure Combinations
⊞　　ØUT[2,7]ØZZ
⊞　　ØUT[4,C][Ø,4,7,8]ZZ
⊞　　ØUTGØZZ
⊞　　ØUT9[Ø,4,7,8,F]ZZ
⊞　　ØUTM[Ø,X]ZZ

Ø   **Medical and Surgical**
U   **Female Reproductive System**
U   **Supplement**   Definition: Putting in or on biological or synthetic material that physically reinforces and/or augments the function of a portion of a body part

                 Explanation: The biological material is non-living, or is living and from the same individual. The body part may have been previously replaced, and the SUPPLEMENT procedure is performed to physically reinforce and/or augment the function of the replaced body part.

Body Part Character 4	Approach Character 5	Device Character 6	Qualifier Character 7

4 Uterine Supporting Structure ♀
   Broad ligament
   Infundibulopelvic ligament
   Ovarian ligament
   Round ligament of uterus
	Ø Open
	4 Percutaneous Endoscopic
		7 Autologous Tissue Substitute
		J Synthetic Substitute
		K Nonautologous Tissue Substitute
			Z No Qualifier

5 Fallopian Tube, Right ♀
   Oviduct
   Salpinx
   Uterine tube
6 Fallopian Tube, Left ♀
   See 5 Fallopian Tube, Right
7 Fallopian Tubes, Bilateral ♀
F Cul-de-sac ♀
	Ø Open
	4 Percutaneous Endoscopic
	7 Via Natural or Artificial Opening
	8 Via Natural or Artificial Opening Endoscopic
		7 Autologous Tissue Substitute
		J Synthetic Substitute
		K Nonautologous Tissue Substitute
			Z No Qualifier

G Vagina ♀ **K** Hymen ♀	**Ø** Open **4** Percutaneous Endoscopic **7** Via Natural or Artificial Opening **8** Via Natural or Artificial Opening Endoscopic **X** External	**7** Autologous Tissue Substitute **J** Synthetic Substitute **K** Nonautologous Tissue Substitute	**Z** No Qualifier

J Clitoris ♀
M Vulva ♀
   Labia majora
   Labia minora
	Ø Open
	X External
		7 Autologous Tissue Substitute
		J Synthetic Substitute
		K Nonautologous Tissue Substitute
			Z No Qualifier

♀   All body part, approach, device, and qualifier values

Ø   **Medical and Surgical**
U   **Female Reproductive System**
V   **Restriction**   Definition: Partially closing an orifice or the lumen of a tubular body part

                 Explanation: The orifice can be a natural orifice or an artificially created orifice

Body Part Character 4	Approach Character 5	Device Character 6	Qualifier Character 7
C Cervix ♀	**Ø** Open **3** Percutaneous **4** Percutaneous Endoscopic	**C** Extraluminal Device **D** Intraluminal Device **Z** No Device	**Z** No Qualifier
C Cervix ♀	**7** Via Natural or Artificial Opening **8** Via Natural or Artificial Opening Endoscopic	**D** Intraluminal Device **Z** No Device	**Z** No Qualifier

♀   All body part, approach, device, and qualifier values

NC Noncovered Procedure   **LC** Limited Coverage   **QA** Questionable OB Admit   **NT** New Tech Add-on   ⊞ Combination Member   ♂ Male   ♀ Female

ICD-10-PCS 2022   653

Female Reproductive System

Ø   **Medical and Surgical**
U   **Female Reproductive System**
W   **Revision**   Definition: Correcting, to the extent possible, a portion of a malfunctioning device or the position of a displaced device
                 Explanation: Revision can include correcting a malfunctioning or displaced device by taking out or putting in components of the device such as a screw or pin

Body Part Character 4		Approach Character 5	Device Character 6	Qualifier Character 7
3 Ovary	♀	**Ø** Open **3** Percutaneous **4** Percutaneous Endoscopic	**Ø** Drainage Device **3** Infusion Device **Y** Other Device	**Z** No Qualifier
3 Ovary	♀	**7** Via Natural or Artificial Opening **8** Via Natural or Artificial Opening Endoscopic	**Y** Other Device	**Z** No Qualifier
3 Ovary	♀	**X** External	**Ø** Drainage Device **3** Infusion Device	**Z** No Qualifier
8 Fallopian Tube	♀	**Ø** Open **3** Percutaneous **4** Percutaneous Endoscopic **7** Via Natural or Artificial Opening **8** Via Natural or Artificial Opening Endoscopic	**Ø** Drainage Device **3** Infusion Device **7** Autologous Tissue Substitute **C** Extraluminal Device **D** Intraluminal Device **J** Synthetic Substitute **K** Nonautologous Tissue Substitute **Y** Other Device	**Z** No Qualifier
8 Fallopian Tube	♀	**X** External	**Ø** Drainage Device **3** Infusion Device **7** Autologous Tissue Substitute **C** Extraluminal Device **D** Intraluminal Device **J** Synthetic Substitute **K** Nonautologous Tissue Substitute	**Z** No Qualifier
D Uterus and Cervix	♀	**Ø** Open **3** Percutaneous **4** Percutaneous Endoscopic **7** Via Natural or Artificial Opening **8** Via Natural or Artificial Opening Endoscopic	**Ø** Drainage Device **1** Radioactive Element **3** Infusion Device **7** Autologous Tissue Substitute **C** Extraluminal Device **D** Intraluminal Device **H** Contraceptive Device **J** Synthetic Substitute **K** Nonautologous Tissue Substitute **Y** Other Device	**Z** No Qualifier
D Uterus and Cervix	♀	**X** External	**Ø** Drainage Device **3** Infusion Device **7** Autologous Tissue Substitute **C** Extraluminal Device **D** Intraluminal Device **H** Contraceptive Device **J** Synthetic Substitute **K** Nonautologous Tissue Substitute	**Z** No Qualifier
H Vagina and Cul-de-sac	♀	**Ø** Open **3** Percutaneous **4** Percutaneous Endoscopic **7** Via Natural or Artificial Opening **8** Via Natural or Artificial Opening Endoscopic	**Ø** Drainage Device **1** Radioactive Element **3** Infusion Device **7** Autologous Tissue Substitute **D** Intraluminal Device **J** Synthetic Substitute **K** Nonautologous Tissue Substitute **Y** Other Device	**Z** No Qualifier
H Vagina and Cul-de-sac	♀	**X** External	**Ø** Drainage Device **3** Infusion Device **7** Autologous Tissue Substitute **D** Intraluminal Device **J** Synthetic Substitute **K** Nonautologous Tissue Substitute	**Z** No Qualifier

M   Vulva
     Labia majora
     Labia minora
	♀	**Ø** Open
		X External
			Ø Drainage Device
			7 Autologous Tissue Substitute
			J Synthetic Substitute
			K Nonautologous Tissue Substitute
				Z No Qualifier

Non-OR	ØUW3[3,4]YZ		Non-OR	ØUWDX[Ø,3,7,C,D,H,J,K]Z
Non-OR	ØUW3[7,8]YZ		Non-OR	ØUWH[3,4,7,8]YZ
Non-OR	ØUW3X[Ø,3]Z		Non-OR	ØUWHX[Ø,3,7,D,J,K]Z
Non-OR	ØUW8[3,4,7,8]YZ		Non-OR	ØUWMX[Ø,7,J,K]Z
Non-OR	ØUW8X[Ø,3,7,C,D,J,K]Z		♀	All body part, approach, device, and qualifier values
Non-OR	ØUWD[3,4,7,8]YZ			

Ø   **Medical and Surgical**
U   **Female Reproductive System**
Y   **Transplantation**   Definition: Putting in or on all or a portion of a living body part taken from another individual or animal to physically take the place and/or function of all or a portion of a similar body part

Explanation: The native body part may or may not be taken out, and the transplanted body part may take over all or a portion of its function

Body Part Character 4		Approach Character 5	Device Character 6	Qualifier Character 7
Ø Ovary, Right	♀	**Ø** Open	**Z** No Device	**Ø** Allogeneic
1 Ovary, Left	♀			**1** Syngeneic
9 Uterus	♀			**2** Zooplastic

  ♀   All body part, approach, device, and qualifier values

Male Reproductive System ØV1–ØVX

Character Meanings

This Character Meaning table is provided as a guide to assist the user in the identification of character members that may be found in this section of code tables. It **SHOULD NOT** be used to build a PCS code.

Operation–Character 3	Body Part–Character 4	Approach–Character 5	Device–Character 6	Qualifier–Character 7
1 Bypass	Ø Prostate	Ø Open	Ø Drainage Device	Ø Allogeneic
2 Change	1 Seminal Vesicle, Right	3 Percutaneous	1 Radioactive Element	1 Syngeneic
5 Destruction	2 Seminal Vesicle, Left	4 Percutaneous Endoscopic	3 Infusion Device	2 Zooplastic
7 Dilation	3 Seminal Vesicles, Bilateral	7 Via Natural or Artificial Opening	7 Autologous Tissue Substitute	D Urethra
9 Drainage	4 Prostate and Seminal Vesicles	8 Via Natural or Artificial Opening Endoscopic	C Extraluminal Device	J Epididymis, Right
B Excision	5 Scrotum	X External	D Intraluminal Device	K Epididymis, Left
C Extirpation	6 Tunica Vaginalis, Right		J Synthetic Substitute	N Vas Deferens, Right
H Insertion	7 Tunica Vaginalis, Left		K Nonautologous Tissue Substitute	P Vas Deferens, Left
J Inspection	8 Scrotum and Tunica Vaginalis		Y Other Device	S Penis
L Occlusion	9 Testis, Right		Z No Device	X Diagnostic
M Reattachment	B Testis, Left			Z No Qualifier
N Release	C Testes, Bilateral			
P Removal	D Testis			
Q Repair	F Spermatic Cord, Right			
R Replacement	G Spermatic Cord, Left			
S Reposition	H Spermatic Cords, Bilateral			
T Resection	J Epididymis, Right			
U Supplement	K Epididymis, Left			
W Revision	L Epididymis, Bilateral			
X Transfer	M Epididymis and Spermatic Cord			
Y Transplantation	N Vas Deferens, Right			
	P Vas Deferens, Left			
	Q Vas Deferens, Bilateral			
	R Vas Deferens			
	S Penis			
	T Prepuce			

AHA Coding Clinic for table ØV1
2018, 3Q, 12   Al-Ghorab distal penile shunt surgery

AHA Coding Clinic for table ØV9
2018, 3Q, 12   Al-Ghorab distal penile shunt surgery

AHA Coding Clinic for table ØVB
2020, 1Q, 31   Repair of buried penis
2019, 3Q, 18   Radical prostatectomy and lymph node dissection with biopsy of neurovascular bundle
2016, 1Q, 23   Transurethral resection of ejaculatory ducts
2014, 4Q, 33   Radical prostatectomy

AHA Coding Clinic for table ØVH
2020, 4Q, 43-44 Insertion of radioactive element

AHA Coding Clinic for table ØVP
2016, 2Q, 28   Removal of multi-component inflatable penile prosthesis with placement of new malleable device

AHA Coding Clinic for table ØVQ
2018, 3Q, 12   Al-Ghorab distal penile shunt surgery

AHA Coding Clinic for table ØVT
2020, 4Q, 99   Robotic-assisted prostatectomy with extension of incision for specimen removal
2019, 3Q, 18   Radical prostatectomy and lymph node dissection with biopsy of neurovascular bundle
2014, 4Q, 33   Radical prostatectomy

AHA Coding Clinic for table ØVU
2020, 1Q, 31   Repair of buried penis
2016, 2Q, 28   Removal of multi-component inflatable penile prosthesis with placement of new malleable device
2015, 3Q, 25   Placement of inflatable penile prosthesis

AHA Coding Clinic for table ØVX
2018, 4Q, 40   Transfer of prepuce

AHA Coding Clinic for table ØVY
2020, 4Q, 58   Male reproductive organ transplant

Male Reproductive System

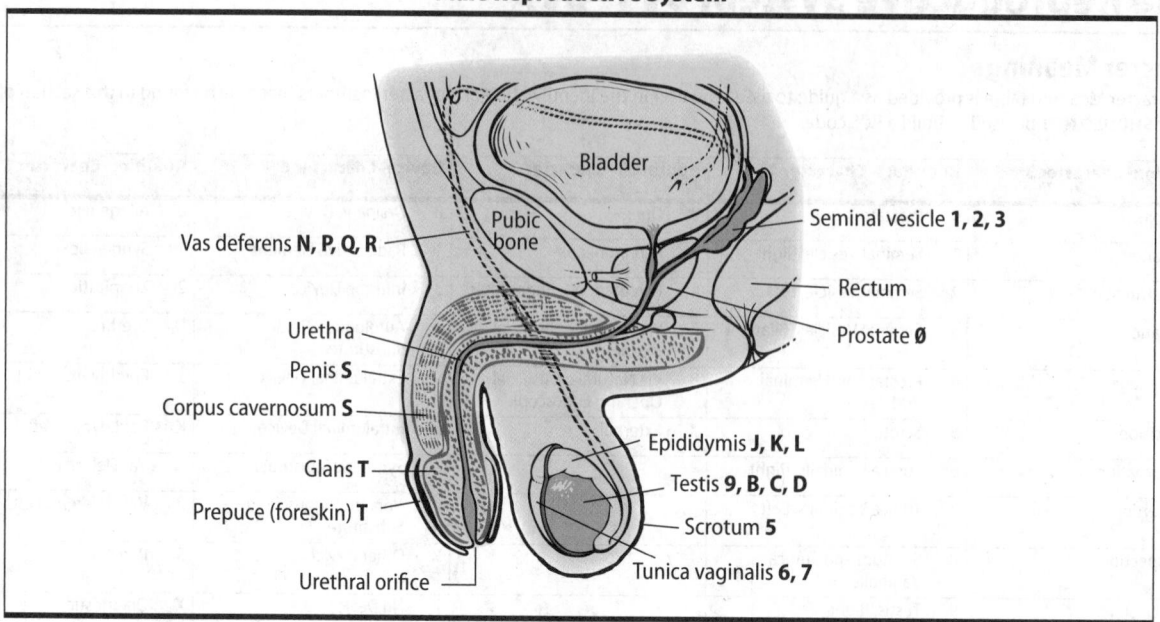

- Vas deferens **N, P, Q, R**
- Bladder
- Pubic bone
- Seminal vesicle **1, 2, 3**
- Rectum
- Prostate **Ø**
- Urethra
- Penis **S**
- Corpus cavernosum **S**
- Glans **T**
- Prepuce (foreskin) **T**
- Epididymis **J, K, L**
- Testis **9, B, C, D**
- Scrotum **5**
- Tunica vaginalis **6, 7**
- Urethral orifice

Penis

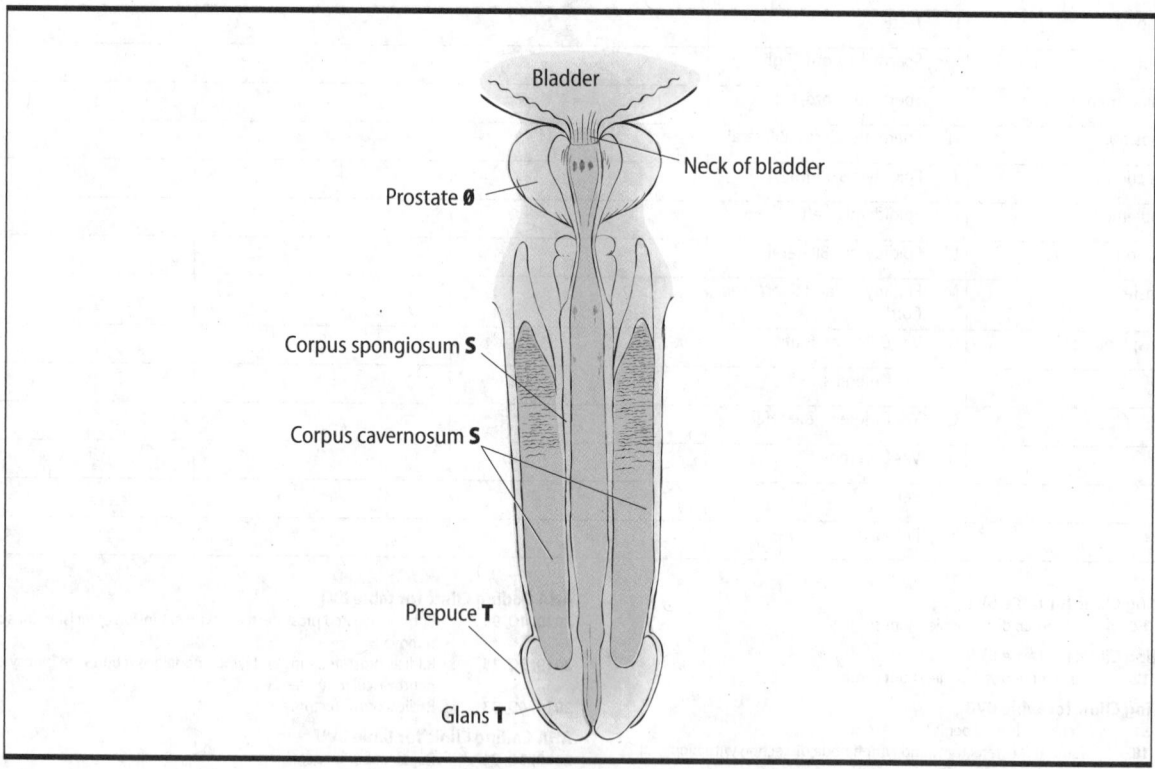

- Bladder
- Prostate **Ø**
- Neck of bladder
- Corpus spongiosum **S**
- Corpus cavernosum **S**
- Prepuce **T**
- Glans **T**

Male Reproductive System

Ø   **Medical and Surgical**
V   **Male Reproductive System**
1   **Bypass**   Definition: Altering the route of passage of the contents of a tubular body part
    Explanation: Rerouting contents of a body part to a downstream area of the normal route, to a similar route and body part, or to an abnormal route and dissimilar body part. Includes one or more anastomoses, with or without the use of a device.

Body Part Character 4	Approach Character 5	Device Character 6	Qualifier Character 7

N Vas Deferens, Right ♂
    Ductus deferens
    Ejaculatory duct
P Vas Deferens, Left ♂
    See N Vas Deferens, Right
Q Vas Deferens, Bilateral ♂
    See N Vas Deferens, Right
	Ø Open
	4 Percutaneous Endoscopic
		7 Autologous Tissue Substitute
		J Synthetic Substitute
		K Nonautologous Tissue Substitute
		Z No Device
			J Epididymis, Right
			K Epididymis, Left
			N Vas Deferens, Right
			P Vas Deferens, Left

♂   All body part, approach, device, and qualifier values

Ø   **Medical and Surgical**
V   **Male Reproductive System**
2   **Change**   Definition: Taking out or off a device from a body part and putting back an identical or similar device in or on the same body part without cutting or puncturing the skin or a mucous membrane
    Explanation: All CHANGE procedures are coded using the approach EXTERNAL

Body Part Character 4	Approach Character 5	Device Character 6	Qualifier Character 7

4 Prostate and Seminal Vesicles ♂
8 Scrotum and Tunica Vaginalis ♂
D Testis ♂
M Epididymis and Spermatic Cord ♂
R Vas Deferens ♂
    Ductus deferens
    Ejaculatory duct
S Penis ♂
    Corpus cavernosum
    Corpus spongiosum
	X External	Ø Drainage Device
		Y Other Device
			Z No Qualifier

Non-OR   All body part, approach, device, and qualifier values   ♂   All body part, approach, device, and qualifier values

Ø   **Medical and Surgical**
V   **Male Reproductive System**
5   **Destruction**   Definition: Physical eradication of all or a portion of a body part by the direct use of energy, force, or a destructive agent
    Explanation: None of the body part is physically taken out

Body Part Character 4	Approach Character 5	Device Character 6	Qualifier Character 7
Ø Prostate ♂	Ø Open 3 Percutaneous 4 Percutaneous Endoscopic 7 Via Natural or Artificial Opening 8 Via Natural or Artificial Opening Endoscopic	Z No Device	Z No Qualifier
1 Seminal Vesicle, Right ♂ 2 Seminal Vesicle, Left ♂ 3 Seminal Vesicles, Bilateral ♂ 6 Tunica Vaginalis, Right ♂ 7 Tunica Vaginalis, Left ♂ 9 Testis, Right ♂ B Testis, Left ♂ C Testes, Bilateral ♂	Ø Open 3 Percutaneous 4 Percutaneous Endoscopic	Z No Device	Z No Qualifier

5 Scrotum ♂
S Penis ♂
    Corpus cavernosum
    Corpus spongiosum
T Prepuce ♂
    Foreskin
    Glans penis
	Ø Open
	3 Percutaneous
	4 Percutaneous Endoscopic
	X External
		Z No Device	Z No Qualifier

F Spermatic Cord, Right ♂
G Spermatic Cord, Left ♂
H Spermatic Cords, Bilateral ♂
J Epididymis, Right ♂
K Epididymis, Left ♂
L Epididymis, Bilateral ♂
N Vas Deferens, Right [NC]♂
    Ductus deferens
    Ejaculatory duct
P Vas Deferens, Left [NC]♂
    See N Vas Deferens, Right
Q Vas Deferens, Bilateral [NC]♂
    See N Vas Deferens, Right
	Ø Open
	3 Percutaneous
	4 Percutaneous Endoscopic
	8 Via Natural or Artificial Opening Endoscopic
		Z No Device	Z No Qualifier

Non-OR   ØV55[Ø,3,4,X]ZZ
Non-OR   ØV5[N,P,Q][Ø,3,4,8]ZZ

[NC]   ØV5[N,P,Q][Ø,3,4]ZZ with principal or secondary diagnosis of Z3Ø.2
♂   All body part, approach, device, and qualifier values

[NC] Noncovered Procedure   [LC] Limited Coverage   [QA] Questionable OB Admit   [NT] New Tech Add-on   ⊞ Combination Member   ♂ Male   ♀ Female

Male Reproductive System

Ø   Medical and Surgical
V   Male Reproductive System
7   Dilation   Definition: Expanding an orifice or the lumen of a tubular body part

Explanation: The orifice can be a natural orifice or an artificially created orifice. Accomplished by stretching a tubular body part using intraluminal pressure or by cutting part of the orifice or wall of the tubular body part.

Body Part Character 4	Approach Character 5	Device Character 6	Qualifier Character 7

N   Vas Deferens, Right   ♂
     Ductus deferens
     Ejaculatory duct
P   Vas Deferens, Left   ♂
     See N Vas Deferens, Right
Q   Vas Deferens, Bilateral   ♂
     See N Vas Deferens, Right
	Ø Open
	3 Percutaneous
	4 Percutaneous Endoscopic
		D Intraluminal Device
		Z No Device
			Z No Qualifier

♂   All body part, approach, device, and qualifier values

Ø   Medical and Surgical
V   Male Reproductive System
9   Drainage   Definition: Taking or letting out fluids and/or gases from a body part

Explanation: The qualifier DIAGNOSTIC is used to identify drainage procedures that are biopsies

Body Part Character 4	Approach Character 5	Device Character 6	Qualifier Character 7
Ø Prostate ♂	Ø Open 3 Percutaneous 4 Percutaneous Endoscopic 7 Via Natural or Artificial Opening 8 Via Natural or Artificial Opening Endoscopic	Ø Drainage Device	Z No Qualifier
Ø Prostate ♂	Ø Open 3 Percutaneous 4 Percutaneous Endoscopic 7 Via Natural or Artificial Opening 8 Via Natural or Artificial Opening Endoscopic	Z No Device	X Diagnostic Z No Qualifier

1   Seminal Vesicle, Right   ♂
2   Seminal Vesicle, Left   ♂
3   Seminal Vesicles, Bilateral   ♂
6   Tunica Vaginalis, Right   ♂
7   Tunica Vaginalis, Left   ♂
9   Testis, Right   ♂
B   Testis, Left   ♂
C   Testes, Bilateral   ♂
F   Spermatic Cord, Right   ♂
G   Spermatic Cord, Left   ♂
H   Spermatic Cords, Bilateral   ♂
J   Epididymis, Right   ♂
K   Epididymis, Left   ♂
L   Epididymis, Bilateral   ♂
N   Vas Deferens, Right   ♂
     Ductus deferens
     Ejaculatory duct
P   Vas Deferens, Left   ♂
     See N Vas Deferens, Right
Q   Vas Deferens, Bilateral   ♂
     See N Vas Deferens, Right
	Ø Open
	3 Percutaneous
	4 Percutaneous Endoscopic
		Ø Drainage Device	Z No Qualifier

Non-OR	ØV9Ø[3,4]ØZ
Non-OR	ØV9Ø[3,4]Z[X,Z]
Non-OR	ØV9Ø[7,8]ZX
Non-OR	ØV9[1,2,3,9,B,C][3,4]ØZ

Non-OR	ØV9[6,7,F,G,H,N,P,Q][Ø,3,4]ØZ
Non-OR	ØV9[J,K,L]3ØZ
♂	All body part, approach, device, and qualifier values

ØV9 Continued on next page

Non-OR Procedure   DRG Non-OR Procedure   Valid OR Procedure   HAC Associated Procedure   Combination Only   New/Revised GREEN

ØV9 Continued

Ø   **Medical and Surgical**
V   **Male Reproductive System**
9   **Drainage**   Definition: Taking or letting out fluids and/or gases from a body part
               Explanation: The qualifier DIAGNOSTIC is used to identify drainage procedures that are biopsies

Body Part Character 4	Approach Character 5	Device Character 6	Qualifier Character 7

1   Seminal Vesicle, Right   ♂
2   Seminal Vesicle, Left   ♂
3   Seminal Vesicles, Bilateral   ♂
6   Tunica Vaginalis, Right   ♂
7   Tunica Vaginalis, Left   ♂
9   Testis, Right   ♂
B   Testis, Left   ♂
C   Testes, Bilateral   ♂
F   Spermatic Cord, Right   ♂
G   Spermatic Cord, Left   ♂
H   Spermatic Cords, Bilateral   ♂
J   Epididymis, Right   ♂
K   Epididymis, Left   ♂
L   Epididymis, Bilateral   ♂
N   Vas Deferens, Right   ♂
     Ductus deferens
     Ejaculatory duct
P   Vas Deferens, Left   ♂
     See N Vas Deferens, Right
Q   Vas Deferens, Bilateral   ♂
     See N Vas Deferens, Right
	Ø Open
	3 Percutaneous
	4 Percutaneous Endoscopic
		Z No Device	X Diagnostic
			Z No Qualifier

5   Scrotum   ♂
S   Penis   ♂
     Corpus cavernosum
     Corpus spongiosum
T   Prepuce   ♂
     Foreskin
     Glans penis
	Ø Open
	3 Percutaneous
	4 Percutaneous Endoscopic
	X External
		Ø Drainage Device	Z No Qualifier

5   Scrotum   ♂
S   Penis   ♂
     Corpus cavernosum
     Corpus spongiosum
T   Prepuce   ♂
     Foreskin
     Glans penis
	Ø Open
	3 Percutaneous
	4 Percutaneous Endoscopic
	X External
		Z No Device	X Diagnostic
			Z No Qualifier

Non-OR ØV9[1,2,3,9,B,C][3,4]Z[X,Z]		**Non-OR** ØV9[S,T]3ØZ	
Non-OR ØV9[6,7,F,G,H,J,K,L,N,P,Q][Ø,3,4]ZX		**Non-OR** ØV95ØZX	
Non-OR ØV9[6,7,F,G,H,N,P,Q][Ø,3,4]ZZ		**Non-OR** ØV95[3,4,X]Z[X,Z]	
Non-OR ØV9[J,K,L]3ZZ		**Non-OR** ØV9[S,T]3ZZ	
Non-OR ØV95[Ø,3,4,X]ØZ		♂ All body part, approach, device, and qualifier values	

NC Noncovered Procedure   LC Limited Coverage   QA Questionable OB Admit   NT New Tech Add-on   ⊞ Combination Member   ♂ Male   ♀ Female

ICD-10-PCS 2022   **661**

Ø   **Medical and Surgical**
V   **Male Reproductive System**
B   **Excision**   Definition: Cutting out or off, without replacement, a portion of a body part
                       Explanation: The qualifier DIAGNOSTIC is used to identify excision procedures that are biopsies

Body Part Character 4	Approach Character 5	Device Character 6	Qualifier Character 7
Ø Prostate ♂	**Ø** Open **3** Percutaneous **4** Percutaneous Endoscopic **7** Via Natural or Artificial Opening **8** Via Natural or Artificial Opening Endoscopic	**Z** No Device	**X** Diagnostic **Z** No Qualifier
1 Seminal Vesicle, Right ♂ **2** Seminal Vesicle, Left ♂ **3** Seminal Vesicles, Bilateral ♂ **6** Tunica Vaginalis, Right ♂ **7** Tunica Vaginalis, Left ♂ **9** Testis, Right ♂ **B** Testis, Left ♂ **C** Testes, Bilateral ♂	**Ø** Open **3** Percutaneous **4** Percutaneous Endoscopic	**Z** No Device	**X** Diagnostic **Z** No Qualifier

5 Scrotum   ♂
S Penis   ♂
    Corpus cavernosum
    Corpus spongiosum
T Prepuce   ♂
    Foreskin
    Glans penis
	Ø Open
	3 Percutaneous
	4 Percutaneous Endoscopic
	X External
		Z No Device	**X** Diagnostic
			Z No Qualifier

F Spermatic Cord, Right   ♂
G Spermatic Cord, Left   ♂
H Spermatic Cords, Bilateral   ♂
J Epididymis, Right   ♂
K Epididymis, Left   ♂
L Epididymis, Bilateral   ♂
N Vas Deferens, Right   NC ♂
    Ductus deferens
    Ejaculatory duct
P Vas Deferens, Left   NC ♂
    See N Vas Deferens, Right
Q Vas Deferens, Bilateral   NC ♂
    See N Vas Deferens, Right
	Ø Open
	3 Percutaneous
	4 Percutaneous Endoscopic
	8 Via Natural or Artificial Opening
	    Endoscopic
		Z No Device	**X** Diagnostic
			Z No Qualifier

Non-OR ØVBØ[3,4,7,8]ZX		**Non-OR** ØVB[F,G,H,J,K,L][Ø,3,4,8]ZX	
Non-OR ØVB[1,2,3,9,B,C][3,4]ZX		**Non-OR** ØVB[N,P,Q][Ø,3,4,8]Z[X,Z]	
Non-OR ØVB[6,7][Ø,3,4]ZX		**NC** ØVB[N,P,Q][Ø,3,4]ZZ with principal or secondary diagnosis of Z3Ø.2	
Non-OR ØVB5ØZX		♂ All body part, approach, device, and qualifier values	
Non-OR ØVB5[3,4,X]Z[X,Z]			

Ø Medical and Surgical
V Male Reproductive System
C Extirpation   Definition: Taking or cutting out solid matter from a body part

Explanation: The solid matter may be an abnormal byproduct of a biological function or a foreign body; it may be imbedded in a body part or in the lumen of a tubular body part. The solid matter may or may not have been previously broken into pieces.

Body Part Character 4	Approach Character 5	Device Character 6	Qualifier Character 7
Ø Prostate ♂	**Ø** Open **3** Percutaneous **4** Percutaneous Endoscopic **7** Via Natural or Artificial Opening **8** Via Natural or Artificial Opening Endoscopic	**Z** No Device	**Z** No Qualifier

1 Seminal Vesicle, Right ♂
2 Seminal Vesicle, Left ♂
3 Seminal Vesicles, Bilateral ♂
6 Tunica Vaginalis, Right ♂
7 Tunica Vaginalis, Left ♂
9 Testis, Right ♂
B Testis, Left ♂
C Testes, Bilateral ♂
F Spermatic Cord, Right ♂
G Spermatic Cord, Left ♂
H Spermatic Cords, Bilateral ♂
J Epididymis, Right ♂
K Epididymis, Left ♂
L Epididymis, Bilateral ♂
N Vas Deferens, Right ♂
   Ductus deferens
   Ejaculatory duct
P Vas Deferens, Left ♂
   See N Vas Deferens, Right
Q Vas Deferens, Bilateral ♂
   See N Vas Deferens, Right
	Ø Open
	3 Percutaneous
	4 Percutaneous Endoscopic
		Z No Device	**Z** No Qualifier

5 Scrotum ♂
S Penis ♂
   Corpus cavernosum
   Corpus spongiosum
T Prepuce ♂
   Foreskin
   Glans penis
	Ø Open
	3 Percutaneous
	4 Percutaneous Endoscopic
	X External
		Z No Device	**Z** No Qualifier

Non-OR ØVC[6,7,N,P,Q][Ø,3,4]ZZ
Non-OR ØVC5[3,4,X]ZZ

Non-OR ØVCSXZZ
♂   All body part, approach, device, and qualifier values

Ø Medical and Surgical
V Male Reproductive System
H Insertion Definition: Putting in a nonbiological appliance that monitors, assists, performs, or prevents a physiological function but does not physically take the place of a body part
Explanation: None

Body Part Character 4	Approach Character 5	Device Character 6	Qualifier Character 7
Ø Prostate ♂	Ø Open 3 Percutaneous 4 Percutaneous Endoscopic 7 Via Natural or Artificial Opening 8 Via Natural or Artificial Opening Endoscopic	1 Radioactive Element	Z No Qualifier

4 Prostate and Seminal Vesicles ♂
8 Scrotum and Tunica Vaginalis ♂
M Epididymis and Spermatic Cord ♂
R Vas Deferens ♂
  Ductus deferens
  Ejaculatory duct
	Ø Open
	3 Percutaneous
	4 Percutaneous Endoscopic
	7 Via Natural or Artificial Opening
	8 Via Natural or Artificial Opening Endoscopic
		3 Infusion Device
		Y Other Device
			Z No Qualifier

D Testis ♂	Ø Open 3 Percutaneous 4 Percutaneous Endoscopic 7 Via Natural or Artificial Opening 8 Via Natural or Artificial Opening Endoscopic	1 Radioactive Element 3 Infusion Device Y Other Device	Z No Qualifier

S Penis ♂
  Corpus cavernosum
  Corpus spongiosum
	Ø Open
	3 Percutaneous
	4 Percutaneous Endoscopic
		3 Infusion Device
		Y Other Device
			Z No Qualifier

S Penis ♂
  Corpus cavernosum
  Corpus spongiosum
	7 Via Natural or Artificial Opening
	8 Via Natural or Artificial Opening Endoscopic
		Y Other Device	Z No Qualifier

S Penis ♂
  Corpus cavernosum
  Corpus spongiosum
	X External	3 Infusion Device	Z No Qualifier

Non-OR ØVH[4,8,M,R][Ø,3,4,7,8][3,Y]Z
Non-OR ØVHD[Ø,3,4,7,8][1,3,Y]Z
Non-OR ØVHS[Ø,3,4][3,Y]Z
Non-OR ØVHS[7,8]YZ
Non-OR ØVHSX3Z
♂ All body part, approach, device, and qualifier values

Ø Medical and Surgical
V Male Reproductive System
J Inspection Definition: Visually and/or manually exploring a body part
Explanation: Visual exploration may be performed with or without optical instrumentation. Manual exploration may be performed directly or through intervening body layers.

Body Part Character 4	Approach Character 5	Device Character 6	Qualifier Character 7

4 Prostate and Seminal Vesicles ♂
8 Scrotum and Tunica Vaginalis ♂
D Testis ♂
M Epididymis and Spermatic Cord ♂
R Vas Deferens ♂
  Ductus deferens
  Ejaculatory duct
S Penis ♂
  Corpus cavernosum
  Corpus spongiosum
	Ø Open
	3 Percutaneous
	4 Percutaneous Endoscopic
	X External
		Z No Device	Z No Qualifier

Non-OR ØVJ[4,D,M,R][3,X]ZZ
Non-OR ØVJ8[Ø,3,4,X]ZZ
Non-OR ØVJS[3,4,X]ZZ
♂ All body part, approach, device, and qualifier values

Ø   **Medical and Surgical**
V   **Male Reproductive System**
L   **Occlusion**   Definition: Completely closing an orifice or the lumen of a tubular body part
                 Explanation: The orifice can be a natural orifice or an artificially created orifice

Body Part Character 4	Approach Character 5	Device Character 6	Qualifier Character 7

F   Spermatic Cord, Right   NC ♂
G   Spermatic Cord, Left   NC ♂
H   Spermatic Cords, Bilateral   NC ♂
N   Vas Deferens, Right   NC ♂
      Ductus deferens
      Ejaculatory duct
P   Vas Deferens, Left   NC ♂
      See N Vas Deferens, Right
Q   Vas Deferens, Bilateral   NC ♂
      See N Vas Deferens, Right
	Ø Open
	3 Percutaneous
	4 Percutaneous Endoscopic
	8 Via Natural or Artificial Opening
	      Endoscopic
		C Extraluminal Device
		D Intraluminal Device
		Z No Device
			Z No Qualifier

Non-OR ØVL[F,G,H][Ø,3,4,8][C,D,Z]Z Non-OR ØVL[N,P,Q][Ø,3,4,8][C,Z]Z	NC NC ♂	ØVL[F,G,H][Ø,3,4][C,D,Z]Z with principal or secondary diagnosis of Z3Ø.2 ØVL[N,P,Q][Ø,3,4][C,Z]Z with principal or secondary diagnosis of Z3Ø.2 All body part, approach, device, and qualifier values

Ø   **Medical and Surgical**
V   **Male Reproductive System**
M   **Reattachment**   Definition: Putting back in or on all or a portion of a separated body part to its normal location or other suitable location
                   Explanation: Vascular circulation and nervous pathways may or may not be reestablished

Body Part Character 4	Approach Character 5	Device Character 6	Qualifier Character 7

5   Scrotum   ♂
S   Penis   ♂
      Corpus cavernosum
      Corpus spongiosum
	X External	**Z** No Device	**Z** No Qualifier

6 Tunica Vaginalis, Right ♂ **7** Tunica Vaginalis, Left ♂ **9** Testis, Right ♂ **B** Testis, Left ♂ **C** Testes, Bilateral ♂ **F** Spermatic Cord, Right ♂ **G** Spermatic Cord, Left ♂ **H** Spermatic Cords, Bilateral ♂	**Ø** Open **4** Percutaneous Endoscopic	**Z** No Device	**Z** No Qualifier

♂	All body part, approach, device, and qualifier values

NC Noncovered Procedure   LC Limited Coverage   OA Questionable OB Admit   NT New Tech Add-on   ⊞ Combination Member   ♂ Male   ♀ Female

ICD-10-PCS 2022   **665**

Ø   Medical and Surgical
V   Male Reproductive System
N   Release   Definition: Freeing a body part from an abnormal physical constraint by cutting or by the use of force
                          Explanation: Some of the restraining tissue may be taken out but none of the body part is taken out

Body Part Character 4		Approach Character 5	Device Character 6	Qualifier Character 7
Ø Prostate	♂	Ø Open 3 Percutaneous 4 Percutaneous Endoscopic 7 Via Natural or Artificial Opening 8 Via Natural or Artificial Opening Endoscopic	Z No Device	Z No Qualifier
1 Seminal Vesicle, Right 2 Seminal Vesicle, Left 3 Seminal Vesicles, Bilateral 6 Tunica Vaginalis, Right 7 Tunica Vaginalis, Left 9 Testis, Right B Testis, Left C Testes, Bilateral	♂ ♂ ♂ ♂ ♂ ♂ ♂ ♂	Ø Open 3 Percutaneous 4 Percutaneous Endoscopic	Z No Device	Z No Qualifier

5 Scrotum
S Penis
  Corpus cavernosum
  Corpus spongiosum
T Prepuce
  Foreskin
  Glans penis
	♂
	♂
	
	♂
		Ø Open
		3 Percutaneous
		4 Percutaneous Endoscopic
		X External
			Z No Device	Z No Qualifier

F Spermatic Cord, Right
G Spermatic Cord, Left
H Spermatic Cords, Bilateral
J Epididymis, Right
K Epididymis, Left
L Epididymis, Bilateral
N Vas Deferens, Right
  Ductus deferens
  Ejaculatory duct
P Vas Deferens, Left
  See N Vas Deferens, Right
Q Vas Deferens, Bilateral
  See N Vas Deferens, Right
	♂
	♂
	♂
	♂
	♂
	♂
	♂
	
	♂
	
	♂
		Ø Open
		3 Percutaneous
		4 Percutaneous Endoscopic
		8 Via Natural or Artificial Opening Endoscopic
			Z No Device	Z No Qualifier

Non-OR   ØVN[9,B,C][Ø,3,4]ZZ   ♂   All body part, approach, device, and qualifier values
Non-OR   ØVNT[Ø,3,4,X]ZZ

Ø   Medical and Surgical
V   Male Reproductive System
P   Removal   Definition: Taking out or off a device from a body part

Explanation: If a device is taken out and a similar device put in without cutting or puncturing the skin or mucous membrane, the procedure is coded to the root operation CHANGE. Otherwise, the procedure for taking out the device is coded to the root operation REMOVAL.

Body Part Character 4		Approach Character 5	Device Character 6	Qualifier Character 7
4 Prostate and Seminal Vesicles ♂		Ø Open 3 Percutaneous 4 Percutaneous Endoscopic 7 Via Natural or Artificial Opening 8 Via Natural or Artificial Opening Endoscopic	Ø Drainage Device 1 Radioactive Element 3 Infusion Device 7 Autologous Tissue Substitute J Synthetic Substitute K Nonautologous Tissue Substitute Y Other Device	Z No Qualifier
4 Prostate and Seminal Vesicles ♂	X	External	Ø Drainage Device 1 Radioactive Element 3 Infusion Device	Z No Qualifier

8   Scrotum and Tunica Vaginalis   ♂
D   Testis   ♂
S   Penis   ♂
    Corpus cavernosum
    Corpus spongiosum
		Ø Open
		3 Percutaneous
		4 Percutaneous Endoscopic
		7 Via Natural or Artificial Opening
		8 Via Natural or Artificial Opening
		    Endoscopic
			Ø Drainage Device
			3 Infusion Device
			7 Autologous Tissue Substitute
			J Synthetic Substitute
			K Nonautologous Tissue Substitute
			Y Other Device
				Z No Qualifier

8   Scrotum and Tunica Vaginalis   ♂
D   Testis   ♂
S   Penis   ♂
    Corpus cavernosum
    Corpus spongiosum
	X	External	Ø Drainage Device
			3 Infusion Device
				Z No Qualifier

M Epididymis and Spermatic Cord ♂		Ø Open 3 Percutaneous 4 Percutaneous Endoscopic 7 Via Natural or Artificial Opening 8 Via Natural or Artificial Opening Endoscopic	Ø Drainage Device 3 Infusion Device 7 Autologous Tissue Substitute C Extraluminal Device J Synthetic Substitute K Nonautologous Tissue Substitute Y Other Device	Z No Qualifier
M Epididymis and Spermatic Cord ♂	X	External	Ø Drainage Device 3 Infusion Device	Z No Qualifier

R   Vas Deferens   ♂
    Ductus deferens
    Ejaculatory duct
		Ø Open
		3 Percutaneous
		4 Percutaneous Endoscopic
		7 Via Natural or Artificial Opening
		8 Via Natural or Artificial Opening
		    Endoscopic
			Ø Drainage Device
			3 Infusion Device
			7 Autologous Tissue Substitute
			C Extraluminal Device
			D Intraluminal Device
			J Synthetic Substitute
			K Nonautologous Tissue Substitute
			Y Other Device
				Z No Qualifier

R   Vas Deferens   ♂
    Ductus deferens
    Ejaculatory duct
	X	External	Ø Drainage Device
			3 Infusion Device
			D Intraluminal Device
				Z No Qualifier

Non-OR	ØVP4[3,4]YZ		**Non-OR**	ØVPM[3,4]YZ
Non-OR	ØVP4[7,8][Ø,3,Y]Z		**Non-OR**	ØVPM[7,8][Ø,3,Y]Z
Non-OR	ØVP4X[Ø,1,3]Z		**Non-OR**	ØVPMX[Ø,3]Z
Non-OR	ØVP8[Ø,3,4,7,8][Ø,3,7,J,K,Y]Z		**Non-OR**	ØVPR[Ø,3,4][Ø,3,7,C,J,K,Y]Z
Non-OR	ØVP[D,S][3,4]YZ		**Non-OR**	ØVPR[7,8][Ø,3,7,C,D,J,K,Y]Z
Non-OR	ØVP[D,S][7,8][Ø,3,Y]Z		**Non-OR**	ØVPRX[Ø,3,D]Z
Non-OR	ØVP[8,D,S]X[Ø,3]Z		♂	All body part, approach, device, and qualifier values

NC Noncovered Procedure   LC Limited Coverage   QA Questionable OB Admit   NT New Tech Add-on   ⊞ Combination Member   ♂ Male   ♀ Female

ICD-10-PCS 2022   667

ØVP–ØVP

Male Reproductive System

Ø Medical and Surgical
V Male Reproductive System
Q Repair Definition: Restoring, to the extent possible, a body part to its normal anatomic structure and function

Explanation: Used only when the method to accomplish the repair is not one of the other root operations

Body Part Character 4		Approach Character 5	Device Character 6	Qualifier Character 7
Ø Prostate	♂	Ø Open 3 Percutaneous 4 Percutaneous Endoscopic 7 Via Natural or Artificial Opening 8 Via Natural or Artificial Opening Endoscopic	Z No Device	Z No Qualifier
1 Seminal Vesicle, Right 2 Seminal Vesicle, Left 3 Seminal Vesicles, Bilateral 6 Tunica Vaginalis, Right 7 Tunica Vaginalis, Left 9 Testis, Right B Testis, Left C Testes, Bilateral	♂ ♂ ♂ ♂ ♂ ♂ ♂ ♂	Ø Open 3 Percutaneous 4 Percutaneous Endoscopic	Z No Device	Z No Qualifier

5 Scrotum
S Penis
  Corpus cavernosum
  Corpus spongiosum
T Prepuce
  Foreskin
  Glans penis
	♂
	♂
	
	♂
		Ø Open
		3 Percutaneous
		4 Percutaneous Endoscopic
		X External
			Z No Device	Z No Qualifier

F Spermatic Cord, Right
G Spermatic Cord, Left
H Spermatic Cords, Bilateral
J Epididymis, Right
K Epididymis, Left
L Epididymis, Bilateral
N Vas Deferens, Right
  Ductus deferens
  Ejaculatory duct
P Vas Deferens, Left
  See N Vas Deferens, Right
Q Vas Deferens, Bilateral
  See N Vas Deferens, Right
	♂
	♂
	♂
	♂
	♂
	♂
	♂
	
	♂
	
	♂
		Ø Open
		3 Percutaneous
		4 Percutaneous Endoscopic
		8 Via Natural or Artificial Opening Endoscopic
			Z No Device	Z No Qualifier

Non-OR	ØVQ[6,7][Ø,3,4]ZZ	♂	All body part, approach, device, and qualifier values	
Non-OR	ØVQ5[Ø,3,4,X]ZZ			

Ø Medical and Surgical
V Male Reproductive System
R Replacement Definition: Putting in or on biological or synthetic material that physically takes the place and/or function of all or a portion of a body part

Explanation: The body part may have been taken out or replaced, or may be taken out, physically eradicated, or rendered nonfunctional during the REPLACEMENT procedure. A REMOVAL procedure is coded for taking out the device used in a previous replacement procedure.

Body Part Character 4		Approach Character 5	Device Character 6	Qualifier Character 7
9 Testis, Right B Testis, Left C Testes, Bilateral	♂ ♂ ♂	Ø Open	J Synthetic Substitute	Z No Qualifier

♂	All body part, approach, device, and qualifier values	

Ø Medical and Surgical
V Male Reproductive System
S Reposition Definition: Moving to its normal location, or other suitable location, all or a portion of a body part

Explanation: The body part is moved to a new location from an abnormal location, or from a normal location where it is not functioning correctly. The body part may or may not be cut out or off to be moved to the new location.

Body Part Character 4		Approach Character 5	Device Character 6	Qualifier Character 7
9 Testis, Right B Testis, Left C Testes, Bilateral F Spermatic Cord, Right G Spermatic Cord, Left H Spermatic Cords, Bilateral	♂ ♂ ♂ ♂ ♂ ♂	Ø Open 3 Percutaneous 4 Percutaneous Endoscopic 8 Via Natural or Artificial Opening Endoscopic	Z No Device	Z No Qualifier

♂	All body part, approach, device, and qualifier values	

Ø   Medical and Surgical
V   Male Reproductive System
T   Resection   Definition: Cutting out or off, without replacement, all of a body part
                Explanation: None

Body Part Character 4	Approach Character 5	Device Character 6	Qualifier Character 7
Ø Prostate ⊞♂	Ø Open 4 Percutaneous Endoscopic 7 Via Natural or Artificial Opening 8 Via Natural or Artificial Opening Endoscopic	Z No Device	Z No Qualifier

1 Seminal Vesicle, Right ♂
2 Seminal Vesicle, Left ♂
3 Seminal Vesicles, Bilateral ⊞♂
6 Tunica Vaginalis, Right ♂
7 Tunica Vaginalis, Left ♂
9 Testis, Right ♂
B Testis, Left ♂
C Testes, Bilateral ♂
F Spermatic Cord, Right ♂
G Spermatic Cord, Left ♂
H Spermatic Cords, Bilateral ♂
J Epididymis, Right ♂
K Epididymis, Left ♂
L Epididymis, Bilateral ♂
N Vas Deferens, Right NC♂
     Ductus deferens
     Ejaculatory duct
P Vas Deferens, Left NC♂
     See N Vas Deferens, Right
Q Vas Deferens, Bilateral NC♂
     See N Vas Deferens, Right
	Ø Open
	4 Percutaneous Endoscopic
		Z No Device	Z No Qualifier

5 Scrotum ♂
S Penis ♂
     Corpus cavernosum
     Corpus spongiosum
T Prepuce ♂
     Foreskin
     Glans penis
	Ø Open
	4 Percutaneous Endoscopic
	X External
		Z No Device	Z No Qualifier

Non-OR ØVT[N,P,Q][Ø,4]ZZ		
Non-OR ØVT[5,T][Ø,4,X]ZZ	**See Appendix L for Procedure Combinations**	
NC ØVT[N,P,Q][Ø,4]ZZ with principal or secondary diagnosis of Z3Ø.2	⊞ ØVTØ[Ø,4,7,8]ZZ	
♂ All body part, approach, device, and qualifier values	⊞ ØVT3[Ø,4]ZZ	

NC Noncovered Procedure   **LC** Limited Coverage   **QA** Questionable OB Admit   **NT** New Tech Add-on   ⊞ Combination Member   ♂ Male   ♀ Female

ICD-10-PCS 2022   669

Ø Medical and Surgical
V Male Reproductive System
U Supplement　　Definition: Putting in or on biological or synthetic material that physically reinforces and/or augments the function of a portion of a body part
　　　　　　　　Explanation: The biological material is non-living, or is living and from the same individual. The body part may have been previously replaced, and the SUPPLEMENT procedure is performed to physically reinforce and/or augment the function of the replaced body part.

Body Part Character 4	Approach Character 5	Device Character 6	Qualifier Character 7
1 Seminal Vesicle, Right ♂ 2 Seminal Vesicle, Left ♂ 3 Seminal Vesicles, Bilateral ♂ 6 Tunica Vaginalis, Right ♂ 7 Tunica Vaginalis, Left ♂ F Spermatic Cord, Right ♂ G Spermatic Cord, Left ♂ H Spermatic Cords, Bilateral ♂ J Epididymis, Right ♂ K Epididymis, Left ♂ L Epididymis, Bilateral ♂ N Vas Deferens, Right ♂ 　Ductus deferens 　Ejaculatory duct P Vas Deferens, Left ♂ 　*See N Vas Deferens, Right* Q Vas Deferens, Bilateral ♂ 　*See N Vas Deferens, Right*	Ø Open 4 Percutaneous Endoscopic 8 Via Natural or Artificial Opening Endoscopic	7 Autologous Tissue Substitute J Synthetic Substitute K Nonautologous Tissue Substitute	Z No Qualifier
5 Scrotum ♂ S Penis ♂ 　Corpus cavernosum 　Corpus spongiosum T Prepuce ♂ 　Foreskin 　Glans penis	Ø Open 4 Percutaneous Endoscopic X External	7 Autologous Tissue Substitute J Synthetic Substitute K Nonautologous Tissue Substitute	Z No Qualifier
9 Testis, Right ♂ B Testis, Left ♂ C Testes, Bilateral ♂	Ø Open	7 Autologous Tissue Substitute J Synthetic Substitute K Nonautologous Tissue Substitute	Z No Qualifier

Non-OR　ØVUSX[7,J,K]Z　　　　　　　♂　　All body part, approach, device, and qualifier values

Ø Medical and Surgical
V Male Reproductive System
W Revision   Definition: Correcting, to the extent possible, a portion of a malfunctioning device or the position of a displaced device

Explanation: Revision can include correcting a malfunctioning or displaced device by taking out or putting in components of the device such as a screw or pin

Body Part Character 4	Approach Character 5	Device Character 6	Qualifier Character 7

4 Prostate and Seminal Vesicles ♂
8 Scrotum and Tunica Vaginalis ♂
D Testis ♂
S Penis ♂
    Corpus cavernosum
    Corpus spongiosum
	Ø Open
	3 Percutaneous
	4 Percutaneous Endoscopic
	7 Via Natural or Artificial Opening
	8 Via Natural or Artificial Opening
	    Endoscopic
		Ø Drainage Device
		3 Infusion Device
		7 Autologous Tissue Substitute
		J Synthetic Substitute
		K Nonautologous Tissue Substitute
		Y Other Device
			Z No Qualifier

4 Prostate and Seminal Vesicles ♂
8 Scrotum and Tunica Vaginalis ♂
D Testis ♂
S Penis ♂
    Corpus cavernosum
    Corpus spongiosum
	X External	**Ø** Drainage Device
		3 Infusion Device
		7 Autologous Tissue Substitute
		J Synthetic Substitute
		K Nonautologous Tissue Substitute
			Z No Qualifier

M Epididymis and Spermatic Cord ♂	**Ø** Open **3** Percutaneous **4** Percutaneous Endoscopic **7** Via Natural or Artificial Opening **8** Via Natural or Artificial Opening Endoscopic	**Ø** Drainage Device **3** Infusion Device **7** Autologous Tissue Substitute **C** Extraluminal Device **J** Synthetic Substitute **K** Nonautologous Tissue Substitute **Y** Other Device	**Z** No Qualifier
M Epididymis and Spermatic Cord ♂	**X** External	**Ø** Drainage Device **3** Infusion Device **7** Autologous Tissue Substitute **C** Extraluminal Device **J** Synthetic Substitute **K** Nonautologous Tissue Substitute	**Z** No Qualifier

R Vas Deferens ♂
    Ductus deferens
    Ejaculatory duct
	Ø Open
	3 Percutaneous
	4 Percutaneous Endoscopic
	7 Via Natural or Artificial Opening
	8 Via Natural or Artificial Opening
	    Endoscopic
		Ø Drainage Device
		3 Infusion Device
		7 Autologous Tissue Substitute
		C Extraluminal Device
		D Intraluminal Device
		J Synthetic Substitute
		K Nonautologous Tissue Substitute
		Y Other Device
			Z No Qualifier

R Vas Deferens ♂
    Ductus deferens
    Ejaculatory duct
	X External	**Ø** Drainage Device
		3 Infusion Device
		7 Autologous Tissue Substitute
		C Extraluminal Device
		D Intraluminal Device
		J Synthetic Substitute
		K Nonautologous Tissue Substitute
			Z No Qualifier

Non-OR	ØVW[4,D,S][3,4,7,8]YZ	Non-OR	ØVWMX[Ø,3,7,C,J,K]Z
Non-OR	ØVW8[Ø,3,4,7,8][Ø,3,7,J,K,Y]Z	Non-OR	ØVWR[Ø,3,4,7,8][Ø,3,7,C,D,J,K,Y]Z
Non-OR	ØVW[4,8,D,S]X[Ø,3,7,J,K]Z	Non-OR	ØVWRX[Ø,3,7,C,D,J,K]Z
Non-OR	ØVWM[3,4,7,8]YZ	♂	All body part, approach, device, and qualifier values

Ø Medical and Surgical
V Male Reproductive System
X Transfer   Definition: Moving, without taking out, all or a portion of a body part to another location to take over the function of all or a portion of a body part

Explanation: The body part transferred remains connected to its vascular and nervous supply

Body Part Character 4	Approach Character 5	Device Character 6	Qualifier Character 7

T Prepuce
    Foreskin
    Glans penis
	Ø Open
	X External
		Z No Device	**D** Urethra
			S Penis

NC Noncovered Procedure   **LC** Limited Coverage   **QA** Questionable OB Admit   **NT** New Tech Add-on   ✚ Combination Member   ♂ Male   ♀ Female

ICD-10-PCS 2022   671

Ø **Medical and Surgical**
V **Male Reproductive System**
Y **Transplantation** Definition: Putting in or on all or a portion of a living body part taken from another individual or animal to physically take the place and/or function of all or a portion of a similar body part
　　　　Explanation: The native body part may or may not be taken out, and the transplanted body part may take over all or a portion of its function

Body Part Character 4	Approach Character 5	Device Character 6	Qualifier Character 7
5　Scrotum　♂ S　Penis　♂ 　　Corpus cavernosum 　　Corpus spongiosum	Ø　Open	Z　No Device	Ø　Allogeneic 1　Syngeneic 2　Zooplastic

♂　　All body part, approach, device, and qualifier values

Anatomical Regions, General ØWØ–ØWY

Character Meanings

This Character Meaning table is provided as a guide to assist the user in the identification of character members that may be found in this section of code tables. It **SHOULD NOT** be used to build a PCS code.

Operation–Character 3		Body Region–Character 4		Approach–Character 5		Device–Character 6		Qualifier–Character 7	
Ø	Alteration	Ø	Head	Ø	Open	Ø	Drainage Device	Ø	Vagina OR Allogeneic
1	Bypass	1	Cranial Cavity	3	Percutaneous	1	Radioactive Element	1	Penis OR Syngeneic
2	Change	2	Face	4	Percutaneous Endoscopic	3	Infusion Device	2	Stoma
3	Control	3	Oral Cavity and Throat	7	Via Natural or Artificial Opening	7	Autologous Tissue Substitute	4	Cutaneous
4	Creation	4	Upper Jaw	8	Via Natural or Artificial Opening Endoscopic	J	Synthetic Substitute	6	Bladder
8	Division	5	Lower Jaw	X	External	K	Nonautologous Tissue Substitute	9	Pleural Cavity, Right
9	Drainage	6	Neck			Y	Other Device	B	Pleural Cavity, Left
B	Excision	8	Chest Wall			Z	No Device	G	Peritoneal Cavity
C	Extirpation	9	Pleural Cavity, Right					J	Pelvic Cavity
F	Fragmentation	B	Pleural Cavity, Left					W	Upper Vein
H	Insertion	C	Mediastinum					X	Diagnostic
J	Inspection	D	Pericardial Cavity					Y	Lower Vein
M	Reattachment	F	Abdominal Wall					Z	No Qualifier
P	Removal	G	Peritoneal Cavity						
Q	Repair	H	Retroperitoneum						
U	Supplement	J	Pelvic Cavity						
W	Revision	K	Upper Back						
Y	Transplantation	L	Lower Back						
		M	Perineum, Male						
		N	Perineum, Female						
		P	Gastrointestinal Tract						
		Q	Respiratory Tract						
		R	Genitourinary Tract						

AHA Coding Clinic for table ØWØ
2015, 1Q, 31   Bilateral browpexy

AHA Coding Clinic for table ØW1
2020, 4Q, 55   Insertion of subcutaneous pump system for ascites drainage
2018, 4Q, 41-42   Anatomical regions bypass qualifiers
2015, 2Q, 36   Insertion of infusion device into peritoneal cavity
2013, 4Q, 126-127 Creation of percutaneous cutaneoperitoneal fistula

AHA Coding Clinic for table ØW3
2019, 3Q, 4   Evacuation of subdural hematoma and control of bleeding artery
2018, 4Q, 38   Control of epistaxis
2018, 1Q, 19   Argon plasma coagulation of duodenal arteriovenous malformation
2018, 1Q, 19   Control of epistaxis via silver nitrate cauterization
2017, 4Q, 57-58   Added approach values - Transorifice esophageal vein banding
2017, 4Q, 105   Control of gastrointestinal bleeding
2017, 4Q, 106   Control of bleeding of external naris using suture
2017, 4Q, 106   Nasal packing for epistaxis
2016, 4Q, 99-100 Root operation Control
2014, 4Q, 44   Bakri balloon for control of postpartum hemorrhage
2013, 3Q, 23   Control of intraoperative bleeding

AHA Coding Clinic for table ØW4
2019, 4Q, 30   Transfer large intestine to vagina
2016, 4Q, 101   Root operation Creation

AHA Coding Clinic for table ØW9
2020, 4Q, 56   Transvaginal drainage of pelvis
2017, 3Q, 12   Therapeutic and diagnostic paracentesis
2017, 2Q, 16   Incision and drainage of floor of mouth

AHA Coding Clinic for table ØWB
2019, 1Q, 27   Excision of pelvic sidewall mass
2017, 2Q, 16   Excision of floor of mouth
2016, 1Q, 21   Excision of urachal mass
2013, 4Q, 119   Excision of inclusion cyst of perineum

AHA Coding Clinic for table ØWC
2019, 4Q, 35   Extirpation of jaw
2017, 2Q, 16   Excision of floor of mouth

AHA Coding Clinic for table ØWH
2021, 2Q, 14   Peritoneal dialysis catheter placement
2019, 4Q, 43   Unidirectional source brachytherapy
2018, 1Q, 25   Intrauterine brachytherapy & placement of tandems & ovoids
2017, 4Q, 104   Intrauterine brachytherapy & placement of tandems & ovoids
2016, 2Q, 14   Insertion of peritoneal totally implantable venous access device
2015, 2Q, 36   Insertion of infusion device into peritoneal cavity

AHA Coding Clinic for table ØWJ
2021, 2Q, 19   Electromagnetic stealth guided ventriculoperitoneal shunt insertion with endoscopy
2019, 1Q, 3-8   Whipple procedure
2019, 1Q, 25   Laparoscopic appendectomy converted to open procedure
2018, 3Q, 29   Decommissioning of left ventricular assist device with exploration of mediastinum
2016, 4Q, 58   Longitudinal vaginal septum
2013, 2Q, 36   Insertion of ventriculoperitoneal shunt with laparoscopic assistance

AHA Coding Clinic for table ØWP
2021, 2Q, 14   Removal of peritoneal dialysis catheter

AHA Coding Clinic for table ØWQ
2017, 4Q, 106   Control of bleeding of external naris using suture
2017, 3Q, 8   Removal of silo and closure of gastroschisis
2016, 3Q, 3-7   Stoma creation & takedown procedures
2014, 4Q, 38   Abdominoplasty and abdominal wall plication for hernia repair
2014, 3Q, 28   Ileostomy takedown and parastomal hernia repair

AHA Coding Clinic for table ØWU
2017, 3Q, 8   First stage of gastroschisis repair with silo placement
2016, 3Q, 40   Omentoplasty
2015, 2Q, 29   Placement of Ioban™ antimicrobial drape over surgical wound
2014, 4Q, 39   Abdominal component release with placement of mesh for hernia repair
2012, 4Q, 101   Rib resection with reconstruction of anterior chest wall

AHA Coding Clinic for table ØWW
2015, 2Q, 9   Revision of ventriculoperitoneal (VP) shunt

AHA Coding Clinic for table ØWY
2016, 4Q, 112-113 Transplantation

Ø   **Medical and Surgical**
W   **Anatomical Regions, General**
Ø   **Alteration**   Definition: Modifying the anatomic structure of a body part without affecting the function of the body part

                 Explanation: Principal purpose is to improve appearance

Body Part Character 4	Approach Character 5	Device Character 6	Qualifier Character 7

Ø Head
2 Face
4 Upper Jaw
5 Lower Jaw
6 Neck
    Parapharyngeal space
    Retropharyngeal space
8 Chest Wall
F Abdominal Wall
K Upper Back
L Lower Back
M Perineum, Male   ♂
N Perineum, Female   ♀
	Ø Open
	3 Percutaneous
	4 Percutaneous Endoscopic
		7 Autologous Tissue Substitute
		J Synthetic Substitute
		K Nonautologous Tissue Substitute
		Z No Device
			Z No Qualifier

♂   ØWØM[Ø,3,4][7,J,K,Z]Z
♀   ØWØN[Ø,3,4][7,J,K,Z]Z

Ø   **Medical and Surgical**
W   **Anatomical Regions, General**
1   **Bypass**   Definition: Altering the route of passage of the contents of a tubular body part

                 Explanation: Rerouting contents of a body part to a downstream area of the normal route, to a similar route and body part, or to an abnormal route and dissimilar body part. Includes one or more anastomoses, with or without the use of a device.

Body Part Character 4	Approach Character 5	Device Character 6	Qualifier Character 7
1 Cranial Cavity	Ø Open	J Synthetic Substitute	9 Pleural Cavity, Right B Pleural Cavity, Left G Peritoneal Cavity J Pelvic Cavity
9 Pleural Cavity, Right B Pleural Cavity, Left J Pelvic Cavity Retropubic space	Ø Open 3 Percutaneous 4 Percutaneous Endoscopic	J Synthetic Substitute	4 Cutaneous 9 Pleural Cavity, Right B Pleural Cavity, Left G Peritoneal Cavity J Pelvic Cavity W Upper Vein Y Lower Vein
G Peritoneal Cavity	Ø Open 3 Percutaneous 4 Percutaneous Endoscopic	J Synthetic Substitute	4 Cutaneous 6 Bladder 9 Pleural Cavity, Right B Pleural Cavity, Left G Peritoneal Cavity J Pelvic Cavity W Upper Vein Y Lower Vein

Non-OR   ØW1[9,B][Ø,3,4]J[4,G,W,Y]
Non-OR   ØW1J[Ø,3,4]J[4,W,Y]
Non-OR   ØW1G[Ø,3,4]J[9,B,G,J]

Ø   Medical and Surgical
W   Anatomical Regions, General
2   Change   Definition: Taking out or off a device from a body part and putting back an identical or similar device in or on the same body part without cutting or puncturing the skin or a mucous membrane

               Explanation: All CHANGE procedures are coded using the approach EXTERNAL

Body Part Character 4	Approach Character 5	Device Character 6	Qualifier Character 7
Ø Head	X External	Ø Drainage Device	Z No Qualifier
1 Cranial Cavity		Y Other Device	
2 Face			
4 Upper Jaw			
5 Lower Jaw			
6 Neck			
Parapharyngeal space			
Retropharyngeal space			
8 Chest Wall			
9 Pleural Cavity, Right			
B Pleural Cavity, Left			
C Mediastinum			
Mediastinal cavity			
Mediastinal space			
D Pericardial Cavity			
F Abdominal Wall			
G Peritoneal Cavity			
H Retroperitoneum			
Retroperitoneal cavity			
Retroperitoneal space			
J Pelvic Cavity			
Retropubic space			
K Upper Back			
L Lower Back			
M Perineum, Male ♂			
N Perineum, Female ♀			

Non-OR	All body part, approach, device, and qualifier values	♂	ØW2MX[Ø,Y]Z
		♀	ØW2NX[Ø,Y]Z

NC Noncovered Procedure   **LC** Limited Coverage   **QA** Questionable OB Admit   **NT** New Tech Add-on   ⊞ Combination Member   ♂ Male   ♀ Female

ICD-10-PCS 2022   675

Ø   **Medical and Surgical**
W   **Anatomical Regions, General**
3   **Control**   Definition: Stopping, or attempting to stop, postprocedural or other acute bleeding
                     Explanation: None

Body Part Character 4	Approach Character 5	Device Character 6	Qualifier Character 7

Ø   Head
1   Cranial Cavity
2   Face
4   Upper Jaw
5   Lower Jaw
6   Neck
     Parapharyngeal space
     Retropharyngeal space
8   Chest Wall
9   Pleural Cavity, Right
B   Pleural Cavity, Left
C   Mediastinum
     Mediastinal cavity
     Mediastinal space
D   Pericardial Cavity
F   Abdominal Wall
G   Peritoneal Cavity
H   Retroperitoneum
     Retroperitoneal cavity
     Retroperitoneal space
J   Pelvic Cavity
     Retropubic space
K   Upper Back
L   Lower Back
M   Perineum, Male   ♂
N   Perineum, Female   ♀
	Ø Open
	3 Percutaneous
	4 Percutaneous Endoscopic
		Z No Device	Z No Qualifier

3 Oral Cavity and Throat	Ø Open 3 Percutaneous 4 Percutaneous Endoscopic 7 Via Natural or Artificial Opening 8 Via Natural or Artificial Opening Endoscopic X External	Z No Device	Z No Qualifier
P Gastrointestinal Tract Q Respiratory Tract R Genitourinary Tract	Ø Open 3 Percutaneous 4 Percutaneous Endoscopic 7 Via Natural or Artificial Opening 8 Via Natural or Artificial Opening Endoscopic	Z No Device	Z No Qualifier

Non-OR   ØW3P8ZZ
♂   ØW3M[Ø,3,4]ZZ
♀   ØW3N[Ø,3,4]ZZ

Ø   **Medical and Surgical**
W   **Anatomical Regions, General**
4   **Creation**   Definition: Putting in or on biological or synthetic material to form a new body part that to the extent possible replicates the anatomic structure or function of an absent body part
                     Explanation: Used for gender reassignment surgery and corrective procedures in individuals with congenital anomalies

Body Part Character 4	Approach Character 5	Device Character 6	Qualifier Character 7
M Perineum, Male ♂	Ø Open	7 Autologous Tissue Substitute J Synthetic Substitute K Nonautologous Tissue Substitute	Ø Vagina
N Perineum, Female ♀	Ø Open	7 Autologous Tissue Substitute J Synthetic Substitute K Nonautologous Tissue Substitute	1 Penis

♂   ØW4MØ[7,J,K]Ø
♀   ØW4NØ[7,J,K]1

Ø   **Medical and Surgical**
W   **Anatomical Regions, General**
8   **Division**   Definition: Cutting into a body part, without draining fluids and/or gases from the body part, in order to separate or transect a body part
                     Explanation: All or a portion of the body part is separated into two or more portions

Body Part Character 4	Approach Character 5	Device Character 6	Qualifier Character 7
N Perineum, Female ♀	X External	Z No Device	Z No Qualifier

Non-OR   ØW8NXZZ
♀   ØW8NXZZ

Ø   Medical and Surgical
W   Anatomical Regions, General
9   Drainage   Definition: Taking or letting out fluids and/or gases from a body part
                      Explanation: The qualifier DIAGNOSTIC is used to identify drainage procedures that are biopsies

Body Part Character 4	Approach Character 5	Device Character 6	Qualifier Character 7

Ø   Head
1   Cranial Cavity
2   Face
3   Oral Cavity and Throat
4   Upper Jaw
5   Lower Jaw
6   Neck
     Parapharyngeal space
     Retropharyngeal space
8   Chest Wall
9   Pleural Cavity, Right
B   Pleural Cavity, Left
C   Mediastinum
     Mediastinal cavity
     Mediastinal space
D   Pericardial Cavity
F   Abdominal Wall
G   Peritoneal Cavity
H   Retroperitoneum
     Retroperitoneal cavity
     Retroperitoneal space
K   Upper Back
L   Lower Back
M   Perineum, Male   ♂
N   Perineum, Female   ♀
	Ø Open
	3 Percutaneous
	4 Percutaneous Endoscopic
		Ø Drainage Device	Z No Qualifier

Ø   Head
1   Cranial Cavity
2   Face
3   Oral Cavity and Throat
4   Upper Jaw
5   Lower Jaw
6   Neck
     Parapharyngeal space
     Retropharyngeal space
8   Chest Wall
9   Pleural Cavity, Right
B   Pleural Cavity, Left
C   Mediastinum
     Mediastinal cavity
     Mediastinal space
D   Pericardial Cavity
F   Abdominal Wall
G   Peritoneal Cavity
H   Retroperitoneum
     Retroperitoneal cavity
     Retroperitoneal space
K   Upper Back
L   Lower Back
M   Perineum, Male   ♂
N   Perineum, Female   ♀
	Ø Open
	3 Percutaneous
	4 Percutaneous Endoscopic
		Z No Device	X Diagnostic
			Z No Qualifier

J   Pelvic Cavity
     Retropubic space
	Ø Open
	3 Percutaneous
	4 Percutaneous Endoscopic
	7 Via Natural or Artificial Opening
	8 Via Natural or Artificial Opening
	     Endoscopic
		Ø Drainage Device	Z No Qualifier

J   Pelvic Cavity
     Retropubic space
	Ø Open
	3 Percutaneous
	4 Percutaneous Endoscopic
	7 Via Natural or Artificial Opening
	8 Via Natural or Artificial Opening
	     Endoscopic
		Z No Device	X Diagnostic
			Z No Qualifier

Non-OR ØW9[Ø,8,9,B,K,L,M]ØØZ	**Non-OR** ØW9[Ø,1,8,F,K,L,M]4ZZ
Non-OR ØW9[Ø,1,2,3,4,5,6,8,9,B,C,D,F,G,H,K,L,M,N]3ØZ	**Non-OR** ØW9J[3,7,8]ØZ
Non-OR ØW9[Ø,1,8,F,K,L,M]4ØZ	**Non-OR** ØW9J[3,7,8]Z[X,Z]
Non-OR ØW9[Ø,2,3,4,5,6,8,9,B,K,L,M,N]ØZX	
Non-OR ØW9[Ø,1,2,3,4,5,6,8,9,B,C,D,G,K,L,M,N]3ZX	♂ ØW9M[Ø,3,4]ØZ
Non-OR ØW9[Ø,1,2,3,4,5,6,8,C,K,L,M,N]4ZX	♂ ØW9M[Ø,3,4]Z[X,Z]
Non-OR ØW9[Ø,8,9,B,K,L,M]ØZZ	♀ ØW9N[Ø,3,4]ØZ
Non-OR ØW9[Ø,1,2,3,4,5,6,8,9,B,C,D,F,G,H,K,L,M,N]3ZZ	♀ ØW9N[Ø,3]Z[X,Z]
	♀ ØW9N4ZZ

NC Noncovered Procedure   **LC** Limited Coverage   **QA** Questionable OB Admit   **NT** New Tech Add-on   ⊞ Combination Member   ♂Male   ♀Female

ICD-10-PCS 2022   **677**

Anatomical Regions, General

Ø **Medical and Surgical**
W **Anatomical Regions, General**
B **Excision**   Definition: Cutting out or off, without replacement, a portion of a body part
                 Explanation: The qualifier DIAGNOSTIC is used to identify excision procedures that are biopsies

Body Part Character 4	Approach Character 5	Device Character 6	Qualifier Character 7
Ø Head 2 Face 3 Oral Cavity and Throat 4 Upper Jaw 5 Lower Jaw 8 Chest Wall K Upper Back L Lower Back M Perineum, Male ♂ N Perineum, Female ♀	Ø Open 3 Percutaneous 4 Percutaneous Endoscopic X External	Z No Device	X Diagnostic Z No Qualifier

6 Neck
  Parapharyngeal space
  Retropharyngeal space
F Abdominal Wall
	Ø Open
	3 Percutaneous
	4 Percutaneous Endoscopic
		Z No Device	X Diagnostic
			Z No Qualifier

6 Neck
  Parapharyngeal space
  Retropharyngeal space
F Abdominal Wall
	X External	Z No Device	2 Stoma
			X Diagnostic
			Z No Qualifier

C Mediastinum
  Mediastinal cavity
  Mediastinal space
H Retroperitoneum
  Retroperitoneal cavity
  Retroperitoneal space
	Ø Open
	3 Percutaneous
	4 Percutaneous Endoscopic
		Z No Device	X Diagnostic
			Z No Qualifier

Non-OR	ØWB[Ø,2,4,5,8,K,L,M][Ø,3,4,X]ZX
Non-OR	ØWB6[Ø,3,4]ZX
Non-OR	ØWB6XZX
Non-OR	ØWBH[3,4]ZX

♂ ØWBM[Ø,3,4,X]Z[X,Z]
♀ ØWBN[Ø,3,4,X]Z[X,Z]

Ø **Medical and Surgical**
W **Anatomical Regions, General**
C **Extirpation**   Definition: Taking or cutting out solid matter from a body part
                 Explanation: The solid matter may be an abnormal byproduct of a biological function or a foreign body; it may be imbedded in a body part or in the lumen of a tubular body part. The solid matter may or may not have been previously broken into pieces.

Body Part Character 4	Approach Character 5	Device Character 6	Qualifier Character 7

1 Cranial Cavity
3 Oral Cavity and Throat
9 Pleural Cavity, Right
B Pleural Cavity, Left
C Mediastinum
  Mediastinal cavity
  Mediastinal space
D Pericardial Cavity
G Peritoneal Cavity
H Retroperitoneum
  Retroperitoneal cavity
  Retroperitoneal space
J Pelvic Cavity
  Retropubic space
	Ø Open
	3 Percutaneous
	4 Percutaneous Endoscopic
	X External
		Z No Device	Z No Qualifier

4 Upper Jaw 5 Lower Jaw	Ø Open 3 Percutaneous 4 Percutaneous Endoscopic	Z No Device	Z No Qualifier
P Gastrointestinal Tract Q Respiratory Tract R Genitourinary Tract	Ø Open 3 Percutaneous 4 Percutaneous Endoscopic 7 Via Natural or Artificial Opening 8 Via Natural or Artificial Opening Endoscopic X External	Z No Device	Z No Qualifier

Non-OR	ØWC[1,3]XZZ
Non-OR	ØWC[9,B][Ø,3,4,X]ZZ
Non-OR	ØWC[C,D,G,H,J]XZZ
Non-OR	ØWC[4,5][Ø,3,4]ZZ
Non-OR	ØWC[P,R][7,8,X]ZZ
Non-OR	ØWCQ[Ø,3,4,X]ZZ

Non-OR Procedure   DRG Non-OR Procedure   Valid OR Procedure   HAC Associated Procedure   Combination Only   New/Revised GREEN

Ø   **Medical and Surgical**
W   **Anatomical Regions, General**
F   **Fragmentation**   Definition: Breaking solid matter in a body part into pieces

Explanation: Physical force (e.g., manual, ultrasonic) applied directly or indirectly is used to break the solid matter into pieces. The solid matter may be an abnormal byproduct of a biological function or a foreign body. The pieces of solid matter are not taken out.

Body Part Character 4	Approach Character 5	Device Character 6	Qualifier Character 7

1   Cranial Cavity   NC
3   Oral Cavity and Throat   NC
9   Pleural Cavity, Right   NC
B   Pleural Cavity, Left   NC
C   Mediastinum   NC
    Mediastinal cavity
    Mediastinal space
D   Pericardial Cavity
G   Peritoneal Cavity   NC
J   Pelvic Cavity   NC
    Retropubic space
	Ø Open
	3 Percutaneous
	4 Percutaneous Endoscopic
	X External
		Z No Device	Z No Qualifier

P Gastrointestinal Tract NC Q Respiratory Tract NC R Genitourinary Tract	Ø Open 3 Percutaneous 4 Percutaneous Endoscopic 7 Via Natural or Artificial Opening 8 Via Natural or Artificial Opening Endoscopic X External	Z No Device	Z No Qualifier

Non-OR ØWF[1,3,9,B,C,G]XZZ		NC ØWF[1,3,9,B,C,G,J]XZZ
Non-OR ØWFJ[Ø,3,4,X]ZZ		NC ØWF[P,Q]XZZ
Non-OR ØWFP[Ø,3,4,7,8,X]ZZ		
Non-OR ØWFQXZZ		
Non-OR ØWFR[Ø,3,4,7,8,X]ZZ		

Ø   **Medical and Surgical**
W   **Anatomical Regions, General**
H   **Insertion**   Definition: Putting in a nonbiological appliance that monitors, assists, performs, or prevents a physiological function but does not physically take the place of a body part

Explanation: None

Body Part Character 4	Approach Character 5	Device Character 6	Qualifier Character 7

Ø   Head
1   Cranial Cavity
2   Face
3   Oral Cavity and Throat
4   Upper Jaw
5   Lower Jaw
6   Neck
    Parapharyngeal space
    Retropharyngeal space
8   Chest Wall
9   Pleural Cavity, Right
B   Pleural Cavity, Left
C   Mediastinum
    Mediastinal cavity
    Mediastinal space
D   Pericardial Cavity
F   Abdominal Wall
G   Peritoneal Cavity
H   Retroperitoneum
    Retroperitoneal cavity
    Retroperitoneal space
J   Pelvic Cavity
    Retropubic space
K   Upper Back
L   Lower Back
M   Perineum, Male
N   Perineum, Female   ♀
	Ø Open
	3 Percutaneous
	4 Percutaneous Endoscopic
		1 Radioactive Element
		3 Infusion Device
		Y Other Device
			Z No Qualifier

P Gastrointestinal Tract Q Respiratory Tract R Genitourinary Tract	Ø Open 3 Percutaneous 4 Percutaneous Endoscopic 7 Via Natural or Artificial Opening 8 Via Natural or Artificial Opening Endoscopic	1 Radioactive Element 3 Infusion Device Y Other Device	Z No Qualifier

DRG Non-OR ØWH[Ø,2,4,5,6,K,L,M][Ø,3,4][3,Y]Z	Non-OR ØWHP[3,4,7,8][3,Y]Z
Non-OR ØWH1[Ø,3,4]3Z	Non-OR ØWHQ[Ø,7,8][3,Y]Z
Non-OR ØWH[8,9,B][Ø,3,4][3,Y]Z	Non-OR ØWHR[Ø,3,4,7,8][3,Y]Z
Non-OR ØWHPØYZ	♀ ØWHN[Ø,3,4][3,Y]Z

NC Noncovered Procedure   LC Limited Coverage   QA Questionable OB Admit   NT New Tech Add-on   ⊞ Combination Member   ♂ Male   ♀ Female

Anatomical Regions, General

Ø   **Medical and Surgical**
W   **Anatomical Regions, General**
J   **Inspection**   Definition: Visually and/or manually exploring a body part

Explanation: Visual exploration may be performed with or without optical instrumentation. Manual exploration may be performed directly or through intervening body layers.

Body Part Character 4	Approach Character 5	Device Character 6	Qualifier Character 7

Ø Head
2 Face
3 Oral Cavity and Throat
4 Upper Jaw
5 Lower Jaw
6 Neck
  Parapharyngeal space
  Retropharyngeal space
8 Chest Wall
F Abdominal Wall
K Upper Back
L Lower Back
M Perineum, Male   ♂
N Perineum, Female   ♀
	Ø Open
	3 Percutaneous
	4 Percutaneous Endoscopic
	X External
		Z No Device	Z No Qualifier

1 Cranial Cavity
9 Pleural Cavity, Right
B Pleural Cavity, Left
C Mediastinum
  Mediastinal cavity
  Mediastinal space
D Pericardial Cavity
G Peritoneal Cavity
H Retroperitoneum
  Retroperitoneal cavity
  Retroperitoneal space
J Pelvic Cavity
  Retropubic space
	Ø Open
	3 Percutaneous
	4 Percutaneous Endoscopic
		Z No Device	Z No Qualifier

P Gastrointestinal Tract Q Respiratory Tract R Genitourinary Tract	Ø Open 3 Percutaneous 4 Percutaneous Endoscopic 7 Via Natural or Artificial Opening 8 Via Natural or Artificial Opening Endoscopic	Z No Device	Z No Qualifier

DRG Non-OR	ØWJ[Ø,2,4,5,K,L]ØZZ	♂	ØWJM[Ø,3,4,X]ZZ
DRG Non-OR	ØWJM[Ø,4]ZZ	♀	ØWJN[Ø,3,4,X]ZZ
Non-OR	ØWJ3ØZZ		
Non-OR	ØWJ[Ø,2,3,4,5,6,8,F,K,L,M,N][3,X]ZZ		
Non-OR	ØWJ[Ø,2,3,4,5,K,L]4ZZ		
Non-OR	ØWJDØZZ		
Non-OR	ØWJ[1,9,B,C,D,G,H,J]3ZZ ·		
Non-OR	ØWJ[P,Q,R][3,7,8]ZZ		

Ø   **Medical and Surgical**
W   **Anatomical Regions, General**
M   **Reattachment**   Definition: Putting back in or on all or a portion of a separated body part to its normal location or other suitable location

Explanation: Vascular circulation and nervous pathways may or may not be reestablished

Body Part Character 4	Approach Character 5	Device Character 6	Qualifier Character 7

2 Face
4 Upper Jaw
5 Lower Jaw
6 Neck
  Parapharyngeal space
  Retropharyngeal space
8 Chest Wall
F Abdominal Wall
K Upper Back
L Lower Back
M Perineum, Male   ♂
N Perineum, Female   ♀
	Ø Open	Z No Device	Z No Qualifier

♂ ØWMMØZZ	
♀ ØWMNØZZ	

Ø   Medical and Surgical
W   Anatomical Regions, General
P   Removal   Definition: Taking out or off a device from a body part

Explanation: If a device is taken out and a similar device put in without cutting or puncturing the skin or mucous membrane, the procedure is coded to the root operation CHANGE. Otherwise, the procedure for taking out the device is coded to the root operation REMOVAL.

Body Part Character 4	Approach Character 5	Device Character 6	Qualifier Character 7

Ø Head
2 Face
4 Upper Jaw
5 Lower Jaw
6 Neck
  Parapharyngeal space
  Retropharyngeal space
8 Chest Wall
C Mediastinum
  Mediastinal cavity
  Mediastinal space
F Abdominal Wall
K Upper Back
L Lower Back
M Perineum, Male   ♂
N Perineum, Female   ♀
	Ø Open
	3 Percutaneous
	4 Percutaneous Endoscopic
	X External
		Ø Drainage Device
		1 Radioactive Element
		3 Infusion Device
		7 Autologous Tissue Substitute
		J Synthetic Substitute
		K Nonautologous Tissue Substitute
		Y Other Device
			Z No Qualifier

1 Cranial Cavity 9 Pleural Cavity, Right B Pleural Cavity, Left G Peritoneal Cavity J Pelvic Cavity Retropubic space	Ø Open 3 Percutaneous 4 Percutaneous Endoscopic	Ø Drainage Device 1 Radioactive Element 3 Infusion Device J Synthetic Substitute Y Other Device	Z No Qualifier
1 Cranial Cavity 9 Pleural Cavity, Right B Pleural Cavity, Left G Peritoneal Cavity J Pelvic Cavity Retropubic space	X External	Ø Drainage Device 1 Radioactive Element 3 Infusion Device	Z No Qualifier

D Pericardial Cavity
H Retroperitoneum
  Retroperitoneal cavity
  Retroperitoneal space
	Ø Open
	3 Percutaneous
	4 Percutaneous Endoscopic
		Ø Drainage Device
		1 Radioactive Element
		3 Infusion Device
		Y Other Device
			Z No Qualifier

D Pericardial Cavity
H Retroperitoneum
  Retroperitoneal cavity
  Retroperitoneal space
	X External	Ø Drainage Device
		1 Radioactive Element
		3 Infusion Device
			Z No Qualifier

P Gastrointestinal Tract Q Respiratory Tract R Genitourinary Tract	Ø Open 3 Percutaneous 4 Percutaneous Endoscopic 7 Via Natural or Artificial Opening 8 Via Natural or Artificial Opening Endoscopic X External	1 Radioactive Element 3 Infusion Device Y Other Device	Z No Qualifier

Non-OR	ØWP[Ø,2,4,5,6,8][Ø,3,4,X][Ø,1,3,7,J,K,Y]Z	♂	ØWPM[Ø,3,4,X][Ø,1,3,7,J,K,Y]Z
Non-OR	ØWP[C,F]X[Ø,1,3,7,J,K,Y]Z	♀	ØWPN[Ø,3,4,X][Ø,1,3,7,J,K,Y]Z
Non-OR	ØWP[K,L][Ø,3,4,X][Ø,1,3,7,J,K,Y]Z		
Non-OR	ØWPM[Ø,3,4][Ø,1,3,J,Y]Z		
Non-OR	ØWPMX[Ø,1,3,Y]Z		
Non-OR	ØWPNX[Ø,1,3,7,J,K,Y]Z		
Non-OR	ØWP1[Ø,3,4]3Z		
Non-OR	ØWP[9,B,J][Ø,3,4][Ø,1,3,J,Y]Z		
Non-OR	ØWP[1,9,B,G,J]X[Ø,1,3]Z		
Non-OR	ØWP[D,H]X[Ø,1,3]Z		
Non-OR	ØWPP[3,4,7,8,X][1,3,Y]Z		
Non-OR	ØWPQ73Z		
Non-OR	ØWPQ8[3,Y]Z		
Non-OR	ØWPQ[Ø,X][1,3,Y]Z		
Non-OR	ØWPR[Ø,3,4,7,8,X][1,3,Y]Z		

NC Noncovered Procedure   LC Limited Coverage   QA Questionable OB Admit   NT New Tech Add-on   ⊞ Combination Member   ♂ Male   ♀ Female

ICD-10-PCS 2022   681

Ø   **Medical and Surgical**
W   **Anatomical Regions, General**
Q   **Repair**   Definition: Restoring, to the extent possible, a body part to its normal anatomic structure and function
                     Explanation: Used only when the method to accomplish the repair is not one of the other root operations

Body Part Character 4	Approach Character 5	Device Character 6	Qualifier Character 7
Ø Head **2** Face **3** Oral Cavity and Throat **4** Upper Jaw **5** Lower Jaw **8** Chest Wall **K** Upper Back **L** Lower Back **M** Perineum, Male ♂ **N** Perineum, Female ♀	**Ø** Open **3** Percutaneous **4** Percutaneous Endoscopic **X** External	**Z** No Device	**Z** No Qualifier

6 Neck
     Parapharyngeal space
     Retropharyngeal space
F Abdominal Wall
	Ø Open
	3 Percutaneous
	4 Percutaneous Endoscopic
		Z No Device	**Z** No Qualifier

6 Neck
     Parapharyngeal space
     Retropharyngeal space
F Abdominal Wall   ⊞
	X External	**Z** No Device	**2** Stoma
			Z No Qualifier

C Mediastinum
     Mediastinal cavity
     Mediastinal space
	Ø Open
	3 Percutaneous
	4 Percutaneous Endoscopic
		Z No Device	**Z** No Qualifier

Non-OR   ØWQNXZZ
♂   ØWQM[Ø,3,4,X]ZZ
♀   ØWQN[Ø,3,4,X]ZZ

See Appendix L for Procedure Combinations
⊞   ØWQFXZ[2,Z]

Ø   **Medical and Surgical**
W   **Anatomical Regions, General**
U   **Supplement**   Definition: Putting in or on biological or synthetic material that physically reinforces and/or augments the function of a portion of a body part
                     Explanation: The biological material is non-living, or is living and from the same individual. The body part may have been previously replaced, and the SUPPLEMENT procedure is performed to physically reinforce and/or augment the function of the replaced body part.

Body Part Character 4	Approach Character 5	Device Character 6	Qualifier Character 7

Ø Head
2 Face
4 Upper Jaw
5 Lower Jaw
6 Neck
     Parapharyngeal space
     Retropharyngeal space
8 Chest Wall
C Mediastinum
     Mediastinal cavity
     Mediastinal space
F Abdominal Wall
K Upper Back
L Lower Back
M Perineum, Male   ♂
N Perineum, Female   ♀
	Ø Open
	4 Percutaneous Endoscopic
		7 Autologous Tissue Substitute
		J Synthetic Substitute
		K Nonautologous Tissue Substitute
			Z No Qualifier

♂   ØWUM[Ø,4][7,J,K]Z
♀   ØWUN[Ø,4][7,J,K]Z

Ø   Medical and Surgical
W   Anatomical Regions, General
W   Revision   Definition: Correcting, to the extent possible, a portion of a malfunctioning device or the position of a displaced device

                   Explanation: Revision can include correcting a malfunctioning or displaced device by taking out or putting in components of the device such as a screw or pin

Body Part Character 4	Approach Character 5	Device Character 6	Qualifier Character 7

Ø Head
2 Face
4 Upper Jaw
5 Lower Jaw
6 Neck
   Parapharyngeal space
   Retropharyngeal space
8 Chest Wall
C Mediastinum
   Mediastinal cavity
   Mediastinal space
F Abdominal Wall
K Upper Back
L Lower Back
M Perineum, Male   ♂
N Perineum, Female ♀
	Ø Open
	3 Percutaneous
	4 Percutaneous Endoscopic
	X External
		Ø Drainage Device
		1 Radioactive Element
		3 Infusion Device
		7 Autologous Tissue Substitute
		J Synthetic Substitute
		K Nonautologous Tissue Substitute
		Y Other Device
			Z No Qualifier

1 Cranial Cavity 9 Pleural Cavity, Right B Pleural Cavity, Left G Peritoneal Cavity J Pelvic Cavity Retropubic space	Ø Open 3 Percutaneous 4 Percutaneous Endoscopic X External	Ø Drainage Device 1 Radioactive Element 3 Infusion Device J Synthetic Substitute Y Other Device	Z No Qualifier

D Pericardial Cavity
H Retroperitoneum
   Retroperitoneal cavity
   Retroperitoneal space
	Ø Open
	3 Percutaneous
	4 Percutaneous Endoscopic
	X External
		Ø Drainage Device
		1 Radioactive Element
		3 Infusion Device
		Y Other Device
			Z No Qualifier

P Gastrointestinal Tract Q Respiratory Tract R Genitourinary Tract	Ø Open 3 Percutaneous 4 Percutaneous Endoscopic 7 Via Natural or Artificial Opening 8 Via Natural or Artificial Opening Endoscopic X External	1 Radioactive Element 3 Infusion Device Y Other Device	Z No Qualifier

DRG Non-OR	ØWW[Ø,2,4,5,6,K,L][Ø,3,4][Ø,1,3,7,J,K,Y]Z	♂ ØWWM[Ø,3,4,X][Ø,1,3,7,K,Y]Z
DRG Non-OR	ØWWM[Ø,3,4][Ø,1,3,J,Y]Z	♀ ØWWN[Ø,3,4,X][Ø,1,3,7,K,Y]Z
Non-OR	ØWW[Ø,2,4,5,6,C,F,K,L,M,N]X[Ø,1,3,7,J,K,Y]Z	
Non-OR	ØWW8[Ø,3,4,X][Ø,1,3,7,J,K,Y]Z	
Non-OR	ØWW[1,G,J]X[Ø,1,3,J,Y]Z	
Non-OR	ØWW[9,B][Ø,3,4,X][Ø,1,3,J,Y]Z	
Non-OR	ØWW[D,H]X[Ø,1,3,Y]Z	
Non-OR	ØWWP[3,4,7,8,X][1,3,Y]Z	
Non-OR	ØWWQ[Ø,X][1,3,Y]Z	
Non-OR	ØWWR[Ø,3,4,7,8,X][1,3,Y]Z	

Ø   Medical and Surgical
W   Anatomical Regions, General
Y   Transplantation   Definition: Putting in or on all or a portion of a living body part taken from another individual or animal to physically take the place and/or function of all or a portion of a similar body part

                    Explanation: The native body part may or may not be taken out, and the transplanted body part may take over all or a portion of its function

Body Part Character 4	Approach Character 5	Device Character 6	Qualifier Character 7
2 Face	Ø Open	Z No Device	Ø Allogeneic 1 Syngeneic

NC Noncovered Procedure   **LC** Limited Coverage   **QA** Questionable OB Admit   **NT** New Tech Add-on   ⊞ Combination Member   ♂ Male   ♀ Female

ICD-10-PCS 2022   683

ØWW–ØWY

Anatomical Regions, Upper Extremities ØXØ–ØXY

Character Meanings

This Character Meaning table is provided as a guide to assist the user in the identification of character members that may be found in this section of code tables. It **SHOULD NOT** be used to build a PCS code.

Operation–Character 3	Body Part–Character 4	Approach–Character 5	Device–Character 6	Qualifier–Character 7
Ø Alteration	Ø Forequarter, Right	Ø Open	Ø Drainage Device	Ø Allogeneic OR Complete
2 Change	1 Forequarter, Left	3 Percutaneous	1 Radioactive Element	1 High OR Syngeneic
3 Control	2 Shoulder Region, Right	4 Percutaneous Endoscopic	3 Infusion Device	2 Mid
6 Detachment	3 Shoulder Region, Left	X External	7 Autologous Tissue Substitute	3 Low
9 Drainage	4 Axilla, Right		J Synthetic Substitute	4 Complete 1st Ray
B Excision	5 Axilla, Left		K Nonautologous Tissue Substitute	5 Complete 2nd Ray
H Insertion	6 Upper Extremity, Right		Y Other Device	6 Complete 3rd Ray
J Inspection	7 Upper Extremity, Left		Z No Device	7 Complete 4th Ray
M Reattachment	8 Upper Arm, Right			8 Complete 5th Ray
P Removal	9 Upper Arm, Left			9 Partial 1st Ray
Q Repair	B Elbow Region, Right			B Partial 2nd Ray
R Replacement	C Elbow Region, Left			C Partial 3rd Ray
U Supplement	D Lower Arm, Right			D Partial 4th Ray
W Revision	F Lower Arm, Left			F Partial 5th Ray
X Transfer	G Wrist Region, Right			L Thumb, Right
Y Transplantation	H Wrist Region, Left			M Thumb, Left
	J Hand, Right			N Toe, Right
	K Hand, Left			P Toe, Left
	L Thumb, Right			X Diagnostic
	M Thumb, Left			Z No Qualifier
	N Index Finger, Right			
	P Index Finger, Left			
	Q Middle Finger, Right			
	R Middle Finger, Left			
	S Ring Finger, Right			
	T Ring Finger, Left			
	V Little Finger, Right			
	W Little Finger, Left			

AHA Coding Clinic for table ØX3
2016, 4Q, 99   Root operation Control
2015, 1Q, 35   Evacuation of hematoma for control of postprocedural bleeding
2013, 3Q, 23   Control of intraoperative bleeding

AHA Coding Clinic for table ØX6
2017, 2Q, 3-4   Qualifiers for the root operation detachment
2017, 2Q, 18   Removal of polydactyl digits
2017, 1Q, 52   Further distal phalangeal amputation
2016, 3Q, 33   Traumatic amputation of fingers with further revision amputation

AHA Coding Clinic for table ØXH
2017, 2Q, 20   Exchange of intramedullary antibiotic impregnated spacer

AHA Coding Clinic for table ØXP
2017, 2Q, 20   Exchange of intramedullary antibiotic impregnated spacer

AHA Coding Clinic for table ØXY
2016, 4Q, 112-113 Transplantation

Detachment Qualifier Descriptions

Qualifier Definition	Upper Arm	Lower Arm
1 **High:** Amputation at the proximal portion of the shaft of the:	Humerus	Radius/Ulna
2 **Mid:** Amputation at the middle portion of the shaft of the:	Humerus	Radius/Ulna
3 **Low:** Amputation at the distal portion of the shaft of the:	Humerus	Radius/Ulna

Qualifier Definition	Hand
Ø Complete 1st through 5th Rays Ray: digit of hand or foot with corresponding metacarpus or metatarsus	Through carpo-metacarpal joint, **Wrist**
4 Complete 1st Ray	Through carpo-metacarpal joint, **Thumb**
5 Complete 2nd Ray	Through carpo-metacarpal joint, **Index Finger**
6 Complete 3rd Ray	Through carpo-metacarpal joint, **Middle Finger**
7 Complete 4th Ray	Through carpo-metacarpal joint, **Ring Finger**
8 Complete 5th Ray	Through carpo-metacarpal joint, **Little Finger**
9 Partial 1st Ray	Anywhere along shaft or head of metacarpal bone, **Thumb**
B Partial 2nd Ray	Anywhere along shaft or head of metacarpal bone, **Index Finger**
C Partial 3rd Ray	Anywhere along shaft or head of metacarpal bone, **Middle Finger**
D Partial 4th Ray	Anywhere along shaft or head of metacarpal bone, **Ring Finger**
F Partial 5th Ray	Anywhere along shaft or head of metacarpal bone, **Little Finger**

Qualifier Definition	Thumb/Finger
Ø Complete	At the metacarpophalangeal joint
1 High	Anywhere along the proximal phalanx
2 Mid	Through the proximal interphalangeal joint or anywhere along the middle phalanx
3 Low	Through the distal interphalangeal joint or anywhere along the distal phalanx

Ø   Medical and Surgical
X   Anatomical Regions, Upper Extremities
Ø   Alteration   Definition: Modifying the anatomic structure of a body part without affecting the function of the body part
                Explanation: Principal purpose is to improve appearance

Body Part Character 4	Approach Character 5	Device Character 6	Qualifier Character 7
2 Shoulder Region, Right	Ø Open	7 Autologous Tissue Substitute	Z No Qualifier
3 Shoulder Region, Left	3 Percutaneous	J Synthetic Substitute	
4 Axilla, Right	4 Percutaneous Endoscopic	K Nonautologous Tissue Substitute	
5 Axilla, Left		Z No Device	
6 Upper Extremity, Right			
7 Upper Extremity, Left			
8 Upper Arm, Right			
9 Upper Arm, Left			
B Elbow Region, Right			
C Elbow Region, Left			
D Lower Arm, Right			
F Lower Arm, Left			
G Wrist Region, Right			
H Wrist Region, Left			

Ø   Medical and Surgical
X   Anatomical Regions, Upper Extremities
2   Change   Definition: Taking out or off a device from a body part and putting back an identical or similar device in or on the same body part without cutting or puncturing the skin or a mucous membrane
                Explanation: All CHANGE procedures are coded using the approach EXTERNAL

Body Part Character 4	Approach Character 5	Device Character 6	Qualifier Character 7
6 Upper Extremity, Right	X External	Ø Drainage Device	Z No Qualifier
7 Upper Extremity, Left		Y Other Device	

    Non-OR   All body part, approach, device, and qualifier values

Ø   Medical and Surgical
X   Anatomical Regions, Upper Extremities
3   Control   Definition: Stopping, or attempting to stop, postprocedural or other acute bleeding
                Explanation: None

Body Part Character 4	Approach Character 5	Device Character 6	Qualifier Character 7
2 Shoulder Region, Right	Ø Open	Z No Device	Z No Qualifier
3 Shoulder Region, Left	3 Percutaneous		
4 Axilla, Right	4 Percutaneous Endoscopic		
5 Axilla, Left			
6 Upper Extremity, Right			
7 Upper Extremity, Left			
8 Upper Arm, Right			
9 Upper Arm, Left			
B Elbow Region, Right			
C Elbow Region, Left			
D Lower Arm, Right			
F Lower Arm, Left			
G Wrist Region, Right			
H Wrist Region, Left			
J Hand, Right			
K Hand, Left			

Anatomical Regions, Upper Extremities *(side margin)*

Ø   **Medical and Surgical**
X   **Anatomical Regions, Upper Extremities**
6   **Detachment**   Definition: Cutting off all or a portion of the upper or lower extremities

                                Explanation: The body part value is the site of the detachment, with a qualifier if applicable to further specify the level where the extremity was detached

Body Part Character 4	Approach Character 5	Device Character 6	Qualifier Character 7
Ø Forequarter, Right **1** Forequarter, Left **2** Shoulder Region, Right **3** Shoulder Region, Left **B** Elbow Region, Right **C** Elbow Region, Left	**Ø** Open	**Z** No Device	**Z** No Qualifier
8 Upper Arm, Right **9** Upper Arm, Left **D** Lower Arm, Right **F** Lower Arm, Left	**Ø** Open	**Z** No Device	**1** High **2** Mid **3** Low
J Hand, Right **K** Hand, Left	**Ø** Open	**Z** No Device	**Ø** Complete **4** Complete 1st Ray **5** Complete 2nd Ray **6** Complete 3rd Ray **7** Complete 4th Ray **8** Complete 5th Ray **9** Partial 1st Ray **B** Partial 2nd Ray **C** Partial 3rd Ray **D** Partial 4th Ray **F** Partial 5th Ray
L Thumb, Right **M** Thumb, Left **N** Index Finger, Right **P** Index Finger, Left **Q** Middle Finger, Right **R** Middle Finger, Left **S** Ring Finger, Right **T** Ring Finger, Left **V** Little Finger, Right **W** Little Finger, Left	**Ø** Open	**Z** No Device	**Ø** Complete **1** High **2** Mid **3** Low

Ø   Medical and Surgical
X   Anatomical Regions, Upper Extremities
9   Drainage   Definition: Taking or letting out fluids and/or gases from a body part

           Explanation: The qualifier DIAGNOSTIC is used to identify drainage procedures that are biopsies

Body Part Character 4	Approach Character 5	Device Character 6	Qualifier Character 7
2 Shoulder Region, Right 3 Shoulder Region, Left 4 Axilla, Right 5 Axilla, Left 6 Upper Extremity, Right 7 Upper Extremity, Left 8 Upper Arm, Right 9 Upper Arm, Left B Elbow Region, Right C Elbow Region, Left D Lower Arm, Right F Lower Arm, Left G Wrist Region, Right H Wrist Region, Left J Hand, Right K Hand, Left	Ø Open 3 Percutaneous 4 Percutaneous Endoscopic	Ø Drainage Device	Z No Qualifier
2 Shoulder Region, Right 3 Shoulder Region, Left 4 Axilla, Right 5 Axilla, Left 6 Upper Extremity, Right 7 Upper Extremity, Left 8 Upper Arm, Right 9 Upper Arm, Left B Elbow Region, Right C Elbow Region, Left D Lower Arm, Right F Lower Arm, Left G Wrist Region, Right H Wrist Region, Left J Hand, Right K Hand, Left	Ø Open 3 Percutaneous 4 Percutaneous Endoscopic	Z No Device	X Diagnostic Z No Qualifier

Non-OR   All body part, approach, device, and qualifier values

Ø   Medical and Surgical
X   Anatomical Regions, Upper Extremities
B   Excision   Definition: Cutting out or off, without replacement, a portion of a body part

           Explanation: The qualifier DIAGNOSTIC is used to identify excision procedures that are biopsies

Body Part Character 4	Approach Character 5	Device Character 6	Qualifier Character 7
2 Shoulder Region, Right 3 Shoulder Region, Left 4 Axilla, Right 5 Axilla, Left 6 Upper Extremity, Right 7 Upper Extremity, Left 8 Upper Arm, Right 9 Upper Arm, Left B Elbow Region, Right C Elbow Region, Left D Lower Arm, Right F Lower Arm, Left G Wrist Region, Right H Wrist Region, Left J Hand, Right K Hand, Left	Ø Open 3 Percutaneous 4 Percutaneous Endoscopic	Z No Device	X Diagnostic Z No Qualifier

Non-OR   ØXB[2,3,4,5,6,7,8,9,B,C,D,F,G,H,J,K][Ø,3,4]ZX

Ø   Medical and Surgical
X   Anatomical Regions, Upper Extremities
H   Insertion   Definition: Putting in a nonbiological appliance that monitors, assists, performs, or prevents a physiological function but does not physically take the place of a body part

Explanation: None

Body Part Character 4	Approach Character 5	Device Character 6	Qualifier Character 7
2 Shoulder Region, Right 3 Shoulder Region, Left 4 Axilla, Right 5 Axilla, Left 6 Upper Extremity, Right 7 Upper Extremity, Left 8 Upper Arm, Right 9 Upper Arm, Left B Elbow Region, Right C Elbow Region, Left D Lower Arm, Right F Lower Arm, Left G Wrist Region, Right H Wrist Region, Left J Hand, Right K Hand, Left	Ø Open 3 Percutaneous 4 Percutaneous Endoscopic	1 Radioactive Element 3 Infusion Device Y Other Device	Z No Qualifier

DRG Non-OR   ØXH[2,3,4,5,6,7,8,9,B,C,D,F,G,H,J,K][Ø,3,4][3,Y]Z

Ø   Medical and Surgical
X   Anatomical Regions, Upper Extremities
J   Inspection   Definition: Visually and/or manually exploring a body part

Explanation: Visual exploration may be performed with or without optical instrumentation. Manual exploration may be performed directly or through intervening body layers.

Body Part Character 4	Approach Character 5	Device Character 6	Qualifier Character 7
2 Shoulder Region, Right 3 Shoulder Region, Left 4 Axilla, Right 5 Axilla, Left 6 Upper Extremity, Right 7 Upper Extremity, Left 8 Upper Arm, Right 9 Upper Arm, Left B Elbow Region, Right C Elbow Region, Left D Lower Arm, Right F Lower Arm, Left G Wrist Region, Right H Wrist Region, Left J Hand, Right K Hand, Left	Ø Open 3 Percutaneous 4 Percutaneous Endoscopic X External	Z No Device	Z No Qualifier

DRG Non-OR   ØXJ[2,3,4,5,6,7,8,9,B,C,D,F,G,H,J,K]ØZZ
Non-OR   ØXJ[2,3,4,5,6,7,8,9,B,C,D,F,G,H][3,4,X]ZZ
Non-OR   ØXJ[J,K][3,X]ZZ

Ø   **Medical and Surgical**
X   **Anatomical Regions, Upper Extremities**
M   **Reattachment**   Definition: Putting back in or on all or a portion of a separated body part to its normal location or other suitable location
                        Explanation: Vascular circulation and nervous pathways may or may not be reestablished

Body Part Character 4	Approach Character 5	Device Character 6	Qualifier Character 7
Ø Forequarter, Right	Ø Open	Z No Device	Z No Qualifier
1 Forequarter, Left			
2 Shoulder Region, Right			
3 Shoulder Region, Left			
4 Axilla, Right			
5 Axilla, Left			
6 Upper Extremity, Right			
7 Upper Extremity, Left			
8 Upper Arm, Right			
9 Upper Arm, Left			
B Elbow Region, Right			
C Elbow Region, Left			
D Lower Arm, Right			
F Lower Arm, Left			
G Wrist Region, Right			
H Wrist Region, Left			
J Hand, Right			
K Hand, Left			
L Thumb, Right			
M Thumb, Left			
N Index Finger, Right			
P Index Finger, Left			
Q Middle Finger, Right			
R Middle Finger, Left			
S Ring Finger, Right			
T Ring Finger, Left			
V Little Finger, Right			
W Little Finger, Left			

Ø   **Medical and Surgical**
X   **Anatomical Regions, Upper Extremities**
P   **Removal**   Definition: Taking out or off a device from a body part
                    Explanation: If a device is taken out and a similar device put in without cutting or puncturing the skin or mucous membrane, the procedure is coded to the root operation CHANGE. Otherwise, the procedure for taking out the device is coded to the root operation REMOVAL.

Body Part Character 4	Approach Character 5	Device Character 6	Qualifier Character 7
6 Upper Extremity, Right	Ø Open	Ø Drainage Device	Z No Qualifier
7 Upper Extremity, Left	3 Percutaneous	1 Radioactive Element	
	4 Percutaneous Endoscopic	3 Infusion Device	
	X External	7 Autologous Tissue Substitute	
		J Synthetic Substitute	
		K Nonautologous Tissue Substitute	
		Y Other Device	

Non-OR   All body part, approach, device, and qualifier values

NC Noncovered Procedure   **LC** Limited Coverage   **QA** Questionable OB Admit   **NT** New Tech Add-on   ⊞ Combination Member   ♂ Male   ♀ Female

ICD-10-PCS 2022   **691**

Ø   **Medical and Surgical**
X   **Anatomical Regions, Upper Extremities**
Q   **Repair**   Definition: Restoring, to the extent possible, a body part to its normal anatomic structure and function
                             Explanation: Used only when the method to accomplish the repair is not one of the other root operations

Body Part Character 4	Approach Character 5	Device Character 6	Qualifier Character 7
2 Shoulder Region, Right	Ø Open	Z No Device	Z No Qualifier
3 Shoulder Region, Left	3 Percutaneous		
4 Axilla, Right	4 Percutaneous Endoscopic		
5 Axilla, Left	X External		
6 Upper Extremity, Right			
7 Upper Extremity, Left			
8 Upper Arm, Right			
9 Upper Arm, Left			
B Elbow Region, Right			
C Elbow Region, Left			
D Lower Arm, Right			
F Lower Arm, Left			
G Wrist Region, Right			
H Wrist Region, Left			
J Hand, Right			
K Hand, Left			
L Thumb, Right			
M Thumb, Left			
N Index Finger, Right			
P Index Finger, Left			
Q Middle Finger, Right			
R Middle Finger, Left			
S Ring Finger, Right			
T Ring Finger, Left			
V Little Finger, Right			
W Little Finger, Left			

Ø   **Medical and Surgical**
X   **Anatomical Regions, Upper Extremities**
R   **Replacement**   Definition: Putting in or on biological or synthetic material that physically takes the place and/or function of all or a portion of a body part
                             Explanation: The body part may have been taken out or replaced, or may be taken out, physically eradicated, or rendered nonfunctional during the REPLACEMENT procedure. A REMOVAL procedure is coded for taking out the device used in a previous replacement procedure.

Body Part Character 4	Approach Character 5	Device Character 6	Qualifier Character 7
L Thumb, Right	Ø Open	7 Autologous Tissue Substitute	N Toe, Right
M Thumb, Left	4 Percutaneous Endoscopic		P Toe, Left

Ø   **Medical and Surgical**
X   **Anatomical Regions, Upper Extremities**
U   **Supplement**   Definition: Putting in or on biological or synthetic material that physically reinforces and/or augments the function of a portion of a body part

         Explanation: The biological material is non-living, or is living and from the same individual. The body part may have been previously replaced, and the SUPPLEMENT procedure is performed to physically reinforce and/or augment the function of the replaced body part.

Body Part Character 4	Approach Character 5	Device Character 6	Qualifier Character 7
2 Shoulder Region, Right 3 Shoulder Region, Left 4 Axilla, Right 5 Axilla, Left 6 Upper Extremity, Right 7 Upper Extremity, Left 8 Upper Arm, Right 9 Upper Arm, Left B Elbow Region, Right C Elbow Region, Left D Lower Arm, Right F Lower Arm, Left G Wrist Region, Right H Wrist Region, Left J Hand, Right K Hand, Left L Thumb, Right M Thumb, Left N Index Finger, Right P Index Finger, Left Q Middle Finger, Right R Middle Finger, Left S Ring Finger, Right T Ring Finger, Left V Little Finger, Right W Little Finger, Left	Ø Open 4 Percutaneous Endoscopic	7 Autologous Tissue Substitute J Synthetic Substitute K Nonautologous Tissue Substitute	Z No Qualifier

Ø   **Medical and Surgical**
X   **Anatomical Regions, Upper Extremities**
W   **Revision**   Definition: Correcting, to the extent possible, a portion of a malfunctioning device or the position of a displaced device

         Explanation: Revision can include correcting a malfunctioning or displaced device by taking out or putting in components of the device such as a screw or pin

Body Part Character 4	Approach Character 5	Device Character 6	Qualifier Character 7
6 Upper Extremity, Right 7 Upper Extremity, Left	Ø Open 3 Percutaneous 4 Percutaneous Endoscopic X External	Ø Drainage Device 3 Infusion Device 7 Autologous Tissue Substitute J Synthetic Substitute K Nonautologous Tissue Substitute Y Other Device	Z No Qualifier

DRG Non-OR	ØXW[6,7][Ø,3,4][Ø,3,7,J,K,Y]Z
Non-OR	ØXW[6,7]X[Ø,3,7,J,K,Y]Z

Ø   **Medical and Surgical**
X   **Anatomical Regions, Upper Extremities**
X   **Transfer**   Definition: Moving, without taking out, all or a portion of a body part to another location to take over the function of all or a portion of a body part

         Explanation: The body part transferred remains connected to its vascular and nervous supply

Body Part Character 4	Approach Character 5	Device Character 6	Qualifier Character 7
N Index Finger, Right	Ø Open	Z No Device	L Thumb, Right
P Index Finger, Left	Ø Open	Z No Device	M Thumb, Left

Ø   **Medical and Surgical**
X   **Anatomical Regions, Upper Extremities**
Y   **Transplantation**   Definition: Putting in or on all or a portion of a living body part taken from another individual or animal to physically take the place and/or function of all or a portion of a similar body part

         Explanation: The native body part may or may not be taken out, and the transplanted body part may take over all or a portion of its function

Body Part Character 4	Approach Character 5	Device Character 6	Qualifier Character 7
J Hand, Right K Hand, Left	Ø Open	Z No Device	Ø Allogeneic 1 Syngeneic

NC Noncovered Procedure   **LC** Limited Coverage   **QA** Questionable OB Admit   **NT** New Tech Add-on   ⊞ Combination Member   ♂ Male   ♀ Female

ICD-10-PCS 2022   693

Anatomical Regions, Lower Extremities ØYØ–ØYW

Character Meanings

This Character Meaning table is provided as a guide to assist the user in the identification of character members that may be found in this section of code tables. It **SHOULD NOT** be used to build a PCS code.

Operation–Character 3		Body Part–Character 4		Approach–Character 5		Device–Character 6		Qualifier–Character 7	
Ø	Alteration	Ø	Buttock, Right	Ø	Open	Ø	Drainage Device	Ø	Complete
2	Change	1	Buttock, Left	3	Percutaneous	1	Radioactive Element	1	High
3	Control	2	Hindquarter, Right	4	Percutaneous Endoscopic	3	Infusion Device	2	Mid
6	Detachment	3	Hindquarter, Left	X	External	7	Autologous Tissue Substitute	3	Low
9	Drainage	4	Hindquarter, Bilateral			J	Synthetic Substitute	4	Complete 1st Ray
B	Excision	5	Inguinal Region, Right			K	Nonautologous Tissue Substitute	5	Complete 2nd Ray
H	Insertion	6	Inguinal Region, Left			Y	Other Device	6	Complete 3rd Ray
J	Inspection	7	Femoral Region, Right			Z	No Device	7	Complete 4th Ray
M	Reattachment	8	Femoral Region, Left					8	Complete 5th Ray
P	Removal	9	Lower Extremity, Right					9	Partial 1st Ray
Q	Repair	A	Inguinal Region, Bilateral					B	Partial 2nd Ray
U	Supplement	B	Lower Extremity, Left					C	Partial 3rd Ray
W	Revision	C	Upper Leg, Right					D	Partial 4th Ray
		D	Upper Leg, Left					F	Partial 5th Ray
		E	Femoral Region, Bilateral					X	Diagnostic
		F	Knee Region, Right					Z	No Qualifier
		G	Knee Region, Left						
		H	Lower Leg, Right						
		J	Lower Leg, Left						
		K	Ankle Region, Right						
		L	Ankle Region, Left						
		M	Foot, Right						
		N	Foot, Left						
		P	1st Toe, Right						
		Q	1st Toe, Left						
		R	2nd Toe, Right						
		S	2nd Toe, Left						
		T	3rd Toe, Right						
		U	3rd Toe, Left						
		V	4th Toe, Right						
		W	4th Toe, Left						
		X	5th Toe, Right						
		Y	5th Toe, Left						

AHA Coding Clinic for table ØY3

2016, 4Q, 99	Root operation Control
2013, 3Q, 23	Control of intraoperative bleeding

AHA Coding Clinic for table ØY6

2019, 2Q, 17	Cryoamputation of lower leg
2017, 2Q, 3-4	Qualifiers for the root operation detachment
2017, 1Q, 22	Chopart amputation of foot
2015, 2Q, 28	Partial amputation of hallux at interphalangeal Joint
2015, 1Q, 28	Mid-foot amputation

AHA Coding Clinic for table ØY9

2015, 1Q, 22	Incision and drainage of abscess of femoropopliteal bypass site
2015, 1Q, 22	Incision and drainage of groin abscess

Detachment Qualifier Descriptions

Qualifier Definition		Upper Leg	Lower Leg
1	**High:** Amputation at the proximal portion of the shaft of the:	Femur	Tibia/Fibula
2	**Mid:** Amputation at the middle portion of the shaft of the:	Femur	Tibia/Fibula
3	**Low:** Amputation at the distal portion of the shaft of the:	Femur	Tibia/Fibula

Qualifier Definition		Foot
Ø	Complete 1st through 5th Rays Ray: digit of hand or foot with corresponding metacarpus or metatarsus	Through tarso-metatarsal Joint, **Ankle**
4	Complete 1st Ray	Through tarso-metatarsal joint, **Great Toe**
5	Complete 2nd Ray	Through tarso-metatarsal joint, **2nd Toe**
6	Complete 3rd Ray	Through tarso-metatarsal joint, **3rd Toe**
7	Complete 4th Ray	Through tarso-metatarsal joint, **4th Toe**
8	Complete 5th Ray	Through tarso-metatarsal joint, **Little Toe**
9	Partial 1st Ray	Anywhere along shaft or head of metatarsal bone, **Great Toe**
B	Partial 2nd Ray	Anywhere along shaft or head of metatarsal bone, **2nd Toe**
C	Partial 3rd Ray	Anywhere along shaft or head of metatarsal bone, **3rd Toe**
D	Partial 4th Ray	Anywhere along shaft or head of metatarsal bone, **4th Toe**
F	Partial 5th Ray	Anywhere along shaft or head of metatarsal bone, **Little Toe**

Qualifier Definition	Toe
Ø Complete	At the metatarsal-phalangeal joint
1 High	Anywhere along the proximal phalanx
2 Mid	Through the proximal interphalangeal joint or anywhere along the middle phalanx
3 Low	Through the distal interphalangeal joint or anywhere along the distal phalanx

Ø   Medical and Surgical
Y   Anatomical Regions, Lower Extremities
Ø   Alteration   Definition: Modifying the anatomic structure of a body part without affecting the function of the body part
                     Explanation: Principal purpose is to improve appearance

Body Part Character 4	Approach Character 5	Device Character 6	Qualifier Character 7
Ø Buttock, Right 1 Buttock, Left 9 Lower Extremity, Right B Lower Extremity, Left C Upper Leg, Right D Upper Leg, Left F Knee Region, Right G Knee Region, Left H Lower Leg, Right J Lower Leg, Left K Ankle Region, Right L Ankle Region, Left	Ø Open 3 Percutaneous 4 Percutaneous Endoscopic	7 Autologous Tissue Substitute J Synthetic Substitute K Nonautologous Tissue Substitute Z No Device	Z No Qualifier

Ø   Medical and Surgical
Y   Anatomical Regions, Lower Extremities
2   Change   Definition: Taking out or off a device from a body part and putting back an identical or similar device in or on the same body part without cutting or puncturing the skin or a mucous membrane
                     Explanation: All CHANGE procedures are coded using the approach EXTERNAL

Body Part Character 4	Approach Character 5	Device Character 6	Qualifier Character 7
9 Lower Extremity, Right B Lower Extremity, Left	X External	Ø Drainage Device Y Other Device	Z No Qualifier

Non-OR   All body part, approach, device, and qualifier values

Ø   Medical and Surgical
Y   Anatomical Regions, Lower Extremities
3   Control   Definition: Stopping, or attempting to stop, postprocedural or other acute bleeding
                     Explanation: None

Body Part Character 4	Approach Character 5	Device Character 6	Qualifier Character 7

Ø Buttock, Right
1 Buttock, Left
5 Inguinal Region, Right
   Inguinal canal
   Inguinal triangle
6 Inguinal Region, Left
   See 5 Inguinal Region, Right
7 Femoral Region, Right
8 Femoral Region, Left
9 Lower Extremity, Right
B Lower Extremity, Left
C Upper Leg, Right
D Upper Leg, Left
F Knee Region, Right
G Knee Region, Left
H Lower Leg, Right
J Lower Leg, Left
K Ankle Region, Right
L Ankle Region, Left
M Foot, Right
N Foot, Left
	Ø Open
	3 Percutaneous
	4 Percutaneous Endoscopic
		Z No Device	Z No Qualifier

NC Noncovered Procedure   **LC** Limited Coverage   **QA** Questionable OB Admit   **NT** New Tech Add-on   ⊞ Combination Member   ♂ Male   ♀ Female

ICD-10-PCS 2022   **697**

Ø   Medical and Surgical
Y   Anatomical Regions, Lower Extremities
6   Detachment   Definition: Cutting off all or a portion of the upper or lower extremities

Explanation: The body part value is the site of the detachment, with a qualifier if applicable to further specify the level where the extremity was detached

Body Part Character 4	Approach Character 5	Device Character 6	Qualifier Character 7
2 Hindquarter, Right 3 Hindquarter, Left 4 Hindquarter, Bilateral 7 Femoral Region, Right 8 Femoral Region, Left F Knee Region, Right G Knee Region, Left	Ø Open	Z No Device	Z No Qualifier
C Upper Leg, Right D Upper Leg, Left H Lower Leg, Right J Lower Leg, Left	Ø Open	Z No Device	1 High 2 Mid 3 Low
M Foot, Right N Foot, Left	Ø Open	Z No Device	Ø Complete 4 Complete 1st Ray 5 Complete 2nd Ray 6 Complete 3rd Ray 7 Complete 4th Ray 8 Complete 5th Ray 9 Partial 1st Ray B Partial 2nd Ray C Partial 3rd Ray D Partial 4th Ray F Partial 5th Ray

P 1st Toe, Right
   Hallux
Q 1st Toe, Left
   See 1st Toe, Right
R 2nd Toe, Right
S 2nd Toe, Left
T 3rd Toe, Right
U 3rd Toe, Left
V 4th Toe, Right
W 4th Toe, Left
X 5th Toe, Right
Y 5th Toe, Left
	Ø Open	Z No Device	Ø Complete
			1 High
			2 Mid
			3 Low

Non-OR Procedure   DRG Non-OR Procedure   Valid OR Procedure   HAC Associated Procedure   Combination Only   New/Revised GREEN

Ø   **Medical and Surgical**
Y   **Anatomical Regions, Lower Extremities**
9   **Drainage**   Definition: Taking or letting out fluids and/or gases from a body part
                   Explanation: The qualifier DIAGNOSTIC is used to identify drainage procedures that are biopsies

Body Part Character 4	Approach Character 5	Device Character 6	Qualifier Character 7

Ø Buttock, Right
1 Buttock, Left
5 Inguinal Region, Right
    Inguinal canal
    Inguinal triangle
6 Inguinal Region, Left
    See 5 Inguinal Region, Right
7 Femoral Region, Right
8 Femoral Region, Left
9 Lower Extremity, Right
B Lower Extremity, Left
C Upper Leg, Right
D Upper Leg, Left
F Knee Region, Right
G Knee Region, Left
H Lower Leg, Right
J Lower Leg, Left
K Ankle Region, Right
L Ankle Region, Left
M Foot, Right
N Foot, Left
	Ø Open
	3 Percutaneous
	4 Percutaneous Endoscopic
		Ø Drainage Device	**Z** No Qualifier

Ø Buttock, Right
1 Buttock, Left
5 Inguinal Region, Right
    Inguinal canal
    Inguinal triangle
6 Inguinal Region, Left
    See 5 Inguinal Region, Right
7 Femoral Region, Right
8 Femoral Region, Left
9 Lower Extremity, Right
B Lower Extremity, Left
C Upper Leg, Right
D Upper Leg, Left
F Knee Region, Right
G Knee Region, Left
H Lower Leg, Right
J Lower Leg, Left
K Ankle Region, Right
L Ankle Region, Left
M Foot, Right
N Foot, Left
	Ø Open
	3 Percutaneous
	4 Percutaneous Endoscopic
		Z No Device	**X** Diagnostic
			Z No Qualifier

Non-OR   ØY9[Ø,1,7,8,9,B,C,D,F,G,H,J,K,L,M,N][Ø,3,4]ØZ
Non-OR   ØY9[5,6]3ØZ
Non-OR   ØY9[Ø,1,7,8,9,B,C,D,F,G,H,J,K,L,M,N][Ø,3,4]Z[X,Z]
Non-OR   ØY9[5,6]3ZZ

NC Noncovered Procedure   **LC** Limited Coverage   **QA** Questionable OB Admit   **NT** New Tech Add-on   ⊞ Combination Member   ♂ Male   ♀ Female

ICD-10-PCS 2022   **699**

Ø Medical and Surgical
Y Anatomical Regions, Lower Extremities
B Excision   Definition: Cutting out or off, without replacement, a portion of a body part
                  Explanation: The qualifier DIAGNOSTIC is used to identify excision procedures that are biopsies

Body Part Character 4	Approach Character 5	Device Character 6	Qualifier Character 7

Ø Buttock, Right
1 Buttock, Left
5 Inguinal Region, Right
   Inguinal canal
   Inguinal triangle
6 Inguinal Region, Left
   See 5 Inguinal Region, Right
7 Femoral Region, Right
8 Femoral Region, Left
9 Lower Extremity, Right
B Lower Extremity, Left
C Upper Leg, Right
D Upper Leg, Left
F Knee Region, Right
G Knee Region, Left
H Lower Leg, Right
J Lower Leg, Left
K Ankle Region, Right
L Ankle Region, Left
M Foot, Right
N Foot, Left
	Ø Open
	3 Percutaneous
	4 Percutaneous Endoscopic
		Z No Device	X Diagnostic
			Z No Qualifier

Non-OR   ØYB[Ø,1,9,B,C,D,F,G,H,J,K,L,M,N][Ø,3,4]ZX

Ø Medical and Surgical
Y Anatomical Regions, Lower Extremities
H Insertion   Definition: Putting in a nonbiological appliance that monitors, assists, performs, or prevents a physiological function but does not physically
                  take the place of a body part
                  Explanation: None

Body Part Character 4	Approach Character 5	Device Character 6	Qualifier Character 7

Ø Buttock, Right
1 Buttock, Left
5 Inguinal Region, Right
   Inguinal canal
   Inguinal triangle
6 Inguinal Region, Left
   See 5 Inguinal Region, Right
7 Femoral Region, Right
8 Femoral Region, Left
9 Lower Extremity, Right
B Lower Extremity, Left
C Upper Leg, Right
D Upper Leg, Left
F Knee Region, Right
G Knee Region, Left
H Lower Leg, Right
J Lower Leg, Left
K Ankle Region, Right
L Ankle Region, Left
M Foot, Right
N Foot, Left
	Ø Open
	3 Percutaneous
	4 Percutaneous Endoscopic
		1 Radioactive Element
		3 Infusion Device
		Y Other Device
			Z No Qualifier

DRG Non-OR   ØYH[Ø,1,5,6,7,8,9,B,C,D,F,G,H,J,K,L,M,N][Ø,3,4][3,Y]Z

Ø   Medical and Surgical
Y   Anatomical Regions, Lower Extremities
J   Inspection   Definition: Visually and/or manually exploring a body part

Explanation: Visual exploration may be performed with or without optical instrumentation. Manual exploration may be performed directly or through intervening body layers.

Body Part Character 4	Approach Character 5	Device Character 6	Qualifier Character 7
Ø Buttock, Right	**Ø** Open	**Z** No Device	**Z** No Qualifier
1 Buttock, Left	**3** Percutaneous		
5 Inguinal Region, Right	**4** Percutaneous Endoscopic		
Inguinal canal	**X** External		
Inguinal triangle			
6 Inguinal Region, Left			
See 5 Inguinal Region, Right			
7 Femoral Region, Right			
8 Femoral Region, Left			
9 Lower Extremity, Right			
A Inguinal Region, Bilateral			
See 5 Inguinal Region, Right			
B Lower Extremity, Left			
C Upper Leg, Right			
D Upper Leg, Left			
E Femoral Region, Bilateral			
F Knee Region, Right			
G Knee Region, Left			
H Lower Leg, Right			
J Lower Leg, Left			
K Ankle Region, Right			
L Ankle Region, Left			
M Foot, Right			
N Foot, Left			

DRG Non-OR   ØYJ[Ø,1,8,9,B,C,D,E,F,G,H,J,K,L,M,N]ØZZ
Non-OR   ØYJ[Ø,1,9,B,C,D,F,G,H,J,K,L,M,N][3,4,X]ZZ
Non-OR   ØYJ[5,6,7,8,A,E][3,X]ZZ

Ø   **Medical and Surgical**
Y   **Anatomical Regions, Lower Extremities**
M   **Reattachment**   Definition: Putting back in or on all or a portion of a separated body part to its normal location or other suitable location
                      Explanation: Vascular circulation and nervous pathways may or may not be reestablished

Body Part Character 4	Approach Character 5	Device Character 6	Qualifier Character 7

Ø   Buttock, Right
1   Buttock, Left
2   Hindquarter, Right
3   Hindquarter, Left
4   Hindquarter, Bilateral
5   Inguinal Region, Right
     Inguinal canal
     Inguinal triangle
6   Inguinal Region, Left
     See 5 Inguinal Region, Right
7   Femoral Region, Right
8   Femoral Region, Left
9   Lower Extremity, Right
B   Lower Extremity, Left
C   Upper Leg, Right
D   Upper Leg, Left
F   Knee Region, Right
G   Knee Region, Left
H   Lower Leg, Right
J   Lower Leg, Left
K   Ankle Region, Right
L   Ankle Region, Left
M   Foot, Right
N   Foot, Left
P   1st Toe, Right
     Hallux
Q   1st Toe, Left
     See 1st Toe, Right
R   2nd Toe, Right
S   2nd Toe, Left
T   3rd Toe, Right
U   3rd Toe, Left
V   4th Toe, Right
W   4th Toe, Left
X   5th Toe, Right
Y   5th Toe, Left
	Ø Open	Z No Device	Z No Qualifier

Ø   **Medical and Surgical**
Y   **Anatomical Regions, Lower Extremities**
P   **Removal**   Definition: Taking out or off a device from a body part
                      Explanation: If a device is taken out and a similar device put in without cutting or puncturing the skin or mucous membrane, the procedure is coded to the root operation CHANGE. Otherwise, the procedure for taking out the device is coded to the root operation REMOVAL.

Body Part Character 4	Approach Character 5	Device Character 6	Qualifier Character 7
9 Lower Extremity, Right B Lower Extremity, Left	Ø Open 3 Percutaneous 4 Percutaneous Endoscopic X External	Ø Drainage Device 1 Radioactive Element 3 Infusion Device 7 Autologous Tissue Substitute J Synthetic Substitute K Nonautologous Tissue Substitute Y Other Device	Z No Qualifier

Non-OR   All body part, approach, device, and qualifier values

Ø   **Medical and Surgical**
Y   **Anatomical Regions, Lower Extremities**
Q   **Repair**   Definition: Restoring, to the extent possible, a body part to its normal anatomic structure and function

Explanation: Used only when the method to accomplish the repair is not one of the other root operations

Body Part Character 4	Approach Character 5	Device Character 6	Qualifier Character 7

Ø Buttock, Right
1 Buttock, Left
5 Inguinal Region, Right
     Inguinal canal
     Inguinal triangle
6 Inguinal Region, Left
     See 5 Inguinal Region, Right
7 Femoral Region, Right
8 Femoral Region, Left
9 Lower Extremity, Right
A Inguinal Region, Bilateral
     See 5 Inguinal Region, Right
B Lower Extremity, Left
C Upper Leg, Right
D Upper Leg, Left
E Femoral Region, Bilateral
F Knee Region, Right
G Knee Region, Left
H Lower Leg, Right
J Lower Leg, Left
K Ankle Region, Right
L Ankle Region, Left
M Foot, Right
N Foot, Left
P 1st Toe, Right
     Hallux
Q 1st Toe, Left
     See 1st Toe, Right
R 2nd Toe, Right
S 2nd Toe, Left
T 3rd Toe, Right
U 3rd Toe, Left
V 4th Toe, Right
W 4th Toe, Left
X 5th Toe, Right
Y 5th Toe, Left
	Ø Open
	3 Percutaneous
	4 Percutaneous Endoscopic
	X External
		Z No Device	Z No Qualifier

Non-OR   ØYQ[5,6,7,8,A,E]XZZ

NC Noncovered Procedure   **LC** Limited Coverage   **QA** Questionable OB Admit   **NT** New Tech Add-on   ⊞ Combination Member   ♂ Male   ♀ Female

ICD-10-PCS 2022   **703**

Ø Medical and Surgical
Y Anatomical Regions, Lower Extremities
U Supplement   Definition: Putting in or on biological or synthetic material that physically reinforces and/or augments the function of a portion of a body part

Explanation: The biological material is non-living, or is living and from the same individual. The body part may have been previously replaced, and the SUPPLEMENT procedure is performed to physically reinforce and/or augment the function of the replaced body part.

Body Part Character 4	Approach Character 5	Device Character 6	Qualifier Character 7
Ø Buttock, Right	Ø Open	7 Autologous Tissue Substitute	Z No Qualifier
1 Buttock, Left	4 Percutaneous Endoscopic	J Synthetic Substitute	
5 Inguinal Region, Right		K Nonautologous Tissue Substitute	
Inguinal canal			
Inguinal triangle			
6 Inguinal Region, Left			
See 5 Inguinal Region, Right			
7 Femoral Region, Right			
8 Femoral Region, Left			
9 Lower Extremity, Right			
A Inguinal Region, Bilateral			
See 5 Inguinal Region, Right			
B Lower Extremity, Left			
C Upper Leg, Right			
D Upper Leg, Left			
E Femoral Region, Bilateral			
F Knee Region, Right			
G Knee Region, Left			
H Lower Leg, Right			
J Lower Leg, Left			
K Ankle Region, Right			
L Ankle Region, Left			
M Foot, Right			
N Foot, Left			
P 1st Toe, Right			
Hallux			
Q 1st Toe, Left			
See 1st Toe, Right			
R 2nd Toe, Right			
S 2nd Toe, Left			
T 3rd Toe, Right			
U 3rd Toe, Left			
V 4th Toe, Right			
W 4th Toe, Left			
X 5th Toe, Right			
Y 5th Toe, Left			

Ø Medical and Surgical
Y Anatomical Regions, Lower Extremities
W Revision   Definition: Correcting, to the extent possible, a portion of a malfunctioning device or the position of a displaced device

Explanation: Revision can include correcting a malfunctioning or displaced device by taking out or putting in components of the device such as a screw or pin

Body Part Character 4	Approach Character 5	Device Character 6	Qualifier Character 7
9 Lower Extremity, Right	Ø Open	Ø Drainage Device	Z No Qualifier
B Lower Extremity, Left	3 Percutaneous	3 Infusion Device	
	4 Percutaneous Endoscopic	7 Autologous Tissue Substitute	
	X External	J Synthetic Substitute	
		K Nonautologous Tissue Substitute	
		Y Other Device	

DRG Non-OR   ØYW[9,B][Ø,3,4][Ø,3,7,J,K,Y]Z
Non-OR   ØYW[9,B]X[Ø,3,7,J,K,Y]Z

Obstetrics 1Ø2–1ØY

Character Meanings

This Character Meaning table is provided as a guide to assist the user in the identification of character members that may be found in this section of code tables. It **SHOULD NOT** be used to build a PCS code.

Ø: Pregnancy

Operation–Character 3	Body Part–Character 4	Approach–Character 5	Device–Character 6	Qualifier–Character 7
2 Change	Ø Products of Conception	Ø Open	3 Monitoring Electrode	Ø High
9 Drainage	1 Products of Conception, Retained	3 Percutaneous	Y Other Device	1 Low
A Abortion	2 Products of Conception, Ectopic	4 Percutaneous Endoscopic	Z No Device	2 Extraperitoneal
D Extraction		7 Via Natural or Artificial Opening		3 Low Forceps
E Delivery		8 Via Natural or Artificial Opening Endoscopic		4 Mid Forceps
H Insertion		X External		5 High Forceps
J Inspection				6 Vacuum
P Removal				7 Internal Version
Q Repair				8 Other
S Reposition				9 Fetal Blood OR Manual
T Resection				A Fetal Cerebrospinal Fluid
Y Transplantation				B Fetal Fluid, Other
				C Amniotic Fluid, Therapeutic
				D Fluid, Other
				E Nervous System
				F Cardiovascular System
				G Lymphatics & Hemic
				H Eye
				J Ear, Nose & Sinus
				K Respiratory System
				L Mouth & Throat
				M Gastrointestinal System
				N Hepatobiliary & Pancreas
				P Endocrine System
				Q Skin
				R Musculoskeletal System
				S Urinary System
				T Female Reproductive System
				U Amniotic Fluid, Diagnostic
				V Male Reproductive System
				W Laminaria
				X Abortifacient
				Y Other Body System
				Z No Qualifier

AHA Coding Clinic for table 1Ø9

| 2014, 3Q, 12 | Fetoscopic laser photocoagulation and laser microseptostomy for twin-twin transfusion syndrome |
| 2014, 2Q, 9 | Pitocin administration to augment labor |

AHA Coding Clinic for table 1ØD

2021, 1Q, 52	Removal of ectopic pregnancy via laparotomy
2020, 4Q, 59-60	Extraction of ectopic products of conception
2018, 4Q, 49-51	Revised qualifier values for root operation "extraction" (cesarean delivery)
2018, 2Q, 17	High transverse cesarean section
2016, 1Q, 9	Vaginal delivery assisted by vacuum and low forceps extraction
2014, 4Q, 43	Cesarean delivery assisted by vacuum extraction
2014, 4Q, 43	Vacuum dilation and curettage for blighted ovum

AHA Coding Clinic for table 1ØE

2017, 3Q, 5	Delivery of placenta
2016, 2Q, 34	Assisted vaginal delivery
2014, 4Q, 17	RH (D) alloimmunization (sensitization)
2014, 2Q, 9	Pitocin administration to augment labor

AHA Coding Clinic for table 1ØH

| 2013, 2Q, 36 | Intrauterine pressure monitor |

AHA Coding Clinic for table 1ØQ

| 2021, 2Q, 21 | Ex Utero intrapartum treatment procedure |
| 2014, 3Q, 12 | Fetoscopic laser photocoagulation and laser microseptostomy for twin-twin transfusion syndrome |

AHA Coding Clinic for table 1ØT

| 2020, 3Q, 47 | Removal of ectopic cornual pregnancy |
| 2015, 3Q, 31 | Laparoscopic partial salpingectomy for ectopic pregnancy |

1 Obstetrics
Ø Pregnancy
2 Change Definition: Taking out or off a device from a body part and putting back an identical or similar device in or on the same body part without cutting or puncturing the skin or a mucous membrane
Explanation: None

Body Part Character 4	Approach Character 5	Device Character 6	Qualifier Character 7
Ø Products of Conception ♀	7 Via Natural or Artificial Opening	3 Monitoring Electrode Y Other Device	Z No Qualifier

Non-OR	All body part, approach, device, and qualifier values	♀ All body part, approach, device, and qualifier values

1 Obstetrics
Ø Pregnancy
9 Drainage Definition: Taking or letting out fluids and/or gases from a body part
Explanation: None

Body Part Character 4	Approach Character 5	Device Character 6	Qualifier Character 7
Ø Products of Conception ♀	Ø Open 3 Percutaneous 4 Percutaneous Endoscopic 7 Via Natural or Artificial Opening 8 Via Natural or Artificial Opening Endoscopic	Z No Device	9 Fetal Blood A Fetal Cerebrospinal Fluid B Fetal Fluid, Other C Amniotic Fluid, Therapeutic D Fluid, Other U Amniotic Fluid, Diagnostic

Non-OR	All body part, approach, device, and qualifier values	♀ All body part, approach, device, and qualifier values

1 Obstetrics
Ø Pregnancy
A Abortion Definition: Artificially terminating a pregnancy
Explanation: None

Body Part Character 4	Approach Character 5	Device Character 6	Qualifier Character 7
Ø Products of Conception ♀	Ø Open 3 Percutaneous 4 Percutaneous Endoscopic 8 Via Natural or Artificial Opening Endoscopic	Z No Device	Z No Qualifier
Ø Products of Conception ♀	7 Via Natural or Artificial Opening	Z No Device	6 Vacuum W Laminaria X Abortifacient Z No Qualifier

Non-OR	10A07Z[6,W,X]	♀ All body part, approach, device, and qualifier values

1 Obstetrics
Ø Pregnancy
D Extraction Definition: Pulling or stripping out or off all or a portion of a body part by the use of force
Explanation: None

Body Part Character 4	Approach Character 5	Device Character 6	Qualifier Character 7
Ø Products of Conception 【QA】♀	Ø Open	Z No Device	Ø High 1 Low 2 Extraperitoneal
Ø Products of Conception 【QA】♀	7 Via Natural or Artificial Opening	Z No Device	3 Low Forceps 4 Mid Forceps 5 High Forceps 6 Vacuum 7 Internal Version 8 Other
1 Products of Conception, Retained ♀	7 Via Natural or Artificial Opening 8 Via Natural or Artificial Opening Endoscopic	Z No Device	9 Manual Z No Qualifier
2 Products of Conception, Ectopic ♀	Ø Open 4 Percutaneous Endoscopic 7 Via Natural or Artificial Opening 8 Via Natural or Artificial Opening Endoscopic	Z No Device	Z No Qualifier

DRG Non-OR 【QA】 【QA】	10D07Z[3,4,5,6,7,8] 10D00Z[Ø,1,2] except when a corresponding SDX of Z37.Ø-Z37.9 is also reported 10D07Z[3,4,5,7] except when a corresponding SDX of Z37.Ø-Z37.9 is also reported	♀ All body part, approach, device, and qualifier values

1 Obstetrics
Ø Pregnancy
E Delivery

Definition: Assisting the passage of the products of conception from the genital canal

Explanation: None

Body Part Character 4		Approach Character 5	Device Character 6	Qualifier Character 7
Ø Products of Conception QA ♀	X	External	Z No Device	Z No Qualifier

DRG Non-OR	10EØXZZ	♀ All body part, approach, device, and qualifier values
QA	10EØXZZ except when a corresponding SDX of Z37.Ø-Z37.9 is also reported	

1 Obstetrics
Ø Pregnancy
H Insertion

Definition: Putting in a nonbiological appliance that monitors, assists, performs, or prevents a physiological function but does not physically take the place of a body part

Explanation: None

Body Part Character 4		Approach Character 5	Device Character 6	Qualifier Character 7
Ø Products of Conception ♀	Ø 7	Open Via Natural or Artificial Opening	3 Monitoring Electrode Y Other Device	Z No Qualifier

Non-OR	All body part, approach, device, and qualifier values	♀ All body part, approach, device, and qualifier values

1 Obstetrics
Ø Pregnancy
J Inspection

Definition: Visually and/or manually exploring a body part

Explanation: Visual exploration may be performed with or without optical instrumentation. Manual exploration may be performed directly or through intervening body layers.

Body Part Character 4		Approach Character 5	Device Character 6	Qualifier Character 7
Ø Products of Conception ♀ 1 Products of Conception, Retained ♀ 2 Products of Conception, Ectopic ♀	Ø 3 4 7 8 X	Open Percutaneous Percutaneous Endoscopic Via Natural or Artificial Opening Via Natural or Artificial Opening Endoscopic External	Z No Device	Z No Qualifier

Non-OR	All body part, approach, device, and qualifier values	♀ All body part, approach, device, and qualifier values

1 Obstetrics
Ø Pregnancy
P Removal

Definition: Taking out or off a device from a body part, region or orifice

Explanation: If a device is taken out and a similar device put in without cutting or puncturing the skin or mucous membrane, the procedure is coded to the root operation CHANGE. Otherwise, the procedure for taking out a device is coded to the root operation REMOVAL.

Body Part Character 4		Approach Character 5	Device Character 6	Qualifier Character 7
Ø Products of Conception ♀	Ø 7	Open Via Natural or Artificial Opening	3 Monitoring Electrode Y Other Device	Z No Qualifier

Non-OR	All body part, approach, device, and qualifier values	♀ All body part, approach, device, and qualifier values

1 Obstetrics
Ø Pregnancy
Q Repair

Definition: Restoring, to the extent possible, a body part to its normal anatomic structure and function

Explanation: Used only when the method to accomplish the repair is not one of the other root operations

Body Part Character 4		Approach Character 5	Device Character 6	Qualifier Character 7
Ø Products of Conception ♀	Ø 3 4 7 8	Open Percutaneous Percutaneous Endoscopic Via Natural or Artificial Opening Via Natural or Artificial Opening Endoscopic	Y Other Device Z No Device	E Nervous System F Cardiovascular System G Lymphatics and Hemic H Eye J Ear, Nose and Sinus K Respiratory System L Mouth and Throat M Gastrointestinal System N Hepatobiliary and Pancreas P Endocrine System Q Skin R Musculoskeletal System S Urinary System T Female Reproductive System V Male Reproductive System Y Other Body System

Non-OR	All body part, approach, device, and qualifier values	♀ All body part, approach, device, and qualifier values

NC Noncovered Procedure   **LC** Limited Coverage   **QA** Questionable OB Admit   **NT** New Tech Add-on   ⊞ Combination Member   ♂ Male   ♀ Female

1   Obstetrics
Ø   Pregnancy
S   Reposition   Definition: Moving to its normal location, or other suitable location, all or a portion of a body part

Explanation: The body part is moved to a new location from an abnormal location, or from a normal location where it is not functioning correctly. The body part may or may not be cut out or off to be moved to the new location.

Body Part Character 4	Approach Character 5	Device Character 6	Qualifier Character 7
Ø Products of Conception ♀	7 Via Natural or Artificial Opening X External	Z No Device	Z No Qualifier
2 Products of Conception, Ectopic ♀	Ø Open 3 Percutaneous 4 Percutaneous Endoscopic 7 Via Natural or Artificial Opening 8 Via Natural or Artificial Opening Endoscopic	Z No Device	Z No Qualifier

Non-OR	1ØS0[7,X]ZZ	♀	All body part, approach, device, and qualifier values

1   Obstetrics
Ø   Pregnancy
T   Resection   Definition: Cutting out or off, without replacement, all of a body part

Explanation: None

Body Part Character 4	Approach Character 5	Device Character 6	Qualifier Character 7
2 Products of Conception, Ectopic ♀	Ø Open 3 Percutaneous 4 Percutaneous Endoscopic 7 Via Natural or Artificial Opening 8 Via Natural or Artificial Opening Endoscopic	Z No Device	Z No Qualifier

♀	All body part, approach, device, and qualifier values

1   Obstetrics
Ø   Pregnancy
Y   Transplantation   Definition: Putting in or on all or a portion of a living body part taken from another individual or animal to physically take the place and/or function of all or a portion of a similar body part

Explanation: The native body part may or may not be taken out, and the transplanted body part may take over all or a portion of its function

Body Part Character 4	Approach Character 5	Device Character 6	Qualifier Character 7
Ø Products of Conception ♀	3 Percutaneous 4 Percutaneous Endoscopic 7 Via Natural or Artificial Opening	Z No Device	E Nervous System F Cardiovascular System G Lymphatics and Hemic H Eye J Ear, Nose and Sinus K Respiratory System L Mouth and Throat M Gastrointestinal System N Hepatobiliary and Pancreas P Endocrine System Q Skin R Musculoskeletal System S Urinary System T Female Reproductive System V Male Reproductive System Y Other Body System

Non-OR	All body part, approach, device, and qualifier values	♀	All body part, approach, device, and qualifier values

Placement 2WØ–2Y5

AHA Coding Clinic for table 2W6

2015, 2Q, 35	Application of tongs to reduce and stabilize cervical fracture
2013, 2Q, 39	Application of cervical tongs for reduction of cervical fracture

AHA Coding Clinic for table 2Y4

2018, 4Q, 38	Control of epistaxis
2017, 4Q, 106	Nasal packing for epistaxis

2   Placement
W   Anatomical Regions
Ø   Change   Definition: Taking out or off a device from a body part and putting back an identical or similar device in or on the same body part without cutting or puncturing the skin or a mucous membrane

Body Region Character 4	Approach Character 5	Device Character 6	Qualifier Character 7
Ø Head 2 Neck 3 Abdominal Wall 4 Chest Wall 5 Back 6 Inguinal Region, Right 7 Inguinal Region, Left 8 Upper Extremity, Right 9 Upper Extremity, Left A Upper Arm, Right B Upper Arm, Left C Lower Arm, Right D Lower Arm, Left E Hand, Right F Hand, Left G Thumb, Right H Thumb, Left J Finger, Right K Finger, Left L Lower Extremity, Right M Lower Extremity, Left N Upper Leg, Right P Upper Leg, Left Q Lower Leg, Right R Lower Leg, Left S Foot, Right T Foot, Left U Toe, Right V Toe, Left	X External	Ø Traction Apparatus 1 Splint 2 Cast 3 Brace 4 Bandage 5 Packing Material 6 Pressure Dressing 7 Intermittent Pressure Device Y Other Device	Z No Qualifier
1 Face	X External	Ø Traction Apparatus 1 Splint 2 Cast 3 Brace 4 Bandage 5 Packing Material 6 Pressure Dressing 7 Intermittent Pressure Device 9 Wire Y Other Device	Z No Qualifier

NC Noncovered Procedure   LC Limited Coverage   QA Questionable OB Admit   NT New Tech Add-on   ⊞ Combination Member   ♂ Male   ♀ Female

ICD-10-PCS 2022   709

2   Placement
W   Anatomical Regions
1   Compression   Definition: Putting pressure on a body region

Body Region Character 4	Approach Character 5	Device Character 6	Qualifier Character 7
Ø Head 1 Face 2 Neck 3 Abdominal Wall 4 Chest Wall 5 Back 6 Inguinal Region, Right 7 Inguinal Region, Left 8 Upper Extremity, Right 9 Upper Extremity, Left A Upper Arm, Right B Upper Arm, Left C Lower Arm, Right D Lower Arm, Left E Hand, Right F Hand, Left G Thumb, Right H Thumb, Left J Finger, Right K Finger, Left L Lower Extremity, Right M Lower Extremity, Left N Upper Leg, Right P Upper Leg, Left Q Lower Leg, Right R Lower Leg, Left S Foot, Right T Foot, Left U Toe, Right V Toe, Left	X External	6 Pressure Dressing 7 Intermittent Pressure Device	Z No Qualifier

2   Placement
W   Anatomical Regions
2   Dressing   Definition: Putting material on a body region for protection

Body Region Character 4	Approach Character 5	Device Character 6	Qualifier Character 7
Ø Head 1 Face 2 Neck 3 Abdominal Wall 4 Chest Wall 5 Back 6 Inguinal Region, Right 7 Inguinal Region, Left 8 Upper Extremity, Right 9 Upper Extremity, Left A Upper Arm, Right B Upper Arm, Left C Lower Arm, Right D Lower Arm, Left E Hand, Right F Hand, Left G Thumb, Right H Thumb, Left J Finger, Right K Finger, Left L Lower Extremity, Right M Lower Extremity, Left N Upper Leg, Right P Upper Leg, Left Q Lower Leg, Right R Lower Leg, Left S Foot, Right T Foot, Left U Toe, Right V Toe, Left	X External	4 Bandage	Z No Qualifier

2 Placement
W Anatomical Regions
3 Immobilization Definition: Limiting or preventing motion of a body region

Body Region Character 4	Approach Character 5	Device Character 6	Qualifier Character 7
Ø Head	X External	1 Splint	Z No Qualifier
2 Neck		2 Cast	
3 Abdominal Wall		3 Brace	
4 Chest Wall		Y Other Device	
5 Back			
6 Inguinal Region, Right			
7 Inguinal Region, Left			
8 Upper Extremity, Right			
9 Upper Extremity, Left			
A Upper Arm, Right			
B Upper Arm, Left			
C Lower Arm, Right			
D Lower Arm, Left			
E Hand, Right			
F Hand, Left			
G Thumb, Right			
H Thumb, Left			
J Finger, Right			
K Finger, Left			
L Lower Extremity, Right			
M Lower Extremity, Left			
N Upper Leg, Right			
P Upper Leg, Left			
Q Lower Leg, Right			
R Lower Leg, Left			
S Foot, Right			
T Foot, Left			
U Toe, Right			
V Toe, Left			
1 Face	X External	1 Splint	Z No Qualifier
		2 Cast	
		3 Brace	
		9 Wire	
		Y Other Device	

2 Placement
W Anatomical Regions
4 Packing Definition: Putting material in a body region or orifice

Body Region Character 4	Approach Character 5	Device Character 6	Qualifier Character 7
Ø Head	X External	5 Packing Material	Z No Qualifier
1 Face			
2 Neck			
3 Abdominal Wall			
4 Chest Wall			
5 Back			
6 Inguinal Region, Right			
7 Inguinal Region, Left			
8 Upper Extremity, Right			
9 Upper Extremity, Left			
A Upper Arm, Right			
B Upper Arm, Left			
C Lower Arm, Right			
D Lower Arm, Left			
E Hand, Right			
F Hand, Left			
G Thumb, Right			
H Thumb, Left			
J Finger, Right			
K Finger, Left			
L Lower Extremity, Right			
M Lower Extremity, Left			
N Upper Leg, Right			
P Upper Leg, Left			
Q Lower Leg, Right			
R Lower Leg, Left			
S Foot, Right			
T Foot, Left			
U Toe, Right			
V Toe, Left			

NC Noncovered Procedure   LC Limited Coverage   QA Questionable OB Admit   NT New Tech Add-on   ⊞ Combination Member   ♂Male   ♀Female

ICD-10-PCS 2022   711   2W3–2W4

Placement *(side tab)*

2   Placement
W   Anatomical Regions
5   Removal   Definition: Taking out or off a device from a body part

Body Region Character 4	Approach Character 5	Device Character 6	Qualifier Character 7
Ø Head	X External	Ø Traction Apparatus	Z No Qualifier
2 Neck		1 Splint	
3 Abdominal Wall		2 Cast	
4 Chest Wall		3 Brace	
5 Back		4 Bandage	
6 Inguinal Region, Right		5 Packing Material	
7 Inguinal Region, Left		6 Pressure Dressing	
8 Upper Extremity, Right		7 Intermittent Pressure Device	
9 Upper Extremity, Left		Y Other Device	
A Upper Arm, Right			
B Upper Arm, Left			
C Lower Arm, Right			
D Lower Arm, Left			
E Hand, Right			
F Hand, Left			
G Thumb, Right			
H Thumb, Left			
J Finger, Right			
K Finger, Left			
L Lower Extremity, Right			
M Lower Extremity, Left			
N Upper Leg, Right			
P Upper Leg, Left			
Q Lower Leg, Right			
R Lower Leg, Left			
S Foot, Right			
T Foot, Left			
U Toe, Right			
V Toe, Left			
1 Face	X External	Ø Traction Apparatus	Z No Qualifier
		1 Splint	
		2 Cast	
		3 Brace	
		4 Bandage	
		5 Packing Material	
		6 Pressure Dressing	
		7 Intermittent Pressure Device	
		9 Wire	
		Y Other Device	

2 Placement
W Anatomical Regions
6 Traction   Definition: Exerting a pulling force on a body region in a distal direction

Body Region Character 4	Approach Character 5	Device Character 6	Qualifier Character 7
Ø Head 1 Face 2 Neck 3 Abdominal Wall 4 Chest Wall 5 Back 6 Inguinal Region, Right 7 Inguinal Region, Left 8 Upper Extremity, Right 9 Upper Extremity, Left A Upper Arm, Right B Upper Arm, Left C Lower Arm, Right D Lower Arm, Left E Hand, Right F Hand, Left G Thumb, Right H Thumb, Left J Finger, Right K Finger, Left L Lower Extremity, Right M Lower Extremity, Left N Upper Leg, Right P Upper Leg, Left Q Lower Leg, Right R Lower Leg, Left S Foot, Right T Foot, Left U Toe, Right V Toe, Left	X External	Ø Traction Apparatus Z No Device	Z No Qualifier

2 Placement
Y Anatomical Orifices
Ø Change   Definition: Taking out or off a device from a body part and putting back an identical or similar device in or on the same body part without cutting or puncturing the skin or a mucous membrane

Body Region Character 4	Approach Character 5	Device Character 6	Qualifier Character 7
Ø Mouth and Pharynx 1 Nasal 2 Ear 3 Anorectal 4 Female Genital Tract ♀ 5 Urethra	X External	5 Packing Material	Z No Qualifier

    ♀   2YØ4X5Z

2 Placement
Y Anatomical Orifices
4 Packing   Definition: Putting material in a body region or orifice

Body Region Character 4	Approach Character 5	Device Character 6	Qualifier Character 7
Ø Mouth and Pharynx 1 Nasal 2 Ear 3 Anorectal 4 Female Genital Tract ♀ 5 Urethra	X External	5 Packing Material	Z No Qualifier

    ♀   2Y44X5Z

2 Placement
Y Anatomical Orifices
5 Removal   Definition: Taking out or off a device from a body part

Body Region Character 4	Approach Character 5	Device Character 6	Qualifier Character 7
Ø Mouth and Pharynx 1 Nasal 2 Ear 3 Anorectal 4 Female Genital Tract ♀ 5 Urethra	X External	5 Packing Material	Z No Qualifier

    ♀   2Y54X5Z

NC Noncovered Procedure   LC Limited Coverage   QA Questionable OB Admit   NT New Tech Add-on   ⊞ Combination Member   ♂ Male   ♀ Female

ICD-10-PCS 2022   713

2W6–2Y5

Administration 302–3E1

AHA Coding Clinic for table 302

2020, 4Q, 60-61	Transfusion stem cell progenitor cells
2019, 4Q, 35	Transfusion of blood products
2019, 4Q, 36	T-cell depleted hematopoietic stem cells for transplantation
2016, 4Q, 113	Bone marrow and stem cell transfusion (Transplantation)

AHA Coding Clinic for table 3E0

2021, 1Q, 49	Frequently asked questions regarding ICD-10-CM and ICD-10-PCS coding for COVID-19
2020, 4Q, 49-50	Intravascular ultrasound assisted thrombolysis
2020, 4Q, 95	Frequently Asked Questions Regarding ICD-10-PCS Coding for COVID-19
2020, 3Q, 17-21	New procedure codes for introduction or infusion of therapeutics
2019, 4Q, 36-37	Hyperthermic antineoplastic chemotherapy
2018, 3Q, 7	Coronary brachytherapy with angioplasty
2018, 1Q, 8	Placement of bone morphogenetic protein & spinal fusion surgery
2017, 2Q, 14	Infusion of tPA into pleural cavity
2017, 1Q, 37	Injection of glue into enteric fistula tract
2016, 4Q, 113-114	Substances applied to cranial cavity and brain
2016, 3Q, 29	Closure of bilateral alveolar clefts
2016, 1Q, 20	Metatarsophalangeal joint resection arthroplasty
2015, 3Q, 24	Esophagogastroduodenoscopy with epinephrine injection for control of bleeding

AHA Coding Clinic for table 3E0 (Continued)

2015, 3Q, 29	Placement of adhesion barrier
2015, 2Q, 29	Insertion of nasogastric tube for drainage and feeding
2015, 2Q, 31	Thoracoscopic talc pleurodesis
2015, 1Q, 31	Intrathecal chemotherapy
2015, 1Q, 38	Chemoembolization of the hepatic artery
2014, 4Q, 16	Administration of RH (D) immunoglobulin
2014, 4Q, 17	RH (D) alloimmunization (sensitization)
2014, 4Q, 19	Ultrasound accelerated thrombolysis
2014, 4Q, 34	Resection of brain malignancy with implantation of chemotherapeutic wafer
2014, 4Q, 38	Placement of saline and seprafilm solution into abdominal cavity
2014, 3Q, 26	Coil embolization of gastroduodenal artery with chemoembolization of hepatic artery
2014, 2Q, 8	Medical induction of labor with Cervidil tampon insertion
2014, 2Q, 10	Prophylactic Neulasta injection for infection prevention
2013, 4Q, 124	Administration of tPA for stroke treatment prior to transfer
2013, 1Q, 27	Injection of sclerosing agent into an esophageal varix

AHA Coding Clinic for table 3E1

2019, 4Q, 38	Irrigation of joint using irrigating substance
2017, 3Q, 14	Bronchoscopy with suctioning and washings for removal of mucus plug

3　Administration
0　Circulatory
2　Transfusion　　Definition: Putting in blood or blood products

Body System/Region Character 4	Approach Character 5	Substance Character 6	Qualifier Character 7
3　Peripheral Vein　NC 4　Central Vein　NC	3　Percutaneous	A　Stem Cells, Embryonic	Z　No Qualifier
3　Peripheral Vein 4　Central Vein	3　Percutaneous	C　Hematopoietic Stem/Progenitor Cells, Genetically Modified	0　Autologous
3　Peripheral Vein 4　Central Vein	3　Percutaneous	D　Pathogen Reduced Cryoprecipitated Fibrinogen Complex	1　Nonautologous
3　Peripheral Vein　NC 4　Central Vein　NC	3　Percutaneous	G　Bone Marrow X　Stem Cells, Cord Blood Y　Stem Cells, Hematopoietic	0　Autologous 2　Allogeneic, Related 3　Allogeneic, Unrelated 4　Allogeneic, Unspecified
3　Peripheral Vein 4　Central Vein	3　Percutaneous	H　Whole Blood J　Serum Albumin K　Frozen Plasma L　Fresh Plasma M　Plasma Cryoprecipitate N　Red Blood Cells P　Frozen Red Cells Q　White Cells R　Platelets S　Globulin T　Fibrinogen V　Antihemophilic Factors W　Factor IX	0　Autologous 1　Nonautologous
3　Peripheral Vein 4　Central Vein	3　Percutaneous	U　Stem Cells, T-cell Depleted Hematopoietic	2　Allogeneic, Related 3　Allogeneic, Unrelated 4　Allogeneic, Unspecified
7　Products of Conception, Circulatory　♀	3　Percutaneous 7　Via Natural or Artificial Opening	H　Whole Blood J　Serum Albumin K　Frozen Plasma L　Fresh Plasma M　Plasma Cryoprecipitate N　Red Blood Cells P　Frozen Red Cells Q　White Cells R　Platelets S　Globulin T　Fibrinogen V　Antihemophilic Factors W　Factor IX	1　Nonautologous
8　Vein	3　Percutaneous	B　4-Factor Prothrombin Complex Concentrate	1　Nonautologous

DRG Non-OR　302[3,4]3AZ
DRG Non-OR　302[3,4]3C0
DRG Non-OR　302[3,4]3[G,X,Y][0,2,3,4]
DRG Non-OR　302[3,4]3U[2,3,4]

NC　302[3,4]3AZ Only when reported with PDx or SDx of C91.00, C92.00, C92.11, C92.40, C92.50, C92.60, C92.A0, C93.00, C94.00, C95.00
NC　302[3,4]3[G,Y]0 Only when reported with PDx or SDx of C91.00, C92.00, C92.10, C92.11, C92.40, C92.50, C92.60, C92.A0, C93.00, C94.00, C95.00
♀　3027[3,7][H,J,K,L,M,N,P,Q,R,S,T,V,W]1

NC Noncovered Procedure　　LC Limited Coverage　　QA Questionable OB Admit　　NT New Tech Add-on　　＋ Combination Member　　♂ Male　　♀ Female

ICD-10-PCS 2022　　　　　　　　　　　　　　　　　　　　　　　　　　　715

302–302

Administration

3   **Administration**
C   **Indwelling Device**
1   **Irrigation**   Definition: Putting in or on a cleansing substance

Body System/Region Character 4	Approach Character 5	Substance Character 6	Qualifier Character 7
Z None	X External	8 Irrigating Substance	Z No Qualifier

3   **Administration**
E   **Physiological Systems and Anatomical Regions**
Ø   **Introduction**   Definition: Putting in or on a therapeutic, diagnostic, nutritional, physiological, or prophylactic substance except blood or blood products

Body System/Region Character 4	Approach Character 5	Substance Character 6	Qualifier Character 7
Ø Skin and Mucous Membranes	X External	Ø Antineoplastic	5 Other Antineoplastic M Monoclonal Antibody
Ø Skin and Mucous Membranes	X External	2 Anti-infective	8 Oxazolidinones 9 Other Anti-infective
Ø Skin and Mucous Membranes	X External	3 Anti-inflammatory 4 Serum, Toxoid and Vaccine B Anesthetic Agent K Other Diagnostic Substance M Pigment N Analgesics, Hypnotics, Sedatives T Destructive Agent	Z No Qualifier
Ø Skin and Mucous Membranes	X External	G Other Therapeutic Substance	C Other Substance
1 Subcutaneous Tissue	Ø Open	2 Anti-infective	A Anti-Infective Envelope
1 Subcutaneous Tissue	3 Percutaneous	Ø Antineoplastic	5 Other Antineoplastic M Monoclonal Antibody
1 Subcutaneous Tissue	3 Percutaneous	2 Anti-infective	8 Oxazolidinones 9 Other Anti-infective A Anti-Infective Envelope
1 Subcutaneous Tissue	3 Percutaneous	3 Anti-inflammatory 6 Nutritional Substance 7 Electrolytic and Water Balance Substance B Anesthetic Agent H Radioactive Substance K Other Diagnostic Substance N Analgesics, Hypnotics, Sedatives T Destructive Agent	Z No Qualifier
1 Subcutaneous Tissue	3 Percutaneous	4 Serum, Toxoid and Vaccine	Ø Influenza Vaccine Z No Qualifier
1 Subcutaneous Tissue	3 Percutaneous	G Other Therapeutic Substance	C Other Substance
1 Subcutaneous Tissue	3 Percutaneous	V Hormone	G Insulin J Other Hormone
2 Muscle	3 Percutaneous	Ø Antineoplastic	5 Other Antineoplastic M Monoclonal Antibody
2 Muscle	3 Percutaneous	2 Anti-infective	8 Oxazolidinones 9 Other Anti-infective
2 Muscle	3 Percutaneous	3 Anti-inflammatory 6 Nutritional Substance 7 Electrolytic and Water Balance Substance B Anesthetic Agent H Radioactive Substance K Other Diagnostic Substance N Analgesics, Hypnotics, Sedatives T Destructive Agent	Z No Qualifier
2 Muscle	3 Percutaneous	4 Serum, Toxoid and Vaccine	Ø Influenza Vaccine Z No Qualifier
2 Muscle	3 Percutaneous	G Other Therapeutic Substance	C Other Substance
3 Peripheral Vein	Ø Open	Ø Antineoplastic	2 High-dose Interleukin-2 3 Low-dose Interleukin-2 5 Other Antineoplastic M Monoclonal Antibody P Clofarabine
3 Peripheral Vein	Ø Open	1 Thrombolytic	6 Recombinant Human- activated Protein C 7 Other Thrombolytic
3 Peripheral Vein	Ø Open	2 Anti-infective	8 Oxazolidinones 9 Other Anti-infective

DRG Non-OR	3E03002
DRG Non-OR	3E03017

3EØ Continued on next page

3 Administration
E Physiological Systems and Anatomical Regions
Ø Introduction   Definition: Putting in or on a therapeutic, diagnostic, nutritional, physiological, or prophylactic substance except blood or blood products

3EØ Continued

Body System/Region Character 4	Approach Character 5	Substance Character 6	Qualifier Character 7
3 Peripheral Vein	Ø Open	3 Anti-inflammatory 4 Serum, Toxoid and Vaccine 6 Nutritional Substance 7 Electrolytic and Water Balance Substance F Intracirculatory Anesthetic H Radioactive Substance K Other Diagnostic Substance N Analgesics, Hypnotics, Sedatives P Platelet Inhibitor R Antiarrhythmic T Destructive Agent X Vasopressor	Z No Qualifier
3 Peripheral Vein	Ø Open	G Other Therapeutic Substance	C Other Substance N Blood Brain Barrier Disruption
3 Peripheral Vein	Ø Open	U Pancreatic Islet Cells	Ø Autologous 1 Nonautologous
3 Peripheral Vein	Ø Open	V Hormone	G Insulin H Human B-type Natriuretic Peptide J Other Hormone
3 Peripheral Vein	Ø Open	W Immunotherapeutic	K Immunostimulator L Immunosuppressive
3 Peripheral Vein	3 Percutaneous	Ø Antineoplastic	2 High-dose Interleukin-2 3 Low-dose Interleukin-2 5 Other Antineoplastic M Monoclonal Antibody P Clofarabine
3 Peripheral Vein	3 Percutaneous	1 Thrombolytic	6 Recombinant Human- activated Protein C 7 Other Thrombolytic
3 Peripheral Vein	3 Percutaneous	2 Anti-infective	8 Oxazolidinones 9 Other Anti-infective
3 Peripheral Vein	3 Percutaneous	3 Anti-inflammatory 4 Serum, Toxoid and Vaccine 6 Nutritional Substance 7 Electrolytic and Water Balance Substance F Intracirculatory Anesthetic H Radioactive Substance K Other Diagnostic Substance N Analgesics, Hypnotics, Sedatives P Platelet Inhibitor R Antiarrhythmic T Destructive Agent X Vasopressor	Z No Qualifier
3 Peripheral Vein	3 Percutaneous	G Other Therapeutic Substance	C Other Substance N Blood Brain Barrier Disruption Q Glucarpidase
3 Peripheral Vein	3 Percutaneous	U Pancreatic Islet Cells	Ø Autologous 1 Nonautologous
3 Peripheral Vein	3 Percutaneous	V Hormone	G Insulin H Human B-type Natriuretic Peptide J Other Hormone
3 Peripheral Vein	3 Percutaneous	W Immunotherapeutic	K Immunostimulator L Immunosuppressive
4 Central Vein	Ø Open	Ø Antineoplastic	2 High-dose Interleukin-2 3 Low-dose Interleukin-2 5 Other Antineoplastic M Monoclonal Antibody P Clofarabine
4 Central Vein	Ø Open	1 Thrombolytic	6 Recombinant Human- activated Protein C 7 Other Thrombolytic

Valid OR	3EØ3ØTZ	**DRG Non-OR**	3EØ33U[Ø,1]
DRG Non-OR	3EØ3ØU[Ø,1]	**DRG Non-OR**	3EØ4ØØ2
DRG Non-OR	3EØ33Ø2	**DRG Non-OR**	3EØ4Ø17
DRG Non-OR	3EØ3317		

3EØ Continued on next page

NC Noncovered Procedure   LC Limited Coverage   QA Questionable OB Admit   NT New Tech Add-on   ⊞ Combination Member   ♂ Male   ♀ Female

ICD-10-PCS 2022   717

3   Administration
E   Physiological Systems and Anatomical Regions
0   Introduction   Definition: Putting in or on a therapeutic, diagnostic, nutritional, physiological, or prophylactic substance except blood or blood products

3E0 Continued

Body System/Region Character 4	Approach Character 5	Substance Character 6	Qualifier Character 7
4 Central Vein	0 Open	2 Anti-infective	8 Oxazolidinones 9 Other Anti-infective
4 Central Vein	0 Open	3 Anti-inflammatory 4 Serum, Toxoid and Vaccine 6 Nutritional Substance 7 Electrolytic and Water Balance Substance F Intracirculatory Anesthetic H Radioactive Substance K Other Diagnostic Substance N Analgesics, Hypnotics, Sedatives P Platelet Inhibitor R Antiarrhythmic T Destructive Agent X Vasopressor	Z No Qualifier
4 Central Vein	0 Open	G Other Therapeutic Substance	C Other Substance N Blood Brain Barrier Disruption
4 Central Vein	0 Open	V Hormone	G Insulin H Human B-type Natriuretic Peptide J Other Hormone
4 Central Vein	0 Open	W Immunotherapeutic	K Immunostimulator L Immunosuppressive
4 Central Vein	3 Percutaneous	0 Antineoplastic	2 High-dose Interleukin-2 3 Low-dose Interleukin-2 5 Other Antineoplastic M Monoclonal Antibody P Clofarabine
4 Central Vein	3 Percutaneous	1 Thrombolytic	6 Recombinant Human- activated Protein C 7 Other Thrombolytic
4 Central Vein	3 Percutaneous	2 Anti-infective	8 Oxazolidinones 9 Other Anti-infective
4 Central Vein	3 Percutaneous	3 Anti-inflammatory 4 Serum, Toxoid and Vaccine 6 Nutritional Substance 7 Electrolytic and Water Balance Substance F Intracirculatory Anesthetic H Radioactive Substance K Other Diagnostic Substance N Analgesics, Hypnotics, Sedatives P Platelet Inhibitor R Antiarrhythmic T Destructive Agent X Vasopressor	Z No Qualifier
4 Central Vein	3 Percutaneous	G Other Therapeutic Substance	C Other Substance N Blood Brain Barrier Disruption Q Glucarpidase
4 Central Vein	3 Percutaneous	V Hormone	G Insulin H Human B-type Natriuretic Peptide J Other Hormone
4 Central Vein	3 Percutaneous	W Immunotherapeutic	K Immunostimulator L Immunosuppressive
5 Peripheral Artery 6 Central Artery	0 Open 3 Percutaneous	0 Antineoplastic	2 High-dose Interleukin-2 3 Low-dose Interleukin-2 5 Other Antineoplastic M Monoclonal Antibody P Clofarabine
5 Peripheral Artery 6 Central Artery	0 Open 3 Percutaneous	1 Thrombolytic	6 Recombinant Human- activated Protein C 7 Other Thrombolytic
5 Peripheral Artery 6 Central Artery	0 Open 3 Percutaneous	2 Anti-infective	8 Oxazolidinones 9 Other Anti-infective

Valid OR	3E040TZ		DRG Non-OR	3E0[5,6][0,3]02
DRG Non-OR	3E04302		DRG Non-OR	3E0[5,6][0,3]17
DRG Non-OR	3E04317			

3E0 Continued on next page

3EØ Continued

3   **Administration**
E   **Physiological Systems and Anatomical Regions**
Ø   **Introduction**   Definition: Putting in or on a therapeutic, diagnostic, nutritional, physiological, or prophylactic substance except blood or blood products

Body System/Region Character 4	Approach Character 5	Substance Character 6	Qualifier Character 7
5 Peripheral Artery 6 Central Artery	Ø Open 3 Percutaneous	3 Anti-inflammatory 4 Serum, Toxoid and Vaccine 6 Nutritional Substance 7 Electrolytic and Water Balance Substance F Intracirculatory Anesthetic H Radioactive Substance K Other Diagnostic Substance N Analgesics, Hypnotics, Sedatives P Platelet Inhibitor R Antiarrhythmic T Destructive Agent X Vasopressor	Z No Qualifier
5 Peripheral Artery 6 Central Artery	Ø Open 3 Percutaneous	G Other Therapeutic Substance	C Other Substance N Blood Brain Barrier Disruption
5 Peripheral Artery 6 Central Artery	Ø Open 3 Percutaneous	V Hormone	G Insulin H Human B-type Natriuretic Peptide J Other Hormone
5 Peripheral Artery 6 Central Artery	Ø Open 3 Percutaneous	W Immunotherapeutic	K Immunostimulator L Immunosuppressive
7 Coronary Artery 8 Heart	Ø Open 3 Percutaneous	1 Thrombolytic	6 Recombinant Human- activated Protein C 7 Other Thrombolytic
7 Coronary Artery 8 Heart	Ø Open 3 Percutaneous	G Other Therapeutic Substance	C Other Substance
7 Coronary Artery 8 Heart	Ø Open 3 Percutaneous	K Other Diagnostic Substance P Platelet Inhibitor	Z No Qualifier
7 Coronary Artery 8 Heart	4 Percutaneous Endoscopic	G Other Therapeutic Substance	C Other Substance
9 Nose	3 Percutaneous 7 Via Natural or Artificial Opening X External	Ø Antineoplastic	5 Other Antineoplastic M Monoclonal Antibody
9 Nose	3 Percutaneous 7 Via Natural or Artificial Opening X External	2 Anti-infective	8 Oxazolidinones 9 Other Anti-infective
9 Nose	3 Percutaneous 7 Via Natural or Artificial Opening X External	3 Anti-inflammatory 4 Serum, Toxoid and Vaccine B Anesthetic Agent H Radioactive Substance K Other Diagnostic Substance N Analgesics, Hypnotics, Sedatives T Destructive Agent	Z No Qualifier
9 Nose	3 Percutaneous 7 Via Natural or Artificial Opening X External	G Other Therapeutic Substance	C Other Substance
A Bone Marrow	3 Percutaneous	Ø Antineoplastic	5 Other Antineoplastic M Monoclonal Antibody
A Bone Marrow	3 Percutaneous	G Other Therapeutic Substance	C Other Substance
B Ear	3 Percutaneous 7 Via Natural or Artificial Opening X External	Ø Antineoplastic	4 Liquid Brachytherapy Radioisotope 5 Other Antineoplastic M Monoclonal Antibody
B Ear	3 Percutaneous 7 Via Natural or Artificial Opening X External	2 Anti-infective	8 Oxazolidinones 9 Other Anti-infective
B Ear	3 Percutaneous 7 Via Natural or Artificial Opening X External	3 Anti-inflammatory B Anesthetic Agent H Radioactive Substance K Other Diagnostic Substance N Analgesics, Hypnotics, Sedatives T Destructive Agent	Z No Qualifier
B Ear	3 Percutaneous 7 Via Natural or Artificial Opening X External	G Other Therapeutic Substance	C Other Substance

DRG Non-OR   3EØ8[Ø,3]17

3EØ Continued on next page

NC Noncovered Procedure   **LC** Limited Coverage   **QA** Questionable OB Admit   **NT** New Tech Add-on   ⊞ Combination Member   ♂ Male   ♀ Female

ICD-10-PCS 2022   719

Administration

3   Administration
E   Physiological Systems and Anatomical Regions
Ø   Introduction   Definition: Putting in or on a therapeutic, diagnostic, nutritional, physiological, or prophylactic substance except blood or blood products

3EØ Continued

Body System/Region Character 4	Approach Character 5	Substance Character 6	Qualifier Character 7
C Eye	3 Percutaneous 7 Via Natural or Artificial Opening X External	Ø Antineoplastic	4 Liquid Brachytherapy Radioisotope 5 Other Antineoplastic M Monoclonal Antibody
C Eye	3 Percutaneous 7 Via Natural or Artificial Opening X External	2 Anti-infective	8 Oxazolidinones 9 Other Anti-infective
C Eye	3 Percutaneous 7 Via Natural or Artificial Opening X External	3 Anti-inflammatory B Anesthetic Agent H Radioactive Substance K Other Diagnostic Substance M Pigment N Analgesics, Hypnotics, Sedatives T Destructive Agent	Z No Qualifier
C Eye	3 Percutaneous 7 Via Natural or Artificial Opening X External	G Other Therapeutic Substance	C Other Substance
C Eye	3 Percutaneous 7 Via Natural or Artificial Opening X External	S Gas	F Other Gas
D Mouth and Pharynx	3 Percutaneous 7 Via Natural or Artificial Opening X External	Ø Antineoplastic	4 Liquid Brachytherapy Radioisotope 5 Other Antineoplastic M Monoclonal Antibody
D Mouth and Pharynx	3 Percutaneous 7 Via Natural or Artificial Opening X External	2 Anti-infective	8 Oxazolidinones 9 Other Anti-infective
D Mouth and Pharynx	3 Percutaneous 7 Via Natural or Artificial Opening X External	3 Anti-inflammatory 4 Serum, Toxoid and Vaccine 6 Nutritional Substance 7 Electrolytic and Water Balance Substance B Anesthetic Agent H Radioactive Substance K Other Diagnostic Substance N Analgesics, Hypnotics, Sedatives R Antiarrhythmic T Destructive Agent	Z No Qualifier
D Mouth and Pharynx	3 Percutaneous 7 Via Natural or Artificial Opening X External	G Other Therapeutic Substance	C Other Substance
E Products of Conception ♀ G Upper GI H Lower GI K Genitourinary Tract N Male Reproductive ♂	3 Percutaneous 7 Via Natural or Artificial Opening 8 Via Natural or Artificial Opening Endoscopic	Ø Antineoplastic	4 Liquid Brachytherapy Radioisotope 5 Other Antineoplastic M Monoclonal Antibody
E Products of Conception ♀ G Upper GI H Lower GI K Genitourinary Tract N Male Reproductive ♂	3 Percutaneous 7 Via Natural or Artificial Opening 8 Via Natural or Artificial Opening Endoscopic	2 Anti-infective	8 Oxazolidinones 9 Other Anti-infective
E Products of Conception ♀ G Upper GI H Lower GI K Genitourinary Tract N Male Reproductive ♂	3 Percutaneous 7 Via Natural or Artificial Opening 8 Via Natural or Artificial Opening Endoscopic	3 Anti-inflammatory 6 Nutritional Substance 7 Electrolytic and Water Balance Substance B Anesthetic Agent H Radioactive Substance K Other Diagnostic Substance N Analgesics, Hypnotics, Sedatives T Destructive Agent	Z No Qualifier
E Products of Conception ♀ G Upper GI H Lower GI K Genitourinary Tract N Male Reproductive ♂	3 Percutaneous 7 Via Natural or Artificial Opening 8 Via Natural or Artificial Opening Endoscopic	G Other Therapeutic Substance	C Other Substance

♂   All approach, substance, and qualifier values for body system/region (character 4) with this icon
♀   All approach, substance, and qualifier values for body system/region (character 4) with this icon

3EØ Continued on next page

3   **Administration**
E   **Physiological Systems and Anatomical Regions**
0   **Introduction**   Definition: Putting in or on a therapeutic, diagnostic, nutritional, physiological, or prophylactic substance except blood or blood products

Body System/Region Character 4	Approach Character 5	Substance Character 6	Qualifier Character 7
E Products of Conception ♀ **G** Upper GI **H** Lower GI **K** Genitourinary Tract **N** Male Reproductive ♂	**3** Percutaneous **7** Via Natural or Artificial Opening **8** Via Natural or Artificial Opening Endoscopic	**S** Gas	**F** Other Gas
E Products of Conception ♀ **G** Upper GI **H** Lower GI **K** Genitourinary Tract **N** Male Reproductive ♂	**4** Percutaneous Endoscopic	**G** Other Therapeutic Substance	**C** Other Substance
F Respiratory Tract	**3** Percutaneous **7** Via Natural or Artificial Opening **8** Via Natural or Artificial Opening Endoscopic	**0** Antineoplastic	**4** Liquid Brachytherapy Radioisotope **5** Other Antineoplastic **M** Monoclonal Antibody
F Respiratory Tract	**3** Percutaneous **7** Via Natural or Artificial Opening **8** Via Natural or Artificial Opening Endoscopic	**2** Anti-infective	**8** Oxazolidinones **9** Other Anti-infective
F Respiratory Tract	**3** Percutaneous **7** Via Natural or Artificial Opening **8** Via Natural or Artificial Opening Endoscopic	**3** Anti-inflammatory **6** Nutritional Substance **7** Electrolytic and Water Balance Substance **B** Anesthetic Agent **H** Radioactive Substance **K** Other Diagnostic Substance **N** Analgesics, Hypnotics, Sedatives **T** Destructive Agent	**Z** No Qualifier
F Respiratory Tract	**3** Percutaneous **7** Via Natural or Artificial Opening **8** Via Natural or Artificial Opening Endoscopic	**G** Other Therapeutic Substance	**C** Other Substance
F Respiratory Tract	**3** Percutaneous **7** Via Natural or Artificial Opening **8** Via Natural or Artificial Opening Endoscopic	**S** Gas	**D** Nitric Oxide **F** Other Gas
F Respiratory Tract	**4** Percutaneous Endoscopic	**G** Other Therapeutic Substance	**C** Other Substance
J Biliary and Pancreatic Tract	**3** Percutaneous **7** Via Natural or Artificial Opening **8** Via Natural or Artificial Opening Endoscopic	**0** Antineoplastic	**4** Liquid Brachytherapy Radioisotope **5** Other Antineoplastic **M** Monoclonal Antibody
J Biliary and Pancreatic Tract	**3** Percutaneous **7** Via Natural or Artificial Opening **8** Via Natural or Artificial Opening Endoscopic	**2** Anti-infective	**8** Oxazolidinones **9** Other Anti-infective
J Biliary and Pancreatic Tract	**3** Percutaneous **7** Via Natural or Artificial Opening **8** Via Natural or Artificial Opening Endoscopic	**3** Anti-inflammatory **6** Nutritional Substance **7** Electrolytic and Water Balance Substance **B** Anesthetic Agent **H** Radioactive Substance **K** Other Diagnostic Substance **N** Analgesics, Hypnotics, Sedatives **T** Destructive Agent	**Z** No Qualifier
J Biliary and Pancreatic Tract	**3** Percutaneous **7** Via Natural or Artificial Opening **8** Via Natural or Artificial Opening Endoscopic	**G** Other Therapeutic Substance	**C** Other Substance
J Biliary and Pancreatic Tract	**3** Percutaneous **7** Via Natural or Artificial Opening **8** Via Natural or Artificial Opening Endoscopic	**S** Gas	**F** Other Gas

♂   All approach, substance, and qualifier values for body system/region (character 4) with this icon
♀   All approach, substance, and qualifier values for body system/region (character 4) with this icon

3E0 Continued on next page

NC Noncovered Procedure   **LC** Limited Coverage   **QA** Questionable OB Admit   **NT** New Tech Add-on   ⊞ Combination Member   ♂ Male   ♀ Female

ICD-10-PCS 2022   721

3   **Administration**
E   **Physiological Systems and Anatomical Regions**
Ø   **Introduction**   Definition: Putting in or on a therapeutic, diagnostic, nutritional, physiological, or prophylactic substance except blood or blood products

3EØ Continued

Body System/Region Character 4		Approach Character 5		Substance Character 6		Qualifier Character 7	
J	Biliary and Pancreatic Tract	3 7 8	Percutaneous Via Natural or Artificial Opening Via Natural or Artificial Opening Endoscopic	U	Pancreatic Islet Cells	Ø 1	Autologous Nonautologous
J	Biliary and Pancreatic Tract	4	Percutaneous Endoscopic	G	Other Therapeutic Substance	C	Other Substance
L	Pleural Cavity	Ø	Open	5	Adhesion Barrier	Z	No Qualifier
L	Pleural Cavity	3	Percutaneous	Ø	Antineoplastic	4 5 M	Liquid Brachytherapy Radioisotope Other Antineoplastic Monoclonal Antibody
L	Pleural Cavity	3	Percutaneous	2	Anti-infective	8 9	Oxazolidinones Other Anti-infective
L	Pleural Cavity	3	Percutaneous	3 5 6 7 B H K N T	Anti-inflammatory Adhesion Barrier Nutritional Substance Electrolytic and Water Balance Substance Anesthetic Agent Radioactive Substance Other Diagnostic Substance Analgesics, Hypnotics, Sedatives Destructive Agent	Z	No Qualifier
L	Pleural Cavity	3	Percutaneous	G	Other Therapeutic Substance	C	Other Substance
L	Pleural Cavity	3	Percutaneous	S	Gas	F	Other Gas
L	Pleural Cavity	4	Percutaneous Endoscopic	5	Adhesion Barrier	Z	No Qualifier
L	Pleural Cavity	4	Percutaneous Endoscopic	G	Other Therapeutic Substance	C	Other Substance
L	Pleural Cavity	7	Via Natural or Artificial Opening	Ø	Antineoplastic	4 5 M	Liquid Brachytherapy Radioisotope Other Antineoplastic Monoclonal Antibody
L	Pleural Cavity	7	Via Natural or Artificial Opening	S	Gas	F	Other Gas
M	Peritoneal Cavity	Ø	Open	5	Adhesion Barrier	Z	No Qualifier
M	Peritoneal Cavity	3	Percutaneous	Ø	Antineoplastic	4 5 M Y	Liquid Brachytherapy Radioisotope Other Antineoplastic Monoclonal Antibody Hyperthermic
M	Peritoneal Cavity	3	Percutaneous	2	Anti-infective	8 9	Oxazolidinones Other Anti-infective
M	Peritoneal Cavity	3	Percutaneous	3 5 6 7 B H K N T	Anti-inflammatory Adhesion Barrier Nutritional Substance Electrolytic and Water Balance Substance Anesthetic Agent Radioactive Substance Other Diagnostic Substance Analgesics, Hypnotics, Sedatives Destructive Agent	Z	No Qualifier
M	Peritoneal Cavity	3	Percutaneous	G	Other Therapeutic Substance	C	Other Substance
M	Peritoneal Cavity	3	Percutaneous	S	Gas	F	Other Gas
M	Peritoneal Cavity	4	Percutaneous Endoscopic	5	Adhesion Barrier	Z	No Qualifier
M	Peritoneal Cavity	4	Percutaneous Endoscopic	G	Other Therapeutic Substance	C	Other Substance
M	Peritoneal Cavity	7	Via Natural or Artificial Opening	Ø	Antineoplastic	4 5 M	Liquid Brachytherapy Radioisotope Other Antineoplastic Monoclonal Antibody
M	Peritoneal Cavity	7	Via Natural or Artificial Opening	S	Gas	F	Other Gas
P	Female Reproductive ♀	Ø	Open	5	Adhesion Barrier	Z	No Qualifier
P	Female Reproductive ♀	3	Percutaneous	Ø	Antineoplastic	4 5 M	Liquid Brachytherapy Radioisotope Other Antineoplastic Monoclonal Antibody
P	Female Reproductive ♀	3	Percutaneous	2	Anti-infective	8 9	Oxazolidinones Other Anti-infective

Valid OR   3EØL4GC
DRG Non-OR   3EØJ[3,7,8]U[Ø,1]
♀   All approach, substance, and qualifier values for body system/region (character 4) with this icon

3EØ Continued on next page

Administration *(side tab)*

3E0 Continued

3   **Administration**
E   **Physiological Systems and Anatomical Regions**
0   **Introduction**   Definition: Putting in or on a therapeutic, diagnostic, nutritional, physiological, or prophylactic substance except blood or blood products

Body System/Region Character 4	Approach Character 5	Substance Character 6	Qualifier Character 7
P Female Reproductive ♀	3 Percutaneous	3 Anti-inflammatory 5 Adhesion Barrier 6 Nutritional Substance 7 Electrolytic and Water Balance Substance B Anesthetic Agent H Radioactive Substance K Other Diagnostic Substance L Sperm N Analgesics, Hypnotics, Sedatives T Destructive Agent V Hormone	Z No Qualifier
P Female Reproductive ♀	3 Percutaneous	G Other Therapeutic Substance	C Other Substance
P Female Reproductive ♀	3 Percutaneous	Q Fertilized Ovum	0 Autologous 1 Nonautologous
P Female Reproductive ♀	3 Percutaneous	S Gas	F Other Gas
P Female Reproductive ♀	4 Percutaneous Endoscopic	5 Adhesion Barrier	Z No Qualifier
P Female Reproductive ♀	4 Percutaneous Endoscopic	G Other Therapeutic Substance	C Other Substance
P Female Reproductive ♀	7 Via Natural or Artificial Opening	0 Antineoplastic	4 Liquid Brachytherapy Radioisotope 5 Other Antineoplastic M Monoclonal Antibody
P Female Reproductive ♀	7 Via Natural or Artificial Opening	2 Anti-infective	8 Oxazolidinones 9 Other Anti-infective
P Female Reproductive ♀	7 Via Natural or Artificial Opening	3 Anti-inflammatory 6 Nutritional Substance 7 Electrolytic and Water Balance Substance B Anesthetic Agent H Radioactive Substance K Other Diagnostic Substance L Sperm N Analgesics, Hypnotics, Sedatives T Destructive Agent V Hormone	Z No Qualifier
P Female Reproductive ♀	7 Via Natural or Artificial Opening	G Other Therapeutic Substance	C Other Substance
P Female Reproductive ♀	7 Via Natural or Artificial Opening	Q Fertilized Ovum	0 Autologous 1 Nonautologous
P Female Reproductive ♀	7 Via Natural or Artificial Opening	S Gas	F Other Gas
P Female Reproductive ♀	8 Via Natural or Artificial Opening Endoscopic	0 Antineoplastic	4 Liquid Brachytherapy Radioisotope 5 Other Antineoplastic M Monoclonal Antibody
P Female Reproductive ♀	8 Via Natural or Artificial Opening Endoscopic	2 Anti-infective	8 Oxazolidinones 9 Other Anit-infection
P Female Reproductive ♀	8 Via Natural or Artificial Opening Endoscopic	3 Anti-inflammatory 6 Nutritional Substance 7 Electrolytic and Water Balance Substance B Anesthetic Agent H Radioactive Substance K Other Diagnostic Substance N Analgesics, Hypnotics, Sedative T Destructive Agent	Z No Qualifier
P Female Reproductive ♀	8 Via Natural or Artificial Opening Endoscopic	G Other Therapeutic Substance	C Other Substance
P Female Reproductive ♀	8 Via Natural or Artificial Opening Endoscopic	S Gas	F Other Gas
Q Cranial Cavity and Brain	0 Open 3 Percutaneous	0 Antineoplastic	4 Liquid Brachytherapy Radioisotope 5 Other Antineoplastic M Monoclonal Antibody
Q Cranial Cavity and Brain	0 Open 3 Percutaneous	2 Anti-infective	8 Oxazolidinones 9 Other Anti-infective

Valid OR   3E0P3Q[0,1]
Valid OR   3E0P7Q[0,1]
DRG Non-OR   3E0Q[0,3]05
♀   All approach, substance, and qualifier values for body system/region (character 4) with this icon

3E0 Continued on next page

3E0–3E0 (side tab)

3 **Administration**   *3E0 Continued*
E **Physiological Systems and Anatomical Regions**
0 **Introduction**   Definition: Putting in or on a therapeutic, diagnostic, nutritional, physiological, or prophylactic substance except blood or blood products

Body System/Region Character 4	Approach Character 5	Substance Character 6	Qualifier Character 7
Q Cranial Cavity and Brain	**0** Open **3** Percutaneous	**3** Anti-inflammatory **6** Nutritional Substance **7** Electrolytic and Water Balance Substance **A** Stem Cells, Embryonic **B** Anesthetic Agent **H** Radioactive Substance **K** Other Diagnostic Substance **N** Analgesics, Hypnotics, Sedatives **T** Destructive Agent	**Z** No Qualifier
Q Cranial Cavity and Brain	**0** Open **3** Percutaneous	**E** Stem Cells, Somatic	**0** Autologous **1** Nonautologous
Q Cranial Cavity and Brain	**0** Open **3** Percutaneous	**G** Other Therapeutic Substance	**C** Other Substance
Q Cranial Cavity and Brain	**0** Open **3** Percutaneous	**S** Gas	**F** Other Gas
Q Cranial Cavity and Brain	**7** Via Natural or Artificial Opening	**0** Antineoplastic	**4** Liquid Brachytherapy Radioisotope **5** Other Antineoplastic **M** Monoclonal Antibody
Q Cranial Cavity and Brain	**7** Via Natural or Artificial Opening	**S** Gas	**F** Other Gas
R Spinal Canal	**0** Open	**A** Stem Cells, Embryonic	**Z** No Qualifier
R Spinal Canal	**0** Open	**E** Stem Cells, Somatic	**0** Autologous **1** Nonautologous
R Spinal Canal	**3** Percutaneous	**0** Antineoplastic	**2** High-dose Interleukin-2 **3** Low-dose Interleukin-2 **4** Liquid Brachytherapy Radioisotope **5** Other Antineoplastic **M** Monoclonal Antibody
R Spinal Canal	**3** Percutaneous	**2** Anti-infective	**8** Oxazolidinones **9** Other Anti-infective
R Spinal Canal	**3** Percutaneous	**3** Anti-inflammatory **6** Nutritional Substance **7** Electrolytic and Water Balance Substance **A** Stem Cells, Embryonic **B** Anesthetic Agent **H** Radioactive Substance **K** Other Diagnostic Substance **N** Analgesics, Hypnotics, Sedatives **T** Destructive Agent	**Z** No Qualifier
R Spinal Canal	**3** Percutaneous	**E** Stem Cells, Somatic	**0** Autologous **1** Nonautologous
R Spinal Canal	**3** Percutaneous	**G** Other Therapeutic Substance	**C** Other Substance
R Spinal Canal	**3** Percutaneous	**S** Gas	**F** Other Gas
R Spinal Canal	**7** Via Natural or Artificial Opening	**S** Gas	**F** Other Gas
S Epidural Space	**3** Percutaneous	**0** Antineoplastic	**2** High-dose Interleukin-2 **3** Low-dose Interleukin-2 **4** Liquid Brachytherapy Radioisotope **5** Other Antineoplastic **M** Monoclonal Antibody
S Epidural Space	**3** Percutaneous	**2** Anti-infective	**8** Oxazolidinones **9** Other Anti-infective
S Epidural Space	**3** Percutaneous	**3** Anti-inflammatory **6** Nutritional Substance **7** Electrolytic and Water Balance Substance **B** Anesthetic Agent **H** Radioactive Substance **K** Other Diagnostic Substance **N** Analgesics, Hypnotics, Sedatives **T** Destructive Agent	**Z** No Qualifier

DRG Non-OR   3E0Q705
DRG Non-OR   3E0R302
DRG Non-OR   3E0S302

3E0 Continued on next page

Non-OR Procedure   DRG Non-OR Procedure   Valid OR Procedure   HAC Associated Procedure   Combination Only   New/Revised GREEN

3   Administration
E   Physiological Systems and Anatomical Regions
Ø   Introduction   Definition: Putting in or on a therapeutic, diagnostic, nutritional, physiological, or prophylactic substance except blood or blood products

3EØ Continued

Body System/Region Character 4	Approach Character 5	Substance Character 6	Qualifier Character 7
S Epidural Space	3 Percutaneous	G Other Therapeutic Substance	C Other Substance
S Epidural Space	3 Percutaneous	S Gas	F Other Gas
S Epidural Space	7 Via Natural or Artificial Opening	S Gas	F Other Gas
T Peripheral Nerves and Plexi X Cranial Nerves	3 Percutaneous	3 Anti-inflammatory B Anesthetic Agent T Destructive Agent	Z No Qualifier
T Peripheral Nerves and Plexi X Cranial Nerves	3 Percutaneous	G Other Therapeutic Substance	C Other Substance
U Joints	Ø Open	2 Anti-infective	8 Oxazolidinones 9 Other Anti-infective
U Joints	Ø Open	G Other Therapeutic Substance	B Recombinant Bone Morphogenetic Protein
U Joints	3 Percutaneous	Ø Antineoplastic	4 Liquid Brachytherapy Radioisotope 5 Other Antineoplastic M Monoclonal Antibody
U Joints	3 Percutaneous	2 Anti-infective	8 Oxazolidinones 9 Other Anti-infective
U Joints	3 Percutaneous	3 Anti-inflammatory 6 Nutritional Substance 7 Electrolytic and Water Balance Substance B Anesthetic Agent H Radioactive Substance K Other Diagnostic Substance N Analgesics, Hypnotics, Sedatives T Destructive Agent	Z No Qualifier
U Joints	3 Percutaneous	G Other Therapeutic Substance	B Recombinant Bone Morphogenetic Protein C Other Substance
U Joints	3 Percutaneous	S Gas	F Other Gas
U Joints	4 Percutaneous Endoscopic	G Other Therapeutic Substance	C Other Substance
V Bones	Ø Open	G Other Therapeutic Substance	B Recombinant Bone Morphogenetic Protein
V Bones	3 Percutaneous	Ø Antineoplastic	5 Other Antineoplastic M Monoclonal Antibody
V Bones	3 Percutaneous	2 Anti-infective	8 Oxazolidinones 9 Other Anti-infective
V Bones	3 Percutaneous	3 Anti-inflammatory 6 Nutritional Substance 7 Electrolytic and Water Balance Substance B Anesthetic Agent H Radioactive Substance K Other Diagnostic Substance N Analgesics, Hypnotics, Sedatives T Destructive Agent	Z No Qualifier
V Bones	3 Percutaneous	G Other Therapeutic Substance	B Recombinant Bone Morphogenetic Protein C Other Substance
W Lymphatics	3 Percutaneous	Ø Antineoplastic	5 Other Antineoplastic M Monoclonal Antibody
W Lymphatics	3 Percutaneous	2 Anti-infective	8 Oxazolidinones 9 Other Anti-infective
W Lymphatics	3 Percutaneous	3 Anti-inflammatory 6 Nutritional Substance 7 Electrolytic and Water Balance Substance B Anesthetic Agent H Radioactive Substance K Other Diagnostic Substance N Analgesics, Hypnotics, Sedatives T Destructive Agent	Z No Qualifier
W Lymphatics	3 Percutaneous	G Other Therapeutic Substance	C Other Substance

3EØ Continued on next page

NC Noncovered Procedure   LC Limited Coverage   QA Questionable OB Admit   NT New Tech Add-on   ⊞ Combination Member   ♂ Male   ♀ Female

Administration

3   **Administration**

E   **Physiological Systems and Anatomical Regions**

Ø   **Introduction**   Definition: Putting in or on a therapeutic, diagnostic, nutritional, physiological, or prophylactic substance except blood or blood products

Body System/Region Character 4	Approach Character 5	Substance Character 6	Qualifier Character 7
Y Pericardial Cavity	3 Percutaneous	Ø Antineoplastic	4 Liquid Brachytherapy Radioisotope 5 Other Antineoplastic M Monoclonal Antibody
Y Pericardial Cavity	3 Percutaneous	2 Anti-infective	8 Oxazolidinones 9 Other Anti-infective
Y Pericardial Cavity	3 Percutaneous	3 Anti-inflammatory 6 Nutritional Substance 7 Electrolytic and Water Balance Substance B Anesthetic Agent H Radioactive Substance K Other Diagnostic Substance N Analgesics, Hypnotics, Sedatives T Destructive Agent	Z No Qualifier
Y Pericardial Cavity	3 Percutaneous	G Other Therapeutic Substance	C Other Substance
Y Pericardial Cavity	3 Percutaneous	S Gas	F Other Gas
Y Pericardial Cavity	4 Percutaneous Endoscopic	G Other Therapeutic Substance	C Other Substance
Y Pericardial Cavity	7 Via Natural or Artificial Opening	Ø Antineoplastic	4 Liquid Brachytherapy Radioisotope 5 Other Antineoplastic M Monoclonal Antibody
Y Pericardial Cavity	7 Via Natural or Artificial Opening	S Gas	F Other Gas

3   **Administration**

E   **Physiological Systems and Anatomical Regions**

1   **Irrigation**   Definition: Putting in or on a cleansing substance

Body System/Region Character 4	Approach Character 5	Substance Character 6	Qualifier Character 7
Ø Skin and Mucous Membranes C Eye	3 Percutaneous X External	8 Irrigating Substance	X Diagnostic Z No Qualifier
9 Nose B Ear F Respiratory Tract G Upper GI H Lower GI J Biliary and Pancreatic Tract K Genitourinary Tract N Male Reproductive ♂ P Female Reproductive ♀	3 Percutaneous 7 Via Natural or Artificial Opening 8 Via Natural or Artificial Opening Endoscopic	8 Irrigating Substance	X Diagnostic Z No Qualifier
L Pleural Cavity Q Cranial Cavity and Brain R Spinal Canal S Epidural Space Y Pericardial Cavity	3 Percutaneous	8 Irrigating Substance	X Diagnostic Z No Qualifier
M Peritoneal Cavity	3 Percutaneous	8 Irrigating Substance	X Diagnostic Z No Qualifier
M Peritoneal Cavity	3 Percutaneous	9 Dialysate	Z No Qualifier
M Peritoneal Cavity	4 Percutaneous Endoscopic	8 Irrigating Substance	X Diagnostic Z No Qualifier
U Joints	3 Percutaneous 4 Percutaneous Endoscopic	8 Irrigating Substance	X Diagnostic Z No Qualifier

♂   3E1N[3,7,8]8[X,Z]

♀   3E1P[3,7,8]8[X,Z]

Measurement and Monitoring 4AØ–4BØ

AHA Coding Clinic for table 4AØ

2020, 4Q, 62	Measurement of intracranial arterial flow
2020, 4Q, 62	Percutaneous endoscopic measurement of portal venous pressure
2020, 4Q, 63	Intercompartmental pressure measurement
2019, 3Q, 32	Endomyocardial biopsy and right heart catheterization
2018, 1Q, 12	Percutaneous balloon valvuloplasty & cardiac catheterization with ventriculogram
2016, 3Q, 37	Fractional flow reserve
2015, 3Q, 29	Approach value for esophageal electrophysiology study

AHA Coding Clinic for table 4A1

2019, 4Q, 38-39	Intraoperative fluorescence lymphatic mapping using Indocyanine green dye
2016, 4Q, 114	Fluorescence vascular angiography
2016, 2Q, 29	Decompressive craniectomy with cryopreservation and storage of bone flap
2016, 2Q, 33	Monitoring of arterial pressure & pulse
2015, 3Q, 35	Swan Ganz catheterization
2015, 2Q, 14	Intraoperative EMG monitoring via endotracheal tube
2015, 1Q, 26	Intraoperative monitoring using Sentio MMG®
2014, 4Q, 28	Removal and replacement of displaced growing rods

4   Measurement and Monitoring
A   Physiological Systems
Ø   Measurement   Definition: Determining the level of a physiological or physical function at a point in time

Body System Character 4	Approach Character 5	Function/Device Character 6	Qualifier Character 7
Ø Central Nervous	Ø Open	2 Conductivity 4 Electrical Activity B Pressure	Z No Qualifier
Ø Central Nervous	3 Percutaneous 7 Via Natural or Artificial Opening 8 Via Natural or Artificial Opening Endoscopic	4 Electrical Activity	Z No Qualifier
Ø Central Nervous	3 Percutaneous 7 Via Natural or Artificial Opening 8 Via Natural or Artificial Opening Endoscopic	B Pressure K Temperature R Saturation	D Intracranial
Ø Central Nervous	X External	2 Conductivity 4 Electrical Activity	Z No Qualifier
1 Peripheral Nervous	Ø Open 3 Percutaneous 7 Via Natural or Artificial Opening 8 Via Natural or Artificial Opening Endoscopic X External	2 Conductivity	9 Sensory B Motor
1 Peripheral Nervous	Ø Open 3 Percutaneous 7 Via Natural or Artificial Opening 8 Via Natural or Artificial Opening Endoscopic X External	4 Electrical Activity	Z No Qualifier
2 Cardiac	Ø Open 3 Percutaneous 7 Via Natural or Artificial Opening 8 Via Natural or Artificial Opening Endoscopic	4 Electrical Activity 9 Output C Rate F Rhythm H Sound P Action Currents	Z No Qualifier
2 Cardiac	Ø Open 3 Percutaneous 7 Via Natural or Artificial Opening 8 Via Natural or Artificial Opening Endoscopic	N Sampling and Pressure	6 Right Heart 7 Left Heart 8 Bilateral
2 Cardiac	X External	4 Electrical Activity	A Guidance Z No Qualifier
2 Cardiac	X External	9 Output C Rate F Rhythm H Sound P Action Currents	Z No Qualifier
2 Cardiac	X External	M Total Activity	4 Stress
3 Arterial	Ø Open 3 Percutaneous	5 Flow J Pulse	1 Peripheral 3 Pulmonary C Coronary
3 Arterial	Ø Open 3 Percutaneous	B Pressure	1 Peripheral 3 Pulmonary C Coronary F Other Thoracic

DRG Non-OR	4AØ2[3,7,8]FZ
DRG Non-OR	4AØ2[Ø,3,7,8]N[6,7,8]

4AØ Continued on next page

NC Noncovered Procedure   LC Limited Coverage   QA Questionable OB Admit   NT New Tech Add-on   ⊞ Combination Member   ♂ Male   ♀ Female

ICD-10-PCS 2022   727

4AØ–4AØ

Measurement and Monitoring

4A0 Continued

4   **Measurement and Monitoring**
A   **Physiological Systems**
0   **Measurement**   Definition: Determining the level of a physiological or physical function at a point in time

Body System Character 4		Approach Character 5		Function/Device Character 6		Qualifier Character 7	
3	Arterial	Ø 3	Open Percutaneous	H R	Sound Saturation	1	Peripheral
3	Arterial	X	External	5	Flow NT	1 D	Peripheral Intracranial
3	Arterial	X	External	B H J R	Pressure Sound Pulse Saturation	1	Peripheral
4	Venous	Ø 3	Open Percutaneous	5 B J	Flow Pressure Pulse	Ø 1 2 3	Central Peripheral Portal Pulmonary
4	Venous	Ø 3	Open Percutaneous	R	Saturation	1	Peripheral
4	Venous	4	Percutaneous Endoscopic	B	Pressure	2	Portal
4	Venous	X	External	5 B J R	Flow Pressure Pulse Saturation	1	Peripheral
5	Circulatory	X	External	L	Volume	Z	No Qualifier
6	Lymphatic	Ø 3 7 8	Open Percutaneous Via Natural or Artificial Opening Via Natural or Artificial Opening Endoscopic	5 B	Flow Pressure	Z	No Qualifier
7	Visual	X	External	Ø 7 B	Acuity Mobility Pressure	Z	No Qualifier
8	Olfactory	X	External	Ø	Acuity	Z	No Qualifier
9	Respiratory	7 8 X	Via Natural or Artificial Opening Via Natural or Artificial Opening Endoscopic External	1 5 C D L M	Capacity Flow Rate Resistance Volume Total Activity	Z	No Qualifier
B	Gastrointestinal	7 8	Via Natural or Artificial Opening Via Natural or Artificial Opening Endoscopic	8 B G	Motility Pressure Secretion	Z	No Qualifier
C	Biliary	3 4 7 8	Percutaneous Percutaneous Endoscopic Via Natural or Artificial Opening Via Natural or Artificial Opening Endoscopic	5 B	Flow Pressure	Z	No Qualifier
D	Urinary	7 8	Via Natural or Artificial Opening Via Natural or Artificial Opening Endoscopic	3 5 B D L	Contractility Flow Pressure Resistance Volume	Z	No Qualifier
F	Musculoskeletal	3	Percutaneous	3	Contractility	Z	No Qualifier
F	Musculoskeletal	3	Percutaneous	B	Pressure	E	Compartment
F	Musculoskeletal	X	External	3	Contractility	Z	No Qualifier
H	Products of Conception, Cardiac ♀	7 8 X	Via Natural or Artificial Opening Via Natural or Artificial Opening Endoscopic External	4 C F H	Electrical Activity Rate Rhythm Sound	Z	No Qualifier
J	Products of Conception, Nervous ♀	7 8 X	Via Natural or Artificial Opening Via Natural or Artificial Opening Endoscopic External	2 4 B	Conductivity Electrical Activity Pressure	Z	No Qualifier
Z	None	7	Via Natural or Artificial Opening	6 K	Metabolism Temperature	Z	No Qualifier
Z	None	X	External	6 K Q	Metabolism Temperature Sleep	Z	No Qualifier

Valid OR	4A060[5,B]Z	♀	4A0H[7,8,X][4,C,F,H]Z
Valid OR	4A0C4[5,B]Z	♀	4A0J[7,8,X][2,4,B]Z
NT	4A03X5D for use of ContaCT		

4 Measurement and Monitoring
A Physiological Systems
1 Monitoring

Definition: Determining the level of a physiological or physical function repetitively over a period of time

Body System Character 4	Approach Character 5	Function/Device Character 6	Qualifier Character 7
Ø Central Nervous	Ø Open	2 Conductivity B Pressure	Z No Qualifier
Ø Central Nervous	Ø Open	4 Electrical Activity	G Intraoperative Z No Qualifier
Ø Central Nervous	3 Percutaneous 7 Via Natural or Artificial Opening 8 Via Natural or Artificial Opening Endoscopic	4 Electrical Activity	G Intraoperative Z No Qualifier
Ø Central Nervous	3 Percutaneous 7 Via Natural or Artificial Opening 8 Via Natural or Artificial Opening Endoscopic	B Pressure K Temperature R Saturation	D Intracranial
Ø Central Nervous	X External	2 Conductivity	Z No Qualifier
Ø Central Nervous	X External	4 Electrical Activity	G Intraoperative Z No Qualifier
1 Peripheral Nervous	Ø Open 3 Percutaneous 7 Via Natural or Artificial Opening 8 Via Natural or Artificial Opening Endoscopic X External	2 Conductivity	9 Sensory B Motor
1 Peripheral Nervous	Ø Open 3 Percutaneous 7 Via Natural or Artificial Opening 8 Via Natural or Artificial Opening Endoscopic X External	4 Electrical Activity	G Intraoperative Z No Qualifier
2 Cardiac	Ø Open 3 Percutaneous 7 Via Natural or Artificial Opening 8 Via Natural or Artificial Opening Endoscopic	4 Electrical Activity 9 Output C Rate F Rhythm H Sound	Z No Qualifier
2 Cardiac	X External	4 Electrical Activity	5 Ambulatory Z No Qualifier
2 Cardiac	X External	9 Output C Rate F Rhythm H Sound	Z No Qualifier
2 Cardiac	X External	M Total Activity	4 Stress
2 Cardiac	X External	S Vascular Perfusion	H Indocyanine Green Dye
3 Arterial	Ø Open 3 Percutaneous	5 Flow B Pressure J Pulse	1 Peripheral 3 Pulmonary C Coronary
3 Arterial	Ø Open 3 Percutaneous	H Sound R Saturation	1 Peripheral
3 Arterial	X External	5 Flow B Pressure H Sound J Pulse R Saturation	1 Peripheral
4 Venous	Ø Open 3 Percutaneous	5 Flow B Pressure J Pulse	Ø Central 1 Peripheral 2 Portal 3 Pulmonary
4 Venous	Ø Open 3 Percutaneous	R Saturation	Ø Central 2 Portal 3 Pulmonary
4 Venous	X External	5 Flow B Pressure J Pulse	1 Peripheral
6 Lymphatic	Ø Open 3 Percutaneous 7 Via Natural or Artificial Opening 8 Via Natural or Artificial Opening Endoscopic	5 Flow	H Indocyanine Green Dye Z No Qualifier

Valid OR   4A1605Z

4A1 Continued on next page

NC Noncovered Procedure   LC Limited Coverage   QA Questionable OB Admit   NT New Tech Add-on   ⊞ Combination Member   ♂ Male   ♀ Female

4A1 Continued

4 Measurement and Monitoring
A Physiological Systems
1 Monitoring Definition: Determining the level of a physiological or physical function repetitively over a period of time

Body System Character 4	Approach Character 5	Function/Device Character 6	Qualifier Character 7
6 Lymphatic	Ø Open 3 Percutaneous 7 Via Natural or Artificial Opening 8 Via Natural or Artificial Opening Endoscopic	B Pressure	Z No Qualifier
9 Respiratory	7 Via Natural or Artificial Opening X External	1 Capacity 5 Flow C Rate D Resistance L Volume	Z No Qualifier
B Gastrointestinal	7 Via Natural or Artificial Opening 8 Via Natural or Artificial Opening Endoscopic	8 Motility B Pressure G Secretion	Z No Qualifier
B Gastrointestinal	X External	S Vascular Perfusion	H Indocyanine Green Dye
D Urinary	7 Via Natural or Artificial Opening 8 Via Natural or Artificial Opening Endoscopic	3 Contractility 5 Flow B Pressure D Resistance L Volume	Z No Qualifier
G Skin and Breast	X External	S Vascular Perfusion	H Indocyanine Green Dye
H Products of Conception, Cardiac ♀	7 Via Natural or Artificial Opening 8 Via Natural or Artificial Opening Endoscopic X External	4 Electrical Activity C Rate F Rhythm H Sound	Z No Qualifier
J Products of Conception, Nervous ♀	7 Via Natural or Artificial Opening 8 Via Natural or Artificial Opening Endoscopic X External	2 Conductivity 4 Electrical Activity B Pressure	Z No Qualifier
Z None	7 Via Natural or Artificial Opening	K Temperature	Z No Qualifier
Z None	X External	K Temperature Q Sleep	Z No Qualifier

Valid OR 4A16ØBZ
♀   4A1H[7,8,X][4,C,F,H]Z
♀   4A1J[7,8,X][2,4,B]Z

4 Measurement and Monitoring
B Physiological Devices
Ø Measurement Definition: Determining the level of a physiological or physical function at a point in time

Body System Character 4	Approach Character 5	Function/Device Character 6	Qualifier Character 7
Ø Central Nervous	X External	V Stimulator	Z No Qualifier
Ø Central Nervous	X External	W Cerebrospinal Fluid Shunt	Ø Wireless Sensor
1 Peripheral Nervous F Musculoskeletal	X External	V Stimulator	Z No Qualifier
2 Cardiac	X External	S Pacemaker T Defibrillator	Z No Qualifier
9 Respiratory	X External	S Pacemaker	Z No Qualifier

Extracorporeal or Systemic Assistance and Performance 5A0–5A2

AHA Coding Clinic for table 5A0

2021, 2Q, 12	Repositioning of displaced intra-aortic balloon pump
2020, 4Q, 64-65	Ventilatory assistance by high flow or high velocity nasal cannula devices
2020, 1Q, 10	Intermittent use of continuous positive airway pressure
2018, 2Q, 3-5	Intra-aortic balloon pump
2017, 4Q, 43-44	Insertion of external heart assist devices
2017, 3Q, 18	Intra-aortic balloon pump removal
2017, 1Q, 10-11	External heart assist device
2017, 1Q, 29	Newborn resuscitation using positive pressure ventilation
2017, 1Q, 29	Newborn noninvasive ventilation
2016, 4Q, 137-139	Heart assist device systems
2014, 4Q, 9	Mechanical ventilation
2014, 3Q, 19	Ablation of ventricular tachycardia with Impella® support
2013, 3Q, 18	Heart transplant surgery

AHA Coding Clinic for table 5A1

2019, 4Q, 39-41	Intraoperative extracorporeal membrane oxygenation
2019, 3Q, 19	Insertion of left ventricular catheter
2019, 3Q, 20	Removal and revision of ECMO component
2019, 3Q, 21	Exchange of extracorporeal membrane oxygenation component (oxygenator)
2019, 2Q, 36	Veno-arterial extracorporeal membrane oxygenation via sternotomy
2019, 3Q, 22	Extracorporeal membrane oxygenation and Centrimag™ pump
2019, 3Q, 22	Extracorporeal membrane oxygenation transfers
2018, 4Q, 52-54	Percutaneous extracorporeal membrane oxygenation
2018, 1Q, 13	Mechanical ventilation using patient's equipment
2017, 4Q, 71-73	Hemodialysis and renal replacement therapy
2017, 3Q, 7	Senning procedure (arterial switch)
2017, 1Q, 19	Norwood Sano procedure
2016, 1Q, 27	Aortocoronary bypass graft utilizing Y-graft
2016, 1Q, 28	Extracorporeal liver assist device
2016, 1Q, 29	Duration of hemodialysis
2015, 4Q, 22-24	Congenital heart corrective procedures
2014, 4Q, 3-10	Mechanical ventilation
2014, 4Q, 11-15	Sequencing of mechanical ventilation with other procedures
2014, 3Q, 16	Repair of Tetralogy of Fallot
2014, 3Q, 20	MAZE procedure performed with coronary artery bypass graft
2014, 1Q, 10	Repair of thoracic aortic aneurysm & coronary artery bypass graft
2013, 3Q, 18	Heart transplant surgery

5   **Extracorporeal or Systemic Assistance and Performance**
A   **Physiological Systems**
0   **Assistance**   Definition: Taking over a portion of a physiological function by extracorporeal means

Body System Character 4	Duration Character 5	Function Character 6	Qualifier Character 7
2 Cardiac	**1** Intermittent **2** Continuous	**1** Output	**0** Balloon Pump **5** Pulsatile Compression **6** Other Pump **D** Impeller Pump
5 Circulatory	**1** Intermittent **2** Continuous	**2** Oxygenation	**1** Hyperbaric **C** Supersaturated
9 Respiratory	**2** Continuous	**0** Filtration	**Z** No Qualifier
9 Respiratory	**3** Less than 24 Consecutive Hours **4** 24-96 Consecutive Hours **5** Greater than 96 Consecutive Hours	**5** Ventilation	**7** Continuous Positive Airway Pressure **8** Intermittent Positive Airway Pressure **9** Continuous Negative Airway Pressure **A** High Nasal Flow/Velocity **B** Intermittent Negative Airway Pressure **Z** No Qualifier

Valid OR   5A02[1,2]1[0,6,D]

NC Noncovered Procedure   LC Limited Coverage   QA Questionable OB Admit   NT New Tech Add-on   ⊞ Combination Member   ♂ Male   ♀ Female

ICD-10-PCS 2022   731

5   Extracorporeal or Systemic Assistance and Performance
A   Physiological Systems
1   Performance   Definition: Completely taking over a physiological function by extracorporeal means

Body System Character 4	Duration Character 5	Function Character 6	Qualifier Character 7
2 Cardiac	**Ø** Single	**1** Output	**2** Manual
2 Cardiac	**1** Intermittent	**3** Pacing	**Z** No Qualifier
2 Cardiac	**2** Continuous	**1** Output	**J** Automated **Z** No Qualifier
2 Cardiac	**2** Continuous	**3** Pacing	**Z** No Qualifier
5 Circulatory	**2** Continuous **A** Intraoperative	**2** Oxygenation	**F** Membrane, Central **G** Membrane, Peripheral Veno-arterial **H** Membrane, Peripheral Veno-venous
9 Respiratory	**Ø** Single	**5** Ventilation	**4** Nonmechanical
9 Respiratory	**3** Less than 24 Consecutive Hours **4** 24-96 Consecutive Hours **5** Greater than 96 Consecutive Hours	**5** Ventilation	**Z** No Qualifier
C Biliary	**Ø** Single **6** Multiple	**Ø** Filtration	**Z** No Qualifier
D Urinary	**7** Intermittent, Less than 6 Hours per day **8** Prolonged Intermittent, 6-18 Hours per day **9** Continuous, Greater than 18 Hours per day	**Ø** Filtration	**Z** No Qualifier

Valid OR   5A1522F
DRG Non-OR   5A1522[G,H]
DRG Non-OR   5A19[3,4]5Z
DRG Non-OR   5A1955Z Length of stay must be > 4 consecutive days.
DRG Non-OR   5A1D[7,8,9]ØZ

5   Extracorporeal or Systemic Assistance and Performance
A   Physiological Systems
2   Restoration   Definition: Returning, or attempting to return, a physiological function to its original state by extracorporeal means.

Body System Character 4	Duration Character 5	Function Character 6	Qualifier Character 7
2 Cardiac	**Ø** Single	**4** Rhythm	**Z** No Qualifier

Extracorporeal or Systemic Therapies 6A0–6AB

AHA Coding Clinic for table 6A4
2019, 2Q, 17   Cryoamputation of lower leg

AHA Coding Clinic for table 6A7
2014, 4Q, 19   Ultrasound accelerated thrombolysis

AHA Coding Clinic for table 6AB
2016, 4Q, 115   Donor organ perfusion

6   Extracorporeal or Systemic Therapies
A   Physiological Systems
0   Atmospheric Control   Definition: Extracorporeal control of atmospheric pressure and composition

Body System Character 4	Duration Character 5	Qualifier Character 6	Qualifier Character 7
Z None	0 Single 1 Multiple	Z No Qualifier	Z No Qualifier

6   Extracorporeal or Systemic Therapies
A   Physiological Systems
1   Decompression   Definition: Extracorporeal elimination of undissolved gas from body fluids

Body System Character 4	Duration Character 5	Qualifier Character 6	Qualifier Character 7
5 Circulatory	0 Single 1 Multiple	Z No Qualifier	Z No Qualifier

6   Extracorporeal or Systemic Therapies
A   Physiological Systems
2   Electromagnetic Therapy   Definition: Extracorporeal treatment by electromagnetic rays

Body System Character 4	Duration Character 5	Qualifier Character 6	Qualifier Character 7
1 Urinary 2 Central Nervous	0 Single 1 Multiple	Z No Qualifier	Z No Qualifier

6   Extracorporeal or Systemic Therapies
A   Physiological Systems
3   Hyperthermia   Definition: Extracorporeal raising of body temperature

Body System Character 4	Duration Character 5	Qualifier Character 6	Qualifier Character 7
Z None	0 Single 1 Multiple	Z No Qualifier	Z No Qualifier

6   Extracorporeal or Systemic Therapies
A   Physiological Systems
4   Hypothermia   Definition: Extracorporeal lowering of body temperature

Body System Character 4	Duration Character 5	Qualifier Character 6	Qualifier Character 7
Z None	0 Single 1 Multiple	Z No Qualifier	Z No Qualifier

6   Extracorporeal or Systemic Therapies
A   Physiological Systems
5   Pheresis   Definition: Extracorporeal separation of blood products

Body System Character 4	Duration Character 5	Qualifier Character 6	Qualifier Character 7
5 Circulatory	0 Single 1 Multiple	Z No Qualifier	0 Erythrocytes 1 Leukocytes 2 Platelets 3 Plasma T Stem Cells, Cord Blood V Stem Cells, Hematopoietic

6   Extracorporeal or Systemic Therapies
A   Physiological Systems
6   Phototherapy   Definition: Extracorporeal treatment by light rays

Body System Character 4	Duration Character 5	Qualifier Character 6	Qualifier Character 7
0 Skin 5 Circulatory	0 Single 1 Multiple	Z No Qualifier	Z No Qualifier

NC Noncovered Procedure   LC Limited Coverage   QA Questionable OB Admit   NT New Tech Add-on   ⊞ Combination Member   ♂ Male   ♀ Female

ICD-10-PCS 2022   733

Extracorporeal or Systemic Therapies

6   Extracorporeal or Systemic Therapies
A   Physiological Systems
7   Ultrasound Therapy   Definition: Extracorporeal treatment by ultrasound

Body System Character 4	Duration Character 5	Qualifier Character 6	Qualifier Character 7
5 Circulatory	Ø Single 1 Multiple	Z No Qualifier	4 Head and Neck Vessels 5 Heart 6 Peripheral Vessels 7 Other Vessels Z No Qualifier

6   Extracorporeal or Systemic Therapies
A   Physiological Systems
8   Ultraviolet Light Therapy   Definition: Extracorporeal treatment by ultraviolet light

Body System Character 4	Duration Character 5	Qualifier Character 6	Qualifier Character 7
Ø Skin	Ø Single 1 Multiple	Z No Qualifier	Z No Qualifier

6   Extracorporeal or Systemic Therapies
A   Physiological Systems
9   Shock Wave Therapy   Definition: Extracorporeal treatment by shock waves

Body System Character 4	Duration Character 5	Qualifier Character 6	Qualifier Character 7
3 Musculoskeletal	Ø Single 1 Multiple	Z No Qualifier	Z No Qualifier

6   Extracorporeal or Systemic Therapies
A   Physiological Systems
B   Perfusion   Definition: Extracorporeal treatment by diffusion of therapeutic fluid

Body System Character 4	Duration Character 5	Qualifier Character 6	Qualifier Character 7
5 Circulatory B Respiratory System F Hepatobiliary System and Pancreas T Urinary System	Ø Single	B Donor Organ	Z No Qualifier

Osteopathic 7WØ

7   **Osteopathic**
W   **Anatomical Regions**
Ø   **Treatment**   Definition: Manual treatment to eliminate or alleviate somatic dysfunction and related disorders

Body Region Character 4	Approach Character 5	Method Character 6	Qualifier Character 7
Ø Head	**X** External	**Ø** Articulatory-Raising	**Z** None
1 Cervical		**1** Fascial Release	
2 Thoracic		**2** General Mobilization	
3 Lumbar		**3** High Velocity-Low Amplitude	
4 Sacrum		**4** Indirect	
5 Pelvis		**5** Low Velocity-High Amplitude	
6 Lower Extremities		**6** Lymphatic Pump	
7 Upper Extremities		**7** Muscle Energy-Isometric	
8 Rib Cage		**8** Muscle Energy-Isotonic	
9 Abdomen		**9** Other Method	

NC Noncovered Procedure   **LC** Limited Coverage   **QA** Questionable OB Admit   **NT** New Tech Add-on   ⊞ Combination Member   ♂ Male   ♀ Female

ICD-10-PCS 2022   **735**

Other Procedures 8C0–8E0

AHA Coding Clinic for table 8E0

2021, 2Q, 19	Electromagnetic stealth guided ventriculoperitoneal shunt insertion with endoscopy
2020, 4Q, 53	Bypass pancreatic duct to stomach
2020, 4Q, 65-66	Near infrared spectroscopy for tissue viability assessment
2020, 4Q, 99	Robotic-assisted prostatectomy with extension of incision for specimen removal
2020, 4Q, 100	Robotic-assisted sigmoid colectomy with extension of incision for specimen removal
2019, 4Q, 41-42	Intraoperative fluorescence guidance
2019, 1Q, 30	Laparoscopic-assisted rectopexy with manual reduction of prolapse
2015, 1Q, 33	Robotic-assisted laparoscopic hysterectomy converted to open procedure
2014, 4Q, 33	Radical prostatectomy

8   Other Procedures
C   Indwelling Device
0   Other Procedures   Definition: Methodologies which attempt to remediate or cure a disorder or disease

Body Region Character 4	Approach Character 5	Method Character 6	Qualifier Character 7
1 Nervous System	**X** External	**6** Collection	**J** Cerebrospinal Fluid **L** Other Fluid
2 Circulatory System	**X** External	**6** Collection	**K** Blood **L** Other Fluid

8   Other Procedures
E   Physiological Systems and Anatomical Regions
0   Other Procedures   Definition: Methodologies which attempt to remediate or cure a disorder or disease

Body Region Character 4	Approach Character 5	Method Character 6	Qualifier Character 7
1 Nervous System **U** Female Reproductive System ♀	**X** External	**Y** Other Method	**7** Examination
2 Circulatory System	**3** Percutaneous **X** External	**D** Near Infrared Spectroscopy	**Z** No Qualifier
9 Head and Neck Region	**0** Open	**C** Robotic Assisted Procedure	**Z** No Qualifier
9 Head and Neck Region	**0** Open	**E** Fluorescence Guided Procedure	**M** Aminolevulinic Acid **Z** No Qualifier
9 Head and Neck Region	**3** Percutaneous **4** Percutaneous Endoscopic **7** Via Natural or Artificial Opening **8** Via Natural or Artificial Opening Endoscopic	**C** Robotic Assisted Procedure **E** Fluorescence Guided Procedure	**Z** No Qualifier
9 Head and Neck Region	**X** External	**B** Computer Assisted Procedure	**F** With Fluoroscopy **G** With Computerized Tomography **H** With Magnetic Resonance Imaging **Z** No Qualifier
9 Head and Neck Region	**X** External	**C** Robotic Assisted Procedure	**Z** No Qualifier
9 Head and Neck Region	**X** External	**Y** Other Method	**8** Suture Removal
H Integumentary System and Breast	**3** Percutaneous	**0** Acupuncture	**0** Anesthesia **Z** No Qualifier
H Integumentary System and Breast ♀	**X** External	**6** Collection	**2** Breast Milk
H Integumentary System and Breast	**X** External	**Y** Other Method	**9** Piercing
K Musculoskeletal System	**X** External	**1** Therapeutic Massage	**Z** No Qualifier
K Musculoskeletal System	**X** External	**Y** Other Method	**7** Examination
V Male Reproductive System ♂	**X** External	**1** Therapeutic Massage	**C** Prostate **D** Rectum
V Male Reproductive System ♂	**X** External	**6** Collection	**3** Sperm
W Trunk Region	**0** Open **3** Percutaneous **4** Percutaneous Endoscopic **7** Via Natural or Artificial Opening **8** Via Natural or Artificial Opening Endoscopic	**C** Robotic Assisted Procedure **E** Fluorescence Guided Procedure	**Z** No Qualifier
W Trunk Region	**X** External	**B** Computer Assisted Procedure	**F** With Fluoroscopy **G** With Computerized Tomography **H** With Magnetic Resonance Imaging **Z** No Qualifier
W Trunk Region	**X** External	**C** Robotic Assisted Procedure	**Z** No Qualifier
W Trunk Region	**X** External	**Y** Other Method	**8** Suture Removal
X Upper Extremity **Y** Lower Extremity	**0** Open **3** Percutaneous **4** Percutaneous Endoscopic	**C** Robotic Assisted Procedure **E** Fluorescence Guided Procedure	**Z** No Qualifier

♂	8E0VX1C	♀	8E0UXY7
♂	8E0VX63	♀	8E0HX62

8E0 Continued on next page

NC Noncovered Procedure   **LC** Limited Coverage   **UA** Questionable OB Admit   **NT** New Tech Add-on   ⊞ Combination Member   ♂ Male   ♀ Female

ICD-10-PCS 2022   737

8C0–8E0

8   **Other Procedures**
E   **Physiological Systems and Anatomical Regions**
Ø   **Other Procedures**   Definition: Methodologies which attempt to remediate or cure a disorder or disease

Body Region Character 4		Approach Character 5		Method Character 6		Qualifier Character 7	
X	Upper Extremity	**X**	External	**B**	Computer Assisted Procedure	**F**	With Fluoroscopy
Y	Lower Extremity					**G**	With Computerized Tomography
						H	With Magnetic Resonance Imaging
						Z	No Qualifier
X	Upper Extremity	**X**	External	**C**	Robotic Assisted Procedure	**Z**	No Qualifier
Y	Lower Extremity						
X	Upper Extremity	**X**	External	**Y**	Other Method	**8**	Suture Removal
Y	Lower Extremity						
Z	None	**X**	External	**Y**	Other Method	**1**	In Vitro Fertilization
						4	Yoga Therapy
						5	Meditation
						6	Isolation

Chiropractic 9WB

9   Chiropractic
W   Anatomical Regions
B   Manipulation   Definition: Manual procedure that involves a directed thrust to move a joint past the physiological range of motion, without exceeding the anatomical limit

Body Region Character 4	Approach Character 5	Method Character 6	Qualifier Character 7
Ø Head	X External	B Non-Manual	Z None
1 Cervical		C Indirect Visceral	
2 Thoracic		D Extra-Articular	
3 Lumbar		F Direct Visceral	
4 Sacrum		G Long Lever Specific Contact	
5 Pelvis		H Short Lever Specific Contact	
6 Lower Extremities		J Long and Short Lever Specific Contact	
7 Upper Extremities		K Mechanically Assisted	
8 Rib Cage		L Other Method	
9 Abdomen			

NC Noncovered Procedure   LC Limited Coverage   QA Questionable OB Admit   NT New Tech Add-on   ⊞ Combination Member   ♂ Male   ♀ Female

ICD-10-PCS 2022   739

Imaging BØØ–BY4

AHA Coding Clinic for table B21

2018, 1Q, 12	Percutaneous balloon valvuloplasty & cardiac catheterization with ventriculogram
2016, 3Q, 36	Type of contrast medium for angiography (high osmolar, low osmolar, and other)

AHA Coding Clinic for table B41

2015, 3Q, 9	Aborted endovascular stenting of superficial femoral artery

AHA Coding Clinic for table B51

2015, 4Q, 30	Vascular access devices

AHA Coding Clinic for table BF4

2014, 3Q, 15	Drainage of pancreatic pseudocyst
2020, 4Q, 66	Other imaging type

AHA Coding Clinic for table BF5

2020, 4Q, 66	Other imaging type
2020, 4Q, 66-67	Fluorescence imaging of hepatobiliary system

AHA Coding Clinic for table BW5

2020, 4Q, 66	Other imaging type
2020, 4Q, 68	Bacterial autofluorescence detection

B　Imaging
Ø　Central Nervous System
Ø　Plain Radiography　Definition: Planar display of an image developed from the capture of external ionizing radiation on photographic or photoconductive plate

Body Part Character 4	Contrast Character 5	Qualifier Character 6	Qualifier Character 7
B　Spinal Cord	Ø　High Osmolar 1　Low Osmolar Y　Other Contrast Z　None	Z　None	Z　None

B　Imaging
Ø　Central Nervous System
1　Fluoroscopy　Definition: Single plane or bi-plane real time display of an image developed from the capture of external ionizing radioation on a fluorescent screen. The image may also be stored by either digital or analog means.

Body Part Character 4	Contrast Character 5	Qualifier Character 6	Qualifier Character 7
B　Spinal Cord	Ø　High Osmolar 1　Low Osmolar Y　Other Contrast Z　None	Z　None	Z　None

B　Imaging
Ø　Central Nervous System
2　Computerized Tomography (CT Scan) Definition: Computer reformatted digital display of multiplanar images developed from the capture of multiple exposures of external ionizing radiation

Body Part Character 4	Contrast Character 5	Qualifier Character 6	Qualifier Character 7
Ø　Brain 7　Cisterna 8　Cerebral Ventricle(s) 9　Sella Turcica/Pituitary Gland B　Spinal Cord	Ø　High Osmolar 1　Low Osmolar Y　Other Contrast	Ø　Unenhanced and Enhanced Z　None	Z　None
Ø　Brain 7　Cisterna 8　Cerebral Ventricle(s) 9　Sella Turcica/Pituitary Gland B　Spinal Cord	Z　None	Z　None	Z　None

B　Imaging
Ø　Central Nervous System
3　Magnetic Resonance Imaging (MRI)　Definition: Computer reformatted digital display of multiplanar images developed from the capture of radio-frequency signals emitted by nuclei in a body site excited within a magnetic field

Body Part Character 4	Contrast Character 5	Qualifier Character 6	Qualifier Character 7
Ø　Brain 9　Sella Turcica/Pituitary Gland B　Spinal Cord C　Acoustic Nerves	Y　Other Contrast	Ø　Unenhanced and Enhanced Z　None	Z　None
Ø　Brain 9　Sella Turcica/Pituitary Gland B　Spinal Cord C　Acoustic Nerves	Z　None	Z　None	Z　None

NC Noncovered Procedure　　**LC** Limited Coverage　　**QA** Questionable OB Admit　　**NT** New Tech Add-on　　⊞ Combination Member　　♂ Male　　♀ Female

ICD-10-PCS 2022　　741

B0Ø–B03

B   **Imaging**
0   **Central Nervous System**
4   **Ultrasonography**   Definition: Real time display of images of anatomy or flow information developed from the capture of reflected and attenuated high frequency sound waves

Body Part Character 4	Contrast Character 5	Qualifier Character 6	Qualifier Character 7
0 Brain B Spinal Cord	Z None	Z None	Z None

B   **Imaging**
2   **Heart**
0   **Plain Radiography**   Definition: Planar display of an image developed from the capture of external ionizing radiation on photographic or photoconductive plate

Body Part Character 4	Contrast Character 5	Qualifier Character 6	Qualifier Character 7
0 Coronary Artery, Single 1 Coronary Arteries, Multiple 2 Coronary Artery Bypass Graft, Single 3 Coronary Artery Bypass Grafts, Multiple 4 Heart, Right 5 Heart, Left 6 Heart, Right and Left 7 Internal Mammary Bypass Graft, Right 8 Internal Mammary Bypass Graft, Left F Bypass Graft, Other	0 High Osmolar 1 Low Osmolar Y Other Contrast	Z None	Z None

DRG Non-OR All body part, contrast, and qualifier values

B   **Imaging**
2   **Heart**
1   **Fluoroscopy**   Definition: Single plane or bi-plane real time display of an image developed from the capture of external ionizing radioation on a fluorescent screen. The image may also be stored by either digital or analog means.

Body Part Character 4	Contrast Character 5	Qualifier Character 6	Qualifier Character 7
0 Coronary Artery, Single 1 Coronary Arteries, Multiple 2 Coronary Artery Bypass Graft, Single 3 Coronary Artery Bypass Grafts, Multiple	0 High Osmolar 1 Low Osmolar Y Other Contrast	1 Laser	0 Intraoperative
0 Coronary Artery, Single 1 Coronary Arteries, Multiple 2 Coronary Artery Bypass Graft, Single 3 Coronary Artery Bypass Grafts, Multiple	0 High Osmolar 1 Low Osmolar Y Other Contrast	Z None	Z None
4 Heart, Right 5 Heart, Left 6 Heart, Right and Left 7 Internal Mammary Bypass Graft, Right 8 Internal Mammary Bypass Graft, Left F Bypass Graft, Other	0 High Osmolar 1 Low Osmolar Y Other Contrast	Z None	Z None

DRG Non-OR B21[0,1,2,3][0,1,Y]ZZ
DRG Non-OR B21[4,5,6,7,8,F][0,1,Y]ZZ

B   **Imaging**
2   **Heart**
2   **Computerized Tomography (CT Scan)** Definition: Computer reformatted digital display of multiplanar images developed from the capture of multiple exposures of external ionizing radiation

Body Part Character 4	Contrast Character 5	Qualifier Character 6	Qualifier Character 7
1 Coronary Arteries, Multiple 3 Coronary Artery Bypass Grafts, Multiple 6 Heart, Right and Left	0 High Osmolar 1 Low Osmolar Y Other Contrast	0 Unenhanced and Enhanced Z None	Z None
1 Coronary Arteries, Multiple 3 Coronary Artery Bypass Grafts, Multiple 6 Heart, Right and Left	Z None	2 Intravascular Optical Coherence Z None	Z None

B Imaging
2 Heart
3 Magnetic Resonance Imaging (MRI)   Definition: Computer reformatted digital display of multiplanar images developed from the capture of radio-frequency signals emitted by nuclei in a body site excited within a magnetic field

Body Part Character 4	Contrast Character 5	Qualifier Character 6	Qualifier Character 7
1 Coronary Arteries, Multiple 3 Coronary Artery Bypass Grafts, Multiple 6 Heart, Right and Left	Y Other Contrast	Ø Unenhanced and Enhanced Z None	Z None
1 Coronary Arteries, Multiple 3 Coronary Artery Bypass Grafts, Multiple 6 Heart, Right and Left	Z None	Z None	Z None

B Imaging
2 Heart
4 Ultrasonography   Definition: Real time display of images of anatomy or flow information developed from the capture of reflected and attenuated high frequency sound waves

Body Part Character 4	Contrast Character 5	Qualifier Character 6	Qualifier Character 7
Ø Coronary Artery, Single 1 Coronary Arteries, Multiple 4 Heart, Right 5 Heart, Left 6 Heart, Right and Left B Heart with Aorta C Pericardium D Pediatric Heart	Y Other Contrast	Z None	Z None
Ø Coronary Artery, Single 1 Coronary Arteries, Multiple 4 Heart, Right 5 Heart, Left 6 Heart, Right and Left B Heart with Aorta C Pericardium D Pediatric Heart	Z None	Z None	3 Intravascular 4 Transesophageal Z None

B Imaging
3 Upper Arteries
Ø Plain Radiography   Definition: Planar display of an image developed from the capture of external ionizing radiation on photographic or photoconductive plate

Body Part Character 4	Contrast Character 5	Qualifier Character 6	Qualifier Character 7
Ø Thoracic Aorta 1 Brachiocephalic-Subclavian Artery, Right 2 Subclavian Artery, Left 3 Common Carotid Artery, Right 4 Common Carotid Artery, Left 5 Common Carotid Arteries, Bilateral 6 Internal Carotid Artery, Right 7 Internal Carotid Artery, Left 8 Internal Carotid Arteries, Bilateral 9 External Carotid Artery, Right B External Carotid Artery, Left C External Carotid Arteries, Bilateral D Vertebral Artery, Right F Vertebral Artery, Left G Vertebral Arteries, Bilateral H Upper Extremity Arteries, Right J Upper Extremity Arteries, Left K Upper Extremity Arteries, Bilateral L Intercostal and Bronchial Arteries M Spinal Arteries N Upper Arteries, Other P Thoraco-Abdominal Aorta Q Cervico-Cerebral Arch R Intracranial Arteries S Pulmonary Artery, Right T Pulmonary Artery, Left	Ø High Osmolar 1 Low Osmolar Y Other Contrast Z None	Z None	Z None

Imaging

B **Imaging**
3 **Upper Arteries**
1 **Fluoroscopy**   Definition: Single plane or bi-plane real time display of an image developed from the capture of external ionizing radiation on a fluorescent screen. The image may also be stored by either digital or analog means.

Body Part Character 4	Contrast Character 5	Qualifier Character 6	Qualifier Character 7
Ø Thoracic Aorta	**Ø** High Osmolar	**1** Laser	**Ø** Intraoperative
1 Brachiocephalic-Subclavian Artery, Right	**1** Low Osmolar		
2 Subclavian Artery, Left	**Y** Other Contrast		
3 Common Carotid Artery, Right			
4 Common Carotid Artery, Left			
5 Common Carotid Arteries, Bilateral			
6 Internal Carotid Artery, Right			
7 Internal Carotid Artery, Left			
8 Internal Carotid Arteries, Bilateral			
9 External Carotid Artery, Right			
B External Carotid Artery, Left			
C External Carotid Arteries, Bilateral			
D Vertebral Artery, Right			
F Vertebral Artery, Left			
G Vertebral Arteries, Bilateral			
H Upper Extremity Arteries, Right			
J Upper Extremity Arteries, Left			
K Upper Extremity Arteries, Bilateral			
L Intercostal and Bronchial Arteries			
M Spinal Arteries			
N Upper Arteries, Other			
P Thoraco-Abdominal Aorta			
Q Cervico-Cerebral Arch			
R Intracranial Arteries			
S Pulmonary Artery, Right			
T Pulmonary Artery, Left			
U Pulmonary Trunk			
Ø Thoracic Aorta	**Ø** High Osmolar	**Z** None	**Z** None
1 Brachiocephalic-Subclavian Artery, Right	**1** Low Osmolar		
2 Subclavian Artery, Left	**Y** Other Contrast		
3 Common Carotid Artery, Right			
4 Common Carotid Artery, Left			
5 Common Carotid Arteries, Bilateral			
6 Internal Carotid Artery, Right			
7 Internal Carotid Artery, Left			
8 Internal Carotid Arteries, Bilateral			
9 External Carotid Artery, Right			
B External Carotid Artery, Left			
C External Carotid Arteries, Bilateral			
D Vertebral Artery, Right			
F Vertebral Artery, Left			
G Vertebral Arteries, Bilateral			
H Upper Extremity Arteries, Right			
J Upper Extremity Arteries, Left			
K Upper Extremity Arteries, Bilateral			
L Intercostal and Bronchial Arteries			
M Spinal Arteries			
N Upper Arteries, Other			
P Thoraco-Abdominal Aorta			
Q Cervico-Cerebral Arch			
R Intracranial Arteries			
S Pulmonary Artery, Right			
T Pulmonary Artery, Left			
U Pulmonary Trunk			

B31 Continued on next page

Non-OR Procedure   DRG Non-OR Procedure   Valid OR Procedure   HAC Associated Procedure   Combination Only   New/Revised GREEN

B31 Continued

B   **Imaging**
3   **Upper Arteries**
1   **Fluoroscopy**   Definition: Single plane or bi-plane real time display of an image developed from the capture of external ionizing radiation on a fluorescent screen. The image may also be stored by either digital or analog means.

Body Part Character 4	Contrast Character 5	Qualifier Character 6	Qualifier Character 7
Ø Thoracic Aorta	**Z** None	**Z** None	**Z** None
1 Brachiocephalic-Subclavian Artery, Right			
2 Subclavian Artery, Left			
3 Common Carotid Artery, Right			
4 Common Carotid Artery, Left			
5 Common Carotid Arteries, Bilateral			
6 Internal Carotid Artery, Right			
7 Internal Carotid Artery, Left			
8 Internal Carotid Arteries, Bilateral			
9 External Carotid Artery, Right			
B External Carotid Artery, Left			
C External Carotid Arteries, Bilateral			
D Vertebral Artery, Right			
F Vertebral Artery, Left			
G Vertebral Arteries, Bilateral			
H Upper Extremity Arteries, Right			
J Upper Extremity Arteries, Left			
K Upper Extremity Arteries, Bilateral			
L Intercostal and Bronchial Arteries			
M Spinal Arteries			
N Upper Arteries, Other			
P Thoraco-Abdominal Aorta			
Q Cervico-Cerebral Arch			
R Intracranial Arteries			
S Pulmonary Artery, Right			
T Pulmonary Artery, Left			
U Pulmonary Trunk			

B   **Imaging**
3   **Upper Arteries**
2   **Computerized Tomography (CT Scan)**   Definition: Computer reformatted digital display of multiplanar images developed from the capture of multiple exposures of external ionizing radiation

Body Part Character 4	Contrast Character 5	Qualifier Character 6	Qualifier Character 7
Ø Thoracic Aorta	**Ø** High Osmolar	**Z** None	**Z** None
5 Common Carotid Arteries, Bilateral	**1** Low Osmolar		
8 Internal Carotid Arteries, Bilateral	**Y** Other Contrast		
G Vertebral Arteries, Bilateral			
R Intracranial Arteries			
S Pulmonary Artery, Right			
T Pulmonary Artery, Left			
Ø Thoracic Aorta	**Z** None	**2** Intravascular Optical Coherence	**Z** None
5 Common Carotid Arteries, Bilateral		**Z** None	
8 Internal Carotid Arteries, Bilateral			
G Vertebral Arteries, Bilateral			
R Intracranial Arteries			
S Pulmonary Artery, Right			
T Pulmonary Artery, Left			

NC Noncovered Procedure   **LC** Limited Coverage   **QA** Questionable OB Admit   **NT** New Tech Add-on   ⊞ Combination Member   ♂ Male   ♀ Female

ICD-10-PCS 2022   745

B31–B32

B   **Imaging**
3   **Upper Arteries**
3   **Magnetic Resonance Imaging (MRI)**   Definition: Computer reformatted digital display of multiplanar images developed from the capture of radio-frequency signals emitted by nuclei in a body site excited within a magnetic field

Body Part Character 4	Contrast Character 5	Qualifier Character 6	Qualifier Character 7
Ø Thoracic Aorta **5** Common Carotid Arteries, Bilateral **8** Internal Carotid Arteries, Bilateral **G** Vertebral Arteries, Bilateral **H** Upper Extremity Arteries, Right **J** Upper Extremity Arteries, Left **K** Upper Extremity Arteries, Bilateral **M** Spinal Arteries **Q** Cervico-Cerebral Arch **R** Intracranial Arteries	**Y** Other Contrast	**Ø** Unenhanced and Enhanced **Z** None	**Z** None
Ø Thoracic Aorta **5** Common Carotid Arteries, Bilateral **8** Internal Carotid Arteries, Bilateral **G** Vertebral Arteries, Bilateral **H** Upper Extremity Arteries, Right **J** Upper Extremity Arteries, Left **K** Upper Extremity Arteries, Bilateral **M** Spinal Arteries **Q** Cervico-Cerebral Arch **R** Intracranial Arteries	**Z** None	**Z** None	**Z** None

B   **Imaging**
3   **Upper Arteries**
4   **Ultrasonography**   Definition: Real time display of images of anatomy or flow information developed from the capture of reflected and attenuated high frequency sound waves

Body Part Character 4	Contrast Character 5	Qualifier Character 6	Qualifier Character 7
Ø Thoracic Aorta **1** Brachiocephalic-Subclavian Artery, Right **2** Subclavian Artery, Left **3** Common Carotid Artery, Right **4** Common Carotid Artery, Left **5** Common Carotid Arteries, Bilateral **6** Internal Carotid Artery, Right **7** Internal Carotid Artery, Left **8** Internal Carotid Arteries, Bilateral **H** Upper Extremity Arteries, Right **J** Upper Extremity Arteries, Left **K** Upper Extremity Arteries, Bilateral **R** Intracranial Arteries **S** Pulmonary Artery, Right **T** Pulmonary Artery, Left **V** Ophthalmic Arteries	**Z** None	**Z** None	**3** Intravascular **Z** None

B   **Imaging**
4   **Lower Arteries**
Ø   **Plain Radiography**   Definition: Planar display of an image developed from the capture of external ionizing radiation on photographic or photoconductive plate

Body Part Character 4	Contrast Character 5	Qualifier Character 6	Qualifier Character 7
Ø Abdominal Aorta **2** Hepatic Artery **3** Splenic Arteries **4** Superior Mesenteric Artery **5** Inferior Mesenteric Artery **6** Renal Artery, Right **7** Renal Artery, Left **8** Renal Arteries, Bilateral **9** Lumbar Arteries **B** Intra-Abdominal Arteries, Other **C** Pelvic Arteries **D** Aorta and Bilateral Lower Extremity Arteries **F** Lower Extremity Arteries, Right **G** Lower Extremity Arteries, Left **J** Lower Arteries, Other **M** Renal Artery Transplant	**Ø** High Osmolar **1** Low Osmolar **Y** Other Contrast	**Z** None	**Z** None

B   **Imaging**
4   **Lower Arteries**
1   **Fluoroscopy**   Definition: Single plane or bi-plane real time display of an image developed from the capture of external ionizing radiation on a fluorescent screen. The image may also be stored by either digital or analog means.

Body Part Character 4	Contrast Character 5	Qualifier Character 6	Qualifier Character 7
Ø Abdominal Aorta **2** Hepatic Artery **3** Splenic Arteries **4** Superior Mesenteric Artery **5** Inferior Mesenteric Artery **6** Renal Artery, Right **7** Renal Artery, Left **8** Renal Arteries, Bilateral **9** Lumbar Arteries **B** Intra-Abdominal Arteries, Other **C** Pelvic Arteries **D** Aorta and Bilateral Lower Extremity Arteries **F** Lower Extremity Arteries, Right **G** Lower Extremity Arteries, Left **J** Lower Arteries, Other	**Ø** High Osmolar **1** Low Osmolar **Y** Other Contrast	**1** Laser	**Ø** Intraoperative
Ø Abdominal Aorta **2** Hepatic Artery **3** Splenic Arteries **4** Superior Mesenteric Artery **5** Inferior Mesenteric Artery **6** Renal Artery, Right **7** Renal Artery, Left **8** Renal Arteries, Bilateral **9** Lumbar Arteries **B** Intra-Abdominal Arteries, Other **C** Pelvic Arteries **D** Aorta and Bilateral Lower Extremity Arteries **F** Lower Extremity Arteries, Right **G** Lower Extremity Arteries, Left **J** Lower Arteries, Other	**Ø** High Osmolar **1** Low Osmolar **Y** Other Contrast	**Z** None	**Z** None
Ø Abdominal Aorta **2** Hepatic Artery **3** Splenic Arteries **4** Superior Mesenteric Artery **5** Inferior Mesenteric Artery **6** Renal Artery, Right **7** Renal Artery, Left **8** Renal Arteries, Bilateral **9** Lumbar Arteries **B** Intra-Abdominal Arteries, Other **C** Pelvic Arteries **D** Aorta and Bilateral Lower Extremity Arteries **F** Lower Extremity Arteries, Right **G** Lower Extremity Arteries, Left **J** Lower Arteries, Other	**Z** None	**Z** None	**Z** None

NC Noncovered Procedure   LC Limited Coverage   QA Questionable OB Admit   NT New Tech Add-on   ⊞ Combination Member   ♂ Male   ♀ Female

ICD-10-PCS 2022   747

B41–B41

B   **Imaging**
4   **Lower Arteries**
2   **Computerized Tomography (CT Scan)** Definition: Computer reformatted digital display of multiplanar images developed from the capture of multiple exposures of external ionizing radiation

Body Part Character 4	Contrast Character 5	Qualifier Character 6	Qualifier Character 7
Ø Abdominal Aorta 1 Celiac Artery 4 Superior Mesenteric Artery 8 Renal Arteries, Bilateral C Pelvic Arteries F Lower Extremity Arteries, Right G Lower Extremity Arteries, Left H Lower Extremity Arteries, Bilateral M Renal Artery Transplant	Ø High Osmolar 1 Low Osmolar Y Other Contrast	Z None	Z None
Ø Abdominal Aorta 1 Celiac Artery 4 Superior Mesenteric Artery 8 Renal Arteries, Bilateral C Pelvic Arteries F Lower Extremity Arteries, Right G Lower Extremity Arteries, Left H Lower Extremity Arteries, Bilateral M Renal Artery Transplant	Z None	2 Intravascular Optical Coherence Z None	Z None

B   **Imaging**
4   **Lower Arteries**
3   **Magnetic Resonance Imaging (MRI)** Definition: Computer reformatted digital display of multiplanar images developed from the capture of radio-frequency signals emitted by nuclei in a body site excited within a magnetic field

Body Part Character 4	Contrast Character 5	Qualifier Character 6	Qualifier Character 7
Ø Abdominal Aorta 1 Celiac Artery 4 Superior Mesenteric Artery 8 Renal Arteries, Bilateral C Pelvic Arteries F Lower Extremity Arteries, Right G Lower Extremity Arteries, Left H Lower Extremity Arteries, Bilateral	Y Other Contrast	Ø Unenhanced and Enhanced Z None	Z None
Ø Abdominal Aorta 1 Celiac Artery 4 Superior Mesenteric Artery 8 Renal Arteries, Bilateral C Pelvic Arteries F Lower Extremity Arteries, Right G Lower Extremity Arteries, Left H Lower Extremity Arteries, Bilateral	Z None	Z None	Z None

B   **Imaging**
4   **Lower Arteries**
4   **Ultrasonography** Definition: Real time display of images of anatomy or flow information developed from the capture of reflected and attenuated high frequency sound waves

Body Part Character 4	Contrast Character 5	Qualifier Character 6	Qualifier Character 7
Ø Abdominal Aorta 4 Superior Mesenteric Artery 5 Inferior Mesenteric Artery 6 Renal Artery, Right 7 Renal Artery, Left 8 Renal Arteries, Bilateral B Intra-Abdominal Arteries, Other F Lower Extremity Arteries, Right G Lower Extremity Arteries, Left H Lower Extremity Arteries, Bilateral K Celiac and Mesenteric Arteries L Femoral Artery N Penile Arteries	Z None	Z None	3 Intravascular Z None

B Imaging
5 Veins
Ø Plain Radiography   Definition: Planar display of an image developed from the capture of external ionizing radiation on photographic or photoconductive plate

Body Part Character 4	Contrast Character 5	Qualifier Character 6	Qualifier Character 7
Ø Epidural Veins	Ø High Osmolar	Z None	Z None
1 Cerebral and Cerebellar Veins	1 Low Osmolar		
2 Intracranial Sinuses	Y Other Contrast		
3 Jugular Veins, Right			
4 Jugular Veins, Left			
5 Jugular Veins, Bilateral			
6 Subclavian Vein, Right			
7 Subclavian Vein, Left			
8 Superior Vena Cava			
9 Inferior Vena Cava			
B Lower Extremity Veins, Right			
C Lower Extremity Veins, Left			
D Lower Extremity Veins, Bilateral			
F Pelvic (Iliac) Veins, Right			
G Pelvic (Iliac) Veins, Left			
H Pelvic (Iliac) Veins, Bilateral			
J Renal Vein, Right			
K Renal Vein, Left			
L Renal Veins, Bilateral			
M Upper Extremity Veins, Right			
N Upper Extremity Veins, Left			
P Upper Extremity Veins, Bilateral			
Q Pulmonary Vein, Right			
R Pulmonary Vein, Left			
S Pulmonary Veins, Bilateral			
T Portal and Splanchnic Veins			
V Veins, Other			
W Dialysis Shunt/Fistula			

B Imaging
5 Veins
1 Fluoroscopy   Definition: Single plane or bi-plane real time display of an image developed from the capture of external ionizing radioation on a fluorescent screen. The image may also be stored by either digital or analog means.

Body Part Character 4	Contrast Character 5	Qualifier Character 6	Qualifier Character 7
Ø Epidural Veins	Ø High Osmolar	Z None	A Guidance
1 Cerebral and Cerebellar Veins	1 Low Osmolar		Z None
2 Intracranial Sinuses	Y Other Contrast		
3 Jugular Veins, Right	Z None		
4 Jugular Veins, Left			
5 Jugular Veins, Bilateral			
6 Subclavian Vein, Right			
7 Subclavian Vein, Left			
8 Superior Vena Cava			
9 Inferior Vena Cava			
B Lower Extremity Veins, Right			
C Lower Extremity Veins, Left			
D Lower Extremity Veins, Bilateral			
F Pelvic (Iliac) Veins, Right			
G Pelvic (Iliac) Veins, Left			
H Pelvic (Iliac) Veins, Bilateral			
J Renal Vein, Right			
K Renal Vein, Left			
L Renal Veins, Bilateral			
M Upper Extremity Veins, Right			
N Upper Extremity Veins, Left			
P Upper Extremity Veins, Bilateral			
Q Pulmonary Vein, Right			
R Pulmonary Vein, Left			
S Pulmonary Veins, Bilateral			
T Portal and Splanchnic Veins			
V Veins, Other			
W Dialysis Shunt/Fistula			

NC Noncovered Procedure   **LC** Limited Coverage   **QA** Questionable OB Admit   **NT** New Tech Add-on   ⊞ Combination Member   ♂ Male   ♀ Female

ICD-10-PCS 2022   **749**

B5Ø–B51

B Imaging
5 Veins
2 Computerized Tomography (CT Scan) Definition: Computer reformatted digital display of multiplanar images developed from the capture of multiple exposures of external ionizing radiation

Body Part Character 4	Contrast Character 5	Qualifier Character 6	Qualifier Character 7
2 Intracranial Sinuses 8 Superior Vena Cava 9 Inferior Vena Cava F Pelvic (Iliac) Veins, Right G Pelvic (Iliac) Veins, Left H Pelvic (Iliac) Veins, Bilateral J Renal Vein, Right K Renal Vein, Left L Renal Veins, Bilateral Q Pulmonary Vein, Right R Pulmonary Vein, Left S Pulmonary Veins, Bilateral T Portal and Splanchnic Veins	Ø High Osmolar 1 Low Osmolar Y Other Contrast	Ø Unenhanced and Enhanced Z None	Z None
2 Intracranial Sinuses 8 Superior Vena Cava 9 Inferior Vena Cava F Pelvic (Iliac) Veins, Right G Pelvic (Iliac) Veins, Left H Pelvic (Iliac) Veins, Bilateral J Renal Vein, Right K Renal Vein, Left L Renal Veins, Bilateral Q Pulmonary Vein, Right R Pulmonary Vein, Left S Pulmonary Veins, Bilateral T Portal and Splanchnic Veins	Z None	2 Intravascular Optical Coherence Z None	Z None

B Imaging
5 Veins
3 Magnetic Resonance Imaging (MRI) Definition: Computer reformatted digital display of multiplanar images developed from the capture of radio-frequency signals emitted by nuclei in a body site excited within a magnetic field

Body Part Character 4	Contrast Character 5	Qualifier Character 6	Qualifier Character 7
1 Cerebral and Cerebellar Veins 2 Intracranial Sinuses 5 Jugular Veins, Bilateral 8 Superior Vena Cava 9 Inferior Vena Cava B Lower Extremity Veins, Right C Lower Extremity Veins, Left D Lower Extremity Veins, Bilateral H Pelvic (Iliac) Veins, Bilateral L Renal Veins, Bilateral M Upper Extremity Veins, Right N Upper Extremity Veins, Left P Upper Extremity Veins, Bilateral S Pulmonary Veins, Bilateral T Portal and Splanchnic Veins V Veins, Other	Y Other Contrast	Ø Unenhanced and Enhanced Z None	Z None
1 Cerebral and Cerebellar Veins 2 Intracranial Sinuses 5 Jugular Veins, Bilateral 8 Superior Vena Cava 9 Inferior Vena Cava B Lower Extremity Veins, Right C Lower Extremity Veins, Left D Lower Extremity Veins, Bilateral H Pelvic (Iliac) Veins, Bilateral L Renal Veins, Bilateral M Upper Extremity Veins, Right N Upper Extremity Veins, Left P Upper Extremity Veins, Bilateral S Pulmonary Veins, Bilateral T Portal and Splanchnic Veins V Veins, Other	Z None	Z None	Z None

B   **Imaging**
5   **Veins**
4   **Ultrasonography**   Definition: Real time display of images of anatomy or flow information developed from the capture of reflected and attenuated high frequency sound waves

Body Part Character 4	Contrast Character 5	Qualifier Character 6	Qualifier Character 7
3 Jugular Veins, Right 4 Jugular Veins, Left 6 Subclavian Vein, Right 7 Subclavian Vein, Left 8 Superior Vena Cava 9 Inferior Vena Cava B Lower Extremity Veins, Right C Lower Extremity Veins, Left D Lower Extremity Veins, Bilateral J Renal Vein, Right K Renal Vein, Left L Renal Veins, Bilateral M Upper Extremity Veins, Right N Upper Extremity Veins, Left P Upper Extremity Veins, Bilateral T Portal and Splanchnic Veins	Z None	Z None	3 Intravascular A Guidance Z None

B   **Imaging**
7   **Lymphatic System**
Ø   **Plain Radiography**   Definition: Planar display of an image developed from the capture of external ionizing radiation on photographic or photoconductive plate

Body Part Character 4	Contrast Character 5	Qualifier Character 6	Qualifier Character 7

Ø Abdominal/Retroperitoneal
    Lymphatics, Unilateral
1 Abdominal/Retroperitoneal
    Lymphatics, Bilateral
4 Lymphatics, Head and Neck
5 Upper Extremity Lymphatics, Right
6 Upper Extremity Lymphatics, Left
7 Upper Extremity Lymphatics,
    Bilateral
8 Lower Extremity Lymphatics, Right
9 Lower Extremity Lymphatics, Left
B Lower Extremity Lymphatics,
    Bilateral
C Lymphatics, Pelvic
	Ø High Osmolar
	1 Low Osmolar
	Y Other Contrast
		Z None	Z None

B   **Imaging**
8   **Eye**
Ø   **Plain Radiography**   Definition: Planar display of an image developed from the capture of external ionizing radiation on photographic or photoconductive plate

Body Part Character 4	Contrast Character 5	Qualifier Character 6	Qualifier Character 7
Ø Lacrimal Duct, Right 1 Lacrimal Duct, Left 2 Lacrimal Ducts, Bilateral	Ø High Osmolar 1 Low Osmolar Y Other Contrast	Z None	Z None
3 Optic Foramina, Right 4 Optic Foramina, Left 5 Eye, Right 6 Eye, Left 7 Eyes, Bilateral	Z None	Z None	Z None

B   **Imaging**
8   **Eye**
2   **Computerized Tomography (CT Scan)**   Definition: Computer reformatted digital display of multiplanar images developed from the capture of multiple exposures of external ionizing radiation

Body Part Character 4	Contrast Character 5	Qualifier Character 6	Qualifier Character 7
5 Eye, Right 6 Eye, Left 7 Eyes, Bilateral	Ø High Osmolar 1 Low Osmolar Y Other Contrast	Ø Unenhanced and Enhanced Z None	Z None
5 Eye, Right 6 Eye, Left 7 Eyes, Bilateral	Z None	Z None	Z None

NC Noncovered Procedure   LC Limited Coverage   QA Questionable OB Admit   NT New Tech Add-on   ⊞ Combination Member   ♂ Male   ♀ Female

ICD-10-PCS 2022   751

B54–B82

Imaging

B　Imaging
8　Eye
3　Magnetic Resonance Imaging (MRI)　Definition: Computer reformatted digital display of multiplanar images developed from the capture of radio-frequency signals emitted by nuclei in a body site excited within a magnetic field

Body Part Character 4	Contrast Character 5	Qualifier Character 6	Qualifier Character 7
5　Eye, Right 6　Eye, Left 7　Eyes, Bilateral	Y　Other Contrast	Ø　Unenhanced and Enhanced Z　None	Z　None
5　Eye, Right 6　Eye, Left 7　Eyes, Bilateral	Z　None	Z　None	Z　None

B　Imaging
8　Eye
4　Ultrasonography　Definition: Real time display of images of anatomy or flow information developed from the capture of reflected and attenuated high frequency sound waves

Body Part Character 4	Contrast Character 5	Qualifier Character 6	Qualifier Character 7
5　Eye, Right 6　Eye, Left 7　Eyes, Bilateral	Z　None	Z　None	Z　None

B　Imaging
9　Ear, Nose, Mouth and Throat
Ø　Plain Radiography　Definition: Planar display of an image developed from the capture of external ionizing radiation on photographic or photoconductive plate

Body Part Character 4	Contrast Character 5	Qualifier Character 6	Qualifier Character 7
2　Paranasal Sinuses F　Nasopharynx/Oropharynx H　Mastoids	Z　None	Z　None	Z　None
4　Parotid Gland, Right 5　Parotid Gland, Left 6　Parotid Glands, Bilateral 7　Submandibular Gland, Right 8　Submandibular Gland, Left 9　Submandibular Glands, Bilateral B　Salivary Gland, Right C　Salivary Gland, Left D　Salivary Glands, Bilateral	Ø　High Osmolar 1　Low Osmolar Y　Other Contrast	Z　None	Z　None

B　Imaging
9　Ear, Nose, Mouth and Throat
1　Fluoroscopy　Definition: Single plane or bi-plane real time display of an image developed from the capture of external ionizing radioation on a fluorescent screen. The image may also be stored by either digital or analog means.

Body Part Character 4	Contrast Character 5	Qualifier Character 6	Qualifier Character 7
G　Pharynx and Epiglottis J　Larynx	Y　Other Contrast Z　None	Z　None	Z　None

B　Imaging
9　Ear, Nose, Mouth and Throat
2　Computerized Tomography (CT Scan)　Definition: Computer reformatted digital display of multiplanar images developed from the capture of multiple exposures of external ionizing radiation

Body Part Character 4	Contrast Character 5	Qualifier Character 6	Qualifier Character 7
Ø　Ear 2　Paranasal Sinuses 6　Parotid Glands, Bilateral 9　Submandibular Glands, Bilateral D　Salivary Glands, Bilateral F　Nasopharynx/Oropharynx J　Larynx	Ø　High Osmolar 1　Low Osmolar Y　Other Contrast	Ø　Unenhanced and Enhanced Z　None	Z　None
Ø　Ear 2　Paranasal Sinuses 6　Parotid Glands, Bilateral 9　Submandibular Glands, Bilateral D　Salivary Glands, Bilateral F　Nasopharynx/Oropharynx J　Larynx	Z　None	Z　None	Z　None

Non-OR Procedure　　　DRG Non-OR Procedure　　　Valid OR Procedure　　　HAC Associated Procedure　　　Combination Only　　　New/Revised GREEN

B　Imaging
9　Ear, Nose, Mouth and Throat
3　Magnetic Resonance Imaging (MRI)　Definition: Computer reformatted digital display of multiplanar images developed from the capture of radio-frequency signals emitted by nuclei in a body site excited within a magnetic field

Body Part Character 4	Contrast Character 5	Qualifier Character 6	Qualifier Character 7
Ø　Ear 2　Paranasal Sinuses 6　Parotid Glands, Bilateral 9　Submandibular Glands, Bilateral D　Salivary Glands, Bilateral F　Nasopharynx/Oropharynx J　Larynx	Y　Other Contrast	Ø　Unenhanced and Enhanced Z　None	Z　None
Ø　Ear 2　Paranasal Sinuses 6　Parotid Glands, Bilateral 9　Submandibular Glands, Bilateral D　Salivary Glands, Bilateral F　Nasopharynx/Oropharynx J　Larynx	Z　None	Z　None	Z　None

B　Imaging
B　Respiratory System
Ø　Plain Radiography　Definition: Planar display of an image developed from the capture of external ionizing radiation on photographic or photoconductive plate

Body Part Character 4	Contrast Character 5	Qualifier Character 6	Qualifier Character 7
7　Tracheobronchial Tree, Right 8　Tracheobronchial Tree, Left 9　Tracheobronchial Trees, Bilateral	Y　Other Contrast	Z　None	Z　None
D　Upper Airways	Z　None	Z　None	Z　None

B　Imaging
B　Respiratory System
1　Fluoroscopy　Definition: Single plane or bi-plane real time display of an image developed from the capture of external ionizing radioation on a fluorescent screen. The image may also be stored by either digital or analog means.

Body Part Character 4	Contrast Character 5	Qualifier Character 6	Qualifier Character 7
2　Lung, Right 3　Lung, Left 4　Lungs, Bilateral 6　Diaphragm C　Mediastinum D　Upper Airways	Z　None	Z　None	Z　None
7　Tracheobronchial Tree, Right 8　Tracheobronchial Tree, Left 9　Tracheobronchial Trees, Bilateral	Y　Other Contrast	Z　None	Z　None

B　Imaging
B　Respiratory System
2　Computerized Tomography (CT Scan)　Definition: Computer reformatted digital display of multiplanar images developed from the capture of multiple exposures of external ionizing radiation

Body Part Character 4	Contrast Character 5	Qualifier Character 6	Qualifier Character 7
4　Lungs, Bilateral 7　Tracheobronchial Tree, Right 8　Tracheobronchial Tree, Left 9　Tracheobronchial Trees, Bilateral F　Trachea/Airways	Ø　High Osmolar 1　Low Osmolar Y　Other Contrast	Ø　Unenhanced and Enhanced Z　None	Z　None
4　Lungs, Bilateral 7　Tracheobronchial Tree, Right 8　Tracheobronchial Tree, Left 9　Tracheobronchial Trees, Bilateral F　Trachea/Airways	Z　None	Z　None	Z　None

NC Noncovered Procedure　　LC Limited Coverage　　QA Questionable OB Admit　　NT New Tech Add-on　　⊞ Combination Member　　♂ Male　　♀ Female

ICD-10-PCS 2022　　　753

B93–BB2

B   Imaging
B   Respiratory System
3   Magnetic Resonance Imaging (MRI)   Definition: Computer reformatted digital display of multiplanar images developed from the capture of radio-frequency signals emitted by nuclei in a body site excited within a magnetic field

Body Part Character 4	Contrast Character 5	Qualifier Character 6	Qualifier Character 7
G Lung Apices	Y Other Contrast	Ø Unenhanced and Enhanced Z None	Z None
G Lung Apices	Z None	Z None	Z None

B   Imaging
B   Respiratory System
4   Ultrasonography   Definition: Real time display of images of anatomy or flow information developed from the capture of reflected and attenuated high frequency sound waves

Body Part Character 4	Contrast Character 5	Qualifier Character 6	Qualifier Character 7
B Pleura C Mediastinum	Z None	Z None	Z None

B   Imaging
D   Gastrointestinal System
1   Fluoroscopy   Definition: Single plane or bi-plane real time display of an image developed from the capture of external ionizing radioation on a fluorescent screen. The image may also be stored by either digital or analog means.

Body Part Character 4	Contrast Character 5	Qualifier Character 6	Qualifier Character 7
1 Esophagus 2 Stomach 3 Small Bowel 4 Colon 5 Upper GI 6 Upper GI and Small Bowel 9 Duodenum B Mouth/Oropharynx	Y Other Contrast Z None	Z None	Z None

B   Imaging
D   Gastrointestinal System
2   Computerized Tomography (CT Scan)   Definition: Computer reformatted digital display of multiplanar images developed from the capture of multiple exposures of external ionizing radiation

Body Part Character 4	Contrast Character 5	Qualifier Character 6	Qualifier Character 7
4 Colon	Ø High Osmolar 1 Low Osmolar Y Other Contrast	Ø Unenhanced and Enhanced Z None	Z None
4 Colon	Z None	Z None	Z None

B   Imaging
D   Gastrointestinal System
4   Ultrasonography   Definition: Real time display of images of anatomy or flow information developed from the capture of reflected and attenuated high frequency sound waves

Body Part Character 4	Contrast Character 5	Qualifier Character 6	Qualifier Character 7
1 Esophagus 2 Stomach 7 Gastrointestinal Tract 8 Appendix 9 Duodenum C Rectum	Z None	Z None	Z None

B   Imaging
F   Hepatobiliary System and Pancreas
Ø   Plain Radiography   Definition: Planar display of an image developed from the capture of external ionizing radiation on photographic or photoconductive plate

Body Part Character 4	Contrast Character 5	Qualifier Character 6	Qualifier Character 7
Ø Bile Ducts 3 Gallbladder and Bile Ducts C Hepatobiliary System, All	Ø High Osmolar 1 Low Osmolar Y Other Contrast	Z None	Z None

B   Imaging
F   Hepatobiliary System and Pancreas
1   Fluoroscopy   Definition: Single plane or bi-plane real time display of an image developed from the capture of external ionizing radioation on a fluorescent screen. The image may also be stored by either digital or analog means.

Body Part Character 4	Contrast Character 5	Qualifier Character 6	Qualifier Character 7
Ø Bile Ducts 1 Biliary and Pancreatic Ducts 2 Gallbladder 3 Gallbladder and Bile Ducts 4 Gallbladder, Bile Ducts and Pancreatic Ducts 8 Pancreatic Ducts	Ø High Osmolar 1 Low Osmolar Y Other Contrast	Z None	Z None
5 Liver	Ø High Osmolar 1 Low Osmolar Y Other Contrast	Z None	Z None
5 Liver	Z None	Z None	A Guidance

B   Imaging
F   Hepatobiliary System and Pancreas
2   Computerized Tomography (CT Scan)   Definition: Computer reformatted digital display of multiplanar images developed from the capture of multiple exposures of external ionizing radiation

Body Part Character 4	Contrast Character 5	Qualifier Character 6	Qualifier Character 7
5 Liver 6 Liver and Spleen 7 Pancreas C Hepatobiliary System, All	Ø High Osmolar 1 Low Osmolar Y Other Contrast	Ø Unenhanced and Enhanced Z None	Z None
5 Liver 6 Liver and Spleen 7 Pancreas C Hepatobiliary System, All	Z None	Z None	Z None

B   Imaging
F   Hepatobiliary System and Pancreas
3   Magnetic Resonance Imaging (MRI)   Definition: Computer reformatted digital display of multiplanar images developed from the capture of radio-frequency signals emitted by nuclei in a body site excited within a magnetic field

Body Part Character 4	Contrast Character 5	Qualifier Character 6	Qualifier Character 7
5 Liver 6 Liver and Spleen 7 Pancreas	Y Other Contrast	Ø Unenhanced and Enhanced Z None	Z None
5 Liver 6 Liver and Spleen 7 Pancreas	Z None	Z None	Z None

B   Imaging
F   Hepatobiliary System and Pancreas
4   Ultrasonography   Definition: Real time display of images of anatomy or flow information developed from the capture of reflected and attenuated high frequency sound waves

Body Part Character 4	Contrast Character 5	Qualifier Character 6	Qualifier Character 7
Ø Bile Ducts 2 Gallbladder 3 Gallbladder and Bile Ducts 5 Liver 6 Liver and Spleen 7 Pancreas C Hepatobiliary System, All	Z None	Z None	Z None

B   Imaging
F   Hepatobiliary System and Pancreas
5   Other Imaging   Definition: Other specified modality for visualizing a body part

Body Part Character 4	Contrast Character 5	Qualifier Character 6	Qualifier Character 7
Ø Bile Ducts 2 Gallbladder 3 Gallbladder and Bile Ducts 5 Liver 6 Liver and Spleen 7 Pancreas C Hepatobiliary System, All	2 Fluorescing Agent	Ø Indocyanine Green Dye Z None	Ø Intraoperative Z None

NC Noncovered Procedure   LC Limited Coverage   QA Questionable OB Admit   NT New Tech Add-on   ⊞ Combination Member   ♂ Male   ♀ Female

ICD-10-PCS 2022   755

BF1–BF5

B   **Imaging**
G   **Endocrine System**
2   **Computerized Tomography (CT Scan)** Definition: Computer reformatted digital display of multiplanar images developed from the capture of multiple exposures of external ionizing radiation

Body Part Character 4	Contrast Character 5	Qualifier Character 6	Qualifier Character 7
2 Adrenal Glands, Bilateral 3 Parathyroid Glands 4 Thyroid Gland	Ø High Osmolar 1 Low Osmolar Y Other Contrast	Ø Unenhanced and Enhanced Z None	Z None
2 Adrenal Glands, Bilateral 3 Parathyroid Glands 4 Thyroid Gland	Z None	Z None	Z None

B   **Imaging**
G   **Endocrine System**
3   **Magnetic Resonance Imaging (MRI)**   Definition: Computer reformatted digital display of multiplanar images developed from the capture of radio-frequency signals emitted by nuclei in a body site excited within a magnetic field

Body Part Character 4	Contrast Character 5	Qualifier Character 6	Qualifier Character 7
2 Adrenal Glands, Bilateral 3 Parathyroid Glands 4 Thyroid Gland	Y Other Contrast	Ø Unenhanced and Enhanced Z None	Z None
2 Adrenal Glands, Bilateral 3 Parathyroid Glands 4 Thyroid Gland	Z None	Z None	Z None

B   **Imaging**
G   **Endocrine System**
4   **Ultrasonography**   Definition: Real time display of images of anatomy or flow information developed from the capture of reflected and attenuated high frequency sound waves

Body Part Character 4	Contrast Character 5	Qualifier Character 6	Qualifier Character 7
Ø Adrenal Gland, Right 1 Adrenal Gland, Left 2 Adrenal Glands, Bilateral 3 Parathyroid Glands 4 Thyroid Gland	Z None	Z None	Z None

B   **Imaging**
H   **Skin, Subcutaneous Tissue and Breast**
Ø   **Plain Radiography**   Definition: Planar display of an image developed from the capture of external ionizing radiation on photographic or photoconductive plate

Body Part Character 4	Contrast Character 5	Qualifier Character 6	Qualifier Character 7
Ø Breast, Right 1 Breast, Left 2 Breasts, Bilateral	Z None	Z None	Z None
3 Single Mammary Duct, Right 4 Single Mammary Duct, Left 5 Multiple Mammary Ducts, Right 6 Multiple Mammary Ducts, Left	Ø High Osmolar 1 Low Osmolar Y Other Contrast Z None	Z None	Z None

Non-OR Procedure   DRG Non-OR Procedure   Valid OR Procedure   HAC Associated Procedure   Combination Only   New/Revised GREEN
756   ICD-10-PCS 2022

BG2–BHØ

B   **Imaging**
H   **Skin, Subcutaneous Tissue and Breast**
3   **Magnetic Resonance Imaging (MRI)**   Definition: Computer reformatted digital display of multiplanar images developed from the capture of radio-frequency signals emitted by nuclei in a body site excited within a magnetic field

Body Part Character 4	Contrast Character 5	Qualifier Character 6	Qualifier Character 7
Ø Breast, Right **1** Breast, Left **2** Breasts, Bilateral **D** Subcutaneous Tissue, Head/Neck **F** Subcutaneous Tissue, Upper Extremity **G** Subcutaneous Tissue, Thorax **H** Subcutaneous Tissue, Abdomen and Pelvis **J** Subcutaneous Tissue, Lower Extremity	**Y** Other Contrast	**Ø** Unenhanced and Enhanced **Z** None	**Z** None
Ø Breast, Right **1** Breast, Left **2** Breasts, Bilateral **D** Subcutaneous Tissue, Head/Neck **F** Subcutaneous Tissue, Upper Extremity **G** Subcutaneous Tissue, Thorax **H** Subcutaneous Tissue, Abdomen and Pelvis **J** Subcutaneous Tissue, Lower Extremity	**Z** None	**Z** None	**Z** None

B   **Imaging**
H   **Skin, Subcutaneous Tissue and Breast**
4   **Ultrasonography**   Definition: Real time display of images of anatomy or flow information developed from the capture of reflected and attenuated high frequency sound waves

Body Part Character 4	Contrast Character 5	Qualifier Character 6	Qualifier Character 7
Ø Breast, Right **1** Breast, Left **2** Breasts, Bilateral **7** Extremity, Upper **8** Extremity, Lower **9** Abdominal Wall **B** Chest Wall **C** Head and Neck	**Z** None	**Z** None	**Z** None

B   **Imaging**
L   **Connective Tissue**
3   **Magnetic Resonance Imaging (MRI)**   Definition: Computer reformatted digital display of multiplanar images developed from the capture of radio-frequency signals emitted by nuclei in a body site excited within a magnetic field

Body Part Character 4	Contrast Character 5	Qualifier Character 6	Qualifier Character 7
Ø Connective Tissue, Upper Extremity **1** Connective Tissue, Lower Extremity **2** Tendons, Upper Extremity **3** Tendons, Lower Extremity	**Y** Other Contrast	**Ø** Unenhanced and Enhanced **Z** None	**Z** None
Ø Connective Tissue, Upper Extremity **1** Connective Tissue, Lower Extremity **2** Tendons, Upper Extremity **3** Tendons, Lower Extremity	**Z** None	**Z** None	**Z** None

B   **Imaging**
L   **Connective Tissue**
4   **Ultrasonography**   Definition: Real time display of images of anatomy or flow information developed from the capture of reflected and attenuated high frequency sound waves

Body Part Character 4	Contrast Character 5	Qualifier Character 6	Qualifier Character 7
Ø Connective Tissue, Upper Extremity **1** Connective Tissue, Lower Extremity **2** Tendons, Upper Extremity **3** Tendons, Lower Extremity	**Z** None	**Z** None	**Z** None

NC Noncovered Procedure   **LC** Limited Coverage   **QA** Questionable OB Admit   **NT** New Tech Add-on   ⊞ Combination Member   ♂ Male   ♀ Female

ICD-10-PCS 2022   **757**

BH3–BL4

B　Imaging
N　Skull and Facial Bones
Ø　Plain Radiography　Definition: Planar display of an image developed from the capture of external ionizing radiation on photographic or photoconductive plate

Body Part Character 4	Contrast Character 5	Qualifier Character 6	Qualifier Character 7
Ø　Skull 1　Orbit, Right 2　Orbit, Left 3　Orbits, Bilateral 4　Nasal Bones 5　Facial Bones 6　Mandible B　Zygomatic Arch, Right C　Zygomatic Arch, Left D　Zygomatic Arches, Bilateral G　Tooth, Single H　Teeth, Multiple J　Teeth, All	Z　None	Z　None	Z　None
7　Temporomandibular Joint, Right 8　Temporomandibular Joint, Left 9　Temporomandibular Joints, 　　Bilateral	Ø　High Osmolar 1　Low Osmolar Y　Other Contrast Z　None	Z　None	Z　None

B　Imaging
N　Skull and Facial Bones
1　Fluoroscopy　Definition: Single plane or bi-plane real time display of an image developed from the capture of external ionizing radioation on a fluorescent screen. The image may also be stored by either digital or analog means.

Body Part Character 4	Contrast Character 5	Qualifier Character 6	Qualifier Character 7
7　Temporomandibular Joint, Right 8　Temporomandibular Joint, Left 9　Temporomandibular Joints, 　　Bilateral	Ø　High Osmolar 1　Low Osmolar Y　Other Contrast Z　None	Z　None	Z　None

B　Imaging
N　Skull and Facial Bones
2　Computerized Tomography (CT Scan)　Definition: Computer reformatted digital display of multiplanar images developed from the capture of multiple exposures of external ionizing radiation

Body Part Character 4	Contrast Character 5	Qualifier Character 6	Qualifier Character 7
Ø　Skull 3　Orbits, Bilateral 5　Facial Bones 6　Mandible 9　Temporomandibular Joints, 　　Bilateral F　Temporal Bones	Ø　High Osmolar 1　Low Osmolar Y　Other Contrast Z　None	Z　None	Z　None

B　Imaging
N　Skull and Facial Bones
3　Magnetic Resonance Imaging (MRI)　Definition: Computer reformatted digital display of multiplanar images developed from the capture of radio-frequency signals emitted by nuclei in a body site excited within a magnetic field

Body Part Character 4	Contrast Character 5	Qualifier Character 6	Qualifier Character 7
9　Temporomandibular Joints, 　　Bilateral	Y　Other Contrast Z　None	Z　None	Z　None

B Imaging
P Non-Axial Upper Bones
Ø Plain Radiography　Definition: Planar display of an image developed from the capture of external ionizing radiation on photographic or photoconductive plate

Body Part Character 4	Contrast Character 5	Qualifier Character 6	Qualifier Character 7
Ø Sternoclavicular Joint, Right 1 Sternoclavicular Joint, Left 2 Sternoclavicular Joints, Bilateral 3 Acromioclavicular Joints, Bilateral 4 Clavicle, Right 5 Clavicle, Left 6 Scapula, Right 7 Scapula, Left A Humerus, Right B Humerus, Left E Upper Arm, Right F Upper Arm, Left J Forearm, Right K Forearm, Left N Hand, Right P Hand, Left R Finger(s), Right S Finger(s), Left X Ribs, Right Y Ribs, Left	Z None	Z None	Z None
8 Shoulder, Right 9 Shoulder, Left C Hand/Finger Joint, Right D Hand/Finger Joint, Left G Elbow, Right H Elbow, Left L Wrist, Right M Wrist, Left	Ø High Osmolar 1 Low Osmolar Y Other Contrast Z None	Z None	Z None

B Imaging
P Non-Axial Upper Bones
1 Fluoroscopy　Definition: Single plane or bi-plane real time display of an image developed from the capture of external ionizing radioation on a fluorescent screen. The image may also be stored by either digital or analog means.

Body Part Character 4	Contrast Character 5	Qualifier Character 6	Qualifier Character 7
Ø Sternoclavicular Joint, Right 1 Sternoclavicular Joint, Left 2 Sternoclavicular Joints, Bilateral 3 Acromioclavicular Joints, Bilateral 4 Clavicle, Right 5 Clavicle, Left 6 Scapula, Right 7 Scapula, Left A Humerus, Right B Humerus, Left E Upper Arm, Right F Upper Arm, Left J Forearm, Right K Forearm, Left N Hand, Right P Hand, Left R Finger(s), Right S Finger(s), Left X Ribs, Right Y Ribs, Left	Z None	Z None	Z None
8 Shoulder, Right 9 Shoulder, Left L Wrist, Right M Wrist, Left	Ø High Osmolar 1 Low Osmolar Y Other Contrast Z None	Z None	Z None
C Hand/Finger Joint, Right D Hand/Finger Joint, Left G Elbow, Right H Elbow, Left	Ø High Osmolar 1 Low Osmolar Y Other Contrast	Z None	Z None

NC Noncovered Procedure　**LC** Limited Coverage　**QA** Questionable OB Admit　**NT** New Tech Add-on　⊞ Combination Member　♂ Male　♀ Female

ICD-10-PCS 2022　　　　　　　　　　　　　　　　　　　　　　　　　　　　759

BP0–BP1

B   **Imaging**
P   **Non-Axial Upper Bones**
2   **Computerized Tomography (CT Scan)** Definition: Computer reformatted digital display of multiplanar images developed from the capture of multiple exposures of external ionizing radiation

Body Part Character 4	Contrast Character 5	Qualifier Character 6	Qualifier Character 7
0 Sternoclavicular Joint, Right **1** Sternoclavicular Joint, Left **W** Thorax	**0** High Osmolar **1** Low Osmolar **Y** Other Contrast	**Z** None	**Z** None
2 Sternoclavicular Joints, Bilateral **3** Acromioclavicular Joints, Bilateral **4** Clavicle, Right **5** Clavicle, Left **6** Scapula, Right **7** Scapula, Left **8** Shoulder, Right **9** Shoulder, Left **A** Humerus, Right **B** Humerus, Left **E** Upper Arm, Right **F** Upper Arm, Left **G** Elbow, Right **H** Elbow, Left **J** Forearm, Right **K** Forearm, Left **L** Wrist, Right **M** Wrist, Left **N** Hand, Right **P** Hand, Left **Q** Hands and Wrists, Bilateral **R** Finger(s), Right **S** Finger(s), Left **T** Upper Extremity, Right **U** Upper Extremity, Left **V** Upper Extremities, Bilateral **X** Ribs, Right **Y** Ribs, Left	**0** High Osmolar **1** Low Osmolar **Y** Other Contrast **Z** None	**Z** None	**Z** None
C Hand/Finger Joint, Right **D** Hand/Finger Joint, Left	**Z** None	**Z** None	**Z** None

B   **Imaging**
P   **Non-Axial Upper Bones**
3   **Magnetic Resonance Imaging (MRI)** Definition: Computer reformatted digital display of multiplanar images developed from the capture of radio-frequency signals emitted by nuclei in a body site excited within a magnetic field

Body Part Character 4	Contrast Character 5	Qualifier Character 6	Qualifier Character 7
8 Shoulder, Right **9** Shoulder, Left **C** Hand/Finger Joint, Right **D** Hand/Finger Joint, Left **E** Upper Arm, Right **F** Upper Arm, Left **G** Elbow, Right **H** Elbow, Left **J** Forearm, Right **K** Forearm, Left **L** Wrist, Right **M** Wrist, Left	**Y** Other Contrast	**0** Unenhanced and Enhanced **Z** None	**Z** None
8 Shoulder, Right **9** Shoulder, Left **C** Hand/Finger Joint, Right **D** Hand/Finger Joint, Left **E** Upper Arm, Right **F** Upper Arm, Left **G** Elbow, Right **H** Elbow, Left **J** Forearm, Right **K** Forearm, Left **L** Wrist, Right **M** Wrist, Left	**Z** None	**Z** None	**Z** None

B   **Imaging**
P   **Non-Axial Upper Bones**
4   **Ultrasonography**   Definition: Real time display of images of anatomy or flow information developed from the capture of reflected and attenuated high frequency sound waves

Body Part Character 4	Contrast Character 5	Qualifier Character 6	Qualifier Character 7
8 Shoulder, Right 9 Shoulder, Left G Elbow, Right H Elbow, Left L Wrist, Right M Wrist, Left N Hand, Right P Hand, Left	Z None	Z None	1 Densitometry Z None

B   **Imaging**
Q   **Non-Axial Lower Bones**
Ø   **Plain Radiography**   Definition: Planar display of an image developed from the capture of external ionizing radiation on photographic or photoconductive plate

Body Part Character 4	Contrast Character 5	Qualifier Character 6	Qualifier Character 7
Ø Hip, Right 1 Hip, Left	Ø High Osmolar 1 Low Osmolar Y Other Contrast	Z None	Z None
Ø Hip, Right 1 Hip, Left	Z None	Z None	1 Densitometry Z None
3 Femur, Right 4 Femur, Left	Z None	Z None	1 Densitometry Z None
7 Knee, Right 8 Knee, Left G Ankle, Right H Ankle, Left	Ø High Osmolar 1 Low Osmolar Y Other Contrast Z None	Z None	Z None
D Lower Leg, Right F Lower Leg, Left J Calcaneus, Right K Calcaneus, Left L Foot, Right M Foot, Left P Toe(s), Right Q Toe(s), Left V Patella, Right W Patella, Left	Z None	Z None	Z None
X Foot/Toe Joint, Right Y Foot/Toe Joint, Left	Ø High Osmolar 1 Low Osmolar Y Other Contrast	Z None	Z None

B   **Imaging**
Q   **Non-Axial Lower Bones**
1   **Fluoroscopy**   Definition: Single plane or bi-plane real time display of an image developed from the capture of external ionizing radioation on a fluorescent screen. The image may also be stored by either digital or analog means.

Body Part Character 4	Contrast Character 5	Qualifier Character 6	Qualifier Character 7
Ø Hip, Right 1 Hip, Left 7 Knee, Right 8 Knee, Left G Ankle, Right H Ankle, Left X Foot/Toe Joint, Right Y Foot/Toe Joint, Left	Ø High Osmolar 1 Low Osmolar Y Other Contrast Z None	Z None	Z None
3 Femur, Right 4 Femur, Left D Lower Leg, Right F Lower Leg, Left J Calcaneus, Right K Calcaneus, Left L Foot, Right M Foot, Left P Toe(s), Right Q Toe(s), Left V Patella, Right W Patella, Left	Z None	Z None	Z None

NC Noncovered Procedure   **LC** Limited Coverage   **QA** Questionable OB Admit   **NT** New Tech Add-on   ⊞ Combination Member   ♂ Male   ♀ Female

ICD-10-PCS 2022   761

BP4–BQ1

Imaging

B   **Imaging**
Q   **Non-Axial Lower Bones**
2   **Computerized Tomography (CT Scan)** Definition: Computer reformatted digital display of multiplanar images developed from the capture of multiple exposures of external ionizing radiation

Body Part Character 4	Contrast Character 5	Qualifier Character 6	Qualifier Character 7
Ø Hip, Right 1 Hip, Left 3 Femur, Right 4 Femur, Left 7 Knee, Right 8 Knee, Left D Lower Leg, Right F Lower Leg, Left G Ankle, Right H Ankle, Left J Calcaneus, Right K Calcaneus, Left L Foot, Right M Foot, Left P Toe(s), Right Q Toe(s), Left R Lower Extremity, Right S Lower Extremity, Left V Patella, Right W Patella, Left X Foot/Toe Joint, Right Y Foot/Toe Joint, Left	Ø High Osmolar 1 Low Osmolar Y Other Contrast Z None	Z None	Z None
B Tibia/Fibula, Right C Tibia/Fibula, Left	Ø High Osmolar 1 Low Osmolar Y Other Contrast	Z None	Z None

B   **Imaging**
Q   **Non-Axial Lower Bones**
3   **Magnetic Resonance Imaging (MRI)** Definition: Computer reformatted digital display of multiplanar images developed from the capture of radio-frequency signals emitted by nuclei in a body site excited within a magnetic field

Body Part Character 4	Contrast Character 5	Qualifier Character 6	Qualifier Character 7
Ø Hip, Right 1 Hip, Left 3 Femur, Right 4 Femur, Left 7 Knee, Right 8 Knee, Left D Lower Leg, Right F Lower Leg, Left G Ankle, Right H Ankle, Left J Calcaneus, Right K Calcaneus, Left L Foot, Right M Foot, Left P Toe(s), Right Q Toe(s), Left V Patella, Right W Patella, Left	Y Other Contrast	Ø Unenhanced and Enhanced Z None	Z None
Ø Hip, Right 1 Hip, Left 3 Femur, Right 4 Femur, Left 7 Knee, Right 8 Knee, Left D Lower Leg, Right F Lower Leg, Left G Ankle, Right H Ankle, Left J Calcaneus, Right K Calcaneus, Left L Foot, Right M Foot, Left P Toe(s), Right Q Toe(s), Left V Patella, Right W Patella, Left	Z None	Z None	Z None

B   Imaging
Q   **Non-Axial Lower Bones**
4   **Ultrasonography**   Definition: Real time display of images of anatomy or flow information developed from the capture of reflected and attenuated high frequency sound waves

Body Part Character 4	Contrast Character 5	Qualifier Character 6	Qualifier Character 7
Ø Hip, Right 1 Hip, Left 2 Hips, Bilateral 7 Knee, Right 8 Knee, Left 9 Knees, Bilateral	Z None	Z None	Z None

B   Imaging
R   **Axial Skeleton, Except Skull and Facial Bones**
Ø   **Plain Radiography**   Definition: Planar display of an image developed from the capture of external ionizing radiation on photographic or photoconductive plate

Body Part Character 4	Contrast Character 5	Qualifier Character 6	Qualifier Character 7
Ø Cervical Spine 7 Thoracic Spine 9 Lumbar Spine G Whole Spine	Z None	Z None	1 Densitometry Z None
1 Cervical Disc(s) 2 Thoracic Disc(s) 3 Lumbar Disc(s) 4 Cervical Facet Joint(s) 5 Thoracic Facet Joint(s) 6 Lumbar Facet Joint(s) D Sacroiliac Joints	Ø High Osmolar 1 Low Osmolar Y Other Contrast Z None	Z None	Z None
8 Thoracolumbar Joint B Lumbosacral Joint C Pelvis F Sacrum and Coccyx H Sternum	Z None	Z None	Z None

B   Imaging
R   **Axial Skeleton, Except Skull and Facial Bones**
1   **Fluoroscopy**   Definition: Single plane or bi-plane real time display of an image developed from the capture of external ionizing radiation on a fluorescent screen. The image may also be stored by either digital or analog means.

Body Part Character 4	Contrast Character 5	Qualifier Character 6	Qualifier Character 7
Ø Cervical Spine 1 Cervical Disc(s) 2 Thoracic Disc(s) 3 Lumbar Disc(s) 4 Cervical Facet Joint(s) 5 Thoracic Facet Joint(s) 6 Lumbar Facet Joint(s) 7 Thoracic Spine 8 Thoracolumbar Joint 9 Lumbar Spine B Lumbosacral Joint C Pelvis D Sacroiliac Joints F Sacrum and Coccyx G Whole Spine H Sternum	Ø High Osmolar 1 Low Osmolar Y Other Contrast Z None	Z None	Z None

B   Imaging
R   **Axial Skeleton, Except Skull and Facial Bones**
2   **Computerized Tomography (CT Scan)**   Definition: Computer reformatted digital display of multiplanar images developed from the capture of multiple exposures of external ionizing radiation

Body Part Character 4	Contrast Character 5	Qualifier Character 6	Qualifier Character 7
Ø Cervical Spine 7 Thoracic Spine 9 Lumbar Spine C Pelvis D Sacroiliac Joints F Sacrum and Coccyx	Ø High Osmolar 1 Low Osmolar Y Other Contrast Z None	Z None	Z None

NC Noncovered Procedure   LC Limited Coverage   QA Questionable OB Admit   NT New Tech Add-on   ⊞ Combination Member   ♂ Male   ♀ Female

ICD-10-PCS 2022   763   BQ4–BR2

B   **Imaging**
R   **Axial Skeleton, Except Skull and Facial Bones**
3   **Magnetic Resonance Imaging (MRI)**   Definition: Computer reformatted digital display of multiplanar images developed from the capture of radio-frequency signals emitted by nuclei in a body site excited within a magnetic field

Body Part Character 4	Contrast Character 5	Qualifier Character 6	Qualifier Character 7
Ø Cervical Spine 1 Cervical Disc(s) 2 Thoracic Disc(s) 3 Lumbar Disc(s) 7 Thoracic Spine 9 Lumbar Spine C Pelvis F Sacrum and Coccyx	Y Other Contrast	Ø Unenhanced and Enhanced Z None	Z None
Ø Cervical Spine 1 Cervical Disc(s) 2 Thoracic Disc(s) 3 Lumbar Disc(s) 7 Thoracic Spine 9 Lumbar Spine C Pelvis F Sacrum and Coccyx	Z None	Z None	Z None

B   **Imaging**
R   **Axial Skeleton, Except Skull and Facial Bones**
4   **Ultrasonography**   Definition: Real time display of images of anatomy or flow information developed from the capture of reflected and attenuated high frequency sound waves

Body Part Character 4	Contrast Character 5	Qualifier Character 6	Qualifier Character 7
Ø Cervical Spine 7 Thoracic Spine 9 Lumbar Spine F Sacrum and Coccyx	Z None	Z None	Z None

B   **Imaging**
T   **Urinary System**
Ø   **Plain Radiography**   Definition: Planar display of an image developed from the capture of external ionizing radiation on photographic or photoconductive plate

Body Part Character 4	Contrast Character 5	Qualifier Character 6	Qualifier Character 7
Ø Bladder 1 Kidney, Right 2 Kidney, Left 3 Kidneys, Bilateral 4 Kidneys, Ureters and Bladder 5 Urethra 6 Ureter, Right 7 Ureter, Left 8 Ureters, Bilateral B Bladder and Urethra C Ileal Diversion Loop	Ø High Osmolar 1 Low Osmolar Y Other Contrast Z None	Z None	Z None

B   **Imaging**
T   **Urinary System**
1   **Fluoroscopy**   Definition: Single plane or bi-plane real time display of an image developed from the capture of external ionizing radioation on a fluorescent screen. The image may also be stored by either digital or analog means.

Body Part Character 4	Contrast Character 5	Qualifier Character 6	Qualifier Character 7
Ø Bladder 1 Kidney, Right 2 Kidney, Left 3 Kidneys, Bilateral 4 Kidneys, Ureters and Bladder 5 Urethra 6 Ureter, Right 7 Ureter, Left B Bladder and Urethra C Ileal Diversion Loop D Kidney, Ureter and Bladder, Right F Kidney, Ureter and Bladder, Left G Ileal Loop, Ureters and Kidneys	Ø High Osmolar 1 Low Osmolar Y Other Contrast Z None	Z None	Z None

B　Imaging
T　Urinary System
2　Computerized Tomography (CT Scan)　Definition: Computer reformatted digital display of multiplanar images developed from the capture of multiple exposures of external ionizing radiation

Body Part Character 4	Contrast Character 5	Qualifier Character 6	Qualifier Character 7
Ø Bladder 1 Kidney, Right 2 Kidney, Left 3 Kidneys, Bilateral 9 Kidney Transplant	Ø High Osmolar 1 Low Osmolar Y Other Contrast	Ø Unenhanced and Enhanced Z None	Z None
Ø Bladder 1 Kidney, Right 2 Kidney, Left 3 Kidneys, Bilateral 9 Kidney Transplant	Z None	Z None	Z None

B　Imaging
T　Urinary System
3　Magnetic Resonance Imaging (MRI)　Definition: Computer reformatted digital display of multiplanar images developed from the capture of radio-frequency signals emitted by nuclei in a body site excited within a magnetic field

Body Part Character 4	Contrast Character 5	Qualifier Character 6	Qualifier Character 7
Ø Bladder 1 Kidney, Right 2 Kidney, Left 3 Kidneys, Bilateral 9 Kidney Transplant	Y Other Contrast	Ø Unenhanced and Enhanced Z None	Z None
Ø Bladder 1 Kidney, Right 2 Kidney, Left 3 Kidneys, Bilateral 9 Kidney Transplant	Z None	Z None	Z None

B　Imaging
T　Urinary System
4　Ultrasonography　Definition: Real time display of images of anatomy or flow information developed from the capture of reflected and attenuated high frequency sound waves

Body Part Character 4	Contrast Character 5	Qualifier Character 6	Qualifier Character 7
Ø Bladder 1 Kidney, Right 2 Kidney, Left 3 Kidneys, Bilateral 5 Urethra 6 Ureter, Right 7 Ureter, Left 8 Ureters, Bilateral 9 Kidney Transplant J Kidneys and Bladder	Z None	Z None	Z None

B　Imaging
U　Female Reproductive System
Ø　Plain Radiography　Definition: Planar display of an image developed from the capture of external ionizing radiation on photographic or photoconductive plate

Body Part Character 4	Contrast Character 5	Qualifier Character 6	Qualifier Character 7
Ø Fallopian Tube, Right ♀ 1 Fallopian Tube, Left ♀ 2 Fallopian Tubes, Bilateral ♀ 6 Uterus ♀ 8 Uterus and Fallopian Tubes ♀ 9 Vagina ♀	Ø High Osmolar 1 Low Osmolar Y Other Contrast	Z None	Z None
♀　All body part, contrast, and qualifier values			

NC Noncovered Procedure　**LC** Limited Coverage　**OA** Questionable OB Admit　**NT** New Tech Add-on　⊞ Combination Member　♂ Male　♀ Female

ICD-10-PCS 2022　　　　　　　　　　　　　　　　　　　　　　　　　　　　　　　**765**

BT2–BUØ

B Imaging
U Female Reproductive System
1 Fluoroscopy Definition: Single plane or bi-plane real time display of an image developed from the capture of external ionizing radiation on a fluorescent screen. The image may also be stored by either digital or analog means.

Body Part Character 4		Contrast Character 5	Qualifier Character 6	Qualifier Character 7
Ø Fallopian Tube, Right ♀	Ø High Osmolar ♀	Z None	Z None
1 Fallopian Tube, Left ♀	1 Low Osmolar ♀		
2 Fallopian Tubes, Bilateral ♀	Y Other Contrast ♀		
6 Uterus ♀	Z None ♀		
8 Uterus and Fallopian Tubes ♀			
9 Vagina ♀			

♀ All body part, contrast, and qualifier values

B Imaging
U Female Reproductive System
3 Magnetic Resonance Imaging (MRI) Definition: Computer reformatted digital display of multiplanar images developed from the capture of radio-frequency signals emitted by nuclei in a body site excited within a magnetic field

Body Part Character 4		Contrast Character 5	Qualifier Character 6	Qualifier Character 7
3 Ovary, Right ♀	Y Other Contrast	Ø Unenhanced and Enhanced	Z None
4 Ovary, Left ♀		Z None	
5 Ovaries, Bilateral ♀			
6 Uterus ♀			
9 Vagina ♀			
B Pregnant Uterus ♀			
C Uterus and Ovaries ♀			
3 Ovary, Right ♀	Z None	Z None	Z None
4 Ovary, Left ♀			
5 Ovaries, Bilateral ♀			
6 Uterus ♀			
9 Vagina ♀			
B Pregnant Uterus ♀			
C Uterus and Ovaries ♀			

♀ All body part, contrast, and qualifier values

B Imaging
U Female Reproductive System
4 Ultrasonography Definition: Real time display of images of anatomy or flow information developed from the capture of reflected and attenuated high frequency sound waves

Body Part Character 4		Contrast Character 5	Qualifier Character 6	Qualifier Character 7
Ø Fallopian Tube, Right ♀	Y Other Contrast	Z None	Z None
1 Fallopian Tube, Left ♀	Z None		
2 Fallopian Tubes, Bilateral ♀			
3 Ovary, Right ♀			
4 Ovary, Left ♀			
5 Ovaries, Bilateral ♀			
6 Uterus ♀			
C Uterus and Ovaries ♀			

♀ All body part, contrast, and qualifier values

B Imaging
V Male Reproductive System
Ø Plain Radiography Definition: Planar display of an image developed from the capture of external ionizing radiation on photographic or photoconductive plate

Body Part Character 4		Contrast Character 5	Qualifier Character 6	Qualifier Character 7
Ø Corpora Cavernosa ♂	Ø High Osmolar ♂	Z None	Z None
1 Epididymis, Right ♂	1 Low Osmolar ♂		
2 Epididymis, Left ♂	Y Other Contrast ♂		
3 Prostate ♂			
5 Testicle, Right ♂			
6 Testicle, Left ♂			
8 Vasa Vasorum ♂			

♂ All body part, contrast, and qualifier values

B   **Imaging**
V   **Male Reproductive System**
1   **Fluoroscopy**   Definition: Single plane or bi-plane real time display of an image developed from the capture of external ionizing radioation on a fluorescent screen. The image may also be stored by either digital or analog means.

Body Part Character 4		Contrast Character 5	Qualifier Character 6	Qualifier Character 7
Ø Corpora Cavernosa	♂	Ø High Osmolar	Z None	Z None
8 Vasa Vasorum	♂	1 Low Osmolar		
		Y Other Contrast		
		Z None		

♂   All body part, contrast, and qualifier values

B   **Imaging**
V   **Male Reproductive System**
2   **Computerized Tomography (CT Scan)**   Definition: Computer reformatted digital display of multiplanar images developed from the capture of multiple exposures of external ionizing radiation

Body Part Character 4		Contrast Character 5	Qualifier Character 6	Qualifier Character 7
3 Prostate	♂	Ø High Osmolar	Ø Unenhanced and Enhanced	Z None
		1 Low Osmolar	Z None	
		Y Other Contrast		
3 Prostate	♂	Z None	Z None	Z None

♂   BV23[Ø,Y][Ø,Z]Z   ♂   BV23ZZZ
♂   BV231ØZ

B   **Imaging**
V   **Male Reproductive System**
3   **Magnetic Resonance Imaging (MRI)**   Definition: Computer reformatted digital display of multiplanar images developed from the capture of radio-frequency signals emitted by nuclei in a body site excited within a magnetic field

Body Part Character 4		Contrast Character 5	Qualifier Character 6	Qualifier Character 7
Ø Corpora Cavernosa	♂	Y Other Contrast	Ø Unenhanced and Enhanced	Z None
3 Prostate	♂		Z None	
4 Scrotum	♂			
5 Testicle, Right	♂			
6 Testicle, Left	♂			
7 Testicles, Bilateral	♂			
Ø Corpora Cavernosa	♂	Z None	Z None	Z None
3 Prostate	♂			
4 Scrotum	♂			
5 Testicle, Right	♂			
6 Testicle, Left	♂			
7 Testicles, Bilateral	♂			

♂   All body part, contrast, and qualifier values

B   **Imaging**
V   **Male Reproductive System**
4   **Ultrasonography**   Definition: Real time display of images of anatomy or flow information developed from the capture of reflected and attenuated high frequency sound waves

Body Part Character 4		Contrast Character 5	Qualifier Character 6	Qualifier Character 7
4 Scrotum	♂	Z None	Z None	Z None
9 Prostate and Seminal Vesicles	♂			
B Penis	♂			

♂   All body part, contrast, and qualifier values

B   **Imaging**
W   **Anatomical Regions**
Ø   **Plain Radiography**   Definition: Planar display of an image developed from the capture of external ionizing radiation on photographic or photoconductive plate

Body Part Character 4	Contrast Character 5	Qualifier Character 6	Qualifier Character 7
Ø Abdomen	Z None	Z None	Z None
1 Abdomen and Pelvis			
3 Chest			
B Long Bones, All			
C Lower Extremity			
J Upper Extremity			
K Whole Body			
L Whole Skeleton			
M Whole Body, Infant			

NC Noncovered Procedure   LC Limited Coverage   QA Questionable OB Admit   NT New Tech Add-on   ⊞ Combination Member   ♂ Male   ♀ Female

B   **Imaging**
W   **Anatomical Regions**
1   **Fluoroscopy**   Definition: Single plane or bi-plane real time display of an image developed from the capture of external ionizing radioation on a fluorescent screen. The image may also be stored by either digital or analog means.

Body Part Character 4	Contrast Character 5	Qualifier Character 6	Qualifier Character 7
1 Abdomen and Pelvis 9 Head and Neck C Lower Extremity J Upper Extremity	0 High Osmolar 1 Low Osmolar Y Other Contrast Z None	Z None	Z None

B   **Imaging**
W   **Anatomical Regions**
2   **Computerized Tomography (CT Scan)**   Definition: Computer reformatted digital display of multiplanar images developed from the capture of multiple exposures of external ionizing radiation

Body Part Character 4	Contrast Character 5	Qualifier Character 6	Qualifier Character 7
0 Abdomen 1 Abdomen and Pelvis 4 Chest and Abdomen 5 Chest, Abdomen and Pelvis 8 Head 9 Head and Neck F Neck G Pelvic Region	0 High Osmolar 1 Low Osmolar Y Other Contrast	0 Unenhanced and Enhanced Z None	Z None
0 Abdomen 1 Abdomen and Pelvis 4 Chest and Abdomen 5 Chest, Abdomen and Pelvis 8 Head 9 Head and Neck F Neck G Pelvic Region	Z None	Z None	Z None

B   **Imaging**
W   **Anatomical Regions**
3   **Magnetic Resonance Imaging (MRI)**   Definition: Computer reformatted digital display of multiplanar images developed from the capture of radio-frequency signals emitted by nuclei in a body site excited within a magnetic field

Body Part Character 4	Contrast Character 5	Qualifier Character 6	Qualifier Character 7
0 Abdomen 8 Head F Neck G Pelvic Region H Retroperitoneum P Brachial Plexus	Y Other Contrast	0 Unenhanced and Enhanced Z None	Z None
0 Abdomen 8 Head F Neck G Pelvic Region H Retroperitoneum P Brachial Plexus	Z None	Z None	Z None
3 Chest	Y Other Contrast	0 Unenhanced and Enhanced Z None	Z None

B   **Imaging**
W   **Anatomical Regions**
4   **Ultrasonography**   Definition: Real time display of images of anatomy or flow information developed from the capture of reflected and attenuated high frequency sound waves

Body Part Character 4	Contrast Character 5	Qualifier Character 6	Qualifier Character 7
0 Abdomen 1 Abdomen and Pelvis F Neck G Pelvic Region	Z None	Z None	Z None

B   **Imaging**
W   **Anatomical Regions**
5   **Other Imaging**   Definition: Other specified modality for visualizing a body part

Body Part Character 4	Contrast Character 5	Qualifier Character 6	Qualifier Character 7
2 Trunk 9 Head and Neck C Lower Extremity J Upper Extremity	Z None	1 Bacterial Autofluorescence	Z None

B   **Imaging**
Y   **Fetus and Obstetrical**
3   **Magnetic Resonance Imaging (MRI)**   Definition: Computer reformatted digital display of multiplanar images developed from the capture of radio-frequency signals emitted by nuclei in a body site excited within a magnetic field

Body Part Character 4	Contrast Character 5	Qualifier Character 6	Qualifier Character 7
Ø Fetal Head ♀ 1 Fetal Heart ♀ 2 Fetal Thorax ♀ 3 Fetal Abdomen ♀ 4 Fetal Spine ♀ 5 Fetal Extremities ♀ 6 Whole Fetus ♀	Y Other Contrast	Ø Unenhanced and Enhanced Z None	Z None
Ø Fetal Head ♀ 1 Fetal Heart ♀ 2 Fetal Thorax ♀ 3 Fetal Abdomen ♀ 4 Fetal Spine ♀ 5 Fetal Extremities ♀ 6 Whole Fetus ♀	Z None	Z None	Z None

♀   BY3[Ø,1,2,3,5,6]Y[Ø,Z]Z
♀   BY34YZZ
♀   BY3[Ø,1,2,3,4,5,6]ZZZ

B   **Imaging**
Y   **Fetus and Obstetrical**
4   **Ultrasonography**   Definition: Real time display of images of anatomy or flow information developed from the capture of reflected and attenuated high frequency sound waves

Body Part Character 4	Contrast Character 5	Qualifier Character 6	Qualifier Character 7
7 Fetal Umbilical Cord ♀ 8 Placenta ♀ 9 First Trimester, Single Fetus ♀ B First Trimester, Multiple Gestation ♀ C Second Trimester, Single Fetus ♀ D Second Trimester, Multiple Gestation ♀ F Third Trimester, Single Fetus ♀ G Third Trimester, Multiple Gestation ♀	Z None	Z None	Z None

♀   All body part, contrast, and qualifier values

Nuclear Medicine CØ1–CW7

C   **Nuclear Medicine**
Ø   **Central Nervous System**
1   **Planar Nuclear Medicine Imaging**   Definition: Introduction of radioactive materials into the body for single plane display of images developed from the capture of radioactive emissions

Body Part Character 4	Radionuclide Character 5	Qualifier Character 6	Qualifier Character 7
Ø Brain	**1** Technetium 99m (Tc-99m) **Y** Other Radionuclide	**Z** None	**Z** None
5 Cerebrospinal Fluid	**D** Indium 111 (In-111) **Y** Other Radionuclide	**Z** None	**Z** None
Y Central Nervous System	**Y** Other Radionuclide	**Z** None	**Z** None

C   **Nuclear Medicine**
Ø   **Central Nervous System**
2   **Tomographic (Tomo) Nuclear Medicine Imaging**   Definition: Introduction of radioactive materials into the body for three dimensional display of images developed from the capture of radioactive emissions

Body Part Character 4	Radionuclide Character 5	Qualifier Character 6	Qualifier Character 7
Ø Brain	**1** Technetium 99m (Tc-99m) **F** Iodine 123 (I-123) **S** Thallium 201 (Tl-201) **Y** Other Radionuclide	**Z** None	**Z** None
5 Cerebrospinal Fluid	**D** Indium 111 (In-111) **Y** Other Radionuclide	**Z** None	**Z** None
Y Central Nervous System	**Y** Other Radionuclide	**Z** None	**Z** None

C   **Nuclear Medicine**
Ø   **Central Nervous System**
3   **Positron Emission Tomographic (PET) Imaging**   Definition: Introduction of radioactive materials into the body for three dimensional display of images developed from the simultaneous capture, 180 degrees apart, of radioactive emissions

Body Part Character 4	Radionuclide Character 5	Qualifier Character 6	Qualifier Character 7
Ø Brain	**B** Carbon 11 (C-11) **K** Fluorine 18 (F-18) **M** Oxygen 15 (O-15) **Y** Other Radionuclide	**Z** None	**Z** None
Y Central Nervous System	**Y** Other Radionuclide	**Z** None	**Z** None

C   **Nuclear Medicine**
Ø   **Central Nervous System**
5   **Nonimaging Nuclear Medicine Probe**   Definition: Introduction of radioactive materials into the body for the study of distribution and fate of certain substances by the detection of radioactive emissions; or, alternatively, measurement of absorption of radioactive emissions from an external source

Body Part Character 4	Radionuclide Character 5	Qualifier Character 6	Qualifier Character 7
Ø Brain	**V** Xenon 133 (Xe-133) **Y** Other Radionuclide	**Z** None	**Z** None
Y Central Nervous System	**Y** Other Radionuclide	**Z** None	**Z** None

C   **Nuclear Medicine**
2   **Heart**
1   **Planar Nuclear Medicine Imaging**   Definition: Introduction of radioactive materials into the body for single plane display of images developed from the capture of radioactive emissions

Body Part Character 4	Radionuclide Character 5	Qualifier Character 6	Qualifier Character 7
6 Heart, Right and Left	**1** Technetium 99m (Tc-99m) **Y** Other Radionuclide	**Z** None	**Z** None
G Myocardium	**1** Technetium 99m (Tc-99m) **D** Indium 111 (In-111) **S** Thallium 201 (Tl-201) **Y** Other Radionuclide **Z** None	**Z** None	**Z** None
Y Heart	**Y** Other Radionuclide	**Z** None	**Z** None

NC Noncovered Procedure   **LC** Limited Coverage   **QA** Questionable OB Admit   **NT** New Tech Add-on   ⊞ Combination Member   ♂ Male   ♀ Female

ICD-10-PCS 2022   771

C   **Nuclear Medicine**
2   **Heart**
2   **Tomographic (Tomo) Nuclear Medicine Imaging**   Definition: Introduction of radioactive materials into the body for three dimensional display of images developed from the capture of radioactive emissions

Body Part Character 4	Radionuclide Character 5	Qualifier Character 6	Qualifier Character 7
6 Heart, Right and Left	1 Technetium 99m (Tc-99m) Y Other Radionuclide	Z None	Z None
G Myocardium	1 Technetium 99m (Tc-99m) D Indium 111 (In-111) K Fluorine 18 (F-18) S Thallium 201 (Tl-201) Y Other Radionuclide Z None	Z None	Z None
Y Heart	Y Other Radionuclide	Z None	Z None

C   **Nuclear Medicine**
2   **Heart**
3   **Positron Emission Tomographic (PET) Imaging**   Definition: Introduction of radioactive materials into the body for three dimensional display of images developed from the simultaneous capture, 180 degrees apart, of radioactive emissions

Body Part Character 4	Radionuclide Character 5	Qualifier Character 6	Qualifier Character 7
G Myocardium	K Fluorine 18 (F-18) M Oxygen 15 (O-15) Q Rubidium 82 (Rb-82) R Nitrogen 13 (N-13) Y Other Radionuclide	Z None	Z None
Y Heart	Y Other Radionuclide	Z None	Z None

C   **Nuclear Medicine**
2   **Heart**
5   **Nonimaging Nuclear Medicine Probe**   Definition: Introduction of radioactive materials into the body for the study of distribution and fate of certain substances by the detection of radioactive emissions; or, alternatively, measurement of absorption of radioactive emissions from an external source

Body Part Character 4	Radionuclide Character 5	Qualifier Character 6	Qualifier Character 7
6 Heart, Right and Left	1 Technetium 99m (Tc-99m) Y Other Radionuclide	Z None	Z None
Y Heart	Y Other Radionuclide	Z None	Z None

C   **Nuclear Medicine**
5   **Veins**
1   **Planar Nuclear Medicine Imaging**   Definition: Introduction of radioactive materials into the body for single plane display of images developed from the capture of radioactive emissions

Body Part Character 4	Radionuclide Character 5	Qualifier Character 6	Qualifier Character 7
B Lower Extremity Veins, Right C Lower Extremity Veins, Left D Lower Extremity Veins, Bilateral N Upper Extremity Veins, Right P Upper Extremity Veins, Left Q Upper Extremity Veins, Bilateral R Central Veins	1 Technetium 99m (Tc-99m) Y Other Radionuclide	Z None	Z None
Y Veins	Y Other Radionuclide	Z None	Z None

C **Nuclear Medicine**
7 **Lymphatic and Hematologic System**
1 **Planar Nuclear Medicine Imaging**   Definition: Introduction of radioactive materials into the body for single plane display of images developed from the capture of radioactive emissions

Body Part Character 4	Radionuclide Character 5	Qualifier Character 6	Qualifier Character 7
Ø Bone Marrow	1 Technetium 99m (Tc-99m) D Indium 111 (In-111) Y Other Radionuclide	Z None	Z None
2 Spleen 5 Lymphatics, Head and Neck D Lymphatics, Pelvic J Lymphatics, Head K Lymphatics, Neck L Lymphatics, Upper Chest M Lymphatics, Trunk N Lymphatics, Upper Extremity P Lymphatics, Lower Extremity	1 Technetium 99m (Tc-99m) Y Other Radionuclide	Z None	Z None
3 Blood	D Indium 111 (In-111) Y Other Radionuclide	Z None	Z None
Y Lymphatic and Hematologic System	Y Other Radionuclide	Z None	Z None

C **Nuclear Medicine**
7 **Lymphatic and Hematologic System**
2 **Tomographic (Tomo) Nuclear Medicine Imaging**   Definition: Introduction of radioactive materials into the body for three dimensional display of images developed from the capture of radioactive emissions

Body Part Character 4	Radionuclide Character 5	Qualifier Character 6	Qualifier Character 7
2 Spleen	1 Technetium 99m (Tc-99m) Y Other Radionuclide	Z None	Z None
Y Lymphatic and Hematologic System	Y Other Radionuclide	Z None	Z None

C **Nuclear Medicine**
7 **Lymphatic and Hematologic System**
5 **Nonimaging Nuclear Medicine Probe**   Definition: Introduction of radioactive materials into the body for the study of distribution and fate of certain substances by the detection of radioactive emissions; or, alternatively, measurement of absorption of radioactive emissions from an external source

Body Part Character 4	Radionuclide Character 5	Qualifier Character 6	Qualifier Character 7
5 Lymphatics, Head and Neck D Lymphatics, Pelvic J Lymphatics, Head K Lymphatics, Neck L Lymphatics, Upper Chest M Lymphatics, Trunk N Lymphatics, Upper Extremity P Lymphatics, Lower Extremity	1 Technetium 99m (Tc-99m) Y Other Radionuclide	Z None	Z None
Y Lymphatic and Hematologic System	Y Other Radionuclide	Z None	Z None

C **Nuclear Medicine**
7 **Lymphatic and Hematologic System**
6 **Nonimaging Nuclear Medicine Assay**   Definition: Introduction of radioactive materials into the body for the study of body fluids and blood elements, by the detection of radioactive emissions

Body Part Character 4	Radionuclide Character 5	Qualifier Character 6	Qualifier Character 7
3 Blood	1 Technetium 99m (Tc-99m) 7 Cobalt 58 (Co-58) C Cobalt 57 (Co-57) D Indium 111 (In-111) H Iodine 125 (I-125) W Chromium (Cr-51) Y Other Radionuclide	Z None	Z None
Y Lymphatic and Hematologic System	Y Other Radionuclide	Z None	Z None

NC Noncovered Procedure   **LC** Limited Coverage   **QA** Questionable OB Admit   **NT** New Tech Add-on   ⊞ Combination Member   ♂ Male   ♀ Female

ICD-10-PCS 2022   773

Nuclear Medicine

C Nuclear Medicine
8 Eye
1 Planar Nuclear Medicine Imaging   Definition: Introduction of radioactive materials into the body for single plane display of images developed from the capture of radioactive emissions

Body Part Character 4	Radionuclide Character 5	Qualifier Character 6	Qualifier Character 7
9 Lacrimal Ducts, Bilateral	1 Technetium 99m (Tc-99m) Y Other Radionuclide	Z None	Z None
Y Eye	Y Other Radionuclide	Z None	Z None

C Nuclear Medicine
9 Ear, Nose, Mouth and Throat
1 Planar Nuclear Medicine Imaging   Definition: Introduction of radioactive materials into the body for single plane display of images developed from the capture of radioactive emissions

Body Part Character 4	Radionuclide Character 5	Qualifier Character 6	Qualifier Character 7
B Salivary Glands, Bilateral	1 Technetium 99m (Tc-99m) Y Other Radionuclide	Z None	Z None
Y Ear, Nose, Mouth and Throat	Y Other Radionuclide	Z None	Z None

C Nuclear Medicine
B Respiratory System
1 Planar Nuclear Medicine Imaging   Definition: Introduction of radioactive materials into the body for single plane display of images developed from the capture of radioactive emissions

Body Part Character 4	Radionuclide Character 5	Qualifier Character 6	Qualifier Character 7
2 Lungs and Bronchi	1 Technetium 99m (Tc-99m) 9 Krypton (Kr-81m) T Xenon 127 (Xe-127) V Xenon 133 (Xe-133) Y Other Radionuclide	Z None	Z None
Y Respiratory System	Y Other Radionuclide	Z None	Z None

C Nuclear Medicine
B Respiratory System
2 Tomographic (Tomo) Nuclear Medicine Imaging   Definition: Introduction of radioactive materials into the body for three dimensional display of images developed from the capture of radioactive emissions

Body Part Character 4	Radionuclide Character 5	Qualifier Character 6	Qualifier Character 7
2 Lungs and Bronchi	1 Technetium 99m (Tc-99m) 9 Krypton (Kr-81m) Y Other Radionuclide	Z None	Z None
Y Respiratory System	Y Other Radionuclide	Z None	Z None

C Nuclear Medicine
B Respiratory System
3 Positron Emission Tomographic (PET) Imaging   Definition: Introduction of radioactive materials into the body for three dimensional display of images developed from the simultaneous capture, 180 degrees apart, of radioactive emissions

Body Part Character 4	Radionuclide Character 5	Qualifier Character 6	Qualifier Character 7
2 Lungs and Bronchi	K Fluorine 18 (F-18) Y Other Radionuclide	Z None	Z None
Y Respiratory System	Y Other Radionuclide	Z None	Z None

C Nuclear Medicine
D Gastrointestinal System
1 Planar Nuclear Medicine Imaging   Definition: Introduction of radioactive materials into the body for single plane display of images developed from the capture of radioactive emissions

Body Part Character 4	Radionuclide Character 5	Qualifier Character 6	Qualifier Character 7
5 Upper Gastrointestinal Tract 7 Gastrointestinal Tract	1 Technetium 99m (Tc-99m) D Indium 111 (In-111) Y Other Radionuclide	Z None	Z None
Y Digestive System	Y Other Radionuclide	Z None	Z None

C   **Nuclear Medicine**
D   **Gastrointestinal System**
2   **Tomographic (Tomo) Nuclear Medicine Imaging**   Definition: Introduction of radioactive materials into the body for three dimensional display of images developed from the capture of radioactive emissions

Body Part Character 4	Radionuclide Character 5	Qualifier Character 6	Qualifier Character 7
7 Gastrointestinal Tract	1 Technetium 99m (Tc-99m) D Indium 111 (In-111) Y Other Radionuclide	Z None	Z None
Y Digestive System	Y Other Radionuclide	Z None	Z None

C   **Nuclear Medicine**
F   **Hepatobiliary System and Pancreas**
1   **Planar Nuclear Medicine Imaging**   Definition: Introduction of radioactive materials into the body for single plane display of images developed from the capture of radioactive emissions

Body Part Character 4	Radionuclide Character 5	Qualifier Character 6	Qualifier Character 7
4 Gallbladder 5 Liver 6 Liver and Spleen C Hepatobiliary System, All	1 Technetium 99m (Tc-99m) Y Other Radionuclide	Z None	Z None
Y Hepatobiliary System and Pancreas	Y Other Radionuclide	Z None	Z None

C   **Nuclear Medicine**
F   **Hepatobiliary System and Pancreas**
2   **Tomographic (Tomo) Nuclear Medicine Imaging**   Definition: Introduction of radioactive materials into the body for three dimensional display of images developed from the capture of radioactive emissions

Body Part Character 4	Radionuclide Character 5	Qualifier Character 6	Qualifier Character 7
4 Gallbladder 5 Liver 6 Liver and Spleen	1 Technetium 99m (Tc-99m) Y Other Radionuclide	Z None	Z None
Y Hepatobiliary System and Pancreas	Y Other Radionuclide	Z None	Z None

C   **Nuclear Medicine**
G   **Endocrine System**
1   **Planar Nuclear Medicine Imaging**   Definition: Introduction of radioactive materials into the body for single plane display of images developed from the capture of radioactive emissions

Body Part Character 4	Radionuclide Character 5	Qualifier Character 6	Qualifier Character 7
1 Parathyroid Glands	1 Technetium 99m (Tc-99m) S Thallium 201 (Tl-201) Y Other Radionuclide	Z None	Z None
2 Thyroid Gland	1 Technetium 99m (Tc-99m) F Iodine 123 (I-123) G Iodine 131 (I-131) Y Other Radionuclide	Z None	Z None
4 Adrenal Glands, Bilateral	G Iodine 131 (I-131) Y Other Radionuclide	Z None	Z None
Y Endocrine System	Y Other Radionuclide	Z None	Z None

C   **Nuclear Medicine**
G   **Endocrine System**
2   **Tomographic (Tomo) Nuclear Medicine Imaging**   Definition: Introduction of radioactive materials into the body for three dimensional display of images developed from the capture of radioactive emissions

Body Part Character 4	Radionuclide Character 5	Qualifier Character 6	Qualifier Character 7
1 Parathyroid Glands	1 Technetium 99m (Tc-99m) S Thallium 201 (Tl-201) Y Other Radionuclide	Z None	Z None
Y Endocrine System	Y Other Radionuclide	Z None	Z None

NC Noncovered Procedure   LC Limited Coverage   QA Questionable OB Admit   NT New Tech Add-on   ⊞ Combination Member   ♂ Male   ♀ Female

ICD-10-PCS 2022   775

Nuclear Medicine

C   Nuclear Medicine
G   Endocrine System
4   Nonimaging Nuclear Medicine Uptake   Definition: Introduction of radioactive materials into the body for measurements of organ function, from the detection of radioactive emmissions

Body Part Character 4	Radionuclide Character 5	Qualifier Character 6	Qualifier Character 7
2 Thyroid Gland	1 Technetium 99m (Tc-99m) F Iodine 123 (I-123) G Iodine 131 (I-131) Y Other Radionuclide	Z None	Z None
Y Endocrine System	Y Other Radionuclide	Z None	Z None

C   Nuclear Medicine
H   Skin, Subcutaneous Tissue and Breast
1   Planar Nuclear Medicine Imaging   Definition: Introduction of radioactive materials into the body for single plane display of images developed from the capture of radioactive emissions

Body Part Character 4	Radionuclide Character 5	Qualifier Character 6	Qualifier Character 7
Ø Breast, Right 1 Breast, Left 2 Breasts, Bilateral	1 Technetium 99m (Tc-99m) S Thallium 201 (Tl-201) Y Other Radionuclide	Z None	Z None
Y Skin, Subcutaneous Tissue and Breast	Y Other Radionuclide	Z None	Z None

C   Nuclear Medicine
H   Skin, Subcutaneous Tissue and Breast
2   Tomographic (Tomo) Nuclear Medicine Imaging   Definition: Introduction of radioactive materials into the body for three dimensional display of images developed from the capture of radioactive emissions

Body Part Character 4	Radionuclide Character 5	Qualifier Character 6	Qualifier Character 7
Ø Breast, Right 1 Breast, Left 2 Breasts, Bilateral	1 Technetium 99m (Tc-99m) S Thallium 201 (Tl-201) Y Other Radionuclide	Z None	Z None
Y Skin, Subcutaneous Tissue and Breast	Y Other Radionuclide	Z None	Z None

C   Nuclear Medicine
P   Musculoskeletal System
1   Planar Nuclear Medicine Imaging   Definition: Introduction of radioactive materials into the body for single plane display of images developed from the capture of radioactive emissions

Body Part Character 4	Radionuclide Character 5	Qualifier Character 6	Qualifier Character 7
1 Skull 4 Thorax 5 Spine 6 Pelvis 7 Spine and Pelvis 8 Upper Extremity, Right 9 Upper Extremity, Left B Upper Extremities, Bilateral C Lower Extremity, Right D Lower Extremity, Left F Lower Extremities, Bilateral Z Musculoskeletal System, All	1 Technetium 99m (Tc-99m) Y Other Radionuclide	Z None	Z None
Y Musculoskeletal System, Other	Y Other Radionuclide	Z None	Z None

C   Nuclear Medicine
P   Musculoskeletal System
2   Tomographic (Tomo) Nuclear Medicine Imaging   Definition: Introduction of radioactive materials into the body for three dimensional display of images developed from the capture of radioactive emissions

Body Part Character 4	Radionuclide Character 5	Qualifier Character 6	Qualifier Character 7
1 Skull 2 Cervical Spine 3 Skull and Cervical Spine 4 Thorax 6 Pelvis 7 Spine and Pelvis 8 Upper Extremity, Right 9 Upper Extremity, Left B Upper Extremities, Bilateral C Lower Extremity, Right D Lower Extremity, Left F Lower Extremities, Bilateral G Thoracic Spine H Lumbar Spine J Thoracolumbar Spine	1 Technetium 99m (Tc-99m) Y Other Radionuclide	Z None	Z None
Y Musculoskeletal System, Other	Y Other Radionuclide	Z None	Z None

C   Nuclear Medicine
P   Musculoskeletal System
5   Nonimaging Nuclear Medicine Probe   Definition: Introduction of radioactive materials into the body for the study of distribution and fate of certain substances by the detection of radioactive emissions; or, alternatively, measurement of absorption of radioactive emissions from an external source

Body Part Character 4	Radionuclide Character 5	Qualifier Character 6	Qualifier Character 7
5 Spine N Upper Extremities P Lower Extremities	Z None	Z None	Z None
Y Musculoskeletal System, Other	Y Other Radionuclide	Z None	Z None

C   Nuclear Medicine
T   Urinary System
1   Planar Nuclear Medicine Imaging   Definition: Introduction of radioactive materials into the body for single plane display of images developed from the capture of radioactive emissions

Body Part Character 4	Radionuclide Character 5	Qualifier Character 6	Qualifier Character 7
3 Kidneys, Ureters and Bladder	1 Technetium 99m (Tc-99m) F Iodine 123 (I-123) G Iodine 131 (I-131) Y Other Radionuclide	Z None	Z None
H Bladder and Ureters	1 Technetium 99m (Tc-99m) Y Other Radionuclide	Z None	Z None
Y Urinary System	Y Other Radionuclide	Z None	Z None

C   Nuclear Medicine
T   Urinary System
2   Tomographic (Tomo) Nuclear Medicine Imaging   Definition: Introduction of radioactive materials into the body for three dimensional display of images developed from the capture of radioactive emissions

Body Part Character 4	Radionuclide Character 5	Qualifier Character 6	Qualifier Character 7
3 Kidneys, Ureters and Bladder	1 Technetium 99m (Tc-99m) Y Other Radionuclide	Z None	Z None
Y Urinary System	Y Other Radionuclide	Z None	Z None

C   Nuclear Medicine
T   Urinary System
6   Nonimaging Nuclear Medicine Assay   Definition: Introduction of radioactive materials into the body for the study of body fluids and blood elements, by the detection of radioactive emissions

Body Part Character 4	Radionuclide Character 5	Qualifier Character 6	Qualifier Character 7
3 Kidneys, Ureters and Bladder	1 Technetium 99m (Tc-99m) F Iodine 123 (I-123) G Iodine 131 (I-131) H Iodine 125 (I-125) Y Other Radionuclide	Z None	Z None
Y Urinary System	Y Other Radionuclide	Z None	Z None

NC Noncovered Procedure   LC Limited Coverage   QA Questionable OB Admit   NT New Tech Add-on   ⊞ Combination Member   ♂ Male   ♀ Female

ICD-10-PCS 2022   777

CP2–CT6

C   Nuclear Medicine
V   Male Reproductive System
1   Planar Nuclear Medicine Imaging   Definition: Introduction of radioactive materials into the body for single plane display of images developed from the capture of radioactive emissions

Body Part Character 4	Radionuclide Character 5	Qualifier Character 6	Qualifier Character 7
9 Testicles, Bilateral ♂	1 Technetium 99m (Tc-99m) Y Other Radionuclide	Z None	Z None
Y Male Reproductive System ♂	Y Other Radionuclide	Z None	Z None

♂   All body part, radionuclide, and qualifier values

C   Nuclear Medicine
W   Anatomical Regions
1   Planar Nuclear Medicine Imaging   Definition: Introduction of radioactive materials into the body for single plane display of images developed from the capture of radioactive emissions

Body Part Character 4	Radionuclide Character 5	Qualifier Character 6	Qualifier Character 7
Ø Abdomen 1 Abdomen and Pelvis 4 Chest and Abdomen 6 Chest and Neck B Head and Neck D Lower Extremity J Pelvic Region M Upper Extremity N Whole Body	1 Technetium 99m (Tc-99m) D Indium 111 (In-111) F Iodine 123 (I-123) G Iodine 131 (I-131) L Gallium 67 (Ga-67) S Thallium 201 (Tl-201) Y Other Radionuclide	Z None	Z None
3 Chest	1 Technetium 99m (Tc-99m) D Indium 111 (In-111) F Iodine 123 (I-123) G Iodine 131 (I-131) K Fluorine 18 (F-18) L Gallium 67 (Ga-67) S Thallium 201 (Tl-201) Y Other Radionuclide	Z None	Z None
Y Anatomical Regions, Multiple	Y Other Radionuclide	Z None	Z None
Z Anatomical Region, Other	Z None	Z None	Z None

C   Nuclear Medicine
W   Anatomical Regions
2   Tomographic (Tomo) Nuclear Medicine Imaging   Definition: Introduction of radioactive materials into the body for three dimensional display of images developed from the capture of radioactive emissions

Body Part Character 4	Radionuclide Character 5	Qualifier Character 6	Qualifier Character 7
Ø Abdomen 1 Abdomen and Pelvis 3 Chest 4 Chest and Abdomen 6 Chest and Neck B Head and Neck D Lower Extremity J Pelvic Region M Upper Extremity	1 Technetium 99m (Tc-99m) D Indium 111 (In-111) F Iodine 123 (I-123) G Iodine 131 (I-131) K Fluorine 18 (F-18) L Gallium 67 (Ga-67) S Thallium 201 (Tl-201) Y Other Radionuclide	Z None	Z None
Y Anatomical Regions, Multiple	Y Other Radionuclide	Z None	Z None

C   Nuclear Medicine
W   Anatomical Regions
3   Positron Emission Tomographic (PET) Imaging   Definition: Introduction of radioactive materials into the body for three dimensional display of images developed from the simultaneous capture, 180 degrees apart, of radioactive emissions

Body Part Character 4	Radionuclide Character 5	Qualifier Character 6	Qualifier Character 7
N Whole Body	Y Other Radionuclide	Z None	Z None

C   **Nuclear Medicine**
W   **Anatomical Regions**
5   **Nonimaging Nuclear Medicine Probe**   Definition: Introduction of radioactive materials into the body for the study of distribution and fate of certain substances by the detection of radioactive emissions; or, alternatively, measurement of absorption of radioactive emissions from an external source

Body Part Character 4	Radionuclide Character 5	Qualifier Character 6	Qualifier Character 7
Ø Abdomen 1 Abdomen and Pelvis 3 Chest 4 Chest and Abdomen 6 Chest and Neck B Head and Neck D Lower Extremity J Pelvic Region M Upper Extremity	1 Technetium 99m (Tc-99m) D Indium 111 (In-111) Y Other Radionuclide	Z None	Z None

C   **Nuclear Medicine**
W   **Anatomical Regions**
7   **Systemic Nuclear Medicine Therapy**   Definition: Introduction of unsealed radioactive materials into the body for treatment

Body Part Character 4	Radionuclide Character 5	Qualifier Character 6	Qualifier Character 7
Ø Abdomen 3 Chest	N Phosphorus 32 (P-32) Y Other Radionuclide	Z None	Z None
G Thyroid	G Iodine 131 (I-131) Y Other Radionuclide	Z None	Z None
N Whole Body	8 Samarium 153 (Sm-153) G Iodine 131 (I-131) N Phosphorus 32 (P-32) P Strontium 89 (Sr-89) Y Other Radionuclide	Z None	Z None
Y Anatomical Regions, Multiple	Y Other Radionuclide	Z None	Z None

NC Noncovered Procedure   **LC** Limited Coverage   **QA** Questionable OB Admit   **NT** New Tech Add-on   ⊞ Combination Member   ♂ Male   ♀ Female

ICD-10-PCS 2022   **779**

CW5–CW7

Radiation Therapy D00–DWY

AHA Coding Clinic for table D01

2020, 4Q, 43-44	Insertion of radioactive element
2020, 4Q, 69-70	Cesium 131 brachytherapy
2019, 4Q, 42-44	Unidirectional source brachytherapy

AHA Coding Clinic for table D0Y

2020, 4Q, 70	Intraoperative radiation therapy

AHA Coding Clinic for table D71

2020, 4Q, 43-44	Insertion of radioactive element
2020, 4Q, 69-70	Cesium 131 brachytherapy
2019, 4Q, 42-44	Unidirectional source brachytherapy

AHA Coding Clinic for table D81

2020, 4Q, 43-44	Insertion of radioactive element
2020, 4Q, 69-70	Cesium 131 brachytherapy
2019, 4Q, 42-44	Unidirectional source brachytherapy

AHA Coding Clinic for table D91

2020, 4Q, 43-44	Insertion of radioactive element
2020, 4Q, 69-70	Cesium 131 brachytherapy
2019, 4Q, 42-44	Unidirectional source brachytherapy

AHA Coding Clinic for table DB1

2020, 4Q, 43-44	Insertion of radioactive element
2020, 4Q, 69-70	Cesium 131 brachytherapy
2019, 4Q, 42-44	Unidirectional source brachytherapy

AHA Coding Clinic for table DD1

2020, 4Q, 43-44	Insertion of radioactive element
2020, 4Q, 69-70	Cesium 131 brachytherapy
2019, 4Q, 42-44	Unidirectional source brachytherapy

AHA Coding Clinic for table DF1

2020, 4Q, 43-44	Insertion of radioactive element
2020, 4Q, 69-70	Cesium 131 brachytherapy
2019, 4Q, 42-44	Unidirectional source brachytherapy

AHA Coding Clinic for table DG1

2020, 4Q, 43-44	Insertion of radioactive element
2020, 4Q, 69-70	Cesium 131 brachytherapy
2019, 4Q, 42-44	Unidirectional source brachytherapy

AHA Coding Clinic for table DM1

2020, 4Q, 43-44	Insertion of radioactive element
2020, 4Q, 69-70	Cesium 131 brachytherapy
2019, 4Q, 42-44	Unidirectional source brachytherapy

AHA Coding Clinic for table DT1

2020, 4Q, 43-44	Insertion of radioactive element
2020, 4Q, 69-70	Cesium 131 brachytherapy
2019, 4Q, 42-44	Unidirectional source brachytherapy

AHA Coding Clinic for table DU1

2020, 4Q, 43-44	Insertion of radioactive element
2020, 4Q, 69-70	Cesium 131 brachytherapy
2019, 4Q, 42-44	Unidirectional source brachytherapy
2017, 4Q, 104	Intrauterine brachytherapy & placement of tandems & ovoids

AHA Coding Clinic for table DV1

2020, 4Q, 43-44	Insertion of radioactive element
2020, 4Q, 69-70	Cesium 131 brachytherapy
2019, 4Q, 42-44	Unidirectional source brachytherapy

AHA Coding Clinic for table DW1

2020, 4Q, 43-44	Insertion of radioactive element
2020, 4Q, 69-70	Cesium 131 brachytherapy
2019, 4Q, 42-44	Unidirectional source brachytherapy

AHA Coding Clinic for table DWY

2019, 4Q, 37	Hyperthermic antineoplastic chemotherapy

D　Radiation Therapy
0　Central and Peripheral Nervous System
0　Beam Radiation

Treatment Site Character 4	Modality Qualifier Character 5	Isotope Character 6	Qualifier Character 7
0　Brain 1　Brain Stem 6　Spinal Cord 7　Peripheral Nerve	0　Photons <1 MeV 1　Photons 1- 10 MeV 2　Photons >10 MeV 4　Heavy Particles (Protons, Ions) 5　Neutrons 6　Neutron Capture	Z　None	Z　None
0　Brain 1　Brain Stem 6　Spinal Cord 7　Peripheral Nerve	3　Electrons	Z　None	0　Intraoperative Z　None

D　Radiation Therapy
0　Central and Peripheral Nervous System
1　Brachytherapy

Treatment Site Character 4	Modality Qualifier Character 5	Isotope Character 6	Qualifier Character 7
0　Brain 1　Brain Stem 6　Spinal Cord 7　Peripheral Nerve	9　High Dose Rate (HDR)	7　Cesium 137 (Cs-137) 8　Iridium 192 (Ir-192) 9　Iodine 125 (I-125) B　Palladium 103 (Pd-103) C　Californium 252 (Cf-252) Y　Other Isotope	Z　None
0　Brain 1　Brain Stem 6　Spinal Cord 7　Peripheral Nerve	B　Low Dose Rate (LDR)	6　Cesium 131 (Cs-131) 7　Cesium 137 (Cs-137) 8　Iridium 192 (Ir-192) 9　Iodine 125 (I-125) C　Californium 252 (Cf-252) Y　Other Isotope	Z　None
0　Brain 1　Brain Stem 6　Spinal Cord 7　Peripheral Nerve	B　Low Dose Rate (LDR)	B　Palladium 103 (Pd-103)	1　Unidirectional Source Z　None

NC Noncovered Procedure　　**LC** Limited Coverage　　**QA** Questionable OB Admit　　**NT** New Tech Add-on　　**⊞** Combination Member　　♂ Male　　♀ Female

ICD-10-PCS 2022　　　　　　　　　　　　　　　　　　　　　　　　　　**781**

D   Radiation Therapy
Ø   Central and Peripheral Nervous System
2   Stereotactic Radiosurgery

Treatment Site Character 4	Modality Qualifier Character 5	Isotope Character 6	Qualifier Character 7

Ø   Brain
1   Brain Stem
6   Spinal Cord
7   Peripheral Nerve
	D Stereotactic Other Photon
	      Radiosurgery
	H Stereotactic Particulate
	      Radiosurgery
	J Stereotactic Gamma Beam
	      Radiosurgery
		Z None	Z None

DRG Non-OR   All treatment site, modality, isotope, and qualifier values

D   Radiation Therapy
Ø   Central and Peripheral Nervous System
Y   Other Radiation

Treatment Site Character 4	Modality Qualifier Character 5	Isotope Character 6	Qualifier Character 7
Ø Brain 1 Brain Stem 6 Spinal Cord 7 Peripheral Nerve	7 Contact Radiation 8 Hyperthermia C Intraoperative Radiation Therapy (IORT) F Plaque Radiation K Laser Interstitial Thermal Therapy	Z None	Z None

Valid OR   DØY[Ø,1,6,7]KZZ

D   Radiation Therapy
7   Lymphatic and Hematologic System
Ø   Beam Radiation

Treatment Site Character 4	Modality Qualifier Character 5	Isotope Character 6	Qualifier Character 7
Ø Bone Marrow 1 Thymus 2 Spleen 3 Lymphatics, Neck 4 Lymphatics, Axillary 5 Lymphatics, Thorax 6 Lymphatics, Abdomen 7 Lymphatics, Pelvis 8 Lymphatics, Inguinal	Ø Photons <1 MeV 1 Photons 1- 10 MeV 2 Photons >10 MeV 4 Heavy Particles (Protons, Ions) 5 Neutrons 6 Neutron Capture	Z None	Z None
Ø Bone Marrow 1 Thymus 2 Spleen 3 Lymphatics, Neck 4 Lymphatics, Axillary 5 Lymphatics, Thorax 6 Lymphatics, Abdomen 7 Lymphatics, Pelvis 8 Lymphatics, Inguinal	3 Electrons	Z None	Ø Intraoperative Z None

D   Radiation Therapy
7   Lymphatic and Hematologic System
1   Brachytherapy

Treatment Site Character 4	Modality Qualifier Character 5	Isotope Character 6	Qualifier Character 7
Ø Bone Marrow 1 Thymus 2 Spleen 3 Lymphatics, Neck 4 Lymphatics, Axillary 5 Lymphatics, Thorax 6 Lymphatics, Abdomen 7 Lymphatics, Pelvis 8 Lymphatics, Inguinal	9 High Dose Rate (HDR)	7 Cesium 137 (Cs-137) 8 Iridium 192 (Ir-192) 9 Iodine 125 (I-125) B Palladium 103 (Pd-103) C Californium 252 (Cf-252) Y Other Isotope	Z None
Ø Bone Marrow 1 Thymus 2 Spleen 3 Lymphatics, Neck 4 Lymphatics, Axillary 5 Lymphatics, Thorax 6 Lymphatics, Abdomen 7 Lymphatics, Pelvis 8 Lymphatics, Inguinal	B Low Dose Rate (LDR)	6 Cesium 131 (Cs-131) 7 Cesium 137 (Cs-137) 8 Iridium 192 (Ir-192) 9 Iodine 125 (I-125) C Californium 252 (Cf-252) Y Other Isotope	Z None
Ø Bone Marrow 1 Thymus 2 Spleen 3 Lymphatics, Neck 4 Lymphatics, Axillary 5 Lymphatics, Thorax 6 Lymphatics, Abdomen 7 Lymphatics, Pelvis 8 Lymphatics, Inguinal	B Low Dose Rate (LDR)	B Palladium 103 (Pd-103)	1 Unidirectional Source Z None

D   Radiation Therapy
7   Lymphatic and Hematologic System
2   Stereotactic Radiosurgery

Treatment Site Character 4	Modality Qualifier Character 5	Isotope Character 6	Qualifier Character 7

Ø   Bone Marrow
1   Thymus
2   Spleen
3   Lymphatics, Neck
4   Lymphatics, Axillary
5   Lymphatics, Thorax
6   Lymphatics, Abdomen
7   Lymphatics, Pelvis
8   Lymphatics, Inguinal
	D Stereotactic Other Photon
	     Radiosurgery
	H Stereotactic Particulate
	     Radiosurgery
	J Stereotactic Gamma Beam
	     Radiosurgery
		Z None	Z None

DRG Non-OR   All treatment site, modality, isotope, and qualifier values

D   Radiation Therapy
7   Lymphatic and Hematologic System
Y   Other Radiation

Treatment Site Character 4	Modality Qualifier Character 5	Isotope Character 6	Qualifier Character 7
Ø Bone Marrow 1 Thymus 2 Spleen 3 Lymphatics, Neck 4 Lymphatics, Axillary 5 Lymphatics, Thorax 6 Lymphatics, Abdomen 7 Lymphatics, Pelvis 8 Lymphatics, Inguinal	8 Hyperthermia F Plaque Radiation	Z None	Z None

NC Noncovered Procedure   LC Limited Coverage   QA Questionable OB Admit   NT New Tech Add-on   ⊞ Combination Member   ♂ Male   ♀ Female

ICD-10-PCS 2022   783

Radiation Therapy

D   Radiation Therapy
8   Eye
Ø   Beam Radiation

Treatment Site Character 4	Modality Qualifier Character 5	Isotope Character 6	Qualifier Character 7
Ø Eye	Ø Photons <1 MeV 1 Photons 1- 10 MeV 2 Photons >10 MeV 4 Heavy Particles (Protons, Ions) 5 Neutrons 6 Neutron Capture	Z None	Z None
Ø Eye	3 Electrons	Z None	Ø Intraoperative Z None

D   Radiation Therapy
8   Eye
1   Brachytherapy

Treatment Site Character 4	Modality Qualifier Character 5	Isotope Character 6	Qualifier Character 7
Ø Eye	9 High Dose Rate (HDR)	7 Cesium 137 (Cs-137) 8 Iridium 192 (Ir-192) 9 Iodine 125 (I-125) B Palladium 103 (Pd-103) C Californium 252 (Cf-252) Y Other Isotope	Z None
Ø Eye	B Low Dose Rate (LDR)	6 Cesium 131 (Cs-131) 7 Cesium 137 (Cs-137) 8 Iridium 192 (Ir-192) 9 Iodine 125 (I-125) C Californium 252 (Cf-252) Y Other Isotope	Z None
Ø Eye	B Low Dose Rate (LDR)	B Palladium 103 (Pd-103)	1 Unidirectional Source Z None

D   Radiation Therapy
8   Eye
2   Stereotactic Radiosurgery

Treatment Site Character 4	Modality Qualifier Character 5	Isotope Character 6	Qualifier Character 7
Ø Eye	D Stereotactic Other Photon Radiosurgery H Stereotactic Particulate Radiosurgery J Stereotactic Gamma Beam Radiosurgery	Z None	Z None

DRG Non-OR All treatment site, modality, isotope, and qualifier values

D   Radiation Therapy
8   Eye
Y   Other Radiation

Treatment Site Character 4	Modality Qualifier Character 5	Isotope Character 6	Qualifier Character 7
Ø Eye	7 Contact Radiation 8 Hyperthermia F Plaque Radiation	Z None	Z None

D Radiation Therapy
9 Ear, Nose, Mouth and Throat
Ø Beam Radiation

Treatment Site Character 4	Modality Qualifier Character 5	Isotope Character 6	Qualifier Character 7
Ø Ear 1 Nose 3 Hypopharynx 4 Mouth 5 Tongue 6 Salivary Glands 7 Sinuses 8 Hard Palate 9 Soft Palate B Larynx D Nasopharynx F Oropharynx	Ø Photons <1 MeV 1 Photons 1- 10 MeV 2 Photons >10 MeV 4 Heavy Particles (Protons, Ions) 5 Neutrons 6 Neutron Capture	Z None	Z None
Ø Ear 1 Nose 3 Hypopharynx 4 Mouth 5 Tongue 6 Salivary Glands 7 Sinuses 8 Hard Palate 9 Soft Palate B Larynx D Nasopharynx F Oropharynx	3 Electrons	Z None	Ø Intraoperative Z None

D Radiation Therapy
9 Ear, Nose, Mouth and Throat
1 Brachytherapy

Treatment Site Character 4	Modality Qualifier Character 5	Isotope Character 6	Qualifier Character 7
Ø Ear 1 Nose 3 Hypopharynx 4 Mouth 5 Tongue 6 Salivary Glands 7 Sinuses 8 Hard Palate 9 Soft Palate B Larynx D Nasopharynx F Oropharynx	9 High Dose Rate (HDR)	7 Cesium 137 (Cs-137) 8 Iridium 192 (Ir-192) 9 Iodine 125 (I-125) B Palladium 103 (Pd-103) C Californium 252 (Cf-252) Y Other Isotope	Z None
Ø Ear 1 Nose 3 Hypopharynx 4 Mouth 5 Tongue 6 Salivary Glands 7 Sinuses 8 Hard Palate 9 Soft Palate B Larynx D Nasopharynx F Oropharynx	B Low Dose Rate (LDR)	6 Cesium 131 (Cs-131) 7 Cesium 137 (Cs-137) 8 Iridium 192 (Ir-192) 9 Iodine 125 (I-125) C Californium 252 (Cf-252) Y Other Isotope	Z None
Ø Ear 1 Nose 3 Hypopharynx 4 Mouth 5 Tongue 6 Salivary Glands 7 Sinuses 8 Hard Palate 9 Soft Palate B Larynx D Nasopharynx F Oropharynx	B Low Dose Rate (LDR)	B Palladium 103 (Pd-103)	1 Unidirectional Source Z None

NC Noncovered Procedure   LC Limited Coverage   QA Questionable OB Admit   NT New Tech Add-on   ✛ Combination Member   ♂ Male   ♀ Female

Radiation Therapy

D   **Radiation Therapy**
9   **Ear, Nose, Mouth and Throat**
2   **Stereotactic Radiosurgery**

Treatment Site Character 4	Modality Qualifier Character 5	Isotope Character 6	Qualifier Character 7

Ø Ear
1 Nose
4 Mouth
5 Tongue
6 Salivary Glands
7 Sinuses
8 Hard Palate
9 Soft Palate
B Larynx
C Pharynx
D Nasopharynx
	D Stereotactic Other Photon
	   Radiosurgery
	H Stereotactic Particulate
	   Radiosurgery
	J Stereotactic Gamma Beam
	   Radiosurgery
		Z None	Z None

DRG Non-OR All treatment site, modality, isotope, and qualifier values

D   **Radiation Therapy**
9   **Ear, Nose, Mouth and Throat**
Y   **Other Radiation**

Treatment Site Character 4	Modality Qualifier Character 5	Isotope Character 6	Qualifier Character 7
Ø Ear 1 Nose 5 Tongue 6 Salivary Glands 7 Sinuses 8 Hard Palate 9 Soft Palate	7 Contact Radiation 8 Hyperthermia F Plaque Radiation	Z None	Z None
3 Hypopharynx F Oropharynx	7 Contact Radiation 8 Hyperthermia	Z None	Z None
4 Mouth B Larynx D Nasopharynx	7 Contact Radiation 8 Hyperthermia C Intraoperative Radiation Therapy (IORT) F Plaque Radiation	Z None	Z None
C Pharynx	C Intraoperative Radiation Therapy (IORT) F Plaque Radiation	Z None	Z None

D   **Radiation Therapy**
B   **Respiratory System**
Ø   **Beam Radiation**

Treatment Site Character 4	Modality Qualifier Character 5	Isotope Character 6	Qualifier Character 7
Ø Trachea 1 Bronchus 2 Lung 5 Pleura 6 Mediastinum 7 Chest Wall 8 Diaphragm	Ø Photons <1 MeV 1 Photons 1- 10 MeV 2 Photons >10 MeV 4 Heavy Particles (Protons, Ions) 5 Neutrons 6 Neutron Capture	Z None	Z None
Ø Trachea 1 Bronchus 2 Lung 5 Pleura 6 Mediastinum 7 Chest Wall 8 Diaphragm	3 Electrons	Z None	Ø Intraoperative Z None

D   Radiation Therapy
B   Respiratory System
1   Brachytherapy

Treatment Site Character 4	Modality Qualifier Character 5	Isotope Character 6	Qualifier Character 7
Ø Trachea 1 Bronchus 2 Lung 5 Pleura 6 Mediastinum 7 Chest Wall 8 Diaphragm	9 High Dose Rate (HDR)	7 Cesium 137 (Cs-137) 8 Iridium 192 (Ir-192) 9 Iodine 125 (I-125) B Palladium 103 (Pd-103) C Californium 252 (Cf-252) Y Other Isotope	Z None
Ø Trachea 1 Bronchus 2 Lung 5 Pleura 6 Mediastinum 7 Chest Wall 8 Diaphragm	B Low Dose Rate (LDR)	6 Cesium 131 (Cs-131) 7 Cesium 137 (Cs-137) 8 Iridium 192 (Ir-192) 9 Iodine 125 (I-125) C Californium 252 (Cf-252) Y Other Isotope	Z None
Ø Trachea 1 Bronchus 2 Lung 5 Pleura 6 Mediastinum 7 Chest Wall 8 Diaphragm	B Low Dose Rate (LDR)	B Palladium 103 (Pd-103)	1 Unidirectional Source Z None

D   Radiation Therapy
B   Respiratory System
2   Stereotactic Radiosurgery

Treatment Site Character 4	Modality Qualifier Character 5	Isotope Character 6	Qualifier Character 7

Ø Trachea
1 Bronchus
2 Lung
5 Pleura
6 Mediastinum
7 Chest Wall
8 Diaphragm
	D Stereotactic Other Photon
	   Radiosurgery
	H Stereotactic Particulate
	   Radiosurgery
	J Stereotactic Gamma Beam
	   Radiosurgery
		Z None	Z None

DRG Non-OR   All treatment site, modality, isotope, and qualifier values

D   Radiation Therapy
B   Respiratory System
Y   Other Radiation

Treatment Site Character 4	Modality Qualifier Character 5	Isotope Character 6	Qualifier Character 7
Ø Trachea 1 Bronchus 2 Lung 5 Pleura 6 Mediastinum 7 Chest Wall 8 Diaphragm	7 Contact Radiation 8 Hyperthermia F Plaque Radiation K Laser Interstitial Thermal Therapy	Z None	Z None

Valid OR   DBY[Ø,1,2,5,6,7,8]KZZ

NC Noncovered Procedure   **LC** Limited Coverage   **QA** Questionable OB Admit   **NT** New Tech Add-on   ✚ Combination Member   ♂ Male   ♀ Female

ICD-10-PCS 2022   787

D   **Radiation Therapy**
D   **Gastrointestinal System**
Ø   **Beam Radiation**

Treatment Site Character 4	Modality Qualifier Character 5	Isotope Character 6	Qualifier Character 7
Ø Esophagus 1 Stomach 2 Duodenum 3 Jejunum 4 Ileum 5 Colon 7 Rectum	Ø Photons <1 MeV 1 Photons 1- 10 MeV 2 Photons >10 MeV 4 Heavy Particles (Protons, Ions) 5 Neutrons 6 Neutron Capture	Z None	Z None
Ø Esophagus 1 Stomach 2 Duodenum 3 Jejunum 4 Ileum 5 Colon 7 Rectum	3 Electrons	Z None	Ø Intraoperative Z None

D   **Radiation Therapy**
D   **Gastrointestinal System**
1   **Brachytherapy**

Treatment Site Character 4	Modality Qualifier Character 5	Isotope Character 6	Qualifier Character 7
Ø Esophagus 1 Stomach 2 Duodenum 3 Jejunum 4 Ileum 5 Colon 7 Rectum	9 High Dose Rate (HDR)	7 Cesium 137 (Cs-137) 8 Iridium 192 (Ir-192) 9 Iodine 125 (I-125) B Palladium 103 (Pd-103) C Californium 252 (Cf-252) Y Other Isotope	Z None
Ø Esophagus 1 Stomach 2 Duodenum 3 Jejunum 4 Ileum 5 Colon 7 Rectum	B Low Dose Rate (LDR)	6 Cesium 131 (Cs-131) 7 Cesium 137 (Cs-137) 8 Iridium 192 (Ir-192) 9 Iodine 125 (I-125) C Californium 252 (Cf-252) Y Other Isotope	Z None
Ø Esophagus 1 Stomach 2 Duodenum 3 Jejunum 4 Ileum 5 Colon 7 Rectum	B Low Dose Rate (LDR)	B Palladium 103 (Pd-103)	1 Unidirectional Source Z None

D   **Radiation Therapy**
D   **Gastrointestinal System**
2   **Stereotactic Radiosurgery**

Treatment Site Character 4	Modality Qualifier Character 5	Isotope Character 6	Qualifier Character 7
Ø Esophagus 1 Stomach 2 Duodenum 3 Jejunum 4 Ileum 5 Colon 7 Rectum	D Stereotactic Other Photon Radiosurgery H Stereotactic Particulate Radiosurgery J Stereotactic Gamma Beam Radiosurgery	Z None	Z None

DRG Non-OR All treatment site, modality, isotope, and qualifier values

D   **Radiation therapy**
D   **Gastrointestinal System**
Y   **Other Radiation**

Treatment Site Character 4	Modality Qualifier Character 5	Isotope Character 6	Qualifier Character 7
0 Esophagus	**7** Contact Radiation **8** Hyperthermia **F** Plaque Radiation **K** Laser Interstitial Thermal Therapy	**Z** None	**Z** None
1 Stomach **2** Duodenum **3** Jejunum **4** Ileum **5** Colon **7** Rectum	**7** Contact Radiation **8** Hyperthermia **C** Intraoperative Radiation Therapy (IORT) **F** Plaque Radiation **K** Laser Interstitial Thermal Therapy	**Z** None	**Z** None
8 Anus	**C** Intraoperative Radiation Therapy (IORT) **F** Plaque Radiation **K** Laser Interstitial Thermal Therapy	**Z** None	**Z** None

Valid OR	DDY0KZZ
Valid OR	DDY[1,2,3,4,5,7]KZZ
Valid OR	DDY8KZZ

D   **Radiation Therapy**
F   **Hepatobiliary System and Pancreas**
0   **Beam Radiation**

Treatment Site Character 4	Modality Qualifier Character 5	Isotope Character 6	Qualifier Character 7
0 Liver **1** Gallbladder **2** Bile Ducts **3** Pancreas	**0** Photons <1 MeV **1** Photons 1- 10 MeV **2** Photons >10 MeV **4** Heavy Particles (Protons, Ions) **5** Neutrons **6** Neutron Capture	**Z** None	**Z** None
0 Liver **1** Gallbladder **2** Bile Ducts **3** Pancreas	**3** Electrons	**Z** None	**0** Intraoperative **Z** None

D   **Radiation Therapy**
F   **Hepatobiliary System and Pancreas**
1   **Brachytherapy**

Treatment Site Character 4	Modality Qualifier Character 5	Isotope Character 6	Qualifier Character 7
0 Liver **1** Gallbladder **2** Bile Ducts **3** Pancreas	**9** High Dose Rate (HDR)	**7** Cesium 137 (Cs-137) **8** Iridium 192 (Ir-192) **9** Iodine 125 (I-125) **B** Palladium 103 (Pd-103) **C** Californium 252 (Cf-252) **Y** Other Isotope	**Z** None
0 Liver **1** Gallbladder **2** Bile Ducts **3** Pancreas	**B** Low Dose Rate (LDR)	**6** Cesium 131 (Cs-131) **7** Cesium 137 (Cs-137) **8** Iridium 192 (Ir-192) **9** Iodine 125 (I-125) **C** Californium 252 (Cf-252) **Y** Other Isotope	**Z** None
0 Liver **1** Gallbladder **2** Bile Ducts **3** Pancreas	**B** Low Dose Rate (LDR)	**B** Palladium 103 (Pd-103)	**1** Unidirectional Source **Z** None

NC Noncovered Procedure   **LC** Limited Coverage   **QA** Questionable OB Admit   **NT** New Tech Add-on   ⊞ Combination Member   ♂ Male   ♀ Female

ICD-10-PCS 2022   789

D **Radiation Therapy**
F **Hepatobiliary System and Pancreas**
2 **Stereotactic Radiosurgery**

Treatment Site Character 4	Modality Qualifier Character 5	Isotope Character 6	Qualifier Character 7
Ø Liver 1 Gallbladder 2 Bile Ducts 3 Pancreas	**D** Stereotactic Other Photon Radiosurgery **H** Stereotactic Particulate Radiosurgery **J** Stereotactic Gamma Beam Radiosurgery	**Z** None	**Z** None

DRG Non-OR All treatment site, modality, isotope, and qualifier values

D **Radiation Therapy**
F **Hepatobiliary System and Pancreas**
Y **Other Radiation**

Treatment Site Character 4	Modality Qualifier Character 5	Isotope Character 6	Qualifier Character 7
Ø Liver 1 Gallbladder 2 Bile Ducts 3 Pancreas	**7** Contact Radiation **8** Hyperthermia **C** Intraoperative Radiation Therapy (IORT) **F** Plaque Radiation **K** Laser Interstitial Thermal Therapy	**Z** None	**Z** None

Valid OR DFY[Ø,1,2,3]KZZ

D **Radiation Therapy**
G **Endocrine System**
Ø **Beam Radiation**

Treatment Site Character 4	Modality Qualifier Character 5	Isotope Character 6	Qualifier Character 7
Ø Pituitary Gland 1 Pineal Body 2 Adrenal Glands 4 Parathyroid Glands 5 Thyroid	Ø Photons <1 MeV 1 Photons 1- 10 MeV 2 Photons >10 MeV 5 Neutrons 6 Neutron Capture	**Z** None	**Z** None
Ø Pituitary Gland 1 Pineal Body 2 Adrenal Glands 4 Parathyroid Glands 5 Thyroid	3 Electrons	**Z** None	**Ø** Intraoperative **Z** None

D **Radiation Therapy**
G **Endocrine System**
1 **Brachytherapy**

Treatment Site Character 4	Modality Qualifier Character 5	Isotope Character 6	Qualifier Character 7
Ø Pituitary Gland 1 Pineal Body 2 Adrenal Glands 4 Parathyroid Glands 5 Thyroid	9 High Dose Rate (HDR)	7 Cesium 137 (Cs-137) 8 Iridium 192 (Ir-192) 9 Iodine 125 (I-125) B Palladium 103 (Pd-103) C Californium 252 (Cf-252) Y Other Isotope	**Z** None
Ø Pituitary Gland 1 Pineal Body 2 Adrenal Glands 4 Parathyroid Glands 5 Thyroid	B Low Dose Rate (LDR)	6 Cesium 131 (Cs-131) 7 Cesium 137 (Cs-137) 8 Iridium 192 (Ir-192) 9 Iodine 125 (I-125) C Californium 252 (Cf-252) Y Other Isotope	**Z** None
Ø Pituitary Gland 1 Pineal Body 2 Adrenal Glands 4 Parathyroid Glands 5 Thyroid	B Low Dose Rate (LDR)	B Palladium 103 (Pd-103)	**1** Unidirectional Source **Z** None

D   **Radiation Therapy**
G   **Endocrine System**
2   **Stereotactic Radiosurgery**

Treatment Site Character 4	Modality Qualifier Character 5	Isotope Character 6	Qualifier Character 7

Ø Pituitary Gland
1 Pineal Body
2 Adrenal Glands
4 Parathyroid Glands
5 Thyroid
	D Stereotactic Other Photon
	    Radiosurgery
	H Stereotactic Particulate
	    Radiosurgery
	J Stereotactic Gamma Beam
	    Radiosurgery
		Z None	**Z** None

DRG Non-OR   All treatment site, modality, isotope, and qualifier values

D   **Radiation therapy**
G   **Endocrine System**
Y   **Other Radiation**

Treatment Site Character 4	Modality Qualifier Character 5	Isotope Character 6	Qualifier Character 7
Ø Pituitary Gland **1** Pineal Body **2** Adrenal Glands **4** Parathyroid Glands **5** Thyroid	**7** Contact Radiation **8** Hyperthermia **F** Plaque Radiation **K** Laser Interstitial Thermal Therapy	**Z** None	**Z** None

Valid OR   DGY[Ø,1,2,4,5]KZZ

D   **Radiation Therapy**
H   **Skin**
Ø   **Beam Radiation**

Treatment Site Character 4	Modality Qualifier Character 5	Isotope Character 6	Qualifier Character 7
2 Skin, Face **3** Skin, Neck **4** Skin, Arm **6** Skin, Chest **7** Skin, Back **8** Skin, Abdomen **9** Skin, Buttock **B** Skin, Leg	**Ø** Photons <1 MeV **1** Photons 1- 10 MeV **2** Photons >10 MeV **4** Heavy Particles (Protons, Ions) **5** Neutrons **6** Neutron Capture	**Z** None	**Z** None
2 Skin, Face **3** Skin, Neck **4** Skin, Arm **6** Skin, Chest **7** Skin, Back **8** Skin, Abdomen **9** Skin, Buttock **B** Skin, Leg	**3** Electrons	**Z** None	**Ø** Intraoperative **Z** None

D   **Radiation Therapy**
H   **Skin**
Y   **Other Radiation**

Treatment Site Character 4	Modality Qualifier Character 5	Isotope Character 6	Qualifier Character 7
2 Skin, Face **3** Skin, Neck **4** Skin, Arm **6** Skin, Chest **7** Skin, Back **8** Skin, Abdomen **9** Skin, Buttock **B** Skin, Leg	**7** Contact Radiation **8** Hyperthermia **F** Plaque Radiation	**Z** None	**Z** None
5 Skin, Hand **C** Skin, Foot	**F** Plaque Radiation	**Z** None	**Z** None

NC Noncovered Procedure   **LC** Limited Coverage   **QA** Questionable OB Admit   **NT** New Tech Add-on   ⊞ Combination Member   ♂ Male   ♀ Female

ICD-10-PCS 2022   **791**

D　Radiation Therapy
M　Breast
Ø　Beam Radiation

Treatment Site Character 4	Modality Qualifier Character 5	Isotope Character 6	Qualifier Character 7
Ø　Breast, Left 1　Breast, Right	Ø　Photons <1 MeV 1　Photons 1- 10 MeV 2　Photons >10 MeV 4　Heavy Particles (Protons, Ions) 5　Neutrons 6　Neutron Capture	Z　None	Z　None
Ø　Breast, Left 1　Breast, Right	3　Electrons	Z　None	Ø　Intraoperative Z　None

D　Radiation Therapy
M　Breast
1　Brachytherapy

Treatment Site Character 4	Modality Qualifier Character 5	Isotope Character 6	Qualifier Character 7
Ø　Breast, Left 1　Breast, Right	9　High Dose Rate (HDR)	7　Cesium 137 (Cs-137) 8　Iridium 192 (Ir-192) 9　Iodine 125 (I-125) B　Palladium 103 (Pd-103) C　Californium 252 (Cf-252) Y　Other Isotope	Z　None
Ø　Breast, Left 1　Breast, Right	B　Low Dose Rate (LDR)	6　Cesium 131 (Cs-131) 7　Cesium 137 (Cs-137) 8　Iridium 192 (Ir-192) 9　Iodine 125 (I-125) C　Californium 252 (Cf-252) Y　Other Isotope	Z　None
Ø　Breast, Left 1　Breast, Right	B　Low Dose Rate (LDR)	B　Palladium 103 (Pd-103)	1　Unidirectional Source Z　None

D　Radiation Therapy
M　Breast
2　Stereotactic Radiosurgery

Treatment Site Character 4	Modality Qualifier Character 5	Isotope Character 6	Qualifier Character 7
Ø　Breast, Left 1　Breast, Right	D　Stereotactic Other Photon Radiosurgery H　Stereotactic Particulate Radiosurgery J　Stereotactic Gamma Beam Radiosurgery	Z　None	Z　None

DRG Non-OR All treatment site, modality, isotope, and qualifier values

D　Radiation Therapy
M　Breast
Y　Other Radiation

Treatment Site Character 4	Modality Qualifier Character 5	Isotope Character 6	Qualifier Character 7
Ø　Breast, Left 1　Breast, Right	7　Contact Radiation 8　Hyperthermia F　Plaque Radiation K　Laser Interstitial Thermal Therapy	Z　None	Z　None

Valid OR　DMY[Ø,1]KZZ

D   **Radiation Therapy**
P   **Musculoskeletal System**
Ø   **Beam Radiation**

Treatment Site Character 4	Modality Qualifier Character 5	Isotope Character 6	Qualifier Character 7
Ø Skull 2 Maxilla 3 Mandible 4 Sternum 5 Rib(s) 6 Humerus 7 Radius/Ulna 8 Pelvic Bones 9 Femur B Tibia/Fibula C Other Bone	Ø Photons <1 MeV 1 Photons 1- 10 MeV 2 Photons >10 MeV 4 Heavy Particles (Protons, Ions) 5 Neutrons 6 Neutron Capture	Z None	Z None
Ø Skull 2 Maxilla 3 Mandible 4 Sternum 5 Rib(s) 6 Humerus 7 Radius/Ulna 8 Pelvic Bones 9 Femur B Tibia/Fibula C Other Bone	3 Electrons	Z None	Ø Intraoperative Z None

D   **Radiation Therapy**
P   **Musculoskeletal System**
Y   **Other Radiation**

Treatment Site Character 4	Modality Qualifier Character 5	Isotope Character 6	Qualifier Character 7
Ø Skull 2 Maxilla 3 Mandible 4 Sternum 5 Rib(s) 6 Humerus 7 Radius/Ulna 8 Pelvic Bones 9 Femur B Tibia/Fibula C Other Bone	7 Contact Radiation 8 Hyperthermia F Plaque Radiation	Z None	Z None

D   **Radiation Therapy**
T   **Urinary System**
Ø   **Beam Radiation**

Treatment Site Character 4	Modality Qualifier Character 5	Isotope Character 6	Qualifier Character 7
Ø Kidney 1 Ureter 2 Bladder 3 Urethra	Ø Photons <1 MeV 1 Photons 1- 10 MeV 2 Photons >10 MeV 4 Heavy Particles (Protons, Ions) 5 Neutrons 6 Neutron Capture	Z None	Z None
Ø Kidney 1 Ureter 2 Bladder 3 Urethra	3 Electrons	Z None	Ø Intraoperative Z None

NC Noncovered Procedure   **LC** Limited Coverage   **QA** Questionable OB Admit   **NT** New Tech Add-on   ✚ Combination Member   ♂Male   ♀Female

ICD-10-PCS 2022   **793**

Radiation Therapy

D   Radiation Therapy
T   Urinary System
1   Brachytherapy

Treatment Site Character 4	Modality Qualifier Character 5	Isotope Character 6	Qualifier Character 7
Ø Kidney 1 Ureter 2 Bladder 3 Urethra	9 High Dose Rate (HDR)	7 Cesium 137 (Cs-137) 8 Iridium 192 (Ir-192) 9 Iodine 125 (I-125) B Palladium 103 (Pd-103) C Californium 252 (Cf-252) Y Other Isotope	Z None
Ø Kidney 1 Ureter 2 Bladder 3 Urethra	B Low Dose Rate (LDR)	6 Cesium 131 (Cs-131) 7 Cesium 137 (Cs-137) 8 Iridium 192 (Ir-192) 9 Iodine 125 (I-125) C Californium 252 (Cf-252) Y Other Isotope	Z None
Ø Kidney 1 Ureter 2 Bladder 3 Urethra	B Low Dose Rate (LDR)	B Palladium 103 (Pd-103)	1 Unidirectional Source Z None

D   Radiation Therapy
T   Urinary System
2   Stereotactic Radiosurgery

Treatment Site Character 4	Modality Qualifier Character 5	Isotope Character 6	Qualifier Character 7
Ø Kidney 1 Ureter 2 Bladder 3 Urethra	D Stereotactic Other Photon Radiosurgery H Stereotactic Particulate Radiosurgery J Stereotactic Gamma Beam Radiosurgery	Z None	Z None

DRG Non-OR All treatment site, modality, isotope, and qualifier values

D   Radiation Therapy
T   Urinary System
Y   Other Radiation

Treatment Site Character 4	Modality Qualifier Character 5	Isotope Character 6	Qualifier Character 7
Ø Kidney 1 Ureter 2 Bladder 3 Urethra	7 Contact Radiation 8 Hyperthermia C Intraoperative Radiation Therapy (IORT) F Plaque Radiation	Z None	Z None

D   Radiation Therapy
U   Female Reproductive System
Ø   Beam Radiation

Treatment Site Character 4	Modality Qualifier Character 5	Isotope Character 6	Qualifier Character 7
Ø Ovary ♀ 1 Cervix ♀ 2 Uterus ♀	Ø Photons <1 MeV 1 Photons 1- 10 MeV 2 Photons >10 MeV 4 Heavy Particles (Protons, Ions) 5 Neutrons 6 Neutron Capture	Z None	Z None
Ø Ovary ♀ 1 Cervix ♀ 2 Uterus ♀	3 Electrons	Z None	Ø Intraoperative Z None

♀ All treatment site, modality, isotope, and qualifier values

D   Radiation Therapy
U   Female Reproductive System
1   Brachytherapy

Treatment Site Character 4	Modality Qualifier Character 5	Isotope Character 6	Qualifier Character 7
Ø Ovary ♀ 1 Cervix ♀ 2 Uterus ♀	9 High Dose Rate (HDR)	7 Cesium 137 (Cs-137) 8 Iridium 192 (Ir-192) 9 Iodine 125 (I-125) B Palladium 103 (Pd-103) C Californium 252 (Cf-252) Y Other Isotope	Z None
Ø Ovary ♀ 1 Cervix ♀ 2 Uterus ♀	B Low Dose Rate (LDR)	6 Cesium 131 (Cs-131) 7 Cesium 137 (Cs-137) 8 Iridium 192 (Ir-192) 9 Iodine 125 (I-125) C Californium 252 (Cf-252) Y Other Isotope	Z None
Ø Ovary ♀ 1 Cervix ♀ 2 Uterus ♀	B Low Dose Rate (LDR)	B Palladium 103 (Pd-103)	1 Unidirectional Source Z None

  ♀   All treatment site, modality, isotope, and qualifier values

D   Radiation Therapy
U   Female Reproductive System
2   Stereotactic Radiosurgery

Treatment Site Character 4	Modality Qualifier Character 5	Isotope Character 6	Qualifier Character 7

Ø Ovary ♀
1 Cervix ♀
2 Uterus ♀
	D Stereotactic Other Photon
	   Radiosurgery
	H Stereotactic Particulate
	   Radiosurgery
	J Stereotactic Gamma Beam
	   Radiosurgery
		Z None	Z None

  DRG Non-OR   All treatment site, modality, isotope, and qualifier values
  ♀   All treatment site, modality, isotope, and qualifier values

D   Radiation Therapy
U   Female Reproductive System
Y   Other Radiation

Treatment Site Character 4	Modality Qualifier Character 5	Isotope Character 6	Qualifier Character 7
Ø Ovary ♀ 1 Cervix ♀ 2 Uterus ♀	7 Contact Radiation 8 Hyperthermia C Intraoperative Radiation Therapy (IORT) F Plaque Radiation	Z None	Z None

  ♀   All treatment site, modality, isotope, and qualifier values

D   Radiation Therapy
V   Male Reproductive System
Ø   Beam Radiation

Treatment Site Character 4	Modality Qualifier Character 5	Isotope Character 6	Qualifier Character 7
Ø Prostate ♂ 1 Testis ♂	Ø Photons <1 MeV 1 Photons 1- 10 MeV 2 Photons >10 MeV 4 Heavy Particles (Protons, Ions) 5 Neutrons 6 Neutron Capture	Z None	Z None
Ø Prostate ♂ 1 Testis ♂	3 Electrons	Z None	Ø Intraoperative Z None

  ♂   All treatment site, modality, isotope, and qualifier values

---

NC Noncovered Procedure   **LC** Limited Coverage   **QA** Questionable OB Admit   **NT** New Tech Add-on   ✚ Combination Member   ♂ Male   ♀ Female

D Radiation Therapy
V Male Reproductive System
1 Brachytherapy

Treatment Site Character 4	Modality Qualifier Character 5	Isotope Character 6	Qualifier Character 7
0 Prostate ♂ 1 Testis ♂	9 High Dose Rate (HDR)	7 Cesium 137 (Cs-137) 8 Iridium 192 (Ir-192) 9 Iodine 125 (I-125) B Palladium 103 (Pd-103) C Californium 252 (Cf-252) Y Other Isotope	Z None
0 Prostate ♂ 1 Testis ♂	B Low Dose Rate (LDR)	6 Cesium 131 (Cs-131) 7 Cesium 137 (Cs-137) 8 Iridium 192 (Ir-192) 9 Iodine 125 (I-125) C Californium 252 (Cf-252) Y Other Isotope	Z None
0 Prostate ♂ 1 Testis ♂	B Low Dose Rate (LDR)	B Palladium 103 (Pd-103)	1 Unidirectional Source Z None

♂ All treatment site, modality, isotope, and qualifier values

D Radiation Therapy
V Male Reproductive System
2 Stereotactic Radiosurgery

Treatment Site Character 4	Modality Qualifier Character 5	Isotope Character 6	Qualifier Character 7

0 Prostate ♂
1 Testis ♂
	D Stereotactic Other Photon
	   Radiosurgery
	H Stereotactic Particulate
	   Radiosurgery
	J Stereotactic Gamma Beam
	   Radiosurgery
		Z None	Z None

DRG Non-OR All treatment site, modality, isotope, and qualifier values
♂ All treatment site, modality, isotope, and qualifier values

D Radiation Therapy
V Male Reproductive System
Y Other Radiation

Treatment Site Character 4	Modality Qualifier Character 5	Isotope Character 6	Qualifier Character 7
0 Prostate ♂	7 Contact Radiation 8 Hyperthermia C Intraoperative Radiation Therapy (IORT) F Plaque Radiation K Laser Interstitial Thermal Therapy	Z None	Z None
1 Testis ♂	7 Contact Radiation 8 Hyperthermia F Plaque Radiation	Z None	Z None

Valid OR   DVY0KZZ
♂ All treatment site, modality, isotope, and qualifier values

D Radiation Therapy
W Anatomical Regions
0 Beam Radiation

Treatment Site Character 4	Modality Qualifier Character 5	Isotope Character 6	Qualifier Character 7
1 Head and Neck 2 Chest 3 Abdomen 4 Hemibody 5 Whole Body 6 Pelvic Region	0 Photons <1 MeV 1 Photons 1- 10 MeV 2 Photons >10 MeV 4 Heavy Particles (Protons, Ions) 5 Neutrons 6 Neutron Capture	Z None	Z None
1 Head and Neck 2 Chest 3 Abdomen 4 Hemibody 5 Whole Body 6 Pelvic Region	3 Electrons	Z None	0 Intraoperative Z None

D Radiation Therapy
W Anatomical Regions
1 Brachytherapy

Treatment Site Character 4	Modality Qualifier Character 5	Isotope Character 6	Qualifier Character 7
Ø Cranial Cavity K Upper Back L Lower Back P Gastrointestinal Tract Q Respiratory Tract R Genitourinary Tract X Upper Extremity Y Lower Extremity	B Low Dose Rate (LDR)	B Palladium 103 (Pd-103)	1 Unidirectional Source Z None
1 Head and Neck 2 Chest 3 Abdomen 6 Pelvic Region	9 High Dose Rate (HDR)	7 Cesium 137 (Cs-137) 8 Iridium 192 (Ir-192) 9 Iodine 125 (I-125) B Palladium 103 (Pd-103) C Californium 252 (Cf-252) Y Other Isotope	Z None
1 Head and Neck 2 Chest 3 Abdomen 6 Pelvic Region	B Low Dose Rate (LDR)	6 Cesium 131 (Cs-131) 7 Cesium 137 (Cs-137) 8 Iridium 192 (Ir-192) 9 Iodine 125 (I-125) C Californium 252 (Cf-252) Y Other Isotope	Z None
1 Head and Neck 2 Chest 3 Abdomen 6 Pelvic Region	B Low Dose Rate (LDR)	B Palladium 103 (Pd-103)	1 Unidirectional Source Z None

D Radiation Therapy
W Anatomical Regions
2 Stereotactic Radiosurgery

Treatment Site Character 4	Modality Qualifier Character 5	Isotope Character 6	Qualifier Character 7

1 Head and Neck
2 Chest
3 Abdomen
6 Pelvic Region
	D Stereotactic Other Photon
	   Radiosurgery
	H Stereotactic Particulate
	   Radiosurgery
	J Stereotactic Gamma Beam
	   Radiosurgery
		Z None	Z None

DRG Non-OR All treatment site, modality, isotope, and qualifier values

D Radiation Therapy
W Anatomical Regions
Y Other Radiation

Treatment Site Character 4	Modality Qualifier Character 5	Isotope Character 6	Qualifier Character 7
1 Head and Neck 2 Chest 3 Abdomen 4 Hemibody 6 Pelvic Region	7 Contact Radiation 8 Hyperthermia F Plaque Radiation	Z None	Z None
5 Whole Body	7 Contact Radiation 8 Hyperthermia F Plaque Radiation	Z None	Z None
5 Whole Body	G Isotope Administration	D Iodine 131 (I-131) F Phosphorus 32 (P-32) G Strontium 89 (Sr-89) H Strontium 90 (Sr-90) Y Other Isotope	Z None

---

NC Noncovered Procedure   LC Limited Coverage   QA Questionable OB Admit   NT New Tech Add-on   ✛ Combination Member   ♂ Male   ♀ Female

Physical Rehabilitation and Diagnostic Audiology F00–F15

F   **Physical Rehabilitation and Diagnostic Audiology**
0   **Rehabilitation**
0   **Speech Assessment**   Definition: Measurement of speech and related functions

Body System/Region Character 4	Type Qualifier Character 5	Equipment Character 6	Qualifier Character 7
3 Neurological System - Whole Body	**G** Communicative/Cognitive Integration Skills	**K** Audiovisual **M** Augmentative / Alternative Communication **P** Computer **Y** Other Equipment **Z** None	**Z** None
Z None	**0** Filtered Speech **3** Staggered Spondaic Word **Q** Performance Intensity Phonetically Balanced Speech Discrimination **R** Brief Tone Stimuli **S** Distorted Speech **T** Dichotic Stimuli **V** Temporal Ordering of Stimuli **W** Masking Patterns	**1** Audiometer **2** Sound Field / Booth **K** Audiovisual **Z** None	**Z** None
Z None	**1** Speech Threshold **2** Speech/Word Recognition	**1** Audiometer **2** Sound Field / Booth **9** Cochlear Implant **K** Audiovisual **Z** None	**Z** None
Z None	**4** Sensorineural Acuity Level	**1** Audiometer **2** Sound Field / Booth **Z** None	**Z** None
Z None	**5** Synthetic Sentence Identification	**1** Audiometer **2** Sound Field / Booth **9** Cochlear Implant **K** Audiovisual	**Z** None
Z None	**6** Speech and/or Language Screening **7** Nonspoken Language **8** Receptive/Expressive Language **C** Aphasia **G** Communicative/Cognitive Integration Skills **L** Augmentative/Alternative Communication System	**K** Audiovisual **M** Augmentative / Alternative Communication **P** Computer **Y** Other Equipment **Z** None	**Z** None
Z None	**9** Articulation/Phonology	**K** Audiovisual **P** Computer **Q** Speech Analysis **Y** Other Equipment **Z** None	**Z** None
Z None	**B** Motor Speech	**K** Audiovisual **N** Biosensory Feedback **P** Computer **Q** Speech Analysis **T** Aerodynamic Function **Y** Other Equipment **Z** None	**Z** None
Z None	**D** Fluency	**K** Audiovisual **N** Biosensory Feedback **P** Computer **Q** Speech Analysis **S** Voice Analysis **T** Aerodynamic Function **Y** Other Equipment **Z** None	**Z** None
Z None	**F** Voice	**K** Audiovisual **N** Biosensory Feedback **P** Computer **S** Voice Analysis **T** Aerodynamic Function **Y** Other Equipment **Z** None	**Z** None

DRG Non-OR   All body system/region, type qualifier, equipment, and qualifier values

F00 Continued on next page

NC Noncovered Procedure   **LC** Limited Coverage   **QA** Questionable OB Admit   **NT** New Tech Add-on   ⊞ Combination Member   ♂ Male   ♀ Female

F   **Physical Rehabilitation and Diagnostic Audiology**   *F00 Continued*
0   **Rehabilitation**
0   **Speech Assessment**   Definition: Measurement of speech and related functions

Body System/Region Character 4	Type Qualifier Character 5	Equipment Character 6	Qualifier Character 7
Z None	H Bedside Swallowing and Oral Function P Oral Peripheral Mechanism	Y Other Equipment Z None	Z None
Z None	J Instrumental Swallowing and Oral Function	T Aerodynamic Function W Swallowing Y Other Equipment	Z None
Z None	K Orofacial Myofunctional	K Audiovisual P Computer Y Other Equipment Z None	Z None
Z None	M Voice Prosthetic	K Audiovisual P Computer S Voice Analysis V Speech Prosthesis Y Other Equipment Z None	Z None
Z None	N Non-invasive Instrumental Status	N Biosensory Feedback P Computer Q Speech Analysis S Voice Analysis T Aerodynamic Function Y Other Equipment	Z None
Z None	X Other Specified Central Auditory Processing	Z None	Z None

DRG Non-OR   All body system/region, type qualifier, equipment, and qualifier values

F   **Physical Rehabilitation and Diagnostic Audiology**
0   **Rehabilitation**
1   **Motor and/or Nerve Function Assessment**   Definition: Measurement of motor, nerve, and related functions

Body System/Region Character 4	Type Qualifier Character 5	Equipment Character 6	Qualifier Character 7
0 Neurological System - Head and Neck 1 Neurological System - Upper Back/ Upper Extremity 2 Neurological System - Lower Back/ Lower Extremity 3 Neurological System - Whole Body	0 Muscle Performance	E Orthosis F Assistive, Adaptive, Supportive or Protective U Prosthesis Y Other Equipment Z None	Z None
0 Neurological System - Head and Neck 1 Neurological System - Upper Back/ Upper Extremity 2 Neurological System - Lower Back/ Lower Extremity 3 Neurological System - Whole Body	1 Integumentary Integrity 3 Coordination/Dexterity 4 Motor Function G Reflex Integrity	Z None	Z None
0 Neurological System - Head and Neck 1 Neurological System - Upper Back/ Upper Extremity 2 Neurological System - Lower Back/ Lower Extremity 3 Neurological System - Whole Body	5 Range of Motion and Joint Integrity 6 Sensory Awareness/Processing/ Integrity	Y Other Equipment Z None	Z None
D Integumentary System - Head and Neck F Integumentary System - Upper Back/ Upper Extremity G Integumentary System - Lower Back/ Lower Extremity H Integumentary System - Whole Body J Musculoskeletal System - Head and Neck K Musculoskeletal System - Upper Back/ Upper Extremity L Musculoskeletal System - Lower Back/ Lower Extremity M Musculoskeletal System - Whole Body	0 Muscle Performance	E Orthosis F Assistive, Adaptive, Supportive or Protective U Prosthesis Y Other Equipment Z None	Z None

DRG Non-OR   All body system/region, type qualifier, equipment, and qualifier values

F01 Continued on next page

F   Physical Rehabilitation and Diagnostic Audiology
Ø   Rehabilitation
1   Motor and/or Nerve Function Assessment   Definition: Measurement of motor, nerve, and related functions

FØ1 Continued

Body System/Region Character 4	Type Qualifier Character 5	Equipment Character 6	Qualifier Character 7
D Integumentary System - Head and Neck F Integumentary System - Upper Back/ Upper Extremity G Integumentary System - Lower Back/ Lower Extremity H Integumentary System - Whole Body J Musculoskeletal System - Head and Neck K Musculoskeletal System - Upper Back/ Upper Extremity L Musculoskeletal System - Lower Back/ Lower Extremity M Musculoskeletal System - Whole Body	1 Integumentary Integrity	Z None	Z None
D Integumentary System - Head and Neck F Integumentary System - Upper Back/ Upper Extremity G Integumentary System - Lower Back/ Lower Extremity H Integumentary System - Whole Body J Musculoskeletal System - Head and Neck K Musculoskeletal System - Upper Back/ Upper Extremity L Musculoskeletal System - Lower Back/ Lower Extremity M Musculoskeletal System - Whole Body	5 Range of Motion and Joint Integrity 6 Sensory Awareness/Processing/ Integrity	Y Other Equipment Z None	Z None
N Genitourinary System	Ø Muscle Performance	E Orthosis F Assistive, Adaptive, Supportive or Protective U Prosthesis Y Other Equipment Z None	Z None
Z None	2 Visual Motor Integration	K Audiovisual M Augmentative / Alternative Communication N Biosensory Feedback P Computer Q Speech Analysis S Voice Analysis Y Other Equipment Z None	Z None
Z None	7 Facial Nerve Function	7 Electrophysiologic	Z None
Z None	9 Somatosensory Evoked Potentials	J Somatosensory	Z None
Z None	B Bed Mobility C Transfer F Wheelchair Mobility	E Orthosis F Assistive, Adaptive, Supportive or Protective U Prosthesis Z None	Z None
Z None	D Gait and/or Balance	E Orthosis F Assistive, Adaptive, Supportive or Protective U Prosthesis Y Other Equipment Z None	Z None

DRG Non-OR   All body system/region, type qualifier, equipment, and qualifier values

F   **Physical Rehabilitation and Diagnostic Audiology**
0   **Rehabilitation**
2   **Activities of Daily Living Assessment**   Definition: Measurement of functional level for activities of daily living

Body System/Region Character 4	Type Qualifier Character 5	Equipment Character 6	Qualifier Character 7
0 Neurological System - Head and Neck	9 Cranial Nerve Integrity D Neuromotor Development	Y Other Equipment Z None	Z None
1 Neurological System - Upper Back/ Upper Extremity 2 Neurological System - Lower Back/ Lower Extremity 3 Neurological System - Whole Body	D Neuromotor Development	Y Other Equipment Z None	Z None
4 Circulatory System - Head and Neck 5 Circulatory System - Upper Back/ Upper Extremity 6 Circulatory System - Lower Back/ Lower Extremity 8 Respiratory System - Head and Neck 9 Respiratory System - Upper Back/ Upper Extremity B Respiratory System - Lower Back/ Lower Extremity	G Ventilation, Respiration and Circulation	C Mechanical G Aerobic Endurance and Conditioning Y Other Equipment Z None	Z None
7 Circulatory System - Whole Body C Respiratory System - Whole Body	7 Aerobic Capacity and Endurance	E Orthosis G Aerobic Endurance and Conditioning U Prosthesis Y Other Equipment Z None	Z None
7 Circulatory System - Whole Body C Respiratory System - Whole Body	G Ventilation, Respiration and Circulation	C Mechanical G Aerobic Endurance and Conditioning Y Other Equipment Z None	Z None
Z None	0 Bathing/Showering 1 Dressing 3 Grooming/Personal Hygiene 4 Home Management	E Orthosis F Assistive, Adaptive, Supportive or Protective U Prosthesis Z None	Z None
Z None	2 Feeding/Eating 8 Anthropometric Characteristics F Pain	Y Other Equipment Z None	Z None
Z None	5 Perceptual Processing	K Audiovisual M Augmentative / Alternative Communication N Biosensory Feedback P Computer Q Speech Analysis S Voice Analysis Y Other Equipment Z None	Z None
Z None	6 Psychosocial Skills	Z None	Z None
Z None	B Environmental, Home and Work Barriers C Ergonomics and Body Mechanics	E Orthosis F Assistive, Adaptive, Supportive or Protective U Prosthesis Y Other Equipment Z None	Z None
Z None	H Vocational Activities and Functional Community or Work Reintegration Skills	E Orthosis F Assistive, Adaptive, Supportive or Protective G Aerobic Endurance and Conditioning U Prosthesis Y Other Equipment Z None	Z None

DRG Non-OR All body system/region, type qualifier, equipment, and qualifier values

---

Non-OR Procedure   DRG Non-OR Procedure   Valid OR Procedure   HAC Associated Procedure   Combination Only   New/Revised GREEN

F   Physical Rehabilitation and Diagnostic Audiology
Ø   Rehabilitation
6   Speech Treatment   Definition: Application of techniques to improve, augment, or compensate for speech and related functional impairment

Body System/Region Character 4	Type Qualifier Character 5	Equipment Character 6	Qualifier Character 7

3 Neurological System - Whole Body	6 Communicative/Cognitive
	    Integration Skills
		K Audiovisual
		M Augmentative / Alternative
		    Communication
		P Computer
		Y Other Equipment
		Z None
			Z None

Z None	Ø Nonspoken Language
	3 Aphasia
	6 Communicative/Cognitive
	    Integration Skills
		K Audiovisual
		M Augmentative / Alternative
		    Communication
		P Computer
		Y Other Equipment
		Z None
			Z None

Z None	1 Speech-Language Pathology and
	    Related Disorders Counseling
	2 Speech-Language Pathology and
	    Related Disorders Prevention
		K Audiovisual
		Z None
			Z None

Z None	4 Articulation/Phonology	K Audiovisual P Computer Q Speech Analysis T Aerodynamic Function Y Other Equipment Z None	Z None
Z None	5 Aural Rehabilitation	K Audiovisual L Assistive Listening M Augmentative / Alternative Communication N Biosensory Feedback P Computer Q Speech Analysis S Voice Analysis Y Other Equipment Z None	Z None
Z None	7 Fluency	4 Electroacoustic Immitance / Acoustic Reflex K Audiovisual N Biosensory Feedback Q Speech Analysis S Voice Analysis T Aerodynamic Function Y Other Equipment Z None	Z None
Z None	8 Motor Speech	K Audiovisual N Biosensory Feedback P Computer Q Speech Analysis S Voice Analysis T Aerodynamic Function Y Other Equipment Z None	Z None
Z None	9 Orofacial Myofunctional	K Audiovisual P Computer Y Other Equipment Z None	Z None
Z None	B Receptive/Expressive Language	K Audiovisual L Assistive Listening M Augmentative / Alternative Communication P Computer Y Other Equipment Z None	Z None

DRG Non-OR   All body system/region, type qualifier, equipment, and qualifier values

F06 Continued on next page

NC Noncovered Procedure   LC Limited Coverage   QA Questionable OB Admit   NT New Tech Add-on   ⊞ Combination Member   ♂ Male   ♀ Female

ICD-10-PCS 2022   **803**

Physical Rehabilitation and Diagnostic Audiology

F06 Continued

F   **Physical Rehabilitation and Diagnostic Audiology**
Ø   **Rehabilitation**
6   **Speech Treatment**   Definition: Application of techniques to improve, augment, or compensate for speech and related functional impairment

Body System/Region Character 4	Type Qualifier Character 5	Equipment Character 6	Qualifier Character 7
Z None	C Voice	K Audiovisual N Biosensory Feedback P Computer S Voice Analysis T Aerodynamic Function V Speech Prosthesis Y Other Equipment Z None	Z None
Z None	D Swallowing Dysfunction	M Augmentative / Alternative Communication T Aerodynamic Function V Speech Prosthesis Y Other Equipment Z None	Z None

DRG Non-OR   All body system/region, type qualifier, equipment, and qualifier values

F   **Physical Rehabilitation and Diagnostic Audiology**
Ø   **Rehabilitation**
7   **Motor Treatment**   Definition: Exercise or activities to increase or facilitate motor function

Body System/Region Character 4	Type Qualifier Character 5	Equipment Character 6	Qualifier Character 7
Ø Neurological System - Head and Neck 1 Neurological System - Upper Back/ Upper Extremity 2 Neurological System - Lower Back/ Lower Extremity 3 Neurological System - Whole Body D Integumentary System - Head and Neck F Integumentary System - Upper Back/ Upper Extremity G Integumentary System - Lower Back/ Lower Extremity H Integumentary System - Whole Body J Musculoskeletal System - Head and Neck K Musculoskeletal System - Upper Back/ Upper Extremity L Musculoskeletal System - Lower Back/ Lower Extremity M Musculoskeletal System - Whole Body	Ø Range of Motion and Joint Mobility 1 Muscle Performance 2 Coordination/Dexterity 3 Motor Function	E Orthosis F Assistive, Adaptive, Supportive or Protective U Prosthesis Y Other Equipment Z None	Z None
Ø Neurological System - Head and Neck 1 Neurological System - Upper Back/ Upper Extremity 2 Neurological System - Lower Back/ Lower Extremity 3 Neurological System - Whole Body D Integumentary System - Head and Neck F Integumentary System - Upper Back/ Upper Extremity G Integumentary System - Lower Back/ Lower Extremity H Integumentary System - Whole Body J Musculoskeletal System - Head and Neck K Musculoskeletal System - Upper Back/ Upper Extremity L Musculoskeletal System - Lower Back/ Lower Extremity M Musculoskeletal System - Whole Body	6 Therapeutic Exercise	B Physical Agents C Mechanical D Electrotherapeutic E Orthosis F Assistive, Adaptive, Supportive or Protective G Aerobic Endurance and Conditioning H Mechanical or Electromechanical U Prosthesis Y Other Equipment Z None	Z None

DRG Non-OR   All body system/region, type qualifier, equipment, and qualifier values

F07 Continued on next page

F   **Physical Rehabilitation and Diagnostic Audiology**
Ø   **Rehabilitation**
7   **Motor Treatment**   Definition: Exercise or activities to increase or facilitate motor function

F07 Continued

Body System/Region Character 4	Type Qualifier Character 5	Equipment Character 6	Qualifier Character 7
Ø Neurological System - Head and Neck **1** Neurological System - Upper Back/ Upper Extremity **2** Neurological System - Lower Back/ Lower Extremity **3** Neurological System - Whole Body **D** Integumentary System - Head and Neck **F** Integumentary System - Upper Back/ Upper Extremity **G** Integumentary System - Lower Back/ Lower Extremity **H** Integumentary System - Whole Body **J** Musculoskeletal System - Head and Neck **K** Musculoskeletal System - Upper Back/ Upper Extremity **L** Musculoskeletal System - Lower Back/ Lower Extremity **M** Musculoskeletal System - Whole Body	**7** Manual Therapy Techniques	**Z** None	**Z** None
4 Circulatory System - Head and Neck **5** Circulatory System - Upper Back / Upper Extremity **6** Circulatory System - Lower Back / Lower Extremity **7** Circulatory System - Whole Body **8** Respiratory System - Head and Neck **9** Respiratory System - Upper Back / Upper Extremity **B** Respiratory System - Lower Back / Lower Extremity **C** Respiratory System - Whole Body	**6** Therapeutic Exercise	**B** Physical Agents **C** Mechanical **D** Electrotherapeutic **E** Orthosis **F** Assistive, Adaptive, Supportive or Protective **G** Aerobic Endurance and Conditioning **H** Mechanical or Electromechanical **U** Prosthesis **Y** Other Equipment **Z** None	**Z** None
N Genitourinary System	**1** Muscle Performance	**E** Orthosis **F** Assistive, Adaptive, Supportive or Protective **U** Prosthesis **Y** Other Equipment **Z** None	**Z** None
N Genitourinary System	**6** Therapeutic Exercise	**B** Physical Agents **C** Mechanical **D** Electrotherapeutic **E** Orthosis **F** Assistive, Adaptive, Supportive or Protective **G** Aerobic Endurance and Conditioning **H** Mechanical or Electromechanical **U** Prosthesis **Y** Other Equipment **Z** None	**Z** None
Z None	**4** Wheelchair Mobility	**D** Electrotherapeutic **E** Orthosis **F** Assistive, Adaptive, Supportive or Protective **U** Prosthesis **Y** Other Equipment **Z** None	**Z** None
Z None	**5** Bed Mobility	**C** Mechanical **E** Orthosis **F** Assistive, Adaptive, Supportive or Protective **U** Prosthesis **Y** Other Equipment **Z** None	**Z** None
Z None	**8** Transfer Training	**C** Mechanical **D** Electrotherapeutic **E** Orthosis **F** Assistive, Adaptive, Supportive or Protective **U** Prosthesis **Y** Other Equipment **Z** None	**Z** None

DRG Non-OR   All body system/region, type qualifier, equipment, and qualifier values

F07 Continued on next page

F   **Physical Rehabilitation and Diagnostic Audiology**   *F07 Continued*
Ø   **Rehabilitation**
7   **Motor Treatment**   Definition: Exercise or activities to increase or facilitate motor function

Body System/Region Character 4	Type Qualifier Character 5	Equipment Character 6	Qualifier Character 7
Z None	**9** Gait Training/Functional Ambulation	**C** Mechanical **D** Electrotherapeutic **E** Orthosis **F** Assistive, Adaptive, Supportive or Protective **G** Aerobic Endurance and Conditioning **U** Prosthesis **Y** Other Equipment **Z** None	**Z** None

DRG Non-OR   All body system/region, type qualifier, equipment, and qualifier values

F   **Physical Rehabilitation and Diagnostic Audiology**
Ø   **Rehabilitation**
8   **Activities of Daily Living Treatment**   Definition: Exercise or activities to facilitate functional competence for activities of daily living

Body System/Region Character 4	Type Qualifier Character 5	Equipment Character 6	Qualifier Character 7
D Integumentary System - Head and Neck **F** Integumentary System - Upper Back/Upper Extremity **G** Integumentary System - Lower Back/Lower Extremity **H** Integumentary System - Whole Body **J** Musculoskeletal System - Head and Neck **K** Musculoskeletal System - Upper Back/Upper Extremity **L** Musculoskeletal System - Lower Back/Lower Extremity **M** Musculoskeletal System - Whole Body	**5** Wound Management	**B** Physical Agents **C** Mechanical **D** Electrotherapeutic **E** Orthosis **F** Assistive, Adaptive, Supportive or Protective **U** Prosthesis **Y** Other Equipment **Z** None	**Z** None
Z None	**Ø** Bathing/Showering Techniques **1** Dressing Techniques **2** Grooming/Personal Hygiene	**E** Orthosis **F** Assistive, Adaptive, Supportive or Protective **U** Prosthesis **Y** Other Equipment **Z** None	**Z** None
Z None	**3** Feeding/Eating	**C** Mechanical **D** Electrotherapeutic **E** Orthosis **F** Assistive, Adaptive, Supportive or Protective **U** Prosthesis **Y** Other Equipment **Z** None	**Z** None
Z None	**4** Home Management	**D** Electrotherapeutic **E** Orthosis **F** Assistive, Adaptive, Supportive or Protective **U** Prosthesis **Y** Other Equipment **Z** None	**Z** None
Z None	**6** Psychosocial Skills	**Z** None	**Z** None
Z None	**7** Vocational Activities and Functional Community or Work Reintegration Skills	**B** Physical Agents **C** Mechanical **D** Electrotherapeutic **E** Orthosis **F** Assistive, Adaptive, Supportive or Protective **G** Aerobic Endurance and Conditioning **U** Prosthesis **Y** Other Equipment **Z** None	**Z** None

DRG Non-OR   All body system/region, type qualifier, equipment, and qualifier values

Non-OR Procedure   DRG Non-OR Procedure   Valid OR Procedure   HAC Associated Procedure   Combination Only   New/Revised GREEN

F   Physical Rehabilitation and Diagnostic Audiology
0   Rehabilitation
9   Hearing Treatment   Definition: Application of techniques to improve, augment, or compensate for hearing and related functional impairment

Body System/Region Character 4	Type Qualifier Character 5	Equipment Character 6	Qualifier Character 7
Z None	0 Hearing and Related Disorders Counseling 1 Hearing and Related Disorders Prevention	K Audiovisual Z None	Z None
Z None	2 Auditory Processing	K Audiovisual L Assistive Listening P Computer Y Other Equipment Z None	Z None
Z None	3 Cerumen Management	X Cerumen Management Z None	Z None

DRG Non-OR   All body system/region, type qualifier, equipment, and qualifier values

---

F   Physical Rehabilitation and Diagnostic Audiology
0   Rehabilitation
B   Cochlear Implant Treatment   Definition: Application of techniques to improve the communication abilities of individuals with cochlear implant

Body System/Region Character 4	Type Qualifier Character 5	Equipment Character 6	Qualifier Character 7
Z None	0 Cochlear Implant Rehabilitation	1 Audiometer 2 Sound Field / Booth 9 Cochlear Implant K Audiovisual P Computer Y Other Equipment	Z None

DRG Non-OR   All body system/region, type qualifier, equipment, and qualifier values

---

F   Physical Rehabilitation and Diagnostic Audiology
0   Rehabilitation
C   Vestibular Treatment   Definition: Application of techniques to improve, augment, or compensate for vestibular and related functional impairment

Body System/Region Character 4	Type Qualifier Character 5	Equipment Character 6	Qualifier Character 7
3 Neurological System - Whole Body H Integumentary System - Whole Body M Musculoskeletal System - Whole Body	3 Postural Control	E Orthosis F Assistive, Adaptive, Supportive or Protective U Prosthesis Y Other Equipment Z None	Z None
Z None	0 Vestibular	8 Vestibular / Balance Z None	Z None
Z None	1 Perceptual Processing 2 Visual Motor Integration	K Audiovisual L Assistive Listening N Biosensory Feedback P Computer Q Speech Analysis S Voice Analysis T Aerodynamic Function Y Other Equipment Z None	Z None

DRG Non-OR   All body system/region, type qualifier, equipment, and qualifier values

---

NC Noncovered Procedure   LC Limited Coverage   QA Questionable OB Admit   NT New Tech Add-on   ⊞ Combination Member   ♂ Male   ♀ Female

ICD-10-PCS 2022   807

F Physical Rehabilitation and Diagnostic Audiology
0 Rehabilitation
D Device Fitting Definition: Fitting of a device designed to facilitate or support achievement of a higher level of function

Body System/Region Character 4	Type Qualifier Character 5	Equipment Character 6	Qualifier Character 7
Z None	0 Tinnitus Masker	5 Hearing Aid Selection / Fitting / Test Z None	Z None
Z None	1 Monaural Hearing Aid 2 Binaural Hearing Aid 5 Assistive Listening Device	1 Audiometer 2 Sound Field / Booth 5 Hearing Aid Selection / Fitting / Test K Audiovisual L Assistive Listening Z None	Z None

Z None	3 Augmentative/Alternative
	  Communication System
		M Augmentative / Alternative
		  Communication
			Z None

Z None	4 Voice Prosthetic	S Voice Analysis V Speech Prosthesis	Z None

Z None	6 Dynamic Orthosis
	7 Static Orthosis
	8 Prosthesis
	9 Assistive, Adaptive,Supportive or
	  Protective Devices
		E Orthosis
		F Assistive, Adaptive, Supportive or
		  Protective
		U Prosthesis
		Z None
			Z None

DRG Non-OR F0DZ0[5,Z]Z
DRG Non-OR F0DZ[1, 2,5][1,2,5, K,L,Z]Z
DRG Non-OR F0DZ3MZ
DRG Non-OR F0DZ4[S,V]Z
DRG Non-OR F0DZ[6,7][E,F,U,Z]Z
DRG Non-OR F0DZ8[E,F,U]Z

F Physical Rehabilitation and Diagnostic Audiology
0 Rehabilitation
F Caregiver Training Definition: Training in activities to support patient's optimal level of function

Body System/Region Character 4	Type Qualifier Character 5	Equipment Character 6	Qualifier Character 7

Z None	0 Bathing/Showering Technique
	1 Dressing
	2 Feeding and Eating
	3 Grooming/Personal Hygiene
	4 Bed Mobility
	5 Transfer
	6 Wheelchair Mobility
	7 Therapeutic Exercise
	8 Airway Clearance Techniques
	9 Wound Management
	B Vocational Activities and Functional
	  Community or Work Reintegration
	  Skills
	C Gait Training/Functional
	  Ambulation
	D Application, Proper Use and Care of
	  Devices
	F Application, Proper Use and Care of
	  Orthoses
	G Application, Proper Use and Care of
	  Prosthesis
	H Home Management
		E Orthosis
		F Assistive, Adaptive, Supportive or
		  Protective
		U Prosthesis
		Z None
			Z None

Z None	J Communication Skills	K Audiovisual L Assistive Listening M Augmentative / Alternative Communication P Computer Z None	Z None

DRG Non-OR All body system/region, type qualifier, equipment, and qualifier values

Non-OR Procedure DRG Non-OR Procedure Valid OR Procedure HAC Associated Procedure Combination Only New/Revised GREEN

808   ICD-10-PCS 2022

F   Physical Rehabilitation and Diagnostic Audiology
1   Diagnostic Audiology
3   Hearing Assessment   Definition: Measurement of hearing and related functions

Body System/Region Character 4	Type Qualifier Character 5	Equipment Character 6	Qualifier Character 7
Z None	Ø Hearing Screening	Ø Occupational Hearing 1 Audiometer 2 Sound Field / Booth 3 Tympanometer 8 Vestibular / Balance 9 Cochlear Implant Z None	Z None
Z None	1 Pure Tone Audiometry, Air 2 Pure Tone Audiometry, Air and Bone	Ø Occupational Hearing 1 Audiometer 2 Sound Field / Booth Z None	Z None
Z None	3 Bekesy Audiometry 6 Visual Reinforcement Audiometry 9 Short Increment Sensitivity Index B Stenger C Pure Tone Stenger	1 Audiometer 2 Sound Field / Booth Z None	Z None
Z None	4 Conditioned Play Audiometry 5 Select Picture Audiometry	1 Audiometer 2 Sound Field / Booth K Audiovisual Z None	Z None
Z None	7 Alternate Binaural or Monaural Loudness Balance	1 Audiometer K Audiovisual Z None	Z None
Z None	8 Tone Decay D Tympanometry F Eustachian Tube Function G Acoustic Reflex Patterns H Acoustic Reflex Threshold J Acoustic Reflex Decay	3 Tympanometer 4 Electroacoustic Immitance / Acoustic Reflex Z None	Z None
Z None	K Electrocochleography L Auditory Evoked Potentials	7 Electrophysiologic Z None	Z None
Z None	M Evoked Otoacoustic Emissions, Screening N Evoked Otoacoustic Emissions, Diagnostic	6 Otoacoustic Emission (OAE) Z None	Z None
Z None	P Aural Rehabilitation Status	1 Audiometer 2 Sound Field / Booth 4 Electroacoustic Immitance / Acoustic Reflex 9 Cochlear Implant K Audiovisual L Assistive Listening P Computer Z None	Z None
Z None	Q Auditory Processing	K Audiovisual P Computer Y Other Equipment Z None	Z None

NC Noncovered Procedure   **LC** Limited Coverage   **QA** Questionable OB Admit   **NT** New Tech Add-on   ⊞ Combination Member   ♂ Male   ♀ Female

ICD-10-PCS 2022   809

Physical Rehabilitation and Diagnostic Audiology *(vertical side text)*

F   Physical Rehabilitation and Diagnostic Audiology
1   Diagnostic Audiology
4   Hearing Aid Assessment   Definition: Measurement of the appropriateness and/or effectiveness of a hearing device

Body System/Region Character 4	Type Qualifier Character 5	Equipment Character 6	Qualifier Character 7
Z None	Ø Cochlear Implant	1 Audiometer 2 Sound Field / Booth 3 Tympanometer 4 Electroacoustic Immitance / Acoustic Reflex 5 Hearing Aid Selection / Fitting / Test 7 Electrophysiologic 9 Cochlear Implant K Audiovisual L Assistive Listening P Computer Y Other Equipment Z None	Z None

Z None	1 Ear Canal Probe Microphone
	6 Binaural Electroacoustic Hearing
	     Aid Check
	8 Monaural Electroacoustic Hearing
	     Aid Check
		5 Hearing Aid Selection / Fitting / Test
		Z None
			Z None

Z None	2 Monaural Hearing Aid 3 Binaural Hearing Aid	1 Audiometer 2 Sound Field / Booth 3 Tympanometer 4 Electroacoustic Immitance / Acoustic Reflex 5 Hearing Aid Selection / Fitting / Test K Audiovisual L Assistive Listening P Computer Z None	Z None

Z None	4 Assistive Listening System/Device
	     Selection
		1 Audiometer
		2 Sound Field / Booth
		3 Tympanometer
		4 Electroacoustic Immitance /
		     Acoustic Reflex
		K Audiovisual
		L Assistive Listening
		Z None
			Z None

Z None	5 Sensory Aids	1 Audiometer 2 Sound Field / Booth 3 Tympanometer 4 Electroacoustic Immitance / Acoustic Reflex 5 Hearing Aid Selection / Fitting / Test K Audiovisual L Assistive Listening Z None	Z None
Z None	7 Ear Protector Attentuation	Ø Occupational Hearing Z None	Z None

F   Physical Rehabilitation and Diagnostic Audiology
1   Diagnostic Audiology
5   Vestibular Assessment   Definition: Measurement of the vestibular system and related functions

Body System/Region Character 4	Type Qualifier Character 5	Equipment Character 6	Qualifier Character 7

Z None	Ø Bithermal, Binaural Caloric
	     Irrigation
	1 Bithermal, Monaural Caloric
	     Irrigation
	2 Unithermal Binaural Screen
	3 Oscillating Tracking
	4 Sinusoidal Vertical Axis Rotational
	5 Dix-Hallpike Dynamic
	6 Computerized Dynamic
	     Posturography
		8 Vestibular / Balance
		Z None
			Z None

Z None	7 Tinnitus Masker	5 Hearing Aid Selection / Fitting / Test Z None	Z None

Mental Health GZ1–GZJ

G   **Mental Health**
Z   **None**
1   **Psychological Tests**   Definition: The administration and interpretation of standardized psychological tests and measurement instruments for the assessment of psychological function

Qualifier Character 4	Qualifier Character 5	Qualifier Character 6	Qualifier Character 7
Ø Developmental **1** Personality and Behavioral **2** Intellectual and Psychoeducational **3** Neuropsychological **4** Neurobehavioral and Cognitive Status	**Z** None	**Z** None	**Z** None

G   **Mental Health**
Z   **None**
2   **Crisis Intervention**   Definition: Treatment of a traumatized, acutely disturbed or distressed individual for the purpose of short-term stabilization

Qualifier Character 4	Qualifier Character 5	Qualifier Character 6	Qualifier Character 7
Z None	**Z** None	**Z** None	**Z** None

G   **Mental Health**
Z   **None**
3   **Medication Management**   Definition: Monitoring and adjusting the use of medications for the treatment of a mental health disorder

Qualifier Character 4	Qualifier Character 5	Qualifier Character 6	Qualifier Character 7
Z None	**Z** None	**Z** None	**Z** None

G   **Mental Health**
Z   **None**
5   **Individual Psychotherapy**   Definition: Treatment of an individual with a mental health disorder by behavioral, cognitive, psychoanalytic, psychodynamic or psychophysiological means to improve functioning or well-being

Qualifier Character 4	Qualifier Character 5	Qualifier Character 6	Qualifier Character 7
Ø Interactive **1** Behavioral **2** Cognitive **3** Interpersonal **4** Psychoanalysis **5** Psychodynamic **6** Supportive **8** Cognitive-Behavioral **9** Psychophysiological	**Z** None	**Z** None	**Z** None

G   **Mental Health**
Z   **None**
6   **Counseling**   Definition: The application of psychological methods to treat an individual with normal developmental issues and psychological problems in order to increase function, improve well-being, alleviate distress, maladjustment or resolve crises

Qualifier Character 4	Qualifier Character 5	Qualifier Character 6	Qualifier Character 7
Ø Educational **1** Vocational **3** Other Counseling	**Z** None	**Z** None	**Z** None

G   **Mental Health**
Z   **None**
7   **Family Psychotherapy** Definition: Treatment that includes one or more family members of an individual with a mental health disorder by behavioral, cognitive, psychoanalytic, psychodynamic or psychophysiological means to improve functioning or well-being

Explanation: Remediation of emotional or behavioral problems presented by one or more family members in cases where psychotherapy with more than one family member is indicated

Qualifier Character 4	Qualifier Character 5	Qualifier Character 6	Qualifier Character 7
2 Other Family Psychotherapy	**Z** None	**Z** None	**Z** None

NC Noncovered Procedure   **LC** Limited Coverage   **QA** Questionable OB Admit   **NT** New Tech Add-on   ✛ Combination Member   ♂ Male   ♀ Female

ICD-10-PCS 2022   811

GZ1–GZ7

Mental Health

G Mental Health
Z None
B **Electroconvulsive Therapy**   Definition: The application of controlled electrical voltages to treat a mental health disorder

Qualifier Character 4	Qualifier Character 5	Qualifier Character 6	Qualifier Character 7
Ø Unilateral-Single Seizure 1 Unilateral-Multiple Seizure 2 Bilateral-Single Seizure 3 Bilateral-Multiple Seizure 4 Other Electroconvulsive Therapy	Z None	Z None	Z None

G Mental Health
Z None
C **Biofeedback**   Definition: Provision of information from the monitoring and regulating of physiological processes in conjunction with cognitive-behavioral techniques to improve patient functioning or well-being

Qualifier Character 4	Qualifier Character 5	Qualifier Character 6	Qualifier Character 7
9 Other Biofeedback	Z None	Z None	Z None

G Mental Health
Z None
F **Hypnosis**   Definition: Induction of a state of heightened suggestibility by auditory, visual and tactile techniques to elicit an emotional or behavioral response

Qualifier Character 4	Qualifier Character 5	Qualifier Character 6	Qualifier Character 7
Z None	Z None	Z None	Z None

G Mental Health
Z None
G **Narcosynthesis**   Definition: Administration of intravenous barbiturates in order to release suppressed or repressed thoughts

Qualifier Character 4	Qualifier Character 5	Qualifier Character 6	Qualifier Character 7
Z None	Z None	Z None	Z None

G Mental Health
Z None
H **Group Psychotherapy**   Definition: Treatment of two or more individuals with a mental health disorder by behavioral, cognitive, psychoanalytic, psychodynamic or psychophysiological means to improve functioning or well-being

Qualifier Character 4	Qualifier Character 5	Qualifier Character 6	Qualifier Character 7
Z None	Z None	Z None	Z None

G Mental Health
Z None
J **Light Therapy**   Definition: Application of specialized light treatments to improve functioning or well-being

Qualifier Character 4	Qualifier Character 5	Qualifier Character 6	Qualifier Character 7
Z None	Z None	Z None	Z None

Substance Abuse Treatment HZ2–HZ9

AHA Coding Clinic for table HZ2
2020, 1Q, 21   Inpatient detoxification services

AHA Coding Clinic for table HZ9
2020, 1Q, 21   Inpatient detoxification services

H   **Substance Abuse Treatment**
Z   **None**
2   **Detoxification Services**   Definition: Detoxification from alcohol and/or drugs

Explanation: Not a treatment modality, but helps the patient stabilize physically and psychologically until the body becomes free of drugs and the effects of alcohol

Qualifier Character 4	Qualifier Character 5	Qualifier Character 6	Qualifier Character 7
Z None	Z None	Z None	Z None

H   **Substance Abuse Treatment**
Z   **None**
3   **Individual Counseling**   Definition: The application of psychological methods to treat an individual with addictive behavior

Explanation: Comprised of several different techniques, which apply various strategies to address drug addiction

Qualifier Character 4	Qualifier Character 5	Qualifier Character 6	Qualifier Character 7
Ø Cognitive 1 Behavioral 2 Cognitive-Behavioral 3 12-Step 4 Interpersonal 5 Vocational 6 Psychoeducation 7 Motivational Enhancement 8 Confrontational 9 Continuing Care B Spiritual C Pre/Post-Test Infectious Disease	Z None	Z None	Z None

DRG Non-OR   HZ3[Ø,1,2,3,4,5,6,7,8,9,B]ZZZ

H   **Substance Abuse Treatment**
Z   **None**
4   **Group Counseling**   Definition: The application of psychological methods to treat two or more individuals with addictive behavior

Explanation: Provides structured group counseling sessions and healing power through the connection with others

Qualifier Character 4	Qualifier Character 5	Qualifier Character 6	Qualifier Character 7
Ø Cognitive 1 Behavioral 2 Cognitive-Behavioral 3 12-Step 4 Interpersonal 5 Vocational 6 Psychoeducation 7 Motivational Enhancement 8 Confrontational 9 Continuing Care B Spiritual C Pre/Post-Test Infectious Disease	Z None	Z None	Z None

DRG Non-OR   HZ4[Ø,1,2,3,4,5,6,7,8,9,B]ZZZ

NC Noncovered Procedure   LC Limited Coverage   QA Questionable OB Admit   NT New Tech Add-on   ⊞ Combination Member   ♂ Male   ♀ Female

ICD-10-PCS 2022   813

HZ2–HZ4

Substance Abuse Treatment

H Substance Abuse Treatment
Z None
5 Individual Psychotherapy Definition: Treatment of an individual with addictive behavior by behavioral, cognitive, psychoanalytic, psychodynamic or psychophysiological means

Qualifier Character 4	Qualifier Character 5	Qualifier Character 6	Qualifier Character 7
Ø Cognitive	Z None	Z None	Z None
1 Behavioral			
2 Cognitive-Behavioral			
3 12-Step			
4 Interpersonal			
5 Interactive			
6 Psychoeducation			
7 Motivational Enhancement			
8 Confrontational			
9 Supportive			
B Psychoanalysis			
C Psychodynamic			
D Psychophysiological			

DRG Non-OR For all qualifier values

H Substance Abuse Treatment
Z None
6 Family Counseling Definition: The application of psychological methods that includes one or more family members to treat an individual with addictive behavior

Explanation: Provides support and education for family members of addicted individuals. Family member participation is seen as a critical area of substance abuse treatment

Qualifier Character 4	Qualifier Character 5	Qualifier Character 6	Qualifier Character 7
3 Other Family Counseling	Z None	Z None	Z None

H Substance Abuse Treatment
Z None
8 Medication Management Definition: Monitoring or adjusting the use of replacement medications for the treatment of addiction

Qualifier Character 4	Qualifier Character 5	Qualifier Character 6	Qualifier Character 7
Ø Nicotine Replacement	Z None	Z None	Z None
1 Methadone Maintenance			
2 Levo-alpha-acetyl-methadol (LAAM)			
3 Antabuse			
4 Naltrexone			
5 Naloxone			
6 Clonidine			
7 Bupropion			
8 Psychiatric Medication			
9 Other Replacement Medication			

H Substance Abuse Treatment
Z None
9 Pharmacotherapy Definition: The use of replacement medications for the treatment of addiction

Qualifier Character 4	Qualifier Character 5	Qualifier Character 6	Qualifier Character 7
Ø Nicotine Replacement	Z None	Z None	Z None
1 Methadone Maintenance			
2 Levo-alpha-acetyl-methadol (LAAM)			
3 Antabuse			
4 Naltrexone			
5 Naloxone			
6 Clonidine			
7 Bupropion			
8 Psychiatric Medication			
9 Other Replacement Medication			

New Technology X27–XY0

AHA Coding Clinic for all tables in the New Technology Section
2015, 4Q, 8-11   New Section X codes - New Technology procedures

AHA Coding Clinic for table X27
2019, 4Q, 45-46   Sustained released drug-eluting stent

AHA Coding Clinic for table X2A
2021, 1Q, 16   Placement of Sentinel™ embolic protection device with deployment of single filter
2020, 4Q, 70-71   Cerebral embolic filtration extracorporeal flow reversal circuit
2019, 4Q, 46   Cerebral embolic filtration
2016, 4Q, 115-116 Cerebral embolic filtration

AHA Coding Clinic for table X2C
2016, 4Q, 82-83   Coronary artery, number of arteries
2015, 4Q, 8-14   New Section X codes—New Technology procedures

AHA Coding Clinic for table X2R
2016, 4Q, 116   Aortic valve rapid deployment
2015, 4Q, 8-12   New Section X codes—New Technology procedures

AHA Coding Clinic for table XHR
2016, 4Q, 116   Application of wound matrix

AHA Coding Clinic for table XK0
2017, 4Q, 74   Intramuscular autologous bone marrow cell therapy

AHA Coding Clinic for table XNS
2017, 4Q, 74-75   Magnetic growth rods
2016, 4Q, 117   Placement of magnetic growth rods

AHA Coding Clinic for table XNU
2020, 4Q, 72   Implantation of vertebral mechanically expandable device

AHA Coding Clinic for table XRG
2017, 4Q, 76   Radiolucent porous interbody fusion device

AHA Coding Clinic for table XT2
2019, 4Q, 46-47   Renal function monitoring

AHA Coding Clinic for table XV5
2018, 4Q, 55   Robotic waterjet ablation

AHA Coding Clinic for table XW0
2021, 1Q, 49   Frequently asked questions regarding ICD-10-CM and ICD-10-PCS coding for COVID-19
2020, 4Q, 72-76   Introduction of new therapeutic substances
2020, 4Q, 95   Frequently Asked Questions Regarding ICD-10-PCS Coding for COVID-19
2020, 3Q, 17-21   New procedure codes for introduction or infusion of therapeutics
2019, 4Q, 47-50   New therapeutic substances
2018, 4Q, 56   New therapeutic substances
2015, 4Q, 8-15   New Section X codes—New Technology procedures

AHA Coding Clinic for table XW1
2020, 3Q, 17-21   New procedure codes for introduction or infusion of therapeutics

AHA Coding Clinic for table XW2
2020, 4Q, 77-78   Transfusion of chimeric antigen receptor (CAR) T cell immunotherapy

AHA Coding Clinic for table XXE
2020, 4Q, 78-79   Measurement of infection
2020, 4Q, 78-79   Positive blood culture fluorescence hybridization
2020, 4Q, 79   Nucleic acid-base microbial detection
2019, 4Q, 50-51   Whole blood nucleic acid-base microbial detection

AHA Coding Clinic for table XY0
2017, 4Q, 78   Intraoperative treatment of vascular grafts

X   **New Technology**
2   **Cardiovascular System**
7   **Dilation**   Definition: Expanding an orifice or the lumen of a tubular body part
          Explanation: The orifice can be a natural orifice or an artificially created orifice. Accomplished by stretching a tubular body part using intraluminal pressure or by cutting part of the orifice or wall of the tubular body part.

Body Part Character 4	Approach Character 5	Device/Substance/Technology Character 6	Qualifier Character 7

H Femoral Artery, Right
J Femoral Artery, Left
K Popliteal Artery, Proximal Right
L Popliteal Artery, Proximal Left
M Popliteal Artery, Distal Right
N Popliteal Artery, Distal Left
P Anterior Tibial Artery, Right
Q Anterior Tibial Artery, Left
R Posterior Tibial Artery, Right
S Posterior Tibial Artery, Left
T Peroneal Artery, Right
U Peroneal Artery, Left
	3 Percutaneous	8 Intraluminal Device, Sustained [NT]
		   Release Drug-eluting
		9 Intraluminal Device, Sustained [NT]
		   Release Drug-eluting, Two
		B Intraluminal Device, Sustained [NT]
		   Release Drug-eluting, Three
		C Intraluminal Device, Sustained [NT]
		   Release Drug-eluting, Four or
		   More
			5 New Technology Group 5

Valid OR   All body part, approach, device/substance/technology, and qualifier values
[NT]   X27[H,J,K,L]3[8,9,B,C]5 *See* Appendix H for applicable device trade name

---

X   **New Technology**
2   **Cardiovascular System**
A   **Assistance**   Definition: Taking over a portion of a physiological function by extracorporeal means
          Explanation: None

Body Part Character 4	Approach Character 5	Device/Substance/Technology Character 6	Qualifier Character 7

5 Innominate Artery and Left
   Common Carotid Artery
	3 Percutaneous	1 Cerebral Embolic Filtration, Dual
		   Filter
			2 New Technology Group 2

6 Aortic Arch	3 Percutaneous	2 Cerebral Embolic Filtration, Single Deflection Filter	5 New Technology Group 5
H Common Carotid Artery, Right J Common Carotid Artery, Left	3 Percutaneous	3 Cerebral Embolic Filtration, Extracorporeal Flow Reversal Circuit	6 New Technology Group 6

[NC] Noncovered Procedure   [LC] Limited Coverage   [QA] Questionable OB Admit   [NT] New Tech Add-on   ⊞ Combination Member   ♂ Male   ♀ Female

ICD-10-PCS 2022   815

X27–X2A

X New Technology
2 Cardiovascular System
C Extirpation   Definition: Taking or cutting out solid matter from a body part

Explanation: The solid matter may be an abnormal byproduct of a biological function or a foreign body; it may be imbedded in a body part or in the lumen of a tubular body part. The solid matter may or may not have been previously broken into pieces.

Body Part Character 4	Approach Character 5	Device/Substance/Technology Character 6	Qualifier Character 7
P Abdominal Aorta Q Upper Extremity Vein, Right R Upper Extremity Vein, Left S Lower Extremity Artery, Right T Lower Extremity Artery, Left U Lower Extremity Vein, Right V Lower Extremity Vein, Left Y Great Vessel	3 Percutaneous	T Computer-aided Mechanical Aspiration	7 New Technology Group 7

X New Technology
2 Cardiovascular System
J Inspection   Definition: Visually and/or manually exploring a body part

Explanation: None

Body Part Character 4	Approach Character 5	Device/Substance/Technology Character 6	Qualifier Character 7
A Heart	X External	4 Transthoracic Echocardiography, Computer-aided Guidance	7 New Technology Group 7

X New Technology
2 Cardiovascular System
K Bypass   Definition: Altering the route of passage of the contents of a tubular body part

Explanation: None

Body Part Character 4	Approach Character 5	Device/Substance/Technology Character 6	Qualifier Character 7
B Radial Artery, Right C Radial Artery, Left	3 Percutaneous	1 Thermal Resistance Energy	7 New Technology Group 7

X New Technology
2 Cardiovascular System
R Replacement   Definition: Putting in or on biological or synthetic material that physically takes the place and/or function of all or a portion of a body part

Explanation: The body part may have been taken out or replaced, or may be taken out, physically eradicated, or rendered nonfunctional during the REPLACEMENT procedure. A REMOVAL procedure is coded for taking out the device used in a previous replacement procedure

Body Part Character 4	Approach Character 5	Device/Substance/Technology Character 6	Qualifier Character 7
F Aortic Valve	Ø Open 3 Percutaneous 4 Percutaneous Endoscopic	3 Zooplastic Tissue, Rapid Deployment Technique	2 New Technology Group 2
X Thoracic Aorta, Arch	Ø Open	N Branched Synthetic Substitute with Intraluminal Device	7 New Technology Group 7

Valid OR   X2RF[Ø,3,4]32

X New Technology
2 Cardiovascular System
V Restriction   Definition: Partially closing an orifice or the lumen of a tubular body part

Explanation: None

Body Part Character 4	Approach Character 5	Device/Substance/Technology Character 6	Qualifier Character 7
7 Coronary Sinus	3 Percutaneous	Q Reduction Device	7 New Technology Group 7
W Thoracic Aorta, Descending	Ø Open	N Branched Synthetic Substitute with Intraluminal Device	7 New Technology Group 7

Valid OR   X2V73Q7

X New Technology
D Gastrointestinal System
2 Monitoring   Definition: Determining the level of a physiological or physical function repetitively over a period of time

Explanation: None

Body Part Character 4	Approach Character 5	Device/Substance/Technology Character 6	Qualifier Character 7
G Upper GI H Lower GI	4 Percutaneous Endoscopic 8 Via Natural or Artificial Opening Endoscopic	V Oxygen Saturation	7 New Technology Group 7

X　New Technology
D　Gastrointestinal System
P　Irrigation　　Definition: Putting in or on a cleansing substance
　　　　　　　　　Explanation: None

Body Part Character 4	Approach Character 5	Device/Substance/Technology Character 6	Qualifier Character 7
H　Lower GI	8　Via Natural or Artificial Opening Endoscopic	K　Intraoperative Single-use Oversleeve	7　New Technology Group 7

X　New Technology
F　Hepatobiliary System and Pancreas
J　Inspection　　Definition: Visually and/or manually exploring a body part
　　　　　　　　　Explanation: None

Body Part Character 4	Approach Character 5	Device/Substance/Technology Character 6	Qualifier Character 7
B　Hepatobiliary Duct D　Pancreatic Duct	8　Via Natural or Artificial Opening Endoscopic	A　Single-use Duodenoscope	7　New Technology Group 7

X　New Technology
H　Skin, Subcutaneous Tissue, Fascia and Breast
R　Replacement　　Definition: Putting in or on biological or synthetic material that physically takes the place and/or function of all or a portion of a body part
　　　　　　　　　Explanation: The body part may have been taken out or replaced, or may be taken out, physically eradicated, or rendered nonfunctional during the REPLACEMENT procedure. A REMOVAL procedure is coded for taking out the device used in a previous replacement procedure

Body Part Character 4	Approach Character 5	Device/Substance/Technology Character 6	Qualifier Character 7
P　Skin	X　External	F　Bioengineered Allogeneic Construct	7　New Technology Group 7
P　Skin	X　External	L　Skin Substitute, Porcine Liver Derived	2　New Technology Group 2

Valid OR　　XHRPXL2

X　New Technology
K　Muscles, Tendons, Bursae and Ligaments
Ø　Introduction　　Definition: Putting in or on a therapeutic, diagnostic, nutritional, physiological, or prophylactic substance except blood or blood products
　　　　　　　　　Explanation: None

Body Part Character 4	Approach Character 5	Device/Substance/Technology Character 6	Qualifier Character 7
2　Muscle	3　Percutaneous	Ø　Concentrated Bone Marrow Aspirate	3　New Technology Group 3

NC Noncovered Procedure　　LC Limited Coverage　　QA Questionable OB Admit　　NT New Tech Add-on　　⊞ Combination Member　　♂ Male　　♀ Female

ICD-10-PCS 2022　　　　　　　　　　　　　　　　　　　　　　　　　　　　　　　　　　　　817

XDP–XKØ

X   New Technology
N   Bones
S   Reposition

Definition: Moving to its normal location, or other suitable location, all or a portion of a body part

Explanation: The body part is moved to a new location from an abnormal location, or from a normal location where it is not functioning correctly. The body part may or may not be cut out or off to be moved to the new location.

Body Part Character 4	Approach Character 5	Device/Substance/Technology Character 6	Qualifier Character 7
Ø Lumbar Vertebra	Ø Open	3 Magnetically Controlled Growth Rod(s)	2 New Technology Group 2
Ø Lumbar Vertebra	Ø Open	C Posterior (Dynamic) Distraction Device	7 New Technology Group 7
Ø Lumbar Vertebra	3 Percutaneous	3 Magnetically Controlled Growth Rod(s)	2 New Technology Group 2
Ø Lumbar Vertebra	3 Percutaneous	C Posterior (Dynamic) Distraction Device	7 New Technology Group 7
3 Cervical Vertebra	Ø Open 3 Percutaneous	3 Magnetically Controlled Growth Rod(s)	2 New Technology Group 2
4 Thoracic Vertebra	Ø Open	3 Magnetically Controlled Growth Rod(s)	2 New Technology Group 2
4 Thoracic Vertebra	Ø Open	C Posterior (Dynamic) Distraction Device	7 New Technology Group 7
4 Thoracic Vertebra	3 Percutaneous	3 Magnetically Controlled Growth Rod(s)	2 New Technology Group 2
4 Thoracic Vertebra	3 Percutaneous	C Posterior (Dynamic) Distraction Device	7 New Technology Group 7

Valid OR XNS0032
Valid OR XNS0332
Valid OR XNS3[0,3]32
Valid OR XNS4032
Valid OR XNS4332

X   New Technology
N   Bones
U   Supplement

Definition: Putting in or on biological or synthetic material that physically reinforces and/or augments the function of a portion of a body part

Explanation: None

Body Part Character 4	Approach Character 5	Device/Substance/Technology Character 6	Qualifier Character 7
Ø Lumbar Vertebra 4 Thoracic Vertebra	3 Percutaneous	5 Synthetic Substitute, Mechanically Expandable (Paired) NT	6 New Technology Group 6

Valid OR   XNU[0,4]356
NT   XNU[0,4]356 *See* Appendix H for applicable device trade name

X New Technology
R Joints
G Fusion   Definition: Joining together portions of an articular body part rendering the articular body part immobile
         Explanation: The body part is joined together by fixation device, bone graft, or other means

Body Part Character 4	Approach Character 5	Device/Substance/Technology Character 6	Qualifier Character 7
Ø Occipital-cervical Joint	Ø Open	9 Interbody Fusion Device, Nanotextured Surface	2 New Technology Group 2
Ø Occipital-cervical Joint	Ø Open	F Interbody Fusion Device, Radiolucent Porous	3 New Technology Group 3
1 Cervical Vertebral Joint	Ø Open	9 Interbody Fusion Device, Nanotextured Surface	2 New Technology Group 2
1 Cervical Vertebral Joint	Ø Open	F Interbody Fusion Device, Radiolucent Porous	3 New Technology Group 3
2 Cervical Vertebral Joints, 2 or more	Ø Open	9 Interbody Fusion Device, Nanotextured Surface	2 New Technology Group 2
2 Cervical Vertebral Joints, 2 or more	Ø Open	F Interbody Fusion Device, Radiolucent Porous	3 New Technology Group 3
4 Cervicothoracic Vertebral Joint	Ø Open	9 Interbody Fusion Device, Nanotextured Surface	2 New Technology Group 2
4 Cervicothoracic Vertebral Joint	Ø Open	F Interbody Fusion Device, Radiolucent Porous	3 New Technology Group 3
6 Thoracic Vertebral Joint	Ø Open	9 Interbody Fusion Device, Nanotextured Surface	2 New Technology Group 2
6 Thoracic Vertebral Joint	Ø Open	F Interbody Fusion Device, Radiolucent Porous	3 New Technology Group 3
7 Thoracic Vertebral Joints, 2 to 7 ⊞	Ø Open	9 Interbody Fusion Device, Nanotextured Surface	2 New Technology Group 2
7 Thoracic Vertebral Joints, 2 to 7 ⊞	Ø Open	F Interbody Fusion Device, Radiolucent Porous	3 New Technology Group 3
8 Thoracic Vertebral Joints, 8 or more	Ø Open	9 Interbody Fusion Device, Nanotextured Surface	2 New Technology Group 2
8 Thoracic Vertebral Joints, 8 or more	Ø Open	F Interbody Fusion Device, Radiolucent Porous	3 New Technology Group 3
A Thoracolumbar Vertebral Joint	Ø Open	9 Interbody Fusion Device, Nanotextured Surface	2 New Technology Group 2
A Thoracolumbar Vertebral Joint	Ø Open	F Interbody Fusion Device, Radiolucent Porous	3 New Technology Group 3
A Thoracolumbar Vertebral Joint	Ø Open 3 Percutaneous 4 Percutaneous Endoscopic	R Interbody Fusion Device, Customizable	7 New Technology Group 7
B Lumbar Vertebral Joint	Ø Open	9 Interbody Fusion Device, Nanotextured Surface	2 New Technology Group 2
B Lumbar Vertebral Joint	Ø Open	F Interbody Fusion Device, Radiolucent Porous	3 New Technology Group 3
B Lumbar Vertebral Joint	Ø Open 3 Percutaneous 4 Percutaneous Endoscopic	R Interbody Fusion Device, Customizable	7 New Technology Group 7
C Lumbar Vertebral Joints, 2 or more ⊞	Ø Open	9 Interbody Fusion Device, Nanotextured Surface	2 New Technology Group 2
C Lumbar Vertebral Joints, 2 or more ⊞	Ø Open	F Interbody Fusion Device, Radiolucent Porous	3 New Technology Group 3
C Lumbar Vertebral Joints, 2 or more	Ø Open 3 Percutaneous 4 Percutaneous Endoscopic	R Interbody Fusion Device, Customizable	7 New Technology Group 7
D Lumbosacral Joint	Ø Open	9 Interbody Fusion Device, Nanotextured Surface	2 New Technology Group 2
D Lumbosacral Joint	Ø Open	F Interbody Fusion Device, Radiolucent Porous	3 New Technology Group 3
D Lumbosacral Joint	Ø Open 3 Percutaneous 4 Percutaneous Endoscopic	R Interbody Fusion Device, Customizable	7 New Technology Group 7

Valid OR All body part, approach, device/substance/technology, and qualifier values
HAC XRG[Ø,1,2,4,6,7,8,A,B,C,D]Ø92 when reported with SDx K68.11 or T81.4Ø–T81.49, T84.6Ø-T84.619, T84.63-T84.7 with 7th character A
HAC XRG[Ø,1,2,4,6,7,8,A,B,C,D]ØF3 when reported with SDx K68.11 or T81.4Ø–T81.49, T84.6Ø-T84.619, T84.63-T84.7 with 7th character A

See Appendix L for Procedure Combinations
⊞ XRG7092
⊞ XRG7ØF3
⊞ XRGCØ92
⊞ XRGCØF3

X New Technology
T Urinary System
2 Monitoring   Definition: Determining the level of a physiological or physical function repetitively over a period of time
         Explanation: None

Body Part Character 4	Approach Character 5	Device/Substance/Technology Character 6	Qualifier Character 7
5 Kidney	X External	E Fluorescent Pyrazine	5 New Technology Group 5

NC Noncovered Procedure   LC Limited Coverage   QA Questionable OB Admit   NT New Tech Add-on   ⊞ Combination Member   ♂ Male   ♀ Female

X New Technology
V Male Reproductive System
5 Destruction   Definition: Physical eradication of all or a portion of a body part by the direct use of energy, force, or a destructive agent
        Explanation: None of the body part is physically taken out

Body Part Character 4	Approach Character 5	Device/Substance/Technology Character 6	Qualifier Character 7
Ø Prostate	8 Via Natural or Artificial Opening Endoscopic	A Robotic Waterjet Ablation	4 New Technology Group 4

Valid OR   All body part, approach, device/substance/technology, and qualifier values

---

X New Technology
W Anatomical Regions
Ø Introduction   Definition: Putting in or on a therapeutic, diagnostic, nutritional, physiological, or prophylactic substance except blood or blood products
        Explanation: None

Body Part Character 4	Approach Character 5	Device/Substance/Technology Character 6	Qualifier Character 7
Ø Skin	X External	2 Bromelain-enriched Proteolytic Enzyme	7 New Technology Group 7
1 Subcutaneous Tissue	3 Percutaneous	9 Satralizumab-mwge	7 New Technology Group 7
1 Subcutaneous Tissue	3 Percutaneous	F Other New Technology Therapeutic Substance	5 New Technology Group 5
1 Subcutaneous Tissue	3 Percutaneous	H Other New Technology Monoclonal Antibody K Leronlimab Monoclonal Antibody S COVID-19 Vaccine Dose 1 T COVID-19 Vaccine Dose 2 U COVID-19 Vaccine	6 New Technology Group 6
1 Subcutaneous Tissue	3 Percutaneous	W Caplacizumab [NT]	5 New Technology Group 5
1 Subcutaneous Tissue	X External	2 Bromelain-enriched Proteolytic Enzyme	7 New Technology Group 7
2 Muscle	3 Percutaneous	S COVID-19 Vaccine Dose 1 T COVID-19 Vaccine Dose 2 U COVID-19 Vaccine	6 New Technology Group 6
3 Peripheral Vein	3 Percutaneous	Ø Brexanolone 2 Nerinitide 3 Durvalumab Antineoplastic [NT]	6 New Technology Group 6
3 Peripheral Vein	3 Percutaneous	5 Narsoplimab Monoclonal Antibody	7 New Technology Group 7
3 Peripheral Vein	3 Percutaneous	6 Lefamulin Anti-infective [NT]	6 New Technology Group 6
3 Peripheral Vein	3 Percutaneous	6 Terlipressin	7 New Technology Group 7
3 Peripheral Vein	3 Percutaneous	7 Coagulation Factor Xa, Inactivated [NT]	2 New Technology Group 2
3 Peripheral Vein	3 Percutaneous	7 Trilaciclib 8 Lurbinectedin	7 New Technology Group 7
3 Peripheral Vein	3 Percutaneous	9 Defibrotide Sodium Anticoagulant	2 New Technology Group 2
3 Peripheral Vein	3 Percutaneous	9 Ceftolozane/Tazobactam Anti-infective [NT]	6 New Technology Group 6
3 Peripheral Vein	3 Percutaneous	A Bezlotoxumab Monoclonal Antibody	3 New Technology Group 3
3 Peripheral Vein	3 Percutaneous	A Cefiderocol Anti-infective [NT]	6 New Technology Group 6
3 Peripheral Vein	3 Percutaneous	A Ciltacabtagene Autoleucel	7 New Technology Group 7
3 Peripheral Vein	3 Percutaneous	B Cytarabine and Daunorubicin Liposome Antineoplastic	3 New Technology Group 3
3 Peripheral Vein	3 Percutaneous	B Omadacycline Anti-infective [NT]	6 New Technology Group 6
3 Peripheral Vein	3 Percutaneous	B Amivantamab Monoclonal Antibody	7 New Technology Group 7
3 Peripheral Vein	3 Percutaneous	C Eculizumab [NT]	6 New Technology Group 6
3 Peripheral Vein	3 Percutaneous	C Engineered Chimeric Antigen Receptor T-cell Immunotherapy, Autologous	7 New Technology Group 7
3 Peripheral Vein	3 Percutaneous	D Atezolizumab Antineoplastic [NT]	6 New Technology Group 6
3 Peripheral Vein	3 Percutaneous	E Remdesivir Anti-infective [NT]	5 New Technology Group 5
3 Peripheral Vein	3 Percutaneous	E Etesevimab Monoclonal Antibody	6 New Technology Group 6
3 Peripheral Vein	3 Percutaneous	F Other New Technology Therapeutic Substance	3 New Technology Group 3
3 Peripheral Vein	3 Percutaneous	F Other New Technology Therapeutic Substance	5 New Technology Group 5
3 Peripheral Vein	3 Percutaneous	F Bamlanivimab Monoclonal Antibody	6 New Technology Group 6
3 Peripheral Vein	3 Percutaneous	G Plazomicin Anti-infective [NT]	4 New Technology Group 4
3 Peripheral Vein	3 Percutaneous	G Sarilumab	5 New Technology Group 5

DRG Non-OR	XWØ33C7	[NT]	XWØ3366	[NT]	XWØ33A6	[NT]	XWØ33D6
[NT]	XWØ13W5	[NT]	XWØ3372	[NT]	XWØ33B6	[NT]	XWØ33E5
[NT]	XWØ3336	[NT]	XWØ3396	[NT]	XWØ33C6	[NT]	XWØ33G4

* For all codes with NT icon *see* Appendix I for registered or trade name of substance

XWØ Continued on next page

Non-OR Procedure   DRG Non-OR Procedure   Valid OR Procedure   HAC Associated Procedure   Combination Only   New/Revised GREEN

X   New Technology
W   Anatomical Regions
Ø   Introduction   Definition: Putting in or on a therapeutic, diagnostic, nutritional, physiological, or prophylactic substance except blood or blood products
                Explanation: None

XWØ Continued

Body Part Character 4	Approach Character 5	Device/Substance/Technology Character 6	Qualifier Character 7
3 Peripheral Vein	3 Percutaneous	G REGN-COV2 Monoclonal Antibody	6 New Technology Group 6
3 Peripheral Vein	3 Percutaneous	G Engineered Chimeric Antigen Receptor T-cell Immunotherapy, Allogeneic	7 New Technology Group 7
3 Peripheral Vein	3 Percutaneous	H Synthetic Human Angiotensin II	4 New Technology Group 4
3 Peripheral Vein	3 Percutaneous	H Tocilizumab	5 New Technology Group 5
3 Peripheral Vein	3 Percutaneous	H Other New Technology Monoclonal Antibody	6 New Technology Group 6
3 Peripheral Vein	3 Percutaneous	H Axicabtagene Ciloleucel Immunotherapy J Tisagenlecleucel Immunotherapy	7 New Technology Group 7
3 Peripheral Vein	3 Percutaneous	K Fosfomycin Anti-infective	5 New Technology Group 5
3 Peripheral Vein	3 Percutaneous	K Idecabtagene Vicleucel Immunotherapy	7 New Technology Group 7
3 Peripheral Vein	3 Percutaneous	L CD24Fc Immunomodulator	6 New Technology Group 6
3 Peripheral Vein	3 Percutaneous	L Lifileucel Immunotherapy M Brexucabtagene Autoleucel Immunotherapy	7 New Technology Group 7
3 Peripheral Vein	3 Percutaneous	N Meropenem-vaborbactam Anti-infective	5 New Technology Group 5
3 Peripheral Vein	3 Percutaneous	N Lisocabtagene Maraleucel Immunotherapy	7 New Technology Group 7
3 Peripheral Vein	3 Percutaneous	Q Tagraxofusp-erzs Antineoplastic NT S Iobenguane I-131 Antineoplastic NT U Imipenem-cilastatin-relebactam Anti-infective NT W Caplacizumab NT	5 New Technology Group 5
4 Central Vein	3 Percutaneous	Ø Brexanolone 2 Nerinitide 3 Durvalumab Antineoplastic NT	6 New Technology Group 6
4 Central Vein	3 Percutaneous	5 Narsoplimab Monoclonal Antibody	7 New Technology Group 7
4 Central Vein	3 Percutaneous	6 Lefamulin Anti-infective NT	6 New Technology Group 6
4 Central Vein	3 Percutaneous	6 Terlipressin	7 New Technology Group 7
4 Central Vein	3 Percutaneous	7 Coagulation Factor Xa, Inactivated NT	2 New Technology Group 2
4 Central Vein	3 Percutaneous	7 Trilaciclib 8 Lurbinectedin	7 New Technology Group 7
4 Central Vein	3 Percutaneous	9 Defibrotide Sodium Anticoagulant	2 New Technology Group 2
4 Central Vein	3 Percutaneous	9 Ceftolozane/Tazobactam Anti-infective NT	6 New Technology Group 6
4 Central Vein	3 Percutaneous	A Bezlotoxumab Monoclonal Antibody	3 New Technology Group 3
4 Central Vein	3 Percutaneous	A Cefiderocol Anti-infective NT	6 New Technology Group 6
4 Central Vein	3 Percutaneous	A Ciltacabtagene Autoleucel	7 New Technology Group 7
4 Central Vein	3 Percutaneous	B Cytarabine and Daunorubicin Liposome Antineoplastic	3 New Technology Group 3
4 Central Vein	3 Percutaneous	B Omadacycline Anti-infective NT	6 New Technology Group 6
4 Central Vein	3 Percutaneous	B Amivantamab Monoclonal Antibody	7 New Technology Group 7
4 Central Vein	3 Percutaneous	C Eculizumab NT	6 New Technology Group 6
4 Central Vein	3 Percutaneous	C Engineered Chimeric Antigen Receptor T-cell Immunotherapy, Autologous	7 New Technology Group 7
4 Central Vein	3 Percutaneous	D Atezolizumab Antineoplastic NT	6 New Technology Group 6
4 Central Vein	3 Percutaneous	E Remdesivir Anti-infective NT	5 New Technology Group 5
4 Central Vein	3 Percutaneous	E Etesevimab Monoclonal Antibody	6 New Technology Group 6
4 Central Vein	3 Percutaneous	F Other New Technology Therapeutic Substance	3 New Technology Group 3
4 Central Vein	3 Percutaneous	F Other New Technology Therapeutic Substance	5 New Technology Group 5
4 Central Vein	3 Percutaneous	F Bamlanivimab Monoclonal Antibody	6 New Technology Group 6
4 Central Vein	3 Percutaneous	G Plazomicin Anti-infective NT	4 New Technology Group 4

DRG Non-OR XWØ33G7	NT XWØ33[Q,S,U,W]5	NT XWØ4396	NT XWØ43D6
DRG Non-OR XWØ33[H,J]7	NT XWØ4336	NT XWØ43A6	NT XWØ43E5
DRG Non-OR XWØ33K7	NT XWØ4366	NT XWØ43B6	NT XWØ43G4
DRG Non-OR XWØ33[L,M]7	NT XWØ4372	NT XWØ43C6	
DRG Non-OR XWØ33N7			
DRG Non-OR XWØ43C7			

* For all codes with NT icon *see* Appendix I for registered or trade name of substance

XWØ Continued on next page

NC Noncovered Procedure   LC Limited Coverage   QA Questionable OB Admit   NT New Tech Add-on   ⊞ Combination Member   ♂ Male   ♀ Female

New Technology

X   **New Technology**
W   **Anatomical Regions**
Ø   **Introduction**

XWØ Continued

Definition: Putting in or on a therapeutic, diagnostic, nutritional, physiological, or prophylactic substance except blood or blood products
Explanation: None

Body Part Character 4	Approach Character 5	Device/Substance/Technology Character 6	Qualifier Character 7
4 Central Vein	3 Percutaneous	G Sarilumab	5 New Technology Group 5
4 Central Vein	3 Percutaneous	G REGN-COV2 Monoclonal Antibody	6 New Technology Group 6
4 Central Vein	3 Percutaneous	G Engineered Chimeric Antigen Receptor T-cell Immunotherapy, Allogeneic	7 New Technology Group 7
4 Central Vein	3 Percutaneous	H Synthetic Human Angiotensin II	4 New Technology Group 4
4 Central Vein	3 Percutaneous	H Tocilizumab	5 New Technology Group 5
4 Central Vein	3 Percutaneous	H Other New Technology Monoclonal Antibody	6 New Technology Group 6
4 Central Vein	3 Percutaneous	H Axicabtagene Ciloleucel Immunotherapy J Tisagenlecleucel Immunotherapy	7 New Technology Group 7
4 Central Vein	3 Percutaneous	K Fosfomycin Anti-infective	5 New Technology Group 5
4 Central Vein	3 Percutaneous	K Idecabtagene Vicleucel Immunotherapy	7 New Technology Group 7
4 Central Vein	3 Percutaneous	L CD24Fc Immunomodulator	6 New Technology Group 6
4 Central Vein	3 Percutaneous	L Lifileucel Immunotherapy M Brexucabtagene Autoleucel Immunotherapy	7 New Technology Group 7
4 Central Vein	3 Percutaneous	N Meropenem-vaborbactam Anti-infective	5 New Technology Group 5
4 Central Vein	3 Percutaneous	N Lisocabtagene Maraleucel Immunotherapy	7 New Technology Group 7
4 Central Vein	3 Percutaneous	Q Tagraxofusp-erzs Antineoplastic [NT] S Iobenguane I-131 Antineoplastic [NT] U Imipenem-cilastatin-relebactam Anti-infective [NT] W Caplacizumab [NT]	5 New Technology Group 5
9 Nose	7 Via Natural or Artificial Opening	M Esketamine Hydrochloride [NT]	5 New Technology Group 5
D Mouth and Pharynx	X External	6 Lefamulin Anti-infective [NT]	6 New Technology Group 6
D Mouth and Pharynx	X External	8 Uridine Triacetate	2 New Technology Group 2
D Mouth and Pharynx	X External	F Other New Technology Therapeutic Substance J Apalutamide Antineoplastic L Erdafitinib Antineoplastic [NT]	5 New Technology Group 5
D Mouth and Pharynx	X External	M Baricitinib [NT]	6 New Technology Group 6
D Mouth and Pharynx	X External	R Venetoclax Antineoplastic T Ruxolitinib [NT] V Gilteritinib Antineoplastic [NT]	5 New Technology Group 5
G Upper GI H Lower GI	7 Via Natural or Artificial Opening	M Baricitinib [NT]	6 New Technology Group 6
G Upper GI H Lower GI	8 Via Natural or Artificial Opening Endoscopic	8 Mineral-based Topical Hemostatic Agent [NT]	6 New Technology Group 6
Q Cranial Cavity and Brain	3 Percutaneous	1 Eladocagene exuparvovec	6 New Technology Group 6
V Bones	Ø Open	P Antibiotic-eluting Bone Void Filler	7 New Technology Group 7

DRG Non-OR	XWØ43G7	[NT]	XWØ43[Q,S,U,W]5	[NT]	XWØDXL5	[NT]	XWØ[G,H]7M6
DRG Non-OR	XWØ43[H,J]7	[NT]	XWØ97M5	[NT]	XWØDXM6	[NT]	XWØ[G,H]886
DRG Non-OR	XWØ43K7	[NT]	XWØDX66	[NT]	XWØDX[T,V]5		
DRG Non-OR	XWØ43[L,M]7						
DRG Non-OR	XWØ43N7						

* For all codes with NT icon *see* Appendix I for registered or trade name of substance

X New Technology
W Anatomical Regions
1 Transfusion   Definition: Putting in blood or blood products
         Explanation: None

Body Part Character 4	Approach Character 5	Device/Substance/Technology Character 6	Qualifier Character 7
3 Peripheral Vein	**3** Percutaneous	**2** Plasma, Convalescent **NT** (Nonautologous)	**5** New Technology Group 5
3 Peripheral Vein	**3** Percutaneous	**D** High-Dose Intravenous Immune Globulin **E** Hyperimmune Globulin	**7** New Technology Group 7
4 Central Vein	**3** Percutaneous	**2** Plasma, Convalescent **NT** (Nonautologous)	**5** New Technology Group 5
4 Central Vein	**3** Percutaneous	**D** High-Dose Intravenous Immune Globulin **E** Hyperimmune Globulin	**7** New Technology Group 7

> **NT** XW13325
> **NT** XW14325

X New Technology
W Anatomical Regions
H Insertion   Definition: Putting in a nonbiological appliance that monitors, assists, performs, or prevents a physiological function but does not physically take the place of a body part
         Explanation: None

Body Part Character 4	Approach Character 5	Device/Substance/Technology Character 6	Qualifier Character 7
D Mouth and Pharynx	**7** Via Natural or Artificial Opening	**Q** Neurostimulator Lead	**7** New Technology Group 7

X New Technology
X Physiological Systems
E Measurement   Definition: Determining the level of a physiological or physical function at a point in time
         Explanation: None

Body Part Character 4	Approach Character 5	Device/Substance/Technology Character 6	Qualifier Character 7
Ø Central Nervous	**X** External	**Ø** Intracranial Vascular Activity, Computer-aided Assessment	**7** New Technology Group 7
3 Arterial	**X** External	**2** Pulmonary Artery Flow, Computer- aided Triage and Notification	**7** New Technology Group 7
5 Circulatory	**X** External	**M** Infection, Whole Blood Nucleic **NT** Acid-base Microbial Detection	**5** New Technology Group 5
5 Circulatory	**X** External	**N** Infection, Positive Blood Culture Fluorescence Hybridization for Organism Identification, Concentration and Susceptibility	**6** New Technology Group 6
5 Circulatory	**X** External	**R** Infection, Mechanical Initial Specimen Diversion Technique Using Active Negative Pressure **T** Intracranial Arterial Flow, Whole Blood mRNA **V** Infection, Serum/Plasma Nanoparticle Fluorescence SARS- CoV-2 Antibody Detection	**7** New Technology Group 7
9 Nose	**7** Via Natural or Artificial Opening	**U** Infection, Nasopharyngeal Fluid SARS-CoV-2 Polymerase Chain Reaction	**7** New Technology Group 7
B Respiratory	**X** External	**Q** Infection, Lower Respiratory Fluid Nucleic Acid-base Microbial Detection	**6** New Technology Group 6

> **NT** XXE5XM5 for T2 Bacteria Test Panel

X New Technology
Y Extracorporeal
Ø Introduction   Definition: Putting in or on a therapeutic, diagnostic, nutritional, physiological, or prophylactic substance except blood or blood products
         Explanation: None

Body Part Character 4	Approach Character 5	Device/Substance/Technology Character 6	Qualifier Character 7
V Vein Graft	**X** External	**8** Endothelial Damage Inhibitor	**3** New Technology Group 3
Y Extracorporeal	**X** External	**3** Nafamostat Anticoagulant	**7** New Technology Group 7

NC Noncovered Procedure   **LC** Limited Coverage   **QA** Questionable OB Admit   **NT** New Tech Add-on   ⊞ Combination Member   ♂ Male   ♀ Female

ICD-10-PCS 2022   823

XW1–XYØ

Appendixes

Appendix A: Components of the Medical and Surgical Approach Definitions

ICD-10-PCS Value	Definition	Access Location	Method	Type of Instrumentation	Example
Open (Ø)	Cutting through the skin or mucous membrane and any other body layers necessary to expose the site of the procedure	Skin or mucous membrane, any other body layers	Cutting	None	Abdominal hysterectomy
Percutaneous (3)	Entry, by puncture or minor incision, of instrumentation through the skin or mucous membrane and any other body layers necessary to reach the site of the procedure	Skin or mucous membrane, any other body layers	Puncture or minor incision	Without visualization	Needle biopsy of liver, Liposuction
Percutaneous endoscopic (4)	Entry, by puncture or minor incision, of instrumentation through the skin or mucous membrane and any other body layers necessary to reach and visualize the site of the procedure	Skin or mucous membrane, any other body layers	Puncture or minor incision	With visualization	Arthroscopy, Laparoscopic cholecystectomy
Via natural or artificial opening (7)	Entry of instrumentation through a natural or artificial external opening to reach the site of the procedure	Natural or artificial external opening	Direct entry	Without visualization	Endotracheal tube insertion, Foley catheter placement
Via natural or artificial opening endoscopic (8)	Entry of instrumentation through a natural or artificial external opening to reach and visualize the site of the procedure	Natural or artificial external opening	Direct entry	With visualization	Sigmoidoscopy, EGD, ERCP
Via natural or artificial opening with percutaneous endoscopic assistance (F)	Entry of instrumentation through a natural or artificial external opening and entry, by puncture or minor incision, of instrumentation through the skin or mucous membrane and any other body layers necessary to aid in the performance of the procedure	Skin or mucous membrane, any other body layers	Direct entry with puncture or minor incision for instrumentation only	With visualization	Laparoscopic-assisted vaginal hysterectomy
External (X)	Procedures performed directly on the skin or mucous membrane and procedures performed indirectly by the application of external force through the skin or mucous membrane	Skin or mucous membrane	Direct or indirect application	None	Closed fracture reduction, Resection of tonsils

Open (Ø)

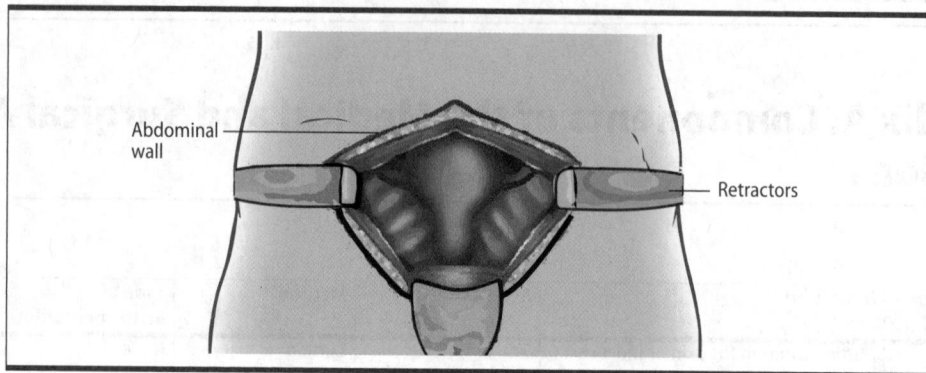

Percutaneous (3)

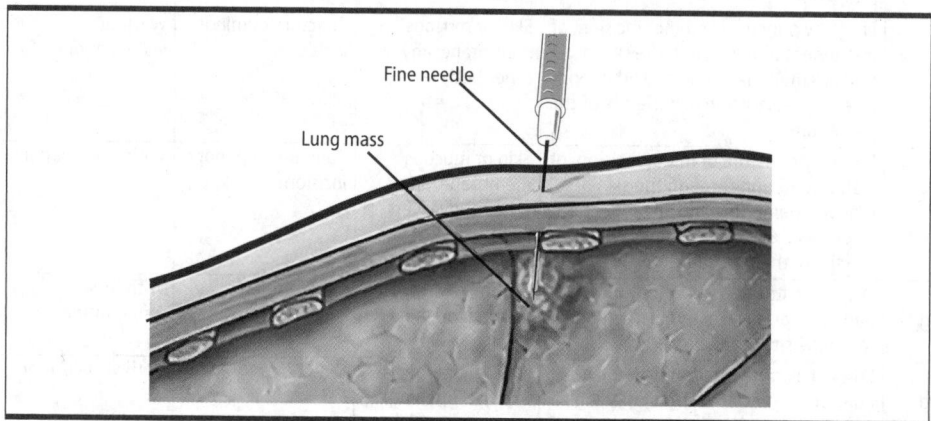

Percutaneous Endoscopic (4)

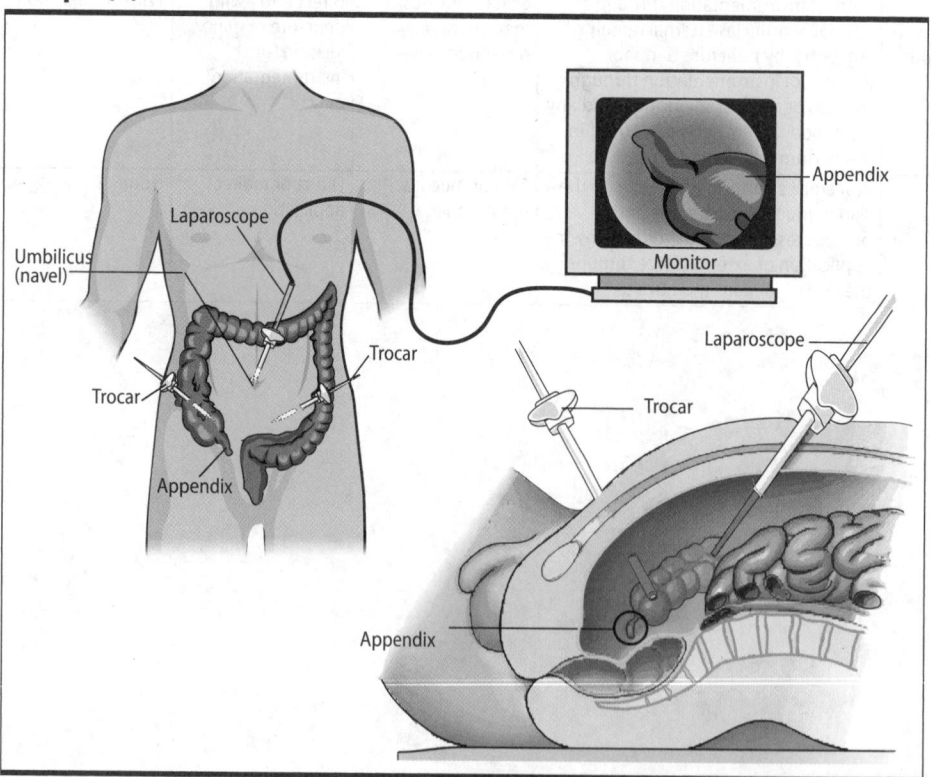

Via Natural or Artificial Opening (7)

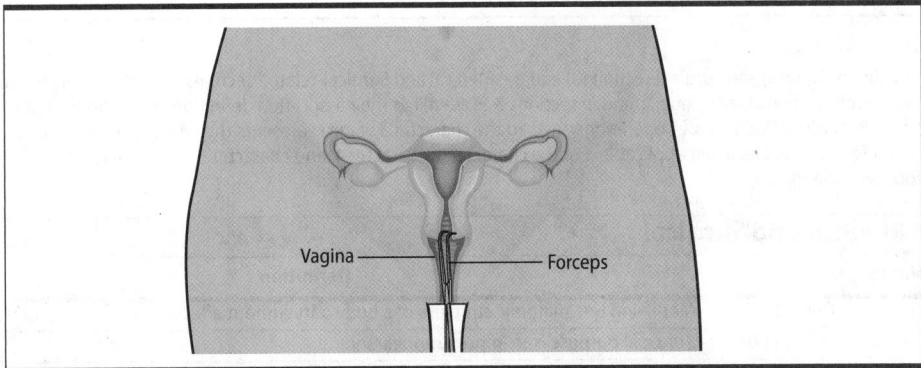

Via Natural or Artificial Opening, Endoscopic (8)

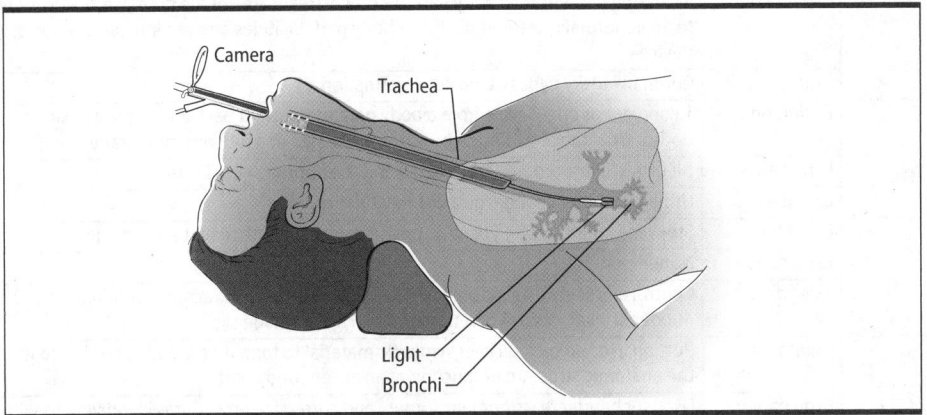

Via Natural or Artificial Opening with Percutaneous Endoscopic Assistance (F)

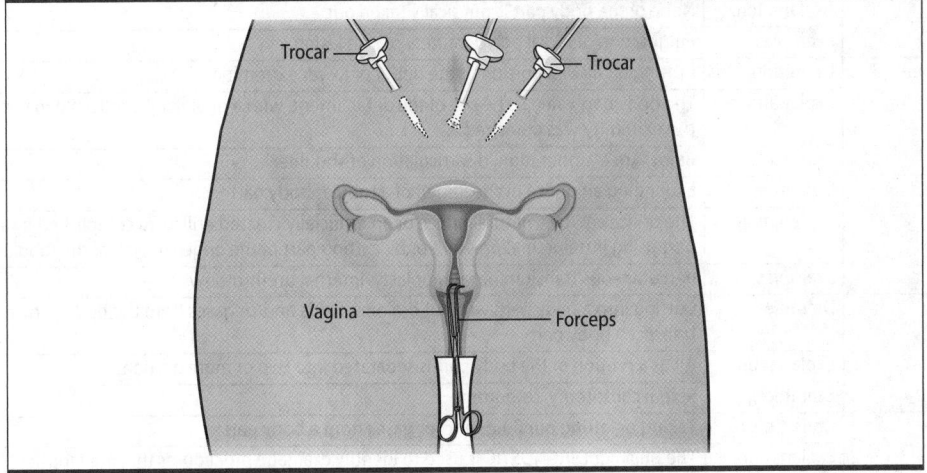

External (X)

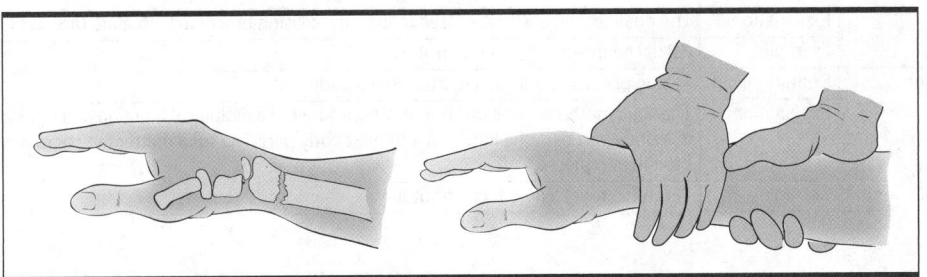

Appendix B: Root Operation Definitions

The character 3 value in the Medical and Surgical section (Ø) and the Medical and Surgical-related sections (1-9) represents the root operation. This resource provides each root operation (character 3) value, found in sections Ø-9, as well as their associated definition, explanation, and examples, where applicable. The Ancillary sections (B-H) do not include root operations; instead the character 3 value represents the type of procedure performed with additional detail provided by the character 4 or 5 value, when applicable. For the character 3, character 4, and character 5 values used in the Ancillary sections of B-H, along with their definitions, see appendix J.

Ø	Medical and Surgical		
ICD-1Ø-PCS Value			**Definition**
Ø	Alteration	Definition:	Modifying the anatomic structure of a body part without affecting the function of the body part
		Explanation:	Principal purpose is to improve appearance
		Examples:	Face lift, breast augmentation
1	Bypass	Definition:	Altering the route of passage of the contents of a tubular body part
		Explanation:	Rerouting contents of a body part to a downstream area of the normal route, to a similar route and body part, or to an abnormal route and dissimilar body part. Includes one or more anastomoses, with or without the use of a device.
		Examples:	Coronary artery bypass, colostomy formation
2	Change	Definition:	Taking out or off a device from a body part and putting back an identical or similar device in or on the same body part without cutting or puncturing the skin or a mucous membrane
		Explanation:	All CHANGE procedures are coded using the approach EXTERNAL
		Example:	Urinary catheter change, gastrostomy tube change
3	Control	Definition:	Stopping, or attempting to stop, postprocedural or other acute bleeding
		Explanation:	None
		Examples:	Control of post-prostatectomy hemorrhage, control of intracranial subdural hemorrhage, control of bleeding duodenal ulcer, control of retroperitoneal hemorrhage
4	Creation	Definition:	Putting in or on biological or synthetic material to form a new body part that to the extent possible replicates the anatomic structure or function of an absent body part
		Explanation:	Used for gender reassignment surgery and corrective procedures in individuals with congenital anomalies
		Examples:	Creation of vagina in a male, creation of right and left atrioventricular valve from common atrioventricular valve
5	Destruction	Definition:	Physical eradication of all or a portion of a body part by the direct use of energy, force, or a destructive agent
		Explanation:	None of the body part is physically taken out
		Examples:	Fulguration of rectal polyp, cautery of skin lesion
6	Detachment	Definition:	Cutting off all or a portion of the upper or lower extremities
		Explanation:	The body part value is the site of the detachment, with a qualifier if applicable to further specify the level where the extremity was detached
		Examples:	Below knee amputation, disarticulation of shoulder
7	Dilation	Definition:	Expanding an orifice or the lumen of a tubular body part
		Explanation:	The orifice can be a natural orifice or an artificially created orifice. Accomplished by stretching a tubular body part using intraluminal pressure or by cutting part of the orifice or wall of the tubular body part.
		Examples:	Percutaneous transluminal angioplasty, internal urethrotomy
8	Division	Definition:	Cutting into a body part, without draining fluids and/or gases from the body part, in order to separate or transect a body part
		Explanation:	All or a portion of the body part is separated into two or more portions
		Examples:	Spinal cordotomy, osteotomy
9	Drainage	Definition:	Taking or letting out fluids and/or gases from a body part
		Explanation:	The qualifier DIAGNOSTIC is used to identify drainage procedures that are biopsies
		Examples:	Thoracentesis, incision and drainage
B	Excision	Definition:	Cutting out or off, without replacement, a portion of a body part
		Explanation:	The qualifier DIAGNOSTIC is used to identify excision procedures that are biopsies
		Examples:	Partial nephrectomy, liver biopsy
C	Extirpation	Definition:	Taking or cutting out solid matter from a body part
		Explanation:	The solid matter may be an abnormal byproduct of a biological function or a foreign body; it may be imbedded in a body part or in the lumen of a tubular body part. The solid matter may or may not have been previously broken into pieces.
		Examples:	Thrombectomy, choledocholithotomy

Continued on next page

Ø	**Medical and Surgical**		*Continued from previous page*
ICD-10-PCS Value			**Definition**
D	Extraction	Definition:	Pulling or stripping out or off all or a portion of a body part by the use of force
		Explanation:	The qualifier DIAGNOSTIC is used to identify extractions that are biopsies
		Examples:	Dilation and curettage, vein stripping
F	Fragmentation	Definition:	Breaking solid matter in a body part into pieces
		Explanation:	Physical force (e.g., manual, ultrasonic) applied directly or indirectly is used to break the solid matter into pieces. The solid matter may be an abnormal byproduct of a biological function or a foreign body. The pieces of solid matter are not taken out.
		Examples:	Extracorporeal shockwave lithotripsy, transurethral lithotripsy
G	Fusion	Definition:	Joining together portions of an articular body part rendering the articular body part immobile
		Explanation:	The body part is joined together by fixation device, bone graft, or other means
		Examples:	Spinal fusion, ankle arthrodesis
H	Insertion	Definition:	Putting in a nonbiological appliance that monitors, assists, performs, or prevents a physiological function but does not physically take the place of a body part
		Explanation:	None
		Examples:	Insertion of radioactive implant, insertion of central venous catheter
J	Inspection	Definition:	Visually and/or manually exploring a body part
		Explanation:	Visual exploration may be performed with or without optical instrumentation. Manual exploration may be performed directly or through intervening body layers.
		Examples:	Diagnostic arthroscopy, exploratory laparotomy
K	Map	Definition:	Locating the route of passage of electrical impulses and/or locating functional areas in a body part
		Explanation:	Applicable only to the cardiac conduction mechanism and the central nervous system
		Examples:	Cardiac mapping, cortical mapping
L	Occlusion	Definition:	Completely closing an orifice or lumen of a tubular body part
		Explanation:	The orifice can be a natural orifice or an artificially created orifice
		Examples:	Fallopian tube ligation, ligation of inferior vena cava
M	Reattachment	Definition:	Putting back in or on all or a portion of a separated body part to its normal location or other suitable location
		Explanation:	Vascular circulation and nervous pathways may or may not be reestablished
		Examples:	Reattachment of hand, reattachment of avulsed kidney
N	Release	Definition:	Freeing a body part from an abnormal physical constraint by cutting or by use of force
		Explanation:	Some of the restraining tissue may be taken out but none of the body part is taken out
		Examples:	Adhesiolysis, carpal tunnel release
P	Removal	Definition:	Taking out or off a device from a body part
		Explanation:	If a device is taken out and a similar device put in without cutting or puncturing the skin or mucous membrane, the procedure is coded to the root operation CHANGE. Otherwise, the procedure for taking out a device is coded to the root operation REMOVAL.
		Examples:	Drainage tube removal, cardiac pacemaker removal
Q	Repair	Definition:	Restoring, to the extent possible, a body part to its normal anatomic structure and function
		Explanation:	Used only when the method to accomplish the repair is not one of the other root operations
		Examples:	Colostomy takedown, suture of laceration
R	Replacement	Definition:	Putting in or on biological or synthetic material that physically takes the place and/or function of all or a portion of a body part
		Explanation:	The body part may have been taken out or replaced, or may be taken out, physically eradicated, or rendered nonfunctional during the REPLACEMENT procedure. A REMOVAL procedure is coded for taking out the device used in a previous replacement procedure.
		Examples:	Total hip replacement, bone graft, free skin graft
S	Reposition	Definition:	Moving to its normal location, or other suitable location, all or a portion of a body part
		Explanation:	The body part is moved to a new location from an abnormal location, or from a normal location where it is not functioning correctly. The body part may or may not be cut out or off to be moved to the new location.
		Examples:	Reposition of undescended testicle, fracture reduction
T	Resection	Definition:	Cutting out or off, without replacement, all of a body part
		Explanation:	None
		Examples:	Total nephrectomy, total lobectomy of lung
V	Restriction	Definition:	Partially closing an orifice or the lumen of a tubular body part
		Explanation:	The orifice can be a natural orifice or an artificially created orifice
		Examples:	Esophagogastric fundoplication, cervical cerclage

Continued on next page

Ø	**Medical and Surgical**		*Continued from previous page*

ICD-10-PCS Value			Definition
W	Revision	Definition:	Correcting, to the extent possible, a portion of a malfunctioning device or the position of a displaced device
		Explanation:	Revision can include correcting a malfunctioning or displaced device by taking out or putting in components of the device such as a screw or pin
		Examples:	Adjustment of position of pacemaker lead, recementing of hip prosthesis
U	Supplement	Definition:	Putting in or on biological or synthetic material that physically reinforces and/or augments the function of a portion of a body part
		Explanation:	The biological material is non-living, or is living and from the same individual. The body part may have been previously replaced, and the SUPPLEMENT procedure is performed to physically reinforce and/or augment the function of the replaced body part.
		Examples:	Herniorrhaphy using mesh, mitral valve ring annuloplasty, put a new acetabular liner in a previous hip replacement
X	Transfer	Definition:	Moving, without taking out, all or a portion of a body part to another location to take over the function of all or a portion of a body part
		Explanation:	The body part transferred remains connected to its vascular and nervous supply
		Examples:	Tendon transfer, skin pedicle flap transfer
Y	Transplantation	Definition:	Putting in or on all or a portion of a living body part taken from another individual or animal to physically take the place and/or function of all or a portion of a similar body part
		Explanation:	The native body part may or may not be taken out, and the transplanted body part may take over all or a portion of its function
		Examples:	Kidney transplant, heart transplant

Root Operation Definitions for Other Sections

1	**Obstetrics**		

ICD-10-PCS Value			Definition
2	Change	Definition:	Taking out or off a device from a body part and putting back an identical or similar device in or on the same body part without cutting or puncturing the skin or a mucous membrane
		Explanation:	None
		Examples:	Replacement of fetal scalp electrode
9	Drainage	Definition:	Taking or letting out fluids and/or gases from a body part
		Explanation:	None
		Examples:	Biopsy of amniotic fluid
A	Abortion	Definition:	Artificially terminating a pregnancy
		Explanation:	None
		Examples:	Transvaginal abortion using vacuum aspiration technique
D	Extraction	Definition:	Pulling or stripping out or off all or a portion of a body part by the use of force
		Explanation:	None
		Examples:	Low-transverse C-section
E	Delivery	Definition:	Assisting the passage of the products of conception from the genital canal
		Explanation:	None
		Examples:	Manually-assisted delivery
H	Insertion	Definition:	Putting in a nonbiological appliance that monitors, assists, performs, or prevents a physiological function but does not physically take the place of a body part
		Explanation:	None
		Examples:	Placement of fetal scalp electrode
J	Inspection	Definition:	Visually and/or manually exploring a body part
		Explanation:	Visual exploration may be performed with or without optical instrumentation. Manual exploration may be performed directly or through intervening body layers.
		Examples:	Bimanual pregnancy exam
P	Removal	Definition:	Taking out or off a device from a body part, region or orifice
		Explanation:	If a device is taken out and a similar device put in without cutting or puncturing the skin or mucous membrane, the procedure is coded to the root operation CHANGE. Otherwise, the procedure for taking out a device is coded to the root operation REMOVAL.
		Examples:	Removal of fetal monitoring electrode

Continued on next page

1   Obstetrics

Continued from previous page

ICD-1Ø-PCS Value			Definition
Q	Repair	Definition:	Restoring, to the extent possible, a body part to its normal anatomic structure and function
		Explanation:	Used only when the method to accomplish the repair is not one of the other root operations
		Examples:	In utero repair of congenital diaphragmatic hernia
S	Reposition	Definition:	Moving to its normal location, or other suitable location, all or a portion of a body part
		Explanation:	The body part is moved to a new location from an abnormal location, or from a normal location where it is not functioning correctly. The body part may or may not be cut out or off to be moved to the new location.
		Examples:	External version of fetus
T	Resection	Definition:	Cutting out or off, without replacement, all of a body part
		Explanation:	None
		Examples:	Total excision of tubal pregnancy
Y	Transplantation	Definition:	Putting in or on all or a portion of a living body part taken from another individual or animal to physically take the place and/or function of all or a portion of a similar body part
		Explanation:	The native body part may or may not be taken out, and the transplanted body part may take over all or a portion of its function
		Examples:	In utero fetal kidney transplant

2   Placement

ICD-1Ø-PCS Value			Definition
Ø	Change	Definition:	Taking out or off a device from a body part and putting back an identical or similar device in or on the same body part without cutting or puncturing the skin or a mucous membrane
		Examples:	Change of vaginal packing
1	Compression	Definition:	Putting pressure on a body region
		Examples:	Placement of pressure dressing on abdominal wall
2	Dressing	Definition:	Putting material on a body region for protection
		Examples:	Application of sterile dressing to head wound
3	Immobilization	Definition:	Limiting or preventing motion of a body region
		Examples:	Placement of splint on left finger
4	Packing	Definition:	Putting material in a body region or orifice
		Examples:	Placement of nasal packing
5	Removal	Definition:	Taking out or off a device from a body part
		Examples:	Removal of stereotactic head frame
6	Traction	Definition:	Exerting a pulling force on a body region in a distal direction
		Examples:	Lumbar traction using motorized split-traction table

3   Administration

ICD-1Ø-PCS Value			Definition
Ø	Introduction	Definition:	Putting in or on a therapeutic, diagnostic, nutritional, physiological, or prophylactic substance except blood or blood products
		Examples:	Nerve block injection to median nerve
1	Irrigation	Definition:	Putting in or on a cleansing substance
		Examples:	Flushing of eye
2	Transfusion	Definition:	Putting in blood or blood products
		Examples:	Transfusion of cell saver red cells into central venous line

4   Measurement and Monitoring

ICD-1Ø-PCS Value			Definition
Ø	Measurement	Definition:	Determining the level of a physiological or physical function at a point in time
		Examples:	External electrocardiogram(EKG), single reading
1	Monitoring	Definition:	Determining the level of a physiological or physical function repetitively over a period of time
		Examples:	Urinary pressure monitoring

5   Extracorporeal or Systemic Assistance and Performance

ICD-1Ø-PCS Value		Definition	
Ø	Assistance	Definition:	Taking over a portion of a physiological function by extracorporeal means
		Examples:	Hyperbaric oxygenation of wound
1	Performance	Definition:	Completely taking over a physiological function by extracorporeal means
		Examples:	Cardiopulmonary bypass in conjunction with CABG
2	Restoration	Definition:	Returning, or attempting to return, a physiological function to its original state by extracorporeal means
		Examples:	Attempted cardiac defibrillation, unsuccessful

6   Extracorporeal or Systemic Therapies

ICD-10-PCS Value		Definition	
Ø	Atmospheric Control	Definition:	Extracorporeal control of atmospheric pressure and composition
		Examples:	Antigen-free air conditioning, series treatment
1	Decompression	Definition:	Extracorporeal elimination of undissolved gas from body fluids
		Examples:	Hyperbaric decompression treatment, single
2	Electromagnetic Therapy	Definition:	Extracorporeal treatment by electromagnetic rays
		Examples:	TMS (transcranial magnetic stimulation), series treatment
3	Hyperthermia	Definition:	Extracorporeal raising of body temperature
		Examples:	None
4	Hypothermia	Definition:	Extracorporeal lowering of body temperature
		Examples:	Whole body hypothermia treatment for temperature imbalances, series
5	Pheresis	Definition:	Extracorporeal separation of blood products
		Examples:	Therapeutic leukopheresis, single treatment
6	Phototherapy	Definition:	Extracorporeal treatment by light rays
		Examples:	Phototherapy of circulatory system, series treatment
7	Ultrasound Therapy	Definition:	Extracorporeal treatment by ultrasound
		Examples:	Therapeutic ultrasound of peripheral vessels, single treatment
8	Ultraviolet Light Therapy	Definition:	Extracorporeal treatment by ultraviolet light
		Examples:	Ultraviolet light phototherapy, series treatment
9	Shock Wave Therapy	Definition:	Extracorporeal treatment by shock waves
		Examples:	Shockwave therapy of plantar fascia, single treatment
B	Perfusion	Definition:	Extracorporeal treatment by diffusion of therapeutic fluid
		Examples:	Perfusion of donor liver while preparing transplant patient

7   Osteopathic

ICD-10-PCS Value		Definition	
Ø	Treatment	Definition:	Manual treatment to eliminate or alleviate somatic dysfunction and related disorders
		Examples:	Fascial release of abdomen, osteopathic treatment

8   Other Procedures

ICD-10-PCS Value		Definition	
Ø	Other Procedures	Definition:	Methodologies which attempt to remediate or cure a disorder or disease
		Examples:	Acupuncture, yoga therapy

9   Chiropractic

ICD-10-PCS Value		Definition	
B	Manipulation	Definition:	Manual procedure that involves a directed thrust to move a joint past the physiological range of motion, without exceeding the anatomical limit
		Examples:	Chiropractic treatment of cervical spine, short lever specific contact

Appendix C: Comparison of Medical and Surgical Root Operations

Note: the character associated with each operation appears in parentheses after its title.

Procedures That Take Out Some or All of a Body Part

Root Operation	Objective of Procedure	Site of Procedure	Example
Destruction (5)	Eradicating without taking out or replacement	Some/all of a body part	Fulguration of endometrium
Detachment (6)	Cutting out/off without replacement	Extremity only, any level	Amputation above elbow
Excision (B)	Cutting out/off without replacement	Some of a body part	Breast lumpectomy
Extraction (D)	Pulling out or off without replacement	Some/all of a body part	Suction D&C
Resection (T)	Cutting out/off without replacement	All of a body part	Total mastectomy

Procedures That Put in/Put Back or Move Some/All of a Body Part

Root Operation	Objective of Procedure	Site of Procedure	Example
Reattachment (M)	Putting back a detached body part	Some/all of a body part	Reattach finger
Reposition (S)	Moving a body part to normal or other suitable location	Some/all of a body part	Move undescended testicle
Transfer (X)	Moving a body part to function for a similar body part	Some/all of a body part	Skin pedicle transfer flap
Transplantation (Y)	Putting in a living body part from a person/animal	Some/all of a body part	Kidney transplant

Procedures That Take Out or Eliminate Solid Matter, Fluids, or Gases From a Body Part

Root Operation	Objective of Procedure	Site of Procedure	Example
Drainage (9)	Taking or letting out	Fluids and/or gases from a body part	Incision and drainage
Extirpation (C)	Taking or cutting out	Solid matter in a body part	Thrombectomy
Fragmentation (F)	Breaking into pieces	Solid matter within a body part	Lithotripsy

Procedures That Involve Only Examination of Body Parts and Regions

Root Operation	Objective of Procedure	Site of Procedure	Example
Inspection (J)	Visual/manual exploration	Some/all of a body part	Diagnostic cystoscopy Exploratory laparoscopy
Map (K)	Locating electrical impulse route/functional areas	Brain/cardiac conduction mechanism	Cardiac mapping

Procedures That Alter the Diameter/Route of a Tubular Body Part

Root Operation	Objective of Procedure	Site of Procedure	Example
Bypass (1)	Altering route of passage of contents	Tubular body part	Coronary artery bypass graft (CABG)
Dilation (7)	Expanding natural or artificially created orifice/lumen	Tubular body part	Percutaneous transluminal coronary angioplasty (PTCA)
Occlusion (L)	Completely closing natural or artificially created orifice/lumen	Tubular body part	Fallopian tube ligation
Restriction (V)	Partially closing natural or artificially created orifice/lumen	Tubular body part	Gastroesophageal fundoplication

Procedures That Always Involve Devices

Root Operation		Objective of Procedure	Site of Procedure	Example
Change (2)	DVC	Exchanging device w/out cutting/puncturing	In/on a body part	Gastrostomy tube change
Insertion (H)	DVC	Putting in nonbiological device	In/on a body part	Central line insertion
Removal (P)	DVC	Taking out device	In/on a body part	Central line removal
Replacement (R)	DVC	Putting in device that replaces a body part	Some/all of a body part	Total hip replacement
Revision (W)	DVC	Correcting a malfunctioning/displaced device	In/on a body part	Revision of pacemaker
Supplement (U)	DVC	Putting in device that reinforces or augments a body part	In/on a body part	Abdominal wall herniorrhaphy using mesh

DVC = Device involved in root operation

Procedures Involving Cutting or Separation Only

Root Operation	Objective of Procedure	Site of Procedure	Example
Division (8)	Cutting into/separating	A body part	Neurotomy
Release (N)	Freeing a body part from constraint	Around a body part	Adhesiolysis

Procedures That Define Other Repairs

Root Operation	Objective of Procedure	Site of Procedure	Example
Control (3)	Stopping/attempting to stop postprocedural or other acute bleeding	Anatomical region or nasal mucosa/soft tissue	Post-prostatectomy bleeding control, control subdural hemorrhage, bleeding ulcer, retroperitoneal hemorrhage
Repair (Q)	Restoring body part to its normal structure/function	Some/all of a body part	Suture laceration

Procedures That Define Other Objectives

Root Operation	Objective of Procedure	Site of Procedure	Example
Alteration (Ø)	Modifying body part for cosmetic purposes without affecting function	Some/all of a body part	Face lift
Creation (4)	Using biological or synthetic material to form a new body part that replicates the anatomic structure or function of a missing body part	Perineum, valve	Sex change/artificial vagina/penis, atrioventricular valve creation
Fusion (G)	Unification or immobilization	Joint or articular body part	Spinal fusion

Appendix D: Body Part Key

Term	ICD-10-PCS Value
Abdominal aortic plexus	Abdominal Sympathetic Nerve
Abdominal esophagus	Esophagus, Lower
Abductor hallucis muscle	Foot Muscle, Right
	Foot Muscle, Left
Accessory cephalic vein	Cephalic Vein, Right
	Cephalic Vein, Left
Accessory obturator nerve	Lumbar Plexus
Accessory phrenic nerve	Phrenic nerve
Accessory spleen	Spleen
Acetabulofemoral joint	Hip Joint, Right
	Hip Joint, Left
Achilles tendon	Lower Leg Tendon, Right
	Lower Leg Tendon, Left
Acromioclavicular ligament	Shoulder Bursa and Ligament, Right
	Shoulder Bursa and Ligament, Left
Acromion (process)	Scapula, Right
	Scapula, Left
Adductor brevis muscle	Upper Leg Muscle, Right
	Upper Leg Muscle, Left
Adductor hallucis muscle	Foot Muscle, Right
	Foot Muscle, Left
Adductor longus muscle	Upper Leg Muscle, Right
	Upper Leg Muscle, Left
Adductor magnus muscle	Upper Leg Muscle, Right
	Upper Leg Muscle, Left
Adenohypophysis	Pituitary Gland
Alar ligament of axis	Head and Neck Bursa and Ligament
Alveolar process of mandible	Mandible, Right
	Mandible, Left
Alveolar process of maxilla	Maxilla
Anal orifice	Anus
Anatomical snuffbox	Lower Arm and Wrist Muscle, Right
	Lower Arm and Wrist Muscle, Left
Angular artery	Face Artery
Angular vein	Face Vein, Right
	Face Vein, Left
Annular ligament	Elbow Bursa and Ligament, Right
	Elbow Bursa and Ligament, Left
Anorectal junction	Rectum
Ansa cervicalis	Cervical Plexus
Antebrachial fascia	Subcutaneous Tissue and Fascia, Right Lower Arm
	Subcutaneous Tissue and Fascia, Left Lower Arm
Anterior (pectoral) lymph node	Lymphatic, Right Axillary
	Lymphatic, Left Axillary
Anterior cerebral artery	Intracranial Artery
Anterior cerebral vein	Intracranial Vein
Anterior choroidal artery	Intracranial Artery
Anterior circumflex humeral artery	Axillary Artery, Right
	Axillary Artery, Left
Anterior communicating artery	Intracranial Artery
Anterior cruciate ligament (ACL)	Knee Bursa and Ligament, Right
	Knee Bursa and Ligament, Left

Term	ICD-10-PCS Value
Anterior crural nerve	Femoral Nerve
Anterior facial vein	Face Vein, Right
	Face Vein, Left
Anterior intercostal artery	Internal Mammary Artery, Right
	Internal Mammary Artery, Left
Anterior interosseous nerve	Median Nerve
Anterior lateral malleolar artery	Anterior Tibial Artery, Right
	Anterior Tibial Artery, Left
Anterior lingual gland	Minor Salivary Gland
Anterior medial malleolar artery	Anterior Tibial Artery, Right
	Anterior Tibial Artery, Left
Anterior spinal artery	Vertebral Artery, Right
	Vertebral Artery, Left
Anterior tibial recurrent artery	Anterior Tibial Artery, Right
	Anterior Tibial Artery, Left
Anterior ulnar recurrent artery	Ulnar Artery, Right
	Ulnar Artery, Left
Anterior vagal trunk	Vagus Nerve
Anterior vertebral muscle	Neck Muscle, Right
	Neck Muscle, Left
Antihelix	External Ear, Right
	External Ear, Left
	External Ear, Bilateral
Antitragus	External Ear, Right
	External Ear, Left
	External Ear, Bilateral
Antrum of Highmore	Maxillary Sinus, Right
	Maxillary Sinus, Left
Aortic annulus	Aortic Valve
Aortic arch	Thoracic Aorta, Ascending/Arch
Aortic intercostal artery	Upper Artery
Apical (subclavicular) lymph node	Lymphatic, Right Axillary
	Lymphatic, Left Axillary
Apneustic center	Pons
Aqueduct of Sylvius	Cerebral Ventricle
Aqueous humour	Anterior Chamber, Right
	Anterior Chamber, Left
Arachnoid mater, intracranial	Cerebral Meninges
Arachnoid mater, spinal	Spinal Meninges
Arcuate artery	Foot Artery, Right
	Foot Artery, Left
Areola	Nipple, Right
	Nipple, Left
Arterial canal (duct)	Pulmonary Artery, Left
Aryepiglottic fold	Larynx
Arytenoid cartilage	Larynx
Arytenoid muscle	Neck Muscle, Right
	Neck Muscle, Left
Ascending aorta	Thoracic Aorta, Ascending/Arch
Ascending palatine artery	Face Artery
Ascending pharyngeal artery	External Carotid Artery, Right
	External Carotid Artery, Left
Atlantoaxial joint	Cervical Vertebral Joint

Appendix D: Body Part Key

Term	ICD-10-PCS Value
Atrioventricular node	Conduction Mechanism
Atrium dextrum cordis	Atrium, Right
Atrium pulmonale	Atrium, Left
Auditory tube	Eustachian Tube, Right
	Eustachian Tube, Left
Auerbach's (myenteric)plexus	Abdominal Sympathetic Nerve
Auricle	External Ear, Right
	External Ear, Left
	External Ear, Bilateral
Auricularis muscle	Head Muscle
Axillary fascia	Subcutaneous Tissue and Fascia, Right Upper Arm
	Subcutaneous Tissue and Fascia, Left Upper Arm
Axillary nerve	Brachial Plexus
Bartholin's (greater vestibular) gland	Vestibular Gland
Basal (internal) cerebral vein	Intracranial Vein
Basal nuclei	Basal Ganglia
Base of tongue	Pharynx
Basilar artery	Intracranial Artery
Basis pontis	Pons
Biceps brachii muscle	Upper Arm Muscle, Right
	Upper Arm Muscle, Left
Biceps femoris muscle	Upper Leg Muscle, Right
	Upper Leg Muscle, Left
Bicipital aponeurosis	Subcutaneous Tissue and Fascia, Right Lower Arm
	Subcutaneous Tissue and Fascia, Left Lower Arm
Bicuspid valve	Mitral Valve
Body of femur	Femoral Shaft, Right
	Femoral Shaft, Left
Body of fibula	Fibula, Right
	Fibula, Left
Bony labyrinth	Inner Ear, Right
	Inner Ear, Left
Bony orbit	Orbit, Right
	Orbit, Left
Bony vestibule	Inner Ear, Right
	Inner Ear, Left
Botallo's duct	Pulmonary Artery, Left
Brachial (lateral) lymph node	Lymphatic, Right Axillary
	Lymphatic, Left Axillary
Brachialis muscle	Upper Arm Muscle, Right
	Upper Arm Muscle, Left
Brachiocephalic artery	Innominate Artery
Brachiocephalic trunk	Innominate Artery
Brachiocephalic vein	Innominate Vein, Right
	Innominate Vein, Left
Brachioradialis muscle	Lower Arm and Wrist Muscle, Right
	Lower Arm and Wrist Muscle, Left
Breast procedures, skin only	Skin, Chest
Broad ligament	Uterine Supporting Structure
Bronchial artery	Upper Artery
Bronchus intermedius	Main Bronchus, Right
Buccal gland	Buccal Mucosa

Term	ICD-10-PCS Value
Buccinator lymph node	Lymphatic, Head
Buccinator muscle	Facial Muscle
Bulbospongiosus muscle	Perineum Muscle
Bulbourethral (Cowper's) gland	Urethra
Bundle of His	Conduction Mechanism
Bundle of Kent	Conduction Mechanism
Calcaneocuboid joint	Tarsal Joint, Right
	Tarsal Joint, Left
Calcaneocuboid ligament	Foot Bursa and Ligament, Right
	Foot Bursa and Ligament, Left
Calcaneofibular ligament	Ankle Bursa and Ligament, Right
	Ankle Bursa and Ligament, Left
Calcaneus	Tarsal, Right
	Tarsal, Left
Capitate bone	Carpal, Right
	Carpal, Left
Cardia	Esophagogastric Junction
Cardiac plexus	Thoracic Sympathetic Nerve
Cardioesophageal junction	Esophagogastric Junction
Caroticotympanic artery	Internal Carotid Artery, Right
	Internal Carotid Artery, Left
Carotid glomus	Carotid Body, Right
	Carotid Body, Left
	Carotid Bodies, Bilateral
Carotid sinus	Internal Carotid Artery, Right
	Internal Carotid Artery, Left
Carotid sinus nerve	Glossopharyngeal Nerve
Carpometacarpal ligament	Hand Bursa and Ligament, Right
	Hand Bursa and Ligament, Left
Cauda equina	Lumbar Spinal Cord
Cavernous plexus	Head and Neck Sympathetic Nerve
Celiac ganglion	Abdominal Sympathetic Nerve
Celiac (solar) plexus	Abdominal Sympathetic Nerve
Celiac lymph node	Lymphatic, Aortic
Celiac trunk	Celiac Artery
Central axillary lymph node	Lymphatic, Right Axillary
	Lymphatic, Left Axillary
Cerebral aqueduct (Sylvius)	Cerebral Ventricle
Cerebrum	Brain
Cervical esophagus	Esophagus, Upper
Cervical facet joint	Cervical Vertebral Joint
	Cervical Vertebral Joints, 2 or more
Cervical ganglion	Head and Neck Sympathetic Nerve
Cervical interspinous ligament	Head and Neck Bursa and Ligament
Cervical intertransverse ligament	Head and Neck Bursa and Ligament
Cervical ligamentum flavum	Head and Neck Bursa and Ligament
Cervical lymph node	Lymphatic, Right Neck
	Lymphatic, Left Neck
Cervicothoracic facet joint	Cervicothoracic Vertebral Joint
Choana	Nasopharynx
Chondroglossus muscle	Tongue, Palate, Pharynx Muscle
Chorda tympani	Facial Nerve
Choroid plexus	Cerebral Ventricle
Ciliary body	Eye, Right
	Eye, Left

Term	ICD-10-PCS Value
Ciliary ganglion	Head and Neck Sympathetic Nerve
Circle of Willis	Intracranial Artery
Circumflex illiac artery	Femoral Artery, Right
	Femoral Artery, Left
Claustrum	Basal Ganglia
Coccygeal body	Coccygeal Glomus
Coccygeus muscle	Trunk Muscle, Right
	Trunk Muscle, Left
Cochlea	Inner Ear, Right
	Inner Ear, Left
Cochlear nerve	Acoustic Nerve
Columella	Nasal Mucosa and Soft Tissue
Common digital vein	Foot Vein, Right
	Foot Vein, Left
Common facial vein	Face Vein, Right
	Face Vein, Left
Common fibular nerve	Peroneal Nerve
Common hepatic artery	Hepatic Artery
Common iliac (subaortic) lymph node	Lymphatic, Pelvis
Common interosseous artery	Ulnar Artery, Right
	Ulnar Artery, Left
Common peroneal nerve	Peroneal Nerve
Condyloid process	Mandible, Right
	Mandible, Left
Conus arteriosus	Ventricle, Right
Conus medullaris	Lumbar Spinal Cord
Coracoacromial ligament	Shoulder Bursa and Ligament, Right
	Shoulder Bursa and Ligament, Left
Coracobrachialis muscle	Upper Arm Muscle, Right
	Upper Arm Muscle, Left
Coracoclavicular ligament	Shoulder Bursa and Ligament, Right
	Shoulder Bursa and Ligament, Left
Coracohumeral ligament	Shoulder Bursa and Ligament, Right
	Shoulder Bursa and Ligament, Left
Coracoid process	Scapula, Right
	Scapula, Left
Corniculate cartilage	Larynx
Corpus callosum	Brain
Corpus cavernosum	Penis
Corpus spongiosum	Penis
Corpus striatum	Basal Ganglia
Corrugator supercilii muscle	Facial Muscle
Costocervical trunk	Subclavian Artery, Right
	Subclavian Artery, Left
Costoclavicular ligament	Shoulder Bursa and Ligament, Right
	Shoulder Bursa and Ligament, Left
Costotransverse joint	Thoracic Vertebral Joint
Costotransverse ligament	Rib(s) Bursa and Ligament
Costovertebral joint	Thoracic Vertebral Joint
Costoxiphoid ligament	Sternum Bursa and Ligament
Cowper's (bulbourethral) gland	Urethra
Cremaster muscle	Perineum Muscle
Cribriform plate	Ethmoid Bone, Right
	Ethmoid Bone, Left
Cricoid cartilage	Trachea

Term	ICD-10-PCS Value
Cricothyroid artery	Thyroid Artery, Right
	Thyroid Artery, Left
Cricothyroid muscle	Neck Muscle, Right
	Neck Muscle, Left
Crural fascia	Subcutaneous Tissue and Fascia, Right Upper Leg
	Subcutaneous Tissue and Fascia, Left Upper Leg
Cubital lymph node	Lymphatic, Right Upper Extremity
	Lymphatic, Left Upper Extremity
Cubital nerve	Ulnar Nerve
Cuboid bone	Tarsal, Right
	Tarsal, Left
Cuboideonavicular joint	Tarsal Joint, Right
	Tarsal Joint, Left
Culmen	Cerebellum
Cuneiform cartilage	Larynx
Cuneonavicular joint	Tarsal Joint, Right
	Tarsal Joint, Left
Cuneonavicular ligament	Foot Bursa and Ligament, Right
	Foot Bursa and Ligament, Left
Cutaneous (transverse) cervical nerve	Cervical Plexus
Deep cervical fascia	Subcutaneous Tissue and Fascia, Right Neck
	Subcutaneous Tissue and Fascia, Left Neck
Deep cervical vein	Vertebral Vein, Right
	Vertebral Vein, Left
Deep circumflex iliac artery	External Iliac Artery, Right
	External Iliac Artery, Left
Deep facial vein	Face Vein, Right
	Face Vein, Left
Deep femoral artery	Femoral Artery, Right
	Femoral Artery, Left
Deep femoral (profunda femoris) vein	Femoral Vein, Right
	Femoral Vein, Left
Deep palmar arch	Hand Artery, Right
	Hand Artery, Left
Deep transverse perineal muscle	Perineum Muscle
Deferential artery	Internal Iliac Artery, Right
	Internal Iliac Artery, Left
Deltoid fascia	Subcutaneous Tissue and Fascia, Right Upper Arm
	Subcutaneous Tissue and Fascia, Left Upper Arm
Deltoid ligament	Ankle Bursa and Ligament, Right
	Ankle Bursa and Ligament, Left
Deltoid muscle	Shoulder Muscle, Right
	Shoulder Muscle, Left
Deltopectoral (infraclavicular) lymph node	Lymphatic, Right Upper Extremity
	Lymphatic, Left Upper Extremity
Dens	Cervical Vertebra
Denticulate (dentate) ligament	Spinal Meninges
Depressor anguli oris muscle	Facial Muscle
Depressor labii inferioris muscle	Facial Muscle

Term	ICD-10-PCS Value
Depressor septi nasi muscle	Facial Muscle
Depressor supercilii muscle	Facial Muscle
Dermis	Skin
Descending genicular artery	Femoral Artery, Right
	Femoral Artery, Left
Diaphragma sellae	Dura Mater
Distal humerus	Humeral Shaft, Right
	Humeral Shaft, Left
Distal humerus, involving joint	Elbow Joint, Right
	Elbow Joint, Left
Distal radioulnar joint	Wrist Joint, Right
	Wrist Joint, Left
Dorsal digital nerve	Radial Nerve
Dorsal metacarpal vein	Hand Vein, Right
	Hand Vein, Left
Dorsal metatarsal artery	Foot Artery, Right
	Foot Artery, Left
Dorsal metatarsal vein	Foot Vein, Right
	Foot Vein, Left
Dorsal root ganglion	Cervical Spinal Cord
	Lumbar Spinal Cord
	Spinal Cord
	Thoracic Spinal Cord
Dorsal scapular artery	Subclavian Artery, Right
	Subclavian Artery, Left
Dorsal scapular nerve	Brachial Plexus
Dorsal venous arch	Foot Vein, Right
	Foot Vein, Left
Dorsalis pedis artery	Anterior Tibial Artery, Right
	Anterior Tibial Artery, Left
Duct of Santorini	Pancreatic Duct, Accessory
Duct of Wirsung	Pancreatic Duct
Ductus deferens	Vas Deferens, Right
	Vas Deferens, Left
	Vas Deferens, Bilateral
	Vas Deferens
Duodenal ampulla	Ampulla of Vater
Duodenojejunal flexure	Jejunum
Dura mater, intracranial	Dura Mater
Dura mater, spinal	Spinal Meninges
Dural venous sinus	Intracranial Vein
Earlobe	External Ear, Right
	External Ear, Left
	External Ear, Bilateral
Eighth cranial nerve	Acoustic Nerve
Ejaculatory duct	Vas Deferens, Right
	Vas Deferens, Left
	Vas Deferens, Bilateral
	Vas Deferens
Eleventh cranial nerve	Accessory Nerve
Encephalon	Brain
Ependyma	Cerebral Ventricle
Epidermis	Skin
Epidural space, spinal	Spinal Canal
Epiploic foramen	Peritoneum
Epithalamus	Thalamus

Term	ICD-10-PCS Value
Epitroclear lymph node	Lymphatic, Right Upper Extremity
	Lymphatic, Left Upper Extremity
Erector spinae muscle	Trunk Muscle, Right
	Trunk Muscle, Left
Esophageal artery	Upper Artery
Esophageal plexus	Thoracic Sympathetic Nerve
Ethmoidal air cell	Ethmoid Sinus, Right
	Ethmoid Sinus, Left
Extensor carpi radialis muscle	Lower Arm and Wrist Muscle, Right
	Lower Arm and Wrist Muscle, Left
Extensor carpi ulnaris muscle	Lower Arm and Wrist Muscle, Right
	Lower Arm and Wrist Muscle, Left
Extensor digitorum brevis muscle	Foot Muscle, Right
	Foot Muscle, Left
Extensor digitorum longus muscle	Lower Leg Muscle, Right
	Lower Leg Muscle, Left
Extensor hallucis brevis muscle	Foot Muscle, Right
	Foot Muscle, Left
Extensor hallucis longus muscle	Lower Leg Muscle, Right
	Lower Leg Muscle, Left
External anal sphincter	Anal Sphincter
External auditory meatus	External Auditory Canal, Right
	External Auditory Canal, Left
External maxillary artery	Face Artery
External naris	Nasal Mucosa and Soft Tissue
External oblique aponeurosis	Subcutaneous Tissue and Fascia, Trunk
External oblique muscle	Abdomen Muscle, Right
	Abdomen Muscle, Left
External popliteal nerve	Peroneal Nerve
External pudendal artery	Femoral Artery, Right
	Femoral Artery, Left
External pudenal vein	Saphenous Vein, Right
	Saphenous Vein, Left
External urethral sphincter	Urethra
Extradural space, intracranial	Epidural Space, Intracranial
Extradural space, spinal	Spinal Canal
Facial artery	Face Artery
False vocal cord	Larynx
Falx cerebri	Dura Mater
Fascia lata	Subcutaneous Tissue and Fascia, Right Upper Leg
	Subcutaneous Tissue and Fascia, Left Upper Leg
Femoral head	Upper Femur, Right
	Upper Femur, Left
Femoral lymph node	Lymphatic, Right Lower Extremity
	Lymphatic, Left Lower Extremity
Femoropatellar joint	Knee Joint, Right
	Knee Joint, Left
	Knee Joint, Femoral Surface, Right
	Knee Joint, Femoral Surface, Left
Femorotibial joint	Knee Joint, Right
	Knee Joint, Left
	Knee Joint, Tibial Surface, Right
	Knee Joint, Tibial Surface, Left
Fibular artery	Peroneal Artery, Right
	Peroneal Artery, Left

Term	ICD-10-PCS Value
Fibular sesamoid	Metatarsal, Right
	Metatarsal, Left
Fibularis brevis muscle	Lower Leg Muscle, Right
	Lower Leg Muscle, Left
Fibularis longus muscle	Lower Leg Muscle, Right
	Lower Leg Muscle, Left
Fifth cranial nerve	Trigeminal Nerve
Filum terminale	Spinal Meninges
First cranial nerve	Olfactory Nerve
First intercostal nerve	Brachial Plexus
Flexor carpi radialis muscle	Lower Arm and Wrist Muscle, Right
	Lower Arm and Wrist Muscle, Left
Flexor carpi ulnaris muscle	Lower Arm and Wrist Muscle, Right
	Lower Arm and Wrist Muscle, Left
Flexor digitorum brevis muscle	Foot Muscle, Right
	Foot Muscle, Left
Flexor digitorum longus muscle	Lower Leg Muscle, Right
	Lower Leg Muscle, Left
Flexor hallucis brevis muscle	Foot Muscle, Right
	Foot Muscle, Left
Flexor hallucis longus muscle	Lower Leg Muscle, Right
	Lower Leg Muscle, Left
Flexor pollicis longus muscle	Lower Arm and Wrist Muscle, Right
	Lower Arm and Wrist Muscle, Left
Foramen magnum	Occipital Bone
Foramen of Monro (intraventricular)	Cerebral Ventricle
Foreskin	Prepuce
Fossa of Rosenmuller	Nasopharynx
Fourth cranial nerve	Trochlear Nerve
Fourth ventricle	Cerebral Ventricle
Fovea	Retina, Right
	Retina, Left
Frenulum labii inferioris	Lower Lip
Frenulum labii superioris	Upper Lip
Frenulum linguae	Tongue
Frontal lobe	Cerebral Hemisphere
Frontal vein	Face Vein, Right
	Face Vein, Left
Fundus uteri	Uterus
Galea aponeurotica	Subcutaneous Tissue and Fascia, Scalp
Ganglion impar (ganglion of Walther)	Sacral Sympathetic Nerve
Gasserian ganglion	Trigeminal Nerve
Gastric lymph node	Lymphatic, Aortic
Gastric plexus	Abdominal Sympathetic Nerve
Gastrocnemius muscle	Lower Leg Muscle, Right
	Lower Leg Muscle, Left
Gastrocolic ligament	Omentum
Gastrocolic omentum	Omentum
Gastroduodenal artery	Hepatic Artery
Gastroesophageal (GE) junction	Esophagogastric Junction
Gastrohepatic omentum	Omentum
Gastrophrenic ligament	Omentum
Gastrosplenic ligament	Omentum
Gemellus muscle	Hip Muscle, Right
	Hip Muscle, Left
Geniculate ganglion	Facial Nerve

Term	ICD-10-PCS Value
Geniculate nucleus	Thalamus
Genioglossus muscle	Tongue, Palate, Pharynx Muscle
Genitofemoral nerve	Lumbar Plexus
Glans penis	Prepuce
Glenohumeral joint	Shoulder Joint, Right
	Shoulder Joint, Left
Glenohumeral ligament	Shoulder Bursa and Ligament, Right
	Shoulder Bursa and Ligament, Left
Glenoid fossa (of scapula)	Glenoid Cavity, Right
	Glenoid Cavity, Left
Glenoid ligament (labrum)	Shoulder Joint, Right
	Shoulder Joint, Left
Globus pallidus	Basal Ganglia
Glossoepiglottic fold	Epiglottis
Glottis	Larynx
Gluteal lymph node	Lymphatic, Pelvis
Gluteal vein	Hypogastric Vein, Right
	Hypogastric Vein, Left
Gluteus maximus muscle	Hip Muscle, Right
	Hip Muscle, Left
Gluteus medius muscle	Hip Muscle, Right
	Hip Muscle, Left
Gluteus minimus muscle	Hip Muscle, Right
	Hip Muscle, Left
Gracilis muscle	Upper Leg Muscle, Right
	Upper Leg Muscle, Left
Great auricular nerve	Cervical Plexus
Great cerebral vein	Intracranial Vein
Great(er) saphenous vein	Saphenous Vein, Right
	Saphenous Vein, Left
Greater alar cartilage	Nasal Mucosa and Soft Tissue
Greater occipital nerve	Cervical Nerve
Greater omentum	Omentum
Greater splanchnic nerve	Thoracic Sympathetic Nerve
Greater superficial petrosal nerve	Facial Nerve
Greater trochanter	Upper Femur, Right
	Upper Femur, Left
Greater tuberosity	Humeral Head, Right
	Humeral Head, Left
Greater vestibular (Bartholin's) gland	Vestibular Gland
Greater wing	Sphenoid Bone
Hallux	1st Toe, Right
	1st Toe, Left
Hamate bone	Carpal, Right
	Carpal, Left
Head of fibula	Fibula, Right
	Fibula, Left
Helix	External Ear, Right
	External Ear, Left
	External Ear, Bilateral
Hepatic artery proper	Hepatic Artery
Hepatic flexure	Transverse Colon
Hepatic lymph node	Lymphatic, Aortic
Hepatic plexus	Abdominal Sympathetic Nerve
Hepatic portal vein	Portal Vein
Hepatogastric ligament	Omentum

Term	ICD-10-PCS Value
Hepatopancreatic ampulla	Ampulla of Vater
Humeroradial joint	Elbow Joint, Right
	Elbow Joint, Left
Humeroulnar joint	Elbow Joint, Right
	Elbow Joint, Left
Humerus, distal	Humeral Shaft, Right
	Humeral Shaft, Left
Hyoglossus muscle	Tongue, Palate, Pharynx Muscle
Hyoid artery	Thyroid Artery, Right
	Thyroid Artery, Left
Hypogastric artery	Internal Iliac Artery, Right
	Internal Iliac Artery, Left
Hypopharynx	Pharynx
Hypophysis	Pituitary Gland
Hypothenar muscle	Hand Muscle, Right
	Hand Muscle, Left
Ileal artery	Superior Mesenteric Artery
Ileocolic artery	Superior Mesenteric Artery
Ileocolic vein	Colic Vein
Iliac crest	Pelvic Bone, Right
	Pelvic Bone, Left
Iliac fascia	Subcutaneous Tissue and Fascia, Right Upper Leg
	Subcutaneous Tissue and Fascia, Left Upper Leg
Iliac lymph node	Lymphatic, Pelvis
Iliacus muscle	Hip Muscle, Right
	Hip Muscle, Left
Iliofemoral ligament	Hip Bursa and Ligament, Right
	Hip Bursa and Ligament, Left
Iliohypogastric nerve	Lumbar Plexus
Ilioinguinal nerve	Lumbar Plexus
Iliolumbar artery	Internal Iliac Artery, Right
	Internal Iliac Artery, Left
Iliolumbar ligament	Lower Spine Bursa and Ligament
Iliotibial tract (band)	Subcutaneous Tissue and Fascia, Right Upper Leg
	Subcutaneous Tissue and Fascia, Left Upper Leg
Ilium	Pelvic Bone, Right
	Pelvic Bone, Left
Incus	Auditory Ossicle, Right
	Auditory Ossicle, Left
Inferior cardiac nerve	Thoracic Sympathetic Nerve
Inferior cerebellar vein	Intracranial Vein
Inferior cerebral vein	Intracranial Vein
Inferior epigastric artery	External Iliac Artery, Right
	External Iliac Artery, Left
Inferior epigastric lymph node	Lymphatic, Pelvis
Inferior genicular artery	Popliteal Artery, Right
	Popliteal Artery, Left
Inferior gluteal artery	Internal Iliac Artery, Right
	Internal Iliac Artery, Left
Inferior gluteal nerve	Sacral Plexus
Inferior hypogastric plexus	Abdominal Sympathetic Nerve
Inferior labial artery	Face Artery
Inferior longitudinal muscle	Tongue, Palate, Pharynx Muscle

Term	ICD-10-PCS Value
Inferior mesenteric ganglion	Abdominal Sympathetic Nerve
Inferior mesenteric lymph node	Lymphatic, Mesenteric
Inferior mesenteric plexus	Abdominal Sympathetic Nerve
Inferior oblique muscle	Extraocular Muscle, Right
	Extraocular Muscle, Left
Inferior pancreaticoduodenal artery	Superior Mesenteric Artery
Inferior phrenic artery	Abdominal Aorta
Inferior rectus muscle	Extraocular Muscle, Right
	Extraocular Muscle, Left
Inferior suprarenal artery	Renal Artery, Right
	Renal Artery, Left
Inferior tarsal plate	Lower Eyelid, Right
	Lower Eyelid, Left
Inferior thyroid vein	Innominate Vein, Right
	Innominate Vein, Left
Inferior tibiofibular joint	Ankle Joint, Right
	Ankle Joint, Left
Inferior turbinate	Nasal Turbinate
Inferior ulnar collateral artery	Brachial Artery, Right
	Brachial Artery, Left
Inferior vesical artery	Internal Iliac Artery, Right
	Internal Iliac Artery, Left
Infraauricular lymph node	Lymphatic, Head
Infraclavicular (deltopectoral) lymph node	Lymphatic, Right Upper Extremity
	Lymphatic, Left Upper Extremity
Infrahyoid muscle	Neck Muscle, Right
	Neck Muscle, Left
Infraparotid lymph node	Lymphatic, Head
Infraspinatus fascia	Subcutaneous Tissue and Fascia, Right Upper Arm
	Subcutaneous Tissue and Fascia, Left Upper Arm
Infraspinatus muscle	Shoulder Muscle, Right
	Shoulder Muscle, Left
Infundibulopelvic ligament	Uterine Supporting Structure
Inguinal canal	Inguinal Region, Right
	Inguinal Region, Left
	Inguinal Region, Bilateral
Inguinal triangle	Inguinal Region, Right
	Inguinal Region, Left
	Inguinal Region, Bilateral
Interatrial septum	Atrial Septum
Intercarpal joint	Carpal Joint, Right
	Carpal Joint, Left
Intercarpal ligament	Hand Bursa and Ligament, Right
	Hand Bursa and Ligament, Left
Interclavicular ligament	Shoulder Bursa and Ligament, Right
	Shoulder Bursa and Ligament, Left
Intercostal lymph node	Lymphatic, Thorax
Intercostal muscle	Thorax Muscle, Right
	Thorax Muscle, Left
Intercostal nerve	Thoracic Nerve
Intercostobrachial nerve	Thoracic Nerve
Intercuneiform joint	Tarsal Joint, Right
	Tarsal Joint, Left

Term	ICD-10-PCS Value
Intercuneiform ligament	Foot Bursa and Ligament, Right
	Foot Bursa and Ligament, Left
Intermediate bronchus	Main Bronchus, Right
Intermediate cuneiform bone	Tarsal, Right
	Tarsal, Left
Internal anal sphincter	Anal Sphincter
Internal (basal) cerebral vein	Intracranial Vein
Internal carotid artery, intracranial portion	Intracranial Artery
Internal carotid plexus	Head and Neck Sympathetic Nerve
Internal iliac vein	Hypogastric Vein, Right
	Hypogastric Vein, Left
Internal maxillary artery	External Carotid Artery, Right
	External Carotid Artery, Left
Internal naris	Nasal Mucosa and Soft Tissue
Internal oblique muscle	Abdomen Muscle, Right
	Abdomen Muscle, Left
Internal pudendal artery	Internal Iliac Artery, Right
	Internal Iliac Artery, Left
Internal pudendal vein	Hypogastric Vein, Right
	Hypogastric Vein, Left
Internal thoracic artery	Internal Mammary Artery, Right
	Internal Mammary Artery, Left
	Subclavian Artery, Right
	Subclavian Artery, Left
Internal urethral sphincter	Urethra
Interphalangeal (IP) joint	Finger Phalangeal Joint, Right
	Finger Phalangeal Joint, Left
	Toe Phalangeal Joint, Right
	Toe Phalangeal Joint, Left
Interphalangeal ligament	Foot Bursa and Ligament, Right
	Foot Bursa and Ligament, Left
	Hand Bursa and Ligament, Right
	Hand Bursa and Ligament, Left
Interspinalis muscle	Trunk Muscle, Right
	Trunk Muscle, Left
Interspinous ligament, cervical	Head and Neck Bursa and Ligament
Interspinous ligament, lumbar	Lower Spine Bursa and Ligament
Interspinous ligament, thoracic	Upper Spine Bursa and Ligament
Intertransversarius muscle	Trunk Muscle, Right
	Trunk Muscle, Left
Intertransverse ligament, cervical	Head and Neck Bursa and Ligament
Intertransverse ligament, lumbar	Lower Spine Bursa and Ligament
Intertransverse ligament, thoracic	Upper Spine Bursa and Ligament
Interventricular foramen (Monro)	Cerebral Ventricle
Interventricular septum	Ventricular Septum
Intestinal lymphatic trunk	Cisterna Chyli
Ischiatic nerve	Sciatic Nerve
Ischiocavernosus muscle	Perineum Muscle
Ischiofemoral ligament	Hip Bursa and Ligament, Right
	Hip Bursa and Ligament, Left

Term	ICD-10-PCS Value
Ischium	Pelvic Bone, Right
	Pelvic Bone, Left
Jejunal artery	Superior Mesenteric Artery
Jugular body	Glomus Jugulare
Jugular lymph node	Lymphatic, Right Neck
	Lymphatic, Left Neck
Labia majora	Vulva
Labia minora	Vulva
Labial gland	Upper Lip
	Lower Lip
Lacrimal canaliculus	Lacrimal Duct, Right
	Lacrimal Duct, Left
Lacrimal punctum	Lacrimal Duct, Right
	Lacrimal Duct, Left
Lacrimal sac	Lacrimal Duct, Right
	Lacrimal Duct, Left
Laryngopharynx	Pharynx
Lateral (brachial) lymph node	Lymphatic, Right Axillary
	Lymphatic, Left Axillary
Lateral canthus	Upper Eyelid, Right
	Upper Eyelid, Left
Lateral collateral ligament (LCL)	Knee Bursa and Ligament, Right
	Knee Bursa and Ligament, Left
Lateral condyle of femur	Lower Femur, Right
	Lower Femur, Left
Lateral condyle of tibia	Tibia, Right
	Tibia, Left
Lateral cuneiform bone	Tarsal, Right
	Tarsal, Left
Lateral epicondyle of femur	Lower Femur, Right
	Lower Femur, Left
Lateral epicondyle of humerus	Humeral Shaft, Right
	Humeral Shaft, Left
Lateral femoral cutaneous nerve	Lumbar Plexus
Lateral malleolus	Fibula, Right
	Fibula, Left
Lateral meniscus	Knee Joint, Right
	Knee Joint, Left
Lateral nasal cartilage	Nasal Mucosa and Soft Tissue
Lateral plantar artery	Foot Artery, Right
	Foot Artery, Left
Lateral plantar nerve	Tibial Nerve
Lateral rectus muscle	Extraocular Muscle, Right
	Extraocular Muscle, Left
Lateral sacral artery	Internal Iliac Artery, Right
	Internal Iliac Artery, Left
Lateral sacral vein	Hypogastric Vein, Right
	Hypogastric Vein, Left
Lateral sural cutaneous nerve	Peroneal Nerve
Lateral tarsal artery	Foot Artery, Right
	Foot Artery, Left
Lateral temporo-mandibular ligament	Head and Neck Bursa and Ligament
Lateral thoracic artery	Axillary Artery, Right
	Axillary Artery, Left
Latissimus dorsi muscle	Trunk Muscle, Right
	Trunk Muscle, Left

Term	ICD-10-PCS Value
Least splanchnic nerve	Thoracic Sympathetic Nerve
Left ascending lumbar vein	Hemiazygos Vein
Left atrioventricular valve	Mitral Valve
Left auricular appendix	Atrium, Left
Left colic vein	Colic Vein
Left coronary sulcus	Heart, Left
Left gastric artery	Gastric Artery
Left gastroepiploic artery	Splenic Artery
Left gastroepiploic vein	Splenic Vein
Left inferior phrenic vein	Renal Vein, Left
Left inferior pulmonary vein	Pulmonary Vein, Left
Left jugular trunk	Thoracic Duct
Left lateral ventricle	Cerebral Ventricle
Left ovarian vein	Renal Vein, Left
Left second lumbar vein	Renal Vein, Left
Left subclavian trunk	Thoracic Duct
Left subcostal vein	Hemiazygos Vein
Left superior pulmonary vein	Pulmonary Vein, Left
Left suprarenal vein	Renal Vein, Left
Left testicular vein	Renal Vein, Left
Leptomeninges, intracranial	Cerebral Meninges
Leptomeninges, spinal	Spinal Meninges
Lesser alar cartilage	Nasal Mucosa and Soft Tissue
Lesser occipital nerve	Cervical Plexus
Lesser omentum	Omentum
Lesser saphenous vein	Saphenous Vein, Right
	Saphenous Vein, Left
Lesser splanchnic nerve	Thoracic Sympathetic Nerve
Lesser trochanter	Upper Femur, Right
	Upper Femur, Left
Lesser tuberosity	Humeral Head, Right
	Humeral Head, Left
Lesser wing	Sphenoid Bone
Levator anguli oris muscle	Facial Muscle
Levator ani muscle	Perineum Muscle
Levator labii superioris alaeque nasi muscle	Facial Muscle
Levator labii superioris muscle	Facial Muscle
Levator palpebrae superioris muscle	Upper Eyelid, Right
	Upper Eyelid, Left
Levator scapulae muscle	Neck Muscle, Right
	Neck Muscle, Left
Levator veli palatini muscle	Tongue, Palate, Pharynx Muscle
Levatores costarum muscle	Thorax Muscle, Right
	Thorax Muscle, Left
Ligament of head of fibula	Knee Bursa and Ligament, Right
	Knee Bursa and Ligament, Left
Ligament of the lateral malleolus	Ankle Bursa and Ligament, Right
	Ankle Bursa and Ligament, Left
Ligamentum flavum, cervical	Head and Neck Bursa and Ligament
Ligamentum flavum, lumbar	Lower Spine Bursa and Ligament
Ligamentum flavum, thoracic	Upper Spine Bursa and Ligament

Term	ICD-10-PCS Value
Lingual artery	External Carotid Artery, Right
	External Carotid Artery, Left
Lingual tonsil	Pharynx
Locus ceruleus	Pons
Long thoracic nerve	Brachial Plexus
Lumbar artery	Abdominal Aorta
Lumbar facet joint	Lumbar Vertebral Joint
Lumbar ganglion	Lumbar Sympathetic Nerve
Lumbar lymph node	Lymphatic, Aortic
Lumbar lymphatic trunk	Cisterna Chyli
Lumbar splanchnic nerve	Lumbar Sympathetic Nerve
Lumbosacral facet joint	Lumbosacral Joint
Lumbosacral trunk	Lumbar Nerve
Lunate bone	Carpal, Right
	Carpal, Left
Lunotriquetral ligament	Hand Bursa and Ligament, Right
	Hand Bursa and Ligament, Left
Macula	Retina, Right
	Retina, Left
Malleus	Auditory Ossicle, Right
	Auditory Ossicle, Left
Mammary duct	Breast, Right
	Breast, Left
	Breast, Bilateral
Mammary gland	Breast, Right
	Breast, Left
	Breast, Bilateral
Mammillary body	Hypothalamus
Mandibular nerve	Trigeminal Nerve
Mandibular notch	Mandible, Right
	Mandible, Left
Manubrium	Sternum
Masseter muscle	Head Muscle
Masseteric fascia	Subcutaneous Tissue and Fascia, Face
Mastoid (postauricular) lymph node	Lymphatic, Right Neck
	Lymphatic, Left Neck
Mastoid air cells	Mastoid Sinus, Right
	Mastoid Sinus, Left
Mastoid process	Temporal Bone, Right
	Temporal Bone, Left
Maxillary artery	External Carotid Artery, Right
	External Carotid Artery, Left
Maxillary nerve	Trigeminal Nerve
Medial canthus	Lower Eyelid, Right
	Lower Eyelid, Left
Medial collateral ligament (MCL)	Knee Bursa and Ligament, Right
	Knee Bursa and Ligament, Left
Medial condyle of femur	Lower Femur, Right
	Lower Femur, Left
Medial condyle of tibia	Tibia, Right
	Tibia, Left
Medial cuneiform bone	Tarsal, Right
	Tarsal, Left
Medial epicondyle of femur	Lower Femur, Right
	Lower Femur, Left
Medial epicondyle of humerus	Humeral Shaft, Right
	Humeral Shaft, Left

Term	ICD-10-PCS Value
Medial malleolus	Tibia, Right
	Tibia, Left
Medial meniscus	Knee Joint, Right
	Knee Joint, Left
Medial plantar artery	Foot Artery, Right
	Foot Artery, Left
Medial plantar nerve	Tibial Nerve
Medial popliteal nerve	Tibial Nerve
Medial rectus muscle	Extraocular Muscle, Right
	Extraocular Muscle, Left
Medial sural cutaneous nerve	Tibial Nerve
Median antebrachial vein	Basilic Vein, Right
	Basilic Vein, Left
Median cubital vein	Basilic Vein, Right
	Basilic Vein, Left
Median sacral artery	Abdominal Aorta
Mediastinal cavity	Mediastinum
Mediastinal lymph node	Lymphatic, Thorax
Mediastinal space	Mediastinum
Meissner's (submucous) plexus	Abdominal Sympathetic Nerve
Membranous urethra	Urethra
Mental foramen	Mandible, Right
	Mandible, Left
Mentalis muscle	Facial Muscle
Mesoappendix	Mesentery
Mesocolon	Mesentery
Metacarpal ligament	Hand Bursa and Ligament, Right
	Hand Bursa and Ligament, Left
Metacarpophalangeal ligament	Hand Bursa and Ligament, Right
	Hand Bursa and Ligament, Left
Metatarsal ligament	Foot Bursa and Ligament, Right
	Foot Bursa and Ligament, Left
Metatarsophalangeal ligament	Foot Bursa and Ligament, Right
	Foot Bursa and Ligament, Left
Metatarsophalangeal (MTP) joint	Metatarsal-Phalangeal Joint, Right
	Metatarsal-Phalangeal Joint, Left
Metathalamus	Thalamus
Midcarpal joint	Carpal Joint, Right
	Carpal Joint, Left
Middle cardiac nerve	Thoracic Sympathetic Nerve
Middle cerebral artery	Intracranial Artery
Middle cerebral vein	Intracranial Vein
Middle colic vein	Colic Vein
Middle genicular artery	Popliteal Artery, Right
	Popliteal Artery, Left
Middle hemorrhoidal vein	Hypogastric Vein, Right
	Hypogastric Vein, Left
Middle rectal artery	Internal Iliac Artery, Right
	Internal Iliac Artery, Left
Middle suprarenal artery	Abdominal Aorta
Middle temporal artery	Temporal Artery, Right
	Temporal Artery, Left
Middle turbinate	Nasal Turbinate
Mitral annulus	Mitral Valve
Molar gland	Buccal Mucosa
Musculocutaneous nerve	Brachial Plexus

Term	ICD-10-PCS Value
Musculophrenic artery	Internal Mammary Artery, Right
	Internal Mammary Artery, Left
Musculospiral nerve	Radial Nerve
Myelencephalon	Medulla Oblongata
Myenteric (Auerbach's) plexus	Abdominal Sympathetic Nerve
Myometrium	Uterus
Nail bed	Finger Nail
	Toe Nail
Nail plate	Finger Nail
	Toe Nail
Nasal cavity	Nasal Mucosa and Soft Tissue
Nasal concha	Nasal Turbinate
Nasalis muscle	Facial Muscle
Nasolacrimal duct	Lacrimal Duct, Right
	Lacrimal Duct, Left
Navicular bone	Tarsal, Right
	Tarsal, Left
Neck of femur	Upper Femur, Right
	Upper Femur, Left
Neck of humerus (anatomical) (surgical)	Humeral Head, Right
	Humeral Head, Left
Nerve to the stapedius	Facial Nerve
Neurohypophysis	Pituitary Gland
Ninth cranial nerve	Glossopharyngeal Nerve
Nostril	Nasal Mucosa and Soft Tissue
Obturator artery	Internal Iliac Artery, Right
	Internal Iliac Artery, Left
Obturator lymph node	Lymphatic, Pelvis
Obturator muscle	Hip Muscle, Right
	Hip Muscle, Left
Obturator nerve	Lumbar Plexus
Obturator vein	Hypogastric Vein, Right
	Hypogastric Vein, Left
Obtuse margin	Heart, Left
Occipital artery	External Carotid Artery, Right
	External Carotid Artery, Left
Occipital lobe	Cerebral Hemisphere
Occipital lymph node	Lymphatic, Right Neck
	Lymphatic, Left Neck
Occipitofrontalis muscle	Facial Muscle
Odontoid process	Cervical Vertebra
Olecranon bursa	Elbow Bursa and Ligament, Right
	Elbow Bursa and Ligament, Left
Olecranon process	Ulna, Right
	Ulna, Left
Olfactory bulb	Olfactory Nerve
Ophthalmic artery	Intracranial Artery
Ophthalmic nerve	Trigeminal Nerve
Ophthalmic vein	Intracranial Vein
Optic chiasma	Optic Nerve
Optic disc	Retina, Right
	Retina, Left
Optic foramen	Sphenoid Bone
Orbicularis oculi muscle	Upper Eyelid, Right
	Upper Eyelid, Left
Orbicularis oris muscle	Facial Muscle
Orbital fascia	Subcutaneous Tissue and Fascia, Face

Term	ICD-10-PCS Value
Orbital portion of ethmoid bone	Orbit, Right
	Orbit, Left
Orbital portion of frontal bone	Orbit, Right
	Orbit, Left
Orbital portion of lacrimal bone	Orbit, Right
	Orbit, Left
Orbital portion of maxilla	Orbit, Right
	Orbit, Left
Orbital portion of palatine bone	Orbit, Right
	Orbit, Left
Orbital portion of sphenoid bone	Orbit, Right
	Orbit, Left
Orbital portion of zygomatic bone	Orbit, Right
	Orbit, Left
Oropharynx	Pharynx
Otic ganglion	Head and Neck Sympathetic Nerve
Oval window	Middle Ear, Right
	Middle Ear, Left
Ovarian artery	Abdominal Aorta
Ovarian ligament	Uterine Supporting Structure
Oviduct	Fallopian Tube, Right
	Fallopian Tube, Left
Palatine gland	Buccal Mucosa
Palatine tonsil	Tonsils
Palatine uvula	Uvula
Palatoglossal muscle	Tongue, Palate, Pharynx Muscle
Palatopharyngeal muscle	Tongue, Palate, Pharynx Muscle
Palmar (volar) digital vein	Hand Vein, Right
	Hand Vein, Left
Palmar (volar) metacarpal vein	Hand Vein, Right
	Hand Vein, Left
Palmar cutaneous nerve	Median Nerve
	Radial Nerve
Palmar fascia (aponeurosis)	Subcutaneous Tissue and Fascia, Right Hand
	Subcutaneous Tissue and Fascia, Left Hand
Palmar interosseous muscle	Hand Muscle, Right
	Hand Muscle, Left
Palmar ulnocarpal ligament	Wrist Bursa and Ligament, Right
	Wrist Bursa and Ligament, Left
Palmaris longus muscle	Lower Arm and Wrist Muscle, Right
	Lower Arm and Wrist Muscle, Left
Pancreatic artery	Splenic Artery
Pancreatic plexus	Abdominal Sympathetic Nerve
Pancreatic vein	Splenic Vein
Pancreaticosplenic lymph node	Lymphatic, Aortic
Paraaortic lymph node	Lymphatic, Aortic
Parapharyngeal space	Neck
Pararectal lymph node	Lymphatic, Mesenteric
Parasternal lymph node	Lymphatic, Thorax
Paratracheal lymph node	Lymphatic, Thorax
Paraurethral (Skene's) gland	Vestibular Gland
Parietal lobe	Cerebral Hemisphere
Parotid lymph node	Lymphatic, Head
Parotid plexus	Facial Nerve

Term	ICD-10-PCS Value
Pars flaccida	Tympanic Membrane, Right
	Tympanic Membrane, Left
Patellar ligament	Knee Bursa and Ligament, Right
	Knee Bursa and Ligament, Left
Patellar tendon	Knee Tendon, Right
	Knee Tendon, Left
Patellofemoral joint	Knee Joint, Right
	Knee Joint, Left
	Knee Joint, Femoral Surface, Right
	Knee Joint, Femoral Surface, Left
Pectineus muscle	Upper Leg Muscle, Right
	Upper Leg Muscle, Left
Pectoral (anterior) lymph node	Lymphatic, Right Axillary
	Lymphatic, Left Axillary
Pectoral fascia	Subcutaneous Tissue and Fascia, Chest
Pectoralis major muscle	Thorax Muscle, Right
	Thorax Muscle, Left
Pectoralis minor muscle	Thorax Muscle, Right
	Thorax Muscle, Left
Pelvic splanchnic nerve	Abdominal Sympathetic Nerve
	Sacral Sympathetic Nerve
Penile urethra	Urethra
Pericardiophrenic artery	Internal Mammary Artery, Right
	Internal Mammary Artery, Left
Perimetrium	Uterus
Peroneus brevis muscle	Lower Leg Muscle, Right
	Lower Leg Muscle, Left
Peroneus longus muscle	Lower Leg Muscle, Right
	Lower Leg Muscle, Left
Petrous part of temporal bone	Temporal Bone, Right
	Temporal Bone, Left
Pharyngeal constrictor muscle	Tongue, Palate, Pharynx Muscle
Pharyngeal plexus	Vagus Nerve
Pharyngeal recess	Nasopharynx
Pharyngeal tonsil	Adenoids
Pharyngotympanic tube	Eustachian Tube, Right
	Eustachian Tube, Left
Pia mater, intracranial	Cerebral Meninges
Pia mater, spinal	Spinal Meninges
Pinna	External Ear, Right
	External Ear, Left
	External Ear, Bilateral
Piriform recess (sinus)	Pharynx
Piriformis muscle	Hip Muscle, Right
	Hip Muscle, Left
Pisiform bone	Carpal, Right
	Carpal, Left
Pisohamate ligament	Hand Bursa and Ligament, Right
	Hand Bursa and Ligament, Left
Pisometacarpal ligament	Hand Bursa and Ligament, Right
	Hand Bursa and Ligament, Left
Plantar digital vein	Foot Vein, Right
	Foot Vein, Left
Plantar fascia (aponeurosis)	Subcutaneous Tissue and Fascia, Right Foot
	Subcutaneous Tissue and Fascia, Left Foot

Term	ICD-10-PCS Value
Plantar metatarsal vein	Foot Vein, Right
	Foot Vein, Left
Plantar venous arch	Foot Vein, Right
	Foot Vein, Left
Platysma muscle	Neck Muscle, Right
	Neck Muscle, Left
Plica semilunaris	Conjunctiva, Right
	Conjunctiva, Left
Pneumogastric nerve	Vagus Nerve
Pneumotaxic center	Pons
Pontine tegmentum	Pons
Popliteal ligament	Knee Bursa and Ligament, Right
	Knee Bursa and Ligament, Left
Popliteallymph node	Lymphatic, Left Lower Extremity
	Lymphatic, Right Lower Extremity
Popliteal vein	Femoral Vein, Right
	Femoral Vein, Left
Popliteus muscle	Lower Leg Muscle, Right
	Lower Leg Muscle, Left
Postauricular (mastoid) lymph node	Lymphatic, Right Neck
	Lymphatic, Left Neck
Postcava	Inferior Vena Cava
Posterior (subscapular) lymph node	Lymphatic, Right Axillary
	Lymphatic, Left Axillary
Posterior auricular artery	External Carotid Artery, Right
	External Carotid Artery, Left
Posterior auricular nerve	Facial Nerve
Posterior auricular vein	External Jugular Vein, Right
	External Jugular Vein, Left
Posterior cerebral artery	Intracranial Artery
Posterior chamber	Eye, Right
	Eye, Left
Posterior circumflex humeral artery	Axillary Artery, Right
	Axillary Artery, Left
Posterior communicating artery	Intracranial Artery
Posterior cruciate ligament (PCL)	Knee Bursa and Ligament, Right
	Knee Bursa and Ligament, Left
Posterior facial (retromandibular) vein	Face Vein, Right
	Face Vein, Left
Posterior femoral cutaneous nerve	Sacral Plexus
Posterior inferior cerebellar artery (PICA)	Intracranial Artery
Posterior interosseous nerve	Radial Nerve
Posterior labial nerve	Pudendal Nerve
Posterior scrotal nerve	Pudendal Nerve
Posterior spinal artery	Vertebral Artery, Right
	Vertebral Artery, Left
Posterior tibial recurrent artery	Anterior Tibial Artery, Right
	Anterior Tibial Artery, Left
Posterior ulnar recurrent artery	Ulnar Artery, Right
	Ulnar Artery, Left
Posterior vagal trunk	Vagus Nerve
Preauricular lymph node	Lymphatic, Head
Precava	Superior Vena Cava
Prepatellar bursa	Knee Bursa and Ligament, Right
	Knee Bursa and Ligament, Left

Term	ICD-10-PCS Value
Pretracheal fascia	Subcutaneous Tissue and Fascia, Right Neck
	Subcutaneous Tissue and Fascia, Left Neck
Prevertebral fascia	Subcutaneous Tissue and Fascia, Right Neck
	Subcutaneous Tissue and Fascia, Left Neck
Princeps pollicis artery	Hand Artery, Right
	Hand Artery, Left
Procerus muscle	Facial Muscle
Profunda brachii	Brachial Artery, Right
	Brachial Artery, Left
Profunda femoris (deep femoral) vein	Femoral Vein, Right
	Femoral Vein, Left
Pronator quadratus muscle	Lower Arm and Wrist Muscle, Right
	Lower Arm and Wrist Muscle, Left
Pronator teres muscle	Lower Arm and Wrist Muscle, Right
	Lower Arm and Wrist Muscle, Left
Prostatic urethra	Urethra
Proximal radioulnar joint	Elbow Joint, Right
	Elbow Joint, Left
Psoas muscle	Hip Muscle, Right
	Hip Muscle, Left
Pterygoid muscle	Head Muscle
Pterygoid process	Sphenoid Bone
Pterygopalatine (sphenopalatine) ganglion	Head and Neck Sympathetic Nerve
Pubis	Pelvic Bone, Right
	Pelvic Bone, Left
Pubofemoral ligament	Hip Bursa and Ligament, Right
	Hip Bursa and Ligament, Left
Pudendal nerve	Sacral Plexus
Pulmoaortic canal	Pulmonary Artery, Left
Pulmonary annulus	Pulmonary Valve
Pulmonary plexus	Thoracic Sympathetic Nerve
	Vagus Nerve
Pulmonic valve	Pulmonary Valve
Pulvinar	Thalamus
Pyloric antrum	Stomach, Pylorus
Pyloric canal	Stomach, Pylorus
Pyloric sphincter	Stomach, Pylorus
Pyramidalis muscle	Abdomen Muscle, Right
	Abdomen Muscle, Left
Quadrangular cartilage	Nasal Septum
Quadrate lobe	Liver
Quadratus femoris muscle	Hip Muscle, Right
	Hip Muscle, Left
Quadratus lumborum muscle	Trunk Muscle, Right
	Trunk Muscle, Left
Quadratus plantae muscle	Foot Muscle, Right
	Foot Muscle, Left
Quadriceps (femoris)	Upper Leg Muscle, Right
	Upper Leg Muscle, Left
Radial collateral carpal ligament	Wrist Bursa and Ligament, Right
	Wrist Bursa and Ligament, Left
Radial collateral ligament	Elbow Bursa and Ligament, Right
	Elbow Bursa and Ligament, Left
Radial notch	Ulna, Right
	Ulna, Left

Term	ICD-10-PCS Value
Radial recurrent artery	Radial Artery, Right
	Radial Artery, Left
Radial vein	Brachial Vein, Right
	Brachial Vein, Left
Radialis indicis	Hand Artery, Right
	Hand Artery, Left
Radiocarpal joint	Wrist Joint, Right
	Wrist Joint, Left
Radiocarpal ligament	Wrist Bursa and Ligament, Right
	Wrist Bursa and Ligament, Left
Radioulnar ligament	Wrist Bursa and Ligament, Right
	Wrist Bursa and Ligament, Left
Rectosigmoid junction	Sigmoid Colon
Rectus abdominis muscle	Abdomen Muscle, Right
	Abdomen Muscle, Left
Rectus femoris muscle	Upper Leg Muscle, Right
	Upper Leg Muscle, Left
Recurrent laryngeal nerve	Vagus Nerve
Renal calyx	Kidney, Right
	Kidney, Left
	Kidneys, Bilateral
	Kidney
Renal capsule	Kidney, Right
	Kidney, Left
	Kidneys, Bilateral
	Kidney
Renal cortex	Kidney, Right
	Kidney, Left
	Kidneys, Bilateral
	Kidney
Renal nerve	Abdominal sympathetic Nerve
Renal plexus	Abdominal Sympathetic Nerve
Renal segment	Kidney, Right
	Kidney, Left
	Kidneys, Bilateral
	Kidney
Renal segmental artery	Renal Artery, Right
	Renal Artery, Left
Retroperitoneal cavity	Retroperitoneum
Retroperitoneal lymph node	Lymphatic, Aortic
Retroperitoneal space	Retroperitoneum
Retropharyngeal lymph node	Lymphatic, Right Neck
	Lymphatic, Left Neck
Retropharyngeal space	Neck
Retropubic space	Pelvic Cavity
Rhinopharynx	Nasopharynx
Rhomboid major muscle	Trunk Muscle, Right
	Trunk Muscle, Left
Rhomboid minor muscle	Trunk Muscle, Right
	Trunk Muscle, Left
Right ascending lumbar vein	Azygos Vein
Right atrioventricular valve	Tricuspid Valve
Right auricular appendix	Atrium, Right
Right colic vein	Colic Vein
Right coronary sulcus	Heart, Right
Right gastric artery	Gastric Artery

Term	ICD-10-PCS Value
Right gastroepiploic vein	Superior Mesenteric Vein
Right inferior phrenic vein	Inferior Vena Cava
Right inferior pulmonary vein	Pulmonary Vein, Right
Right jugular trunk	Lymphatic, Right Neck
Right lateral ventricle	Cerebral Ventricle
Right lymphatic duct	Lymphatic, Right Neck
Right ovarian vein	Inferior Vena Cava
Right second lumbar vein	Inferior Vena Cava
Right subclavian trunk	Lymphatic, Right Neck
Right subcostal vein	Azygos Vein
Right superior pulmonary vein	Pulmonary Vein, Right
Right suprarenal vein	Inferior Vena Cava
Right testicular vein	Inferior Vena Cava
Rima glottidis	Larynx
Risorius muscle	Facial Muscle
Round ligament of uterus	Uterine Supporting Structure
Round window	Inner Ear, Right
	Inner Ear, Left
Sacral ganglion	Sacral Sympathetic Nerve
Sacral lymph node	Lymphatic, Pelvis
Sacral splanchnic nerve	Sacral Sympathetic Nerve
Sacrococcygeal ligament	Lower Spine Bursa and Ligament
Sacrococcygeal symphysis	Sacrococcygeal Joint
Sacroiliac ligament	Lower Spine Bursa and Ligament
Sacrospinous ligament	Lower Spine Bursa and Ligament
Sacrotuberous ligament	Lower Spine Bursa and Ligament
Salpingopharyngeus muscle	Tongue, Palate, Pharynx Muscle
Salpinx	Fallopian Tube, Right
	Fallopian Tube, Left
Saphenous nerve	Femoral Nerve
Sartorius muscle	Upper Leg Muscle, Right
	Upper Leg Muscle, Left
Scalene muscle	Neck Muscle, Right
	Neck Muscle, Left
Scaphoid bone	Carpal, Right
	Carpal, Left
Scapholunate ligament	Wrist Bursa and Ligament, Right
	Wrist Bursa and Ligament, Left
Scaphotrapezium ligament	Hand Bursa and Ligament, Right
	Hand Bursa and Ligament, Left
Scarpa's (vestibular) ganglion	Acoustic Nerve
Sebaceous gland	Skin
Second cranial nerve	Optic Nerve
Sella turcica	Sphenoid Bone
Semicircular canal	Inner Ear, Right
	Inner Ear, Left
Semimembranosus muscle	Upper Leg Muscle, Right
	Upper Leg Muscle, Left
Semitendinosus muscle	Upper Leg Muscle, Right
	Upper Leg Muscle, Left
Septal cartilage	Nasal Septum
Serratus anterior muscle	Thorax Muscle, Right
	Thorax Muscle, Left
Serratus posterior muscle	Trunk Muscle, Right
	Trunk Muscle, Left

Term	ICD-10-PCS Value
Seventh cranial nerve	Facial Nerve
Short gastric artery	Splenic Artery
Sigmoid artery	Inferior Mesenteric Artery
Sigmoid flexure	Sigmoid Colon
Sigmoid vein	Inferior Mesenteric Vein
Sinoatrial node	Conduction Mechanism
Sinus venosus	Atrium, Right
Sixth cranial nerve	Abducens Nerve
Skene's (paraurethral) gland	Vestibular Gland
Small saphenous vein	Saphenous Vein, Right
	Saphenous Vein, Left
Solar (celiac) plexus	Abdominal Sympathetic Nerve
Soleus muscle	Lower Leg Muscle, Right
	Lower Leg Muscle, Left
Sphenomandibular ligament	Head and Neck Bursa and Ligament
Sphenopalatine (pterygopalatine) ganglion	Head and Neck Sympathetic Nerve
Spinal nerve, cervical	Cervical Nerve
Spinal nerve, lumbar	Lumbar Nerve
Spinal nerve, sacral	Sacral Nerve
Spinal nerve, thoracic	Thoracic Nerve
Spinous process	Cervical Vertebra
	Lumbar Vertebra
	Thoracic Vertebra
Spiral ganglion	Acoustic Nerve
Splenic flexure	Transverse Colon
Splenic plexus	Abdominal Sympathetic Nerve
Splenius capitis muscle	Head Muscle
Splenius cervicis muscle	Neck Muscle, Right
	Neck Muscle, Left
Stapes	Auditory Ossicle, Right
	Auditory Ossicle, Left
Stellate ganglion	Head and Neck Sympathetic Nerve
Stensen's duct	Parotid Duct, Right
	Parotid Duct, Left
Sternoclavicular ligament	Shoulder Bursa and Ligament, Right
	Shoulder Bursa and Ligament, Left
Sternocleidomastoid artery	Thyroid Artery, Right
	Thyroid Artery, Left
Sternocleidomastoid muscle	Neck Muscle, Right
	Neck Muscle, Left
Sternocostal ligament	Sternum Bursa and Ligament
Styloglossus muscle	Tongue, Palate, Pharynx Muscle
Stylomandibular ligament	Head and Neck Bursa and Ligament
Stylopharyngeus muscle	Tongue, Palate, Pharynx Muscle
Subacromial bursa	Shoulder Bursa and Ligament, Right
	Shoulder Bursa and Ligament, Left
Subaortic (common iliac) lymph node	Lymphatic, Pelvis
Subarachnoid space, spinal	Spinal Canal
Subclavicular (apical) lymph node	Lymphatic, Right Axillary
	Lymphatic, Left Axillary
Subclavius muscle	Thorax Muscle, Right
	Thorax Muscle, Left
Subclavius nerve	Brachial Plexus
Subcostal artery	Upper Artery

Term	ICD-10-PCS Value
Subcostal muscle	Thorax Muscle, Right
	Thorax Muscle, Left
Subcostal nerve	Thoracic Nerve
Subdural space, spinal	Spinal Canal
Submandibular ganglion	Facial Nerve
	Head and Neck Sympathetic Nerve
Submandibular gland	Submaxillary Gland, Right
	Submaxillary Gland, Left
Submandibular lymph node	Lymphatic, Head
Submandibular space	Subcutaneous Tissue and Fascia, Face
Submaxillary ganglion	Head and Neck Sympathetic Nerve
Submaxillary lymph node	Lymphatic, Head
Submental artery	Face Artery
Submental lymph node	Lymphatic, Head
Submucous (Meissner's) plexus	Abdominal Sympathetic Nerve
Suboccipital nerve	Cervical Nerve
Suboccipital venous plexus	Vertebral Vein, Right
	Vertebral Vein, Left
Subparotid lymph node	Lymphatic, Head
Subscapular aponeurosis	Subcutaneous Tissue and Fascia, Right Upper Arm
	Subcutaneous Tissue and Fascia, Left Upper Arm
Subscapular artery	Axillary Artery, Right
	Axillary Artery, Left
Subscapular (posterior) lymph node	Lymphatic, Right Axillary
	Lymphatic, Left Axillary
Subscapularis muscle	Shoulder Muscle, Right
	Shoulder Muscle, Left
Substantia nigra	Basal Ganglia
Subtalar (talocalcaneal) joint	Tarsal Joint, Right
	Tarsal Joint, Left
Subtalar ligament	Foot Bursa and Ligament, Right
	Foot Bursa and Ligament, Left
Subthalamic nucleus	Basal Ganglia
Superficial circumflex iliac vein	Saphenous Vein, Right
	Saphenous Vein, Left
Superficial epigastric artery	Femoral Artery, Right
	Femoral Artery, Left
Superficial epigastric vein	Saphenous Vein, Right
	Saphenous Vein, Left
Superficial palmar arch	Hand Artery, Right
	Hand Artery, Left
Superficial palmar venous arch	Hand Vein, Right
	Hand Vein, Left
Superficial temporal artery	Temporal Artery, Right
	Temporal Artery, Left
Superficial transverse perineal muscle	Perineum Muscle
Superior cardiac nerve	Thoracic Sympathetic Nerve
Superior cerebellar vein	Intracranial Vein
Superior cerebral vein	Intracranial Vein
Superior clunic (cluneal) nerve	Lumbar Nerve
Superior epigastric artery	Internal Mammary Artery, Right
	Internal Mammary Artery, Left

Term	ICD-10-PCS Value
Superior genicular artery	Popliteal Artery, Right
	Popliteal Artery, Left
Superior gluteal artery	Internal Iliac Artery, Right
	Internal Iliac Artery, Left
Superior gluteal nerve	Lumbar Plexus
Superior hypogastric plexus	Abdominal Sympathetic Nerve
Superior labial artery	Face Artery
Superior laryngeal artery	Thyroid Artery, Right
	Thyroid Artery, Left
Superior laryngeal nerve	Vagus Nerve
Superior longitudinal muscle	Tongue, Palate, Pharynx Muscle
Superior mesenteric ganglion	Abdominal Sympathetic Nerve
Superior mesenteric lymph node	Lymphatic, Mesenteric
Superior mesenteric plexus	Abdominal Sympathetic Nerve
Superior oblique muscle	Extraocular Muscle, Right
	Extraocular Muscle, Left
Superior olivary nucleus	Pons
Superior rectal artery	Inferior Mesenteric Artery
Superior rectal vein	Inferior Mesenteric Vein
Superior rectus muscle	Extraocular Muscle, Right
	Extraocular Muscle, Left
Superior tarsal plate	Upper Eyelid, Right
	Upper Eyelid, Left
Superior thoracic artery	Axillary Artery, Right
	Axillary Artery, Left
Superior thyroid artery	External Carotid Artery, Right
	External Carotid Artery, Left
	Thyroid Artery, Right
	Thyroid Artery, Left
Superior turbinate	Nasal Turbinate
Superior ulnar collateral artery	Brachial Artery, Right
	Brachial Artery, Left
Supraclavicular nerve	Cervical Plexus
Supraclavicular (Virchow's) lymph node	Lymphatic, Right Neck
	Lymphatic, Left Neck
Suprahyoid lymph node	Lymphatic, Head
Suprahyoid muscle	Neck Muscle, Right
	Neck Muscle, Left
Suprainguinal lymph node	Lymphatic, Pelvis
Supraorbital vein	Face Vein, Right
	Face Vein, Left
Suprarenal gland	Adrenal Gland, Right
	Adrenal Gland, Left
	Adrenal Glands, Bilateral
	Adrenal Gland
Suprarenal plexus	Abdominal Sympathetic Nerve
Suprascapular nerve	Brachial Plexus
Supraspinatus fascia	Subcutaneous Tissue and Fascia, Right Upper Arm
	Subcutaneous Tissue and Fascia, Left Upper Arm
Supraspinatus muscle	Shoulder Muscle, Right
	Shoulder Muscle, Left
Supraspinous ligament	Upper Spine Bursa and Ligament
	Lower Spine Bursa and Ligament

Term	ICD-10-PCS Value
Suprasternal notch	Sternum
Supratrochlear lymph node	Lymphatic, Right Upper Extremity
	Lymphatic, Left Upper Extremity
Sural artery	Popliteal Artery, Right
	Popliteal Artery, Left
Sweat gland	Skin
Talocalcaneal ligament	Foot Bursa and Ligament, Right
	Foot Bursa and Ligament, Left
Talocalcaneal (subtalar) joint	Tarsal Joint, Right
	Tarsal Joint, Left
Talocalcaneonavicular joint	Tarsal Joint, Right
	Tarsal Joint, Left
Talocalcaneonavicular ligament	Foot Bursa and Ligament, Right
	Foot Bursa and Ligament, Left
Talocrural joint	Ankle Joint, Right
	Ankle Joint, Left
Talofibular ligament	Ankle Bursa and Ligament, Right
	Ankle Bursa and Ligament, Left
Talus bone	Tarsal, Right
	Tarsal, Left
Tarsometatarsal ligament	Foot Bursa and Ligament, Right
	Foot Bursa and Ligament, Left
Temporal lobe	Cerebral Hemisphere
Temporalis muscle	Head Muscle
Temporoparietalis muscle	Head Muscle
Tensor fasciae latae muscle	Hip Muscle, Right
	Hip Muscle, Left
Tensor veli palatini muscle	Tongue, Palate, Pharynx Muscle
Tenth cranial nerve	Vagus Nerve
Tentorium cerebelli	Dura Mater
Teres major muscle	Shoulder Muscle, Right
	Shoulder Muscle, Left
Teres minor muscle	Shoulder Muscle, Right
	Shoulder Muscle, Left
Testicular artery	Abdominal Aorta
Thenar muscle	Hand Muscle, Right
	Hand Muscle, Left
Third cranial nerve	Oculomotor Nerve
Third occipital nerve	Cervical Nerve
Third ventricle	Cerebral Ventricle
Thoracic aortic plexus	Thoracic Sympathetic Nerve
Thoracic esophagus	Esophagus, Middle
Thoracic facet joint	Thoracic Vertebral Joint
Thoracic ganglion	Thoracic Sympathetic Nerve
Thoracoacromial artery	Axillary Artery, Right
	Axillary Artery, Left
Thoracolumbar facet joint	Thoracolumbar Vertebral Joint
Thymus gland	Thymus
Thyroarytenoid muscle	Neck Muscle, Right
	Neck Muscle, Left
Thyrocervical trunk	Thyroid Artery, Right
	Thyroid Artery, Left
Thyroid cartilage	Larynx
Tibial sesamoid	Metatarsal, Right
	Metatarsal, Left
Tibialis anterior muscle	Lower Leg Muscle, Right
	Lower Leg Muscle, Left

Term	ICD-10-PCS Value
Tibialis posterior muscle	Lower Leg Muscle, Right
	Lower Leg Muscle, Left
Tibiofemoral joint	Knee Joint, Right
	Knee Joint, Left
	Knee Joint, Tibial Surface, Right
	Knee Joint, Tibial Surface, Left
Tibioperoneal trunk	Popliteal Artery, Right
	Popliteal Artery, Left
Tongue, base of	Pharynx
Tracheobronchial lymph node	Lymphatic, Thorax
Tragus	External Ear, Right
	External Ear, Left
	External Ear, Bilateral
Transversalis fascia	Subcutaneous Tissue and Fascia, Trunk
Transverse acetabular ligament	Hip Bursa and Ligament, Right
	Hip Bursa and Ligament, Left
Transverse (cutaneous) cervical nerve	Cervical Plexus
Transverse facial artery	Temporal Artery, Right
	Temporal Artery, Left
Transverse foramen	Cervical Vertebra
Transverse humeral ligament	Shoulder Bursa and Ligament, Right
	Shoulder Bursa and Ligament, Left
Transverse ligament of atlas	Head and Neck Bursa and Ligament
Transverse process	Cervical Vertebra
	Thoracic Vertebra
	Lumbar Vertebra
Transverse scapular ligament	Shoulder Bursa and Ligament, Right
	Shoulder Bursa and Ligament, Left
Transverse thoracis muscle	Thorax Muscle, Right
	Thorax Muscle, Left
Transversospinalis muscle	Trunk Muscle, Right
	Trunk Muscle, Left
Transversus abdominis muscle	Abdomen Muscle, Right
	Abdomen Muscle, Left
Trapezium bone	Carpal, Right
	Carpal, Left
Trapezius muscle	Trunk Muscle, Right
	Trunk Muscle, Left
Trapezoid bone	Carpal, Right
	Carpal, Left
Triceps brachii muscle	Upper Arm Muscle, Right
	Upper Arm Muscle, Left
Tricuspid annulus	Tricuspid Valve
Trifacial nerve	Trigeminal Nerve
Trigone of bladder	Bladder
Triquetral bone	Carpal, Right
	Carpal, Left
Trochantericbursa	Hip Bursa and Ligament, Right
	Hip Bursa and Ligament, Left
Twelfth cranial nerve	Hypoglossal Nerve
Tympanic cavity	Middle Ear, Right
	Middle Ear, Left
Tympanic nerve	Glossopharyngeal Nerve
Tympanic part of temoporal bone	Temporal Bone, Right
	Temporal Bone, Left

Term	ICD-10-PCS Value
Ulnar collateral carpal ligament	Wrist Bursa and Ligament, Right
	Wrist Bursa and Ligament, Left
Ulnar collateral ligament	Elbow Bursa and Ligament, Right
	Elbow Bursa and Ligament, Left
Ulnar notch	Radius, Right
	Radius, Left
Ulnar vein	Brachial Vein, Right
	Brachial Vein, Left
Umbilical artery	Internal Iliac Artery, Right
	Internal Iliac Artery, Left
	Lower Artery
Ureteral orifice	Ureter, Right
	Ureter, Left
	Ureters, Bilateral
	Ureter
Ureteropelvic junction (UPJ)	Kidney Pelvis, Right
	Kidney Pelvis, Left
Ureterovesical orifice	Ureter, Right
	Ureter, Left
	Ureters, Bilateral
	Ureter
Uterine artery	Internal Iliac Artery, Right
	Internal Iliac Artery, Left
Uterine cornu	Uterus
Uterine tube	Fallopian Tube, Right
	Fallopian Tube, Left
Uterine vein	Hypogastric Vein, Right
	Hypogastric Vein, Left
Vaginal artery	Internal Iliac Artery, Right
	Internal Iliac Artery, Left
Vaginal vein	Hypogastric Vein, Right
	Hypogastric Vein, Left
Vastus intermedius muscle	Upper Leg Muscle, Right
	Upper Leg Muscle, Left
Vastus lateralis muscle	Upper Leg Muscle, Right
	Upper Leg Muscle, Left
Vastus medialis muscle	Upper Leg Muscle, Right
	Upper Leg Muscle, Left
Ventricular fold	Larynx
Vermiform appendix	Appendix
Vermilion border	Upper Lip
	Lower Lip
Vertebral arch	Cervical Vertebra
	Lumbar Vertebra
	Thoracic Vertebra
Vertebral body	Cervical Vertebra
	Lumbar Vertebra
	Thoracic Vertebra
Vertebral canal	Spinal Canal
Vertebral foramen	Cervical Vertebra
	Lumbar Vertebra
	Thoracic Vertebra
Vertebral lamina	Cervical Vertebra
	Lumbar Vertebra
	Thoracic Vertebra
Vertebral pedicle	Cervical Vertebra
	Lumbar Vertebra
	Thoracic Vertebra

Term	ICD-10-PCS Value
Vesical vein	Hypogastric Vein, Right
	Hypogastric Vein, Left
Vestibular (Scarpa's) ganglion	Acoustic Nerve
Vestibular nerve	Acoustic Nerve
Vestibulocochlear nerve	Acoustic Nerve
Virchow's (supraclavicular) lymph node	Lymphatic, Right Neck
	Lymphatic, Left Neck
Vitreous body	Vitreous, Right
	Vitreous, Left
Vocal fold	Vocal Cord, Right
	Vocal Cord, Left
Volar (palmar) digital vein	Hand Vein, Right
	Hand Vein, Left
Volar (palmar) metacarpal vein	Hand Vein, Right
	Hand Vein, Left
Vomer bone	Nasal Septum
Vomer of nasal septum	Nasal Bone
Xiphoid process	Sternum
Zonule of Zinn	Lens, Right
	Lens, Left
Zygomatic process of frontal bone	Frontal Bone
Zygomatic process of temporal bone	Temporal Bone, Right
	Temporal Bone, Left
Zygomaticus muscle	Facial Muscle

Appendix E: Body Part Definitions

ICD-10-PCS Value	Definition
1st Toe, Left 1st Toe, Right	**Includes:** Hallux
Abdomen Muscle, Left Abdomen Muscle, Right	**Includes:** External oblique muscle Internal oblique muscle Pyramidalis muscle Rectus abdominis muscle Transversus abdominis muscle
Abdominal Aorta	**Includes:** Inferior phrenic artery Lumbar artery Median sacral artery Middle suprarenal artery Ovarian artery Testicular artery
Abdominal Sympathetic Nerve	**Includes:** Abdominal aortic plexus Auerbach's (myenteric) plexus Celiac (solar) plexus Celiac ganglion Gastric plexus Hepatic plexus Inferior hypogastric plexus Inferior mesenteric ganglion Inferior mesenteric plexus Meissner's (submucous) plexus Myenteric (Auerbach's) plexus Pancreatic plexus Pelvic splanchnic nerve Renal nerve Renal plexus Solar (celiac) plexus Splenic plexus Submucous (Meissner's) plexus Superior hypogastric plexus Superior mesenteric ganglion Superior mesenteric plexus Suprarenal plexus
Abducens Nerve	**Includes:** Sixth cranial nerve
Accessory Nerve	**Includes:** Eleventh cranial nerve
Acoustic Nerve	**Includes:** Cochlear nerve Eighth cranial nerve Scarpa's (vestibular) ganglion Spiral ganglion Vestibular (Scarpa's) ganglion Vestibular nerve Vestibulocochlear nerve
Adenoids	**Includes:** Pharyngeal tonsil
Adrenal Gland Adrenal Gland, Left Adrenal Gland, Right Adrenal Glands, Bilateral	**Includes:** Suprarenal gland
Ampulla of Vater	**Includes:** Duodenal ampulla Hepatopancreatic ampulla
Anal Sphincter	**Includes:** External anal sphincter Internal anal sphincter

ICD-10-PCS Value	Definition
Ankle Bursa and Ligament, Left Ankle Bursa and Ligament, Right	**Includes:** Calcaneofibular ligament Deltoid ligament Ligament of the lateral malleolus Talofibular ligament
Ankle Joint, Left Ankle Joint, Right	**Includes:** Inferior tibiofibular joint Talocrural joint
Anterior Chamber, Left Anterior Chamber, Right	**Includes:** Aqueous humour
Anterior Tibial Artery, Left Anterior Tibial Artery, Right	**Includes:** Anterior lateral malleolar artery Anterior medial malleolar artery Anterior tibial recurrent artery Dorsalis pedis artery Posterior tibial recurrent artery
Anus	**Includes:** Anal orifice
Aortic Valve	**Includes:** Aortic annulus
Appendix	**Includes:** Vermiform appendix
Atrial Septum	**Includes:** Interatrial septum
Atrium, Left	**Includes:** Atrium pulmonale Left auricular appendix
Atrium, Right	**Includes:** Atrium dextrum cordis Right auricular appendix Sinus venosus
Auditory Ossicle, Left Auditory Ossicle, Right	**Includes:** Incus Malleus Stapes
Axillary Artery, Left Axillary Artery, Right	**Includes:** Anterior circumflex humeral artery Lateral thoracic artery Posterior circumflex humeral artery Subscapular artery Superior thoracic artery Thoracoacromial artery
Azygos Vein	**Includes:** Right ascending lumbar vein Right subcostal vein
Basal Ganglia	**Includes:** Basal nuclei Claustrum Corpus striatum Globus pallidus Substantia nigra Subthalamic nucleus
Basilic Vein, Left Basilic Vein, Right	**Includes:** Median antebrachial vein Median cubital vein
Bladder	**Includes:** Trigone of bladder
Brachial Artery, Left Brachial Artery, Right	**Includes:** Inferior ulnar collateral artery Profunda brachii Superior ulnar collateral artery

ICD-10-PCS Value	Definition
Brachial Plexus	**Includes:** Axillary nerve Dorsal scapular nerve First intercostal nerve Long thoracic nerve Musculocutaneous nerve Subclavius nerve Suprascapular nerve
Brachial Vein, Left Brachial Vein, Right	**Includes:** Radial vein Ulnar vein
Brain	**Includes:** Cerebrum Corpus callosum Encephalon
Breast, Bilateral Breast, Left Breast, Right	**Includes:** Mammary duct Mammary gland
Buccal Mucosa	**Includes:** Buccal gland Molar gland Palatine gland
Carotid Bodies, Bilateral Carotid Body, Left Carotid Body, Right	**Includes:** Carotid glomus
Carpal Joint, Left Carpal Joint, Right	**Includes:** Intercarpal joint Midcarpal joint
Carpal, Left Carpal, Right	**Includes:** Capitate bone Hamate bone Lunate bone Pisiform bone Scaphoid bone Trapezium bone Trapezoid bone Triquetral bone
Celiac Artery	**Includes:** Celiac trunk
Cephalic Vein, Left Cephalic Vein, Right	**Includes:** Accessory cephalic vein
Cerebellum	**Includes:** Culmen
Cerebral Hemisphere	**Includes:** Frontal lobe Occipital lobe Parietal lobe Temporal lobe
Cerebral Meninges	**Includes:** Arachnoid mater, intracranial Leptomeninges, intracranial Pia mater, intracranial
Cerebral Ventricle	**Includes:** Aqueduct of Sylvius Cerebral aqueduct (Sylvius) Choroid plexus Ependyma Foramen of Monro (intraventricular) Fourth ventricle Interventricular foramen (Monro) Left lateral ventricle Right lateral ventricle Third ventricle

ICD-10-PCS Value	Definition
Cervical Nerve	**Includes:** Greater occipital nerve Spinal nerve, cervical Suboccipital nerve Third occipital nerve
Cervical Plexus	**Includes:** Ansa cervicalis Cutaneous (transverse) cervical nerve Great auricular nerve Lesser occipital nerve Supraclavicular nerve Transverse (cutaneous) cervical nerve
Cervical Spinal Cord	**Includes:** Dorsal root ganglion
Cervical Vertebra	**Includes:** Dens Odontoid process Spinous process Transverse foramen Transverse process Vertebral arch Vertebral body Vertebral foramen Vertebral lamina Vertebral pedicle
Cervical Vertebral Joint	**Includes:** Atlantoaxial joint Cervical facet joint
Cervical Vertebral Joints, 2 or more	**Includes:** Cervical facet joint
Cervicothoracic Vertebral Joint	**Includes:** Cervicothoracic facet joint
Cisterna Chyli	**Includes:** Intestinal lymphatic trunk Lumbar lymphatic trunk
Coccygeal Glomus	**Includes:** Coccygeal body
Colic Vein	**Includes:** Ileocolic vein Left colic vein Middle colic vein Right colic vein
Conduction Mechanism	**Includes:** Atrioventricular node Bundle of His Bundle of Kent Sinoatrial node
Conjunctiva, Left Conjunctiva, Right	**Includes:** Plica semilunaris
Dura Mater	**Includes:** Diaphragma sellae Dura mater, intracranial Falx cerebri Tentorium cerebelli
Elbow Bursa and Ligament, Left Elbow Bursa and Ligament, Right	**Includes:** Annular ligament Olecranon bursa Radial collateral ligament Ulnar collateral ligament
Elbow Joint, Left Elbow Joint, Right	**Includes:** Distal humerus, involving joint Humeroradial joint Humeroulnar joint Proximal radioulnar joint
Epidural Space, Intracranial	**Includes:** Extradural space, intracranial

ICD-10-PCS Value	Definition
Epiglottis	**Includes:** Glossoepiglottic fold
Esophagogastric Junction	**Includes:** Cardia Cardioesophageal junction Gastroesophageal (GE) junction
Esophagus, Lower	**Includes:** Abdominal esophagus
Esophagus, Middle	**Includes:** Thoracic esophagus
Esophagus, Upper	**Includes:** Cervical esophagus
Ethmoid Bone, Left **Ethmoid Bone, Right**	**Includes:** Cribriform plate
Ethmoid Sinus, Left **Ethmoid Sinus, Right**	**Includes:** Ethmoidal air cell
Eustachian Tube, Left **Eustachian Tube, Right**	**Includes:** Auditory tube Pharyngotympanic tube
External Auditory Canal, Left **External Auditory Canal, Right**	**Includes:** External auditory meatus
External Carotid Artery, Left **External Carotid Artery, Right**	**Includes:** Ascending pharyngeal artery Internal maxillary artery Lingual artery Maxillary artery Occipital artery Posterior auricular artery Superior thyroid artery
External Ear, Bilateral **External Ear, Left** **External Ear, Right**	**Includes:** Antihelix Antitragus Auricle Earlobe Helix Pinna Tragus
External Iliac Artery, Left **External Iliac Artery, Right**	**Includes:** Deep circumflex iliac artery Inferior epigastric artery
External Jugular Vein, Left **External Jugular Vein, Right**	**Includes:** Posterior auricular vein
Extraocular Muscle, Left **Extraocular Muscle, Right**	**Includes:** Inferior oblique muscle Inferior rectus muscle Lateral rectus muscle Medial rectus muscle Superior oblique muscle Superior rectus muscle
Eye, Left **Eye, Right**	**Includes:** Ciliary body Posterior chamber
Face Artery	**Includes:** Angular artery Ascending palatine artery External maxillary artery Facial artery Inferior labial artery Submental artery Superior labial artery

ICD-10-PCS Value	Definition
Face Vein, Left **Face Vein, Right**	**Includes:** Angular vein Anterior facial vein Common facial vein Deep facial vein Frontal vein Posterior facial (retromandibular) vein Supraorbital vein
Facial Muscle	**Includes:** Buccinator muscle Corrugator supercilii muscle Depressor anguli oris muscle Depressor labii inferioris muscle Depressor septi nasi muscle Depressor supercilii muscle Levator anguli oris muscle Levator labii superioris alaeque nasi muscle Levator labii superioris muscle Mentalis muscle Nasalis muscle Occipitofrontalis muscle Orbicularis oris muscle Procerus muscle Risorius muscle Zygomaticus muscle
Facial Nerve	**Includes:** Chorda tympani Geniculate ganglion Greater superficial petrosal nerve Nerve to the stapedius Parotid plexus Posterior auricular nerve Seventh cranial nerve Submandibular ganglion
Fallopian Tube, Left **Fallopian Tube, Right**	**Includes:** Oviduct Salpinx Uterine tube
Femoral Artery, Left **Femoral Artery, Right**	**Includes:** Circumflex iliac artery Deep femoral artery Descending genicular artery External pudendal artery Superficial epigastric artery
Femoral Nerve	**Includes:** Anterior crural nerve Saphenous nerve
Femoral Shaft, Left **Femoral Shaft, Right**	**Includes:** Body of femur
Femoral Vein, Left **Femoral Vein, Right**	**Includes:** Deep femoral (profunda femoris) vein Popliteal vein Profunda femoris (deep femoral) vein
Fibula, Left **Fibula, Right**	**Includes:** Body of fibula Head of fibula Lateral malleolus
Finger Nail	**Includes:** Nail bed Nail plate
Finger Phalangeal Joint, Left **Finger Phalangeal Joint, Right**	**Includes:** Interphalangeal (IP) joint

ICD-10-PCS Value	Definition
Foot Artery, Left Foot Artery, Right	**Includes:** Arcuate artery Dorsal metatarsal artery Lateral plantar artery Lateral tarsal artery Medial plantar artery
Foot Bursa and Ligament, Left Foot Bursa and Ligament, Right	**Includes:** Calcaneocuboid ligament Cuneonavicular ligament Intercuneiform ligament Interphalangeal ligament Metatarsal ligament Metatarsophalangeal ligament Subtalar ligament Talocalcaneal ligament Talocalcaneonavicular ligament Tarsometatarsal ligament
Foot Muscle, Left Foot Muscle, Right	**Includes:** Abductor hallucis muscle Adductor hallucis muscle Extensor digitorum brevis muscle Extensor hallucis brevis muscle Flexor digitorum brevis muscle Flexor hallucis brevis muscle Quadratus plantae muscle
Foot Vein, Left Foot Vein, Right	**Includes:** Common digital vein Dorsal metatarsal vein Dorsal venous arch Plantar digital vein Plantar metatarsal vein Plantar venous arch
Frontal Bone	**Includes:** Zygomatic process of frontal bone
Gastric Artery	**Includes:** Left gastric artery Right gastric artery
Glenoid Cavity, Left Glenoid Cavity, Right	**Includes:** Glenoid fossa (of scapula)
Glomus Jugulare	**Includes:** Jugular body
Glossopharyngeal Nerve	**Includes:** Carotid sinus nerve Ninth cranial nerve Tympanic nerve
Hand Artery, Left Hand Artery, Right	**Includes:** Deep palmar arch Princeps pollicis artery Radialis indicis Superficial palmar arch
Hand Bursa and Ligament, Left Hand Bursa and Ligament, Right	**Includes:** Carpometacarpal ligament Intercarpal ligament Interphalangeal ligament Lunotriquetral ligament Metacarpal ligament Metacarpophalangeal ligament Pisohamate ligament Pisometacarpal ligament Scaphotrapezium ligament
Hand Muscle, Left Hand Muscle, Right	**Includes:** Hypothenar muscle Palmar interosseous muscle Thenar muscle

ICD-10-PCS Value	Definition
Hand Vein, Left Hand Vein, Right	**Includes:** Dorsal metacarpal vein Palmar (volar) digital vein Palmar (volar) metacarpal vein Superficial palmar venous arch Volar (palmar) digital vein Volar (palmar) metacarpal vein
Head and Neck Bursa and Ligament	**Includes:** Alar ligament of axis Cervical interspinous ligament Cervical intertransverse ligament Cervical ligamentum flavum Interspinous ligament, cervical Intertransverse ligament, cervical Lateral temporomandibular ligament Ligamentum flavum, cervical Sphenomandibular ligament Stylomandibular ligament Transverse ligament of atlas
Head and Neck Sympathetic Nerve	**Includes:** Cavernous plexus Cervical ganglion Ciliary ganglion Internal carotid plexus Otic ganglion Pterygopalatine (sphenopalatine) ganglion Sphenopalatine (pterygopalatine) ganglion Stellate ganglion Submandibular ganglion Submaxillary ganglion
Head Muscle	**Includes:** Auricularis muscle Masseter muscle Pterygoid muscle Splenius capitis muscle Temporalis muscle Temporoparietalis muscle
Heart, Left	**Includes:** Left coronary sulcus Obtuse margin
Heart, Right	**Includes:** Right coronary sulcus
Hemiazygos Vein	**Includes:** Left ascending lumbar vein Left subcostal vein
Hepatic Artery	**Includes:** Common hepatic artery Gastroduodenal artery Hepatic artery proper
Hip Bursa and Ligament, Left Hip Bursa and Ligament, Right	**Includes:** Iliofemoral ligament Ischiofemoral ligament Pubofemoral ligament Transverse acetabular ligament Trochanteric bursa
Hip Joint, Left Hip Joint, Right	**Includes:** Acetabulofemoral joint
Hip Muscle, Left Hip Muscle, Right	**Includes:** Gemellus muscle Gluteus maximus muscle Gluteus medius muscle Gluteus minimus muscle Iliacus muscle Obturator muscle Piriformis muscle Psoas muscle Quadratus femoris muscle Tensor fasciae latae muscle

ICD-10-PCS Value	Definition
Humeral Head, Left Humeral Head, Right	**Includes:** Greater tuberosity Lesser tuberosity Neck of humerus (anatomical)(surgical)
Humeral Shaft, Left Humeral Shaft, Right	**Includes:** Distal humerus Humerus, distal Lateral epicondyle of humerus Medial epicondyle of humerus
Hypogastric Vein, Left Hypogastric Vein, Right	**Includes:** Gluteal vein Internal iliac vein Internal pudendal vein Lateral sacral vein Middle hemorrhoidal vein Obturator vein Uterine vein Vaginal vein Vesical vein
Hypoglossal Nerve	**Includes:** Twelfth cranial nerve
Hypothalamus	**Includes:** Mammillary body
Inferior Mesenteric Artery	**Includes:** Sigmoid artery Superior rectal artery
Inferior Mesenteric Vein	**Includes:** Sigmoid vein Superior rectal vein
Inferior Vena Cava	**Includes:** Postcava Right inferior phrenic vein Right ovarian vein Right second lumbar vein Right suprarenal vein Right testicular vein
Inguinal Region, Bilateral Inguinal Region, Left Inguinal Region, Right	**Includes:** Inguinal canal Inguinal triangle
Inner Ear, Left Inner Ear, Right	**Includes:** Bony labyrinth Bony vestibule Cochlea Round window Semicircular canal
Innominate Artery	**Includes:** Brachiocephalic artery Brachiocephalic trunk
Innominate Vein, Left Innominate Vein, Right	**Includes:** Brachiocephalic vein Inferior thyroid vein
Internal Carotid Artery, Left Internal Carotid Artery, Right	**Includes:** Caroticotympanic artery Carotid sinus

ICD-10-PCS Value	Definition
Internal Iliac Artery, Left Internal Iliac Artery, Right	**Includes:** Deferential artery Hypogastric artery Iliolumbar artery Inferior gluteal artery Inferior vesical artery Internal pudendal artery Lateral sacral artery Middle rectal artery Obturator artery Superior gluteal artery Umbilical artery Uterine artery Vaginal artery
Internal Mammary Artery, Left Internal Mammary Artery, Right	**Includes:** Anterior intercostal artery Internal thoracic artery Musculophrenic artery Pericardiophrenic artery Superior epigastric artery
Intracranial Artery	**Includes:** Anterior cerebral artery Anterior choroidal artery Anterior communicating artery Basilar artery Circle of Willis Internal carotid artery, intracranial portion Middle cerebral artery Ophthalmic artery Posterior cerebral artery Posterior communicating artery Posterior inferior cerebellar artery (PICA)
Intracranial Vein	**Includes:** Anterior cerebral vein Basal (internal) cerebral vein Dural venous sinus Great cerebral vein Inferior cerebellar vein Inferior cerebral vein Internal (basal) cerebral vein Middle cerebral vein Ophthalmic vein Superior cerebellar vein Superior cerebral vein
Jejunum	**Includes:** Duodenojejunal flexure
Kidney	**Includes:** Renal calyx Renal capsule Renal cortex Renal segment
Kidney Pelvis, Left Kidney Pelvis, Right	**Includes:** Ureteropelvic junction (UPJ)
Kidney, Left Kidney, Right Kidneys, Bilateral	**Includes:** Renal calyx Renal capsule Renal cortex Renal segment
Knee Bursa and Ligament, Left Knee Bursa and Ligament, Right	**Includes:** Anterior cruciate ligament (ACL) Lateral collateral ligament (LCL) Ligament of head of fibula Medial collateral ligament (MCL) Patellar ligament Popliteal ligament Posterior cruciate ligament (PCL) Prepatellar bursa

ICD-10-PCS Value	Definition
Knee Joint, Femoral Surface, Left Knee Joint, Femoral Surface, Right	**Includes:** Femoropatellar joint Patellofemoral joint
Knee Joint, Left Knee Joint, Right	**Includes:** Femoropatellar joint Femorotibial joint Lateral meniscus Medial meniscus Patellofemoral joint Tibiofemoral joint
Knee Joint, Tibial Surface, Left Knee Joint, Tibial Surface, Right	**Includes:** Femorotibial joint Tibiofemoral joint
Knee Tendon, Left Knee Tendon, Right	**Includes:** Patellar tendon
Lacrimal Duct, Left Lacrimal Duct, Right	**Includes:** Lacrimal canaliculus Lacrimal punctum Lacrimal sac Nasolacrimal duct
Larynx	**Includes:** Aryepiglottic fold Arytenoid cartilage Corniculate cartilage Cuneiform cartilage False vocal cord Glottis Rima glottidis Thyroid cartilage Ventricular fold
Lens, Left Lens, Right	**Includes:** Zonule of Zinn
Liver	**Includes:** Quadrate lobe
Lower Arm and Wrist Muscle, Left Lower Arm and Wrist Muscle, Right	**Includes:** Anatomical snuffbox Brachioradialis muscle Extensor carpi radialis muscle Extensor carpi ulnaris muscle Flexor carpi radialis muscle Flexor carpi ulnaris muscle Flexor pollicis longus muscle Palmaris longus muscle Pronator quadratus muscle Pronator teres muscle
Lower Artery	**Includes:** Umbilical artery
Lower Eyelid, Left Lower Eyelid, Right	**Includes:** Inferior tarsal plate Medial canthus
Lower Femur, Left Lower Femur, Right	**Includes:** Lateral condyle of femur Lateral epicondyle of femur Medial condyle of femur Medial epicondyle of femur

ICD-10-PCS Value	Definition
Lower Leg Muscle, Left Lower Leg Muscle, Right	**Includes:** Extensor digitorum longus muscle Extensor hallucis longus muscle Fibularis brevis muscle Fibularis longus muscle Flexor digitorum longus muscle Flexor hallucis longus muscle Gastrocnemius muscle Peroneus brevis muscle Peroneus longus muscle Popliteus muscle Soleus muscle Tibialis anterior muscle Tibialis posterior muscle
Lower Leg Tendon, Left Lower Leg Tendon, Right	**Includes:** Achilles tendon
Lower Lip	**Includes:** Frenulum labii inferioris Labial gland Vermilion border
Lower Spine Bursa and Ligament	**Includes:** Iliolumbar ligament Interspinous ligament, lumbar Intertransverse ligament, lumbar Ligamentum flavum, lumbar Sacrococcygeal ligament Sacroiliac ligament Sacrospinous ligament Sacrotuberous ligament Supraspinous ligament
Lumbar Nerve	**Includes:** Lumbosacral trunk Spinal nerve, lumbar Superior clunic (cluneal) nerve
Lumbar Plexus	**Includes:** Accessory obturator nerve Genitofemoral nerve Iliohypogastric nerve Ilioinguinal nerve Lateral femoral cutaneous nerve Obturator nerve Superior gluteal nerve
Lumbar Spinal Cord	**Includes:** Cauda equina Conus medullaris Dorsal root ganglion
Lumbar Sympathetic Nerve	**Includes:** Lumbar ganglion Lumbar splanchnic nerve
Lumbar Vertebra	**Includes:** Spinous process Transverse process Vertebral arch Vertebral body Vertebral foramen Vertebral lamina Vertebral pedicle
Lumbar Vertebral Joint	**Includes:** Lumbar facet joint
Lumbosacral Joint	**Includes:** Lumbosacral facet joint

ICD-10-PCS Value	Definition
Lymphatic, Aortic	**Includes:** Celiac lymph node Gastric lymph node Hepatic lymph node Lumbar lymph node Pancreaticosplenic lymph node Paraaortic lymph node Retroperitoneal lymph node
Lymphatic, Head	**Includes:** Buccinator lymph node Infraauricular lymph node Infraparotid lymph node Parotid lymph node Preauricular lymph node Submandibular lymph node Submaxillary lymph node Submental lymph node Subparotid lymph node Suprahyoid lymph node
Lymphatic, Left Axillary	**Includes:** Anterior (pectoral) lymph node Apical (subclavicular) lymph node Brachial (lateral) lymph node Central axillary lymph node Lateral (brachial) lymph node Pectoral (anterior) lymph node Posterior (subscapular) lymph node Subclavicular (apical) lymph node Subscapular (posterior) lymph node
Lymphatic, Left Lower Extremity	**Includes:** Femoral lymph node Popliteal lymph node
Lymphatic, Left Neck	**Includes:** Cervical lymph node Jugular lymph node Mastoid (postauricular) lymph node Occipital lymph node Postauricular (mastoid) lymph node Retropharyngeal lymph node Supraclavicular (Virchow's) lymph node Virchow's (supraclavicular) lymph node
Lymphatic, Left Upper Extremity	**Includes:** Cubital lymph node Deltopectoral (infraclavicular) lymph node Epitrochlear lymph node Infraclavicular (deltopectoral) lymph node Supratrochlear lymph node
Lymphatic, Mesenteric	**Includes:** Inferior mesenteric lymph node Pararectal lymph node Superior mesenteric lymph node
Lymphatic, Pelvis	**Includes:** Common iliac (subaortic) lymph node Gluteal lymph node Iliac lymph node Inferior epigastric lymph node Obturator lymph node Sacral lymph node Subaortic (common iliac) lymph node Suprainguinal lymph node

ICD-10-PCS Value	Definition
Lymphatic, Right Axillary	**Includes:** Anterior (pectoral) lymph node Apical (subclavicular) lymph node Brachial (lateral) lymph node Central axillary lymph node Lateral (brachial) lymph node Pectoral (anterior) lymph node Posterior (subscapular) lymph node Subclavicular (apical) lymph node Subscapular (posterior) lymph node
Lymphatic, Right Lower Extremity	**Includes:** Femoral lymph node Popliteal lymph node
Lymphatic, Right Neck	**Includes:** Cervical lymph node Jugular lymph node Mastoid (postauricular) lymph node Occipital lymph node Postauricular (mastoid) lymph node Retropharyngeal lymph node Right jugular trunk Right lymphatic duct Right subclavian trunk Supraclavicular (Virchow's) lymph node Virchow's (supraclavicular) lymph node
Lymphatic, Right Upper Extremity	**Includes:** Cubital lymph node Deltopectoral (infraclavicular) lymph node Epitrochlear lymph node Infraclavicular (deltopectoral) lymph node Supratrochlear lymph node
Lymphatic, Thorax	**Includes:** Intercostal lymph node Mediastinal lymph node Parasternal lymph node Paratracheal lymph node Tracheobronchial lymph node
Main Bronchus, Right	**Includes:** Bronchus intermedius Intermediate bronchus
Mandible, Left **Mandible, Right**	**Includes:** Alveolar process of mandible Condyloid process Mandibular notch Mental foramen
Mastoid Sinus, Left **Mastoid Sinus, Right**	**Includes:** Mastoid air cells
Metatarsal, Left **Metatarsal, Right**	**Includes:** Fibular sesamoid Tibial sesamoid
Maxilla	**Includes:** Alveolar process of maxilla
Maxillary Sinus, Left **Maxillary Sinus, Right**	**Includes:** Antrum of Highmore
Median Nerve	**Includes:** Anterior interosseous nerve Palmar cutaneous nerve
Mediastinum	**Includes:** Mediastinal cavity Mediastinal space
Medulla Oblongata	**Includes:** Myelencephalon
Mesentery	**Includes:** Mesoappendix Mesocolon

ICD-10-PCS Value	Definition
Metatarsal, Right **Metatarsal, Left**	**Includes:** Fibular sesamoid Tibial sesamoid
Metatarsal-Phalangeal Joint, Left **Metatarsal-Phalangeal Joint, Right**	**Includes:** Metatarsophalangeal (MTP) joint
Middle Ear, Left **Middle Ear, Right**	**Includes:** Oval window Tympanic cavity
Minor Salivary Gland	**Includes:** Anterior lingual gland
Mitral Valve	**Includes:** Bicuspid valve Left atrioventricular valve Mitral annulus
Nasal Bone	**Includes:** Vomer of nasal septum
Nasal Mucosa and Soft Tissue	**Includes:** Columella External naris Greater alar cartilage Internal naris Lateral nasal cartilage Lesser alar cartilage Nasal cavity Nostril
Nasal Septum	**Includes:** Quadrangular cartilage Septal cartilage Vomer bone
Nasal Turbinate	**Includes:** Inferior turbinate Middle turbinate Nasal concha Superior turbinate
Nasopharynx	**Includes:** Choana Fossa of Rosenmuller Pharyngeal recess Rhinopharynx
Neck	**Includes:** Parapharyngeal space Retropharyngeal space
Neck Muscle, Left **Neck Muscle, Right**	**Includes:** Anterior vertebral muscle Arytenoid muscle Cricothyroid muscle Infrahyoid muscle Levator scapulae muscle Platysma muscle Scalene muscle Splenius cervicis muscle Sternocleidomastoid muscle Suprahyoid muscle Thyroarytenoid muscle
Nipple, Left **Nipple, Right**	**Includes:** Areola
Occipital Bone	**Includes:** Foramen magnum
Oculomotor Nerve	**Includes:** Third cranial nerve
Olfactory Nerve	**Includes:** First cranial nerve Olfactory bulb

ICD-10-PCS Value	Definition
Omentum	**Includes:** Gastrocolic ligament Gastrocolic omentum Gastrohepatic omentum Gastrophrenic ligament Gastrosplenic ligament Greater Omentum Hepatogastric ligament Lesser Omentum
Optic Nerve	**Includes:** Optic chiasma Second cranial nerve
Orbit, Left **Orbit, Right**	**Includes:** Bony orbit Orbital portion of ethmoid bone Orbital portion of frontal bone Orbital portion of lacrimal bone Orbital portion of maxilla Orbital portion of palatine bone Orbital portion of sphenoid bone Orbital portion of zygomatic bone
Pancreatic Duct	**Includes:** Duct of Wirsung
Pancreatic Duct, Accessory	**Includes:** Duct of Santorini
Parotid Duct, Left **Parotid Duct, Right**	**Includes:** Stensen's duct
Pelvic Bone, Left **Pelvic Bone, Right**	**Includes:** Iliac crest Ilium Ischium Pubis
Pelvic Cavity	**Includes:** Retropubic space
Penis	**Includes:** Corpus cavernosum Corpus spongiosum
Perineum Muscle	**Includes:** Bulbospongiosus muscle Cremaster muscle Deep transverse perineal muscle Ischiocavernosus muscle Levator ani muscle Superficial transverse perineal muscle
Peritoneum	**Includes:** Epiploic foramen
Peroneal Artery, Left **Peroneal Artery, Right**	**Includes:** Fibular artery
Peroneal Nerve	**Includes:** Common fibular nerve Common peroneal nerve External popliteal nerve Lateral sural cutaneous nerve
Pharynx	**Includes:** Base of Tongue Hypopharynx Laryngopharynx Lingual tonsil Oropharynx Piriform recess (sinus) Tongue, base of
Phrenic Nerve	**Includes:** Accessory phrenic nerve
Pituitary Gland	**Includes:** Adenohypophysis Hypophysis Neurohypophysis

ICD-10-PCS Value	Definition
Pons	**Includes:** Apneustic center Basis pontis Locus ceruleus Pneumotaxic center Pontine tegmentum Superior olivary nucleus
Popliteal Artery, Left Popliteal Artery, Right	**Includes:** Inferior genicular artery Middle genicular artery Superior genicular artery Sural artery Tibioperoneal trunk
Portal Vein	**Includes:** Hepatic portal vein
Prepuce	**Includes:** Foreskin Glans penis
Pudendal Nerve	**Includes:** Posterior labial nerve Posterior scrotal nerve
Pulmonary Artery, Left	**Includes:** Arterial canal (duct) Botallo's duct Pulmoaortic canal
Pulmonary Valve	**Includes:** Pulmonary annulus Pulmonic valve
Pulmonary Vein, Left	**Includes:** Left inferior pulmonary vein Left superior pulmonary vein
Pulmonary Vein, Right	**Includes:** Right inferior pulmonary vein Right superior pulmonary vein
Radial Artery, Left Radial Artery, Right	**Includes:** Radial recurrent artery
Radial Nerve	**Includes:** Dorsal digital nerve Musculospiral nerve Palmar cutaneous nerve Posterior interosseous nerve
Radius, Left Radius, Right	**Includes:** Ulnar notch
Rectum	**Includes:** Anorectal junction
Renal Artery, Left Renal Artery, Right	**Includes:** Inferior suprarenal artery Renal segmental artery
Renal Vein, Left	**Includes:** Left inferior phrenic vein Left ovarian vein Left second lumbar vein Left suprarenal vein Left testicular vein
Retina, Left Retina, Right	**Includes:** Fovea Macula Optic disc
Retroperitoneum	**Includes:** Retroperitoneal cavity Retroperitoneal space
Rib(s) Bursa and Ligament	**Includes:** Costotransverse ligament
Sacral Nerve	**Includes:** Spinal nerve, sacral

ICD-10-PCS Value	Definition
Sacral Plexus	**Includes:** Inferior gluteal nerve Posterior femoral cutaneous nerve Pudendal nerve
Sacral Sympathetic Nerve	**Includes:** Ganglion impar (ganglion of Walther) Pelvic splanchnic nerve Sacral ganglion Sacral splanchnic nerve
Sacrococcygeal Joint	**Includes:** Sacrococcygeal symphysis
Saphenous Vein, Left Saphenous Vein, Right	**Includes:** External pudendal vein Great(er) saphenous vein Lesser saphenous vein Small saphenous vein Superficial circumflex iliac vein Superficial epigastric vein
Scapula, Left Scapula, Right	**Includes:** Acromion (process) Coracoid process
Sciatic Nerve	**Includes:** Ischiatic nerve
Shoulder Bursa and Ligament, Left Shoulder Bursa and Ligament, Right	**Includes:** Acromioclavicular ligament Coracoacromial ligament Coracoclavicular ligament Coracohumeral ligament Costoclavicular ligament Glenohumeral ligament Interclavicular ligament Sternoclavicular ligament Subacromial bursa Transverse humeral ligament Transverse scapular ligament
Shoulder Joint, Left Shoulder Joint, Right	**Includes:** Glenohumeral joint Glenoid ligament (labrum)
Shoulder Muscle, Left Shoulder Muscle, Right	**Includes:** Deltoid muscle Infraspinatus muscle Subscapularis muscle Supraspinatus muscle Teres major muscle Teres minor muscle
Sigmoid Colon	**Includes:** Rectosigmoid junction Sigmoid flexure
Skin	**Includes:** Dermis Epidermis Sebaceous gland Sweat gland
Skin, Chest	**Includes:** Breast procedures, skin only
Sphenoid Bone	**Includes:** Greater wing Lesser wing Optic foramen Pterygoid process Sella turcica
Spinal Canal	**Includes:** Epidural space, spinal Extradural space, spinal Subarachnoid space, spinal Subdural space, spinal Vertebral canal

ICD-10-PCS Value	Definition
Spinal Cord	**Includes:** Dorsal root ganglion
Spinal Meninges	**Includes:** Arachnoid mater, spinal Denticulate (dentate) ligament Dura mater, spinal Filum terminale Leptomeninges, spinal Pia mater, spinal
Spleen	**Includes:** Accessory spleen
Splenic Artery	**Includes:** Left gastroepiploic artery Pancreatic artery Short gastric artery
Splenic Vein	**Includes:** Left gastroepiploic vein Pancreatic vein
Sternum	**Includes:** Manubrium Suprasternal notch Xiphoid process
Sternum Bursa and Ligament	**Includes:** Costoxiphoid ligament Sternocostal ligament
Stomach, Pylorus	**Includes:** Pyloric antrum Pyloric canal Pyloric sphincter
Subclavian Artery, Left Subclavian Artery, Right	**Includes:** Costocervical trunk Dorsal scapular artery Internal thoracic artery
Subcutaneous Tissue and Fascia, Chest	**Includes:** Pectoral fascia
Subcutaneous Tissue and Fascia, Face	**Includes:** Masseteric fascia Orbital fascia Submandibular space
Subcutaneous Tissue and Fascia, Left Foot	**Includes:** Plantar fascia (aponeurosis)
Subcutaneous Tissue and Fascia, Left Hand	**Includes:** Palmar fascia (aponeurosis)
Subcutaneous Tissue and Fascia, Left Lower Arm	**Includes:** Antebrachial fascia Bicipital aponeurosis
Subcutaneous Tissue and Fascia, Left Neck	**Includes:** Deep cervical fascia Pretracheal fascia Prevertebral fascia
Subcutaneous Tissue and Fascia, Left Upper Arm	**Includes:** Axillary fascia Deltoid fascia Infraspinatus fascia Subscapular aponeurosis Supraspinatus fascia
Subcutaneous Tissue and Fascia, Left Upper Leg	**Includes:** Crural fascia Fascia lata Iliac fascia Iliotibial tract (band)
Subcutaneous Tissue and Fascia, Right Foot	**Includes:** Plantar fascia (aponeurosis)
Subcutaneous Tissue and Fascia, Right Hand	**Includes:** Palmar fascia (aponeurosis)

ICD-10-PCS Value	Definition
Subcutaneous Tissue and Fascia, Right Lower Arm	**Includes:** Antebrachial fascia Bicipital aponeurosis
Subcutaneous Tissue and Fascia, Right Neck	**Includes:** Deep cervical fascia Pretracheal fascia Prevertebral fascia
Subcutaneous Tissue and Fascia, Right Upper Arm	**Includes:** Axillary fascia Deltoid fascia Infraspinatus fascia Subscapular aponeurosis Supraspinatus fascia
Subcutaneous Tissue and Fascia, Right Upper Leg	**Includes:** Crural fascia Fascia lata Iliac fascia Iliotibial tract (band)
Subcutaneous Tissue and Fascia, Scalp	**Includes:** Galea aponeurotica
Subcutaneous Tissue and Fascia, Trunk	**Includes:** External oblique aponeurosis Transversalis fascia
Submaxillary Gland, Left Submaxillary Gland, Right	**Includes:** Submandibular gland
Superior Mesenteric Artery	**Includes:** Ileal artery Ileocolic artery Inferior pancreaticoduodenal artery Jejunal artery
Superior Mesenteric Vein	**Includes:** Right gastroepiploic vein
Superior Vena Cava	**Includes:** Precava
Tarsal Joint, Left Tarsal Joint, Right	**Includes:** Calcaneocuboid joint Cuboideonavicular joint Cuneonavicular joint Intercuneiform joint Subtalar (talocalcaneal) joint Talocalcaneal (subtalar) joint Talocalcaneonavicular joint
Tarsal, Left Tarsal, Right	**Includes:** Calcaneus Cuboid bone Intermediate cuneiform bone Lateral cuneiform bone Medial cuneiform bone Navicular bone Talus bone
Temporal Artery, Left Temporal Artery, Right	**Includes:** Middle temporal artery Superficial temporal artery Transverse facial artery
Temporal Bone, Left Temporal Bone, Right	**Includes:** Mastoid process Petrous part of temporal bone Tympanic part of temporal bone Zygomatic process of temporal bone
Thalamus	**Includes:** Epithalamus Geniculate nucleus Metathalamus Pulvinar
Thoracic Aorta, Ascending/Arch	**Includes:** Aortic arch Ascending aorta

ICD-10-PCS Value	Definition
Thoracic Duct	**Includes:** Left jugular trunk Left subclavian trunk
Thoracic Nerve	**Includes:** Intercostal nerve Intercostobrachial nerve Spinal nerve, thoracic Subcostal nerve
Thoracic Spinal Cord	**Includes:** Dorsal root ganglion
Thoracic Sympathetic Nerve	**Includes:** Cardiac plexus Esophageal plexus Greater splanchnic nerve Inferior cardiac nerve Least splanchnic nerve Lesser splanchnic nerve Middle cardiac nerve Pulmonary plexus Superior cardiac nerve Thoracic aortic plexus Thoracic ganglion
Thoracic Vertebra	**Includes:** Spinous process Transverse process Vertebral arch Vertebral body Vertebral foramen Vertebral lamina Vertebral pedicle
Thoracic Vertebral Joint	**Includes:** Costotransverse joint Costovertebral joint Thoracic facet joint
Thoracolumbar Vertebral Joint	**Includes:** Thoracolumbar facet joint
Thorax Muscle, Left **Thorax Muscle, Right**	**Includes:** Intercostal muscle Levatores costarum muscle Pectoralis major muscle Pectoralis minor muscle Serratus anterior muscle Subclavius muscle Subcostal muscle Transverse thoracis muscle
Thymus	**Includes:** Thymus gland
Thyroid Artery, Left **Thyroid Artery, Right**	**Includes:** Cricothyroid artery Hyoid artery Sternocleidomastoid artery Superior laryngeal artery Superior thyroid artery Thyrocervical trunk
Tibia, Left **Tibia, Right**	**Includes:** Lateral condyle of tibia Medial condyle of tibia Medial malleolus
Tibial Nerve	**Includes:** Lateral plantar nerve Medial plantar nerve Medial popliteal nerve Medial sural cutaneous nerve
Toe Nail	**Includes:** Nail bed Nail plate

ICD-10-PCS Value	Definition
Toe Phalangeal Joint, Left **Toe Phalangeal Joint, Right**	**Includes:** Interphalangeal (IP) joint
Tongue	**Includes:** Frenulum linguae
Tongue, Palate, Pharynx Muscle	**Includes:** Chondroglossus muscle Genioglossus muscle Hyoglossus muscle Inferior longitudinal muscle Levator veli palatini muscle Palatoglossal muscle Palatopharyngeal muscle Pharyngeal constrictor muscle Salpingopharyngeus muscle Styloglossus muscle Stylopharyngeus muscle Superior longitudinal muscle Tensor veli palatini muscle
Tonsils	**Includes:** Palatine tonsil
Trachea	**Includes:** Cricoid cartilage
Transverse Colon	**Includes:** Hepatic flexure Splenic flexure
Tricuspid Valve	**Includes:** Right atrioventricular valve Tricuspid annulus
Trigeminal Nerve	**Includes:** Fifth cranial nerve Gasserian ganglion Mandibular nerve Maxillary nerve Ophthalmic nerve Trifacial nerve
Trochlear Nerve	**Includes:** Fourth cranial nerve
Trunk Muscle, Left **Trunk Muscle, Right**	**Includes:** Coccygeus muscle Erector spinae muscle Interspinalis muscle Intertransversarius muscle Latissimus dorsi muscle Quadratus lumborum muscle Rhomboid major muscle Rhomboid minor muscle Serratus posterior muscle Transversospinalis muscle Trapezius muscle
Tympanic Membrane, Left **Tympanic Membrane, Right**	**Includes:** Pars flaccida
Ulna, Left **Ulna, Right**	**Includes:** Olecranon process Radial notch
Ulnar Artery, Left **Ulnar Artery, Right**	**Includes:** Anterior ulnar recurrent artery Common interosseous artery Posterior ulnar recurrent artery
Ulnar Nerve	**Includes:** Cubital nerve
Upper Arm Muscle, Left **Upper Arm Muscle, Right**	**Includes:** Biceps brachii muscle Brachialis muscle Coracobrachialis muscle Triceps brachii muscle

ICD-10-PCS Value	Definition
Upper Artery	**Includes:** Aortic intercostal artery Bronchial artery Esophageal artery Subcostal artery
Upper Eyelid, Left **Upper Eyelid, Right**	**Includes:** Lateral canthus Levator palpebrae superioris muscle Orbicularis oculi muscle Superior tarsal plate
Upper Femur, Left **Upper Femur, Right**	**Includes:** Femoral head Greater trochanter Lesser trochanter Neck of femur
Upper Leg Muscle, Left **Upper Leg Muscle, Right**	**Includes:** Adductor brevis muscle Adductor longus muscle Adductor magnus muscle Biceps femoris muscle Gracilis muscle Pectineus muscle Quadriceps (femoris) Rectus femoris muscle Sartorius muscle Semimembranosus muscle Semitendinosus muscle Vastus intermedius muscle Vastus lateralis muscle Vastus medialis muscle
Upper Lip	**Includes:** Frenulum labii superioris Labial gland Vermilion border
Upper Spine Bursa and Ligament	**Includes:** Interspinous ligament, thoracic Intertransverse ligament, thoracic Ligamentum flavum, thoracic Supraspinous ligament
Ureter **Ureter, Left** **Ureter, Right** **Ureters, Bilateral**	**Includes:** Ureteral orifice Ureterovesical orifice
Urethra	**Includes:** Bulbourethral (Cowper's) gland Cowper's (bulbourethral) gland External urethral sphincter Internal urethral sphincter Membranous urethra Penile urethra Prostatic urethra
Uterine Supporting Structure	**Includes:** Broad ligament Infundibulopelvic ligament Ovarian ligament Round ligament of uterus
Uterus	**Includes:** Fundus uteri Myometrium Perimetrium Uterine cornu
Uvula	**Includes:** Palatine uvula

ICD-10-PCS Value	Definition
Vagus Nerve	**Includes:** Anterior vagal trunk Pharyngeal plexus Pneumogastric nerve Posterior vagal trunk Pulmonary plexus Recurrent laryngeal nerve Superior laryngeal nerve Tenth cranial nerve
Vas Deferens **Vas Deferens, Bilateral** **Vas Deferens, Left** **Vas Deferens, Right**	**Includes:** Ductus deferens Ejaculatory duct
Ventricle, Right	**Includes:** Conus arteriosus
Ventricular Septum	**Includes:** Interventricular septum
Vertebral Artery, Left **Vertebral Artery, Right**	**Includes:** Anterior spinal artery Posterior spinal artery
Vertebral Vein, Left **Vertebral Vein, Right**	**Includes:** Deep cervical vein Suboccipital venous plexus
Vestibular Gland	**Includes:** Bartholin's (greater vestibular) gland Greater vestibular (Bartholin's) gland Paraurethral (Skene's) gland Skene's (paraurethral) gland
Vitreous, Left **Vitreous, Right**	**Includes:** Vitreous body
Vocal Cord, Left **Vocal Cord, Right**	**Includes:** Vocal fold
Vulva	**Includes:** Labia majora Labia minora
Wrist Bursa and Ligament, Left **Wrist Bursa and Ligament, Right**	**Includes:** Palmar ulnocarpal ligament Radial collateral carpal ligament Radiocarpal ligament Radioulnar ligament Scapholunate ligament Ulnar collateral carpal ligament
Wrist Joint, Left **Wrist Joint, Right**	**Includes:** Distal radioulnar joint Radiocarpal joint

Appendix F: Device Classification

In most PCS codes, the sixth character of the code classifies the device. The sixth character device value "defines the material or appliance used to accomplish the objective of the procedure that remains in or on the procedure site at the end of the procedure." If the device is the means by which the procedural objective is accomplished, then a specific device value is coded in the sixth character. If no device is used to accomplish the objective of the procedure, the device value No Device is coded in the sixth character. In limited root operations, the classification provides the qualifier values Temporary and Intraoperative, for specific procedures involving clinically significant devices whose purpose is brief use during the procedure or current inpatient stay.

Material that is classified as a PCS device is distinguished from material classified as a PCS substance by its having a specific location. A device is intended to maintain a fixed location at the procedure site where it was put, whereas a substance is intended to disperse or be absorbed in the body. There are circumstances in which a device does not stay where it was put and may need to be "revised" in a subsequent procedure to move the device back to its intended location.

Material classified as a PCS device is also distinguishable by the fact that it is removable. Although it may not be practical to remove some types of devices once they become established at the site, it is physically possible to remove a device for some time after the procedure. A skin graft, for example, once it "takes," may be nearly indistinguishable from the surrounding skin and so is no longer clearly identifiable as a device. Nevertheless, procedures that involve material coded as a device can for the most part be "reversed" by removing the device from the procedure site.

General Device Types

Device Type	Definition	Examples
Grafts	Biological or synthetic material that **takes the place of all or a portion of a body part.**	Full- or partial-thickness skin grafts: • Autologous • Nonautologous • Synthetic • Zooplastic Other tissue grafts: • Bone • Tendon • Vascular
Prosthesis	Biological or synthetic material that **takes the place of all or a portion of a body part.**	Joint prosthesis: • Autologous • Nonautologous • Synthetic
Implants	**Therapeutic** material that is not absorbed by, eliminated by, or incorporated into a body part.	External fixation device Internal fixation device: • Orthopaedic pins • Intramedullary rods Radioactive element implant Mesh
Simple or mechanical appliances	Biological or synthetic material that **assists or prevents a physiological function.**	Drainage device Extraluminal device Endobrachial device Fusion device Intraluminal device (can be temporary) Tracheostomy device IUD
Electronic appliances	Electronic appliances used to **assist, monitor, take the pace of, or prevent a physiological function.**	Cardiac leads Diaphragmatic pacemaker External heart assist system Short-term external heart assist system (Intraoperative) Fetal monitoring Hearing device Monitoring device Neurostimulator
External appliances	Performed without making an incision or a puncture, external appliances are used for the purpose of **protection, immobilization, stretching, compression, or packing.**	Bandage Cast Packing material Pressure dressing Traction apparatus

Transplant/Grafting Tissue Type Terminology

Tissue Type	Terminology
Tissue or organ transferred into a new position in **the body of the same individual**	Autograft Autologous Autoplastic
Having to do with individuals or tissues that have **identical genes**, such as identical twins	Isograft Isologous Syngeneic Syngraft
Tissue or organ taken from **different individuals** of the same species	Allogeneic Allograft Homologous Homograft
Tissue or organ from a **cadaver**	Nonautologous
Tissue or organ from individuals of **different species**	Heterogeneic Heterologous Xenogeneic Xenograft Zooplastic

Appendix G: Device Key and Aggregation Table

This **NT** symbol next to a device in the Term column identifies that the device has been approved for NTAP (new technology add-on payment). CMS provides incremental payment, in addition to the DRG payment, for technologies that have received an NTAP designation.

Device Key

Term	ICD-10-PCS Value
3f (Aortic) Bioprosthesis valve	Zooplastic Tissue in Heart and Great Vessels
AbioCor® Total Replacement Heart	Synthetic Substitute
Absolute Pro Vascular (OTW) Self-Expanding Stent System	Intraluminal Device
Acculink (RX) Carotid Stent System	Intraluminal Device
Acellular Hydrated Dermis	Nonautologous Tissue Substitute
Acetabular cup	Liner in Lower Joints
Activa PC neurostimulator	Stimulator Generator, Multiple Array for Insertion in Subcutaneous Tissue and Fascia
Activa RC neurostimulator	Stimulator Generator, Multiple Array Rechargeable for Insertion in Subcutaneous Tissue and Fascia
Activa SC neurostimulator	Stimulator Generator, Single Array for Insertion in Subcutaneous Tissue and Fascia
ACUITY™ Steerable Lead	Cardiac Lead, Pacemaker for Insertion in Heart and Great Vessels Cardiac Lead, Defibrillator for Insertion in Heart and Great Vessels
Advisa (MRI)	Pacemaker, Dual Chamber for Insertion in Subcutaneous Tissue and Fascia
AFX® Endovascular AAA System	Intraluminal Device
Alfapump® system	Other Device
AMPLATZER® Muscular VSD Occluder	Synthetic Substitute
AMS 800® Urinary Control System	Artificial Sphincter in Urinary System
AneuRx® AAA Advantage®	Intraluminal Device
Annuloplasty ring	Synthetic Substitute
ApiFix® Minimally Invasive Deformity Correction (MID-C) System (C)	Posterior (Dynamic) Distraction Device in New Technology
Aprevo™	Interbody Fusion Device, Customizable in New Technology
Articulating Spacer (Antibiotic)	Articulating Spacer in Lower Joints
Artificial anal sphincter (AAS)	Artificial Sphincter in Gastrointestinal System
Artificial bowel sphincter (neosphincter)	Artificial Sphincter in Gastrointestinal System
Artificial urinary sphincter (AUS)	Artificial Sphincter in Urinary System
Ascenda Intrathecal Catheter	Infusion Device
Assurant (Cobalt) stent	Intraluminal Device
AtriClip LAA Exclusion System	Extraluminal Device
Attain Ability® Lead	Cardiac Lead, Pacemaker for Insertion in Heart and Great Vessels Cardiac Lead, Defibrillator for Insertion in Heart and Great Vessels

Term	ICD-10-PCS Value
Attain StarFix® (OTW) Lead	Cardiac Lead, Pacemaker for Insertion in Heart and Great Vessels Cardiac Lead, Defibrillator for Insertion in Heart and Great Vessels
Autograft	Autologous Tissue Substitute
Autologous artery graft	Autologous Arterial Tissue in Heart and Great Vessels Autologous Arterial Tissue in Upper Arteries Autologous Arterial Tissue in Lower Arteries Autologous Arterial Tissue in Upper Veins Autologous Arterial Tissue in Lower Veins
Autologous vein graft	Autologous Venous Tissue in Heart and Great Vessels Autologous Venous Tissue in Upper Arteries Autologous Venous Tissue in Lower Arteries Autologous Venous Tissue in Upper Veins Autologous Venous Tissue in Lower Veins
Axial Lumbar Interbody Fusion System	Interbody Fusion Device in Lower Joints
AxiaLIF® System	Interbody Fusion Device in Lower Joints
BAK/C® Interbody Cervical Fusion System	Interbody Fusion Device in Upper Joints
Bard® Composix® (E/X)(LP) mesh	Synthetic Substitute
Bard® Composix® Kugel® patch	Synthetic Substitute
Bard® Dulex™ mesh	Synthetic Substitute
Bard® Ventralex™ hernia patch	Synthetic Substitute
Baroreflex Activation Therapy® (BAT®) **NT**	Stimulator Lead in Upper Arteries Stimulator Generator in Subcutaneous Tissue and Fascia
Barricaid® Annular Closure Device (ACD)	Synthetic Substitute
Berlin Heart Ventricular Assist Device	Implantable Heart Assist System in Heart and Great Vessels
Bioactive embolization coil(s)	Intraluminal Device, Bioactive in Upper Arteries
Biventricular external heart assist system	Short-term External Heart Assist System in Heart and Great Vessels
Blood glucose monitoring system	Monitoring Device
Bone anchored hearing device	Hearing Device, Bone Conduction for Insertion in Ear, Nose, Sinus Hearing Device, in Head and Facial Bones
Bone bank bone graft	Nonautologous Tissue Substitute
Bone screw (interlocking)(lag)(pedicle) (recessed)	Internal Fixation Device in Head and Facial Bones Internal Fixation Device in Upper Bones Internal Fixation Device in Lower Bones
Bovine pericardial valve	Zooplastic Tissue in Heart and Great Vessels
Bovine pericardium graft	Zooplastic Tissue in Heart and Great Vessels
Brachytherapy seeds	Radioactive Element

Term	ICD-10-PCS Value
BRYAN® Cervical Disc System	Synthetic Substitute
BVS 5000 Ventricular Assist Device	Short-term External Heart Assist System in Heart and Great Vessels
Cardiac contractility modulation lead [NT]	Cardiac Lead in Heart and Great Vessels
Cardiac event recorder	Monitoring Device
Cardiac resynchronization therapy (CRT) lead	Cardiac Lead, Pacemaker for Insertion in Heart and Great Vessels Cardiac Lead, Defibrillator for Insertion in Heart and Great Vessels
CardioMEMS® pressure sensor	Monitoring Device, Pressure Sensor for Insertion in Heart and Great Vessels
Carmat total artificial heart (TAH)	Biologic with Synthetic Substitute, Autoregulated Electrohydraulic for Replacement in Heart and Great Vessels
Carotid (artery) sinus (baroreceptor) lead	Stimulator Lead in Upper Arteries
Carotid WALLSTENT® Monorail® Endoprosthesis	Intraluminal Device
Centrimag® Blood Pump	Short-term External Heart Assist System in Heart and Great Vessels
Ceramic on ceramic bearing surface	Synthetic Substitute, Ceramic for Replacement in Lower Joints
Cesium-131 Collagen Implant	Radioactive Element, Cesium-131 Collagen Implant for Insertion in Central Nervous System and Cranial Nerves
CivaSheet®	Radioactive Element
Clamp and rod internal fixation system (CRIF)	Internal Fixation Device in Upper Bones Internal Fixation Device in Lower Bones
COALESCE® radiolucent interbody fusion device	Interbody Fusion Device, Radiolucent Porous in New Technology
CoAxia NeuroFlo catheter	Intraluminal Device
Cobalt/chromium head and polyethylene socket	Synthetic Substitute, Metal on Polyethylene for Replacement in Lower Joints
Cobalt/chromium head and socket	Synthetic Substitute, Metal for Replacement in Lower Joints
Cochlear implant (CI), multiple channel (electrode)	Hearing Device, Multiple Channel Cochlear Prosthesis for Insertion in Ear, Nose, Sinus
Cochlear implant (CI), single channel (electrode)	Hearing Device, Single Channel Cochlear Prosthesis for Insertion in Ear, Nose, Sinus
COGNIS® CRT-D	Cardiac Resynchronization Defibrillator Pulse Generator for Insertion in Subcutaneous Tissue and Fascia
COHERE® radiolucent interbody fusion device	Interbody Fusion Device, Radiolucent Porous in New Technology
Colonic Z-Stent®	Intraluminal Device
Complete (SE) stent	Intraluminal Device
Concerto II CRT-D	Cardiac Resynchronization Defibrillator Pulse Generator for Insertion in Subcutaneous Tissue and Fascia
CONSERVE® PLUS Total Resurfacing Hip System	Resurfacing Device in Lower Joints
Consulta CRT-D	Cardiac Resynchronization Defibrillator Pulse Generator for Insertion in Subcutaneous Tissue and Fascia
Consulta CRT-P	Cardiac Resynchronization Pacemaker Pulse Generator for Insertion in Subcutaneous Tissue and Fascia

Term	ICD-10-PCS Value
CONTAK RENEWAL® 3 RF (HE) CRT-D	Cardiac Resynchronization Defibrillator Pulse Generator for Insertion in Subcutaneous Tissue and Fascia
Contegra Pulmonary Valved Conduit	Zooplastic Tissue in Heart and Great Vessels
Continuous Glucose Monitoring (CGM) device	Monitoring Device
Cook Biodesign® Fistula Plug(s)	Nonautologous Tissue Substitute
Cook Biodesign® Hernia Graft(s)	Nonautologous Tissue Substitute
Cook Biodesign® Layered Graft(s)	Nonautologous Tissue Substitute
Cook Zenapro™ Layered Graft(s)	Nonautologous Tissue Substitute
Cook Zenith AAA Endovascular Graft	Intraluminal Device
Cook Zenith® Fenestrated AAA Endovascular Graft	Intraluminal Device, Branched or Fenestrated, One or Two Arteries for Restriction in Lower Arteries Intraluminal Device, Branched or Fenestrated, Three or More Arteries for Restriction in Lower Arteries
CoreValve transcatheter aortic valve	Zooplastic Tissue in Heart and Great Vessels
Cormet Hip Resurfacing System	Resurfacing Device in Lower Joints
CoRoent® XL	Interbody Fusion Device in Lower Joints
Corox (OTW) Bipolar Lead	Cardiac Lead, Pacemaker for Insertion in Heart and Great Vessels Cardiac Lead, Defibrillator for Insertion in Heart and Great Vessels
Cortical strip neurostimulator lead	Neurostimulator Lead in Central Nervous System and Cranial Nerves
Corvia IASD®	Synthetic Substitute
Cultured epidermal cell autograft	Autologous Tissue Substitute
CYPHER® Stent	Intraluminal Device, Drug-eluting in Heart and Great Vessels
Cystostomy tube	Drainage Device
DBS lead	Neurostimulator Lead in Central Nervous System and Cranial Nerves
DeBakey Left Ventricular Assist Device	Implantable Heart Assist System in Heart and Great Vessels
Deep brain neurostimulator lead	Neurostimulator Lead in Central Nervous System and Cranial Nerves
Delta frame external fixator	External Fixation Device, Hybrid for Insertion in Upper Bones External Fixation Device, Hybrid for Reposition in Upper Bones External Fixation Device, Hybrid for Insertion in Lower Bones External Fixation Device, Hybrid for Reposition in Lower Bones
Delta III Reverse shoulder prosthesis	Synthetic Substitute, Reverse Ball and Socket for Replacement in Upper Joints
Diaphragmatic pacemaker generator	Stimulator Generator in Subcutaneous Tissue and Fascia
Direct Lateral Interbody Fusion (DLIF) device	Interbody Fusion Device in Lower Joints
Driver stent (RX) (OTW)	Intraluminal Device
DuraHeart Left Ventricular Assist System	Implantable Heart Assist System in Heart and Great Vessels

Term	ICD-10-PCS Value
Durata® Defibrillation Lead	Cardiac Lead, Defibrillator for Insertion in Heart and Great Vessels
DynaNail®	Internal Fixation Device, Sustained Compression for Fusion in Lower Joints Internal Fixation Device, Sustained Compression for Fusion in Upper Joints
DynaNail Mini®	Internal Fixation Device, Sustained Compression for Fusion in Lower Joints Internal Fixation Device, Sustained Compression for Fusion in Upper Joints
Dynesys® Dynamic Stabilization System	Spinal Stabilization Device, Pedicle-Based for Insertion in Upper Joints Spinal Stabilization Device, Pedicle-Based for Insertion in Lower Joints
E-Luminexx™ (Biliary)(Vascular) Stent	Intraluminal Device
EDWARDS INTUITY Elite valve system	Zooplastic Tissue, Rapid Deployment Technique in New Technology
Electrical bone growth stimulator (EBGS)	Bone Growth Stimulator in Head and Facial Bones Bone Growth Stimulator in Upper Bones Bone Growth Stimulator in Lower Bones
Electrical muscle stimulation (EMS) lead	Stimulator Lead in Muscles
Electronic muscle stimulator lead	Stimulator Lead in Muscles
Eluvia™ Drug-eluting Vascular Stent System NT	Intraluminal Device, Sustained Release Drug-eluting in New Technology Intraluminal Device, Sustained Release Drug-eluting, Two in New Technology Intraluminal Device, Sustained Release Drug-eluting, Three in New Technology Intraluminal Device, Sustained Release Drug-eluting, Four or More in New Technology
Embolization coil(s)	Intraluminal Device
Endeavor® (III)(IV) (Sprint) Zotarolimus-eluting Coronary Stent System	Intraluminal Device, Drug-eluting in Heart and Great Vessels
Endologix AFX® Endovascular AAA System	Intraluminal Device
EndoSure® sensor	Monitoring Device, Pressure Sensor for Insertion in Heart and Great Vessels
ENDOTAK RELIANCE® (G) Defibrillation Lead	Cardiac Lead, Defibrillator for Insertion in Heart and Great Vessels
Endotracheal tube (cuffed)(double-lumen)	Intraluminal Device, Endotracheal Airway in Respiratory System
Endurant® Endovascular Stent Graft	Intraluminal Device
Endurant® II AAA stent graft system	Intraluminal Device
EnRhythm	Pacemaker, Dual Chamber for Insertion in Subcutaneous Tissue and Fascia
Enterra gastric neurostimulator	Stimulator Generator, Multiple Array for Insertion in Subcutaneous Tissue and Fascia
Epic™ Stented Tissue Valve (aortic)	Zooplastic Tissue in Heart and Great Vessels
Epicel® cultured epidermal autograft	Autologous Tissue Substitute

Term	ICD-10-PCS Value
Esophageal obturator airway (EOA)	Intraluminal Device, Airway in Gastrointestinal System
Esteem® implantable hearing system	Hearing Device in Ear, Nose, Sinus
Evera (XT)(S)(DR/VR)	Defibrillator Generator for Insertion in Subcutaneous Tissue and Fascia
Everolimus-eluting coronary stent	Intraluminal Device, Drug-eluting in Heart and Great Vessels
Ex-PRESS™ mini glaucoma shunt	Synthetic Substitute
EXCLUDER® AAA Endoprosthesis	Intraluminal Device Intraluminal Device, Branched or Fenestrated, One or Two Arteries for Restriction in Lower Arteries Intraluminal Device, Branched or Fenestrated, Three or More Arteries for Restriction in Lower Arteries
EXCLUDER® IBE Endoprosthesis	Intraluminal Device, Branched or Fenestrated, One or Two Arteries for Restriction in Lower Arteries
Express® (LD) Premounted Stent System	Intraluminal Device
Express® Biliary SD Monorail® Premounted Stent System	Intraluminal Device
Express® SD Renal Monorail® Premounted Stent System	Intraluminal Device
External fixator	External Fixation Device in Head and Facial Bones External Fixation Device in Upper Bones External Fixation Device in Lower Bones External Fixation Device in Upper Joints External Fixation Device in Lower Joints
EXtreme Lateral Interbody Fusion (XLIF) device	Interbody Fusion Device in Lower Joints
Facet replacement spinal stabilization device	Spinal Stabilization Device, Facet Replacement for Insertion in Upper Joints Spinal Stabilization Device, Facet Replacement for Insertion in Lower Joints
FLAIR® Endovascular Stent Graft	Intraluminal Device
Flexible Composite Mesh	Synthetic Substitute
Flow Diverter embolization device	Intraluminal Device, Flow Diverter for Restriction in Upper Arteries
Foley catheter	Drainage Device
Formula™ Balloon-Expandable Renal Stent System	Intraluminal Device
Freestyle (Stentless) Aortic Root Bioprosthesis	Zooplastic Tissue in Heart and Great Vessels
Fusion screw (compression)(lag)(locking)	Internal Fixation Device in Upper Joints Internal Fixation Device in Lower Joints
GammaTile™	Radioactive Element, Cesium-131 Collagen Implant for Insertion in Central Nervous System and Cranial Nerves
Gastric electrical stimulation (GES) lead	Stimulator Lead in Gastrointestinal System
Gastric pacemaker lead	Stimulator Lead in Gastrointestinal System

Term	ICD-10-PCS Value
GORE EXCLUDER® AAA Endoprosthesis	Intraluminal Device Intraluminal Device, Branched or Fenestrated, One or Two Arteries for Restriction in Lower Arteries Intraluminal Device, Branched or Fenestrated, Three or More Arteries for Restriction in Lower Arteries
GORE EXCLUDER® IBE Endoprosthesis	Intraluminal Device, Branched or Fenestrated, One or Two Arteries for Restriction in Lower Arteries
GORE TAG® Thoracic Endoprosthesis	Intraluminal Device
GORE® DUALMESH®	Synthetic Substitute
Guedel airway	Intraluminal Device, Airway in Mouth and Throat
Hancock Bioprosthesis (aortic)(mitral) valve	Zooplastic Tissue in Heart and Great Vessels
Hancock Bioprosthetic Valved Conduit	Zooplastic Tissue in Heart and Great Vessels
HeartMate 3™ LVAS	Implantable Heart Assist System in Heart and Great Vessels
HeartMate II® Left Ventricular Assist Device (LVAD)	Implantable Heart Assist System in Heart and Great Vessels
HeartMate XVE® Left Ventricular Assist Device (LVAD)	Implantable Heart Assist System in Heart and Great Vessels
Herculink (RX) Elite Renal Stent System	Intraluminal Device
Hip (joint) liner	Liner in Lower Joints
Holter valve ventricular shunt	Synthetic Substitute
IASD® (InterAtrial Shunt Device), Corvia	Synthetic Substitute
Ilizarov external fixator	External Fixation Device, Ring for Insertion in Upper Bones External Fixation Device, Ring for Reposition in Upper Bones External Fixation Device, Ring for Insertion in Lower Bones External Fixation Device, Ring for Reposition in Lower Bones
Ilizarov-Vecklich device	External Fixation Device, Limb Lengthening for Insertion in Upper Bones External Fixation Device, Limb Lengthening for Insertion in Lower Bones
Impella® heart pump	Short-term External Heart Assist System in Heart and Great Vessels
Implantable cardioverter-defibrillator (ICD)	Defibrillator Generator for Insertion in Subcutaneous Tissue and Fascia
Implantable drug infusion pump (anti-spasmodic) (chemotherapy)(pain)	Infusion Device, Pump in Subcutaneous Tissue and Fascia
Implantable glucose monitoring device	Monitoring Device
Implantable hemodynamic monitor (IHM)	Monitoring Device, Hemodynamic for Insertion in Subcutaneous Tissue and Fascia
Implantable hemodynamic monitoring system (IHMS)	Monitoring Device, Hemodynamic for Insertion in Subcutaneous Tissue and Fascia
Implantable Miniature Telescope™ (IMT)	Synthetic Substitute, Intraocular Telescope for Replacement in Eye

Term	ICD-10-PCS Value
Implanted (venous)(access) port	Vascular Access Device, Totally Implantable in Subcutaneous Tissue and Fascia
InDura, intrathecal catheter (1P) (spinal)	Infusion Device
Injection reservoir, port	Vascular Access Device, Totally Implantable in Subcutaneous Tissue and Fascia
Injection reservoir, pump	Infusion Device, Pump in Subcutaneous Tissue and Fascia
InterAtrial Shunt Device IASD®, Corvia	Synthetic Substitute
Interbody fusion (spine) cage	Interbody Fusion Device in Upper Joints Interbody Fusion Device in Lower Joints
Interspinous process spinal stabilization device	Spinal Stabilization Device, Interspinous Process for Insertion in Upper Joints Spinal Stabilization Device, Interspinous Process for Insertion in Lower Joints
InterStim™ Micro Therapy neurostimulator	Stimulator Generator, Single Array Rechargeable for Insertion in Subcutaneous Tissue and Fascia
InterStim® Therapy lead	Neurostimulator Lead in Peripheral Nervous System
InterStim™ II Therapy neurostimulator	Stimulator Generator, Single Array for Insertion in Subcutaneous Tissue and Fascia
Intramedullary (IM) rod (nail)	Internal Fixation Device, Intramedullary in Upper Bones Internal Fixation Device, Intramedullary in Lower Bones
Intramedullary skeletal kinetic distractor (ISKD)	Internal Fixation Device, Intramedullary in Upper Bones Internal Fixation Device, Intramedullary in Lower Bones
Intrauterine Device (IUD)	Contraceptive Device in Female Reproductive System
INTUITY Elite valve system, EDWARDS	Zooplastic Tissue, Rapid Deployment Technique in New Technology
Itrel (3)(4) neurostimulator	Stimulator Generator, Single Array for Insertion in Subcutaneous Tissue and Fascia
Joint fixation plate	Internal Fixation Device in Upper Joints Internal Fixation Device in Lower Joints
Joint liner (insert)	Liner in Lower Joints
Joint spacer (antibiotic)	Spacer in Upper Joints Spacer in Lower Joints
Kappa	Pacemaker, Dual Chamber for Insertion in Subcutaneous Tissue and Fascia
Kirschner wire (K-wire)	Internal Fixation Device in Head and Facial Bones Internal Fixation Device in Upper Bones Internal Fixation Device in Lower Bones Internal Fixation Device in Upper Joints Internal Fixation Device in Lower Joints
Knee (implant) insert	Liner in Lower Joints
Kuntscher nail	Internal Fixation Device, Intramedullary in Upper Bones Internal Fixation Device, Intramedullary in Lower Bones
LAP-BAND® adjustable gastric banding system	Extraluminal Device
LifeStent® (Flexstar)(XL) Vascular Stent System	Intraluminal Device

Term	ICD-10-PCS Value
LIVIAN™ CRT-D	Cardiac Resynchronization Defibrillator Pulse Generator for Insertion in Subcutaneous Tissue and Fascia
Loop recorder, implantable	Monitoring Device
MAGEC® Spinal Bracing and Distraction System	Magnetically Controlled Growth Rod(s) in New Technology
Mark IV Breathing Pacemaker System	Stimulator Generator in Subcutaneous Tissue and Fascia
Maximo II DR (VR)	Defibrillator Generator for Insertion in Subcutaneous Tissue and Fascia
Maximo II DR CRT-D	Cardiac Resynchronization Defibrillator Pulse Generator for Insertion in Subcutaneous Tissue and Fascia
Medtronic Endurant® II AAA stent graft system	Intraluminal Device
Melody® transcatheter pulmonary valve	Zooplastic Tissue in Heart and Great Vessels
Metal on metal bearing surface	Synthetic Substitute, Metal for Replacement in Lower Joints
Micro-Driver stent (RX) (OTW)	Intraluminal Device
MicroMed HeartAssist	Implantable Heart Assist System in Heart and Great Vessels
Micrus CERECYTE microcoil	Intraluminal Device, Bioactive in Upper Arteries
MIRODERM™ Biologic Wound Matrix	Skin Substitute, Porcine Liver Derived in New Technology
MitraClip valve repair system	Synthetic Substitute
Mitroflow® Aortic Pericardial Heart Valve	Zooplastic Tissue in Heart and Great Vessels
Mosaic Bioprosthesis (aortic) (mitral) valve	Zooplastic Tissue in Heart and Great Vessels
MULTI-LINK (VISION)(MINI-VISION)(ULTRA) Coronary Stent System	Intraluminal Device
nanoLOCK™ interbody fusion device	Interbody Fusion Device, Nanotextured Surface in New Technology
Nasopharyngeal airway (NPA)	Intraluminal Device, Airway in Ear, Nose, Sinus
Neovasc Reducer™	Reduction Device in New Technology
Neuromuscular electrical stimulation (NEMS) lead	Stimulator Lead in Muscles
Neurostimulator generator, multiple channel	Stimulator Generator, Multiple Array for Insertion in Subcutaneous Tissue and Fascia
Neurostimulator generator, multiple channel rechargeable	Stimulator Generator, Multiple Array Rechargeable for Insertion in Subcutaneous Tissue and Fascia
Neurostimulator generator, single channel	Stimulator Generator, Single Array for Insertion in Subcutaneous Tissue and Fascia
Neurostimulator generator, single channel rechargeable	Stimulator Generator, Single Array Rechargeable for Insertion in Subcutaneous Tissue and Fascia
Neutralization plate	Internal Fixation Device in Head and Facial Bones Internal Fixation Device in Upper Bones Internal Fixation Device in Lower Bones
Nitinol framed polymer mesh	Synthetic Substitute
Non-tunneled central venous catheter	Infusion Device
Novacor Left Ventricular Assist Device	Implantable Heart Assist System in Heart and Great Vessels

Term	ICD-10-PCS Value
Novation® Ceramic AHS® (Articulation Hip System)	Synthetic Substitute, Ceramic for Replacement in Lower Joints
Omnilink Elite Vascular Balloon Expandable Stent System	Intraluminal Device
Open Pivot Aortic Valve Graft (AVG)	Synthetic Substitute
Open Pivot (mechanical) Valve	Synthetic Substitute
Optimizer™ III implantable NT pulse generator	Contractility Modulation Device for Insertion in Subcutaneous Tissue and Fascia
Oropharyngeal airway (OPA)	Intraluminal Device, Airway in Mouth and Throat
Ovatio™ CRT-D	Cardiac Resynchronization Defibrillator Pulse Generator for Insertion in Subcutaneous Tissue and Fascia
OXINIUM	Synthetic Substitute, Oxidized Zirconium on Polyethylene for Replacement in Lower Joints
Paclitaxel-eluting coronary stent	Intraluminal Device, Drug-eluting in Heart and Great Vessels
Paclitaxel-eluting peripheral stent	Intraluminal Device, Drug-eluting in Upper Arteries Intraluminal Device, Drug-eluting in Lower Arteries
Partially absorbable mesh	Synthetic Substitute
Pedicle-based dynamic stabilization device	Spinal Stabilization Device, Pedicle-Based for Insertion in Upper Joints Spinal Stabilization Device, Pedicle-Based for Insertion in Lower Joints
PERCEPT™ PC neurostimulator	Stimulator Generator, Multiple Array for Insertion in Subcutaneous Tissue and Fascia
Perceval sutureless valve	Zooplastic Tissue, Rapid Deployment Technique in New Technology
Percutaneous endoscopic gastrojejunostomy (PEG/J) tube	Feeding Device in Gastrointestinal System
Percutaneous endoscopic gastrostomy (PEG) tube	Feeding Device in Gastrointestinal System
Percutaneous nephrostomy catheter	Drainage Device
Peripherally inserted central catheter (PICC)	Infusion Device
Pessary ring	Intraluminal Device, Pessary in Female Reproductive System
Phrenic nerve stimulator generator	Stimulator Generator in Subcutaneous Tissue and Fascia
Phrenic nerve stimulator lead	Diaphragmatic Pacemaker Lead in Respiratory System
PHYSIOMESH™ Flexible Composite Mesh	Synthetic Substitute
Pipeline™ (Flex) embolization device	Intraluminal Device, Flow Diverter for Restriction in Upper Arteries
Polyethylene socket	Synthetic Substitute, Polyethylene for Replacement in Lower Joints
Polymethylmethacrylate (PMMA)	Synthetic Substitute
Polypropylene mesh	Synthetic Substitute
Porcine (bioprosthetic) valve	Zooplastic Tissue in Heart and Great Vessels

Term	ICD-10-PCS Value
PRECICE intramedullary limb lengthening system	Internal Fixation Device, Intramedullary Limb Lengthening for Insertion in Upper Bones Internal Fixation Device, Intramedullary Limb Lengthening for Insertion in Lower Bones
PRESTIGE® Cervical Disc	Synthetic Substitute
PrimeAdvanced neurostimulator (SureScan)(MRI Safe)	Stimulator Generator, Multiple Array for Insertion in Subcutaneous Tissue and Fascia
PROCEED™ Ventral Patch	Synthetic Substitute
Prodisc-C	Synthetic Substitute
Prodisc-L	Synthetic Substitute
PROLENE Polypropylene Hernia System (PHS)	Synthetic Substitute
Protecta XT CRT-D	Cardiac Resynchronization Defibrillator Pulse Generator for Insertion in Subcutaneous Tissue and Fascia
Protecta XT DR (XT VR)	Defibrillator Generator for Insertion in Subcutaneous Tissue and Fascia
Protégé® RX Carotid Stent System	Intraluminal Device
Pump reservoir	Infusion Device, Pump in Subcutaneous Tissue and Fascia
REALIZE® Adjustable Gastric Band	Extraluminal Device
Rebound HRD® (Hernia Repair Device)	Synthetic Substitute
Reducer™ System	Reduction Device in New Technology
RestoreAdvanced neurostimulator (SureScan)(MRI Safe)	Stimulator Generator, Multiple Array Rechargeable for Insertion in Subcutaneous Tissue and Fascia
RestoreSensor neurostimulator (SureScan)(MRI Safe)	Stimulator Generator, Multiple Array Rechargeable for Insertion in Subcutaneous Tissue and Fascia
RestoreUltra neurostimulator (SureScan)(MRI Safe)	Stimulator Generator, Multiple Array Rechargeable for Insertion in Subcutaneous Tissue and Fascia
Reveal (LINQ)(DX)(XT)	Monitoring Device
Reverse® Shoulder Prosthesis	Synthetic Substitute, Reverse Ball and Socket for Replacement in Upper Joints
Revo MRI™ SureScan® pacemaker	Pacemaker, Dual Chamber for Insertion in Subcutaneous Tissue and Fascia
Rheos® System device	Stimulator Generator in Subcutaneous Tissue and Fascia
Rheos® System lead	Stimulator Lead in Upper Arteries
RNS System lead	Neurostimulator Lead in Central Nervous System and Cranial Nerves
RNS system neurostimulator generator	Neurostimulator Generator in Head and Facial Bones
S-ICD™ lead	Subcutaneous Defibrillator Lead in Subcutaneous Tissue and Fascia
Sacral nerve modulation (SNM) lead	Stimulator Lead in Urinary System
Sacral neuromodulation lead	Stimulator Lead in Urinary System
SAPIEN transcatheter aortic valve	Zooplastic Tissue in Heart and Great Vessels

Term	ICD-10-PCS Value
SAVAL below-the-knee (BTK) drug-eluting stent system	Intraluminal Device, Sustained Release Drug-eluting in New Technology Intraluminal Device, Sustained Release Drug-eluting, Two in New Technology Intraluminal Device, Sustained Release Drug-eluting, Three in New Technology Intraluminal Device, Sustained Release Drug-eluting, Four or More in New Technology
Secura (DR) (VR)	Defibrillator Generator for Insertion in Subcutaneous Tissue and Fascia
Sheffield hybrid external fixator	External Fixation Device, Hybrid for Insertion in Upper Bones External Fixation Device, Hybrid for Reposition in Upper Bones External Fixation Device, Hybrid for Insertion in Lower Bones External Fixation Device, Hybrid for Reposition in Lower Bones
Sheffield ring external fixator	External Fixation Device, Ring for Insertion in Upper Bones External Fixation Device, Ring for Reposition in Upper Bones External Fixation Device, Ring for Insertion in Lower Bones External Fixation Device, Ring for Reposition in Lower Bones
Single lead pacemaker (atrium)(ventricle)	Pacemaker, Single Chamber for Insertion in Subcutaneous Tissue and Fascia
Single lead rate responsive pacemaker (atrium)(ventricle)	Pacemaker, Single Chamber Rate Responsive for Insertion in Subcutaneous Tissue and Fascia
Sirolimus-eluting coronary stent	Intraluminal Device, Drug-eluting in Heart and Great Vessels
SJM Biocor® Stented Valve System	Zooplastic Tissue in Heart and Great Vessels
Spacer, Articulating (Antibiotic)	Articulating Spacer in Lower Joints
Spacer, Static (Antibiotic)	Spacer in Lower Joints
Spinal cord neurostimulator lead	Neurostimulator Lead in Central Nervous System and Cranial Nerves
Spinal growth rods, magnetically controlled	Magnetically Controlled Growth Rod(s) in New Technology
SpineJack® system **NT**	Synthetic Substitute, Mechanically Expandable (Paired) in New Technology
Spiration IBV™ Valve System	Intraluminal Device, Endobronchial Valve in Respiratory System
Static Spacer (Antibiotic)	Spacer in Lower Joints
Stent, intraluminal (cardiovascular) (gastrointestinal) (hepatobiliary)(urinary)	Intraluminal Device
Stented tissue valve	Zooplastic Tissue in Heart and Great Vessels
Stratos LV	Cardiac Resynchronization Pacemaker Pulse Generator for Insertion in Subcutaneous Tissue and Fascia
Subcutaneous injection reservoir, port	Vascular Access Device, Totally Implantable in Subcutaneous Tissue and Fascia
Subcutaneous injection reservoir, pump	Infusion Device, Pump in Subcutaneous Tissue and Fascia

Term	ICD-10-PCS Value
Subdermal progesterone implant	Contraceptive Device in Subcutaneous Tissue and Fascia
Surpass Streamline™ Flow Diverter	Intraluminal Device, Flow Diverter for Restriction in Upper Arteries
Sutureless valve, Perceval	Zooplastic Tissue, Rapid Deployment Technique in New Technology
SynCardia (temporary) Total Artificial Heart (TAH)	Synthetic Substitute, Pneumatic for Replacement in Heart and Great Vessels
SynCardia Total Artificial Heart	Synthetic Substitute
Synchra CRT-P	Cardiac Resynchronization Pacemaker Pulse Generator for Insertion in Subcutaneous Tissue and Fascia
SyncroMed Pump	Infusion Device, Pump in Subcutaneous Tissue and Fascia
Talent® Converter	Intraluminal Device
Talent® Occluder	Intraluminal Device
Talent® Stent Graft (abdominal)(thoracic)	Intraluminal Device
TandemHeart® System	Short-term External Heart Assist System in Heart and Great Vessels
TAXUS® Liberté® Paclitaxel-eluting Coronary Stent System	Intraluminal Device, Drug-eluting in Heart and Great Vessels
Therapeutic occlusion coil(s)	Intraluminal Device
Thoracostomy tube	Drainage Device
Thoraflex™ Hybrid device	Branched Synthetic Substitute with Intraluminal Device in New Technology
Thoratec IVAD (Implantable Ventricular Assist Device)	Implantable Heart Assist System in Heart and Great Vessels
Thoratec Paracorporeal Ventricular Assist Device	Short-term External Heart Assist System in Heart and Great Vessels
Tibial insert	Liner in Lower Joints
Tissue bank graft	Nonautologous Tissue Substitute
Tissue expander (inflatable)(injectable)	Tissue Expander in Skin and Breast Tissue Expander in Subcutaneous Tissue and Fascia
Titanium Sternal Fixation System (TSFS)	Internal Fixation Device, Rigid Plate for Insertion in Upper Bones Internal Fixation Device, Rigid Plate for Reposition in Upper Bones
Total artificial (replacement) heart	Synthetic Substitute
Tracheostomy tube	Tracheostomy Device in Respiratory System
Trifecta™ Valve (aortic)	Zooplastic Tissue in Heart and Great Vessels
Tunneled central venous catheter	Vascular Access Device, Tunneled in Subcutaneous Tissue and Fascia
Tunneled spinal (intrathecal) catheter	Infusion Device
Two lead pacemaker	Pacemaker, Dual Chamber for Insertion in Subcutaneous Tissue and Fascia
Ultraflex™ Precision Colonic Stent System	Intraluminal Device
ULTRAPRO Hernia System (UHS)	Synthetic Substitute
ULTRAPRO Partially Absorbable Lightweight Mesh	Synthetic Substitute
ULTRAPRO Plug	Synthetic Substitute

Term	ICD-10-PCS Value
Ultrasonic osteogenic stimulator	Bone Growth Stimulator in Head and Facial Bones Bone Growth Stimulator in Upper Bones Bone Growth Stimulator in Lower Bones
Ultrasound bone healing system	Bone Growth Stimulator in Head and Facial Bones Bone Growth Stimulator in Upper Bones Bone Growth Stimulator in Lower Bones
Uniplanar external fixator	External Fixation Device, Monoplanar for Insertion in Upper Bones External Fixation Device, Monoplanar for Reposition in Upper Bones External Fixation Device, Monoplanar for Insertion in Lower Bones External Fixation Device, Monoplanar for Reposition in Lower Bones
Urinary incontinence stimulator lead	Stimulator Lead in Urinary System
V-Wave Interatrial Shunt System	Synthetic Substitute
Vaginal pessary	Intraluminal Device, Pessary in Female Reproductive System
Valiant Thoracic Stent Graft	Intraluminal Device
Vectra® Vascular Access Graft	Vascular Access Device, Tunneled in Subcutaneous Tissue and Fascia
Ventrio™ Hernia Patch	Synthetic Substitute
Versa	Pacemaker, Dual Chamber for Insertion in Subcutaneous Tissue and Fascia
Virtuoso (II) (DR) (VR)	Defibrillator Generator for Insertion in Subcutaneous Tissue and Fascia
Viva(XT)(S)	Cardiac Resynchronization Defibrillator Pulse Generator for Insertion in Subcutaneous Tissue and Fascia
WALLSTENT® Endoprosthesis	Intraluminal Device
X-STOP® Spacer	Spinal Stabilization Device, Interspinous Process for Insertion in Upper Joints Spinal Stabilization Device, Interspinous Process for Insertion in Lower Joints
Xact Carotid Stent System	Intraluminal Device
Xenograft	Zooplastic Tissue in Heart and Great Vessels
XIENCE Everolimus Eluting Coronary Stent System	Intraluminal Device, Drug-eluting in Heart and Great Vessels
XLIF® System	Interbody Fusion Device in Lower Joints
Zenith® Fenestrated AAA Endovascular Graft	Intraluminal Device, Branched or Fenestrated, One or Two Arteries for Restriction in Lower Arteries Intraluminal Device, Branched or Fenestrated, Three or More Arteries for Restriction in Lower Arteries Intraluminal Device
Zenith Flex® AAA Endovascular Graft	Intraluminal Device
Zenith TX2® TAA Endovascular Graft	Intraluminal Device
Zenith® Renu™ AAA Ancillary Graft	Intraluminal Device
Zilver® PTX® (paclitaxel) Drug-Eluting Peripheral Stent	Intraluminal Device, Drug-eluting in Upper Arteries Intraluminal Device, Drug-eluting in Lower Arteries
Zimmer® NexGen® LPS Mobile Bearing Knee	Synthetic Substitute

Term	ICD-10-PCS Value
Zimmer® NexGen® LPS-Flex Mobile Knee	Synthetic Substitute
Zotarolimus-eluting coronary stent	Intraluminal Device, Drug-eluting in Heart and Great Vessels

Device Aggregation Table

This table crosswalks specific device character value definitions for specific root operations in a specific body system to the more general device character value to be used when the root operation covers a wide range of body parts and the device character represents an entire family of devices.

Specific Device	for Operation	in Body System	General Device	
Autologous Arterial Tissue (A)	All applicable	Heart and Great Vessels Lower Arteries Lower Veins Upper Arteries Upper Veins	7	Autologous Tissue Substitute
Autologous Venous Tissue (9)	All applicable	Heart and Great Vessels Lower Arteries Lower Veins Upper Arteries Upper Veins	7	Autologous Tissue Substitute
Cardiac Lead, Defibrillator (K)	Insertion	Heart and Great Vessels	M	Cardiac Lead
Cardiac Lead, Pacemaker (J)	Insertion	Heart and Great Vessels	M	Cardiac Lead
Cardiac Resynchronization Defibrillator Pulse Generator (9)	Insertion	Subcutaneous Tissue and Fascia	P	Cardiac Rhythm Related Device
Cardiac Resynchronization Pacemaker Pulse Generator (7)	Insertion	Subcutaneous Tissue and Fascia	P	Cardiac Rhythm Related Device
Contractility Modulation Device (A)	Insertion	Subcutaneous Tissue and Fascia	P	Cardiac Rhythm Related Device
Defibrillator Generator (8)	Insertion	Subcutaneous Tissue and Fascia	P	Cardiac Rhythm Related Device
Epiretinal Visual Prosthesis (5)	All applicable	Eye	J	Synthetic Substitute
External Fixation Device, Hybrid (D)	Insertion	Lower Bones Upper Bones	5	External Fixation Device
External Fixation Device, Hybrid (D)	Reposition	Lower Bones Upper Bones	5	External Fixation Device
External Fixation Device, Limb Lengthening (8)	Insertion	Lower Bones Upper Bones	5	External Fixation Device
External Fixation Device, Monoplanar (B)	Insertion	Lower Bones Upper Bones	5	External Fixation Device
External Fixation Device, Monoplanar (B)	Reposition	Lower Bones Upper Bones	5	External Fixation Device
External Fixation Device, Ring (C)	Insertion	Lower Bones Upper Bones	5	External Fixation Device
External Fixation Device, Ring (C)	Reposition	Lower Bones Upper Bones	5	External Fixation Device
Hearing Device, Bone Conduction (4)	Insertion	Ear, Nose, Sinus	S	Hearing Device
Hearing Device, Multiple Channel Cochlear Prosthesis (6)	Insertion	Ear, Nose, Sinus	S	Hearing Device
Hearing Device, Single Channel Cochlear Prosthesis (5)	Insertion	Ear, Nose, Sinus	S	Hearing Device
Internal Fixation Device, Intramedullary (6)	All applicable	Lower Bones Upper Bones	4	Internal Fixation Device
Internal Fixation Device, Intramedullary Limb Lengthening (7)	Insertion	Lower Bones Upper Bones	6	Internal Fixation Device, Intramedullary
Internal Fixation Device, Rigid Plate (Ø)	Insertion	Upper Bones	4	Internal Fixation Device
Internal Fixation Device, Rigid Plate (Ø)	Reposition	Upper Bones	4	Internal Fixation Device
Intraluminal Device, Airway (B)	All applicable	Ear, Nose, Sinus Gastrointestinal System Mouth and Throat	D	Intraluminal Device
Intraluminal Device, Bioactive (B)	All applicable	Upper Arteries	D	Intraluminal Device
Intraluminal Device, Branched or Fenestrated, One or Two Arteries (E)	Restriction	Heart and Great Vessels Lower Arteries	D	Intraluminal Device

Specific Device	for Operation	in Body System	General Device	
Intraluminal Device, Branched or Fenestrated, Three or More Arteries (F)	Restriction	Heart and Great Vessels Lower Arteries	D	Intraluminal Device
Intraluminal Device, Drug-eluting (4)	All applicable	Heart and Great Vessels Lower Arteries Upper Arteries	D	Intraluminal Device
Intraluminal Device, Drug-eluting, Four or More (7)	All applicable	Heart and Great Vessels Lower Arteries Upper Arteries	D	Intraluminal Device
Intraluminal Device, Drug-eluting, Three (6)	All applicable	Heart and Great Vessels Lower Arteries Upper Arteries	D	Intraluminal Device
Intraluminal Device, Drug-eluting, Two (5)	All applicable	Heart and Great Vessels Lower Arteries Upper Arteries	D	Intraluminal Device
Intraluminal Device, Endobronchial Valve (G)	All applicable	Respiratory System	D	Intraluminal Device
Intraluminal Device, Endotracheal Airway (E)	All applicable	Respiratory System	D	Intraluminal Device
Intraluminal Device, Flow Diverter (H)	Restriction	Upper Arteries	D	Intraluminal Device
Intraluminal Device, Four or More (G)	All applicable	Heart and Great Vessels Lower Arteries Upper Arteries	D	Intraluminal Device
Intraluminal Device, Pessary (G)	All applicable	Female Reproductive System	D	Intraluminal Device
Intraluminal Device, Radioactive (T)	All applicable	Heart and Great Vessels	D	Intraluminal Device
Intraluminal Device, Three (F)	All applicable	Heart and Great Vessels Lower Arteries Upper Arteries	D	Intraluminal Device
Intraluminal Device, Two (E)	All applicable	Heart and Great Vessels Lower Arteries Upper Arteries	D	Intraluminal Device
Monitoring Device, Hemodynamic (Ø)	Insertion	Subcutaneous Tissue and Fascia	2	Monitoring Device
Monitoring Device, Pressure Sensor (Ø)	Insertion	Heart and Great Vessels	2	Monitoring Device
Pacemaker, Dual Chamber (6)	Insertion	Subcutaneous Tissue and Fascia	P	Cardiac Rhythm Related Device
Pacemaker, Single Chamber (4)	Insertion	Subcutaneous Tissue and Fascia	P	Cardiac Rhythm Related Device
Pacemaker, Single Chamber Rate Responsive (5)	Insertion	Subcutaneous Tissue and Fascia	P	Cardiac Rhythm Related Device
Spinal Stabilization Device, Facet Replacement (D)	Insertion	Lower Joints Upper Joints	4	Internal Fixation Device
Spinal Stabilization Device, Interspinous Process (B)	Insertion	Lower Joints Upper Joints	4	Internal Fixation Device
Spinal Stabilization Device, Pedicle-Based (C)	Insertion	Lower Joints Upper Joints	4	Internal Fixation Device
Spinal Stabilization Device, Vertebral Body Tether (3)	Reposition	Lower Bones Upper Bones	4	Internal Fixation Device
Stimulator Generator, Multiple Array (D)	Insertion	Subcutaneous Tissue and Fascia	M	Stimulator Generator
Stimulator Generator, Multiple Array Rechargeable (E)	Insertion	Subcutaneous Tissue and Fascia	M	Stimulator Generator
Stimulator Generator, Single Array (B)	Insertion	Subcutaneous Tissue and Fascia	M	Stimulator Generator
Stimulator Generator, Single Array Rechargeable (C)	Insertion	Subcutaneous Tissue and Fascia	M	Stimulator Generator
Synthetic Substitute, Ceramic (3)	Replacement	Lower Joints	J	Synthetic Substitute
Synthetic Substitute, Ceramic on Polyethylene (4)	Replacement	Lower Joints	J	Synthetic Substitute
Synthetic Substitute, Intraocular Telescope (Ø)	Replacement	Eye	J	Synthetic Substitute
Synthetic Substitute, Metal (1)	Replacement	Lower Joints	J	Synthetic Substitute
Synthetic Substitute, Metal on Polyethylene (2)	Replacement	Lower Joints	J	Synthetic Substitute
Synthetic Substitute, Oxidized Zirconium on Polyethylene (6)	Replacement	Lower Joints	J	Synthetic Substitute
Synthetic Substitute, Polyethylene (Ø)	Replacement	Lower Joints	J	Synthetic Substitute
Synthetic Substitute, Reverse Ball and Socket (Ø)	Replacement	Upper Joints	J	Synthetic Substitute

Appendix G: Device Key and Aggregation Table

Appendix H: Device Definitions

This **NT** symbol next to a device in the Definition column identifies that the device has been approved for NTAP (new technology add-on payment). CMS provides incremental payment, in addition to the DRG payment, for technologies that have received an NTAP designation.

ICD-10-PCS Value	Definition
Articulating Spacer in Lower Joints	**Includes:** Articulating Spacer (Antibiotic) Spacer, Articulating (Antibiotic)
Artificial Sphincter in Gastrointestinal System	**Includes:** Artificial anal sphincter (AAS) Artificial bowel sphincter (neosphincter)
Artificial Sphincter in Urinary System	**Includes:** AMS 800® Urinary Control System Artificial urinary sphincter (AUS)
Autologous Arterial Tissue in Heart and Great Vessels	**Includes:** Autologous artery graft
Autologous Arterial Tissue in Lower Arteries	**Includes:** Autologous artery graft
Autologous Arterial Tissue in Lower Veins	**Includes:** Autologous artery graft
Autologous Arterial Tissue in Upper Arteries	**Includes:** Autologous artery graft
Autologous Arterial Tissue in Upper Veins	**Includes:** Autologous artery graft
Autologous Tissue Substitute	**Includes:** Autograft Cultured epidermal cell autograft Epicel® cultured epidermal autograft
Autologous Venous Tissue in Heart and Great Vessels	**Includes:** Autologous vein graft
Autologous Venous Tissue in Lower Arteries	**Includes:** Autologous vein graft
Autologous Venous Tissue in Lower Veins	**Includes:** Autologous vein graft
Autologous Venous Tissue in Upper Arteries	**Includes:** Autologous vein graft
Autologous Venous Tissue in Upper Veins	**Includes:** Autologous vein graft
Biologic with Synthetic Substitute, Autoregulated Electrohydraulic for Replacement in Heart and Great Vessels	**Includes:** Carmat total artificial heart (TAH)
Bone Growth Stimulator in Head and Facial Bones	**Includes:** Electrical bone growth stimulator (EBGS) Ultrasonic osteogenic stimulator Ultrasound bone healing system
Bone Growth Stimulator in Lower Bones	**Includes:** Electrical bone growth stimulator (EBGS) Ultrasonic osteogenic stimulator Ultrasound bone healing system
Bone Growth Stimulator in Upper Bones	**Includes:** Electrical bone growth stimulator (EBGS) Ultrasonic osteogenic stimulator Ultrasound bone healing system
Branched Synthetic Substitute with Intraluminal Device in New Technology	**Includes:** Thoraflex™ Hybrid device

ICD-10-PCS Value	Definition
Cardiac Lead in Heart and Great Vessels	**Includes:** Cardiac contractility modulation lead **NT**
Cardiac Lead, Defibrillator for Insertion in Heart and Great Vessels	**Includes:** ACUITY™ Steerable Lead Attain Ability® lead Attain StarFix® (OTW) lead Cardiac resynchronization therapy (CRT) lead Corox (OTW) Bipolar Lead Durata® Defibrillation Lead ENDOTAK RELIANCE® (G) Defibrillation Lead
Cardiac Lead, Pacemaker for Insertion in Heart and Great Vessels	**Includes:** ACUITY™ Steerable Lead Attain Ability® lead Attain StarFix® (OTW) lead Cardiac resynchronization therapy (CRT) lead Corox (OTW) Bipolar Lead
Cardiac Resynchronization Defibrillator Pulse Generator for Insertion in Subcutaneous Tissue and Fascia	**Includes:** COGNIS® CRT-D Concerto II CRT-D Consulta CRT-D CONTAK RENEWA® 3 RF (HE) CRT-D LIVIAN™ CRT-D Maximo II DR CRT-D Ovatio™ CRT-D Protecta XT CRT-D Viva (XT)(S)
Cardiac Resynchronization Pacemaker Pulse Generator for Insertion in Subcutaneous Tissue and Fascia	**Includes:** Consulta CRT-P Stratos LV Synchra CRT-P
Contraceptive Device in Female Reproductive System	**Includes:** Intrauterine device (IUD)
Contraceptive Device in Subcutaneous Tissue and Fascia	**Includes:** Subdermal progesterone implant
Contractility Modulation Device for Insertion in Subcutaneous Tissue and Fascia	**Includes:** Optimizer™ III implantable pulse generator **NT**
Defibrillator Generator for Insertion in Subcutaneous Tissue and Fascia	**Includes:** Evera (XT)(S)(DR/VR) Implantable cardioverter-defibrillator (ICD) Maximo II DR (VR) Protecta XT DR (XT VR) Secura (DR) (VR) Virtuoso (II) (DR) (VR)
Diaphragmatic Pacemaker Lead in Respiratory System	**Includes:** Phrenic nerve stimulator lead
Drainage Device	**Includes:** Cystostomy tube Foley catheter Percutaneous nephrostomy catheter Thoracostomy tube

ICD-10-PCS Value	Definition
External Fixation Device in Head and Facial Bones	Includes: External fixator
External Fixation Device in Lower Bones	Includes: External fixator
External Fixation Device in Lower Joints	Includes: External fixator
External Fixation Device in Upper Bones	Includes: External fixator
External Fixation Device in Upper Joints	Includes: External fixator
External Fixation Device, Hybrid for Insertion in Lower Bones	Includes: Delta frame external fixator Sheffield hybrid external fixator
External Fixation Device, Hybrid for Insertion in Upper Bones	Includes: Delta frame external fixator Sheffield hybrid external fixator
External Fixation Device, Hybrid for Reposition in Lower Bones	Includes: Delta frame external fixator Sheffield hybrid external fixator
External Fixation Device, Hybrid for Reposition in Upper Bones	Includes: Delta frame external fixator Sheffield hybrid external fixator
External Fixation Device, Limb Lengthening for Insertion in Lower Bones	Includes: Ilizarov-Vecklich device
External Fixation Device, Limb Lengthening for Insertion in Upper Bones	Includes: Ilizarov-Vecklich device
External Fixation Device, Monoplanar for Insertion in Lower Bones	Includes: Uniplanar external fixator
External Fixation Device, Monoplanar for Insertion in Upper Bones	Includes: Uniplanar external fixator
External Fixation Device, Monoplanar for Reposition in Lower Bones	Includes: Uniplanar external fixator
External Fixation Device, Monoplanar for Reposition in Upper Bones	Includes: Uniplanar external fixator
External Fixation Device, Ring for Insertion in Lower Bones	Includes: Ilizarov external fixator Sheffield ring external fixator
External Fixation Device, Ring for Insertion in Upper Bones	Includes: Ilizarov external fixator Sheffield ring external fixator
External Fixation Device, Ring for Reposition in Lower Bones	Includes: Ilizarov external fixator Sheffield ring external fixator
External Fixation Device, Ring for Reposition in Upper Bones	Includes: Ilizarov external fixator Sheffield ring external fixator
Extraluminal Device	Includes: AtriClip LAA Exclusion System LAP-BAND® adjustable gastric banding system REALIZE® Adjustable Gastric Band
Feeding Device in Gastrointestinal System	Includes: Percutaneous endoscopic gastrojejunostomy (PEG/J) tube Percutaneous endoscopic gastrostomy (PEG) tube

ICD-10-PCS Value	Definition
Hearing Device in Ear, Nose, Sinus	Includes: Esteem® implantable hearing system
Hearing Device in Head and Facial Bones	Includes: Bone anchored hearing device
Hearing Device, Bone Conduction for Insertion in Ear, Nose, Sinus	Includes: Bone anchored hearing device
Hearing Device, Multiple Channel Cochlear Prosthesis for Insertion in Ear, Nose, Sinus	Includes: Cochlear implant (CI), multiple channel (electrode)
Hearing Device, Single Channel Cochlear Prosthesis for Insertion in Ear, Nose, Sinus	Includes: Cochlear implant (CI), single channel (electrode)
Implantable Heart Assist System in Heart and Great Vessels	Includes: Berlin Heart Ventricular Assist Device DeBakey Left Ventricular Assist Device DuraHeart Left Ventricular Assist System HeartMate 3™ LVAS HeartMate II® Left Ventricular Assist Device (LVAD) HeartMate XVE® Left Ventricular Assist Device (LVAD) MicroMed HeartAssist Novacor Left Ventricular Assist Device Thoratec IVAD (Implantable Ventricular Assist Device)
Infusion Device	Includes: Ascenda Intrathecal Catheter InDura, intrathecal catheter (1P) (spinal) Non-tunneled central venous catheter Peripherally inserted central catheter (PICC) Tunneled spinal (intrathecal) catheter
Infusion Device, Pump in Subcutaneous Tissue and Fascia	Includes: Implantable drug infusion pump (anti-spasmodic)(chemotherapy) (pain) Injection reservoir, pump Pump reservoir Subcutaneous injection reservoir, pump SynchroMed pump
Interbody Fusion Device, Customizable in New Technology	Includes: aprevo™
Interbody Fusion Device in Lower Joints	Includes: Axial Lumbar Interbody Fusion System AxiaLIF® System CoRoent® XL Direct Lateral Interbody Fusion (DLIF) device EXtreme Lateral Interbody Fusion (XLIF) device Interbody fusion (spine) cage XLIF® System
Interbody Fusion Device in Upper Joints	Includes: BAK/C® Interbody Cervical Fusion System Interbody fusion (spine) cage
Interbody Fusion Device, Customizable in New Technology	Includes: aprevo™
Interbody Fusion Device, Nanotextured Surface in New Technology	Includes: nanoLOCK™ interbody fusion device

Appendix H: Device Definitions

ICD-10-PCS Value	Definition
Interbody Fusion Device, Radiolucent Porous in New Technology	Includes: COALESCE® radiolucent interbody fusion device COHERE® radiolucent interbody fusion device
Internal Fixation Device in Head and Facial Bones	**Includes:** Bone screw (interlocking)(lag)(pedicle) (recessed) Kirschner wire (K-wire) Neutralization plate
Internal Fixation Device in Lower Bones	**Includes:** Bone screw (interlocking)(lag)(pedicle) (recessed) Clamp and rod internal fixation system (CRIF) Kirschner wire (K-wire) Neutralization plate
Internal Fixation Device in Lower Joints	**Includes:** Fusion screw (compression)(lag)(locking) Joint fixation plate Kirschner wire (K-wire)
Internal Fixation Device in Upper Bones	**Includes:** Bone screw (interlocking)(lag)(pedicle) (recessed) Clamp and rod internal fixation system (CRIF) Kirschner wire (K-wire) Neutralization plate
Internal Fixation Device in Upper Joints	**Includes:** Fusion screw (compression)(lag)(locking) Joint fixation plate Kirschner wire (K-wire)
Internal Fixation Device, Intramedullary in Lower Bones	**Includes:** Intramedullary (IM) rod (nail) Intramedullary skeletal kinetic distractor (ISKD) Kuntscher nail
Internal Fixation Device, Intramedullary in Upper Bones	**Includes:** Intramedullary (IM) rod (nail) Intramedullary skeletal kinetic distractor (ISKD) Kuntscher nail
Internal Fixation Device Intramedullary Limb Lengthening for Insertion in Lower Bones	**Includes:** PRECICE intramedullary limb lengthening system
Internal Fixation Device Intramedullary Limb Lengthening for Insertion in Upper Bones	**Includes:** PRECICE intramedullary limb lengthening system
Internal Fixation Device, Rigid Plate for Insertion in Upper Bones	**Includes:** Titanium Sternal Fixation System (TSFS)
Internal Fixation Device, Rigid Plate for Reposition in Upper Bones	**Includes:** Titanium Sternal Fixation System (TSFS)
Internal Fixation Device, Sustained Compression for Fusion in Lower Joints	**Includes:** DynaNail® DynaNail Mini®
Internal Fixation Device, Sustained Compression for Fusion in Upper Joints	**Includes:** DynaNail® DynaNail Mini®

ICD-10-PCS Value	Definition
Intraluminal Device	**Includes:** Absolute Pro Vascular (OTW) Self-Expanding Stent System Acculink (RX) Carotid Stent System AFX® Endovascular AAA System AneuRx® AAA Advantage® Assurant (Cobalt) stent Carotid WALLSTENT® Monorail® Endoprosthesis CoAxia NeuroFlo catheter Colonic Z-Stent® Complete (SE) stent Cook Zenith AAA Endovascular Graft Driver stent (RX) (OTW) E-Luminexx™ (Biliary)(Vascular) Stent Embolization coil(s) Endologix AFX® Endovascular AAA System Endurant® Endovascular Stent Graft Endurant® II AAA stent graft system EXCLUDER® AAA Endoprosthesis Express® (LD) Premounted Stent System Express® Biliary SD Monorail® Premounted Stent System Express® SD Renal Monorail® Premounted Stent System FLAIR® Endovascular Stent Graft Formula™ Balloon-Expandable Renal Stent System GORE EXCLUDER® AAA Endoprosthesis GORE TAG® Thoracic Endoprosthesis Herculink (RX) Elite Renal Stent System LifeStent® (Flexstar)(XL) Vascular Stent System Medtronic Endurant® II AAA stent graft system Micro-Driver stent (RX) (OTW) MULTI-LINK (VISION)(MINI-VISION)(ULTRA) Coronary Stent System Omnilink Elite Vascular Balloon Expandable Stent System Protege® RX Carotid Stent System Stent, intraluminal (cardiovascular) (gastrointestinal)(hepatobiliary) (urinary) Talent® Converter Talent® Occluder Talent® Stent Graft (abdominal)(thoracic) Therapeutic occlusion coil(s) Ultraflex™ Precision Colonic Stent System Valiant Thoracic Stent Graft WALLSTENT® Endoprosthesis Xact Carotid Stent System Zenith AAA Endovascular Graft Zenith Flex® AAA Endovascular Graft Zenith TX2® TAA Endovascular Graft Zenith® Renu™ AAA Ancillary Graft
Intraluminal Device, Airway in Ear, Nose, Sinus	**Includes:** Nasopharyngeal airway (NPA)
Intraluminal Device, Airway in Gastrointestinal System	**Includes:** Esophageal obturator airway (EOA)
Intraluminal Device, Airway in Mouth and Throat	**Includes:** Guedel airway Oropharyngeal airway (OPA)
Intraluminal Device, Bioactive in Upper Arteries	**Includes:** Bioactive embolization coil(s) Micrus CERECYTE microcoil

ICD-10-PCS Value	Definition
Intraluminal Device, Branched or Fenestrated, One or Two Arteries for Restriction in Lower Arteries	**Includes:** Cook Zenith® Fenestrated AAA Endovascular Graft EXCLUDER® AAA Endoprosthesis EXCLUDER® IBE Endoprosthesis GORE EXCLUDER® AAA Endoprosthesis GORE EXCLUDER®IBE Endoprosthesis Zenith® Fenestrated AAA Endovascular Graft
Intraluminal Device, Branched or Fenestrated, Three or More Arteries for Restriction in Lower Arteries	**Includes:** Cook Zenith® Fenestrated AAA Endovascular Graft EXCLUDER® AAA Endoprosthesis GORE EXCLUDER® AAA Endoprosthesis Zenith® Fenestrated AAA Endovascular Graft
Intraluminal Device, Drug-eluting in Heart and Great Vessels	**Includes:** CYPHER® Stent Endeavor® (III)(IV) (Sprint) Zotarolimus-eluting Coronary Stent System Everolimus-eluting coronary stent Paclitaxel-eluting coronary stent Sirolimus-eluting coronary stent TAXUS® Liberte® Paclitaxel-eluting Coronary Stent System XIENCE Everolimus Eluting Coronary Stent System Zotarolimus-eluting coronary stent
Intraluminal Device, Drug-eluting in Lower Arteries	**Includes:** Paclitaxel-eluting peripheral stent Zilver® PTX® (paclitaxel) Drug-Eluting Peripheral Stent
Intraluminal Device, Drug-eluting in Upper Arteries	**Includes:** Paclitaxel-eluting peripheral stent Zilver® PTX® (paclitaxel) Drug-Eluting Peripheral Stent
Intraluminal Device, Endobronchial Valve in Respiratory System	**Includes:** Spiration IBV™ Valve System
Intraluminal Device, Endotracheal Airway in Respiratory System	**Includes:** Endotracheal tube (cuffed)(double-lumen)
Intraluminal Device, Flow Diverter for Restriction in Upper Arteries	**Includes:** Flow Diverter embolization device Pipeline™ (Flex) embolization device Surpass Streamline™ Flow Diverter
Intraluminal Device, Pessary in Female Reproductive System	**Includes:** Pessary ring Vaginal pessary
Intraluminal Device, Sustained Release Drug-eluting in New Technology	**Includes:** Eluvia™ Drug-eluting Vascular Stent System **NT** SAVAL below-the-knee (BTK) drug-eluting stent system
Intraluminal Device, Sustained Release Drug-eluting, Four or More in New Technology	**Includes:** Eluvia™ Drug-eluting Vascular Stent System **NT** SAVAL below-the-knee (BTK) drug-eluting stent system
Intraluminal Device, Sustained Release Drug-eluting, Three in New Technology	**Includes:** Eluvia™ Drug-eluting Vascular Stent System **NT** SAVAL below-the-knee (BTK) drug-eluting stent system

ICD-10-PCS Value	Definition
Intraluminal Device, Sustained Release Drug-eluting, Two in New Technology	**Includes:** Eluvia™ Drug-eluting Vascular Stent System **NT** SAVAL below-the-knee (BTK) drug-eluting stent system
Liner in Lower Joints	**Includes:** Acetabular cup Hip (joint) liner Joint liner (insert) Knee (implant) insert Tibial insert
Magnetically Controlled Growth Rod(s) in New Technology	**Includes:** MAGEC® Spinal Bracing and Distraction System Spinal growth rods, magnetically controlled
Monitoring Device	**Includes:** Blood glucose monitoring system Cardiac event recorder Continuous Glucose Monitoring (CGM) device Implantable glucose monitoring device Loop recorder, implantable Reveal (LINQ)(DX)(XT)
Monitoring Device, Hemodynamic for Insertion in Subcutaneous Tissue and Fascia	**Includes:** Implantable hemodynamic monitor (IHM) Implantable hemodynamic monitoring system (IHMS)
Monitoring Device, Pressure Sensor for Insertion in Heart and Great Vessels	**Includes:** CardioMEMS® pressure sensor EndoSure® sensor
Neurostimulator Generator in Head and Facial Bones	**Includes:** RNS system neurostimulator generator
Neurostimulator Lead in Central Nervous System and Cranial Nerves	**Includes:** Cortical strip neurostimulator lead DBS lead Deep brain neurostimulator lead RNS System lead Spinal cord neurostimulator lead
Neurostimulator Lead in Peripheral Nervous System	**Includes:** InterStim® Therapy lead
Nonautologous Tissue Substitute	**Includes:** Acellular Hydrated Dermis Bone bank bone graft Cook Biodesign® Fistula Plug(s) Cook Biodesign® Hernia Graft(s) Cook Biodesign® Layered Graft(s) Cook Zenapro™ Layered Graft(s) Tissue bank graft
Other Device	**Includes:** Alfapump® system
Pacemaker, Dual Chamber for Insertion in Subcutaneous Tissue and Fascia	**Includes:** Advisa (MRI) EnRhythm Kappa Revo MRI™ SureScan® pacemaker Two lead pacemaker Versa
Pacemaker, Single Chamber for Insertion in Subcutaneous Tissue and Fascia	**Includes:** Single lead pacemaker (atrium)(ventricle)

ICD-10-PCS Value	Definition
Pacemaker, Single Chamber Rate Responsive for Insertion in Subcutaneous Tissue and Fascia	**Includes:** Single lead rate responsive pacemaker (atrium)(ventricle)
Posterior (Dynamic) Distraction Device in New Technology	**Includes:** ApiFix® Minimally Invasive Deformity Correction (MID-C) System
Radioactive Element	**Includes:** Brachytherapy seeds CivaSheet®
Radioactive Element, Cesium-131 Collagen Implant for Insertion in Central Nervous System and Cranial Nerves	**Includes:** Cesium-131 Collagen Implant GammaTile™
Reduction Device in New Technology	**Includes:** Neovasc Reducer™ Reducer™ System
Resurfacing Device in Lower Joints	**Includes:** CONSERVE® PLUS Total Resurfacing Hip System Cormet Hip Resurfacing System
Short-term External Heart Assist System in Heart and Great Vessels	**Includes:** Biventricular external heart assist system BVS 5000 Ventricular Assist Device Centrimag® Blood Pump Impella® heart pump TandemHeart® System Thoratec Paracorporeal Ventricular Assist Device
Skin Substitute, Porcine Liver Derived in New Technology	**Includes:** MIRODERM™ Biologic Wound Matrix
Spacer in Lower Joints	**Includes:** Joint spacer (antibiotic) Spacer, Static (Antibiotic) Static Spacer (Antibiotic)
Spacer in Upper Joints	**Includes:** Joint spacer (antibiotic)
Spinal Stabilization Device, Facet Replacement for Insertion in Lower Joints	**Includes:** Facet replacement spinal stabilization device
Spinal Stabilization Device, Facet Replacement for Insertion in Upper Joints	**Includes:** Facet replacement spinal stabilization device
Spinal Stabilization Device, Interspinous Process for Insertion in Lower Joints	**Includes:** Interspinous process spinal stabilization device X-STOP® Spacer
Spinal Stabilization Device, Interspinous Process for Insertion in Upper Joints	**Includes:** Interspinous process spinal stabilization device X-STOP® Spacer
Spinal Stabilization Device, Pedicle- Based for Insertion in Lower Joints	**Includes:** Dynesys® Dynamic Stabilization System Pedicle-based dynamic stabilization device
Spinal Stabilization Device, Pedicle-Based for Insertion in Upper Joints	**Includes:** Dynesys® Dynamic Stabilization System Pedicle-based dynamic stabilization device

ICD-10-PCS Value	Definition
Stimulator Generator in Subcutaneous Tissue and Fascia	**Includes:** Baroreflex Activation Therapy® (BAT®) [NT] Diaphragmatic pacemaker generator Mark IV Breathing Pacemaker System Phrenic nerve stimulator generator Rheos® System device
Stimulator Generator, Multiple Array for Insertion in Subcutaneous Tissue and Fascia	**Includes:** Activa PC neurostimulator Enterra gastric neurostimulator Neurostimulator generator, multiple channel PERCEPT™ PC neurostimulator PrimeAdvanced neurostimulator (SureScan)(MRI Safe)
Stimulator Generator, Multiple Array Rechargeable for Insertion in Subcutaneous Tissue and Fascia	**Includes:** Activa RC neurostimulator Neurostimulator generator, multiple channel rechargeable RestoreAdvanced neurostimulator (SureScan)(MRI Safe) RestoreSensor neurostimulator (SureScan)(MRI Safe) RestoreUltra neurostimulator (SureScan)(MRI Safe)
Stimulator Generator, Single Array for Insertion in Subcutaneous Tissue and Fascia	**Includes:** Activa SC neurostimulator InterStim™ II Therapy neurostimulator Itrel (3)(4) neurostimulator Neurostimulator generator, single channel
Stimulator Generator, Single Array Rechargeable for Insertion in Subcutaneous Tissue and Fascia	**Includes:** InterStim™ Micro Therapy neurostimulator Neurostimulator generator, single channel rechargeable
Stimulator Lead in Gastrointestinal System	**Includes:** Gastric electrical stimulation (GES) lead Gastric pacemaker lead
Stimulator Lead in Muscles	**Includes:** Electrical muscle stimulation (EMS) lead Electronic muscle stimulator lead Neuromuscular electrical stimulation (NEMS) lead
Stimulator Lead in Upper Arteries	**Includes:** Baroreflex Activation Therapy® (BAT®) [NT] Carotid (artery) sinus (baroreceptor) lead Rheos® System lead
Stimulator Lead in Urinary System	**Includes:** Sacral nerve modulation (SNM) lead Sacral neuromodulation lead Urinary incontinence stimulator lead
Subcutaneous Defibrillator Lead in Subcutaneous Tissue and Fascia	**Includes:** S-ICD™ lead

ICD-10-PCS Value	Definition
Synthetic Substitute	**Includes:** AbioCor® Total Replacement Heart AMPLATZER® Muscular VSD Occluder Annuloplasty ring Bard® Composix® (E/X) (LP) mesh Bard® Composix® Kugel® patch Bard® Dulex™ mesh Bard® Ventralex™ hernia patch Barricaid® Annular Closure Device (ACD) BRYAN® Cervical Disc System Corvia IASD® Ex-PRESS™ mini glaucoma shunt Flexible Composite Mesh GORE® DUALMESH® Holter valve ventricular shunt IASD® (InterAtrial Shunt Device), Corvia InterAtrial Shunt Device IASD®, Corvia MitraClip valve repair system Nitinol framed polymer mesh Open Pivot (mechanical) valve Open Pivot Aortic Valve Graft (AVG) Partially absorbable mesh PHYSIOMESH™ Flexible Composite Mesh Polymethylmethacrylate (PMMA) Polypropylene mesh PRESTIGE® Cervical Disc PROCEED™ Ventral Patch Prodisc-C Prodisc-L PROLENE Polypropylene Hernia System (PHS) Rebound HRD® (Hernia Repair Device) SynCardia Total Artificial Heart Total artificial (replacement) heart ULTRAPRO Hernia System (UHS) ULTRAPRO Partially Absorbable Lightweight Mesh ULTRAPRO Plug V-Wave Interatrial Shunt System Ventrio™ Hernia Patch Zimmer® NexGen® LPS Mobile Bearing Knee Zimmer® NexGen® LPS-Flex Mobile Knee
Synthetic Substitute, Ceramic for Replacement in Lower Joints	**Includes:** Ceramic on ceramic bearing surface Novation® Ceramic AHS® (Articulation Hip System)
Synthetic Substitute, Intraocular Telescope for Replacement in Eye	**Includes:** Implantable Miniature Telescope™ (IMT)
Synthetic Substitute, Mechanically Expandable (Paired) in New Technology	**Includes:** SpineJack® system `NT`
Synthetic Substitute, Metal for Replacement in Lower Joints	**Includes:** Cobalt/chromium head and socket Metal on metal bearing surface
Synthetic Substitute, Metal on Polyethylene for Replacement in Lower Joints	**Includes:** Cobalt/chromium head and polyethylene socket
Synthetic Substitute, Oxidized Zirconium on Polyethylene for Replacement in Lower Joints	**Includes:** OXINIUM
Synthetic Substitute, Pneumatic for Replacement in Heart and Great Vessels	**Includes:** SynCardia (temporary) total artificial heart (TAH)

ICD-10-PCS Value	Definition
Synthetic Substitute, Polyethylene for Replacement in Lower Joints	**Includes:** Polyethylene socket
Synthetic Substitute, Reverse Ball and Socket for Replacement in Upper Joints	**Includes:** Delta III Reverse shoulder prosthesis Reverse® Shoulder Prosthesis
Tissue Expander in Skin and Breast	**Includes:** Tissue expander (inflatable) (injectable)
Tissue Expander in Subcutaneous Tissue and Fascia	**Includes:** Tissue expander (inflatable) (injectable)
Tracheostomy Device in Respiratory System	**Includes:** Tracheostomy tube
Vascular Access Device, Totally Implantable in Subcutaneous Tissue and Fascia	**Includes:** Implanted (venous)(access) port Injection reservoir, port Subcutaneous injection reservoir, port
Vascular Access Device, Tunneled in Subcutaneous Tissue and Fascia	**Includes:** Tunneled central venous catheter Vectra® Vascular Access Graft
Zooplastic Tissue in Heart and Great Vessels	**Includes:** 3f (Aortic) Bioprosthesis valve Bovine pericardial valve Bovine pericardium graft Contegra Pulmonary Valved Conduit CoreValve transcatheter aortic valve Epic™ Stented Tissue Valve (aortic) Freestyle (Stentless) Aortic Root Bioprosthesis Hancock Bioprosthesis (aortic) (mitral) valve Hancock Bioprosthetic Valved Conduit Melody® transcatheter pulmonary valve Mitroflow® Aortic Pericardial Heart Valve Mosaic Bioprosthesis (aortic) (mitral) valve Porcine (bioprosthetic) valve SAPIEN transcatheter aortic valve SJM Biocor® Stented Valve System Stented tissue valve Trifecta™ Valve (aortic) Xenograft
Zooplastic Tissue, Rapid Deployment Technique in New Technology	**Includes:** EDWARDS INTUITY Elite valve system INTUITY Elite valve system, EDWARDS Perceval sutureless valve Sutureless valve, Perceval

Appendix I: Substance Key/Substance Definitions

Substance Key

This table crosswalks a specific substance, listed by trade name or synonym, to the PCS value that would be used to represent that substance in either the Administration or New Technology section. The ICD-10-PCS value may be located in either the 6th-character Substance column or the 7th-character Qualifier column depending on the section/table to which it is classified. The most specific character is listed in the table.

This **NT** symbol next to a substance/technology in the Trade Name or Synonym column identifies that the substance/technology has been approved for NTAP (new technology add-on payment). CMS provides incremental payment, in addition to the DRG payment, for technologies that have received an NTAP designation.

Substances denoted by an asterisk (*) in the Trade Name or Synonym column, although not included in the official ICD-10-PCS classification, were added based on information provided in the FY 2022 IPPS proposed rule.

Trade Name or Synonym	ICD-10-PCS Value	PCS Section
ABECMA®	Idecabtagene Vicleucel Immunotherapy (K)	New Technology (X)
ACTEMRA®	Tocilizumab (H)	New Technology (X)
AIGISRx Antibacterial Envelope	Anti-Infective Envelope (A)	Administration (3)
Andexanet Alfa, Factor Xa Inhibitor Reversal Agent	Coagulation Factor Xa, Inactivated (7)	New Technology (X)
Andexxa **NT**	Coagulation Factor Xa, Inactivated (7)	New Technology (X)
Angiotensin II	Synthetic Human Angiotensin II (H)	New Technology (X)
Antibacterial Envelope (TYRX) (AIGISRx)	Anti-Infective Envelope (A)	Administration (3)
Antimicrobial envelope	Anti-Infective Envelope (A)	Administration (3)
Anti-SARS-CoV-2 hyperimmune globulin	Hyperimmune Globulin (E)	New Technology (X)
AVYCAZ® (ceftazidime-avibactam)	Other Anti-infective (9)	Administration (3)
Axicabtagene Ciloeucel	Axicabtagene Ciloeucel Immunotherapy (H)	New Technology (X)
AZEDRA® **NT**	Iobenguane I-131 Antineoplastic (S)	New Technology (X)
*Balversa™ **NT**	Erdafitinib Antineoplastic (L)	New Technology (X)
Blinatumomab	Other Antineoplastic (5)	Administration (3)
BLINCYTO® (blinatumomab)	Other Antineoplastic (5)	Administration (3)
Bone morphogenetic protein 2 (BMP 2)	Recombinant Bone Morphogenetic Protein (B)	Administration (3)
Brexucabtagene Autoleucel	Brexucabtagene Autoleucel Immunotherapy (4)	New Technology (X)
*CABLIVI® **NT**	Caplacizumab (W)	New Technology (X)
Casirivimab (REGN10933) and Imdevimab (REGN10987)	REGN-COV2 Monoclonal Antibody (G)	New Technology (X)
CBMA (Concentrated Bone Marrow Aspirate)	Concentrated Bone Marrow Aspirate (Ø)	New Technology (X)
Ceftazidime-avibactam	Other Anti-infective (9)	Administration (3)
CERAMENT® G	Antibiotic-eluting Bone Void Filler (P)	New Technology (X)
cilta-cel	Ciltacabtagene Autoleucel (A)	New Technology (X)
Clolar	Clofarabine (P)	Administration (3)
Coagulation Factor Xa, (Recombinant) Inactivated	Coagulation Factor Xa, Inactivated (7)	New Technology (X)
CONTEPO™	Fosfomycin Anti-infective (K)	New Technology (X)
COSELA™	Trilaciclib (7)	New Technology (X)
CRESEMBA® (isavuconazonium sulfate)	Other Anti-infective (9)	Administration (3)
Defitelio	Defibrotide Sodium Anticoagulant (9)	New Technology (X)
DuraGraft® Endothelial Damage Inhibitor	Endothelial Damage Inhibitor (8)	New Technology (X)
ELZONRIS™ **NT**	Tagraxofusp-erzs Antineoplastic (Q)	New Technology (X)
ENSPRYNG™	Satralizumab-mwge (9)	New Technology (X)
ERLEADA™	Apalutamide Antineoplastic (J)	New Technology (X)
Factor Xa Inhibitor Reversal Agent, Andexanet Alfa	Coagulation Factor Xa, Inactivated (7)	New Technology (X)
FETROJA® **NT**	Cefiderocol Anti-infective (A)	New Technology (X)
Fosfomycin injection	Fosfomycin Anti-infective (K)	New Technology (X)
Gammaglobulin	Globulin (S)	Administration (3)
GAMUNEX-C, for COVID-19 treatment	High-Dose Intravenous Immune Globulin (D)	New Technology (X)
GIAPREZA™	Synthetic Human Angiotensin II (H)	New Technology (X)
GS-5734	Remdesivir Anti-infective (E)	New Technology (X)
hdIVIG (high-dose intravenous immunoglobulin), for COVID-19 treatment	High-Dose Intravenous Immune Globulin (D)	New Technology (X)
Hemospray® Endoscopic Hemostat **NT**	Mineral-based Topical Hemostatic Agent (8)	New Technology (X)
HIG (hyperimmune globulin), for COVID-19 treatment	Hyperimmune Globulin (E)	New Technology (X)

Trade Name or Synonym	ICD-10-PCS Value	PCS Section
High-dose intravenous immunoglobulin (hdIVIG), for COVID-19 treatment	Hyperimmune Globulin (E)	New Technology (X)
hIVIG (hyperimmune intravenous immunoglobulin), for COVID-19 treatment	Hyperimmune Globulin (E)	New Technology (X)
Human angiotensin II, synthetic	Synthetic Human Angiotensin II (H)	New Technology (X)
Hyperimmune globulin	Globulin (S)	Administration (3)
Hyperimmune intravenous immunoglobulin (hIVIG), for COVID-19 treatment	Hyperimmune Globulin (E)	New Technology (X)
Idarucizumab, Pradaxa® (dabigatran) reversal agent	Other Therapeutic Substance (G)	Administration (3)
Idecabtagene Vicleucel	Idecabtagene Vicleucel Immunotherapy (K)	New Technology (X)
Ide-cel	Idecabtagene Vicleucel Immunotherapy (K)	New Technology (X)
IGIV-C, for COVID-19 treatment	Hyperimmune Globulin (E)	New Technology (X)
Imdevimab (REGN10987) and Casirivimab (REGN10933)	REGN-COV2 Monoclonal Antibody (G)	New Technology (X)
IMFINZI®　ᴺᵀ	Durvalumab Antineoplastic (3)	New Technology (X)
IMI/REL	Imipenem-cilastatin-relebactam Anti-infective (U)	New Technology (X)
Immunoglobulin	Globulin (S)	Administration (3)
INTERCEPT Blood System for Plasma Pathogen Reduced Cryoprecipitated Fibrinogen Complex	Pathogen Reduced Cryoprecipitated Fibrinogen Complex (D)	Administration (3)
INTERCEPT Fibrinogen Complex	Pathogen Reduced Cryoprecipitated Fibrinogen Complex (D)	Administration (3)
Iobenguane I-131, High Specific Activity (HSA)	Iobenguane I-131 Antineoplastic (S)	New Technology (X)
Isavuconazole (isavuconazonium sulfate)	Other Anti-infective (9)	Administration (3)
Jakafi®　ᴺᵀ	Ruxolitinib (T)	New Technology (X)
Kcentra	4-Factor Prothrombin Complex Concentrate (B)	Administration (3)
KEVZARA®	Sarilumab (G)	New Technology (X)
KYMRIAH	Tisagenlecleucel Immunotherapy (J)	New Technology (X)
Lifileucel	Lifileucel Immunotherapy (L)	New Technology (X)
Lisocabtagene Maraleucel	Lisocabtagene Maraleucel Immunotherapy (7)	New Technology (X)
LTX Regional Anticoagulant	Nafamostat Anticoagulant (3)	New Technology (X)
NA-1 (Nerinitide)	Nerinitide (2)	New Technology (X)
Nesiritide	Human B-type Natriuretic Peptide (H)	Administration (3)
NexoBrid™	Bromelain-enriched Proteolytic Enzyme (2)	New Technology (X)
Niyad™	Nafamostat Anticoagulant (3)	New Technology (X)
NUZYRA™　ᴺᵀ	Omadacycline Anti-infective (B)	New Technology (X)
Octagam 10%, for COVID-19 treatment	High-Dose Intravenous Immune Globulin (D)	New Technology (X)
Olumiant®　ᴺᵀ	Baricitinib (M)	New Technology (X)
OTL-101	Hematopoietic Stem/Progenitor Cells, Genetically Modified (C)	Administration (3)
OTL-103	Hematopoietic Stem/Progenitor Cells, Genetically Modified (C)	Administration (3)
OTL-200	Hematopoietic Stem/Progenitor Cells, Genetically Modified (C)	Administration (3)
Polyclonal hyperimmune globulin	Globulin (S)	Administration (3)
Praxbind® (idarucizumab), Pradaxa® (dabigatran) reversal agent	Other Therapeutic Substance (G)	Administration (3)
*RECARBRIO™　ᴺᵀ	Imipenem-cilastatin-relebactam Anti-infective (U)	New Technology (X)
rhBMP-2	Recombinant Bone Morphogenetic Protein (B)	Administration (3)
Seprafilm	Adhesion Barrier (5)	Administration (3)
Soliris®　ᴺᵀ	Eculizumab (C)	New Technology (X)
SPRAVATO™　ᴺᵀ	Esketamine Hydrochloride (M)	New Technology (X)
STELARA®	Other New Technology Therapeutic Substance (F)	New Technology (X)
StrataGraft®	Bioengineered Allogeneic Construct (F)	New Technology (X)
Tecartus™	Brexucabtagene Autoleucel Immunotherapy (M)	New Technology (X)
TECENTRIQ®　ᴺᵀ	Atezolizumab Antineoplastic (D)	New Technology (X)
TERLIVAZ®	Terlipressin (6)	New Technology (X)
Tisagenlecleucel	Tisagenlecleucel Immunotherapy (J)	New Technology (X)
Tissue Plasminogen Activator (tPA)(r- tPA)	Other Thrombolytic (7)	Administration (3)
TYRX Antibacterial Envelope	Anti-Infective Envelope (A)	Administration (3)
Ustekinumab	Other New Technology Therapeutic Substance (F)	New Technology (X)
Vabomere™	Meropenem-vaborbactam Anti-infective (N)	New Technology (X)
Veklury　ᴺᵀ	Remdesivir Anti-infective (E)	New Technology (X)
Venclexta®	Ventoclax Antineoplastic (R)	New Technology (X)

Trade Name or Synonym		ICD-10-PCS Value	PCS Section
Vistogard®		Uridine Triacetate (8)	New Technology (X)
Voraxaze		Glucarpidase (Q)	Administration (3)
VYXEOS™		Cytarabine and Daunorubicin Liposome Antineoplastic (B)	New Technology (X)
XENLETA™	NT	Lefamulin Anti-infective (6)	New Technology (X)
XOSPATA®	NT	Gilteritinib Antineoplastic (V)	New Technology (X)
*ZEMDRI™	NT	Plazomicin Anti-infective (6)	New Technology (X)
ZEPZELCA™		Lurbinectedin (8)	New Technology (X)
ZERBAXA®	NT	Ceftolozane/Tazobactam Anti-infective (9)	New Technology (X)
ZINPLAVA™		Bezlotoxumab Monoclonal Antibody (A)	New Technology (X)
ZULRESSO™		Brexanolone (Ø)	New Technology (X)
Zyvox		Oxazolidinones (8)	Administration (3)

Substance Definitions

This table crosswalks a PCS value, used in the Administration or New Technology section, to a specific substance. The specific substances are listed by trade name or synonym. The ICD-10-PCS value may be located in either the 6th-character Substance column or the 7th-character Qualifier column depending on the section/table to which it is classified.

This NT symbol next to a substance/technology in the Trade Name or Synonym column identifies that the substance/technology has been approved for NTAP (new technology add-on payment). CMS provides incremental payment, in addition to the DRG payment, for technologies that have received an NTAP designation.

Substances denoted by an asterisk (*) in the Trade Name or Synonym column, although not included in the official ICD-1Ø-PCS classification, were added based on information provided in the FY 2022 IPPS proposed rule.

ICD-10-PCS Value	Trade Name or Synonym		PCS Section
4-Factor Prothrombin Complex Concentrate (B)	Includes:	Kcentra	Administration (3)
Adhesion Barrier (5)	Includes:	Seprafilm	Administration (3)
Antibiotic-eluting Bone Void Filler (P)	Includes:	CERAMENT® G	New Technology (X)
Anti-Infective Envelope (A)	Includes:	AIGISRx Antibacterial Envelope Antimicrobial envelope Antibacterial Envelope (TYRX) (AIGISRx) TYRX Antibacterial Envelope	Administration (3)
Apalutamide Antineoplastic (J)	Includes:	ERLEADA™	New Technology (X)
Atezolizumab Antineoplastic (D)	Includes:	TECENTRIQ® NT	New Technology (X)
Axicabtagene Ciloleucel Immunotherapy (H)	Includes:	Axicabtagene Ciloleucel Yescarta®	New Technology (X)
Baricitinib (M)	Includes:	Olumiant® NT	New Technology (X)
Bezlotoxumab Monoclonal Antibody (A)	Includes:	ZINPLAVA™	New Technology (X)
Bioengineered Allogeneic Construct (F)	Includes:	StrataGraft®	New Technology (X)
Brexanolone (Ø)	Includes:	ZULRESSO™	New Technology (X)
Brexucabtagene Autoleucel Immunotherapy (M)	Includes:	Tecartus™	New Technology (X)
Bromelain-enriched Proteolytic Enzyme (2)	Includes:	NexoBrid™	New Technology (X)
Caplacizumab (W)	Includes:	*CABLIVI® NT	New Technology (X)
Cefiderocol Anti-infective (A)	Includes:	FETROJA® NT	New Technology (X)
Ceftolozane/Tazobactam Anti- infective (9)	Includes:	ZERBAXA® NT	New Technology (X)
Ciltacabtagene Autoleucel (A)	Includes:	cilta-cel	New Technology (X)
Clofarabine (P)	Includes:	Clolar	Administration (3)
Coagulation Factor Xa, Inactivated (7)	Includes:	Andexanet Alfa, Factor Xa Inhibitor Reversal Agent Andexxa NT Coagulation Factor Xa, (Recombinant) Inactivated Factor Xa Inhibitor Reversal Agent, Andexanet Alfa	New Technology (X)
Concentrated Bone Marrow Aspirate (Ø)	Includes:	CBMA (Concentrated Bone Marrow Aspirate)	New Technology (X)
Cytarabine and Daunorubicin Liposome Antineoplastic (B)	Includes:	VYXEOS™	New Technology (X)
Defibrotide Sodium Anticoagulant (9)	Includes:	Defitelio	New Technology (X)
Durvalumab Antineoplastic (3)	Includes:	IMFINZI® NT	New Technology (X)
Eculizumab (C)	Includes:	Soliris® NT	New Technology (X)
Endothelial Damage Inhibitor (8)	Includes:	DuraGraft® Endothelial Damage Inhibitor	New Technology (X)
Erdafitinib Antineoplastic (L)	Includes:	*Balversa™ NT	New Technology (X)
Esketamine Hydrochloride (M)	Includes:	SPRAVATO™ NT	New Technology (X)

ICD-10-PCS Value	Trade Name or Synonym		PCS Section
Fosfomycin Anti-infective (K)	**Includes:**	CONTEPO™ Fosfomycin injection	New Technology (X)
Gilteritinib Antineoplastic (V)	**Includes:**	XOSPATA® `NT`	New Technology (X)
Globulin (S)	**Includes:**	Gammaglobulin Hyperimmune globulin Immunoglobulin Polyclonal hyperimmune globulin	Administration (3)
Glucarpidase (Q)	**Includes:**	Voraxaze	Administration (3)
Hematopoietic Stem/Progenitor Cells, Genetically Modified (C)	**Includes:**	OTL-101 OTL-103 OTL-200	Administration (3)
High-Dose Intravenous Immune Globulin (D)	**Includes:**	GAMUNEX-C, for COVID-19 treatment hdIVIG (high-dose intravenous immunoglobulin), for COVID-19 treatment High-dose intravenous immunoglobulin (hdIVIG), for COVID-19 treatment Octagam 10%, for COVID-19 treatment	New Technology (X)
Human B-type Natriuretic Peptide (H)	**Includes:**	Nesiritide	Administration (3)
Hyperimmune Globulin (E)	**Includes:**	Anti-SARS-CoV-2 hyperimmune globulin HIG (hyperimmune globulin), for COVID-19 treatment hIVIG (hyperimmune intravenous immunoglobulin), for COVID-19 treatment Hyperimmune intravenous immunoglobulin (hIVIG), for COVID-19 treatment IGIV-C, for COVID-19 treatment	New Technology (X)
Idecabtagene Vicleucel Immunotherapy (K)	**Includes:**	ABECMA® Idecabtagene Vicleucel Ide-cel	New Technology (X)
Imipenem-cilastatin-relebactam Anti-infective (U)	**Includes:**	IMI/REL *RECARBRIO™ `NT`	New Technology (X)
Iobenguane I-131 Antineoplastic (S)	**Includes:**	AZEDRA® `NT` Iobenguane I-131, High Specific Activity (HSA)	New Technology (X)
Lefamulin Anti-infective (6)	**Includes:**	XENLETA™ `NT`	New Technology (X)
Lifileucel Immunotherapy (L)	**Includes:**	Lifileucel	New Technology (X)
Lisocabtagene Maraleucel Immunotherapy (7)	**Includes:**	Lisocabtagene Maraleucel	New Technology (X)
Lurbinectedin (8)	**Includes:**	ZEPZELCA™	New Technology (X)
Meropenem-vaborbactam Anti-infective (N)	**Includes:**	Vabomere™	New Technology (X)
Mineral-based Topical Hemostatic Agent (8)	**Includes:**	Hemospray® Endoscopic Hemostat `NT`	New Technology (X)
Nafamostat Anticoagulant (3)	**Includes:**	LTX Regional Anticoagulant Niyad™	New Technology (X)
Nerinitide (2)	**Includes:**	NA-1 (Nerinitide)	New Technology (X)
Omadacycline Anti-infective (B)	**Includes:**	NUZYRA™ `NT`	New Technology (X)
Other Anti-infective (9)	**Includes:**	AVYCAZ® (ceftazidime-avibactam) Ceftazidime-avibactam CRESEMBA® (isavuconazonium sulfate) Isavuconazole (isavuconazonium sulfate)	Administration (3)
Other Antineoplastic (5)	**Includes:**	Blinatumomab BLINCYTO® (blinatumomab)	Administration (3)
Other New Technology Therapeutic Substance (F)	**Includes:**	STELARA® Ustekinumab	New Technology (X)
Other Therapeutic Substance (G)	**Includes:**	Idarucizumab, Pradaxa® (dabigatran) reversal agent Praxbind® (idarucizumab), Pradaxa® (dabigatran) reversal agent	Administration (3)
Other Thrombolytic (7)	**Includes:**	Tissue Plasminogen Activator (tPA)(r-tPA)	Administration (3)
Oxazolidinones (8)	**Includes:**	Zyvox	Administration (3)
Pathogen Reduced Cryoprecipitated Fibrinogen Complex (D)	**Includes:**	INTERCEPT Blood System for Plasma Pathogen Reduced Cryoprecipitated Fibrinogen Complex INTERCEPT Fibrinogen Complex	Administration (3)
Plazomicin Anti-infective (G)	**Includes:**	*ZEMDRI™ `NT`	New Technology (X)
Recombinant Bone Morphogenetic Protein (B)	**Includes:**	Bone morphogenetic protein 2 (BMP 2) rhBMP-2	Administration (3)
REGN-COV2 Monoclonal Antibody (G)	**Includes:**	Casirivimab (REGN10933) and Imdevimab (REGN10987) Imdevimab (REGN10987) and Casirivimab (REGN10933)	New Technology (X)

ICD-10-PCS Value	Trade Name or Synonym		PCS Section
Remdesivir Anti-infective (E)	**Includes:**	GS-5734 Veklury `NT`	New Technology (X)
Ruxolitinib (T)	**Includes:**	Jakafi® `NT`	New Technology (X)
Sarilumab (G)	**Includes:**	KEVZARA®	New Technology (X)
Satralizumab-mwge (9)	**Includes:**	ENSPRYNG™	New Technology (X)
Synthetic Human Angiotensin II (H)	**Includes:**	Angiotensin II GIAPREZA™ Human angiotensin II, synthetic	New Technology (X)
Tagraxofusp-erzs Antineoplastic (Q)	**Includes:**	ELZONRIS™ `NT`	New Technology (X)
Terlipressin (6)	**Includes:**	TERLIVAZ®	New Technology (X)
Tisagenlecleucel Immunotherapy (J)	**Includes:**	KYMRIAH® Tisagenlecleucel	New Technology (X)
Tocilizumab (H)	**Includes:**	ACTEMRA®	New Technology (X)
Trilaciclib (7)	**Includes:**	COSELA™	New Technology (X)
Uridine Triacetate (8)	**Includes:**	Vistogard®	New Technology (X)
Venetoclax Antineoplastic (R)	**Includes:**	Venclexta®	New Technology (X)

Appendix J: Sections B–H Character Definitions

Sections B-H (Imaging through Substance Abuse Treatment) do not include root operations. Instead, the character 3 value represents the type of procedure performed with additional details about that procedure provided by the character 4 or 5 value, when appropriate. This resource provides the specific ICD-10-PCS value and its associated definition for the character 3, character 4, and character 5 values in the ancillary sections of B-H.

Section B–Imaging

ICD-10-PCS Value (Character 3)	Definition
Computerized Tomography (CT Scan) (2)	Computer reformatted digital display of multiplanar images developed from the capture of multiple exposures of external ionizing radiation
Fluoroscopy (1)	Single plane or bi-plane real time display of an image developed from the capture of external ionizing radiation on a fluorescent screen. The image may also be stored by either digital or analog means.
Magnetic Resonance Imaging (MRI) (3)	Computer reformatted digital display of multiplanar images developed from the capture of radiofrequency signals emitted by nuclei in a body site excited within a magnetic field
Other Imaging (5)	Other specified modality for visualizing a body part
Plain Radiography (Ø)	Planar display of an image developed from the capture of external ionizing radiation on photographic or photoconductive plate
Ultrasonography (4)	Real time display of images of anatomy or flow information developed from the capture of reflected and attenuated high frequency sound waves

Section C–Nuclear Medicine

ICD-10-PCS Value (Character 3)	Definition
Nonimaging Nuclear Medicine Assay (6)	Introduction of radioactive materials into the body for the study of body fluids and blood elements, by the detection of radioactive emissions
Nonimaging Nuclear Medicine Probe (5)	Introduction of radioactive materials into the body for the study of distribution and fate of certain substances by the detection of radioactive emissions; or, alternatively, measurement of absorption of radioactive emissions from an external source
Nonimaging Nuclear Medicine Uptake (4)	Introduction of radioactive materials into the body for measurements of organ function, from the detection of radioactive emissions
Planar Nuclear Medicine Imaging (1)	Introduction of radioactive materials into the body for single plane display of images developed from the capture of radioactive emissions
Positron Emission Tomographic (PET) Imaging (3)	Introduction of radioactive materials into the body for three dimensional display of images developed from the simultaneous capture, 18Ø degrees apart, of radioactive emissions
Systemic Nuclear Medicine Therapy (7)	Introduction of unsealed radioactive materials into the body for treatment
Tomographic (Tomo) Nuclear Medicine Imaging (2)	Introduction of radioactive materials into the body for three dimensional display of images developed from the capture of radioactive emissions

Section F–Physical Rehabilitation and Diagnostic Audiology

ICD-10-PCS Value (Character 3)	Definition
Activities of Daily Living Assessment (2)	Measurement of functional level for activities of daily living
Activities of Daily Living Treatment (8)	Exercise or activities to facilitate functional competence for activities of daily living
Caregiver Training (F)	Training in activities to support patient's optimal level of function
Cochlear Implant Treatment (B)	Application of techniques to improve the communication abilities of individuals with cochlear implant
Device Fitting (D)	Fitting of a device designed to facilitate or support achievement of a higher level of function
Hearing Aid Assessment (4)	Measurement of the appropriateness and/or effectiveness of a hearing device
Hearing Assessment (3)	Measurement of hearing and related functions
Hearing Treatment (9)	Application of techniques to improve, augment, or compensate for hearing and related functional impairment
Motor and/or Nerve Function Assessment (1)	Measurement of motor, nerve, and related functions

Continued on next page

Section F–Physical Rehabilitation and Diagnostic Audiology

Continued from previous page

ICD-10-PCS Value (Character 3)	Definition
Motor Treatment (7)	Exercise or activities to increase or facilitate motor function
Speech Assessment (Ø)	Measurement of speech and related functions
Speech Treatment (6)	Application of techniques to improve, augment, or compensate for speech and related functional impairment
Vestibular Assessment (5)	Measurement of the vestibular system and related functions
Vestibular Treatment (C)	Application of techniques to improve, augment, or compensate for vestibular and related functional impairment

Section F–Physical Rehabilitation and Diagnostic Audiology

ICD-10-PCS Value Qualifier (Character 5)	Definition
Acoustic Reflex Decay (J)	Measures reduction in size/strength of acoustic reflex over time Includes/Examples: Includes site of lesion test
Acoustic Reflex Patterns (G)	Defines site of lesion based upon presence/absence of acoustic reflexes with ipsilateral vs. contralateral stimulation
Acoustic Reflex Threshold (H)	Determines minimal intensity that acoustic reflex occurs with ipsilateral and/or contralateral stimulation
Aerobic Capacity and Endurance (7)	Measures autonomic responses to positional changes; perceived exertion, dyspnea or angina during activity; performance during exercise protocols; standard vital signs; and blood gas analysis or oxygen consumption
Alternate Binaural or Monaural Loudness Balance (7)	Determines auditory stimulus parameter that yields the same objective sensation Includes/Examples: Sound intensities that yield same loudness perception
Anthropometric Characteristics (B)	Measures edema, body fat composition, height, weight, length and girth
Aphasia (Assessment) (C)	Measures expressive and receptive speech and language function including reading and writing
Aphasia (Treatment) (3)	Applying techniques to improve, augment, or compensate for receptive/ expressive language impairments
Articulation/Phonology (Assessment) (9)	Measures speech production
Articulation/Phonology (Treatment) (4)	Applying techniques to correct, improve, or compensate for speech productive impairment
Assistive Listening Device (5)	Assists in use of effective and appropriate assistive listening device/system
Assistive Listening System/Device Selection (4)	Measures the effectiveness and appropriateness of assistive listening systems/devices
Assistive, Adaptive, Supportive or Protective Devices (9)	Explanation: Devices to facilitate or support achievement of a higher level of function in wheelchair mobility; bed mobility; transfer or ambulation ability; bath and showering ability; dressing; grooming; personal hygiene; play or leisure
Auditory Evoked Potentials (L)	Measures electric responses produced by the VIIIth cranial nerve and brainstem following auditory stimulation
Auditory Processing (Assessment) (Q)	Evaluates ability to receive and process auditory information and comprehension of spoken language
Auditory Processing (Treatment) (2)	Applying techniques to improve the receiving and processing of auditory information and comprehension of spoken language
Augmentative/Alternative Communication System (Assessment) (L)	Determines the appropriateness of aids, techniques, symbols, and/or strategies to augment or replace speech and enhance communication Includes/Examples: Includes the use of telephones, writing equipment, emergency equipment, and TDD
Augmentative/Alternative Communication System (Treatment) (3)	Includes/Examples: Includes augmentative communication devices and aids
Aural Rehabilitation (5)	Applying techniques to improve the communication abilities associated with hearing loss
Aural Rehabilitation Status (P)	Measures impact of a hearing loss including evaluation of receptive and expressive communication skills
Bathing/Showering (Ø)	Includes/Examples: Includes obtaining and using supplies; soaping, rinsing, and drying body parts; maintaining bathing position; and transferring to and from bathing positions

Continued on next page

Section F–Physical Rehabilitation and Diagnostic Audiology　　*Continued from previous page*

ICD-10-PCS Value Qualifier (Character 5)	Definition
Bathing/Showering Techniques (Ø)	Activities to facilitate obtaining and using supplies, soaping, rinsing and drying body parts, maintaining bathing position, and transferring to and from bathing positions
Bed Mobility (Assessment) (B)	Transitional movement within bed
Bed Mobility (Treatment) (5)	Exercise or activities to facilitate transitional movements within bed
Bedside Swallowing and Oral Function (H)	Includes/Examples: Bedside swallowing includes assessment of sucking, masticating, coughing, and swallowing. Oral function includes assessment of musculature for controlled movements, structures, and functions to determine coordination and phonation.
Bekesy Audiometry (3)	Uses an instrument that provides a choice of discrete or continuously varying pure tones; choice of pulsed or continuous signal
Binaural Electroacoustic Hearing Aid Check (6)	Determines mechanical and electroacoustic function of bilateral hearing aids using hearing aid test box
Binaural Hearing Aid (Assessment) (3)	Measures the candidacy, effectiveness, and appropriateness of a hearing aid Explanation: Measures bilateral fit
Binaural Hearing Aid (Treatment) (2)	Explanation: Assists in achieving maximum understanding and performance
Bithermal, Binaural Caloric Irrigation (Ø)	Measures the rhythmic eye movements stimulated by changing the temperature of the vestibular system
Bithermal, Monaural Caloric Irrigation (1)	Measures the rhythmic eye movements stimulated by changing the temperature of the vestibular system in one ear
Brief Tone Stimuli (R)	Measures specific central auditory process
Cerumen Management (3)	Includes examination of external auditory canal and tympanic membrane and removal of cerumen from external ear canal
Cochlear Implant (Ø)	Measures candidacy for cochlear implant
Cochlear Implant Rehabilitation (Ø)	Applying techniques to improve the communication abilities of individuals with cochlear implant; includes programming the device, providing patients/families with information
Communicative/Cognitive Integration Skills (Assessment) (G)	Measures ability to use higher cortical functions Includes/Examples: Includes orientation, recognition, attention span, initiation and termination of activity, memory, sequencing, categorizing, concept formation, spatial operations, judgment, problem solving, generalization and pragmatic communication
Communicative/Cognitive Integration Skills (Treatment) (6)	Activities to facilitate the use of higher cortical functions Includes/Examples: Includes level of arousal, orientation, recognition, attention span, initiation and termination of activity, memory sequencing, judgment and problem solving, learning and generalization, and pragmatic communication
Computerized Dynamic Posturography (6)	Measures the status of the peripheral and central vestibular system and the sensory/motor component of balance; evaluates the efficacy of vestibular rehabilitation
Conditioned Play Audiometry (4)	Behavioral measures using nonspeech and speech stimuli to obtain frequency-specific and ear-specific information on auditory status from the patient Explanation: Obtains speech reception threshold by having patient point to pictures of spondaic words
Coordination/Dexterity (Assessment) (3)	Measures large and small muscle groups for controlled goal-directed movements Explanation: Dexterity includes object manipulation
Coordination/Dexterity (Treatment) (2)	Exercise or activities to facilitate gross coordination and fine coordination
Cranial Nerve Integrity (9)	Measures cranial nerve sensory and motor functions, including tastes, smell and facial expression
Dichotic Stimuli (T)	Measures specific central auditory process
Distorted Speech (S)	Measures specific central auditory process
Dix-Hallpike Dynamic (5)	Measures nystagmus following Dix-Hallpike maneuver
Dressing (1)	Includes/Examples: Includes selecting clothing and accessories, obtaining clothing from storage, dressing, fastening and adjusting clothing and shoes, and applying and removing personal devices, prosthesis or orthosis
Dressing Techniques (1)	Activities to facilitate selecting clothing and accessories, dressing and undressing, adjusting clothing and shoes, applying and removing devices, prostheses or orthoses
Dynamic Orthosis (6)	Includes/Examples: Includes customized and prefabricated splints, inhibitory casts, spinal and other braces, and protective devices; allows motion through transfer of movement from other body parts or by use of outside forces

Continued on next page

Section F–Physical Rehabilitation and Diagnostic Audiology

Continued from previous page

ICD-10-PCS Value Qualifier (Character 5)	Definition
Ear Canal Probe Microphone (1)	Real ear measures
Ear Protector Attentuation (7)	Measures ear protector fit and effectiveness
Electrocochleography (K)	Measures the VIIIth cranial nerve action potential
Environmental, Home, Work Barriers (B)	Measures current and potential barriers to optimal function, including safety hazards, access problems and home or office design
Ergonomics and Body Mechanics (C)	Ergonomic measurement of job tasks, work hardening or work conditioning needs; functional capacity; and body mechanics
Eustachian Tube Function (F)	Measures eustachian tube function and patency of eustachian tube
Evoked Otoacoustic Emissions, Diagnostic (N)	Measures auditory evoked potentials in a diagnostic format
Evoked Otoacoustic Emissions, Screening (M)	Measures auditory evoked potentials in a screening format
Facial Nerve Function (7)	Measures electrical activity of the VIIth cranial nerve (facial nerve)
Feeding/Eating (Assessment) (2)	Includes/Examples: Includes setting up food, selecting and using utensils and tableware, bringing food or drink to mouth, cleaning face, hands, and clothing, and management of alternative methods of nourishment
Feeding/Eating (Treatment) (3)	Exercise or activities to facilitate setting up food, selecting and using utensils and tableware, bringing food or drink to mouth, cleaning face, hands, and clothing, and management of alternative methods of nourishment
Filtered Speech (Ø)	Uses high or low pass filtered speech stimuli to assess central auditory processing disorders, site of lesion testing
Fluency (Assessment) (D)	Measures speech fluency or stuttering
Fluency (Treatment) (7)	Applying techniques to improve and augment fluent speech
Gait and/or Balance (D)	Measures biomechanical, arthrokinematic and other spatial and temporal characteristics of gait and balance
Gait Training/Functional Ambulation (9)	Exercise or activities to facilitate ambulation on a variety of surfaces and in a variety of environments
Grooming/Personal Hygiene (Assessment) (3)	Includes/Examples: Includes ability to obtain and use supplies in a sequential fashion, general grooming, oral hygiene, toilet hygiene, personal care devices, including care for artificial airways
Grooming/Personal Hygiene (Treatment) (2)	Activities to facilitate obtaining and using supplies in a sequential fashion: general grooming, oral hygiene, toilet hygiene, cleaning body, and personal care devices, including artificial airways
Hearing and Related Disorders Counseling (Ø)	Provides patients/families/caregivers with information, support, referrals to facilitate recovery from a communication disorder Includes/Examples: Includes strategies for psychosocial adjustment to hearing loss for clients and families/caregivers
Hearing and Related Disorders Prevention (1)	Provides patients/families/caregivers with information and support to prevent communication disorders
Hearing Screening (Ø)	Pass/refer measures designed to identify need for further audiologic assessment
Home Management (Assessment) (4)	Obtaining and maintaining personal and household possessions and environment Includes/Examples: Includes clothing care, cleaning, meal preparation and cleanup, shopping, money management, household maintenance, safety procedures, and childcare/parenting
Home Management (Treatment) (4)	Activities to facilitate obtaining and maintaining personal household possessions and environment Includes/Examples: Includes clothing care, cleaning, meal preparation and clean-up, shopping, money management, household maintenance, safety procedures, childcare/parenting
Instrumental Swallowing and Oral Function (J)	Measures swallowing function using instrumental diagnostic procedures Explanation: Methods include videofluoroscopy, ultrasound, manometry, endoscopy
Integumentary Integrity (1)	Includes/Examples: Includes burns, skin conditions, ecchymosis, bleeding, blisters, scar tissue, wounds and other traumas, tissue mobility, turgor and texture
Manual Therapy Techniques (7)	Techniques in which the therapist uses his/her hands to administer skilled movements Includes/Examples: Includes connective tissue massage, joint mobilization and manipulation, manual lymph drainage, manual traction, soft tissue mobilization and manipulation
Masking Patterns (W)	Measures central auditory processing status

Continued on next page

Section F–Physical Rehabilitation and Diagnostic Audiology   *Continued from previous page*

ICD-10-PCS Value Qualifier (Character 5)	Definition
Monaural Electroacoustic Hearing Aid Check (8)	Determines mechanical and electroacoustic function of one hearing aid using hearing aid test box
Monaural Hearing Aid (Assessment) (2)	Measures the candidacy, effectiveness, and appropriateness of a hearing aid Explanation: Measures unilateral fit
Monaural Hearing Aid (Treatment) (1)	Explanation: Assists in achieving maximum understanding and performance
Motor Function (Assessment) (4)	Measures the body's functional and versatile movement patterns Includes/Examples: Includes motor assessment scales, analysis of head, trunk and limb movement, and assessment of motor learning
Motor Function (Treatment) (3)	Exercise or activities to facilitate crossing midline, laterality, bilateral integration, praxis, neuromuscular relaxation, inhibition, facilitation, motor function and motor learning
Motor Speech (Assessment) (B)	Measures neurological motor aspects of speech production
Motor Speech (Treatment) (8)	Applying techniques to improve and augment the impaired neurological motor aspects of speech production
Muscle Performance (Assessment) (Ø)	Measures muscle strength, power and endurance using manual testing, dynamometry or computer-assisted electromechanical muscle test; functional muscle strength, power and endurance; muscle pain, tone, or soreness; or pelvic-floor musculature Explanation: Muscle endurance refers to the ability to contract a muscle repeatedly over time
Muscle Performance (Treatment) (1)	Exercise or activities to increase the capacity of a muscle to do work in terms of strength, power, and/or endurance Explanation: Muscle strength is the force exerted to overcome resistance in one maximal effort. Muscle power is work produced per unit of time, or the product of strength and speed. Muscle endurance is the ability to contract a muscle repeatedly over time.
Neuromotor Development (D)	Measures motor development, righting and equilibrium reactions, and reflex and equilibrium reactions
Non-invasive Instrumental Status (N)	Instrumental measures of oral, nasal, vocal, and velopharyngeal functions as they pertain to speech production
Nonspoken Language (Assessment) (7)	Measures nonspoken language (print, sign, symbols) for communication
Nonspoken Language (Treatment) (Ø)	Applying techniques that improve, augment, or compensate spoken communication
Oral Peripheral Mechanism (P)	Structural measures of face, jaw, lips, tongue, teeth, hard and soft palate, pharynx as related to speech production
Orofacial Myofunctional (Assessment) (K)	Measures orofacial myofunctional patterns for speech and related functions
Orofacial Myofunctional (Treatment) (9)	Applying techniques to improve, alter, or augment impaired orofacial myofunctional patterns and related speech production errors
Oscillating Tracking (3)	Measures ability to visually track
Pain (F)	Measures muscle soreness, pain and soreness with joint movement, and pain perception Includes/Examples: Includes questionnaires, graphs, symptom magnification scales or visual analog scales
Perceptual Processing (Assessment) (5)	Measures stereognosis, kinesthesia, body schema, right-left discrimination, form constancy, position in space, visual closure, figure-ground, depth perception, spatial relations and topographical orientation
Perceptual Processing (Treatment) (1)	Exercise and activities to facilitate perceptual processing Explanation: Includes stereognosis, kinesthesia, body schema, right-left discrimination, form constancy, position in space, visual closure, figure-ground, depth perception, spatial relations, and topographical orientation Includes/Examples: Includes stereognosis, kinesthesia, body schema, right-left discrimination, form constancy, position in space, visual closure, figure-ground, depth perception, spatial relations, and topographical orientation
Performance Intensity Phonetically Balanced Speech Discrimination (Q)	Measures word recognition over varying intensity levels
Postural Control (3)	Exercise or activities to increase postural alignment and control
Prosthesis (8)	Explanation: Artificial substitutes for missing body parts that augment performance or function Includes/Examples: Limb prosthesis, ocular prosthesis

Continued on next page

Section F–Physical Rehabilitation and Diagnostic Audiology

Continued from previous page

ICD-10-PCS Value Qualifier (Character 5)	Definition
Psychosocial Skills (Assessment) (6)	The ability to interact in society and to process emotions Includes/Examples: Includes psychological (values, interests, self-concept); social (role performance, social conduct, interpersonal skills, self expression); self-management (coping skills, time management, self-control)
Psychosocial Skills (Treatment) (6)	The ability to interact in society and to process emotions Includes/Examples: Includes psychological (values, interests, self-concept); social (role performance, social conduct, interpersonal skills, self expression); self-management (coping skills, time management, self-control)
Pure Tone Audiometry, Air (1)	Air-conduction pure tone threshold measures with appropriate masking
Pure Tone Audiometry, Air and Bone (2)	Air-conduction and bone-conduction pure tone threshold measures with appropriate masking
Pure Tone Stenger (C)	Measures unilateral nonorganic hearing loss based on simultaneous presentation of pure tones of differing volume
Range of Motion and Joint Integrity (5)	Measures quantity, quality, grade, and classification of joint movement and/or mobility Explanation: Range of Motion is the space, distance or angle through which movement occurs at a joint or series of joints. Joint integrity is the conformance of joints to expected anatomic, biomechanical and kinematic norms.
Range of Motion and Joint Mobility (Ø)	Exercise or activities to increase muscle length and joint mobility
Receptive/Expressive Language (Assessment) (8)	Measures receptive and expressive language
Receptive/Expressive Language (Treatment) (B)	Applying techniques to improve and augment receptive/expressive language
Reflex Integrity (G)	Measures the presence, absence, or exaggeration of developmentally appropriate, pathologic or normal reflexes
Select Picture Audiometry (5)	Establishes hearing threshold levels for speech using pictures
Sensorineural Acuity Level (4)	Measures sensorineural acuity masking presented via bone conduction
Sensory Aids (5)	Determines the appropriateness of a sensory prosthetic device, other than a hearing aid or assistive listening system/device
Sensory Awareness/ Processing/ Integrity (6)	Includes/Examples: Includes light touch, pressure, temperature, pain, sharp/dull, proprioception, vestibular, visual, auditory, gustatory, and olfactory
Short Increment Sensitivity Index (9)	Measures the ear's ability to detect small intensity changes; site of lesion test requiring a behavioral response
Sinusoidal Vertical Axis Rotational (4)	Measures nystagmus following rotation
Somatosensory Evoked Potentials (9)	Measures neural activity from sites throughout the body
Speech/Language Screening (6)	Identifies need for further speech and/or language evaluation
Speech Threshold (1)	Measures minimal intensity needed to repeat spondaic words
Speech-Language Pathology and Related Disorders Counseling (1)	Provides patients/families with information, support, referrals to facilitate recovery from a communication disorder
Speech-Language Pathology and Related Disorders Prevention (2)	Applying techniques to avoid or minimize onset and/or development of a communication disorder
Speech/Word Recognition (2)	Measures ability to repeat/identify single syllable words; scores given as a percentage; includes word recognition/speech discrimination
Staggered Spondaic Word (3)	Measures central auditory processing site of lesion based upon dichotic presentation of spondaic words
Static Orthosis (7)	Includes/Examples: Includes customized and prefabricated splints, inhibitory casts, spinal and other braces, and protective devices; has no moving parts, maintains joint(s) in desired position
Stenger (B)	Measures unilateral nonorganic hearing loss based on simultaneous presentation of signals of differing volume
Swallowing Dysfunction (D)	Activities to improve swallowing function in coordination with respiratory function Includes/Examples: Includes function and coordination of sucking, mastication, coughing, swallowing
Synthetic Sentence Identification (5)	Measures central auditory dysfunction using identification of third order approximations of sentences and competing messages

Continued on next page

Section F–Physical Rehabilitation and Diagnostic Audiology　　　*Continued from previous page*

ICD-10-PCS Value Qualifier (Character 5)	Definition
Temporal Ordering of Stimuli (V)	Measures specific central auditory process
Therapeutic Exercise (6)	Exercise or activities to facilitate sensory awareness, sensory processing, sensory integration, balance training, conditioning, reconditioning Includes/Examples: Includes developmental activities, breathing exercises, aerobic endurance activities, aquatic exercises, stretching and ventilatory muscle training
Tinnitus Masker (Assessment) (7)	Determines candidacy for tinnitus masker
Tinnitus Masker (Treatment) (Ø)	Explanation: Used to verify physical fit, acoustic appropriateness, and benefit; assists in achieving maximum benefit
Tone Decay (8)	Measures decrease in hearing sensitivity to a tone; site of lesion test requiring a behavioral response
Transfer (C)	Transitional movement from one surface to another
Transfer Training (8)	Exercise or activities to facilitate movement from one surface to another
Tympanometry (D)	Measures the integrity of the middle ear; measures ease at which sound flows through the tympanic membrane while air pressure against the membrane is varied
Unithermal Binaural Screen (2)	Measures the rhythmic eye movements stimulated by changing the temperature of the vestibular system in both ears using warm water, screening format
Ventilation/Respiration/Circulation (G)	Measures ventilatory muscle strength, power and endurance, pulmonary function and ventilatory mechanics Includes/Examples: Includes ability to clear airway, activities that aggravate or relieve edema, pain, dyspnea or other symptoms, chest wall mobility, cardiopulmonary response to performance of ADL and IAD, cough and sputum, standard vital signs
Vestibular (Ø)	Applying techniques to compensate for balance disorders; includes habituation, exercise therapy, and balance retraining
Visual Motor Integration (Assessment) (2)	Coordinating the interaction of information from the eyes with body movement during activity
Visual Motor Integration (Treatment) (2)	Exercise or activities to facilitate coordinating the interaction of information from eyes with body movement during activity
Visual Reinforcement Audiometry (6)	Behavioral measures using nonspeech and speech stimuli to obtain frequency/ear-specific information on auditory status Includes/Examples: Includes a conditioned response of looking toward a visual reinforcer (e.g., lights, animated toy) every time auditory stimuli are heard
Vocational Activities and Functional Community or Work Reintegration Skills (Assessment) (H)	Measures environmental, home, work (job/school/play) barriers that keep patients from functioning optimally in their environment Includes/Examples: Includes assessment of vocational skills and interests, environment of work (job/school/play), injury potential and injury prevention or reduction, ergonomic stressors, transportation skills, and ability to access and use community resources
Vocational Activities and Functional Community or Work Reintegration Skills (Treatment) (7)	Activities to facilitate vocational exploration, body mechanics training, job acquisition, and environmental or work (job/school/play) task adaptation Includes/Examples: Includes injury prevention and reduction, ergonomic stressor reduction, job coaching and simulation, work hardening and conditioning, driving training, transportation skills, and use of community resources
Voice (Assessment) (F)	Measures vocal structure, function and production
Voice (Treatment) (C)	Applying techniques to improve voice and vocal function
Voice Prosthetic (Assessment) (M)	Determines the appropriateness of voice prosthetic/adaptive device to enhance or facilitate communication
Voice Prosthetic (Treatment) (4)	Includes/Examples: Includes electrolarynx, and other assistive, adaptive, supportive devices
Wheelchair Mobility (Assessment) (F)	Measures fit and functional abilities within wheelchair in a variety of environments
Wheelchair Mobility (Treatment) (4)	Management, maintenance and controlled operation of a wheelchair, scooter or other device, in and on a variety of surfaces and environments
Wound Management (5)	Includes/Examples: Includes non-selective and selective debridement (enzymes, autolysis, sharp debridement), dressings (wound coverings, hydrogel, vacuum-assisted closure), topical agents, etc.

Section G–Mental Health

ICD-10-PCS Value (Character 3)	Definition
Biofeedback (C)	Provision of information from the monitoring and regulating of physiological processes in conjunction with cognitive-behavioral techniques to improve patient functioning or well-being Includes/Examples: Includes EEG, blood pressure, skin temperature or peripheral blood flow, ECG, electrooculogram, EMG, respirometry or capnometry, GSR/EDR, perineometry to monitor/regulate bowel/bladder activity, electrogastrogram to monitor/regulate gastric motility
Counseling (6)	The application of psychological methods to treat an individual with normal developmental issues and psychological problems in order to increase function, improve well-being, alleviate distress, maladjustment or resolve crises
Crisis Intervention (2)	Treatment of a traumatized, acutely disturbed or distressed individual for the purpose of short-term stabilization Includes/Examples: Includes defusing, debriefing, counseling, psychotherapy and/or coordination of care with other providers or agencies
Electroconvulsive Therapy (B)	The application of controlled electrical voltages to treat a mental health disorder Includes/Examples: Includes appropriate sedation and other preparation of the individual
Family Psychotherapy (7)	Treatment that includes one or more family members of an individual with a mental health disorder by behavioral, cognitive, psychoanalytic, psychodynamic or psychophysiological means to improve functioning or well-being Explanation: Remediation of emotional or behavioral problems presented by one or more family members in cases where psychotherapy with more than one family member is indicated
Group Psychotherapy (H)	Treatment of two or more individuals with a mental health disorder by behavioral, cognitive, psychoanalytic, psychodynamic or psychophysiological means to improve functioning or well-being
Hypnosis (F)	Induction of a state of heightened suggestibility by auditory, visual and tactile techniques to elicit an emotional or behavioral response
Individual Psychotherapy (5)	Treatment of an individual with a mental health disorder by behavioral, cognitive, psychoanalytic, psychodynamic or psychophysiological means to improve functioning or well-being
Light Therapy (J)	Application of specialized light treatments to improve functioning or well-being
Medication Management (3)	Monitoring and adjusting the use of medications for the treatment of a mental health disorder
Narcosynthesis (G)	Administration of intravenous barbiturates in order to release suppressed or repressed thoughts
Psychological Tests (1)	The administration and interpretation of standardized psychological tests and measurement instruments for the assessment of psychological function
Behavioral (1)	Primarily to modify behavior Includes/Examples: Includes modeling and role playing, positive reinforcement of target behaviors, response cost, and training of self-management skills
Cognitive (2)	Primarily to correct cognitive distortions and errors
Cognitive-Behavioral (8)	Combining cognitive and behavioral treatment strategies to improve functioning Explanation: Maladaptive responses are examined to determine how cognitions relate to behavior patterns in response to an event. Uses learning principles and information-processing models.
Developmental (Ø)	Age-normed developmental status of cognitive, social and adaptive behavior skills
Intellectual and Psychoeducational (2)	Intellectual abilities, academic achievement and learning capabilities (including behaviors and emotional factors affecting learning)
Interactive (Ø)	Uses primarily physical aids and other forms of non-oral interaction with a patient who is physically, psychologically or developmentally unable to use ordinary language for communication Includes/Examples: Includes the use of toys in symbolic play
Interpersonal (3)	Helps an individual make changes in interpersonal behaviors to reduce psychological dysfunction Includes/Examples: Includes exploratory techniques, encouragement of affective expression, clarification of patient statements, analysis of communication patterns, use of therapy relationship and behavior change techniques
Neurobehavioral and Cognitive Status (4)	Includes neurobehavioral status exam, interview(s), and observation for the clinical assessment of thinking, reasoning and judgment, acquired knowledge, attention, memory, visual spatial abilities, language functions, and planning
Neuropsychological (3)	Thinking, reasoning and judgment, acquired knowledge, attention, memory, visual spatial abilities, language functions, planning
Personality and Behavioral (1)	Mood, emotion, behavior, social functioning, psychopathological conditions, personality traits and characteristics

Continued on next page

Section G–Mental Health

Continued from previous page

ICD-10-PCS Value (Character 3)	Definition
Psychoanalysis (4)	Methods of obtaining a detailed account of past and present mental and emotional experiences to determine the source and eliminate or diminish the undesirable effects of unconscious conflicts Explanation: Accomplished by making the individual aware of their existence, origin, and inappropriate expression in emotions and behavior
Psychodynamic (5)	Exploration of past and present emotional experiences to understand motives and drives using insight-oriented techniques to reduce the undesirable effects of internal conflicts on emotions and behavior Explanation: Techniques include empathetic listening, clarifying self-defeating behavior patterns, and exploring adaptive alternatives
Psychophysiological (9)	Monitoring and alteration of physiological processes to help the individual associate physiological reactions combined with cognitive and behavioral strategies to gain improved control of these processes to help the individual cope more effectively
Supportive (6)	Formation of therapeutic relationship primarily for providing emotional support to prevent further deterioration in functioning during periods of particular stress Explanation: Often used in conjunction with other therapeutic approaches
Vocational (1)	Exploration of vocational interests, aptitudes and required adaptive behavior skills to develop and carry out a plan for achieving a successful vocational placement Includes/Examples: Includes enhancing work related adjustment and/or pursuing viable options in training education or preparation

Section H–Substance Abuse Treatment

ICD-10-PCS Value (Character 3)	Definition
Detoxification Services (2)	Detoxification from alcohol and/or drugs Explanation: Not a treatment modality, but helps the patient stabilize physically and psychologically until the body becomes free of drugs and the effects of alcohol
Family Counseling (6)	The application of psychological methods that includes one or more family members to treat an individual with addictive behavior Explanation: Provides support and education for family members of addicted individuals. Family member participation is seen as a critical area of substance abuse treatment.
Group Counseling (4)	The application of psychological methods to treat two or more individuals with addictive behavior Explanation: Provides structured group counseling sessions and healing power through the connection with others
Individual Counseling (3)	The application of psychological methods to treat an individual with addictive behavior Explanation: Comprised of several different techniques, which apply various strategies to address drug addiction
Individual Psychotherapy (5)	Treatment of an individual with addictive behavior by behavioral, cognitive, psychoanalytic, psychodynamic or psychophysiological means
Medication Management (8)	Monitoring and adjusting the use of replacement medications for the treatment of addiction
Pharmacotherapy (9)	The use of replacement medications for the treatment of addiction

Appendix K: Hospital Acquired Conditions

Hospital acquired conditions (HACs) are conditions considered reasonably preventable through the application of evidence-based guidelines. Although it is the ICD-10-CM diagnosis code that drives a HAC designation, in some cases a specific ICD-10-PCS procedure code must also be present before that diagnosis code can be considered a HAC. This resource provides only those HAC categories that require both an ICD-10-PCS code and an ICD-10-CM diagnosis code. The official descriptions for each code are also provided. To see all 14 HAC categories and their corresponding codes, refer to Optum360's *ICD-10-CM Expert for Hospitals*.

Note: The resource used to compile this list is the proposed, version 39, MS-DRG Grouper software and Definitions Manual files published with the fiscal 2022 IPPS proposed rule. For the final, version 39, MS-DRG Grouper software and Definitions Manual files, refer to the following: https://www.cms.gov/Medicare/Medicare-Fee-for-Service-Payment/AcuteInpatientPPS/MS-DRG-Classifications-and-Software.

HAC 08: Surgical Site Infection of Mediastinitis After Coronary Bypass Graft (CABG) Procedures

Secondary diagnosis not POA:

J98.51	Mediastinitis
J98.59	Other diseases of mediastinum, not elsewhere classified

AND

Any of the following procedures:

0210083	Bypass Coronary Artery, One Artery from Coronary Artery with Zooplastic Tissue, Open Approach
0210088	Bypass Coronary Artery, One Artery from Right Internal Mammary with Zooplastic Tissue, Open Approach
0210089	Bypass Coronary Artery, One Artery from Left Internal Mammary with Zooplastic Tissue, Open Approach
021008C	Bypass Coronary Artery, One Artery from Thoracic Artery with Zooplastic Tissue, Open Approach
021008F	Bypass Coronary Artery, One Artery from Abdominal Artery with Zooplastic Tissue, Open Approach
021008W	Bypass Coronary Artery, One Artery from Aorta with Zooplastic Tissue, Open Approach
0210093	Bypass Coronary Artery, One Artery from Coronary Artery with Autologous Venous Tissue, Open Approach
0210098	Bypass Coronary Artery, One Artery from Right Internal Mammary with Autologous Venous Tissue, Open Approach
0210099	Bypass Coronary Artery, One Artery from Left Internal Mammary with Autologous Venous Tissue, Open Approach
021009C	Bypass Coronary Artery, One Artery from Thoracic Artery with Autologous Venous Tissue, Open Approach
021009F	Bypass Coronary Artery, One Artery from Abdominal Artery with Autologous Venous Tissue, Open Approach
021009W	Bypass Coronary Artery, One Artery from Aorta with Autologous Venous Tissue, Open Approach
02100A3	Bypass Coronary Artery, One Artery from Coronary Artery with Autologous Arterial Tissue, Open Approach
02100A8	Bypass Coronary Artery, One Artery from Right Internal Mammary with Autologous Arterial Tissue, Open Approach
02100A9	Bypass Coronary Artery, One Artery from Left Internal Mammary with Autologous Arterial Tissue, Open Approach
02100AC	Bypass Coronary Artery, One Artery from Thoracic Artery with Autologous Arterial Tissue, Open Approach
02100AF	Bypass Coronary Artery, One Artery from Abdominal Artery with Autologous Arterial Tissue, Open Approach
02100AW	Bypass Coronary Artery, One Artery from Aorta with Autologous Arterial Tissue, Open Approach

02100J3	Bypass Coronary Artery, One Artery from Coronary Artery with Synthetic Substitute, Open Approach
02100J8	Bypass Coronary Artery, One Artery from Right Internal Mammary with Synthetic Substitute, Open Approach
02100J9	Bypass Coronary Artery, One Artery from Left Internal Mammary with Synthetic Substitute, Open Approach
02100JC	Bypass Coronary Artery, One Artery from Thoracic Artery with Synthetic Substitute, Open Approach
02100JF	Bypass Coronary Artery, One Artery from Abdominal Artery with Synthetic Substitute, Open Approach
02100JW	Bypass Coronary Artery, One Artery from Aorta with Synthetic Substitute, Open Approach
02100K3	Bypass Coronary Artery, One Artery from Coronary Artery with Nonautologous Tissue Substitute, Open Approach
02100K8	Bypass Coronary Artery, One Artery from Right Internal Mammary with Nonautologous Tissue Substitute, Open Approach
02100K9	Bypass Coronary Artery, One Artery from Left Internal Mammary with Nonautologous Tissue Substitute, Open Approach
02100KC	Bypass Coronary Artery, One Artery from Thoracic Artery with Nonautologous Tissue Substitute, Open Approach
02100KF	Bypass Coronary Artery, One Artery from Abdominal Artery with Nonautologous Tissue Substitute, Open Approach
02100KW	Bypass Coronary Artery, One Artery from Aorta with Nonautologous Tissue Substitute, Open Approach
02100Z3	Bypass Coronary Artery, One Artery from Coronary Artery, Open Approach
02100Z8	Bypass Coronary Artery, One Artery from Right Internal Mammary, Open Approach
02100Z9	Bypass Coronary Artery, One Artery from Left Internal Mammary, Open Approach
02100ZC	Bypass Coronary Artery, One Artery from Thoracic Artery, Open Approach
02100ZF	Bypass Coronary Artery, One Artery from Abdominal Artery, Open Approach
0210483	Bypass Coronary Artery, One Artery from Coronary Artery with Zooplastic Tissue, Percutaneous Endoscopic Approach
0210488	Bypass Coronary Artery, One Artery from Right Internal Mammary with Zooplastic Tissue, Percutaneous Endoscopic Approach
0210489	Bypass Coronary Artery, One Artery from Left Internal Mammary with Zooplastic Tissue, Percutaneous Endoscopic Approach

021048C	Bypass Coronary Artery, One Artery from Thoracic Artery with Zooplastic Tissue, Percutaneous Endoscopic Approach
021048F	Bypass Coronary Artery, One Artery from Abdominal Artery with Zooplastic Tissue, Percutaneous Endoscopic Approach
021048W	Bypass Coronary Artery, One Artery from Aorta with Zooplastic Tissue, Percutaneous Endoscopic Approach
0210493	Bypass Coronary Artery, One Artery from Coronary Artery with Autologous Venous Tissue, Percutaneous Endoscopic Approach
0210498	Bypass Coronary Artery, One Artery from Right Internal Mammary with Autologous Venous Tissue, Percutaneous Endoscopic Approach
0210499	Bypass Coronary Artery, One Artery from Left Internal Mammary with Autologous Venous Tissue, Percutaneous Endoscopic Approach
021049C	Bypass Coronary Artery, One Artery from Thoracic Artery with Autologous Venous Tissue, Percutaneous Endoscopic Approach
021049F	Bypass Coronary Artery, One Artery from Abdominal Artery with Autologous Venous Tissue, Percutaneous Endoscopic Approach
021049W	Bypass Coronary Artery, One Artery from Aorta with Autologous Venous Tissue, Percutaneous Endoscopic Approach
02104A3	Bypass Coronary Artery, One Artery from Coronary Artery with Autologous Arterial Tissue, Percutaneous Endoscopic Approach
02104A8	Bypass Coronary Artery, One Artery from Right Internal Mammary with Autologous Arterial Tissue, Percutaneous Endoscopic Approach
02104A9	Bypass Coronary Artery, One Artery from Left Internal Mammary with Autologous Arterial Tissue, Percutaneous Endoscopic Approach
02104AC	Bypass Coronary Artery, One Artery from Thoracic Artery with Autologous Arterial Tissue, Percutaneous Endoscopic Approach
02104AF	Bypass Coronary Artery, One Artery from Abdominal Artery with Autologous Arterial Tissue, Percutaneous Endoscopic Approach
02104AW	Bypass Coronary Artery, One Artery from Aorta with Autologous Arterial Tissue, Percutaneous Endoscopic Approach
02104J3	Bypass Coronary Artery, One Artery from Coronary Artery with Synthetic Substitute, Percutaneous Endoscopic Approach

HAC 08: Surgical Site Infection of Mediastinitis After Coronary Bypass Graft (CABG) Procedures (continued)

02104J8 Bypass Coronary Artery, One Artery from Right Internal Mammary with Synthetic Substitute, Percutaneous Endoscopic Approach

02104J9 Bypass Coronary Artery, One Artery from Left Internal Mammary with Synthetic Substitute, Percutaneous Endoscopic Approach

02104JC Bypass Coronary Artery, One Artery from Thoracic Artery with Synthetic Substitute, Percutaneous Endoscopic Approach

02104JF Bypass Coronary Artery, One Artery from Abdominal Artery with Synthetic Substitute, Percutaneous Endoscopic Approach

02104JW Bypass Coronary Artery, One Artery from Aorta with Synthetic Substitute, Percutaneous Endoscopic Approach

02104K3 Bypass Coronary Artery, One Artery from Coronary Artery with Nonautologous Tissue Substitute, Percutaneous Endoscopic Approach

02104K8 Bypass Coronary Artery, One Artery from Right Internal Mammary with Nonautologous Tissue Substitute, Percutaneous Endoscopic Approach

02104K9 Bypass Coronary Artery, One Artery from Left Internal Mammary with Nonautologous Tissue Substitute, Percutaneous Endoscopic Approach

02104KC Bypass Coronary Artery, One Artery from Thoracic Artery with Nonautologous Tissue Substitute, Percutaneous Endoscopic Approach

02104KF Bypass Coronary Artery, One Artery from Abdominal Artery with Nonautologous Tissue Substitute, Percutaneous Endoscopic Approach

02104KW Bypass Coronary Artery, One Artery from Aorta with Nonautologous Tissue Substitute, Percutaneous Endoscopic Approach

02104Z3 Bypass Coronary Artery, One Artery from Coronary Artery, Percutaneous Endoscopic Approach

02104Z8 Bypass Coronary Artery, One Artery from Right Internal Mammary, Percutaneous Endoscopic Approach

02104Z9 Bypass Coronary Artery, One Artery from Left Internal Mammary, Percutaneous Endoscopic Approach

02104ZC Bypass Coronary Artery, One Artery from Thoracic Artery, Percutaneous Endoscopic Approach

02104ZF Bypass Coronary Artery, One Artery from Abdominal Artery, Percutaneous Endoscopic Approach

0211083 Bypass Coronary Artery, Two Arteries from Coronary Artery with Zooplastic Tissue, Open Approach

0211088 Bypass Coronary Artery, Two Arteries from Right Internal Mammary with Zooplastic Tissue, Open Approach

0211089 Bypass Coronary Artery, Two Arteries from Left Internal Mammary with Zooplastic Tissue, Open Approach

021108C Bypass Coronary Artery, Two Arteries from Thoracic Artery with Zooplastic Tissue, Open Approach

021108F Bypass Coronary Artery, Two Arteries from Abdominal Artery with Zooplastic Tissue, Open Approach

021108W Bypass Coronary Artery, Two Arteries from Aorta with Zooplastic Tissue, Open Approach

0211093 Bypass Coronary Artery, Two Arteries from Coronary Artery with Autologous Venous Tissue, Open Approach

0211098 Bypass Coronary Artery, Two Arteries from Right Internal Mammary with Autologous Venous Tissue, Open Approach

0211099 Bypass Coronary Artery, Two Arteries from Left Internal Mammary with Autologous Venous Tissue, Open Approach

021109C Bypass Coronary Artery, Two Arteries from Thoracic Artery with Autologous Venous Tissue, Open Approach

021109F Bypass Coronary Artery, Two Arteries from Abdominal Artery with Autologous Venous Tissue, Open Approach

021109W Bypass Coronary Artery, Two Arteries from Aorta with Autologous Venous Tissue, Open Approach

02110A3 Bypass Coronary Artery, Two Arteries from Coronary Artery with Autologous Arterial Tissue, Open Approach

02110A8 Bypass Coronary Artery, Two Arteries from Right Internal Mammary with Autologous Arterial Tissue, Open Approach

02110A9 Bypass Coronary Artery, Two Arteries from Left Internal Mammary with Autologous Arterial Tissue, Open Approach

02110AC Bypass Coronary Artery, Two Arteries from Thoracic Artery with Autologous Arterial Tissue, Open Approach

02110AF Bypass Coronary Artery, Two Arteries from Abdominal Artery with Autologous Arterial Tissue, Open Approach

02110AW Bypass Coronary Artery, Two Arteries from Aorta with Autologous Arterial Tissue, Open Approach

02110J3 Bypass Coronary Artery, Two Arteries from Coronary Artery with Synthetic Substitute, Open Approach

02110J8 Bypass Coronary Artery, Two Arteries from Right Internal Mammary with Synthetic Substitute, Open Approach

02110J9 Bypass Coronary Artery, Two Arteries from Left Internal Mammary with Synthetic Substitute, Open Approach

02110JC Bypass Coronary Artery, Two Arteries from Thoracic Artery with Synthetic Substitute, Open Approach

02110JF Bypass Coronary Artery, Two Arteries from Abdominal Artery with Synthetic Substitute, Open Approach

02110JW Bypass Coronary Artery, Two Arteries from Aorta with Synthetic Substitute, Open Approach

02110K3 Bypass Coronary Artery, Two Arteries from Coronary Artery with Nonautologous Tissue Substitute, Open Approach

02110K8 Bypass Coronary Artery, Two Arteries from Right Internal Mammary with Nonautologous Tissue Substitute, Open Approach

02110K9 Bypass Coronary Artery, Two Arteries from Left Internal Mammary with Nonautologous Tissue Substitute, Open Approach

02110KC Bypass Coronary Artery, Two Arteries from Thoracic Artery with Nonautologous Tissue Substitute, Open Approach

02110KF Bypass Coronary Artery, Two Arteries from Abdominal Artery with Nonautologous Tissue Substitute, Open Approach

02110KW Bypass Coronary Artery, Two Arteries from Aorta with Nonautologous Tissue Substitute, Open Approach

02110Z3 Bypass Coronary Artery, Two Arteries from Coronary Artery, Open Approach

02110Z8 Bypass Coronary Artery, Two Arteries from Right Internal Mammary, Open Approach

02110Z9 Bypass Coronary Artery, Two Arteries from Left Internal Mammary, Open Approach

02110ZC Bypass Coronary Artery, Two Arteries from Thoracic Artery, Open Approach

02110ZF Bypass Coronary Artery, Two Arteries from Abdominal Artery, Open Approach

0211483 Bypass Coronary Artery, Two Arteries from Coronary Artery with Zooplastic Tissue, Percutaneous Endoscopic Approach

0211488 Bypass Coronary Artery, Two Arteries from Right Internal Mammary with Zooplastic Tissue, Percutaneous Endoscopic Approach

0211489 Bypass Coronary Artery, Two Arteries from Left Internal Mammary with Zooplastic Tissue, Percutaneous Endoscopic Approach

021148C Bypass Coronary Artery, Two Arteries from Thoracic Artery with Zooplastic Tissue, Percutaneous Endoscopic Approach

021148F Bypass Coronary Artery, Two Arteries from Abdominal Artery with Zooplastic Tissue, Percutaneous Endoscopic Approach

021148W Bypass Coronary Artery, Two Arteries from Aorta with Zooplastic Tissue, Percutaneous Endoscopic Approach

0211493 Bypass Coronary Artery, Two Arteries from Coronary Artery with Autologous Venous Tissue, Percutaneous Endoscopic Approach

0211498 Bypass Coronary Artery, Two Arteries from Right Internal Mammary with Autologous Venous Tissue, Percutaneous Endoscopic Approach

0211499 Bypass Coronary Artery, Two Arteries from Left Internal Mammary with Autologous Venous Tissue, Percutaneous Endoscopic Approach

021149C Bypass Coronary Artery, Two Arteries from Thoracic Artery with Autologous Venous Tissue, Percutaneous Endoscopic Approach

021149F Bypass Coronary Artery, Two Arteries from Abdominal Artery with Autologous Venous Tissue, Percutaneous Endoscopic Approach

021149W Bypass Coronary Artery, Two Arteries from Aorta with Autologous Venous Tissue, Percutaneous Endoscopic Approach

02114A3 Bypass Coronary Artery, Two Arteries from Coronary Artery with Autologous Arterial Tissue, Percutaneous Endoscopic Approach

02114A8 Bypass Coronary Artery, Two Arteries from Right Internal Mammary with Autologous Arterial Tissue, Percutaneous Endoscopic Approach

02114A9 Bypass Coronary Artery, Two Arteries from Left Internal Mammary with Autologous Arterial Tissue, Percutaneous Endoscopic Approach

02114AC Bypass Coronary Artery, Two Arteries from Thoracic Artery with Autologous Arterial Tissue, Percutaneous Endoscopic Approach

02114AF Bypass Coronary Artery, Two Arteries from Abdominal Artery with Autologous Arterial Tissue, Percutaneous Endoscopic Approach

HAC 08: Surgical Site Infection of Mediastinitis After Coronary Bypass Graft (CABG) Procedures (continued)

02114AW Bypass Coronary Artery, Two Arteries from Aorta with Autologous Arterial Tissue, Percutaneous Endoscopic Approach

02114J3 Bypass Coronary Artery, Two Arteries from Coronary Artery with Synthetic Substitute, Percutaneous Endoscopic Approach

02114J8 Bypass Coronary Artery, Two Arteries from Right Internal Mammary with Synthetic Substitute, Percutaneous Endoscopic Approach

02114J9 Bypass Coronary Artery, Two Arteries from Left Internal Mammary with Synthetic Substitute, Percutaneous Endoscopic Approach

02114JC Bypass Coronary Artery, Two Arteries from Thoracic Artery with Synthetic Substitute, Percutaneous Endoscopic Approach

02114JF Bypass Coronary Artery, Two Arteries from Abdominal Artery with Synthetic Substitute, Percutaneous Endoscopic Approach

02114JW Bypass Coronary Artery, Two Arteries from Aorta with Synthetic Substitute, Percutaneous Endoscopic Approach

02114K3 Bypass Coronary Artery, Two Arteries from Coronary Artery with Nonautologous Tissue Substitute, Percutaneous Endoscopic Approach

02114K8 Bypass Coronary Artery, Two Arteries from Right Internal Mammary with Nonautologous Tissue Substitute, Percutaneous Endoscopic Approach

02114K9 Bypass Coronary Artery, Two Arteries from Left Internal Mammary with Nonautologous Tissue Substitute, Percutaneous Endoscopic Approach

02114KC Bypass Coronary Artery, Two Arteries from Thoracic Artery with Nonautologous Tissue Substitute, Percutaneous Endoscopic Approach

02114KF Bypass Coronary Artery, Two Arteries from Abdominal Artery with Nonautologous Tissue Substitute, Percutaneous Endoscopic Approach

02114KW Bypass Coronary Artery, Two Arteries from Aorta with Nonautologous Tissue Substitute, Percutaneous Endoscopic Approach

02114Z3 Bypass Coronary Artery, Two Arteries from Coronary Artery, Percutaneous Endoscopic Approach

02114Z8 Bypass Coronary Artery, Two Arteries from Right Internal Mammary, Percutaneous Endoscopic Approach

02114Z9 Bypass Coronary Artery, Two Arteries from Left Internal Mammary, Percutaneous Endoscopic Approach

02114ZC Bypass Coronary Artery, Two Arteries from Thoracic Artery, Percutaneous Endoscopic Approach

02114ZF Bypass Coronary Artery, Two Arteries from Abdominal Artery, Percutaneous Endoscopic Approach

0212083 Bypass Coronary Artery, Three Arteries from Coronary Artery with Zooplastic Tissue, Open Approach

0212088 Bypass Coronary Artery, Three Arteries from Right Internal Mammary with Zooplastic Tissue, Open Approach

0212089 Bypass Coronary Artery, Three Arteries from Left Internal Mammary with Zooplastic Tissue, Open Approach

021208C Bypass Coronary Artery, Three Arteries from Thoracic Artery with Zooplastic Tissue, Open Approach

021208F Bypass Coronary Artery, Three Arteries from Abdominal Artery with Zooplastic Tissue, Open Approach

021208W Bypass Coronary Artery, Three Arteries from Aorta with Zooplastic Tissue, Open Approach

0212093 Bypass Coronary Artery, Three Arteries from Coronary Artery with Autologous Venous Tissue, Open Approach

0212098 Bypass Coronary Artery, Three Arteries from Right Internal Mammary with Autologous Venous Tissue, Open Approach

0212099 Bypass Coronary Artery, Three Arteries from Left Internal Mammary with Autologous Venous Tissue, Open Approach

021209C Bypass Coronary Artery, Three Arteries from Thoracic Artery with Autologous Venous Tissue, Open Approach

021209F Bypass Coronary Artery, Three Arteries from Abdominal Artery with Autologous Venous Tissue, Open Approach

021209W Bypass Coronary Artery, Three Arteries from Aorta with Autologous Venous Tissue, Open Approach

02120A3 Bypass Coronary Artery, Three Arteries from Coronary Artery with Autologous Arterial Tissue, Open Approach

02120A8 Bypass Coronary Artery, Three Arteries from Right Internal Mammary with Autologous Arterial Tissue, Open Approach

02120A9 Bypass Coronary Artery, Three Arteries from Left Internal Mammary with Autologous Arterial Tissue, Open Approach

02120AC Bypass Coronary Artery, Three Arteries from Thoracic Artery with Autologous Arterial Tissue, Open Approach

02120AF Bypass Coronary Artery, Three Arteries from Abdominal Artery with Autologous Arterial Tissue, Open Approach

02120AW Bypass Coronary Artery, Three Arteries from Aorta with Autologous Arterial Tissue, Open Approach

02120J3 Bypass Coronary Artery, Three Arteries from Coronary Artery with Synthetic Substitute, Open Approach

02120J8 Bypass Coronary Artery, Three Arteries from Right Internal Mammary with Synthetic Substitute, Open Approach

02120J9 Bypass Coronary Artery, Three Arteries from Left Internal Mammary with Synthetic Substitute, Open Approach

02120JC Bypass Coronary Artery, Three Arteries from Thoracic Artery with Synthetic Substitute, Open Approach

02120JF Bypass Coronary Artery, Three Arteries from Abdominal Artery with Synthetic Substitute, Open Approach

02120JW Bypass Coronary Artery, Three Arteries from Aorta with Synthetic Substitute, Open Approach

02120K3 Bypass Coronary Artery, Three Arteries from Coronary Artery with Nonautologous Tissue Substitute, Open Approach

02120K8 Bypass Coronary Artery, Three Arteries from Right Internal Mammary with Nonautologous Tissue Substitute, Open Approach

02120K9 Bypass Coronary Artery, Three Arteries from Left Internal Mammary with Nonautologous Tissue Substitute, Open Approach

02120KC Bypass Coronary Artery, Three Arteries from Thoracic Artery with Nonautologous Tissue Substitute, Open Approach

02120KF Bypass Coronary Artery, Three Arteries from Abdominal Artery with Nonautologous Tissue Substitute, Open Approach

02120KW Bypass Coronary Artery, Three Arteries from Aorta with Nonautologous Tissue Substitute, Open Approach

02120Z3 Bypass Coronary Artery, Three Arteries from Coronary Artery, Open Approach

02120Z8 Bypass Coronary Artery, Three Arteries from Right Internal Mammary, Open Approach

02120Z9 Bypass Coronary Artery, Three Arteries from Left Internal Mammary, Open Approach

02120ZC Bypass Coronary Artery, Three Arteries from Thoracic Artery, Open Approach

02120ZF Bypass Coronary Artery, Three Arteries from Abdominal Artery, Open Approach

0212483 Bypass Coronary Artery, Three Arteries from Coronary Artery with Zooplastic Tissue, Percutaneous Endoscopic Approach

0212488 Bypass Coronary Artery, Three Arteries from Right Internal Mammary with Zooplastic Tissue, Percutaneous Endoscopic Approach

0212489 Bypass Coronary Artery, Three Arteries from Left Internal Mammary with Zooplastic Tissue, Percutaneous Endoscopic Approach

021248C Bypass Coronary Artery, Three Arteries from Thoracic Artery with Zooplastic Tissue, Percutaneous Endoscopic Approach

021248F Bypass Coronary Artery, Three Arteries from Abdominal Artery with Zooplastic Tissue, Percutaneous Endoscopic Approach

021248W Bypass Coronary Artery, Three Arteries from Aorta with Zooplastic Tissue, Percutaneous Endoscopic Approach

0212493 Bypass Coronary Artery, Three Arteries from Coronary Artery with Autologous Venous Tissue, Percutaneous Endoscopic Approach

0212498 Bypass Coronary Artery, Three Arteries from Right Internal Mammary with Autologous Venous Tissue, Percutaneous Endoscopic Approach

0212499 Bypass Coronary Artery, Three Arteries from Left Internal Mammary with Autologous Venous Tissue, Percutaneous Endoscopic Approach

021249C Bypass Coronary Artery, Three Arteries from Thoracic Artery with Autologous Venous Tissue, Percutaneous Endoscopic Approach

021249F Bypass Coronary Artery, Three Arteries from Abdominal Artery with Autologous Venous Tissue, Percutaneous Endoscopic Approach

021249W Bypass Coronary Artery, Three Arteries from Aorta with Autologous Venous Tissue, Percutaneous Endoscopic Approach

HAC 08: Surgical Site Infection of Mediastinitis After Coronary Bypass Graft (CABG) Procedures (continued)

02124A3   Bypass Coronary Artery, Three Arteries from Coronary Artery with Autologous Arterial Tissue, Percutaneous Endoscopic Approach

02124A8   Bypass Coronary Artery, Three Arteries from Right Internal Mammary with Autologous Arterial Tissue, Percutaneous Endoscopic Approach

02124A9   Bypass Coronary Artery, Three Arteries from Left Internal Mammary with Autologous Arterial Tissue, Percutaneous Endoscopic Approach

02124AC   Bypass Coronary Artery, Three Arteries from Thoracic Artery with Autologous Arterial Tissue, Percutaneous Endoscopic Approach

02124AF   Bypass Coronary Artery, Three Arteries from Abdominal Artery with Autologous Arterial Tissue, Percutaneous Endoscopic Approach

02124AW   Bypass Coronary Artery, Three Arteries from Aorta with Autologous Arterial Tissue, Percutaneous Endoscopic Approach

02124J3   Bypass Coronary Artery, Three Arteries from Coronary Artery with Synthetic Substitute, Percutaneous Endoscopic Approach

02124J8   Bypass Coronary Artery, Three Arteries from Right Internal Mammary with Synthetic Substitute, Percutaneous Endoscopic Approach

02124J9   Bypass Coronary Artery, Three Arteries from Left Internal Mammary with Synthetic Substitute, Percutaneous Endoscopic Approach

02124JC   Bypass Coronary Artery, Three Arteries from Thoracic Artery with Synthetic Substitute, Percutaneous Endoscopic Approach

02124JF   Bypass Coronary Artery, Three Arteries from Abdominal Artery with Synthetic Substitute, Percutaneous Endoscopic Approach

02124JW   Bypass Coronary Artery, Three Arteries from Aorta with Synthetic Substitute, Percutaneous Endoscopic Approach

02124K3   Bypass Coronary Artery, Three Arteries from Coronary Artery with Nonautologous Tissue Substitute, Percutaneous Endoscopic Approach

02124K8   Bypass Coronary Artery, Three Arteries from Right Internal Mammary with Nonautologous Tissue Substitute, Percutaneous Endoscopic Approach

02124K9   Bypass Coronary Artery, Three Arteries from Left Internal Mammary with Nonautologous Tissue Substitute, Percutaneous Endoscopic Approach

02124KC   Bypass Coronary Artery, Three Arteries from Thoracic Artery with Nonautologous Tissue Substitute, Percutaneous Endoscopic Approach

02124KF   Bypass Coronary Artery, Three Arteries from Abdominal Artery with Nonautologous Tissue Substitute, Percutaneous Endoscopic Approach

02124KW   Bypass Coronary Artery, Three Arteries from Aorta with Nonautologous Tissue Substitute, Percutaneous Endoscopic Approach

02124Z3   Bypass Coronary Artery, Three Arteries from Coronary Artery, Percutaneous Endoscopic Approach

02124Z8   Bypass Coronary Artery, Three Arteries from Right Internal Mammary, Percutaneous Endoscopic Approach

02124Z9   Bypass Coronary Artery, Three Arteries from Left Internal Mammary, Percutaneous Endoscopic Approach

02124ZC   Bypass Coronary Artery, Three Arteries from Thoracic Artery, Percutaneous Endoscopic Approach

02124ZF   Bypass Coronary Artery, Three Arteries from Abdominal Artery, Percutaneous Endoscopic Approach

0213083   Bypass Coronary Artery, Four or More Arteries from Coronary Artery with Zooplastic Tissue, Open Approach

0213088   Bypass Coronary Artery, Four or More Arteries from Right Internal Mammary with Zooplastic Tissue, Open Approach

0213089   Bypass Coronary Artery, Four or More Arteries from Left Internal Mammary with Zooplastic Tissue, Open Approach

021308C   Bypass Coronary Artery, Four or More Arteries from Thoracic Artery with Zooplastic Tissue, Open Approach

021308F   Bypass Coronary Artery, Four or More Arteries from Abdominal Artery with Zooplastic Tissue, Open Approach

021308W   Bypass Coronary Artery, Four or More Arteries from Aorta with Zooplastic Tissue, Open Approach

0213093   Bypass Coronary Artery, Four or More Arteries from Coronary Artery with Autologous Venous Tissue, Open Approach

0213098   Bypass Coronary Artery, Four or More Arteries from Right Internal Mammary with Autologous Venous Tissue, Open Approach

0213099   Bypass Coronary Artery, Four or More Arteries from Left Internal Mammary with Autologous Venous Tissue, Open Approach

021309C   Bypass Coronary Artery, Four or More Arteries from Thoracic Artery with Autologous Venous Tissue, Open Approach

021309F   Bypass Coronary Artery, Four or More Arteries from Abdominal Artery with Autologous Venous Tissue, Open Approach

021309W   Bypass Coronary Artery, Four or More Arteries from Aorta with Autologous Venous Tissue, Open Approach

02130A3   Bypass Coronary Artery, Four or More Arteries from Coronary Artery with Autologous Arterial Tissue, Open Approach

02130A8   Bypass Coronary Artery, Four or More Arteries from Right Internal Mammary with Autologous Arterial Tissue, Open Approach

02130A9   Bypass Coronary Artery, Four or More Arteries from Left Internal Mammary with Autologous Arterial Tissue, Open Approach

02130AC   Bypass Coronary Artery, Four or More Arteries from Thoracic Artery with Autologous Arterial Tissue, Open Approach

02130AF   Bypass Coronary Artery, Four or More Arteries from Abdominal Artery with Autologous Arterial Tissue, Open Approach

02130AW   Bypass Coronary Artery, Four or More Arteries from Aorta with Autologous Arterial Tissue, Open Approach

02130J3   Bypass Coronary Artery, Four or More Arteries from Coronary Artery with Synthetic Substitute, Open Approach

02130J8   Bypass Coronary Artery, Four or More Arteries from Right Internal Mammary with Synthetic Substitute, Open Approach

02130J9   Bypass Coronary Artery, Four or More Arteries from Left Internal Mammary with Synthetic Substitute, Open Approach

02130JC   Bypass Coronary Artery, Four or More Arteries from Thoracic Artery with Synthetic Substitute, Open Approach

02130JF   Bypass Coronary Artery, Four or More Arteries from Abdominal Artery with Synthetic Substitute, Open Approach

02130JW   Bypass Coronary Artery, Four or More Arteries from Aorta with Synthetic Substitute, Open Approach

02130K3   Bypass Coronary Artery, Four or More Arteries from Coronary Artery with Nonautologous Tissue Substitute, Open Approach

02130K8   Bypass Coronary Artery, Four or More Arteries from Right Internal Mammary with Nonautologous Tissue Substitute, Open Approach

02130K9   Bypass Coronary Artery, Four or More Arteries from Left Internal Mammary with Nonautologous Tissue Substitute, Open Approach

02130KC   Bypass Coronary Artery, Four or More Arteries from Thoracic Artery with Nonautologous Tissue Substitute, Open Approach

02130KF   Bypass Coronary Artery, Four or More Arteries from Abdominal Artery with Nonautologous Tissue Substitute, Open Approach

02130KW   Bypass Coronary Artery, Four or More Arteries from Aorta with Nonautologous Tissue Substitute, Open Approach

02130Z3   Bypass Coronary Artery, Four or More Arteries from Coronary Artery, Open Approach

02130Z8   Bypass Coronary Artery, Four or More Arteries from Right Internal Mammary, Open Approach

02130Z9   Bypass Coronary Artery, Four or More Arteries from Left Internal Mammary, Open Approach

02130ZC   Bypass Coronary Artery, Four or More Arteries from Thoracic Artery, Open Approach

02130ZF   Bypass Coronary Artery, Four or More Arteries from Abdominal Artery, Open Approach

0213483   Bypass Coronary Artery, Four or More Arteries from Coronary Artery with Zooplastic Tissue, Percutaneous Endoscopic Approach

0213488   Bypass Coronary Artery, Four or More Arteries from Right Internal Mammary with Zooplastic Tissue, Percutaneous Endoscopic Approach

0213489   Bypass Coronary Artery, Four or More Arteries from Left Internal Mammary with Zooplastic Tissue, Percutaneous Endoscopic Approach

021348C   Bypass Coronary Artery, Four or More Arteries from Thoracic Artery with Zooplastic Tissue, Percutaneous Endoscopic Approach

HAC 08: Surgical Site Infection of Mediastinitis After Coronary Bypass Graft (CABG) Procedures (continued)

021348F   Bypass Coronary Artery, Four or More Arteries from Abdominal Artery with Zooplastic Tissue, Percutaneous Endoscopic Approach

021348W   Bypass Coronary Artery, Four or More Arteries from Aorta with Zooplastic Tissue, Percutaneous Endoscopic Approach

0213493   Bypass Coronary Artery, Four or More Arteries from Coronary Artery with Autologous Venous Tissue, Percutaneous Endoscopic Approach

0213498   Bypass Coronary Artery, Four or More Arteries from Right Internal Mammary with Autologous Venous Tissue, Percutaneous Endoscopic Approach

0213499   Bypass Coronary Artery, Four or More Arteries from Left Internal Mammary with Autologous Venous Tissue, Percutaneous Endoscopic Approach

021349C   Bypass Coronary Artery, Four or More Arteries from Thoracic Artery with Autologous Venous Tissue, Percutaneous Endoscopic Approach

021349F   Bypass Coronary Artery, Four or More Arteries from Abdominal Artery with Autologous Venous Tissue, Percutaneous Endoscopic Approach

021349W   Bypass Coronary Artery, Four or More Arteries from Aorta with Autologous Venous Tissue, Percutaneous Endoscopic Approach

02134A3   Bypass Coronary Artery, Four or More Arteries from Coronary Artery with Autologous Arterial Tissue, Percutaneous Endoscopic Approach

02134A8   Bypass Coronary Artery, Four or More Arteries from Right Internal Mammary with Autologous Arterial Tissue, Percutaneous Endoscopic Approach

02134A9   Bypass Coronary Artery, Four or More Arteries from Left Internal Mammary with Autologous Arterial Tissue, Percutaneous Endoscopic Approach

02134AC   Bypass Coronary Artery, Four or More Arteries from Thoracic Artery with Autologous Arterial Tissue, Percutaneous Endoscopic Approach

02134AF   Bypass Coronary Artery, Four or More Arteries from Abdominal Artery with Autologous Arterial Tissue, Percutaneous Endoscopic Approach

02134AW   Bypass Coronary Artery, Four or More Arteries from Aorta with Autologous Arterial Tissue, Percutaneous Endoscopic Approach

02134J3   Bypass Coronary Artery, Four or More Arteries from Coronary Artery with Synthetic Substitute, Percutaneous Endoscopic Approach

02134J8   Bypass Coronary Artery, Four or More Arteries from Right Internal Mammary with Synthetic Substitute, Percutaneous Endoscopic Approach

02134J9   Bypass Coronary Artery, Four or More Arteries from Left Internal Mammary with Synthetic Substitute, Percutaneous Endoscopic Approach

02134JC   Bypass Coronary Artery, Four or More Arteries from Thoracic Artery with Synthetic Substitute, Percutaneous Endoscopic Approach

02134JF   Bypass Coronary Artery, Four or More Arteries from Abdominal Artery with Synthetic Substitute, Percutaneous Endoscopic Approach

02134JW   Bypass Coronary Artery, Four or More Arteries from Aorta with Synthetic Substitute, Percutaneous Endoscopic Approach

02134K3   Bypass Coronary Artery, Four or More Arteries from Coronary Artery with Nonautologous Tissue Substitute, Percutaneous Endoscopic Approach

02134K8   Bypass Coronary Artery, Four or More Arteries from Right Internal Mammary with Nonautologous Tissue Substitute, Percutaneous Endoscopic Approach

02134K9   Bypass Coronary Artery, Four or More Arteries from Left Internal Mammary with Nonautologous Tissue Substitute, Percutaneous Endoscopic Approach

02134KC   Bypass Coronary Artery, Four or More Arteries from Thoracic Artery with Nonautologous Tissue Substitute, Percutaneous Endoscopic Approach

02134KF   Bypass Coronary Artery, Four or More Arteries from Abdominal Artery with Nonautologous Tissue Substitute, Percutaneous Endoscopic Approach

02134KW   Bypass Coronary Artery, Four or More Arteries from Aorta with Nonautologous Tissue Substitute, Percutaneous Endoscopic Approach

02134Z3   Bypass Coronary Artery, Four or More Arteries from Coronary Artery, Percutaneous Endoscopic Approach

02134Z8   Bypass Coronary Artery, Four or More Arteries from Right Internal Mammary, Percutaneous Endoscopic Approach

02134Z9   Bypass Coronary Artery, Four or More Arteries from Left Internal Mammary, Percutaneous Endoscopic Approach

02134ZC   Bypass Coronary Artery, Four or More Arteries from Thoracic Artery, Percutaneous Endoscopic Approach

02134ZF   Bypass Coronary Artery, Four or More Arteries from Abdominal Artery, Percutaneous Endoscopic Approach

HAC 10: Deep Vein Thrombosis (DVT) or Pulmonary Embolism (PE) with Total Knee or Hip Replacement

Secondary diagnosis not POA:

I26.02   Saddle embolus of pulmonary artery with acute cor pulmonale

I26.09   Other pulmonary embolism with acute cor pulmonale

I26.92   Saddle embolus of pulmonary artery without acute cor pulmonale

I26.93   Single subsegmental pulmonary embolism without acute cor pulmonale

I26.94   Multiple subsegmental pulmonary emboli without acute cor pulmonale

I26.99   Other pulmonary embolism without acute cor pulmonale

I82.401   Acute embolism and thrombosis of unspecified deep veins of right lower extremity

I82.402   Acute embolism and thrombosis of unspecified deep veins of left lower extremity

I82.403   Acute embolism and thrombosis of unspecified deep veins of lower extremity, bilateral

I82.409   Acute embolism and thrombosis of unspecified deep veins of unspecified lower extremity

I82.411   Acute embolism and thrombosis of right femoral vein

I82.412   Acute embolism and thrombosis of left femoral vein

I82.413   Acute embolism and thrombosis of femoral vein, bilateral

I82.419   Acute embolism and thrombosis of unspecified femoral vein

I82.421   Acute embolism and thrombosis of right iliac vein

I82.422   Acute embolism and thrombosis of left iliac vein

I82.423   Acute embolism and thrombosis of iliac vein, bilateral

I82.429   Acute embolism and thrombosis of unspecified iliac vein

I82.431   Acute embolism and thrombosis of right popliteal vein

I82.432   Acute embolism and thrombosis of left popliteal vein

I82.433   Acute embolism and thrombosis of popliteal vein, bilateral

I82.439   Acute embolism and thrombosis of unspecified popliteal vein

I82.441   Acute embolism and thrombosis of right tibial vein

I82.442   Acute embolism and thrombosis of left tibial vein

I82.443   Acute embolism and thrombosis of tibial vein, bilateral

I82.449   Acute embolism and thrombosis of unspecified tibial vein

I82.451   Acute embolism and thrombosis of right peroneal vein

I82.452   Acute embolism and thrombosis of left peroneal vein

I82.453   Acute embolism and thrombosis of peroneal vein, bilateral

I82.459   Acute embolism and thrombosis of unspecified peroneal vein

I82.491   Acute embolism and thrombosis of other specified deep vein of right lower extremity

I82.492   Acute embolism and thrombosis of other specified deep vein of left lower extremity

I82.493   Acute embolism and thrombosis of other specified deep vein of lower extremity, bilateral

I82.499   Acute embolism and thrombosis of other specified deep vein of unspecified lower extremity

I82.4Y1   Acute embolism and thrombosis of unspecified deep veins of right proximal lower extremity

I82.4Y2   Acute embolism and thrombosis of unspecified deep veins of left proximal lower extremity

I82.4Y3   Acute embolism and thrombosis of unspecified deep veins of proximal lower extremity, bilateral

I82.4Y9   Acute embolism and thrombosis of unspecified deep veins of unspecified proximal lower extremity

I82.4Z1   Acute embolism and thrombosis of unspecified deep veins of right distal lower extremity

I82.4Z2   Acute embolism and thrombosis of unspecified deep veins of left distal lower extremity

I82.4Z3   Acute embolism and thrombosis of unspecified deep veins of distal lower extremity, bilateral

I82.4Z9   Acute embolism and thrombosis of unspecified deep veins of unspecified distal lower extremity

HAC 10: Deep Vein Thrombosis (DVT) or Pulmonary Embolism (PE) with Total Knee or Hip Replacement (continued)

AND

Any of the following procedures:

ØSR9Ø19　Replacement of Right Hip Joint with Metal Synthetic Substitute, Cemented, Open Approach

ØSR9Ø1A　Replacement of Right Hip Joint with Metal Synthetic Substitute, Uncemented, Open Approach

ØSR9Ø1Z　Replacement of Right Hip Joint with Metal Synthetic Substitute, Open Approach

ØSR9Ø29　Replacement of Right Hip Joint with Metal on Polyethylene Synthetic Substitute, Cemented, Open Approach

ØSR9Ø2A　Replacement of Right Hip Joint with Metal on Polyethylene Synthetic Substitute, Uncemented, Open Approach

ØSR9Ø2Z　Replacement of Right Hip Joint with Metal on Polyethylene Synthetic Substitute, Open Approach

ØSR9Ø39　Replacement of Right Hip Joint with Ceramic Synthetic Substitute, Cemented, Open Approach

ØSR9Ø3A　Replacement of Right Hip Joint with Ceramic Synthetic Substitute, Uncemented, Open Approach

ØSR9Ø3Z　Replacement of Right Hip Joint with Ceramic Synthetic Substitute, Open Approach

ØSR9Ø49　Replacement of Right Hip Joint with Ceramic on Polyethylene Synthetic Substitute, Cemented, Open Approach

ØSR9Ø4A　Replacement of Right Hip Joint with Ceramic on Polyethylene Synthetic Substitute, Uncemented, Open Approach

ØSR9Ø4Z　Replacement of Right Hip Joint with Ceramic on Polyethylene Synthetic Substitute, Open Approach

ØSR9Ø69　Replacement of Right Hip Joint with Oxidized Zirconium on Polyethylene Synthetic Substitute, Cemented, Open Approach

ØSR9Ø6A　Replacement of Right Hip Joint with Oxidized Zirconium on Polyethylene Synthetic Substitute, Uncemented, Open Approach

ØSR9Ø6Z　Replacement of Right Hip Joint with Oxidized Zirconium on Polyethylene Synthetic Substitute, Open Approach

ØSR9Ø7Z　Replacement of Right Hip Joint with Autologous Tissue Substitute, Open Approach

ØSR9ØEZ　Replacement of Right Hip Joint with Articulating Spacer, Open Approach

ØSR9ØJ9　Replacement of Right Hip Joint with Synthetic Substitute, Cemented, Open Approach

ØSR9ØJA　Replacement of Right Hip Joint with Synthetic Substitute, Uncemented, Open Approach

ØSR9ØJZ　Replacement of Right Hip Joint with Synthetic Substitute, Open Approach

ØSR9ØKZ　Replacement of Right Hip Joint with Nonautologous Tissue Substitute, Open Approach

ØSRAØØ9　Replacement of Right Hip Joint, Acetabular Surface with Polyethylene Synthetic Substitute, Cemented, Open Approach

ØSRAØØA　Replacement of Right Hip Joint, Acetabular Surface with Polyethylene Synthetic Substitute, Uncemented, Open Approach

ØSRAØØZ　Replacement of Right Hip Joint, Acetabular Surface with Polyethylene Synthetic Substitute, Open Approach

ØSRAØ19　Replacement of Right Hip Joint, Acetabular Surface with Metal Synthetic Substitute, Cemented, Open Approach

ØSRAØ1A　Replacement of Right Hip Joint, Acetabular Surface with Metal Synthetic Substitute, Uncemented, Open Approach

ØSRAØ1Z　Replacement of Right Hip Joint, Acetabular Surface with Metal Synthetic Substitute, Open Approach

ØSRAØ39　Replacement of Right Hip Joint, Acetabular Surface with Ceramic Synthetic Substitute, Cemented, Open Approach

ØSRAØ3A　Replacement of Right Hip Joint, Acetabular Surface with Ceramic Synthetic Substitute, Uncemented, Open Approach

ØSRAØ3Z　Replacement of Right Hip Joint, Acetabular Surface with Ceramic Synthetic Substitute, Open Approach

ØSRAØ7Z　Replacement of Right Hip Joint, Acetabular Surface with Autologous Tissue Substitute, Open Approach

ØSRAØJ9　Replacement of Right Hip Joint, Acetabular Surface with Synthetic Substitute, Cemented, Open Approach

ØSRAØJA　Replacement of Right Hip Joint, Acetabular Surface with Synthetic Substitute, Uncemented, Open Approach

ØSRAØJZ　Replacement of Right Hip Joint, Acetabular Surface with Synthetic Substitute, Open Approach

ØSRAØKZ　Replacement of Right Hip Joint, Acetabular Surface with Nonautologous Tissue Substitute, Open Approach

ØSRBØ19　Replacement of Left Hip Joint with Metal Synthetic Substitute, Cemented, Open Approach

ØSRBØ1A　Replacement of Left Hip Joint with Metal Synthetic Substitute, Uncemented, Open Approach

ØSRBØ1Z　Replacement of Left Hip Joint with Metal Synthetic Substitute, Open Approach

ØSRBØ29　Replacement of Left Hip Joint with Metal on Polyethylene Synthetic Substitute, Cemented, Open Approach

ØSRBØ2A　Replacement of Left Hip Joint with Metal on Polyethylene Synthetic Substitute, Uncemented, Open Approach

ØSRBØ2Z　Replacement of Left Hip Joint with Metal on Polyethylene Synthetic Substitute, Open Approach

ØSRBØ39　Replacement of Left Hip Joint with Ceramic Synthetic Substitute, Cemented, Open Approach

ØSRBØ3A　Replacement of Left Hip Joint with Ceramic Synthetic Substitute, Uncemented, Open Approach

ØSRBØ3Z　Replacement of Left Hip Joint with Ceramic Synthetic Substitute, Open Approach

ØSRBØ49　Replacement of Left Hip Joint with Ceramic on Polyethylene Synthetic Substitute, Cemented, Open Approach

ØSRBØ4A　Replacement of Left Hip Joint with Ceramic on Polyethylene Synthetic Substitute, Uncemented, Open Approach

ØSRBØ4Z　Replacement of Left Hip Joint with Ceramic on Polyethylene Synthetic Substitute, Open Approach

ØSRBØ69　Replacement of Left Hip Joint with Oxidized Zirconium on Polyethylene Synthetic Substitute, Cemented, Open Approach

ØSRBØ6A　Replacement of Left Hip Joint with Oxidized Zirconium on Polyethylene Synthetic Substitute, Uncemented, Open Approach

ØSRBØ6Z　Replacement of Left Hip Joint with Oxidized Zirconium on Polyethylene Synthetic Substitute, Open Approach

ØSRBØ7Z　Replacement of Left Hip Joint with Autologous Tissue Substitute, Open Approach

ØSRBØEZ　Replacement of Left Hip Joint with Articulating Spacer, Open Approach

ØSRBØJ9　Replacement of Left Hip Joint with Synthetic Substitute, Cemented, Open Approach

ØSRBØJA　Replacement of Left Hip Joint with Synthetic Substitute, Uncemented, Open Approach

ØSRBØJZ　Replacement of Left Hip Joint with Synthetic Substitute, Open Approach

ØSRBØKZ　Replacement of Left Hip Joint with Nonautologous Tissue Substitute, Open Approach

ØSRCØ69　Replacement of Right Knee Joint with Oxidized Zirconium on Polyethylene Synthetic Substitute, Cemented, Open Approach

ØSRCØ6A　Replacement of Right Knee Joint with Oxidized Zirconium on Polyethylene Synthetic Substitute, Uncemented, Open Approach

ØSRCØ6Z　Replacement of Right Knee Joint with Oxidized Zirconium on Polyethylene Synthetic Substitute, Open Approach

ØSRCØ7Z　Replacement of Right Knee Joint with Autologous Tissue Substitute, Open Approach

ØSRCØEZ　Replacement of Right Knee Joint with Articulating Spacer, Open Approach

ØSRCØJ9　Replacement of Right Knee Joint with Synthetic Substitute, Cemented, Open Approach

ØSRCØJA　Replacement of Right Knee Joint with Synthetic Substitute, Uncemented, Open Approach

ØSRCØJZ　Replacement of Right Knee Joint with Synthetic Substitute, Open Approach

ØSRCØKZ　Replacement of Right Knee Joint with Nonautologous Tissue Substitute, Open Approach

ØSRCØL9　Replacement of Right Knee Joint with Medial Unicondylar Synthetic Substitute, Cemented, Open Approach

ØSRCØLA　Replacement of Right Knee Joint with Medial Unicondylar Synthetic Substitute, Uncemented, Open Approach

ØSRCØLZ　Replacement of Right Knee Joint with Medial Unicondylar Synthetic Substitute, Open Approach

ØSRCØM9　Replacement of Right Knee Joint with Lateral Unicondylar Synthetic Substitute, Cemented, Open Approach

ØSRCØMA　Replacement of Right Knee Joint with Lateral Unicondylar Synthetic Substitute, Uncemented, Open Approach

ØSRCØMZ　Replacement of Right Knee Joint with Lateral Unicondylar Synthetic Substitute, Open Approach

ØSRCØN9　Replacement of Right Knee Joint with Patellofemoral Synthetic Substitute, Cemented, Open Approach

ØSRCØNA　Replacement of Right Knee Joint with Patellofemoral Synthetic Substitute, Uncemented, Open Approach

HAC 10: Deep Vein Thrombosis (DVT) or Pulmonary Embolism (PE) with Total Knee or Hip Replacement (continued)

ØSRCØNZ   Replacement of Right Knee Joint with Patellofemoral Synthetic Substitute, Open Approach

ØSRDØ69   Replacement of Left Knee Joint with Oxidized Zirconium on Polyethylene Synthetic Substitute, Cemented, Open Approach

ØSRDØ6A   Replacement of Left Knee Joint with Oxidized Zirconium on Polyethylene Synthetic Substitute, Uncemented, Open Approach

ØSRDØ6Z   Replacement of Left Knee Joint with Oxidized Zirconium on Polyethylene Synthetic Substitute, Open Approach

ØSRDØ7Z   Replacement of Left Knee Joint with Autologous Tissue Substitute, Open Approach

ØSRDØEZ   Replacement of Left Knee Joint with Articulating Spacer, Open Approach

ØSRDØJ9   Replacement of Left Knee Joint with Synthetic Substitute, Cemented, Open Approach

ØSRDØJA   Replacement of Left Knee Joint with Synthetic Substitute, Uncemented, Open Approach

ØSRDØJZ   Replacement of Left Knee Joint with Synthetic Substitute, Open Approach

ØSRDØKZ   Replacement of Left Knee Joint with Nonautologous Tissue Substitute, Open Approach

ØSRDØL9   Replacement of Left Knee Joint with Medial Unicondylar Synthetic Substitute, Cemented, Open Approach

ØSRDØLA   Replacement of Left Knee Joint with Medial Unicondylar Synthetic Substitute, Uncemented, Open Approach

ØSRDØLZ   Replacement of Left Knee Joint with Medial Unicondylar Synthetic Substitute, Open Approach

ØSRDØM9   Replacement of Left Knee Joint with Lateral Unicondylar Synthetic Substitute, Cemented, Open Approach

ØSRDØMA   Replacement of Left Knee Joint with Lateral Unicondylar Synthetic Substitute, Uncemented, Open Approach

ØSRDØMZ   Replacement of Left Knee Joint with Lateral Unicondylar Synthetic Substitute, Open Approach

ØSRDØN9   Replacement of Left Knee Joint with Patellofemoral Synthetic Substitute, Cemented, Open Approach

ØSRDØNA   Replacement of Left Knee Joint with Patellofemoral Synthetic Substitute, Uncemented, Open Approach

ØSRDØNZ   Replacement of Left Knee Joint with Patellofemoral Synthetic Substitute, Open Approach

ØSREØØ9   Replacement of Left Hip Joint, Acetabular Surface with Polyethylene Synthetic Substitute, Cemented, Open Approach

ØSREØØA   Replacement of Left Hip Joint, Acetabular Surface with Polyethylene Synthetic Substitute, Uncemented, Open Approach

ØSREØØZ   Replacement of Left Hip Joint, Acetabular Surface with Polyethylene Synthetic Substitute, Open Approach

ØSREØ19   Replacement of Left Hip Joint, Acetabular Surface with Metal Synthetic Substitute, Cemented, Open Approach

ØSREØ1A   Replacement of Left Hip Joint, Acetabular Surface with Metal Synthetic Substitute, Uncemented, Open Approach

ØSREØ1Z   Replacement of Left Hip Joint, Acetabular Surface with Metal Synthetic Substitute, Open Approach

ØSREØ39   Replacement of Left Hip Joint, Acetabular Surface with Ceramic Synthetic Substitute, Cemented, Open Approach

ØSREØ3A   Replacement of Left Hip Joint, Acetabular Surface with Ceramic Synthetic Substitute, Uncemented, Open Approach

ØSREØ3Z   Replacement of Left Hip Joint, Acetabular Surface with Ceramic Synthetic Substitute, Open Approach

ØSREØ7Z   Replacement of Left Hip Joint, Acetabular Surface with Autologous Tissue Substitute, Open Approach

ØSREØJ9   Replacement of Left Hip Joint, Acetabular Surface with Synthetic Substitute, Cemented, Open Approach

ØSREØJA   Replacement of Left Hip Joint, Acetabular Surface with Synthetic Substitute, Uncemented, Open Approach

ØSREØJZ   Replacement of Left Hip Joint, Acetabular Surface with Synthetic Substitute, Open Approach

ØSREØKZ   Replacement of Left Hip Joint, Acetabular Surface with Nonautologous Tissue Substitute, Open Approach

ØSRRØ19   Replacement of Right Hip Joint, Femoral Surface with Metal Synthetic Substitute, Cemented, Open Approach

ØSRRØ1A   Replacement of Right Hip Joint, Femoral Surface with Metal Synthetic Substitute, Uncemented, Open Approach

ØSRRØ1Z   Replacement of Right Hip Joint, Femoral Surface with Metal Synthetic Substitute, Open Approach

ØSRRØ39   Replacement of Right Hip Joint, Femoral Surface with Ceramic Synthetic Substitute, Cemented, Open Approach

ØSRRØ3A   Replacement of Right Hip Joint, Femoral Surface with Ceramic Synthetic Substitute, Uncemented, Open Approach

ØSRRØ3Z   Replacement of Right Hip Joint, Femoral Surface with Ceramic Synthetic Substitute, Open Approach

ØSRRØ7Z   Replacement of Right Hip Joint, Femoral Surface with Autologous Tissue Substitute, Open Approach

ØSRRØJ9   Replacement of Right Hip Joint, Femoral Surface with Synthetic Substitute, Cemented, Open Approach

ØSRRØJA   Replacement of Right Hip Joint, Femoral Surface with Synthetic Substitute, Uncemented, Open Approach

ØSRRØJZ   Replacement of Right Hip Joint, Femoral Surface with Synthetic Substitute, Open Approach

ØSRRØKZ   Replacement of Right Hip Joint, Femoral Surface with Nonautologous Tissue Substitute, Open Approach

ØSRSØ19   Replacement of Left Hip Joint, Femoral Surface with Metal Synthetic Substitute, Cemented, Open Approach

ØSRSØ1A   Replacement of Left Hip Joint, Femoral Surface with Metal Synthetic Substitute, Uncemented, Open Approach

ØSRSØ1Z   Replacement of Left Hip Joint, Femoral Surface with Metal Synthetic Substitute, Open Approach

ØSRSØ39   Replacement of Left Hip Joint, Femoral Surface with Ceramic Synthetic Substitute, Cemented, Open Approach

ØSRSØ3A   Replacement of Left Hip Joint, Femoral Surface with Ceramic Synthetic Substitute, Uncemented, Open Approach

ØSRSØ3Z   Replacement of Left Hip Joint, Femoral Surface with Ceramic Synthetic Substitute, Open Approach

ØSRSØ7Z   Replacement of Left Hip Joint, Femoral Surface with Autologous Tissue Substitute, Open Approach

ØSRSØJ9   Replacement of Left Hip Joint, Femoral Surface with Synthetic Substitute, Cemented, Open Approach

ØSRSØJA   Replacement of Left Hip Joint, Femoral Surface with Synthetic Substitute, Uncemented, Open Approach

ØSRSØJZ   Replacement of Left Hip Joint, Femoral Surface with Synthetic Substitute, Open Approach

ØSRSØKZ   Replacement of Left Hip Joint, Femoral Surface with Nonautologous Tissue Substitute, Open Approach

ØSRTØ7Z   Replacement of Right Knee Joint, Femoral Surface with Autologous Tissue Substitute, Open Approach

ØSRTØJ9   Replacement of Right Knee Joint, Femoral Surface with Synthetic Substitute, Cemented, Open Approach

ØSRTØJA   Replacement of Right Knee Joint, Femoral Surface with Synthetic Substitute, Uncemented, Open Approach

ØSRTØJZ   Replacement of Right Knee Joint, Femoral Surface with Synthetic Substitute, Open Approach

ØSRTØKZ   Replacement of Right Knee Joint, Femoral Surface with Nonautologous Tissue Substitute, Open Approach

ØSRUØ7Z   Replacement of Left Knee Joint, Femoral Surface with Autologous Tissue Substitute, Open Approach

ØSRUØJ9   Replacement of Left Knee Joint, Femoral Surface with Synthetic Substitute, Cemented, Open Approach

ØSRUØJA   Replacement of Left Knee Joint, Femoral Surface with Synthetic Substitute, Uncemented, Open Approach

ØSRUØJZ   Replacement of Left Knee Joint, Femoral Surface with Synthetic Substitute, Open Approach

ØSRUØKZ   Replacement of Left Knee Joint, Femoral Surface with Nonautologous Tissue Substitute, Open Approach

ØSRVØ7Z   Replacement of Right Knee Joint, Tibial Surface with Autologous Tissue Substitute, Open Approach

ØSRVØJ9   Replacement of Right Knee Joint, Tibial Surface with Synthetic Substitute, Cemented, Open Approach

ØSRVØJA   Replacement of Right Knee Joint, Tibial Surface with Synthetic Substitute, Uncemented, Open Approach

ØSRVØJZ   Replacement of Right Knee Joint, Tibial Surface with Synthetic Substitute, Open Approach

ØSRVØKZ   Replacement of Right Knee Joint, Tibial Surface with Nonautologous Tissue Substitute, Open Approach

ØSRWØ7Z   Replacement of Left Knee Joint, Tibial Surface with Autologous Tissue Substitute, Open Approach

ØSRWØJ9   Replacement of Left Knee Joint, Tibial Surface with Synthetic Substitute, Cemented, Open Approach

ØSRWØJA   Replacement of Left Knee Joint, Tibial Surface with Synthetic Substitute, Uncemented, Open Approach

ØSRWØJZ   Replacement of Left Knee Joint, Tibial Surface with Synthetic Substitute, Open Approach

HAC 10: Deep Vein Thrombosis (DVT) or Pulmonary Embolism (PE) with Total Knee or Hip Replacement (continued)

ØSRWØKZ   Replacement of Left Knee Joint, Tibial Surface with Nonautologous Tissue Substitute, Open Approach

ØSU9ØBZ   Supplement Right Hip Joint with Resurfacing Device, Open Approach

ØSUAØBZ   Supplement Right Hip Joint, Acetabular Surface with Resurfacing Device, Open Approach

ØSUBØBZ   Supplement Left Hip Joint with Resurfacing Device, Open Approach

ØSUEØBZ   Supplement Left Hip Joint, Acetabular Surface with Resurfacing Device, Open Approach

ØSURØBZ   Supplement Right Hip Joint, Femoral Surface with Resurfacing Device, Open Approach

ØSUSØBZ   Supplement Left Hip Joint, Femoral Surface with Resurfacing Device, Open Approach

HAC 11: Surgical Site Infection-Bariatric Surgery

Principal diagnosis of:

E66.Ø1   Morbid (severe) obesity due to excess calories

AND

Secondary diagnosis not POA:

K68.11   Postprocedural retroperitoneal abscess
K95.Ø1   Infection due to gastric band procedure
K95.81   Infection due to other bariatric procedure
T81.4ØXA   Infection following a procedure, unspecified, initial encounter
T81.41XA   Infection following a procedure, superficial incisional surgical site, initial encounter
T81.42XA   Infection following a procedure, deep incisional surgical site, initial encounter
T81.43XA   Infection following a procedure, organ and space surgical site, initial encounter
T81.44XA   Sepsis following a procedure, initial encounter
T81.49XA   Infection following a procedure, other surgical site, initial encounter

AND

Any of the following procedures:

ØD16Ø79   Bypass Stomach to Duodenum with Autologous Tissue Substitute, Open Approach

ØD16Ø7A   Bypass Stomach to Jejunum with Autologous Tissue Substitute, Open Approach

ØD16Ø7B   Bypass Stomach to Ileum with Autologous Tissue Substitute, Open Approach

ØD16Ø7L   Bypass Stomach to Transverse Colon with Autologous Tissue Substitute, Open Approach

ØD16ØJ9   Bypass Stomach to Duodenum with Synthetic Substitute, Open Approach

ØD16ØJA   Bypass Stomach to Jejunum with Synthetic Substitute, Open Approach

ØD16ØJB   Bypass Stomach to Ileum with Synthetic Substitute, Open Approach

ØD16ØJL   Bypass Stomach to Transverse Colon with Synthetic Substitute, Open Approach

ØD16ØK9   Bypass Stomach to Duodenum with Nonautologous Tissue Substitute, Open Approach

ØD16ØKA   Bypass Stomach to Jejunum with Nonautologous Tissue Substitute, Open Approach

ØD16ØKB   Bypass Stomach to Ileum with Nonautologous Tissue Substitute, Open Approach

ØD16ØKL   Bypass Stomach to Transverse Colon with Nonautologous Tissue Substitute, Open Approach

ØD16ØZ9   Bypass Stomach to Duodenum, Open Approach

ØD16ØZA   Bypass Stomach to Jejunum, Open Approach

ØD16ØZB   Bypass Stomach to Ileum, Open Approach

ØD16ØZL   Bypass Stomach to Transverse Colon, Open Approach

ØD16479   Bypass Stomach to Duodenum with Autologous Tissue Substitute, Percutaneous Endoscopic Approach

ØD1647A   Bypass Stomach to Jejunum with Autologous Tissue Substitute, Percutaneous Endoscopic Approach

ØD1647B   Bypass Stomach to Ileum with Autologous Tissue Substitute, Percutaneous Endoscopic Approach

ØD1647L   Bypass Stomach to Transverse Colon with Autologous Tissue Substitute, Percutaneous Endoscopic Approach

ØD164J9   Bypass Stomach to Duodenum with Synthetic Substitute, Percutaneous Endoscopic Approach

ØD164JA   Bypass Stomach to Jejunum with Synthetic Substitute, Percutaneous Endoscopic Approach

ØD164JB   Bypass Stomach to Ileum with Synthetic Substitute, Percutaneous Endoscopic Approach

ØD164JL   Bypass Stomach to Transverse Colon with Synthetic Substitute, Percutaneous Endoscopic Approach

ØD164K9   Bypass Stomach to Duodenum with Nonautologous Tissue Substitute, Percutaneous Endoscopic Approach

ØD164KA   Bypass Stomach to Jejunum with Nonautologous Tissue Substitute, Percutaneous Endoscopic Approach

ØD164KB   Bypass Stomach to Ileum with Nonautologous Tissue Substitute, Percutaneous Endoscopic Approach

ØD164KL   Bypass Stomach to Transverse Colon with Nonautologous Tissue Substitute, Percutaneous Endoscopic Approach

ØD164Z9   Bypass Stomach to Duodenum, Percutaneous Endoscopic Approach

ØD164ZA   Bypass Stomach to Jejunum, Percutaneous Endoscopic Approach

ØD164ZB   Bypass Stomach to Ileum, Percutaneous Endoscopic Approach

ØD164ZL   Bypass Stomach to Transverse Colon, Percutaneous Endoscopic Approach

ØD16879   Bypass Stomach to Duodenum with Autologous Tissue Substitute, Via Natural or Artificial Opening Endoscopic

ØD1687A   Bypass Stomach to Jejunum with Autologous Tissue Substitute, Via Natural or Artificial Opening Endoscopic

ØD1687B   Bypass Stomach to Ileum with Autologous Tissue Substitute, Via Natural or Artificial Opening Endoscopic

ØD1687L   Bypass Stomach to Transverse Colon with Autologous Tissue Substitute, Via Natural or Artificial Opening Endoscopic

ØD168J9   Bypass Stomach to Duodenum with Synthetic Substitute, Via Natural or Artificial Opening Endoscopic

ØD168JA   Bypass Stomach to Jejunum with Synthetic Substitute, Via Natural or Artificial Opening Endoscopic

ØD168JB   Bypass Stomach to Ileum with Synthetic Substitute, Via Natural or Artificial Opening Endoscopic

ØD168JL   Bypass Stomach to Transverse Colon with Synthetic Substitute, Via Natural or Artificial Opening Endoscopic

ØD168K9   Bypass Stomach to Duodenum with Nonautologous Tissue Substitute, Via Natural or Artificial Opening Endoscopic

ØD168KA   Bypass Stomach to Jejunum with Nonautologous Tissue Substitute, Via Natural or Artificial Opening Endoscopic

ØD168KB   Bypass Stomach to Ileum with Nonautologous Tissue Substitute, Via Natural or Artificial Opening Endoscopic

ØD168KL   Bypass Stomach to Transverse Colon with Nonautologous Tissue Substitute, Via Natural or Artificial Opening Endoscopic

ØD168Z9   Bypass Stomach to Duodenum, Via Natural or Artificial Opening Endoscopic

ØD168ZA   Bypass Stomach to Jejunum, Via Natural or Artificial Opening Endoscopic

ØD168ZB   Bypass Stomach to Ileum, Via Natural or Artificial Opening Endoscopic

ØD168ZL   Bypass Stomach to Transverse Colon, Via Natural or Artificial Opening Endoscopic

ØDV64CZ   Restriction of Stomach with Extraluminal Device, Percutaneous Endoscopic Approach

HAC 12: Surgical Site Infection-Certain Orthopedic Procedures of the Spine, Shoulder, and Elbow

Secondary diagnosis not POA:

K68.11   Postprocedural retroperitoneal abscess
T81.4ØXA   Infection following a procedure, unspecified, initial encounter
T81.41XA   Infection following a procedure, superficial incisional surgical site, initial encounter
T81.42XA   Infection following a procedure, deep incisional surgical site, initial encounter
T81.43XA   Infection following a procedure, organ and space surgical site, initial encounter
T81.44XA   Sepsis following a procedure, initial encounter
T81.49XA   Infection following a procedure, other surgical site, initial encounter
T84.6ØXA   Infection and inflammatory reaction due to internal fixation device of unspecified site, initial encounter
T84.61ØA   Infection and inflammatory reaction due to internal fixation device of right humerus, initial encounter
T84.611A   Infection and inflammatory reaction due to internal fixation device of left humerus, initial encounter
T84.612A   Infection and inflammatory reaction due to internal fixation device of right radius, initial encounter
T84.613A   Infection and inflammatory reaction due to internal fixation device of left radius, initial encounter
T84.614A   Infection and inflammatory reaction due to internal fixation device of right ulna, initial encounter
T84.615A   Infection and inflammatory reaction due to internal fixation device of left ulna, initial encounter
T84.619A   Infection and inflammatory reaction due to internal fixation device of unspecified bone of arm, initial encounter
T84.63XA   Infection and inflammatory reaction due to internal fixation device of spine, initial encounter
T84.69XA   Infection and inflammatory reaction due to internal fixation device of other site, initial encounter

HAC 12: Surgical Site Infection-Certain Orthopedic Procedures of the Spine, Shoulder, and Elbow (continued)

T84.7XXA   Infection and inflammatory reaction due to other internal orthopedic prosthetic devices, implants and grafts, initial encounter

AND

Any of the following procedures:

ØRG0070   Fusion of Occipital-cervical Joint with Autologous Tissue Substitute, Anterior Approach, Anterior Column, Open Approach

ØRG0071   Fusion of Occipital-cervical Joint with Autologous Tissue Substitute, Posterior Approach, Posterior Column, Open Approach

ØRG007J   Fusion of Occipital-cervical Joint with Autologous Tissue Substitute, Posterior Approach, Anterior Column, Open Approach

ØRG00A0   Fusion of Occipital-cervical Joint with Interbody Fusion Device, Anterior Approach, Anterior Column, Open Approach

ØRG00AJ   Fusion of Occipital-cervical Joint with Interbody Fusion Device, Posterior Approach, Anterior Column, Open Approach

ØRG00J0   Fusion of Occipital-cervical Joint with Synthetic Substitute, Anterior Approach, Anterior Column, Open Approach

ØRG00J1   Fusion of Occipital-cervical Joint with Synthetic Substitute, Posterior Approach, Posterior Column, Open Approach

ØRG00JJ   Fusion of Occipital-cervical Joint with Synthetic Substitute, Posterior Approach, Anterior Column, Open Approach

ØRG00K0   Fusion of Occipital-cervical Joint with Nonautologous Tissue Substitute, Anterior Approach, Anterior Column, Open Approach

ØRG00K1   Fusion of Occipital-cervical Joint with Nonautologous Tissue Substitute, Posterior Approach, Posterior Column, Open Approach

ØRG00KJ   Fusion of Occipital-cervical Joint with Nonautologous Tissue Substitute, Posterior Approach, Anterior Column, Open Approach

ØRG0370   Fusion of Occipital-cervical Joint with Autologous Tissue Substitute, Anterior Approach, Anterior Column, Percutaneous Approach

ØRG0371   Fusion of Occipital-cervical Joint with Autologous Tissue Substitute, Posterior Approach, Posterior Column, Percutaneous Approach

ØRG037J   Fusion of Occipital-cervical Joint with Autologous Tissue Substitute, Posterior Approach, Anterior Column, Percutaneous Approach

ØRG03A0   Fusion of Occipital-cervical Joint with Interbody Fusion Device, Anterior Approach, Anterior Column, Percutaneous Approach

ØRG03AJ   Fusion of Occipital-cervical Joint with Interbody Fusion Device, Posterior Approach, Anterior Column, Percutaneous Approach

ØRG03J0   Fusion of Occipital-cervical Joint with Synthetic Substitute, Anterior Approach, Anterior Column, Percutaneous Approach

ØRG03J1   Fusion of Occipital-cervical Joint with Synthetic Substitute, Posterior Approach, Posterior Column, Percutaneous Approach

ØRG03JJ   Fusion of Occipital-cervical Joint with Synthetic Substitute, Posterior Approach, Anterior Column, Percutaneous Approach

ØRG03K0   Fusion of Occipital-cervical Joint with Nonautologous Tissue Substitute, Anterior Approach, Anterior Column, Percutaneous Approach

ØRG03K1   Fusion of Occipital-cervical Joint with Nonautologous Tissue Substitute, Posterior Approach, Posterior Column, Percutaneous Approach

ØRG03KJ   Fusion of Occipital-cervical Joint with Nonautologous Tissue Substitute, Posterior Approach, Anterior Column, Percutaneous Approach

ØRG0470   Fusion of Occipital-cervical Joint with Autologous Tissue Substitute, Anterior Approach, Anterior Column, Percutaneous Endoscopic Approach

ØRG0471   Fusion of Occipital-cervical Joint with Autologous Tissue Substitute, Posterior Approach, Posterior Column, Percutaneous Endoscopic Approach

ØRG047J   Fusion of Occipital-cervical Joint with Autologous Tissue Substitute, Posterior Approach, Anterior Column, Percutaneous Endoscopic Approach

ØRG04A0   Fusion of Occipital-cervical Joint with Interbody Fusion Device, Anterior Approach, Anterior Column, Percutaneous Endoscopic Approach

ØRG04AJ   Fusion of Occipital-cervical Joint with Interbody Fusion Device, Posterior Approach, Anterior Column, Percutaneous Endoscopic Approach

ØRG04J0   Fusion of Occipital-cervical Joint with Synthetic Substitute, Anterior Approach, Anterior Column, Percutaneous Endoscopic Approach

ØRG04J1   Fusion of Occipital-cervical Joint with Synthetic Substitute, Posterior Approach, Posterior Column, Percutaneous Endoscopic Approach

ØRG04JJ   Fusion of Occipital-cervical Joint with Synthetic Substitute, Posterior Approach, Anterior Column, Percutaneous Endoscopic Approach

ØRG04K0   Fusion of Occipital-cervical Joint with Nonautologous Tissue Substitute, Anterior Approach, Anterior Column, Percutaneous Endoscopic Approach

ØRG04K1   Fusion of Occipital-cervical Joint with Nonautologous Tissue Substitute, Posterior Approach, Posterior Column, Percutaneous Endoscopic Approach

ØRG04KJ   Fusion of Occipital-cervical Joint with Nonautologous Tissue Substitute, Posterior Approach, Anterior Column, Percutaneous Endoscopic Approach

ØRG1070   Fusion of Cervical Vertebral Joint with Autologous Tissue Substitute, Anterior Approach, Anterior Column, Open Approach

ØRG1071   Fusion of Cervical Vertebral Joint with Autologous Tissue Substitute, Posterior Approach, Posterior Column, Open Approach

ØRG107J   Fusion of Cervical Vertebral Joint with Autologous Tissue Substitute, Posterior Approach, Anterior Column, Open Approach

ØRG10A0   Fusion of Cervical Vertebral Joint with Interbody Fusion Device, Anterior Approach, Anterior Column, Open Approach

ØRG10AJ   Fusion of Cervical Vertebral Joint with Interbody Fusion Device, Posterior Approach, Anterior Column, Open Approach

ØRG10J0   Fusion of Cervical Vertebral Joint with Synthetic Substitute, Anterior Approach, Anterior Column, Open Approach

ØRG10J1   Fusion of Cervical Vertebral Joint with Synthetic Substitute, Posterior Approach, Posterior Column, Open Approach

ØRG10JJ   Fusion of Cervical Vertebral Joint with Synthetic Substitute, Posterior Approach, Anterior Column, Open Approach

ØRG10K0   Fusion of Cervical Vertebral Joint with Nonautologous Tissue Substitute, Anterior Approach, Anterior Column, Open Approach

ØRG10K1   Fusion of Cervical Vertebral Joint with Nonautologous Tissue Substitute, Posterior Approach, Posterior Column, Open Approach

ØRG10KJ   Fusion of Cervical Vertebral Joint with Nonautologous Tissue Substitute, Posterior Approach, Anterior Column, Open Approach

ØRG1370   Fusion of Cervical Vertebral Joint with Autologous Tissue Substitute, Anterior Approach, Anterior Column, Percutaneous Approach

ØRG1371   Fusion of Cervical Vertebral Joint with Autologous Tissue Substitute, Posterior Approach, Posterior Column, Percutaneous Approach

ØRG137J   Fusion of Cervical Vertebral Joint with Autologous Tissue Substitute, Posterior Approach, Anterior Column, Percutaneous Approach

ØRG13A0   Fusion of Cervical Vertebral Joint with Interbody Fusion Device, Anterior Approach, Anterior Column, Percutaneous Approach

ØRG13AJ   Fusion of Cervical Vertebral Joint with Interbody Fusion Device, Posterior Approach, Anterior Column, Percutaneous Approach

ØRG13J0   Fusion of Cervical Vertebral Joint with Synthetic Substitute, Anterior Approach, Anterior Column, Percutaneous Approach

ØRG13J1   Fusion of Cervical Vertebral Joint with Synthetic Substitute, Posterior Approach, Posterior Column, Percutaneous Approach

ØRG13JJ   Fusion of Cervical Vertebral Joint with Synthetic Substitute, Posterior Approach, Anterior Column, Percutaneous Approach

ØRG13K0   Fusion of Cervical Vertebral Joint with Nonautologous Tissue Substitute, Anterior Approach, Anterior Column, Percutaneous Approach

ØRG13K1   Fusion of Cervical Vertebral Joint with Nonautologous Tissue Substitute, Posterior Approach, Posterior Column, Percutaneous Approach

ØRG13KJ   Fusion of Cervical Vertebral Joint with Nonautologous Tissue Substitute, Posterior Approach, Anterior Column, Percutaneous Approach

ØRG1470   Fusion of Cervical Vertebral Joint with Autologous Tissue Substitute, Anterior Approach, Anterior Column, Percutaneous Endoscopic Approach

HAC 12: Surgical Site Infection-Certain Orthopedic Procedures of the Spine, Shoulder, and Elbow (continued)

ØRG1471 Fusion of Cervical Vertebral Joint with Autologous Tissue Substitute, Posterior Approach, Posterior Column, Percutaneous Endoscopic Approach

ØRG147J Fusion of Cervical Vertebral Joint with Autologous Tissue Substitute, Posterior Approach, Anterior Column, Percutaneous Endoscopic Approach

ØRG14AØ Fusion of Cervical Vertebral Joint with Interbody Fusion Device, Anterior Approach, Anterior Column, Percutaneous Endoscopic Approach

ØRG14AJ Fusion of Cervical Vertebral Joint with Interbody Fusion Device, Posterior Approach, Anterior Column, Percutaneous Endoscopic Approach

ØRG14JØ Fusion of Cervical Vertebral Joint with Synthetic Substitute, Anterior Approach, Anterior Column, Percutaneous Endoscopic Approach

ØRG14J1 Fusion of Cervical Vertebral Joint with Synthetic Substitute, Posterior Approach, Posterior Column, Percutaneous Endoscopic Approach

ØRG14JJ Fusion of Cervical Vertebral Joint with Synthetic Substitute, Posterior Approach, Anterior Column, Percutaneous Endoscopic Approach

ØRG14KØ Fusion of Cervical Vertebral Joint with Nonautologous Tissue Substitute, Anterior Approach, Anterior Column, Percutaneous Endoscopic Approach

ØRG14K1 Fusion of Cervical Vertebral Joint with Nonautologous Tissue Substitute, Posterior Approach, Posterior Column, Percutaneous Endoscopic Approach

ØRG14KJ Fusion of Cervical Vertebral Joint with Nonautologous Tissue Substitute, Posterior Approach, Anterior Column, Percutaneous Endoscopic Approach

ØRG2Ø7Ø Fusion of 2 or more Cervical Vertebral Joints with Autologous Tissue Substitute, Anterior Approach, Anterior Column, Open Approach

ØRG2Ø71 Fusion of 2 or more Cervical Vertebral Joints with Autologous Tissue Substitute, Posterior Approach, Posterior Column, Open Approach

ØRG2Ø7J Fusion of 2 or more Cervical Vertebral Joints with Autologous Tissue Substitute, Posterior Approach, Anterior Column, Open Approach

ØRG2ØAØ Fusion of 2 or more Cervical Vertebral Joints with Interbody Fusion Device, Anterior Approach, Anterior Column, Open Approach

ØRG2ØAJ Fusion of 2 or more Cervical Vertebral Joints with Interbody Fusion Device, Posterior Approach, Anterior Column, Open Approach

ØRG2ØJØ Fusion of 2 or more Cervical Vertebral Joints with Synthetic Substitute, Anterior Approach, Anterior Column, Open Approach

ØRG2ØJ1 Fusion of 2 or more Cervical Vertebral Joints with Synthetic Substitute, Posterior Approach, Posterior Column, Open Approach

ØRG2ØJJ Fusion of 2 or more Cervical Vertebral Joints with Synthetic Substitute, Posterior Approach, Anterior Column, Open Approach

ØRG2ØKØ Fusion of 2 or more Cervical Vertebral Joints with Nonautologous Tissue Substitute, Anterior Approach, Anterior Column, Open Approach

ØRG2ØK1 Fusion of 2 or more Cervical Vertebral Joints with Nonautologous Tissue Substitute, Posterior Approach, Posterior Column, Open Approach

ØRG2ØKJ Fusion of 2 or more Cervical Vertebral Joints with Nonautologous Tissue Substitute, Posterior Approach, Anterior Column, Open Approach

ØRG237Ø Fusion of 2 or more Cervical Vertebral Joints with Autologous Tissue Substitute, Anterior Approach, Anterior Column, Percutaneous Approach

ØRG2371 Fusion of 2 or more Cervical Vertebral Joints with Autologous Tissue Substitute, Posterior Approach, Posterior Column, Percutaneous Approach

ØRG237J Fusion of 2 or more Cervical Vertebral Joints with Autologous Tissue Substitute, Posterior Approach, Anterior Column, Percutaneous Approach

ØRG23AØ Fusion of 2 or more Cervical Vertebral Joints with Interbody Fusion Device, Anterior Approach, Anterior Column, Percutaneous Approach

ØRG23AJ Fusion of 2 or more Cervical Vertebral Joints with Interbody Fusion Device, Posterior Approach, Anterior Column, Percutaneous Approach

ØRG23JØ Fusion of 2 or more Cervical Vertebral Joints with Synthetic Substitute, Anterior Approach, Anterior Column, Percutaneous Approach

ØRG23J1 Fusion of 2 or more Cervical Vertebral Joints with Synthetic Substitute, Posterior Approach, Posterior Column, Percutaneous Approach

ØRG23JJ Fusion of 2 or more Cervical Vertebral Joints with Synthetic Substitute, Posterior Approach, Anterior Column, Percutaneous Approach

ØRG23KØ Fusion of 2 or more Cervical Vertebral Joints with Nonautologous Tissue Substitute, Anterior Approach, Anterior Column, Percutaneous Approach

ØRG23K1 Fusion of 2 or more Cervical Vertebral Joints with Nonautologous Tissue Substitute, Posterior Approach, Posterior Column, Percutaneous Approach

ØRG23KJ Fusion of 2 or more Cervical Vertebral Joints with Nonautologous Tissue Substitute, Posterior Approach, Anterior Column, Percutaneous Approach

ØRG247Ø Fusion of 2 or more Cervical Vertebral Joints with Autologous Tissue Substitute, Anterior Approach, Anterior Column, Percutaneous Endoscopic Approach

ØRG2471 Fusion of 2 or more Cervical Vertebral Joints with Autologous Tissue Substitute, Posterior Approach, Posterior Column, Percutaneous Endoscopic Approach

ØRG247J Fusion of 2 or more Cervical Vertebral Joints with Autologous Tissue Substitute, Posterior Approach, Anterior Column, Percutaneous Endoscopic Approach

ØRG24AØ Fusion of 2 or more Cervical Vertebral Joints with Interbody Fusion Device, Anterior Approach, Anterior Column, Percutaneous Endoscopic Approach

ØRG24AJ Fusion of 2 or more Cervical Vertebral Joints with Interbody Fusion Device, Posterior Approach, Anterior Column, Percutaneous Endoscopic Approach

ØRG24JØ Fusion of 2 or more Cervical Vertebral Joints with Synthetic Substitute, Anterior Approach, Anterior Column, Percutaneous Endoscopic Approach

ØRG24J1 Fusion of 2 or more Cervical Vertebral Joints with Synthetic Substitute, Posterior Approach, Posterior Column, Percutaneous Endoscopic Approach

ØRG24JJ Fusion of 2 or more Cervical Vertebral Joints with Synthetic Substitute, Posterior Approach, Anterior Column, Percutaneous Endoscopic Approach

ØRG24KØ Fusion of 2 or more Cervical Vertebral Joints with Nonautologous Tissue Substitute, Anterior Approach, Anterior Column, Percutaneous Endoscopic Approach

ØRG24K1 Fusion of 2 or more Cervical Vertebral Joints with Nonautologous Tissue Substitute, Posterior Approach, Posterior Column, Percutaneous Endoscopic Approach

ØRG24KJ Fusion of 2 or more Cervical Vertebral Joints with Nonautologous Tissue Substitute, Posterior Approach, Anterior Column, Percutaneous Endoscopic Approach

ØRG4Ø7Ø Fusion of Cervicothoracic Vertebral Joint with Autologous Tissue Substitute, Anterior Approach, Anterior Column, Open Approach

ØRG4Ø71 Fusion of Cervicothoracic Vertebral Joint with Autologous Tissue Substitute, Posterior Approach, Posterior Column, Open Approach

ØRG4Ø7J Fusion of Cervicothoracic Vertebral Joint with Autologous Tissue Substitute, Posterior Approach, Anterior Column, Open Approach

ØRG4ØAØ Fusion of Cervicothoracic Vertebral Joint with Interbody Fusion Device, Anterior Approach, Anterior Column, Open Approach

ØRG4ØAJ Fusion of Cervicothoracic Vertebral Joint with Interbody Fusion Device, Posterior Approach, Anterior Column, Open Approach

ØRG4ØJØ Fusion of Cervicothoracic Vertebral Joint with Synthetic Substitute, Anterior Approach, Anterior Column, Open Approach

ØRG4ØJ1 Fusion of Cervicothoracic Vertebral Joint with Synthetic Substitute, Posterior Approach, Posterior Column, Open Approach

ØRG4ØJJ Fusion of Cervicothoracic Vertebral Joint with Synthetic Substitute, Posterior Approach, Anterior Column, Open Approach

ØRG4ØKØ Fusion of Cervicothoracic Vertebral Joint with Nonautologous Tissue Substitute, Anterior Approach, Anterior Column, Open Approach

ØRG4ØK1 Fusion of Cervicothoracic Vertebral Joint with Nonautologous Tissue Substitute, Posterior Approach, Posterior Column, Open Approach

ØRG4ØKJ Fusion of Cervicothoracic Vertebral Joint with Nonautologous Tissue Substitute, Posterior Approach, Anterior Column, Open Approach

ØRG437Ø Fusion of Cervicothoracic Vertebral Joint with Autologous Tissue Substitute, Anterior Approach, Anterior Column, Percutaneous Approach

HAC 12: Surgical Site Infection-Certain Orthopedic Procedures of the Spine, Shoulder, and Elbow (continued)

ØRG4371 Fusion of Cervicothoracic Vertebral Joint with Autologous Tissue Substitute, Posterior Approach, Posterior Column, Percutaneous Approach

ØRG437J Fusion of Cervicothoracic Vertebral Joint with Autologous Tissue Substitute, Posterior Approach, Anterior Column, Percutaneous Approach

ØRG43AØ Fusion of Cervicothoracic Vertebral Joint with Interbody Fusion Device, Anterior Approach, Anterior Column, Percutaneous Approach

ØRG43AJ Fusion of Cervicothoracic Vertebral Joint with Interbody Fusion Device, Posterior Approach, Anterior Column, Percutaneous Approach

ØRG43JØ Fusion of Cervicothoracic Vertebral Joint with Synthetic Substitute, Anterior Approach, Anterior Column, Percutaneous Approach

ØRG43J1 Fusion of Cervicothoracic Vertebral Joint with Synthetic Substitute, Posterior Approach, Posterior Column, Percutaneous Approach

ØRG43JJ Fusion of Cervicothoracic Vertebral Joint with Synthetic Substitute, Posterior Approach, Anterior Column, Percutaneous Approach

ØRG43KØ Fusion of Cervicothoracic Vertebral Joint with Nonautologous Tissue Substitute, Anterior Approach, Anterior Column, Percutaneous Approach

ØRG43K1 Fusion of Cervicothoracic Vertebral Joint with Nonautologous Tissue Substitute, Posterior Approach, Posterior Column, Percutaneous Approach

ØRG43KJ Fusion of Cervicothoracic Vertebral Joint with Nonautologous Tissue Substitute, Posterior Approach, Anterior Column, Percutaneous Approach

ØRG4470 Fusion of Cervicothoracic Vertebral Joint with Autologous Tissue Substitute, Anterior Approach, Anterior Column, Percutaneous Endoscopic Approach

ØRG4471 Fusion of Cervicothoracic Vertebral Joint with Autologous Tissue Substitute, Posterior Approach, Posterior Column, Percutaneous Endoscopic Approach

ØRG447J Fusion of Cervicothoracic Vertebral Joint with Autologous Tissue Substitute, Posterior Approach, Anterior Column, Percutaneous Endoscopic Approach

ØRG44AØ Fusion of Cervicothoracic Vertebral Joint with Interbody Fusion Device, Anterior Approach, Anterior Column, Percutaneous Endoscopic Approach

ØRG44AJ Fusion of Cervicothoracic Vertebral Joint with Interbody Fusion Device, Posterior Approach, Anterior Column, Percutaneous Endoscopic Approach

ØRG44JØ Fusion of Cervicothoracic Vertebral Joint with Synthetic Substitute, Anterior Approach, Anterior Column, Percutaneous Endoscopic Approach

ØRG44J1 Fusion of Cervicothoracic Vertebral Joint with Synthetic Substitute, Posterior Approach, Posterior Column, Percutaneous Endoscopic Approach

ØRG44JJ Fusion of Cervicothoracic Vertebral Joint with Synthetic Substitute, Posterior Approach, Anterior Column, Percutaneous Endoscopic Approach

ØRG44KØ Fusion of Cervicothoracic Vertebral Joint with Nonautologous Tissue Substitute, Anterior Approach, Anterior Column, Percutaneous Endoscopic Approach

ØRG44K1 Fusion of Cervicothoracic Vertebral Joint with Nonautologous Tissue Substitute, Posterior Approach, Posterior Column, Percutaneous Endoscopic Approach

ØRG44KJ Fusion of Cervicothoracic Vertebral Joint with Nonautologous Tissue Substitute, Posterior Approach, Anterior Column, Percutaneous Endoscopic Approach

ØRG6070 Fusion of Thoracic Vertebral Joint with Autologous Tissue Substitute, Anterior Approach, Anterior Column, Open Approach

ØRG6071 Fusion of Thoracic Vertebral Joint with Autologous Tissue Substitute, Posterior Approach, Posterior Column, Open Approach

ØRG607J Fusion of Thoracic Vertebral Joint with Autologous Tissue Substitute, Posterior Approach, Anterior Column, Open Approach

ØRG60AØ Fusion of Thoracic Vertebral Joint with Interbody Fusion Device, Anterior Approach, Anterior Column, Open Approach

ØRG60AJ Fusion of Thoracic Vertebral Joint with Interbody Fusion Device, Posterior Approach, Anterior Column, Open Approach

ØRG60JØ Fusion of Thoracic Vertebral Joint with Synthetic Substitute, Anterior Approach, Anterior Column, Open Approach

ØRG60J1 Fusion of Thoracic Vertebral Joint with Synthetic Substitute, Posterior Approach, Posterior Column, Open Approach

ØRG60JJ Fusion of Thoracic Vertebral Joint with Synthetic Substitute, Posterior Approach, Anterior Column, Open Approach

ØRG60KØ Fusion of Thoracic Vertebral Joint with Nonautologous Tissue Substitute, Anterior Approach, Anterior Column, Open Approach

ØRG60K1 Fusion of Thoracic Vertebral Joint with Nonautologous Tissue Substitute, Posterior Approach, Posterior Column, Open Approach

ØRG60KJ Fusion of Thoracic Vertebral Joint with Nonautologous Tissue Substitute, Posterior Approach, Anterior Column, Open Approach

ØRG6370 Fusion of Thoracic Vertebral Joint with Autologous Tissue Substitute, Anterior Approach, Anterior Column, Percutaneous Approach

ØRG6371 Fusion of Thoracic Vertebral Joint with Autologous Tissue Substitute, Posterior Approach, Posterior Column, Percutaneous Approach

ØRG637J Fusion of Thoracic Vertebral Joint with Autologous Tissue Substitute, Posterior Approach, Anterior Column, Percutaneous Approach

ØRG63AØ Fusion of Thoracic Vertebral Joint with Interbody Fusion Device, Anterior Approach, Anterior Column, Percutaneous Approach

ØRG63AJ Fusion of Thoracic Vertebral Joint with Interbody Fusion Device, Posterior Approach, Anterior Column, Percutaneous Approach

ØRG63JØ Fusion of Thoracic Vertebral Joint with Synthetic Substitute, Anterior Approach, Anterior Column, Percutaneous Approach

ØRG63J1 Fusion of Thoracic Vertebral Joint with Synthetic Substitute, Posterior Approach, Posterior Column, Percutaneous Approach

ØRG63JJ Fusion of Thoracic Vertebral Joint with Synthetic Substitute, Posterior Approach, Anterior Column, Percutaneous Approach

ØRG63KØ Fusion of Thoracic Vertebral Joint with Nonautologous Tissue Substitute, Anterior Approach, Anterior Column, Percutaneous Approach

ØRG63K1 Fusion of Thoracic Vertebral Joint with Nonautologous Tissue Substitute, Posterior Approach, Posterior Column, Percutaneous Approach

ØRG63KJ Fusion of Thoracic Vertebral Joint with Nonautologous Tissue Substitute, Posterior Approach, Anterior Column, Percutaneous Approach

ØRG6470 Fusion of Thoracic Vertebral Joint with Autologous Tissue Substitute, Anterior Approach, Anterior Column, Percutaneous Endoscopic Approach

ØRG6471 Fusion of Thoracic Vertebral Joint with Autologous Tissue Substitute, Posterior Approach, Posterior Column, Percutaneous Endoscopic Approach

ØRG647J Fusion of Thoracic Vertebral Joint with Autologous Tissue Substitute, Posterior Approach, Anterior Column, Percutaneous Endoscopic Approach

ØRG64AØ Fusion of Thoracic Vertebral Joint with Interbody Fusion Device, Anterior Approach, Anterior Column, Percutaneous Endoscopic Approach

ØRG64AJ Fusion of Thoracic Vertebral Joint with Interbody Fusion Device, Posterior Approach, Anterior Column, Percutaneous Endoscopic Approach

ØRG64JØ Fusion of Thoracic Vertebral Joint with Synthetic Substitute, Anterior Approach, Anterior Column, Percutaneous Endoscopic Approach

ØRG64J1 Fusion of Thoracic Vertebral Joint with Synthetic Substitute, Posterior Approach, Posterior Column, Percutaneous Endoscopic Approach

ØRG64JJ Fusion of Thoracic Vertebral Joint with Synthetic Substitute, Posterior Approach, Anterior Column, Percutaneous Endoscopic Approach

ØRG64KØ Fusion of Thoracic Vertebral Joint with Nonautologous Tissue Substitute, Anterior Approach, Anterior Column, Percutaneous Endoscopic Approach

ØRG64K1 Fusion of Thoracic Vertebral Joint with Nonautologous Tissue Substitute, Posterior Approach, Posterior Column, Percutaneous Endoscopic Approach

ØRG64KJ Fusion of Thoracic Vertebral Joint with Nonautologous Tissue Substitute, Posterior Approach, Anterior Column, Percutaneous Endoscopic Approach

ØRG7070 Fusion of 2 to 7 Thoracic Vertebral Joints with Autologous Tissue Substitute, Anterior Approach, Anterior Column, Open Approach

ØRG7071 Fusion of 2 to 7 Thoracic Vertebral Joints with Autologous Tissue Substitute, Posterior Approach, Posterior Column, Open Approach

ØRG707J Fusion of 2 to 7 Thoracic Vertebral Joints with Autologous Tissue Substitute, Posterior Approach, Anterior Column, Open Approach

HAC 12: Surgical Site Infection-Certain Orthopedic Procedures of the Spine, Shoulder, and Elbow (continued)

ØRG70A0 Fusion of 2 to 7 Thoracic Vertebral Joints with Interbody Fusion Device, Anterior Approach, Anterior Column, Open Approach

ØRG70AJ Fusion of 2 to 7 Thoracic Vertebral Joints with Interbody Fusion Device, Posterior Approach, Anterior Column, Open Approach

ØRG70J0 Fusion of 2 to 7 Thoracic Vertebral Joints with Synthetic Substitute, Anterior Approach, Anterior Column, Open Approach

ØRG70J1 Fusion of 2 to 7 Thoracic Vertebral Joints with Synthetic Substitute, Posterior Approach, Posterior Column, Open Approach

ØRG70JJ Fusion of 2 to 7 Thoracic Vertebral Joints with Synthetic Substitute, Posterior Approach, Anterior Column, Open Approach

ØRG70K0 Fusion of 2 to 7 Thoracic Vertebral Joints with Nonautologous Tissue Substitute, Anterior Approach, Anterior Column, Open Approach

ØRG70K1 Fusion of 2 to 7 Thoracic Vertebral Joints with Nonautologous Tissue Substitute, Posterior Approach, Posterior Column, Open Approach

ØRG70KJ Fusion of 2 to 7 Thoracic Vertebral Joints with Nonautologous Tissue Substitute, Posterior Approach, Anterior Column, Open Approach

ØRG7370 Fusion of 2 to 7 Thoracic Vertebral Joints with Autologous Tissue Substitute, Anterior Approach, Anterior Column, Percutaneous Approach

ØRG7371 Fusion of 2 to 7 Thoracic Vertebral Joints with Autologous Tissue Substitute, Posterior Approach, Posterior Column, Percutaneous Approach

ØRG737J Fusion of 2 to 7 Thoracic Vertebral Joints with Autologous Tissue Substitute, Posterior Approach, Anterior Column, Percutaneous Approach

ØRG73A0 Fusion of 2 to 7 Thoracic Vertebral Joints with Interbody Fusion Device, Anterior Approach, Anterior Column, Percutaneous Approach

ØRG73AJ Fusion of 2 to 7 Thoracic Vertebral Joints with Interbody Fusion Device, Posterior Approach, Anterior Column, Percutaneous Approach

ØRG73J0 Fusion of 2 to 7 Thoracic Vertebral Joints with Synthetic Substitute, Anterior Approach, Anterior Column, Percutaneous Approach

ØRG73J1 Fusion of 2 to 7 Thoracic Vertebral Joints with Synthetic Substitute, Posterior Approach, Posterior Column, Percutaneous Approach

ØRG73JJ Fusion of 2 to 7 Thoracic Vertebral Joints with Synthetic Substitute, Posterior Approach, Anterior Column, Percutaneous Approach

ØRG73K0 Fusion of 2 to 7 Thoracic Vertebral Joints with Nonautologous Tissue Substitute, Anterior Approach, Anterior Column, Percutaneous Approach

ØRG73K1 Fusion of 2 to 7 Thoracic Vertebral Joints with Nonautologous Tissue Substitute, Posterior Approach, Posterior Column, Percutaneous Approach

ØRG73KJ Fusion of 2 to 7 Thoracic Vertebral Joints with Nonautologous Tissue Substitute, Posterior Approach, Anterior Column, Percutaneous Approach

ØRG7470 Fusion of 2 to 7 Thoracic Vertebral Joints with Autologous Tissue Substitute, Anterior Approach, Anterior Column, Percutaneous Endoscopic Approach

ØRG7471 Fusion of 2 to 7 Thoracic Vertebral Joints with Autologous Tissue Substitute, Posterior Approach, Posterior Column, Percutaneous Endoscopic Approach

ØRG747J Fusion of 2 to 7 Thoracic Vertebral Joints with Autologous Tissue Substitute, Posterior Approach, Anterior Column, Percutaneous Endoscopic Approach

ØRG74A0 Fusion of 2 to 7 Thoracic Vertebral Joints with Interbody Fusion Device, Anterior Approach, Anterior Column, Percutaneous Endoscopic Approach

ØRG74AJ Fusion of 2 to 7 Thoracic Vertebral Joints with Interbody Fusion Device, Posterior Approach, Anterior Column, Percutaneous Endoscopic Approach

ØRG74J0 Fusion of 2 to 7 Thoracic Vertebral Joints with Synthetic Substitute, Anterior Approach, Anterior Column, Percutaneous Endoscopic Approach

ØRG74J1 Fusion of 2 to 7 Thoracic Vertebral Joints with Synthetic Substitute, Posterior Approach, Posterior Column, Percutaneous Endoscopic Approach

ØRG74JJ Fusion of 2 to 7 Thoracic Vertebral Joints with Synthetic Substitute, Posterior Approach, Anterior Column, Percutaneous Endoscopic Approach

ØRG74K0 Fusion of 2 to 7 Thoracic Vertebral Joints with Nonautologous Tissue Substitute, Anterior Approach, Anterior Column, Percutaneous Endoscopic Approach

ØRG74K1 Fusion of 2 to 7 Thoracic Vertebral Joints with Nonautologous Tissue Substitute, Posterior Approach, Posterior Column, Percutaneous Endoscopic Approach

ØRG74KJ Fusion of 2 to 7 Thoracic Vertebral Joints with Nonautologous Tissue Substitute, Posterior Approach, Anterior Column, Percutaneous Endoscopic Approach

ØRG8070 Fusion of 8 or More Thoracic Vertebral Joints with Autologous Tissue Substitute, Anterior Approach, Anterior Column, Open Approach

ØRG8071 Fusion of 8 or More Thoracic Vertebral Joints with Autologous Tissue Substitute, Posterior Approach, Posterior Column, Open Approach

ØRG807J Fusion of 8 or More Thoracic Vertebral Joints with Autologous Tissue Substitute, Posterior Approach, Anterior Column, Open Approach

ØRG80A0 Fusion of 8 or More Thoracic Vertebral Joints with Interbody Fusion Device, Anterior Approach, Anterior Column, Open Approach

ØRG80AJ Fusion of 8 or More Thoracic Vertebral Joints with Interbody Fusion Device, Posterior Approach, Anterior Column, Open Approach

ØRG80J0 Fusion of 8 or More Thoracic Vertebral Joints with Synthetic Substitute, Anterior Approach, Anterior Column, Open Approach

ØRG80J1 Fusion of 8 or More Thoracic Vertebral Joints with Synthetic Substitute, Posterior Approach, Posterior Column, Open Approach

ØRG80JJ Fusion of 8 or More Thoracic Vertebral Joints with Synthetic Substitute, Posterior Approach, Anterior Column, Open Approach

ØRG80K0 Fusion of 8 or More Thoracic Vertebral Joints with Nonautologous Tissue Substitute, Anterior Approach, Anterior Column, Open Approach

ØRG80K1 Fusion of 8 or More Thoracic Vertebral Joints with Nonautologous Tissue Substitute, Posterior Approach, Posterior Column, Open Approach

ØRG80KJ Fusion of 8 or More Thoracic Vertebral Joints with Nonautologous Tissue Substitute, Posterior Approach, Anterior Column, Open Approach

ØRG8370 Fusion of 8 or More Thoracic Vertebral Joints with Autologous Tissue Substitute, Anterior Approach, Anterior Column, Percutaneous Approach

ØRG8371 Fusion of 8 or More Thoracic Vertebral Joints with Autologous Tissue Substitute, Posterior Approach, Posterior Column, Percutaneous Approach

ØRG837J Fusion of 8 or More Thoracic Vertebral Joints with Autologous Tissue Substitute, Posterior Approach, Anterior Column, Percutaneous Approach

ØRG83A0 Fusion of 8 or More Thoracic Vertebral Joints with Interbody Fusion Device, Anterior Approach, Anterior Column, Percutaneous Approach

ØRG83AJ Fusion of 8 or More Thoracic Vertebral Joints with Interbody Fusion Device, Posterior Approach, Anterior Column, Percutaneous Approach

ØRG83J0 Fusion of 8 or More Thoracic Vertebral Joints with Synthetic Substitute, Anterior Approach, Anterior Column, Percutaneous Approach

ØRG83J1 Fusion of 8 or More Thoracic Vertebral Joints with Synthetic Substitute, Posterior Approach, Posterior Column, Percutaneous Approach

ØRG83JJ Fusion of 8 or More Thoracic Vertebral Joints with Synthetic Substitute, Posterior Approach, Anterior Column, Percutaneous Approach

ØRG83K0 Fusion of 8 or More Thoracic Vertebral Joints with Nonautologous Tissue Substitute, Anterior Approach, Anterior Column, Percutaneous Approach

ØRG83K1 Fusion of 8 or More Thoracic Vertebral Joints with Nonautologous Tissue Substitute, Posterior Approach, Posterior Column, Percutaneous Approach

ØRG83KJ Fusion of 8 or More Thoracic Vertebral Joints with Nonautologous Tissue Substitute, Posterior Approach, Anterior Column, Percutaneous Approach

ØRG8470 Fusion of 8 or More Thoracic Vertebral Joints with Autologous Tissue Substitute, Anterior Approach, Anterior Column, Percutaneous Endoscopic Approach

ØRG8471 Fusion of 8 or More Thoracic Vertebral Joints with Autologous Tissue Substitute, Posterior Approach, Posterior Column, Percutaneous Endoscopic Approach

ØRG847J Fusion of 8 or More Thoracic Vertebral Joints with Autologous Tissue Substitute, Posterior Approach, Anterior Column, Percutaneous Endoscopic Approach

ØRG84A0 Fusion of 8 or More Thoracic Vertebral Joints with Interbody Fusion Device, Anterior Approach, Anterior Column, Percutaneous Endoscopic Approach

HAC 12: Surgical Site Infection-Certain Orthopedic Procedures of the Spine, Shoulder, and Elbow (continued)

ØRG84AJ Fusion of 8 or More Thoracic Vertebral Joints with Interbody Fusion Device, Posterior Approach, Anterior Column, Percutaneous Endoscopic Approach

ØRG84J0 Fusion of 8 or More Thoracic Vertebral Joints with Synthetic Substitute, Anterior Approach, Anterior Column, Percutaneous Endoscopic Approach

ØRG84J1 Fusion of 8 or More Thoracic Vertebral Joints with Synthetic Substitute, Posterior Approach, Posterior Column, Percutaneous Endoscopic Approach

ØRG84JJ Fusion of 8 or More Thoracic Vertebral Joints with Synthetic Substitute, Posterior Approach, Anterior Column, Percutaneous Endoscopic Approach

ØRG84K0 Fusion of 8 or More Thoracic Vertebral Joints with Nonautologous Tissue Substitute, Anterior Approach, Anterior Column, Percutaneous Endoscopic Approach

ØRG84K1 Fusion of 8 or More Thoracic Vertebral Joints with Nonautologous Tissue Substitute, Posterior Approach, Posterior Column, Percutaneous Endoscopic Approach

ØRG84KJ Fusion of 8 or More Thoracic Vertebral Joints with Nonautologous Tissue Substitute, Posterior Approach, Anterior Column, Percutaneous Endoscopic Approach

ØRGA070 Fusion of Thoracolumbar Vertebral Joint with Autologous Tissue Substitute, Anterior Approach, Anterior Column, Open Approach

ØRGA071 Fusion of Thoracolumbar Vertebral Joint with Autologous Tissue Substitute, Posterior Approach, Posterior Column, Open Approach

ØRGA07J Fusion of Thoracolumbar Vertebral Joint with Autologous Tissue Substitute, Posterior Approach, Anterior Column, Open Approach

ØRGA0A0 Fusion of Thoracolumbar Vertebral Joint with Interbody Fusion Device, Anterior Approach, Anterior Column, Open Approach

ØRGA0AJ Fusion of Thoracolumbar Vertebral Joint with Interbody Fusion Device, Posterior Approach, Anterior Column, Open Approach

ØRGA0J0 Fusion of Thoracolumbar Vertebral Joint with Synthetic Substitute, Anterior Approach, Anterior Column, Open Approach

ØRGA0J1 Fusion of Thoracolumbar Vertebral Joint with Synthetic Substitute, Posterior Approach, Posterior Column, Open Approach

ØRGA0JJ Fusion of Thoracolumbar Vertebral Joint with Synthetic Substitute, Posterior Approach, Anterior Column, Open Approach

ØRGA0K0 Fusion of Thoracolumbar Vertebral Joint with Nonautologous Tissue Substitute, Anterior Approach, Anterior Column, Open Approach

ØRGA0K1 Fusion of Thoracolumbar Vertebral Joint with Nonautologous Tissue Substitute, Posterior Approach, Posterior Column, Open Approach

ØRGA0KJ Fusion of Thoracolumbar Vertebral Joint with Nonautologous Tissue Substitute, Posterior Approach, Anterior Column, Open Approach

ØRGA370 Fusion of Thoracolumbar Vertebral Joint with Autologous Tissue Substitute, Anterior Approach, Anterior Column, Percutaneous Approach

ØRGA371 Fusion of Thoracolumbar Vertebral Joint with Autologous Tissue Substitute, Posterior Approach, Posterior Column, Percutaneous Approach

ØRGA37J Fusion of Thoracolumbar Vertebral Joint with Autologous Tissue Substitute, Posterior Approach, Anterior Column, Percutaneous Approach

ØRGA3A0 Fusion of Thoracolumbar Vertebral Joint with Interbody Fusion Device, Anterior Approach, Anterior Column, Percutaneous Approach

ØRGA3AJ Fusion of Thoracolumbar Vertebral Joint with Interbody Fusion Device, Posterior Approach, Anterior Column, Percutaneous Approach

ØRGA3J0 Fusion of Thoracolumbar Vertebral Joint with Synthetic Substitute, Anterior Approach, Anterior Column, Percutaneous Approach

ØRGA3J1 Fusion of Thoracolumbar Vertebral Joint with Synthetic Substitute, Posterior Approach, Posterior Column, Percutaneous Approach

ØRGA3JJ Fusion of Thoracolumbar Vertebral Joint with Synthetic Substitute, Posterior Approach, Anterior Column, Percutaneous Approach

ØRGA3K0 Fusion of Thoracolumbar Vertebral Joint with Nonautologous Tissue Substitute, Anterior Approach, Anterior Column, Percutaneous Approach

ØRGA3K1 Fusion of Thoracolumbar Vertebral Joint with Nonautologous Tissue Substitute, Posterior Approach, Posterior Column, Percutaneous Approach

ØRGA3KJ Fusion of Thoracolumbar Vertebral Joint with Nonautologous Tissue Substitute, Posterior Approach, Anterior Column, Percutaneous Approach

ØRGA470 Fusion of Thoracolumbar Vertebral Joint with Autologous Tissue Substitute, Anterior Approach, Anterior Column, Percutaneous Endoscopic Approach

ØRGA471 Fusion of Thoracolumbar Vertebral Joint with Autologous Tissue Substitute, Posterior Approach, Posterior Column, Percutaneous Endoscopic Approach

ØRGA47J Fusion of Thoracolumbar Vertebral Joint with Autologous Tissue Substitute, Posterior Approach, Anterior Column, Percutaneous Endoscopic Approach

ØRGA4A0 Fusion of Thoracolumbar Vertebral Joint with Interbody Fusion Device, Anterior Approach, Anterior Column, Percutaneous Endoscopic Approach

ØRGA4AJ Fusion of Thoracolumbar Vertebral Joint with Interbody Fusion Device, Posterior Approach, Anterior Column, Percutaneous Endoscopic Approach

ØRGA4J0 Fusion of Thoracolumbar Vertebral Joint with Synthetic Substitute, Anterior Approach, Anterior Column, Percutaneous Endoscopic Approach

ØRGA4J1 Fusion of Thoracolumbar Vertebral Joint with Synthetic Substitute, Posterior Approach, Posterior Column, Percutaneous Endoscopic Approach

ØRGA4JJ Fusion of Thoracolumbar Vertebral Joint with Synthetic Substitute, Posterior Approach, Anterior Column, Percutaneous Endoscopic Approach

ØRGA4K0 Fusion of Thoracolumbar Vertebral Joint with Nonautologous Tissue Substitute, Anterior Approach, Anterior Column, Percutaneous Endoscopic Approach

ØRGA4K1 Fusion of Thoracolumbar Vertebral Joint with Nonautologous Tissue Substitute, Posterior Approach, Posterior Column, Percutaneous Endoscopic Approach

ØRGA4KJ Fusion of Thoracolumbar Vertebral Joint with Nonautologous Tissue Substitute, Posterior Approach, Anterior Column, Percutaneous Endoscopic Approach

ØRGE04Z Fusion of Right Sternoclavicular Joint with Internal Fixation Device, Open Approach

ØRGE07Z Fusion of Right Sternoclavicular Joint with Autologous Tissue Substitute, Open Approach

ØRGE0JZ Fusion of Right Sternoclavicular Joint with Synthetic Substitute, Open Approach

ØRGE0KZ Fusion of Right Sternoclavicular Joint with Nonautologous Tissue Substitute, Open Approach

ØRGE34Z Fusion of Right Sternoclavicular Joint with Internal Fixation Device, Percutaneous Approach

ØRGE37Z Fusion of Right Sternoclavicular Joint with Autologous Tissue Substitute, Percutaneous Approach

ØRGE3JZ Fusion of Right Sternoclavicular Joint with Synthetic Substitute, Percutaneous Approach

ØRGE3KZ Fusion of Right Sternoclavicular Joint with Nonautologous Tissue Substitute, Percutaneous Approach

ØRGE44Z Fusion of Right Sternoclavicular Joint with Internal Fixation Device, Percutaneous Endoscopic Approach

ØRGE47Z Fusion of Right Sternoclavicular Joint with Autologous Tissue Substitute, Percutaneous Endoscopic Approach

ØRGE4JZ Fusion of Right Sternoclavicular Joint with Synthetic Substitute, Percutaneous Endoscopic Approach

ØRGE4KZ Fusion of Right Sternoclavicular Joint with Nonautologous Tissue Substitute, Percutaneous Endoscopic Approach

ØRGF04Z Fusion of Left Sternoclavicular Joint with Internal Fixation Device, Open Approach

ØRGF07Z Fusion of Left Sternoclavicular Joint with Autologous Tissue Substitute, Open Approach

ØRGF0JZ Fusion of Left Sternoclavicular Joint with Synthetic Substitute, Open Approach

ØRGF0KZ Fusion of Left Sternoclavicular Joint with Nonautologous Tissue Substitute, Open Approach

ØRGF34Z Fusion of Left Sternoclavicular Joint with Internal Fixation Device, Percutaneous Approach

ØRGF37Z Fusion of Left Sternoclavicular Joint with Autologous Tissue Substitute, Percutaneous Approach

ØRGF3JZ Fusion of Left Sternoclavicular Joint with Synthetic Substitute, Percutaneous Approach

ØRGF3KZ Fusion of Left Sternoclavicular Joint with Nonautologous Tissue Substitute, Percutaneous Approach

ØRGF44Z Fusion of Left Sternoclavicular Joint with Internal Fixation Device, Percutaneous Endoscopic Approach

HAC 12: Surgical Site Infection-Certain Orthopedic Procedures of the Spine, Shoulder, and Elbow (continued)

ØRGF47Z Fusion of Left Sternoclavicular Joint with Autologous Tissue Substitute, Percutaneous Endoscopic Approach

ØRGF4JZ Fusion of Left Sternoclavicular Joint with Synthetic Substitute, Percutaneous Endoscopic Approach

ØRGF4KZ Fusion of Left Sternoclavicular Joint with Nonautologous Tissue Substitute, Percutaneous Endoscopic Approach

ØRGG04Z Fusion of Right Acromioclavicular Joint with Internal Fixation Device, Open Approach

ØRGG07Z Fusion of Right Acromioclavicular Joint with Autologous Tissue Substitute, Open Approach

ØRGG0JZ Fusion of Right Acromioclavicular Joint with Synthetic Substitute, Open Approach

ØRGG0KZ Fusion of Right Acromioclavicular Joint with Nonautologous Tissue Substitute, Open Approach

ØRGG34Z Fusion of Right Acromioclavicular Joint with Internal Fixation Device, Percutaneous Approach

ØRGG37Z Fusion of Right Acromioclavicular Joint with Autologous Tissue Substitute, Percutaneous Approach

ØRGG3JZ Fusion of Right Acromioclavicular Joint with Synthetic Substitute, Percutaneous Approach

ØRGG3KZ Fusion of Right Acromioclavicular Joint with Nonautologous Tissue Substitute, Percutaneous Approach

ØRGG44Z Fusion of Right Acromioclavicular Joint with Internal Fixation Device, Percutaneous Endoscopic Approach

ØRGG47Z Fusion of Right Acromioclavicular Joint with Autologous Tissue Substitute, Percutaneous Endoscopic Approach

ØRGG4JZ Fusion of Right Acromioclavicular Joint with Synthetic Substitute, Percutaneous Endoscopic Approach

ØRGG4KZ Fusion of Right Acromioclavicular Joint with Nonautologous Tissue Substitute, Percutaneous Endoscopic Approach

ØRGH04Z Fusion of Left Acromioclavicular Joint with Internal Fixation Device, Open Approach

ØRGH07Z Fusion of Left Acromioclavicular Joint with Autologous Tissue Substitute, Open Approach

ØRGH0JZ Fusion of Left Acromioclavicular Joint with Synthetic Substitute, Open Approach

ØRGH0KZ Fusion of Left Acromioclavicular Joint with Nonautologous Tissue Substitute, Open Approach

ØRGH34Z Fusion of Left Acromioclavicular Joint with Internal Fixation Device, Percutaneous Approach

ØRGH37Z Fusion of Left Acromioclavicular Joint with Autologous Tissue Substitute, Percutaneous Approach

ØRGH3JZ Fusion of Left Acromioclavicular Joint with Synthetic Substitute, Percutaneous Approach

ØRGH3KZ Fusion of Left Acromioclavicular Joint with Nonautologous Tissue Substitute, Percutaneous Approach

ØRGH44Z Fusion of Left Acromioclavicular Joint with Internal Fixation Device, Percutaneous Endoscopic Approach

ØRGH47Z Fusion of Left Acromioclavicular Joint with Autologous Tissue Substitute, Percutaneous Endoscopic Approach

ØRGH4JZ Fusion of Left Acromioclavicular Joint with Synthetic Substitute, Percutaneous Endoscopic Approach

ØRGH4KZ Fusion of Left Acromioclavicular Joint with Nonautologous Tissue Substitute, Percutaneous Endoscopic Approach

ØRGJ04Z Fusion of Right Shoulder Joint with Internal Fixation Device, Open Approach

ØRGJ07Z Fusion of Right Shoulder Joint with Autologous Tissue Substitute, Open Approach

ØRGJ0JZ Fusion of Right Shoulder Joint with Synthetic Substitute, Open Approach

ØRGJ0KZ Fusion of Right Shoulder Joint with Nonautologous Tissue Substitute, Open Approach

ØRGJ34Z Fusion of Right Shoulder Joint with Internal Fixation Device, Percutaneous Approach

ØRGJ37Z Fusion of Right Shoulder Joint with Autologous Tissue Substitute, Percutaneous Approach

ØRGJ3JZ Fusion of Right Shoulder Joint with Synthetic Substitute, Percutaneous Approach

ØRGJ3KZ Fusion of Right Shoulder Joint with Nonautologous Tissue Substitute, Percutaneous Approach

ØRGJ44Z Fusion of Right Shoulder Joint with Internal Fixation Device, Percutaneous Endoscopic Approach

ØRGJ47Z Fusion of Right Shoulder Joint with Autologous Tissue Substitute, Percutaneous Endoscopic Approach

ØRGJ4JZ Fusion of Right Shoulder Joint with Synthetic Substitute, Percutaneous Endoscopic Approach

ØRGJ4KZ Fusion of Right Shoulder Joint with Nonautologous Tissue Substitute, Percutaneous Endoscopic Approach

ØRGK04Z Fusion of Left Shoulder Joint with Internal Fixation Device, Open Approach

ØRGK07Z Fusion of Left Shoulder Joint with Autologous Tissue Substitute, Open Approach

ØRGK0JZ Fusion of Left Shoulder Joint with Synthetic Substitute, Open Approach

ØRGK0KZ Fusion of Left Shoulder Joint with Nonautologous Tissue Substitute, Open Approach

ØRGK34Z Fusion of Left Shoulder Joint with Internal Fixation Device, Percutaneous Approach

ØRGK37Z Fusion of Left Shoulder Joint with Autologous Tissue Substitute, Percutaneous Approach

ØRGK3JZ Fusion of Left Shoulder Joint with Synthetic Substitute, Percutaneous Approach

ØRGK3KZ Fusion of Left Shoulder Joint with Nonautologous Tissue Substitute, Percutaneous Approach

ØRGK44Z Fusion of Left Shoulder Joint with Internal Fixation Device, Percutaneous Endoscopic Approach

ØRGK47Z Fusion of Left Shoulder Joint with Autologous Tissue Substitute, Percutaneous Endoscopic Approach

ØRGK4JZ Fusion of Left Shoulder Joint with Synthetic Substitute, Percutaneous Endoscopic Approach

ØRGK4KZ Fusion of Left Shoulder Joint with Nonautologous Tissue Substitute, Percutaneous Endoscopic Approach

ØRGL03Z Fusion of Right Elbow Joint with Sustained Compression Internal Fixation Device, Open Approach

ØRGL04Z Fusion of Right Elbow Joint with Internal Fixation Device, Open Approach

ØRGL05Z Fusion of Right Elbow Joint with External Fixation Device, Open Approach

ØRGL07Z Fusion of Right Elbow Joint with Autologous Tissue Substitute, Open Approach

ØRGL0JZ Fusion of Right Elbow Joint with Synthetic Substitute, Open Approach

ØRGL0KZ Fusion of Right Elbow Joint with Nonautologous Tissue Substitute, Open Approach

ØRGL33Z Fusion of Right Elbow Joint with Sustained Compression Internal Fixation Device, Percutaneous Approach

ØRGL34Z Fusion of Right Elbow Joint with Internal Fixation Device, Percutaneous Approach

ØRGL35Z Fusion of Right Elbow Joint with External Fixation Device, Percutaneous Approach

ØRGL37Z Fusion of Right Elbow Joint with Autologous Tissue Substitute, Percutaneous Approach

ØRGL3JZ Fusion of Right Elbow Joint with Synthetic Substitute, Percutaneous Approach

ØRGL3KZ Fusion of Right Elbow Joint with Nonautologous Tissue Substitute, Percutaneous Approach

ØRGL43Z Fusion of Right Elbow Joint with Sustained Compression Internal Fixation Device, Percutaneous Endoscopic Approach

ØRGL44Z Fusion of Right Elbow Joint with Internal Fixation Device, Percutaneous Endoscopic Approach

ØRGL45Z Fusion of Right Elbow Joint with External Fixation Device, Percutaneous Endoscopic Approach

ØRGL47Z Fusion of Right Elbow Joint with Autologous Tissue Substitute, Percutaneous Endoscopic Approach

ØRGL4JZ Fusion of Right Elbow Joint with Synthetic Substitute, Percutaneous Endoscopic Approach

ØRGL4KZ Fusion of Right Elbow Joint with Nonautologous Tissue Substitute, Percutaneous Endoscopic Approach

ØRGM03Z Fusion of Left Elbow Joint with Sustained Compression Internal Fixation Device, Open Approach

ØRGM04Z Fusion of Left Elbow Joint with Internal Fixation Device, Open Approach

ØRGM05Z Fusion of Left Elbow Joint with External Fixation Device, Open Approach

ØRGM07Z Fusion of Left Elbow Joint with Autologous Tissue Substitute, Open Approach

ØRGM0JZ Fusion of Left Elbow Joint with Synthetic Substitute, Open Approach

ØRGM0KZ Fusion of Left Elbow Joint with Nonautologous Tissue Substitute, Open Approach

ØRGM33Z Fusion of Left Elbow Joint with Sustained Compression Internal Fixation Device, Percutaneous Approach

ØRGM34Z Fusion of Left Elbow Joint with Internal Fixation Device, Percutaneous Approach

ØRGM35Z Fusion of Left Elbow Joint with External Fixation Device, Percutaneous Approach

ØRGM37Z Fusion of Left Elbow Joint with Autologous Tissue Substitute, Percutaneous Approach

ØRGM3JZ Fusion of Left Elbow Joint with Synthetic Substitute, Percutaneous Approach

ØRGM3KZ Fusion of Left Elbow Joint with Nonautologous Tissue Substitute, Percutaneous Approach

ØRGM43Z Fusion of Left Elbow Joint with Sustained Compression Internal Fixation Device, Percutaneous Endoscopic Approach

HAC 12: Surgical Site Infection-Certain Orthopedic Procedures of the Spine, Shoulder, and Elbow (continued)

ØRGM44Z Fusion of Left Elbow Joint with Internal Fixation Device, Percutaneous Endoscopic Approach

ØRGM45Z Fusion of Left Elbow Joint with External Fixation Device, Percutaneous Endoscopic Approach

ØRGM47Z Fusion of Left Elbow Joint with Autologous Tissue Substitute, Percutaneous Endoscopic Approach

ØRGM4JZ Fusion of Left Elbow Joint with Synthetic Substitute, Percutaneous Endoscopic Approach

ØRGM4KZ Fusion of Left Elbow Joint with Nonautologous Tissue Substitute, Percutaneous Endoscopic Approach

ØRQEØZZ Repair Right Sternoclavicular Joint, Open Approach

ØRQE3ZZ Repair Right Sternoclavicular Joint, Percutaneous Approach

ØRQE4ZZ Repair Right Sternoclavicular Joint, Percutaneous Endoscopic Approach

ØRQEXZZ Repair Right Sternoclavicular Joint, External Approach

ØRQFØZZ Repair Left Sternoclavicular Joint, Open Approach

ØRQF3ZZ Repair Left Sternoclavicular Joint, Percutaneous Approach

ØRQF4ZZ Repair Left Sternoclavicular Joint, Percutaneous Endoscopic Approach

ØRQFXZZ Repair Left Sternoclavicular Joint, External Approach

ØRQGØZZ Repair Right Acromioclavicular Joint, Open Approach

ØRQG3ZZ Repair Right Acromioclavicular Joint, Percutaneous Approach

ØRQG4ZZ Repair Right Acromioclavicular Joint, Percutaneous Endoscopic Approach

ØRQGXZZ Repair Right Acromioclavicular Joint, External Approach

ØRQHØZZ Repair Left Acromioclavicular Joint, Open Approach

ØRQH3ZZ Repair Left Acromioclavicular Joint, Percutaneous Approach

ØRQH4ZZ Repair Left Acromioclavicular Joint, Percutaneous Endoscopic Approach

ØRQHXZZ Repair Left Acromioclavicular Joint, External Approach

ØRQJØZZ Repair Right Shoulder Joint, Open Approach

ØRQJ3ZZ Repair Right Shoulder Joint, Percutaneous Approach

ØRQJ4ZZ Repair Right Shoulder Joint, Percutaneous Endoscopic Approach

ØRQJXZZ Repair Right Shoulder Joint, External Approach

ØRQKØZZ Repair Left Shoulder Joint, Open Approach

ØRQK3ZZ Repair Left Shoulder Joint, Percutaneous Approach

ØRQK4ZZ Repair Left Shoulder Joint, Percutaneous Endoscopic Approach

ØRQKXZZ Repair Left Shoulder Joint, External Approach

ØRQLØZZ Repair Right Elbow Joint, Open Approach

ØRQL3ZZ Repair Right Elbow Joint, Percutaneous Approach

ØRQL4ZZ Repair Right Elbow Joint, Percutaneous Endoscopic Approach

ØRQLXZZ Repair Right Elbow Joint, External Approach

ØRQMØZZ Repair Left Elbow Joint, Open Approach

ØRQM3ZZ Repair Left Elbow Joint, Percutaneous Approach

ØRQM4ZZ Repair Left Elbow Joint, Percutaneous Endoscopic Approach

ØRQMXZZ Repair Left Elbow Joint, External Approach

ØRUEØ7Z Supplement Right Sternoclavicular Joint with Autologous Tissue Substitute, Open Approach

ØRUEØJZ Supplement Right Sternoclavicular Joint with Synthetic Substitute, Open Approach

ØRUEØKZ Supplement Right Sternoclavicular Joint with Nonautologous Tissue Substitute, Open Approach

ØRUE37Z Supplement Right Sternoclavicular Joint with Autologous Tissue Substitute, Percutaneous Approach

ØRUE3JZ Supplement Right Sternoclavicular Joint with Synthetic Substitute, Percutaneous Approach

ØRUE3KZ Supplement Right Sternoclavicular Joint with Nonautologous Tissue Substitute, Percutaneous Approach

ØRUE47Z Supplement Right Sternoclavicular Joint with Autologous Tissue Substitute, Percutaneous Endoscopic Approach

ØRUE4JZ Supplement Right Sternoclavicular Joint with Synthetic Substitute, Percutaneous Endoscopic Approach

ØRUE4KZ Supplement Right Sternoclavicular Joint with Nonautologous Tissue Substitute, Percutaneous Endoscopic Approach

ØRUFØ7Z Supplement Left Sternoclavicular Joint with Autologous Tissue Substitute, Open Approach

ØRUFØJZ Supplement Left Sternoclavicular Joint with Synthetic Substitute, Open Approach

ØRUFØKZ Supplement Left Sternoclavicular Joint with Nonautologous Tissue Substitute, Open Approach

ØRUF37Z Supplement Left Sternoclavicular Joint with Autologous Tissue Substitute, Percutaneous Approach

ØRUF3JZ Supplement Left Sternoclavicular Joint with Synthetic Substitute, Percutaneous Approach

ØRUF3KZ Supplement Left Sternoclavicular Joint with Nonautologous Tissue Substitute, Percutaneous Approach

ØRUF47Z Supplement Left Sternoclavicular Joint with Autologous Tissue Substitute, Percutaneous Endoscopic Approach

ØRUF4JZ Supplement Left Sternoclavicular Joint with Synthetic Substitute, Percutaneous Endoscopic Approach

ØRUF4KZ Supplement Left Sternoclavicular Joint with Nonautologous Tissue Substitute, Percutaneous Endoscopic Approach

ØRUGØ7Z Supplement Right Acromioclavicular Joint with Autologous Tissue Substitute, Open Approach

ØRUGØJZ Supplement Right Acromioclavicular Joint with Synthetic Substitute, Open Approach

ØRUGØKZ Supplement Right Acromioclavicular Joint with Nonautologous Tissue Substitute, Open Approach

ØRUG37Z Supplement Right Acromioclavicular Joint with Autologous Tissue Substitute, Percutaneous Approach

ØRUG3JZ Supplement Right Acromioclavicular Joint with Synthetic Substitute, Percutaneous Approach

ØRUG3KZ Supplement Right Acromioclavicular Joint with Nonautologous Tissue Substitute, Percutaneous Approach

ØRUG47Z Supplement Right Acromioclavicular Joint with Autologous Tissue Substitute, Percutaneous Endoscopic Approach

ØRUG4JZ Supplement Right Acromioclavicular Joint with Synthetic Substitute, Percutaneous Endoscopic Approach

ØRUG4KZ Supplement Right Acromioclavicular Joint with Nonautologous Tissue Substitute, Percutaneous Endoscopic Approach

ØRUHØ7Z Supplement Left Acromioclavicular Joint with Autologous Tissue Substitute, Open Approach

ØRUHØJZ Supplement Left Acromioclavicular Joint with Synthetic Substitute, Open Approach

ØRUHØKZ Supplement Left Acromioclavicular Joint with Nonautologous Tissue Substitute, Open Approach

ØRUH37Z Supplement Left Acromioclavicular Joint with Autologous Tissue Substitute, Percutaneous Approach

ØRUH3JZ Supplement Left Acromioclavicular Joint with Synthetic Substitute, Percutaneous Approach

ØRUH3KZ Supplement Left Acromioclavicular Joint with Nonautologous Tissue Substitute, Percutaneous Approach

ØRUH47Z Supplement Left Acromioclavicular Joint with Autologous Tissue Substitute, Percutaneous Endoscopic Approach

ØRUH4JZ Supplement Left Acromioclavicular Joint with Synthetic Substitute, Percutaneous Endoscopic Approach

ØRUH4KZ Supplement Left Acromioclavicular Joint with Nonautologous Tissue Substitute, Percutaneous Endoscopic Approach

ØRUJØ7Z Supplement Right Shoulder Joint with Autologous Tissue Substitute, Open Approach

ØRUJØJZ Supplement Right Shoulder Joint with Synthetic Substitute, Open Approach

ØRUJØKZ Supplement Right Shoulder Joint with Nonautologous Tissue Substitute, Open Approach

ØRUJ37Z Supplement Right Shoulder Joint with Autologous Tissue Substitute, Percutaneous Approach

ØRUJ3JZ Supplement Right Shoulder Joint with Synthetic Substitute, Percutaneous Approach

ØRUJ3KZ Supplement Right Shoulder Joint with Nonautologous Tissue Substitute, Percutaneous Approach

ØRUJ47Z Supplement Right Shoulder Joint with Autologous Tissue Substitute, Percutaneous Endoscopic Approach

ØRUJ4JZ Supplement Right Shoulder Joint with Synthetic Substitute, Percutaneous Endoscopic Approach

ØRUJ4KZ Supplement Right Shoulder Joint with Nonautologous Tissue Substitute, Percutaneous Endoscopic Approach

ØRUKØ7Z Supplement Left Shoulder Joint with Autologous Tissue Substitute, Open Approach

ØRUKØJZ Supplement Left Shoulder Joint with Synthetic Substitute, Open Approach

ØRUKØKZ Supplement Left Shoulder Joint with Nonautologous Tissue Substitute, Open Approach

ØRUK37Z Supplement Left Shoulder Joint with Autologous Tissue Substitute, Percutaneous Approach

ØRUK3JZ Supplement Left Shoulder Joint with Synthetic Substitute, Percutaneous Approach

ØRUK3KZ Supplement Left Shoulder Joint with Nonautologous Tissue Substitute, Percutaneous Approach

HAC 12: Surgical Site Infection-Certain Orthopedic Procedures of the Spine, Shoulder, and Elbow (continued)

ØRUK47Z Supplement Left Shoulder Joint with Autologous Tissue Substitute, Percutaneous Endoscopic Approach

ØRUK4JZ Supplement Left Shoulder Joint with Synthetic Substitute, Percutaneous Endoscopic Approach

ØRUK4KZ Supplement Left Shoulder Joint with Nonautologous Tissue Substitute, Percutaneous Endoscopic Approach

ØRUL07Z Supplement Right Elbow Joint with Autologous Tissue Substitute, Open Approach

ØRULØJZ Supplement Right Elbow Joint with Synthetic Substitute, Open Approach

ØRULØKZ Supplement Right Elbow Joint with Nonautologous Tissue Substitute, Open Approach

ØRUL37Z Supplement Right Elbow Joint with Autologous Tissue Substitute, Percutaneous Approach

ØRUL3JZ Supplement Right Elbow Joint with Synthetic Substitute, Percutaneous Approach

ØRUL3KZ Supplement Right Elbow Joint with Nonautologous Tissue Substitute, Percutaneous Approach

ØRUL47Z Supplement Right Elbow Joint with Autologous Tissue Substitute, Percutaneous Endoscopic Approach

ØRUL4JZ Supplement Right Elbow Joint with Synthetic Substitute, Percutaneous Endoscopic Approach

ØRUL4KZ Supplement Right Elbow Joint with Nonautologous Tissue Substitute, Percutaneous Endoscopic Approach

ØRUM07Z Supplement Left Elbow Joint with Autologous Tissue Substitute, Open Approach

ØRUMØJZ Supplement Left Elbow Joint with Synthetic Substitute, Open Approach

ØRUMØKZ Supplement Left Elbow Joint with Nonautologous Tissue Substitute, Open Approach

ØRUM37Z Supplement Left Elbow Joint with Autologous Tissue Substitute, Percutaneous Approach

ØRUM3JZ Supplement Left Elbow Joint with Synthetic Substitute, Percutaneous Approach

ØRUM3KZ Supplement Left Elbow Joint with Nonautologous Tissue Substitute, Percutaneous Approach

ØRUM47Z Supplement Left Elbow Joint with Autologous Tissue Substitute, Percutaneous Endoscopic Approach

ØRUM4JZ Supplement Left Elbow Joint with Synthetic Substitute, Percutaneous Endoscopic Approach

ØRUM4KZ Supplement Left Elbow Joint with Nonautologous Tissue Substitute, Percutaneous Endoscopic Approach

ØSG0070 Fusion of Lumbar Vertebral Joint with Autologous Tissue Substitute, Anterior Approach, Anterior Column, Open Approach

ØSG0071 Fusion of Lumbar Vertebral Joint with Autologous Tissue Substitute, Posterior Approach, Posterior Column, Open Approach

ØSG007J Fusion of Lumbar Vertebral Joint with Autologous Tissue Substitute, Posterior Approach, Anterior Column, Open Approach

ØSG00A0 Fusion of Lumbar Vertebral Joint with Interbody Fusion Device, Anterior Approach, Anterior Column, Open Approach

ØSG00AJ Fusion of Lumbar Vertebral Joint with Interbody Fusion Device, Posterior Approach, Anterior Column, Open Approach

ØSG00J0 Fusion of Lumbar Vertebral Joint with Synthetic Substitute, Anterior Approach, Anterior Column, Open Approach

ØSG00J1 Fusion of Lumbar Vertebral Joint with Synthetic Substitute, Posterior Approach, Posterior Column, Open Approach

ØSG00JJ Fusion of Lumbar Vertebral Joint with Synthetic Substitute, Posterior Approach, Anterior Column, Open Approach

ØSG00KØ Fusion of Lumbar Vertebral Joint with Nonautologous Tissue Substitute, Anterior Approach, Anterior Column, Open Approach

ØSG00K1 Fusion of Lumbar Vertebral Joint with Nonautologous Tissue Substitute, Posterior Approach, Posterior Column, Open Approach

ØSG00KJ Fusion of Lumbar Vertebral Joint with Nonautologous Tissue Substitute, Posterior Approach, Anterior Column, Open Approach

ØSG0370 Fusion of Lumbar Vertebral Joint with Autologous Tissue Substitute, Anterior Approach, Anterior Column, Percutaneous Approach

ØSG0371 Fusion of Lumbar Vertebral Joint with Autologous Tissue Substitute, Posterior Approach, Posterior Column, Percutaneous Approach

ØSG037J Fusion of Lumbar Vertebral Joint with Autologous Tissue Substitute, Posterior Approach, Anterior Column, Percutaneous Approach

ØSG03A0 Fusion of Lumbar Vertebral Joint with Interbody Fusion Device, Anterior Approach, Anterior Column, Percutaneous Approach

ØSG03AJ Fusion of Lumbar Vertebral Joint with Interbody Fusion Device, Posterior Approach, Anterior Column, Percutaneous Approach

ØSG03J0 Fusion of Lumbar Vertebral Joint with Synthetic Substitute, Anterior Approach, Anterior Column, Percutaneous Approach

ØSG03J1 Fusion of Lumbar Vertebral Joint with Synthetic Substitute, Posterior Approach, Posterior Column, Percutaneous Approach

ØSG03JJ Fusion of Lumbar Vertebral Joint with Synthetic Substitute, Posterior Approach, Anterior Column, Percutaneous Approach

ØSG03KØ Fusion of Lumbar Vertebral Joint with Nonautologous Tissue Substitute, Anterior Approach, Anterior Column, Percutaneous Approach

ØSG03K1 Fusion of Lumbar Vertebral Joint with Nonautologous Tissue Substitute, Posterior Approach, Posterior Column, Percutaneous Approach

ØSG03KJ Fusion of Lumbar Vertebral Joint with Nonautologous Tissue Substitute, Posterior Approach, Anterior Column, Percutaneous Approach

ØSG0470 Fusion of Lumbar Vertebral Joint with Autologous Tissue Substitute, Anterior Approach, Anterior Column, Percutaneous Endoscopic Approach

ØSG0471 Fusion of Lumbar Vertebral Joint with Autologous Tissue Substitute, Posterior Approach, Posterior Column, Percutaneous Endoscopic Approach

ØSG047J Fusion of Lumbar Vertebral Joint with Autologous Tissue Substitute, Posterior Approach, Anterior Column, Percutaneous Endoscopic Approach

ØSG04A0 Fusion of Lumbar Vertebral Joint with Interbody Fusion Device, Anterior Approach, Anterior Column, Percutaneous Endoscopic Approach

ØSG04AJ Fusion of Lumbar Vertebral Joint with Interbody Fusion Device, Posterior Approach, Anterior Column, Percutaneous Endoscopic Approach

ØSG04J0 Fusion of Lumbar Vertebral Joint with Synthetic Substitute, Anterior Approach, Anterior Column, Percutaneous Endoscopic Approach

ØSG04J1 Fusion of Lumbar Vertebral Joint with Synthetic Substitute, Posterior Approach, Posterior Column, Percutaneous Endoscopic Approach

ØSG04JJ Fusion of Lumbar Vertebral Joint with Synthetic Substitute, Posterior Approach, Anterior Column, Percutaneous Endoscopic Approach

ØSG04KØ Fusion of Lumbar Vertebral Joint with Nonautologous Tissue Substitute, Anterior Approach, Anterior Column, Percutaneous Endoscopic Approach

ØSG04K1 Fusion of Lumbar Vertebral Joint with Nonautologous Tissue Substitute, Posterior Approach, Posterior Column, Percutaneous Endoscopic Approach

ØSG04KJ Fusion of Lumbar Vertebral Joint with Nonautologous Tissue Substitute, Posterior Approach, Anterior Column, Percutaneous Endoscopic Approach

ØSG1070 Fusion of 2 or More Lumbar Vertebral Joints with Autologous Tissue Substitute, Anterior Approach, Anterior Column, Open Approach

ØSG1071 Fusion of 2 or More Lumbar Vertebral Joints with Autologous Tissue Substitute, Posterior Approach, Posterior Column, Open Approach

ØSG107J Fusion of 2 or More Lumbar Vertebral Joints with Autologous Tissue Substitute, Posterior Approach, Anterior Column, Open Approach

ØSG10A0 Fusion of 2 or More Lumbar Vertebral Joints with Interbody Fusion Device, Anterior Approach, Anterior Column, Open Approach

ØSG10AJ Fusion of 2 or More Lumbar Vertebral Joints with Interbody Fusion Device, Posterior Approach, Anterior Column, Open Approach

ØSG10J0 Fusion of 2 or More Lumbar Vertebral Joints with Synthetic Substitute, Anterior Approach, Anterior Column, Open Approach

ØSG10J1 Fusion of 2 or More Lumbar Vertebral Joints with Synthetic Substitute, Posterior Approach, Posterior Column, Open Approach

ØSG10JJ Fusion of 2 or More Lumbar Vertebral Joints with Synthetic Substitute, Posterior Approach, Anterior Column, Open Approach

ØSG10KØ Fusion of 2 or More Lumbar Vertebral Joints with Nonautologous Tissue Substitute, Anterior Approach, Anterior Column, Open Approach

HAC 12: Surgical Site Infection-Certain Orthopedic Procedures of the Spine, Shoulder, and Elbow (continued)

ØSG1ØK1 Fusion of 2 or More Lumbar Vertebral Joints with Nonautologous Tissue Substitute, Posterior Approach, Posterior Column, Open Approach

ØSG1ØKJ Fusion of 2 or More Lumbar Vertebral Joints with Nonautologous Tissue Substitute, Posterior Approach, Anterior Column, Open Approach

ØSG137Ø Fusion of 2 or More Lumbar Vertebral Joints with Autologous Tissue Substitute, Anterior Approach, Anterior Column, Percutaneous Approach

ØSG1371 Fusion of 2 or More Lumbar Vertebral Joints with Autologous Tissue Substitute, Posterior Approach, Posterior Column, Percutaneous Approach

ØSG137J Fusion of 2 or More Lumbar Vertebral Joints with Autologous Tissue Substitute, Posterior Approach, Anterior Column, Percutaneous Approach

ØSG13AØ Fusion of 2 or More Lumbar Vertebral Joints with Interbody Fusion Device, Anterior Approach, Anterior Column, Percutaneous Approach

ØSG13AJ Fusion of 2 or More Lumbar Vertebral Joints with Interbody Fusion Device, Posterior Approach, Anterior Column, Percutaneous Approach

ØSG13JØ Fusion of 2 or More Lumbar Vertebral Joints with Synthetic Substitute, Anterior Approach, Anterior Column, Percutaneous Approach

ØSG13J1 Fusion of 2 or More Lumbar Vertebral Joints with Synthetic Substitute, Posterior Approach, Posterior Column, Percutaneous Approach

ØSG13JJ Fusion of 2 or More Lumbar Vertebral Joints with Synthetic Substitute, Posterior Approach, Anterior Column, Percutaneous Approach

ØSG13KØ Fusion of 2 or More Lumbar Vertebral Joints with Nonautologous Tissue Substitute, Anterior Approach, Anterior Column, Percutaneous Approach

ØSG13K1 Fusion of 2 or More Lumbar Vertebral Joints with Nonautologous Tissue Substitute, Posterior Approach, Posterior Column, Percutaneous Approach

ØSG13KJ Fusion of 2 or More Lumbar Vertebral Joints with Nonautologous Tissue Substitute, Posterior Approach, Anterior Column, Percutaneous Approach

ØSG147Ø Fusion of 2 or More Lumbar Vertebral Joints with Autologous Tissue Substitute, Anterior Approach, Anterior Column, Percutaneous Endoscopic Approach

ØSG1471 Fusion of 2 or More Lumbar Vertebral Joints with Autologous Tissue Substitute, Posterior Approach, Posterior Column, Percutaneous Endoscopic Approach

ØSG147J Fusion of 2 or More Lumbar Vertebral Joints with Autologous Tissue Substitute, Posterior Approach, Anterior Column, Percutaneous Endoscopic Approach

ØSG14AØ Fusion of 2 or More Lumbar Vertebral Joints with Interbody Fusion Device, Anterior Approach, Anterior Column, Percutaneous Endoscopic Approach

ØSG14AJ Fusion of 2 or More Lumbar Vertebral Joints with Interbody Fusion Device, Posterior Approach, Anterior Column, Percutaneous Endoscopic Approach

ØSG14JØ Fusion of 2 or More Lumbar Vertebral Joints with Synthetic Substitute, Anterior Approach, Anterior Column, Percutaneous Endoscopic Approach

ØSG14J1 Fusion of 2 or More Lumbar Vertebral Joints with Synthetic Substitute, Posterior Approach, Posterior Column, Percutaneous Endoscopic Approach

ØSG14JJ Fusion of 2 or More Lumbar Vertebral Joints with Synthetic Substitute, Posterior Approach, Anterior Column, Percutaneous Endoscopic Approach

ØSG14KØ Fusion of 2 or More Lumbar Vertebral Joints with Nonautologous Tissue Substitute, Anterior Approach, Anterior Column, Percutaneous Endoscopic Approach

ØSG14K1 Fusion of 2 or More Lumbar Vertebral Joints with Nonautologous Tissue Substitute, Posterior Approach, Posterior Column, Percutaneous Endoscopic Approach

ØSG14KJ Fusion of 2 or More Lumbar Vertebral Joints with Nonautologous Tissue Substitute, Posterior Approach, Anterior Column, Percutaneous Endoscopic Approach

ØSG3Ø7Ø Fusion of Lumbosacral Joint with Autologous Tissue Substitute, Anterior Approach, Anterior Column, Open Approach

ØSG3Ø71 Fusion of Lumbosacral Joint with Autologous Tissue Substitute, Posterior Approach, Posterior Column, Open Approach

ØSG3Ø7J Fusion of Lumbosacral Joint with Autologous Tissue Substitute, Posterior Approach, Anterior Column, Open Approach

ØSG3ØAØ Fusion of Lumbosacral Joint with Interbody Fusion Device, Anterior Approach, Anterior Column, Open Approach

ØSG3ØAJ Fusion of Lumbosacral Joint with Interbody Fusion Device, Posterior Approach, Anterior Column, Open Approach

ØSG3ØJØ Fusion of Lumbosacral Joint with Synthetic Substitute, Anterior Approach, Anterior Column, Open Approach

ØSG3ØJ1 Fusion of Lumbosacral Joint with Synthetic Substitute, Posterior Approach, Posterior Column, Open Approach

ØSG3ØJJ Fusion of Lumbosacral Joint with Synthetic Substitute, Posterior Approach, Anterior Column, Open Approach

ØSG3ØKØ Fusion of Lumbosacral Joint with Nonautologous Tissue Substitute, Anterior Approach, Anterior Column, Open Approach

ØSG3ØK1 Fusion of Lumbosacral Joint with Nonautologous Tissue Substitute, Posterior Approach, Posterior Column, Open Approach

ØSG3ØKJ Fusion of Lumbosacral Joint with Nonautologous Tissue Substitute, Posterior Approach, Anterior Column, Open Approach

ØSG337Ø Fusion of Lumbosacral Joint with Autologous Tissue Substitute, Anterior Approach, Anterior Column, Percutaneous Approach

ØSG3371 Fusion of Lumbosacral Joint with Autologous Tissue Substitute, Posterior Approach, Posterior Column, Percutaneous Approach

ØSG337J Fusion of Lumbosacral Joint with Autologous Tissue Substitute, Posterior Approach, Anterior Column, Percutaneous Approach

ØSG33AØ Fusion of Lumbosacral Joint with Interbody Fusion Device, Anterior Approach, Anterior Column, Percutaneous Approach

ØSG33AJ Fusion of Lumbosacral Joint with Interbody Fusion Device, Posterior Approach, Anterior Column, Percutaneous Approach

ØSG33JØ Fusion of Lumbosacral Joint with Synthetic Substitute, Anterior Approach, Anterior Column, Percutaneous Approach

ØSG33J1 Fusion of Lumbosacral Joint with Synthetic Substitute, Posterior Approach, Posterior Column, Percutaneous Approach

ØSG33JJ Fusion of Lumbosacral Joint with Synthetic Substitute, Posterior Approach, Anterior Column, Percutaneous Approach

ØSG33KØ Fusion of Lumbosacral Joint with Nonautologous Tissue Substitute, Anterior Approach, Anterior Column, Percutaneous Approach

ØSG33K1 Fusion of Lumbosacral Joint with Nonautologous Tissue Substitute, Posterior Approach, Posterior Column, Percutaneous Approach

ØSG33KJ Fusion of Lumbosacral Joint with Nonautologous Tissue Substitute, Posterior Approach, Anterior Column, Percutaneous Approach

ØSG347Ø Fusion of Lumbosacral Joint with Autologous Tissue Substitute, Anterior Approach, Anterior Column, Percutaneous Endoscopic Approach

ØSG3471 Fusion of Lumbosacral Joint with Autologous Tissue Substitute, Posterior Approach, Posterior Column, Percutaneous Endoscopic Approach

ØSG347J Fusion of Lumbosacral Joint with Autologous Tissue Substitute, Posterior Approach, Anterior Column, Percutaneous Endoscopic Approach

ØSG34AØ Fusion of Lumbosacral Joint with Interbody Fusion Device, Anterior Approach, Anterior Column, Percutaneous Endoscopic Approach

ØSG34AJ Fusion of Lumbosacral Joint with Interbody Fusion Device, Posterior Approach, Anterior Column, Percutaneous Endoscopic Approach

ØSG34JØ Fusion of Lumbosacral Joint with Synthetic Substitute, Anterior Approach, Anterior Column, Percutaneous Endoscopic Approach

ØSG34J1 Fusion of Lumbosacral Joint with Synthetic Substitute, Posterior Approach, Posterior Column, Percutaneous Endoscopic Approach

ØSG34JJ Fusion of Lumbosacral Joint with Synthetic Substitute, Posterior Approach, Anterior Column, Percutaneous Endoscopic Approach

ØSG34KØ Fusion of Lumbosacral Joint with Nonautologous Tissue Substitute, Anterior Approach, Anterior Column, Percutaneous Endoscopic Approach

ØSG34K1 Fusion of Lumbosacral Joint with Nonautologous Tissue Substitute, Posterior Approach, Posterior Column, Percutaneous Endoscopic Approach

HAC 12: Surgical Site Infection-Certain Orthopedic Procedures of the Spine, Shoulder, and Elbow (continued)

ØSG34KJ Fusion of Lumbosacral Joint with Nonautologous Tissue Substitute, Posterior Approach, Anterior Column, Percutaneous Endoscopic Approach

ØSG704Z Fusion of Right Sacroiliac Joint with Internal Fixation Device, Open Approach

ØSG707Z Fusion of Right Sacroiliac Joint with Autologous Tissue Substitute, Open Approach

ØSG70JZ Fusion of Right Sacroiliac Joint with Synthetic Substitute, Open Approach

ØSG70KZ Fusion of Right Sacroiliac Joint with Nonautologous Tissue Substitute, Open Approach

ØSG734Z Fusion of Right Sacroiliac Joint with Internal Fixation Device, Percutaneous Approach

ØSG737Z Fusion of Right Sacroiliac Joint with Autologous Tissue Substitute, Percutaneous Approach

ØSG73JZ Fusion of Right Sacroiliac Joint with Synthetic Substitute, Percutaneous Approach

ØSG73KZ Fusion of Right Sacroiliac Joint with Nonautologous Tissue Substitute, Percutaneous Approach

ØSG744Z Fusion of Right Sacroiliac Joint with Internal Fixation Device, Percutaneous Endoscopic Approach

ØSG747Z Fusion of Right Sacroiliac Joint with Autologous Tissue Substitute, Percutaneous Endoscopic Approach

ØSG74JZ Fusion of Right Sacroiliac Joint with Synthetic Substitute, Percutaneous Endoscopic Approach

ØSG74KZ Fusion of Right Sacroiliac Joint with Nonautologous Tissue Substitute, Percutaneous Endoscopic Approach

ØSG804Z Fusion of Left Sacroiliac Joint with Internal Fixation Device, Open Approach

ØSG807Z Fusion of Left Sacroiliac Joint with Autologous Tissue Substitute, Open Approach

ØSG80JZ Fusion of Left Sacroiliac Joint with Synthetic Substitute, Open Approach

ØSG80KZ Fusion of Left Sacroiliac Joint with Nonautologous Tissue Substitute, Open Approach

ØSG834Z Fusion of Left Sacroiliac Joint with Internal Fixation Device, Percutaneous Approach

ØSG837Z Fusion of Left Sacroiliac Joint with Autologous Tissue Substitute, Percutaneous Approach

ØSG83JZ Fusion of Left Sacroiliac Joint with Synthetic Substitute, Percutaneous Approach

ØSG83KZ Fusion of Left Sacroiliac Joint with Nonautologous Tissue Substitute, Percutaneous Approach

ØSG844Z Fusion of Left Sacroiliac Joint with Internal Fixation Device, Percutaneous Endoscopic Approach

ØSG847Z Fusion of Left Sacroiliac Joint with Autologous Tissue Substitute, Percutaneous Endoscopic Approach

ØSG84JZ Fusion of Left Sacroiliac Joint with Synthetic Substitute, Percutaneous Endoscopic Approach

ØSG84KZ Fusion of Left Sacroiliac Joint with Nonautologous Tissue Substitute, Percutaneous Endoscopic Approach

XRG00922 Fusion of Occipital-cervical Joint using Nanotextured Surface Interbody Fusion Device, Open Approach, New Technology Group 2

XRG00F3 Fusion of Occipital-cervical Joint using Radiolucent Porous Interbody Fusion Device, Open Approach, New Technology Group 3

XRG1092 Fusion of Cervical Vertebral Joint using Nanotextured Surface Interbody Fusion Device, Open Approach, New Technology Group 2

XRG10F3 Fusion of Cervical Vertebral Joint using Radiolucent Porous Interbody Fusion Device, Open Approach, New Technology Group 3

XRG2092 Fusion of 2 or more Cervical Vertebral Joints using Nanotextured Surface Interbody Fusion Device, Open Approach, New Technology Group 2

XRG20F3 Fusion of 2 or more Cervical Vertebral Joints using Radiolucent Porous Interbody Fusion Device, Open Approach, New Technology Group 3

XRG4092 Fusion of Cervicothoracic Vertebral Joint using Nanotextured Surface Interbody Fusion Device, Open Approach, New Technology Group 2

XRG40F3 Fusion of Cervicothoracic Vertebral Joint using Radiolucent Porous Interbody Fusion Device, Open Approach, New Technology Group 3

XRG6092 Fusion of Thoracic Vertebral Joint using Nanotextured Surface Interbody Fusion Device, Open Approach, New Technology Group 2

XRG60F3 Fusion of Thoracic Vertebral Joint using Radiolucent Porous Interbody Fusion Device, Open Approach, New Technology Group 3

XRG7092 Fusion of 2 to 7 Thoracic Vertebral Joints using Nanotextured Surface Interbody Fusion Device, Open Approach, New Technology Group 2

XRG70F3 Fusion of 2 to 7 Thoracic Vertebral Joints using Radiolucent Porous Interbody Fusion Device, Open Approach, New Technology Group 3

XRG8092 Fusion of 8 or more Thoracic Vertebral Joints using Nanotextured Surface Interbody Fusion Device, Open Approach, New Technology Group 2

XRG80F3 Fusion of 8 or more Thoracic Vertebral Joints using Radiolucent Porous Interbody Fusion Device, Open Approach, New Technology Group 3

XRGA092 Fusion of Thoracolumbar Vertebral Joint using Nanotextured Surface Interbody Fusion Device, Open Approach, New Technology Group 2

XRGA0F3 Fusion of Thoracolumbar Vertebral Joint using Radiolucent Porous Interbody Fusion Device, Open Approach, New Technology Group 3

XRGB092 Fusion of Lumbar Vertebral Joint using Nanotextured Surface Interbody Fusion Device, Open Approach, New Technology Group 2

XRGB0F3 Fusion of Lumbar Vertebral Joint using Radiolucent Porous Interbody Fusion Device, Open Approach, New Technology Group 3

XRGC092 Fusion of 2 or more Lumbar Vertebral Joints using Nanotextured Surface Interbody Fusion Device, Open Approach, New Technology Group 2

XRGC0F3 Fusion of 2 or more Lumbar Vertebral Joints using Radiolucent Porous Interbody Fusion Device, Open Approach, New Technology Group 3

XRGD092 Fusion of Lumbosacral Joint using Nanotextured Surface Interbody Fusion Device, Open Approach, New Technology Group 2

XRGD0F3 Fusion of Lumbosacral Joint using Radiolucent Porous Interbody Fusion Device, Open Approach, New Technology Group 3

HAC 13: Surgical Site Infection (SSI) Following Cardiac Implantable Electronic Device (CIED) Procedures

Secondary diagnosis not POA:

K68.11 Postprocedural retroperitoneal abscess

T81.40XA Infection following a procedure, unspecified, initial encounter

T81.41XA Infection following a procedure, superficial incisional surgical site, initial encounter

T81.42XA Infection following a procedure, deep incisional surgical site, initial encounter

T81.43XA Infection following a procedure, organ and space surgical site, initial encounter

T81.44XA Sepsis following a procedure, initial encounter

T81.49XA Infection following a procedure, other surgical site, initial encounter

T82.6XXA Infection and inflammatory reaction due to cardiac valve prosthesis, initial encounter

T82.7XXA Infection and inflammatory reaction due to other internal orthopedic prosthetic devices, implants and grafts, initial encounter

AND

Any of the following procedures:

02H43JZ Insertion of Pacemaker Lead into Coronary Vein, Percutaneous Approach

02H43KZ Insertion of Defibrillator Lead into Coronary Vein, Percutaneous Approach

02H43MZ Insertion of Cardiac Lead into Coronary Vein, Percutaneous Approach

02H63JZ Insertion of Pacemaker Lead into Right Atrium, Percutaneous Approach

02H63MZ Insertion of Cardiac Lead into Right Atrium, Percutaneous Approach

02H73JZ Insertion of Pacemaker Lead into Left Atrium, Percutaneous Approach

02H73MZ Insertion of Cardiac Lead into Left Atrium, Percutaneous Approach

02HK3JZ Insertion of Pacemaker Lead into Right Ventricle, Percutaneous Approach

02HL3JZ Insertion of Pacemaker Lead into Left Ventricle, Percutaneous Approach

02HN0JZ Insertion of Pacemaker Lead into Pericardium, Open Approach

02HN0MZ Insertion of Cardiac Lead into Pericardium, Open Approach

02HN3JZ Insertion of Pacemaker Lead into Pericardium, Percutaneous Approach

02HN3MZ Insertion of Cardiac Lead into Pericardium, Percutaneous Approach

02HN4JZ Insertion of Pacemaker Lead into Pericardium, Percutaneous Endoscopic Approach

02HN4MZ Insertion of Cardiac Lead into Pericardium, Percutaneous Endoscopic Approach

02PA0MZ Removal of Cardiac Lead from Heart, Open Approach

02PA3MZ Removal of Cardiac Lead from Heart, Percutaneous Approach

02PA4MZ Removal of Cardiac Lead from Heart, Percutaneous Endoscopic Approach

HAC 13: Surgical Site Infection (SSI) Following Cardiac Implantable Electronic Device (CIED) Procedures (continued)

02PAXMZ Removal of Cardiac Lead from Heart, External Approach

02WA0MZ Revision of Cardiac Lead in Heart, Open Approach

02WA3MZ Revision of Cardiac Lead in Heart, Percutaneous Approach

02WA4MZ Revision of Cardiac Lead in Heart, Percutaneous Endoscopic Approach

0JH604Z Insertion of Pacemaker, Single Chamber into Chest Subcutaneous Tissue and Fascia, Open Approach

0JH605Z Insertion of Pacemaker, Single Chamber Rate Responsive into Chest Subcutaneous Tissue and Fascia, Open Approach

0JH606Z Insertion of Pacemaker, Dual Chamber into Chest Subcutaneous Tissue and Fascia, Open Approach

0JH607Z Insertion of Cardiac Resynchronization Pacemaker Pulse Generator into Chest Subcutaneous Tissue and Fascia, Open Approach

0JH608Z Insertion of Defibrillator Generator into Chest Subcutaneous Tissue and Fascia, Open Approach

0JH609Z Insertion of Cardiac Resynchronization Defibrillator Pulse Generator into Chest Subcutaneous Tissue and Fascia, Open Approach

0JH60PZ Insertion of Cardiac Rhythm Related Device into Chest Subcutaneous Tissue and Fascia, Open Approach

0JH634Z Insertion of Pacemaker, Single Chamber into Chest Subcutaneous Tissue and Fascia, Percutaneous Approach

0JH635Z Insertion of Pacemaker, Single Chamber Rate Responsive into Chest Subcutaneous Tissue and Fascia, Percutaneous Approach

0JH636Z Insertion of Pacemaker, Dual Chamber into Chest Subcutaneous Tissue and Fascia, Percutaneous Approach

0JH637Z Insertion of Cardiac Resynchronization Pacemaker Pulse Generator into Chest Subcutaneous Tissue and Fascia, Percutaneous Approach

0JH638Z Insertion of Defibrillator Generator into Chest Subcutaneous Tissue and Fascia, Percutaneous Approach

0JH639Z Insertion of Cardiac Resynchronization Defibrillator Pulse Generator into Chest Subcutaneous Tissue and Fascia, Percutaneous Approach

0JH63PZ Insertion of Cardiac Rhythm Related Device into Chest Subcutaneous Tissue and Fascia, Percutaneous Approach

0JH804Z Insertion of Pacemaker, Single Chamber into Abdomen Subcutaneous Tissue and Fascia, Open Approach

0JH805Z Insertion of Pacemaker, Single Chamber Rate Responsive into Abdomen Subcutaneous Tissue and Fascia, Open Approach

0JH806Z Insertion of Pacemaker, Dual Chamber into Abdomen Subcutaneous Tissue and Fascia, Open Approach

0JH807Z Insertion of Cardiac Resynchronization Pacemaker Pulse Generator into Abdomen Subcutaneous Tissue and Fascia, Open Approach

0JH808Z Insertion of Defibrillator Generator into Abdomen Subcutaneous Tissue and Fascia, Open Approach

0JH809Z Insertion of Cardiac Resynchronization Defibrillator Pulse Generator into Abdomen Subcutaneous Tissue and Fascia, Open Approach

0JH80PZ Insertion of Cardiac Rhythm Related Device into Abdomen Subcutaneous Tissue and Fascia, Open Approach

0JH834Z Insertion of Pacemaker, Single Chamber into Abdomen Subcutaneous Tissue and Fascia, Percutaneous Approach

0JH835Z Insertion of Pacemaker, Single Chamber Rate Responsive into Abdomen Subcutaneous Tissue and Fascia, Percutaneous Approach

0JH836Z Insertion of Pacemaker, Dual Chamber into Abdomen Subcutaneous Tissue and Fascia, Percutaneous Approach

0JH837Z Insertion of Cardiac Resynchronization Pacemaker Pulse Generator into Abdomen Subcutaneous Tissue and Fascia, Percutaneous Approach

0JH838Z Insertion of Defibrillator Generator into Abdomen Subcutaneous Tissue and Fascia, Percutaneous Approach

0JH839Z Insertion of Cardiac Resynchronization Defibrillator Pulse Generator into Abdomen Subcutaneous Tissue and Fascia, Percutaneous Approach

0JH83PZ Insertion of Cardiac Rhythm Related Device into Abdomen Subcutaneous Tissue and Fascia, Percutaneous Approach

0JPT0FZ Removal of Subcutaneous Defibrillator Lead from Trunk Subcutaneous Tissue and Fascia, Open Approach

0JPT0PZ Removal of Cardiac Rhythm Related Device from Trunk Subcutaneous Tissue and Fascia, Open Approach

0JPT3FZ Removal of Subcutaneous Defibrillator Lead from Trunk Subcutaneous Tissue and Fascia, Percutaneous Approach

0JPT3PZ Removal of Cardiac Rhythm Related Device from Trunk Subcutaneous Tissue and Fascia, Percutaneous Approach

0JWT0FZ Revision of Subcutaneous Defibrillator Lead in Trunk Subcutaneous Tissue and Fascia, Open Approach

0JWT0PZ Revision of Cardiac Rhythm Related Device in Trunk Subcutaneous Tissue and Fascia, Open Approach

0JWT3FZ Revision of Subcutaneous Defibrillator Lead in Trunk Subcutaneous Tissue and Fascia, Percutaneous Approach

0JWT3PZ Revision of Cardiac Rhythm Related Device in Trunk Subcutaneous Tissue and Fascia, Percutaneous Approach

HAC 14: Iatrogenic Pneumothorax with Venous Catheterization

Secondary diagnosis not POA:

J95.811 Postprocedural pneumothorax

AND

Any of the following procedures:

02H633Z Insertion of Infusion Device into Right Atrium, Percutaneous Approach

02HK33Z Insertion of Infusion Device into Right Ventricle, Percutaneous Approach

02HS33Z Insertion of Infusion Device into Right Pulmonary Vein, Percutaneous Approach

02HS43Z Insertion of Infusion Device into Right Pulmonary Vein, Percutaneous Endoscopic Approach

02HT33Z Insertion of Infusion Device into Left Pulmonary Vein, Percutaneous Approach

02HT43Z Insertion of Infusion Device into Left Pulmonary Vein, Percutaneous Endoscopic Approach

02HV33Z Insertion of Infusion Device into Superior Vena Cava, Percutaneous Approach

02HV43Z Insertion of Infusion Device into Superior Vena Cava, Percutaneous Endoscopic Approach

05H033Z Insertion of Infusion Device into Azygos Vein, Percutaneous Approach

05H043Z Insertion of Infusion Device into Azygos Vein, Percutaneous Endoscopic Approach

05H133Z Insertion of Infusion Device into Hemiazygos Vein, Percutaneous Approach

05H143Z Insertion of Infusion Device into Hemiazygos Vein, Percutaneous Endoscopic Approach

05H333Z Insertion of Infusion Device into Right Innominate Vein, Percutaneous Approach

05H343Z Insertion of Infusion Device into Right Innominate Vein, Percutaneous Endoscopic Approach

05H433Z Insertion of Infusion Device into Left Innominate Vein, Percutaneous Approach

05H443Z Insertion of Infusion Device into Left Innominate Vein, Percutaneous Endoscopic Approach

05H533Z Insertion of Infusion Device into Right Subclavian Vein, Percutaneous Approach

05H543Z Insertion of Infusion Device into Right Subclavian Vein, Percutaneous Endoscopic Approach

05H633Z Insertion of Infusion Device into Left Subclavian Vein, Percutaneous Approach

05H643Z Insertion of Infusion Device into Left Subclavian Vein, Percutaneous Endoscopic Approach

05HM33Z Insertion of Infusion Device into Right Internal Jugular Vein, Percutaneous Approach

05HN33Z Insertion of Infusion Device into Left Internal Jugular Vein, Percutaneous Approach

05HP33Z Insertion of Infusion Device into Right External Jugular Vein, Percutaneous Approach

05HQ33Z Insertion of Infusion Device into Left External Jugular Vein, Percutaneous Approach

0JH63XZ Insertion of Vascular Access Device into Chest Subcutaneous Tissue and Fascia, Percutaneous Approach

Appendix L: Procedure Combination Tables

The tables below were developed to help simplify the relationship between ICD-10-PCS coding and MS-DRG assignment. The Centers for Medicare & Medicaid Services (CMS) has identified in the MS-DRG Definitions Manual certain procedure combinations that must occur in order to assign a specific MS-DRG. There are many factors influencing MS-DRG assignment, including principal and secondary diagnoses, MCC or CC use, sex of the patient, and discharge status. These tables should be used only as a guide. These tables were created based on the proposed, version 39, MS-DRG Grouper software and Definitions Manual files published with the fiscal 2022 IPPS proposed rule. To view the final, version 39, MS-DRG Grouper software and Definitions Manual files, refer to the following: https://www.cms.gov/Medicare/Medicare-Fee-for-Service-Payment/AcuteInpatientPPS/MS-DRG-Classifications-and-Software.

DRG 001-002 Heart Transplant or Implant of Heart Assist System

Heart Transplant
Replacement of Right and Left Ventricle   02RK0JZ and 02RL0JZ

Insertion With Removal of Heart Assist System

Type of Heart Assist System	Code as appropriate Insertion by approach	Code also as appropriate Removal of Heart Assist System by approach
Biventricular External	02HA[0,3,4]RS	02PA[0,3,4]RZ
External	02HA[0,4]RZ	02PA[0,3,4]RZ

Revision With Removal of Heart Assist System

Type of Heart Assist System	Code as appropriate Revision by approach	Code also as appropriate Removal of Heart Assist System by approach
Implantable	02WA[0,3,4]QZ	02PA[0,3,4]RZ
External	02WA[0,3,4]RZ	02PA[0,3,4]RZ

DRG 008 Simultaneous Pancreas/Kidney Transplant

Transplanted Body Part	Code Transplant as appropriate by tissue type			Code also Pancreas Transplant as appropriate by tissue type		
	Allogeneic	Syngeneic	Zooplastic	Allogeneic	Syngeneic	Zooplastic
Kidney, Right	0TY00Z0	0TY00Z1	0TY00Z2	0FYG0Z0	0FYG0Z1	0FYG0Z2
Kidney, Left	0TY10Z0	0TY10Z1	0TY10Z2			

DRG 019 Simultaneous Pancreas/Kidney Transplant with Hemodialysis

Transplanted Body Part	Code Transplant as appropriate by tissue type			Code also Pancreas Transplant as appropriate by tissue type			Code also Hemodialysis		
	Allogeneic	Syngeneic	Zooplastic	Allogeneic	Syngeneic	Zooplastic	< 6 Hours	6-18 Hours	> 18 Hours
Kidney, Right	0TY00Z0	0TY00Z1	0TY00Z2	0FYG0Z0	0FYG0Z1	0FYG0Z2	5A1D07Z	5A1D80Z	5A1D90Z
Kidney, Left	0TY10Z0	0TY10Z1	0TY10Z2						

DRG 023-027 Craniotomy

Site of Neurostimulator Lead	Code as appropriate Insertion of Lead by approach	Code also as appropriate Insertion of Device by type and subcutaneous site						
		Neuro-stimulator Generator	Stimulator Multiple Array Code as appropriate by approach			Stimulator Multiple Array, Rechargeable Code as appropriate by approach		
		Skull	Chest	Back	Abdomen	Chest	Back	Abdomen
Brain	00H0[0,3,4]MZ	0NH00NZ	0JH6[0,3]DZ	0JH7[0,3]DZ	0JH8[0,3]DZ	0JH6[0,3]EZ	0JH7[0,3]EZ	0JH8[0,3]EZ
Cerebral Ventricle	00H6[0,3,4]MZ	0NH00NZ	0JH6[0,3]DZ	0JH7[0,3]DZ	0JH8[0,3]DZ	0JH6[0,3]EZ	0JH7[0,3]EZ	0JH8[0,3]EZ

DRG 028-030 Spinal Procedures

Generator Type	Insertion of Generator by Site			Code also as appropriate Insertion of Neurostimulator Lead by approach	
	Chest	Abdomen	Back	Spinal Canal	Spinal Cord
Single Array	0JH6[0,3]BZ	0JH8[0,3]BZ	0JH7[0,3]BZ	00HU[0,3,4]MZ	00HV[0,3,4]MZ
Single Array, Rechargeable	0JH6[0,3]CZ	0JH8[0,3]CZ	0JH7[0,3]CZ	00HU[0,3,4]MZ	00HV[0,3,4]MZ
Multiple Array	0JH6[0,3]DZ	0JH8[0,3]DZ	0JH7[0,3]DZ	00HU[0,3,4]MZ	00HV[0,3,4]MZ
Multiple Array, Rechargable	0JH6[0,3]EZ	—	0JH7[0,3]EZ	00HU[0,3,4]MZ	00HV[0,3,4]MZ
Multiple Array, Rechargable	—	0JH8[0,3]EZ	—	00HU[0,3,4]MZ	00HV[0,3,4]MZ

DRG 040-042 Peripheral and Cranial Nerve and Other Nervous System Procedures

Insertion of Neurostimulator Lead With Device

Site of Neurostimulator Lead	Code as appropriate Insertion by approach	Code also as appropriate Insertion of Device by type and subcutaneous site					
		Stimulator Single Array Code as appropriate by approach			Stimulator Single Array, Rechargeable Code as appropriate by approach		
		Chest	Back	Abdomen	Chest	Back	Abdomen
Cranial Nerve	00HE[0,3,4]MZ	0JH6[0,3]BZ	0JH7[0,3]BZ	0JH8[0,3]BZ	0JH6[0,3]CZ	0JH7[0,3]CZ	0JH8[0,3]CZ
Peripheral Nerve	01HY[0,3,4]MZ	0JH6[0,3]BZ	0JH7[0,3]BZ	0JH8[0,3]BZ	0JH6[0,3]CZ	0JH7[0,3]CZ	0JH8[0,3]CZ
Stomach	0DH6[0,3,4]MZ	0JH6[0,3]BZ	0JH7[0,3]BZ	0JH8[0,3]BZ	0JH6[0,3]CZ	0JH7[0,3]CZ	0JH8[0,3]CZ
Azygos vein	05H0[0,3,4]MZ	0JH6[0,3]BZ	0JH7[0,S]BZ	0JH8[0,3]BZ	0JH6[0,3]CZ	0JH7[0,S]CZ	0JH8[0,3]CZ
Innominate Vein, Right	05H3[0,3,4]MZ	0JH6[0,3]BZ	0JH7[0,S]BZ	0JH8[0,3]BZ	0JH6[0,3]CZ	0JH7[0,S]CZ	0JH8[0,3]CZ
Innominate Vein, Left	05H4[0,3,4]MZ	0JH6[0,3]BZ	0JH7[0,S]BZ	0JH8[0,3]BZ	0JH6[0,3]CZ	0JH7[0,S]CZ	0JH8[0,3]CZ
		Stimulator Multiple Array Code as appropriate by approach			Stimulator Multiple Array, Rechargeable Code as appropriate by approach		
		Chest	Back	Abdomen	Chest	Back	Abdomen
Cranial Nerve	00HE[0,3,4]MZ	0JH6[0,3]DZ	0JH7[0,3]DZ	0JH8[0,3]DZ	0JH6[0,3]EZ	0JH7[0,3]EZ	0JH8[0,3]EZ
Peripheral Nerve	01HY[0,3,4]MZ	0JH6[0,3]DZ	0JH7[0,3]DZ	0JH8[0,3]DZ	0JH6[0,3]EZ	0JH7[0,3]EZ	0JH8[0,3]EZ
Stomach	0DH6[0,3,4]MZ	0JH6[0,3]DZ	0JH7[0,3]DZ	0JH8[0,3]DZ	0JH6[0,3]EZ	0JH7[0,3]EZ	0JH8[0,3]EZ
Azygos vein	05H0[0,3,4]MZ	0JH6[0,3]DZ	0JH7[0,S]DZ	0JH8[0,3]DZ	0JH6[0,3]EZ	0JH7[0,S]EZ	0JH8[0,3]EZ
Innominate Vein, Right	05H3[0,3,4]MZ	0JH6[0,3]DZ	0JH7[0,S]DZ	0JH8[0,3]DZ	0JH6[0,3]EZ	0JH7[0,S]EZ	0JH8[0,3]EZ
Innominate Vein, Left	05H4[0,3,4]MZ	0JH6[0,3]DZ	0JH7[0,S]DZ	0JH8[0,3]DZ	0JH6[0,3]EZ	0JH7[0,S]EZ	0JH8[0,3]EZ

DRG 222-227 Cardiac Defibrillator Implant

Insertion of Generator With Insertion of Lead(s) into Coronary Vein, Atrium or Ventricle

Generator Type	Insertion of Generator by Site		Code also as appropriate Insertion of Leads by site				
	Chest	Abdomen	Coronary Vein	Atrium		Ventricle	
				Right	Left	Right	Left
Defibrillator	0JH6[0,3]8Z	0JH8[0,3]8Z	02H4[0,4]KZ	02H6[0,3,4]KZ	02H7[0,3,4]KZ	02HK[0,3,4]KZ	02HL[0,3,4]KZ
Cardiac Resynch Defibrillator Pulse Generator	0JH6[0,3]9Z	0JH8[0,3]9Z	02H4[0,3,4]KZ or 02H43[J,M]Z	02H6[0,3,4]KZ	02H7[0,3,4]KZ	02HK[0,3,4]KZ	02HL[0,3,4]KZ
Contractility Modulation Device	0JH6[0,3]AZ	0JH8[0,3]AZ	—	02H6[0,3,4]MZ	—	02HK[0,3,4]MZ	—

Insertion of Generator with Insertion of Lead(s) into Pericardium or Chest

Generator Type	Insertion of Generator by Site		Code also as appropriate Insertion of Leads by Site and Type			
	Chest	Abdomen	Pericardium			Chest
			Pacemaker	Defibrillator	Cardiac	Subcutaneous
Defibrillator	0JH6[0,3]8Z	0JH8[0,3]8Z	02HN[0,3,4]JZ	02HN[0,3,4]KZ	02HN[0,3,4]MZ	0JH6[0,3]FZ
Cardiac Resynch Defibrillator Pulse Generator	0JH6[0,3]9Z	0JH8[0,3]9Z	02HN[0,3,4]JZ	02HN[0,3,4]KZ	02HN[0,3,4]MZ	0JH6[0,3]FZ

DRG 242-244 Permanent Cardiac Pacemaker Implant

Insertion of Generator and Lead(s) Only

Generator Type	Insertion of Generator by Site		Code also as appropriate Insertion of Leads by site					
	Chest	Abdomen	Coronary Vein	Atrium		Ventricle		Pericardium
				Right	Left	Right	Left	
Single Chamber	ØJH6[Ø,3]4Z	ØJH8[Ø,3]4Z	02H4[Ø,3,4][J,M]Z	02H6[Ø,3,4][J,M]Z	02H7[Ø,3,4][J,M]Z	02HK[Ø,3,4][J,M]Z	02HL[Ø,3,4][J,M]Z	02HN[Ø,3,4][J,M]Z
Single Chamber RR	ØJH6[Ø,3]5Z	ØJH8[Ø,3]5Z	02H4[Ø,3,4][J,M]Z	02H6[Ø,3,4][J,M]Z	02H7[Ø,3,4][J,M]Z	02HK[Ø,3,4][J,M]Z	02HL[Ø,3,4][J,M]Z	02HN[Ø,3,4][J,M]Z
Dual Chamber	ØJH6[Ø,3]6Z	ØJH8[Ø,3]6Z	02H4[Ø,3,4][J,M]Z	02H6[Ø,3,4][J,M]Z	02H7[Ø,3,4][J,M]Z	02HK[Ø,3,4][J,M]Z	02HL[Ø,3,4][J,M]Z	02HN[Ø,3,4][J,M]Z
Cardiac Resynch Pulse Generator	ØJH6[Ø,3]7Z	ØJH8[Ø,3]7Z	02H4[Ø,3,4][J,M]Z	02H6[Ø,3,4][J,M]Z	02H7[Ø,3,4][J,M]Z	02HK[Ø,3,4][J,M]Z	02HL[Ø,3,4][J,M]Z	02HN[Ø,3,4][J,M]Z
Cardiac Rhythm Related	ØJH6[Ø,3]PZ	ØJH8[Ø,3]PZ	02H4[Ø,3,4][J,M]Z	02H6[Ø,3,4][J,M]Z	02H7[Ø,3,4][J,M]Z	02HK[Ø,3,4][J,M]Z	02HL[Ø,3,4][J,M]Z	02HN[Ø,3,4][J,M]Z

DRG 326-328 Stomach, Esophageal and Duodenal Procedures

Site	Resection by Open Approach	Code also as appropriate Resection of Pancreas by Open Approach
Duodenum	ØDT9ØZZ	ØFTGØZZ

DRG 344-346 Minor Small and Large Bowel Procedures

Site	Repair by Open Approach	Code also as appropriate Repair by external approach of Abdominal Wall Stoma
Small Intestine	ØDQ8ØZZ	ØWQFXZ2
Duodenum	ØDQ9ØZZ	ØWQFXZ2
Jejunum	ØDQAØZZ	ØWQFXZ2
Ileum	ØDQBØZZ	ØWQFXZ2
Large Intestine	ØDQEØZZ	ØWQFXZ2
Large Intestine, Right	ØDQFØZZ	ØWQFXZ2
Large Intestine, Left	ØDQGØZZ	ØWQFXZ2
Cecum	ØDQHØZZ	ØWQFXZ2
Ascending Colon	ØDQKØZZ	ØWQFXZ2
Transverse Colon	ØDQLØZZ	ØWQFXZ2
Descending Colon	ØDQMØZZ	ØWQFXZ2
Sigmoid Colon	ØDQNØZZ	ØWQFXZ2

DRG 456-458 Spinal Fusion Except Cervical with Spinal Curvature/Malignancy/ Infection or Extensive Fusions

Fusion of Thoracic and Lumbar Vertebra, Anterior Column

2 to 7 Thoracic Vertebra		Code also 2 or more Lumbar Vertebra	
ØRG[Ø,3,4][7,A,J,K]Ø	XRG7ØF3	ØSG1[Ø,3,4][7,A,J,K]Ø	XRGCØF3

Fusion of Thoracic and Lumbar Vertebra, Posterior Column

2 to 7 Thoracic Vertebra			Code also 2 or more Lumbar Vertebra		
Posterior Approach	Anterior Approach	New Technology	Posterior Approach	Anterior Approach	New Technology
ØRG7[Ø,3,4][7,J,K]1	ØRG7[Ø,3,4][7,A,J,K]J	XRG7092 XRG7ØF3	ØSG1[Ø,3,4][7,J,K]1	ØSG1[Ø,3,4][7,A,J,K]J	XRGC092 XRGCØF3

Appendix L: Procedure Combination Tables

DRG 461-462 Bilateral or Multiple Major Joint Procedures of Lower Extremity

For procedures to qualify as bilateral or multiple joint procedures, at least one replacement code or combination removal and replacement code from two different lower extremity sites from the following table(s) must be reported.

Examples: Left hip and right hip codes (bilateral); left hip and left knee codes (multiple); left hip and right ankle codes (multiple); left knee and right knee codes (bilateral); right hip removal and replacement, with right knee replacement

Hip, RT	Hip, LT	Knee, RT	Knee, LT	Ankle, RT	Ankle, LT
ØSR9Ø19	ØSRBØ19	ØSRCØ69	ØSRDØ69	ØSRFØ7Z	ØSRGØ7Z
ØSR9Ø1A	ØSRBØ1A	ØSRCØ6A	ØSRDØ6A	ØSRFØJ9	ØSRGØJ9
ØSR9Ø1Z	ØSRBØ1Z	ØSRCØ6Z	ØSRDØ6Z	ØSRFØJA	ØSRGØJA
ØSR9Ø29	ØSRBØ29	ØSRCØ7Z	ØSRDØ7Z	ØSRFØJZ	ØSRGØJZ
ØSR9Ø2A	ØSRBØ2A	ØSRCØJ9	ØSRDØJ9	ØSRFØKZ	ØSRGØKZ
ØSR9Ø2Z	ØSRBØ2Z	ØSRCØJA	ØSRDØJA		
ØSR9Ø39	ØSRBØ39	ØSRCØJZ	ØSRDØJZ		
ØSR9Ø3A	ØSRBØ3A	ØSRCØKZ	ØSRDØKZ		
ØSR9Ø3Z	ØSRBØ3Z	ØSRCØL9	ØSRDØL9		
ØSR9Ø49	ØSRBØ49	ØSRCØLA	ØSRDØLA		
ØSR9Ø4A	ØSRBØ4A	ØSRCØLZ	ØSRDØLZ		
ØSR9Ø4Z	ØSRBØ4Z	ØSRCØM9	ØSRDØM9		
ØSR9Ø69	ØSRBØ69	ØSRCØMA	ØSRDØMA		
ØSR9Ø6A	ØSRBØ6A	ØSRCØMZ	ØSRDØMZ		
ØSR9Ø6Z	ØSRBØ6Z	ØSRCØN9	ØSRDØN9		
ØSR9Ø7Z	ØSRBØ7Z	ØSRCØNA	ØSRDØNA		
ØSR9ØJ9	ØSRBØJ9	ØSRCØNZ	ØSRDØNZ		
ØSR9ØJA	ØSRBØJA	ØSRTØ7Z	ØSRUØ7Z		
ØSR9ØJZ	ØSRBØJZ	ØSRTØJ9	ØSRUØJ9		
ØSR9ØKZ	ØSRBØKZ	ØSRTØJA	ØSRUØJA		
ØSRAØØ9	ØSREØØ9	ØSRTØJZ	ØSRUØJZ		
ØSRAØØA	ØSREØØA	ØSRTØKZ	ØSRUØKZ		
ØSRAØØZ	ØSREØØZ	ØSRVØ7Z	ØSRWØ7Z		
ØSRAØ19	ØSREØ19	ØSRVØJ9	ØSRWØJ9		
ØSRAØ1A	ØSREØ1A	ØSRVØJA	ØSRWØJA		
ØSRAØ1Z	ØSREØ1Z	ØSRVØJZ	ØSRWØJZ		
ØSRAØ39	ØSREØ39	ØSRVØKZ	ØSRWØKZ		
ØSRAØ3A	ØSREØ3A	ØSPCØJZ	ØSPDØJZ		
ØSRAØ3Z	ØSREØ3Z				
ØSRAØ7Z	ØSREØ7Z				
ØSRAØJ9	ØSREØJ9				
ØSRAØJA	ØSREØJA				
ØSRAØJZ	ØSREØJZ				
ØSRAØKZ	ØSREØKZ				
ØSRRØ19	ØSRSØ19				
ØSRRØ1A	ØSRSØ1A				
ØSRRØ1Z	ØSRSØ1Z				
ØSRRØ39	ØSRSØ39				
ØSRRØ3A	ØSRSØ3A				
ØSRRØ3Z	ØSRSØ3Z				
ØSRRØ7Z	ØSRSØ7Z				
ØSRRØJ9	ØSRSØJ9				
ØSRRØJA	ØSRSØJA				
ØSRRØJZ	ØSRSØJZ				
ØSRRØKZ	ØSRSØKZ				
ØSU9ØBZ	ØSUBØBZ				
ØSUAØBZ	ØSUEØBZ				
ØSURØBZ	ØSUSØBZ				
ØSP9ØJZ	ØSPBØJZ				

Hip Procedure Combinations

Open Removal of Hip Spacer with Replacement

Removal of Spacer		Code also as appropriate Replacement by Device Type					
		Metal	Metal on Poly	Ceramic	Ceramic on Poly	Oxidized Zirc on Poly	Synth Subst
Hip, RT	ØSP9Ø8Z	ØSR9Ø1[9,A,Z]	ØSR9Ø2[9,A,Z]	ØSR9Ø3[9,A,Z]	ØSR9Ø4[9,A,Z]	ØSR9Ø6[9,A,Z]	ØSR9ØJ[9,A,Z]
Hip, LT	ØSPBØ8Z	ØSRBØ1[9,A,Z]	ØSRBØ2[9,A,Z]	ØSRBØ3[9,A,Z]	ØSRBØ4[9,A,Z]	ØSRBØ6[9,A,Z]	ØSRBØJ[9,A,Z]

Open Removal of Hip Spacer with Replacement

Removal of Spacer		Code also as appropriate Replacement by Device Type						
		Acetabular Surface				Femoral Surface		
		Poly	Metal	Ceramic	Synthetic	Metal	Ceramic	Synth
Hip, RT	ØSP9Ø8Z	ØSRAØØ[9,A,Z]	ØSRAØ1[9,A,Z]	ØSRAØ3[9,A,Z]	ØSRAØJ[9,A,Z]	ØSRRØ1[9,A,Z]	ØSRRØ3[9,A,Z]	ØSRRØJ[9,A,Z]
Hip, LT	ØSPBØ8Z	ØSREØØ[9,A,Z]	ØSREØ1[9,A,Z]	ØSREØ3[9,A,Z]	ØSREØJ[9,A,Z]	ØSRSØ1[9,A,Z]	ØSRSØ3[9,A,Z]	ØSRSØJ[9,A,Z]

Open Removal of Hip Liner with Replacement

Removal of Liner		Code also as appropriate Replacement by Device Type					
		Metal	Metal on Poly	Ceramic	Ceramic on Poly	Oxidized Zirc on Poly	Synth Subst
Hip, RT	ØSP9Ø9Z	ØSR9Ø1[9,A,Z]	ØSR9Ø2[9,A,Z]	ØSR9Ø3[9,A,Z]	ØSR9Ø4[9,A,Z]	ØSR9Ø6[9,A,Z]	ØSR9ØJ[9,A,Z]
Hip, LT	ØSPBØ9Z	ØSRBØ1[9,A,Z]	ØSRBØ2[9,A,Z]	ØSRBØ3[9,A,Z]	ØSRBØ4[9,A,Z]	ØSRBØ6[9,A,Z]	ØSRBØJ[9,A,Z]

Open Removal of Hip Liner with Replacement

Removal of Liner		Code also as appropriate Replacement by Device Type						
		Acetabular Surface				Femoral Surface		
		Poly	Metal	Ceramic	Synthetic	Metal	Ceramic	Synth
Hip, RT	ØSP9Ø9Z	ØSRAØØ[9,A,Z]	ØSRAØ1[9,A,Z]	ØSRAØ3[9,A,Z]	ØSRAØJ[9,A,Z]	ØSRRØ1[9,A,Z]	ØSRRØ3[9,A,Z]	ØSRRØJ[9,A,Z]
Hip, LT	ØSPBØ9Z	ØSREØØ[9,A,Z]	ØSREØ1[9,A,Z]	ØSREØ3[9,A,Z]	ØSREØJ[9,A,Z]	ØSRSØ1[9,A,Z]	ØSRSØ3[9,A,Z]	ØSRSØJ[9,A,Z]

Open Removal of Hip Resurfacing Device with Replacement

Removal of Resurfacing Device		Code also as appropriate Replacement by Device Type					
		Metal	Metal on Poly	Ceramic	Ceramic on Poly	Oxidized Zirc on Poly	Synth Subst
Hip, RT	ØSP9ØBZ	ØSR9Ø1[9,A,Z]	ØSR9Ø2[9,A,Z]	ØSR9Ø3[9,A,Z]	ØSR9Ø4[9,A,Z]	ØSR9Ø6[9,A,Z]	ØSR9ØJ[9,A,Z]
Hip, LT	ØSPBØBZ	ØSRBØ1[9,A,Z]	ØSRBØ2[9,A,Z]	ØSRBØ3[9,A,Z]	ØSRBØ4[9,A,Z]	ØSRBØ6[9,A,Z]	ØSRBØJ[9,A,Z]

Open Removal of Hip Resurfacing Device with Replacement

Removal of Resurfacing Device		Code also as appropriate Replacement by Device Type						
		Acetabular Surface				Femoral Surface		
		Poly	Metal	Ceramic	Synthetic	Metal	Ceramic	Synth
Hip, RT	ØSP9ØBZ	ØSRAØØ[9,A,Z]	ØSRAØ1[9,A,Z]	ØSRAØ3[9,A,Z]	ØSRAØJ[9,A,Z]	ØSRRØ1[9,A,Z]	ØSRRØ3[9,A,Z]	ØSRRØJ[9,A,Z]
Hip, LT	ØSPBØBZ	ØSREØØ[9,A,Z]	ØSREØ1[9,A,Z]	ØSREØ3[9,A,Z]	ØSREØJ[9,A,Z]	ØSRSØ1[9,A,Z]	ØSRSØ3[9,A,Z]	ØSRSØJ[9,A,Z]

Open Removal of Hip Articulating Spacer with Replacement

Removal of Articulating Spacer		Code also as appropriate Replacement by Device Type					
		Metal	Metal on Poly	Ceramic	Ceramic on Poly	Oxidized Zirc on Poly	Synth Subst
Hip, RT	ØSP9ØEZ	ØSR9Ø1[9,A,Z]	ØSR9Ø2[9,A,Z]	ØSR9Ø3[9,A,Z]	ØSR9Ø4[9,A,Z]	ØSR9Ø6[9,A,Z]	ØSR9ØJ[9,A,Z]
Hip, LT	ØSPBØEZ	ØSRBØ1[9,A,Z]	ØSRBØ2[9,A,Z]	ØSRBØ3[9,A,Z]	ØSRBØ4[9,A,Z]	ØSRBØ6[9,A,Z]	ØSRBØJ[9,A,Z]

Open Removal of Hip Articulating Spacer with Replacement

Removal of Articulating Spacer		Code also as appropriate Replacement by Device Type						
		Acetabular Surface				Femoral Surface		
		Poly	Metal	Ceramic	Synthetic	Metal	Ceramic	Synth
Hip, RT	ØSP9ØEZ	ØSRAØØ[9,A,Z]	ØSRAØ1[9,A,Z]	ØSRAØ3[9,A,Z]	ØSRAØJ[9,A,Z]	ØSRRØ1[9,A,Z]	ØSRRØ3[9,A,Z]	ØSRRØJ[9,A,Z]
Hip, LT	ØSPBØEZ	ØSREØØ[9,A,Z]	ØSREØ1[9,A,Z]	ØSREØ3[9,A,Z]	ØSREØJ[9,A,Z]	ØSRSØ1[9,A,Z]	ØSRSØ3[9,A,Z]	ØSRSØJ[9,A,Z]

Open Removal of Hip Synthetic Substitute with Replacement

Removal of Synthetic Substitute		Code also as appropriate Replacement by Device Type					
		Metal	Metal on Poly	Ceramic	Ceramic on Poly	Oxidized Zirc on Poly	Synth Subst
Hip, RT	ØSP[9,A,R]ØJZ	ØSR9Ø1[9,A,Z]	ØSR9Ø2[9,A,Z]	ØSR9Ø3[9,A,Z]	ØSR9Ø4[9,A,Z]	ØSR9Ø6[9,A,Z]	ØSR9ØJ[9,A,Z]
Hip, LT	ØSP[B,E,S]ØJZ	ØSRBØ1[9,A,Z]	ØSRBØ2[9,A,Z]	ØSRBØ3[9,A,Z]	ØSRBØ4[9,A,Z]	ØSRBØ6[9,A,Z]	ØSRBØJ[9,A,Z]

Open Removal of Hip Synthetic Substitute with Replacement

Removal of Synthetic Substitute		Code also as appropriate Replacement by Device Type						
		Acetabular Surface				Femoral Surface		
		Poly	Metal	Ceramic	Synthetic	Metal	Ceramic	Synth
Hip, RT	ØSP[9,A,R]ØJZ	ØSRAØØ[9,A,Z]	ØSRAØ1[9,A,Z]	ØSRAØ3[9,A,Z]	ØSRAØJ[9,A,Z]	ØSRRØ1[9,A,Z]	ØSRRØ3[9,A,Z]	ØSRRØJ[9,A,Z]
Hip, LT	ØSP[B,E,S]ØJZ	ØSREØØ[9,A,Z]	ØSREØ1[9,A,Z]	ØSREØ3[9,A,Z]	ØSREØJ[9,A,Z]	ØSRSØ1[9,A,Z]	ØSRSØ3[9,A,Z]	ØSRSØJ[9,A,Z]

Percutaneous Endoscopic Removal of Hip Spacer with Open Replacement

Removal of Spacer		Code also as appropriate Replacement by Device Type					
		Metal	Metal on Poly	Ceramic	Ceramic on Poly	Oxidized Zirc on Poly	Synth Subst
Hip, RT	ØSP948Z	ØSR9Ø1[9,A,Z]	ØSR9Ø2[9,A,Z]	ØSR9Ø3[9,A,Z]	ØSR9Ø4[9,A,Z]	ØSR9Ø6[9,A,Z]	ØSR9ØJ[9,A,Z]
Hip, LT	ØSPB48Z	ØSRBØ1[9,A,Z]	ØSRBØ2[9,A,Z]	ØSRBØ3[9,A,Z]	ØSRBØ4[9,A,Z]	ØSRBØ6[9,A,Z]	ØSRBØJ[9,A,Z]

Percutaneous Endoscopic Removal of Hip Spacer with Open Replacement

Removal of Spacer		Code also as appropriate Replacement by Device Type						
		Acetabular Surface				Femoral Surface		
		Poly	Metal	Ceramic	Synthetic	Metal	Ceramic	Synth
Hip, RT	ØSP948Z	ØSRAØØ[9,A,Z]	ØSRAØ1[9,A,Z]	ØSRAØ3[9,A,Z]	ØSRAØJ[9,A,Z]	ØSRRØ1[9,A,Z]	ØSRRØ3[9,A,Z]	ØSRRØJ[9,A,Z]
Hip, LT	ØSPB48Z	ØSREØØ[9,A,Z]	ØSREØ1[9,A,Z]	ØSREØ3[9,A,Z]	ØSREØJ[9,A,Z]	ØSRSØ1[9,A,Z]	ØSRSØ3[9,A,Z]	ØSRSØJ[9,A,Z]

Percutaneous Endoscopic Removal of Hip Synthetic Substitute with Open Replacement

Removal of Synthetic Substitute		Code also as appropriate Replacement by Device Type					
		Metal	Metal on Poly	Ceramic	Ceramic on Poly	Oxidized Zirc on Poly	Synth Subst
Hip, RT	ØSP[9,A,R]4JZ	ØSR9Ø1[9,A,Z]	ØSR9Ø2[9,A,Z]	ØSR9Ø3[9,A,Z]	ØSR9Ø4[9,A,Z]	ØSR9Ø6[9,A,Z]	ØSR9ØJ[9,A,Z]
Hip, LT	ØSP[B,E,S]4JZ	ØSRBØ1[9,A,Z]	ØSRBØ2[9,A,Z]	ØSRBØ3[9,A,Z]	ØSRBØ4[9,A,Z]	ØSRBØ6[9,A,Z]	ØSRBØJ[9,A,Z]

Percutaneous Endoscopic Removal of Hip Synthetic Substitute with Open Replacement

Removal of Synthetic Substitute		Code also as appropriate Replacement by Device Type						
		Acetabular Surface				Femoral Surface		
		Poly	Metal	Ceramic	Synthetic	Metal	Ceramic	Synth
Hip, RT	ØSP[9,A,R]4JZ	ØSRAØØ[9,A,Z]	ØSRAØ1[9,A,Z]	ØSRAØ3[9,A,Z]	ØSRAØJ[9,A,Z]	ØSRRØ1[9,A,Z]	ØSRRØ3[9,A,Z]	ØSRRØJ[9,A,Z]
Hip, LT	ØSP[B,E,S]4JZ	ØSREØØ[9,A,Z]	ØSREØ1[9,A,Z]	ØSREØ3[9,A,Z]	ØSREØJ[9,A,Z]	ØSRSØ1[9,A,Z]	ØSRSØ3[9,A,Z]	ØSRSØJ[9,A,Z]

Knee Procedure Combinations

Open Removal of Knee Spacer with Synthetic Substitute Replacement

Removal of Spacer		Code also as appropriate Replacement by Type of Synthetic Substitute				
		Oxidized Zircon on Poly	Synth Subst	Patello-femoral	Femoral Surface	Tibial Surface
Knee, RT	ØSPC08Z	ØSRC06[9,A,Z]	ØSRCØJ[9,A,Z]	ØSRCØN[9,A,Z]	ØSRTØJ[9,A,Z]	ØSRVØJ[9,A,Z]
Knee, LT	ØSPD08Z	ØSRD06[9,A,Z]	ØSRDØJ[9,A,Z]	ØSRDØN[9,A,Z]	ØSRUØJ[9,A,Z]	ØSRWØJ[9,A,Z]

Open Removal of Knee Liner with Synthetic Substitute Replacement

Removal of Liner		Code also as appropriate Replacement by Type of Synthetic Substitute						
		Oxidized Zircon on Poly	Synth Subst	Medial Unicondylar	Lateral Unicondylar	Patello-femoral	Femoral Surface	Tibial Surface
Knee, RT	ØSPC09Z	ØSRC06[9,A,Z]	ØSRCØJ[9,A,Z]	ØSRCØL[9,A,Z]	ØSRCØM[9,A,Z]	ØSRCØN[9,A,Z]	ØSRTØJ[9,A,Z]	ØSRVØJ[9,A,Z]
Knee, LT	ØSPD09Z	ØSRD06[9,A,Z]	ØSRDØJ[9,A,Z]	ØSRDØL[9,A,Z]	ØSRDØM[9,A,Z]	ØSRDØN[9,A,Z]	ØSRUØJ[9,A,Z]	ØSRWØJ[9,A,Z]

Open Removal of Knee Articulating Spacer with Synthetic Substitute Replacement

Removal of Articulating Spacer		Code also as appropriate Replacement by Type of Synthetic Substitute			
		Oxidized Zircon on Poly	Synth Subst	Femoral Surface	Tibial Surface
Knee, RT	ØSPCØEZ	ØSRC06[9,A,Z]	ØSRCØJ[9,A,Z]	ØSRTØJ[9,A,Z]	ØSRVØJ[9,A,Z]
Knee, LT	ØSPØDØEZ	ØSRD06[9,A,Z]	ØSRDØJ[9,A,Z]	ØSRUØJ[9,A,Z]	ØSRWØJ[9,A,Z]

Open Removal of Patellar Surface of Knee with Synthetic Substitute Replacement

Removal of Patellar Surface		Code also as appropriate Replacement by Type of Synthetic Substitute				
		Oxidized Zircon on Poly	Synth Subst	Patello-femoral	Femoral Surface	Tibial Surface
Knee, RT	ØSPCØJC	ØSRC06[9,A,Z]	ØSRCØJ[9,A,Z]	ØSRCØN[9,A,Z]	ØSRTØJ[9,A,Z]	ØSRVØJ[9,A,Z]
Knee, LT	ØSPDØJC	ØSRD06[9,A,Z]	ØSRDØJ[9,A,Z]	ØSRDØN[9,A,Z]	ØSRUØJ[9,A,Z]	ØSRWØJ[9,A,Z]

Open Removal of Knee Synthetic Substitute with Synthetic Substitute Replacement

Removal of Synthetic Substitute		Code also as appropriate Replacement by Type of Synthetic Substitute						
		Oxidized Zircon on Poly	Synth Subst	Medial Unicondylar	Lateral Unicondylar	Patello-femoral	Femoral Surface	Tibial Surface
Knee, RT	ØSPCØJZ	ØSRC06[9,A,Z]	ØSRCØJ[9,A,Z]	ØSRCØL[9,A,Z]	ØSRCØM[9,A,Z]	ØSRCØN[9,A,Z]	ØSRTØJ[9,A,Z]	ØSRVØJ[9,A,Z]
Knee, LT	ØSPDØJZ	ØSRD06[9,A,Z]	ØSRDØJ[9,A,Z]	ØSRDØL[9,A,Z]	ØSRDØM[9,A,Z]	ØSRDØN[9,A,Z]	ØSRUØJ[9,A,Z]	ØSRWØJ[9,A,Z]

Open Removal of Medial or Lateral Unicondylar Knee with Synthetic Substitute Replacement

Removal of Medial/Lateral Unicondylar Knee		Code also as appropriate Replacement by Type of Synthetic Substitute				
		Oxidized Zircon on Poly	Synth Subst	Medial Unicondylar	Femoral Surface	Tibial Surface
Knee, RT	ØSPCØ[L,M]Z	ØSRC06[9,A,Z]	ØSRCØJ[9,A,Z]	ØSRCØL[9,A,Z]	ØSRTØJ[9,A,Z]	ØSRVØJ[9,A,Z]
Knee, LT	ØSPDØ[L,M]Z	ØSRD06[9,A,Z]	ØSRDØJ[9,A,Z]	ØSRDØL[9,A,Z]	ØSRUØJ[9,A,Z]	ØSRWØJ[9,A,Z]

Open Removal of Patellofemoral Knee with Synthetic Substitute Replacement

Removal of Patellofemoral Knee		Code also as appropriate Replacement by Type of Synthetic Substitute				
		Oxidized Zircon on Poly	Synth Subst	Medial Unicondylar	Femoral Surface	Tibial Surface
Knee, RT	ØSPCØNZ	ØSRC06[9,A,Z]	ØSRCØJ[9,A,Z]	ØSRCØL[9,A,Z]	ØSRTØJ[9,A,Z]	ØSRVØJ[9,A,Z]
Knee, LT	ØSPDØNZ	ØSRD06[9,A,Z]	ØSRDØJ[9,A,Z]	ØSRDØL[9,A,Z]	ØSRUØJ[9,A,Z]	ØSRWØJ[9,A,Z]

Open Removal of Femoral/Tibial Surface of Knee with Synthetic Substitute Replacement

Removal of Femoral/Tibial Surface of Knee		Code also as appropriate Replacement by Type of Synthetic Substitute					
		Oxidized Zircon on Poly	Synth Subst	Articulating Spacer	Patello-femoral	Femoral Surface	Tibial Surface
Knee, RT	ØSP[T,V]ØJZ	ØSRC06[9,A,Z]	ØSRCØJ[9,A,Z]	ØSRCØEZ	ØSRCØN[9,A,Z]	ØSRTØJ[9,A,Z]	ØSRVØJ[9,A,Z]
Knee, LT	ØSP[U,W]ØJZ	ØSRD06[9,A,Z]	ØSRDØJ[9,A,Z]	ØSRDØEZ	ØSRDØN[9,A,Z]	ØSRUØJ[9,A,Z]	ØSRWØJ[9,A,Z]

Percutaneous/Percutaneous Endoscopic Removal of Knee Spacer with Open Synthetic Substitute Replacement

Removal of Spacer		Code also as appropriate Replacement by Type of Synthetic Substitute				
		Oxidized Zircon on Poly	**Synth Subst**	**Patello-femoral**	**Femoral Surface**	**Tibial Surface**
Knee, RT	ØSPC[3,4]8Z	ØSRC06[9,A,Z]	ØSRCØJ[9,A,Z]	ØSRCØN[9,A,Z]	ØSRTØJ[9,A,Z]	ØSRVØJ[9,A,Z]
Knee, LT	ØSPD[3,4]8Z	ØSRD06[9,A,Z]	ØSRDØJ[9,A,Z]	ØSRDØN[9,A,Z]	ØSRUØJ[9,A,Z]	ØSRWØJ[9,A,Z]

Percutaneous Endoscopic Removal of Patellar Surface of Knee with Synthetic Substitute Replacement

Removal of Patellar Surface		Code also as appropriate Replacement by Type of Synthetic Substitute				
		Oxidized Zircon on Poly	**Synth Subst**	**Patello-femoral**	**Femoral Surface**	**Tibial Surface**
Knee, RT	ØSPC4JC	ØSRC06[9,A,Z]	ØSRCØJ[9,A,Z]	ØSRCØN[9,A,Z]	ØSRTØJ[9,A,Z]	ØSRVØJ[9,A,Z]
Knee, LT	ØSPD4JC	ØSRD06[9,A,Z]	ØSRDØJ[9,A,Z]	ØSRDØN[9,A,Z]	ØSRUØJ[9,A]	ØSRWØJ[9,A,Z]

Percutaneous Endoscopic Removal of Knee Synthetic Substitute with Synthetic Substitute Replacement

Removal of Synthetic Substitute		Code also as appropriate Replacement by Type of Synthetic Substitute						
		Oxidized Zircon on Poly	**Synth Subst**	**Medial Unicondylar**	**Lateral Unicondylar**	**Patello-femoral**	**Femoral Surface**	**Tibial Surface**
Knee, RT	ØSPC4JZ	ØSRC06[9,A,Z]	ØSRCØJ[9,A,Z]	ØSRCØL[9,A,Z]	ØSRCØM[9,A,Z]	ØSRCØN[9,A,Z]	ØSRTØJ[9,A,Z]	ØSRVØJ[9,A,Z]
Knee, LT	ØSPD4JZ	ØSRD06[9,A,Z]	ØSRDØJ[9,A,Z]	ØSRDØL[9,A,Z]	ØSRDØM[9,A,Z]	ØSRDØN[9,A,Z]	ØSRUØJ[9,A,Z]	ØSRWØJ[9,A,Z]

Percutaneous Endoscopic Removal of Medial or Lateral Unicondylar Knee with Synthetic Substitute Replacement

Removal of Medial/Lateral Unicondylar Knee		Code also as appropriate Replacement by Type of Synthetic Substitute				
		Oxidized Zircon on Poly	**Synth Subst**	**Medial Unicondylar**	**Femoral Surface**	**Tibial Surface**
Knee, RT	ØSPC4[L,M]Z	ØSRC06[9,A,Z]	ØSRCØJ[9,A,Z]	ØSRCØL[9,A,Z]	ØSRTØJ[9,A,Z]	ØSRVØJ[9,A,Z]
Knee, LT	ØSPD4[L,M]Z	ØSRD06[9,A,Z]	ØSRDØJ[9,A,Z]	ØSRDØL[9,A,Z]	ØSRUØJ[9,A,Z]	ØSRWØJ[9,A,Z]

Percutaneous Endoscopic Removal of Patellofemoral Knee with Synthetic Substitute Replacement

Removal of Patellofemoral Knee		Code also as appropriate Replacement by Type of Synthetic Substitute				
		Oxidized Zircon on Poly	**Synth Subst**	**Medial Unicondylar**	**Femoral Surface**	**Tibial Surface**
Knee, RT	ØSPC4NZ	ØSRC06[9,A,Z]	ØSRCØJ[9,A,Z]	ØSRCØL[9,A,Z]	ØSRTØJ[9,A,Z]	ØSRVØJ[9,A,Z]
Knee, LT	ØSPD4NZ	ØSRD06[9,A,Z]	ØSRDØJ[9,A,Z]	ØSRDØL[9,A,Z]	ØSRUØJ[9,A,Z]	ØSRWØJ[9,A,Z]

Percutaneous Endoscopic Removal of Femoral/Tibial Surface of Knee with Synthetic Substitute Replacement

Removal of Femoral/Tibial Surface of Knee		Code also as appropriate Replacement by Type of Synthetic Substitute					
		Oxidized Zircon on Poly	**Synth Subst**	**Articulating Spacer**	**Patello-femoral**	**Femoral Surface**	**Tibial Surface**
Knee, RT	ØSP[T,V]4JZ	ØSRC06[9,A,Z]	ØSRCØJ[9,A,Z]	ØSRCØEZ	ØSRCØN[9,A,Z]	ØSRTØJ[9,A,Z]	ØSRVØJ[9,A,Z]
Knee, LT	ØSP[U,W]4JZ	ØSRD06[9,A,Z]	ØSRDØJ[9,A,Z]	ØSRDØEZ	ØSRDØN[9,A,Z]	ØSRUØJ[9,A,Z]	ØSRWØJ[9,A,Z]

466-468 Revision of Hip or Knee Replacement

Hip Procedures

Open Removal of Hip Spacer with Replacement

Removal of Spacer		Code also as appropriate Replacement by Device Type						
		Metal	**Metal on Poly**	**Ceramic**	**Ceramic on Poly**	**Oxidized Zirc on Poly**	**Articulating Spacer**	**Synth Subst**
Hip, RT	ØSP908Z	ØSR901[9,A,Z]	ØSR902[9,A,Z]	ØSR903[9,A,Z]	ØSR904[9,A,Z]	ØSR906[9,A,Z]	ØSR90EZ	ØSR90J[9,A,Z]
Hip, LT	ØSPB08Z	ØSRB01[9,A,Z]	ØSRB02[9,A,Z]	ØSRB03[9,A,Z]	ØSRB04[9,A,Z]	ØSRB06[9,A,Z]	ØSRBØEZ	ØSRBØJ[9,A,Z]

Open Removal of Hip Spacer with Replacement

Removal of Spacer		Code also as appropriate Replacement by Device Type						
		Acetabular Surface				Femoral Surface		
		Poly	Metal	Ceramic	Synthetic	Metal	Ceramic	Synth
Hip, RT	ØSP9Ø8Z	ØSRAØØ[9,A,Z]	ØSRAØ1[9,A,Z]	ØSRAØ3[9,A,Z]	ØSRAØJ[9,A,Z]	ØSRRØ1[9,A,Z]	ØSRRØ3[9,A,Z]	ØSRRØJ[9,A,Z]
Hip, LT	ØSPBØ8Z	ØSREØØ[9,A,Z]	ØSREØ1[9,A,Z]	ØSREØ3[9,A,Z]	ØSREØJ[9,A,Z]	ØSRSØ1[9,A,Z]	ØSRSØ3[9,A,Z]	ØSRSØJ[9,A,Z]

Open Removal of Hip Spacer with Liner Insertion (supplement)

Removal of Spacer		Code also as appropriate Supplement of Body Part by Site		
		Joint	Acetabular Surface	Femoral Surface
Hip, RT	ØSP9Ø8Z	ØSU9Ø9Z	ØSUAØ9Z	ØSURØ9Z
Hip, LT	ØSPBØ8Z	ØSUBØ9Z	ØSUEØ9Z	ØSUSØ9Z

Open Removal of Hip Liner with Replacement

Removal of Liner		Code also as appropriate Replacement by Device Type						
		Metal	Metal on Poly	Ceramic	Ceramic on Poly	Oxidized Zirc on Poly	Articulating Spacer	Synth Subst
Hip, RT	ØSP9Ø9Z	ØSR9Ø1[9,A,Z]	ØSR9Ø2[9,A,Z]	ØSR9Ø3[9,A,Z]	ØSR9Ø4[9,A,Z]	ØSR9Ø6[9,A,Z]	ØSR9ØEZ	ØSR9ØJ[9,A,Z]
Hip, LT	ØSPBØ9Z	ØSRBØ1[9,A,Z]	ØSRBØ2[9,A,Z]	ØSRBØ3[9,A,Z]	ØSRBØ4[9,A,Z]	ØSRBØ6[9,A,Z]	ØSRBØEZ	ØSRBØJ[9,A,Z]

Open Removal of Hip Liner with Replacement

Removal of Liner		Code also as appropriate Replacement by Device Type						
		Acetabular Surface				Femoral Surface		
		Poly	Metal	Ceramic	Synthetic	Metal	Ceramic	Synth
Hip, RT	ØSP9Ø9Z	ØSRAØØ[9,A,Z]	ØSRAØ1[9,A,Z]	ØSRAØ3[9,A,Z]	ØSRAØJ[9,A,Z]	ØSRRØ1[9,A,Z]	ØSRRØ3[9,A,Z]	ØSRRØJ[9,A,Z]
Hip, LT	ØSPBØ9Z	ØSREØØ[9,A,Z]	ØSREØ1[9,A,Z]	ØSREØ3[9,A,Z]	ØSREØJ[9,A,Z]	ØSRSØ1[9,A,Z]	ØSRSØ3[9,A,Z]	ØSRSØJ[9,A,Z]

Open Removal of Hip Liner with Liner Insertion (supplement)

Removal of Liner		Code also as appropriate Supplement of Body Part by Site		
		Joint	Acetabular Surface	Femoral Surface
Hip, RT	ØSP9Ø9Z	ØSU9Ø9Z	ØSUAØ9Z	ØSURØ9Z
Hip, LT	ØSPBØ9Z	ØSUBØ9Z	ØSUEØ9Z	ØSUSØ9Z

Open Removal of Hip Resurfacing Device with Replacement

Removal of Resurfacing Device		Code also as appropriate Replacement by Device Type						
		Metal	Metal on Poly	Ceramic	Ceramic on Poly	Oxidized Zirc on Poly	Articulating Spacer	Synth Subst
Hip, RT	ØSP9ØBZ	ØSR9Ø1[9,A,Z]	ØSR9Ø2[9,A,Z]	ØSR9Ø3[9,A,Z]	ØSR9Ø4[9,A,Z]	ØSR9Ø6[9,A,Z]	ØSR9ØEZ	ØSR9ØJ[9,A,Z]
Hip, LT	ØSPBØBZ	ØSRBØ1[9,A,Z]	ØSRBØ2[9,A,Z]	ØSRBØ3[9,A,Z]	ØSRBØ4[9,A,Z]	ØSRBØ6[9,A,Z]	ØSRBØEZ	ØSRBØJ[9,A,Z]

Open Removal of Hip Resurfacing Device with Replacement

Removal of Resurfacing Device		Code also as appropriate Replacement by Device Type						
		Acetabular Surface				Femoral Surface		
		Poly	Metal	Ceramic	Synthetic	Metal	Ceramic	Synth
Hip, RT	ØSP9ØBZ	ØSRAØØ[9,A,Z]	ØSRAØ1[9,A,Z]	ØSRAØ3[9,A,Z]	ØSRAØJ[9,A,Z]	ØSRRØ1[9,A,Z]	ØSRRØ3[9,A,Z]	ØSRRØJ[9,A,Z]
Hip, LT	ØSPBØBZ	ØSREØØ[9,A,Z]	ØSREØ1[9,A,Z]	ØSREØ3[9,A,Z]	ØSREØJ[9,A,Z]	ØSRSØ1[9,A,Z]	ØSRSØ3[9,A,Z]	ØSRSØJ[9,A,Z]

Open Removal of Hip Resurfacing Device with Liner Insertion (supplement)

Removal of Resurfacing Device		Code also as appropriate Supplement of Body Part by Site		
		Joint	Acetabular Surface	Femoral Surface
Hip, RT	ØSP9ØBZ	ØSU9Ø9Z	ØSUAØ9Z	ØSURØ9Z
Hip, LT	ØSPBØBZ	ØSUBØ9Z	ØSUEØ9Z	ØSUSØ9Z

Appendix L: Procedure Combination Tables

Open Removal of Hip Articulating Spacer with Replacement

Removal of Articulating Spacer		Code also as appropriate Replacement by Device Type					
		Metal	Metal on Poly	Ceramic	Ceramic on Poly	Oxidized Zirc on Poly	Synth Subst
Hip, RT	ØSP9ØEZ	ØSR9Ø1[9,A,Z]	ØSR9Ø2[9,A,Z]	ØSR9Ø3[9,A,Z]	ØSR9Ø4[9,A,Z]	ØSR9Ø6[9,A,Z]	ØSR9ØJ[9,A,Z]
Hip, LT	ØSPBØEZ	ØSRBØ1[9,A,Z]	ØSRBØ2[9,A,Z]	ØSRBØ3[9,A,Z]	ØSRBØ4[9,A,Z]	ØSRBØ6[9,A,Z]	ØSRBØJ[9,A,Z]

Open Removal of Hip Articulating Spacer with Replacement

Removal of Articulating Spacer		Code also as appropriate Replacement by Device Type						
		Acetabular Surface				Femoral Surface		
		Poly	Metal	Ceramic	Synthetic	Metal	Ceramic	Synth
Hip, RT	ØSP9ØEZ	ØSRAØØ[9,A,Z]	ØSRAØ1[9,A,Z]	ØSRAØ3[9,A,Z]	ØSRAØJ[9,A,Z]	ØSRRØ1[9,A,Z]	ØSRRØ3[9,A,Z]	ØSRRØJ[9,A,Z]
Hip, LT	ØSPBØEZ	ØSREØØ[9,A,Z]	ØSREØ1[9,A,Z]	ØSREØ3[9,A,Z]	ØSREØJ[9,A,Z]	ØSRSØ1[9,A,Z]	ØSRSØ3[9,A,Z]	ØSRSØJ[9,A,Z]

Open Removal of Hip Articulating Spacer with Liner Insertion (supplement)

Removal of Articulating Spacer		Code also as appropriate Supplement of Body Part by Site		
		Joint	Acetabular Surface	Femoral Surface
Hip, RT	ØSP9ØEZ	ØSU9Ø9Z	ØSUAØ9Z	ØSURØ9Z
Hip, LT	ØSPBØEZ	ØSUBØ9Z	ØSUEØ9Z	ØSUSØ9Z

Open Removal of Hip Synthetic Substitute with Replacement

Removal of Synthetic Substitute		Code also as appropriate Replacement by Device Type						
		Metal	Metal on Poly	Ceramic	Ceramic on Poly	Oxidized Zirc on Poly	Articulating Spacer	Synth Subst
Hip, RT	ØSP[9,A,R]ØJZ	ØSR9Ø1[9,A,Z]	ØSR9Ø2[9,A,Z]	ØSR9Ø3[9,A,Z]	ØSR9Ø4[9,A,Z]	ØSR9Ø6[9,A,Z]	ØSR9ØEZ	ØSR9ØJ[9,A,Z]
Hip, LT	ØSP[B,E,S]ØJZ	ØSRBØ1[9,A,Z]	ØSRBØ2[9,A,Z]	ØSRBØ3[9,A,Z]	ØSRBØ4[9,A,Z]	ØSRBØ6[9,A,Z]	ØSRBØEZ	ØSRBØJ[9,A,Z]

Open Removal of Hip Synthetic Substitute with Replacement

Removal of Synthetic Substitute		Code also as appropriate Replacement by Device Type						
		Acetabular Surface				Femoral Surface		
		Poly	Metal	Ceramic	Synthetic	Metal	Ceramic	Synth
Hip, RT	ØSP[9,A,R]ØJZ	ØSRAØØ[9,A,Z]	ØSRAØ1[9,A,Z]	ØSRAØ3[9,A,Z]	ØSRAØJ[9,A,Z]	ØSRRØ1[9,A,Z]	ØSRRØ3[9,A,Z]	ØSRRØJ[9,A,Z]
Hip, LT	ØSP[B,E,S]ØJZ	ØSREØØ[9,A,Z]	ØSREØ1[9,A,Z]	ØSREØ3[9,A,Z]	ØSREØJ[9,A,Z]	ØSRSØ1[9,A,Z]	ØSRSØ3[9,A,Z]	ØSRSØJ[9,A,Z]

Percutaneous Endoscopic Removal of Hip Spacer with Open Replacement

Removal of Spacer		Code also as appropriate Replacement by Device Type						
		Metal	Metal on Poly	Ceramic	Ceramic on Poly	Oxidized Zirc on Poly	Articulating Spacer	Synth Subst
Hip, RT	ØSP948Z	ØSR9Ø1[9,A,Z]	ØSR9Ø2[9,A,Z]	ØSR9Ø3[9,A,Z]	ØSR9Ø4[9,A,Z]	ØSR9Ø6[9,A,Z]	ØSR9ØEZ	ØSR9ØJ[9,A,Z]
Hip, LT	ØSPB48Z	ØSRBØ1[9,A,Z]	ØSRBØ2[9,A,Z]	ØSRBØ3[9,A,Z]	ØSRBØ4[9,A,Z]	ØSRBØ6[9,A,Z]	ØSRBØEZ	ØSRBØJ[9,A,Z]

Percutaneous Endoscopic Removal of Hip Spacer with Open Replacement

Removal of Spacer		Code also as appropriate Replacement by Device Type						
		Acetabular Surface				Femoral Surface		
		Poly	Metal	Ceramic	Synthetic	Metal	Ceramic	Synth
Hip, RT	ØSP948Z	ØSRAØØ[9,A,Z]	ØSRAØ1[9,A,Z]	ØSRAØ3[9,A,Z]	ØSRAØJ[9,A,Z]	ØSRRØ1[9,A,Z]	ØSRRØ3[9,A,Z]	ØSRRØJ[9,A,Z]
Hip, LT	ØSPB48Z	ØSREØØ[9,A,Z]	ØSREØ1[9,A,Z]	ØSREØ3[9,A,Z]	ØSREØJ[9,A,Z]	ØSRSØ1[9,A,Z]	ØSRSØ3[9,A,Z]	ØSRSØJ[9,A,Z]

Percutaneous Endoscopic Removal of Hip Spacer with Open Liner Insertion (supplement)

Removal of Spacer		Code also as appropriate Supplement of Body Part by Site		
		Joint	Acetabular Surface	Femoral Surface
Hip, RT	ØSP948Z	ØSU9Ø9Z	ØSUAØ9Z	ØSURØ9Z
Hip, LT	ØSPB48Z	ØSUBØ9Z	ØSUEØ9Z	ØSUSØ9Z

Percutaneous Endoscopic Removal of Hip Synthetic Substitute with Open Replacement

Removal of Synthetic Substitute		Code also as appropriate Replacement by Device Type						
		Metal	Metal on Poly	Ceramic	Ceramic on Poly	Oxidized Zirc on Poly	Articulating Spacer	Synth Subst
Hip, RT	ØSP[9,A,R]4JZ	ØSR9Ø1[9,A,Z]	ØSR9Ø2[9,A,Z]	ØSR9Ø3[9,A,Z]	ØSR9Ø4[9,A,Z]	ØSR9Ø6[9,A,Z]	ØSR9ØEZ	ØSR9ØJ[9,A,Z]
Hip, LT	ØSP[B,E,S]4JZ	ØSRBØ1[9,A,Z]	ØSRBØ2[9,A,Z]	ØSRBØ3[9,A,Z]	ØSRBØ4[9,A,Z]	ØSRBØ6[9,A,Z]	ØSRBØEZ	ØSRBØJ[9,A,Z]

Percutaneous Endoscopic Removal of Hip Synthetic Substitute with Open Replacement

Removal of Synthetic Substitute		Code also as appropriate Replacement by Device Type						
		Acetabular Surface				Femoral Surface		
		Poly	Metal	Ceramic	Synthetic	Metal	Ceramic	Synth
Hip, RT	ØSP[9,A,R]4JZ	ØSRAØØ[9,A,Z]	ØSRAØ1[9,A,Z]	ØSRAØ3[9,A,Z]	ØSRAØJ[9,A,Z]	ØSRRØ1[9,A,Z]	ØSRRØ3[9,A,Z]	ØSRRØJ[9,A,Z]
Hip, LT	ØSP[B,E,S]4JZ	ØSREØØ[9,A,Z]	ØSREØ1[9,A,Z]	ØSREØ3[9,A,Z]	ØSREØJ[9,A,Z]	ØSRSØ1[9,A,Z]	ØSRSØ3[9,A,Z]	ØSRSØJ[9,A,Z]

Percutaneous Endoscopic Removal of Hip Synthetic Substitute with Open Liner Insertion (supplement)

Removal of Synthetic Substitute		Code also as appropriate Supplement of Body Part by Site		
		Joint	Acetabular Surface	Femoral Surface
Hip, RT	ØSP[9,A,R]4JZ	ØSU9Ø9Z	ØSUAØ9Z	ØSURØ9Z
Hip, LT	ØSP[B,E,S]4JZ	ØSUBØ9Z	ØSUEØ9Z	ØSUSØ9Z

Knee Procedures

Open Removal of Knee Spacer with Articulating Spacer Replacement

Removal of Spacer		Code also as appropriate Replacement with Articulating Spacer
Knee, RT	ØSPCØ8Z	ØSRCØEZ
Knee, LT	ØSPDØ8Z	ØSRDØEZ

Open Removal of Knee Spacer with Synthetic Substitute Replacement

Removal of Spacer		Code also as appropriate Replacement by Type of Synthetic Substitute				
		Oxidized Zircon on Poly	Synth Subst	Patello-femoral	Femoral Surface	Tibial Surface
Knee, RT	ØSPCØ8Z	ØSRCØ6[9,A,Z]	ØSRCØJ[9,A,Z]	ØSRCØN[9,A,Z]	ØSRTØJ[9,A,Z]	ØSRVØJ[9,A,Z]
Knee, LT	ØSPDØ8Z	ØSRDØ6[9,A,Z]	ØSRDØJ[9,A,Z]	ØSRDØN[9,A,Z]	ØSRUØJ[9,A,Z]	ØSRWØJ[9,A,Z]

Open Removal of Knee Liner with Articulating Spacer Replacement

Removal of Liner		Code also as appropriate Replacement with Articulating Spacer
Knee, RT	ØSPCØ9Z	ØSRCØEZ
Knee, LT	ØSPDØ9Z	ØSRDØEZ

Open Removal of Knee Liner with Synthetic Substitute Replacement

Removal of Liner		Code also as appropriate Replacement by Type of Synthetic Substitute						
		Oxidized Zircon on Poly	Synth Subst	Medial Unicondylar	Lateral Unicondylar	Patello-femoral	Femoral Surface	Tibial Surface
Knee, RT	ØSPCØ9Z	ØSRCØ6[9,A,Z]	ØSRCØJ[9,A,Z]	ØSRCØL[9,A,Z]	ØSRCØM[9,A,Z]	ØSRCØN[9,A,Z]	ØSRTØJ[9,A,Z]	ØSRVØJ[9,A,Z]
Knee, LT	ØSPDØ9Z	ØSRDØ6[9,A,Z]	ØSRDØJ[9,A,Z]	ØSRDØL[9,A,Z]	ØSRDØM[9,A,Z]	ØSRDØN[9,A,Z]	ØSRUØJ[9,A,Z]	ØSRWØJ[9,A,Z]

Open Removal of Knee Articulating Spacer with Synthetic Substitute Replacement

Removal of Articulating Spacer		Code also as appropriate Replacement by Type of Synthetic Substitute			
		Oxidized Zircon on Poly	Synth Subst	Femoral Surface	Tibial Surface
Knee, RT	ØSPCØEZ	ØSRCØ6[9,A,Z]	ØSRCØJ[9,A,Z]	ØSRTØJ[9,A,Z]	ØSRVØJ[9,A,Z]
Knee, LT	ØSPDØEZ	ØSRDØ6[9,A,Z]	ØSRDØJ[9,A,Z]	ØSRUØJ[9,A,Z]	ØSRWØJ[9,A,Z]

Open Removal of Patellar Surface of Knee with Synthetic Substitute Replacement

Removal of Patellar Surface		Code also as appropriate Replacement by Type of Synthetic Substitute				
		Oxidized Zircon on Poly	Synth Subst	Patello-femoral	Femoral Surface	Tibial Surface
Knee, RT	ØSPCØJC	ØSRCØ6[9,A,Z]	ØSRCØJ[9,A,Z]	ØSRCØN[9,A,Z]	ØSRTØJ[9,A,Z]	ØSRVØJ[9,A,Z]
Knee, LT	ØSPDØJC	ØSRDØ6[9,A,Z]	ØSRDØJ[9,A,Z]	ØSRDØN[9,A,Z]	ØSRUØJ[9,A,Z]	ØSRWØJ[9,A,Z]

Open Removal of Patellar Surface of Knee with Articulating Spacer Replacement

Removal of Patellar Surface		Code also as appropriate Replacement with Articulating Spacer
Knee, RT	ØSPCØJC	ØSRCØEZ
Knee, LT	ØSPDØJC	ØSRDØEZ

Open Removal of Knee Synthetic Substitute with Synthetic Substitute Replacement

Removal of Synthetic Substitute		Code also as appropriate Replacement by Type of Synthetic Substitute						
		Oxidized Zircon on Poly	Synth Subst	Medial Unicondylar	Lateral Unicondylar	Patello-femoral	Femoral Surface	Tibial Surface
Knee, RT	ØSPCØJZ	ØSRCØ6[9,A,Z]	ØSRCØJ[9,A,Z]	ØSRCØL[9,A,Z]	ØSRCØM[9,A,Z]	ØSRCØN[9,A,Z]	ØSRTØJ[9,A,Z]	ØSRVØJ[9,A,Z]
Knee, LT	ØSPDØJZ	ØSRDØ6[9,A,Z]	ØSRDØJ[9,A,Z]	ØSRDØL[9,A,Z]	ØSRDØM[9,A,Z]	ØSRDØN[9,A,Z]	ØSRUØJ[9,A,Z]	ØSRWØJ[9,A,Z]

Open Removal of Knee Synthetic Substitute with Articulating Spacer Replacement

Removal of Synthetic Substitute		Code also as appropriate Replacement with Articulating Spacer
Knee, RT	ØSPCØJZ	ØSRCØEZ
Knee, LT	ØSPDØJZ	ØSRDØEZ

Open Removal of Medial or Lateral Unicondylar Knee with Synthetic Substitute Replacement

Removal of Medial/Lateral Unicondylar Knee		Code also as appropriate Replacement by Type of Synthetic Substitute				
		Oxidized Zircon on Poly	Synth Subst	Medial Unicondylar	Femoral Surface	Tibial Surface
Knee, RT	ØSPCØ[L,M]Z	ØSRCØ6[9,A,Z]	ØSRCØJ[9,A,Z]	ØSRCØL[9,A,Z]	ØSRTØJ[9,A,Z]	ØSRVØJ[9,A,Z]
Knee, LT	ØSPDØ[L,M]Z	ØSRDØ6[9,A,Z]	ØSRDØJ[9,A,Z]	ØSRDØL[9,A,Z]	ØSRUØJ[9,A,Z]	ØSRWØJ[9,A,Z]

Open Removal of Patellofemoral Knee with Synthetic Substitute Replacement

Removal of Patellofemoral Knee		Code also as appropriate Replacement by Type of Synthetic Substitute				
		Oxidized Zircon on Poly	Synth Subst	Medial Unicondylar	Femoral Surface	Tibial Surface
Knee, RT	ØSPCØNZ	ØSRCØ6[9,A,Z]	ØSRCØJ[9,A,Z]	ØSRCØL[9,A,Z]	ØSRTØJ[9,A,Z]	ØSRVØJ[9,A,Z]
Knee, LT	ØSPDØNZ	ØSRDØ6[9,A,Z]	ØSRDØJ[9,A,Z]	ØSRDØL[9,A,Z]	ØSRUØJ[9,A,Z]	ØSRWØJ[9,A,Z]

Open Removal of Femoral/Tibial Surface of Knee with Synthetic Substitute Replacement

Removal of Femoral/Tibial Surface of Knee		Code also as appropriate Replacement by Type of Synthetic Substitute					
		Oxidized Zircon on Poly	Synth Subst	Articulating Spacer	Patello-femoral	Femoral Surface	Tibial Surface
Knee, RT	ØSP[T,V]ØJZ	ØSRCØ6[9,A,Z]	ØSRCØJ[9,A,Z]	ØSRCØEZ	ØSRCØN[9,A,Z]	ØSRTØJ[9,A,Z]	ØSRVØJ[9,A,Z]
Knee, LT	ØSP[U,W]ØJZ	ØSRDØ6[9,A,Z]	ØSRDØJ[9,A,Z]	ØSRDØEZ	ØSRDØN[9,A,Z]	ØSRUØJ[9,A,Z]	ØSRWØJ[9,A,Z]

Percutaneous/Percutaneous Endoscopic Removal of Knee Spacer with Open Synthetic Substitute Replacement

Removal of Spacer		Code also as appropriate Replacement by Type of Synthetic Substitute				
		Oxidized Zircon on Poly	Synth Subst	Patello-femoral	Femoral Surface	Tibial Surface
Knee, RT	ØSPC[3,4]8Z	ØSRCØ6[9,A,Z]	ØSRCØJ[9,A,Z]	ØSRCØN[9,A,Z]	ØSRTØJ[9,A,Z]	ØSRVØJ[9,A,Z]
Knee, LT	ØSPD[3,4]8Z	ØSRDØ6[9,A,Z]	ØSRDØJ[9,A,Z]	ØSRDØN[9,A,Z]	ØSRUØJ[9,A,Z]	ØSRWØJ[9,A,Z]

Percutaneous/Percutaneous Endoscopic Removal of Knee Spacer with Open Articulating Spacer Replacement

Removal of Spacer		Code also as appropriate Replacement with Articulating Spacer
Knee, RT	ØSPC[3,4]8Z	ØSRCØEZ
Knee, LT	ØSPD[3,4]8Z	ØSRDØEZ

Percutaneous Endoscopic Removal of Patellar Surface of Knee with Synthetic Substitute Replacement

Removal of Patellar Surface		Code also as appropriate Replacement by Type of Synthetic Substitute				
		Oxidized Zircon on Poly	Synth Subst	Patello-femoral	Femoral Surface	Tibial Surface
Knee, RT	ØSPC4JC	ØSRCØ6[9,A,Z]	ØSRCØJ[9,A,Z]	ØSRCØN[9,A,Z]	ØSRTØJ[9,A,Z]	ØSRVØJ[9,A,Z]
Knee, LT	ØSPD4JC	ØSRDØ6[9,A,Z]	ØSRDØJ[9,A,Z]	ØSRDØN[9,A,Z]	ØSRUØJ[9,A,Z]	ØSRWØJ[9,A,Z]

Percutaneous Endoscopic Removal of Patellar Surface of Knee with Articulating Spacer Replacement

Removal of Patellar Surface		Code also as appropriate Replacement with Articulating Spacer
Knee, RT	ØSPC4JC	ØSRCØEZ
Knee, LT	ØSPD4JC	ØSRDØEZ

Percutaneous Endoscopic Removal of Knee Synthetic Substitute with Synthetic Substitute Replacement

Removal of Synthetic Substitute		Code also as appropriate Replacement by Type of Synthetic Substitute						
		Oxidized Zircon on Poly	Synth Subst	Medial Unicondylar	Lateral Unicondylar	Patello-femoral	Femoral Surface	Tibial Surface
Knee, RT	ØSPC4JZ	ØSRCØ6[9,A,Z]	ØSRCØJ[9,A,Z]	ØSRCØL[9,A,Z]	ØSRCØM[9,A,Z]	ØSRCØN[9,A,Z]	ØSRTØJ[9,A,Z]	ØSRVØJ[9,A,Z]
Knee, LT	ØSPD4JZ	ØSRDØ6[9,A,Z]	ØSRDØJ[9,A,Z]	ØSRDØL[9,A,Z]	ØSRDØM[9,A,Z]	ØSRDØN[9,A,Z]	ØSRUØJ[9,A,Z]	ØSRWØJ[9,A,Z]

Percutaneous Endoscopic Removal of Knee Synthetic Substitute with Articulating Spacer Replacement

Removal of Synthetic Substitute		Code also as appropriate Replacement with Articulating Spacer
Knee, RT	ØSPC4JZ	ØSRCØEZ
Knee, LT	ØSPD4JZ	ØSRDØEZ

Percutaneous Endoscopic Removal of Medial or Lateral Unicondylar Knee with Synthetic Substitute Replacement

Removal of Medial/Lateral Unicondylar Knee		Code also as appropriate Replacement by Type of Synthetic Substitute				
		Oxidized Zircon on Poly	Synth Subst	Medial Unicondylar	Femoral Surface	Tibial Surface
Knee, RT	ØSPC4[L,M]Z	ØSRCØ6[9,A,Z]	ØSRCØJ[9,A,Z]	ØSRCØL[9,A,Z]	ØSRTØJ[9,A,Z]	ØSRVØJ[9,A,Z]
Knee, LT	ØSPD4[L,M]Z	ØSRDØ6[9,A,Z]	ØSRDØJ[9,A,Z]	ØSRDØL[9,A,Z]	ØSRUØJ[9,A,Z]	ØSRWØJ[9,A,Z]

Percutaneous Endoscopic Removal of Patellofemoral Knee with Synthetic Substitute Replacement

Removal of Patellofemoral Knee		Code also as appropriate Replacement by Type of Synthetic Substitute				
		Oxidized Zircon on Poly	Synth Subst	Medial Unicondylar	Femoral Surface	Tibial Surface
Knee, RT	ØSPC4NZ	ØSRCØ6[9,A,Z]	ØSRCØJ[9,A,Z]	ØSRCØL[9,A,Z]	ØSRTØJ[9,A,Z]	ØSRVØJ[9,A,Z]
Knee, LT	ØSPD4NZ	ØSRDØ6[9,A,Z]	ØSRDØJ[9,A,Z]	ØSRDØL[9,A,Z]	ØSRUØJ[9,A,Z]	ØSRWØJ[9,A,Z]

Percutaneous Endoscopic Removal of Femoral/Tibial Surface of Knee with Synthetic Substitute Replacement

Removal of Femoral/Tibial Surface of Knee		Code also as appropriate Replacement by Type of Synthetic Substitute					
		Oxidized Zircon on Poly	Synth Subst	Articulating Spacer	Patello-femoral	Femoral Surface	Tibial Surface
Knee, RT	ØSP[T,V]4JZ	ØSRCØ6[9,A,Z]	ØSRCØJ[9,A,Z]	ØSRCØEZ	ØSRCØN[9,A,Z]	ØSRTØJ[9,A,Z]	ØSRVØJ[9,A,Z]
Knee, LT	ØSP[U,W]4JZ	ØSRDØ6[9,A,Z]	ØSRDØJ[9,A,Z]	ØSRDØEZ	ØSRDØN[9,A,Z]	ØSRUØJ[9,A,Z]	ØSRWØJ[9,A,Z]

DRG 485-489 Knee Procedures

Joint	Removal of Liner by open approach	Code also as appropriate Supplement of Tibial Surface by Site
Knee, RT	ØSPCØ9Z	ØSUVØ9Z
Knee, LT	ØSPDØ9Z	ØSUWØ9Z

DRG 515-517 Other Musculoskeletal System and Connective Tissue Procedures

Site	Reposition of Vertebra by percutaneous approach	Code also as appropriate Supplement With Synthetic Substitute by Percutaneous Approach at site of Repositioned Vertebra
Cervical	ØPS33ZZ	ØPU33JZ
Coccyx	ØQSS3ZZ	ØQUS3JZ
Lumbar	ØQS03ZZ	ØQU03JZ
Sacrum	ØQS13ZZ	ØQU13JZ
Thoracic	ØPS43ZZ	ØPU43JZ

DRG 518-52Ø Back and Neck Procedures, Except Spinal Fusion, or Disc Devices/Neurostimulators

Generator Type	Insertion of Generator by Site			Code also as appropriate Insertion Neurostimulator Lead by approach and Site	
	Chest	Abdomen	Back	Spinal Canal	Spinal Cord
Single Array	ØJH6[Ø,3]BZ	ØJH8[Ø,3]BZ	ØJH7[Ø,3]BZ	00HU[Ø,3,4]MZ	00HV[Ø,3,4]MZ
Single Array, Rechargeable	ØJH6[Ø,3]CZ	ØJH8[Ø,3]CZ	ØJH7[Ø,3]CZ	00HU[Ø,3,4]MZ	00HV[Ø,3,4]MZ
Multiple Array	ØJH6[Ø,3]DZ	ØJH8[Ø,3]DZ	ØJH7[Ø,3]DZ	00HU[Ø,3,4]MZ	00HV[Ø,3,4]MZ
Multiple Array, Rechargable	ØJH6[Ø,3]EZ	—	ØJH7[Ø,3]EZ	00HU[Ø,3,4]MZ	00HV[Ø,3,4]MZ
Multiple Array, Rechargable	—	ØJH8[Ø,3]EZ	—	00HU[Ø,3,4]MZ	00HV[Ø,3,4]MZ

DRG 582-583 Mastectomy for Malignancy

Site	Resection by Open approach	Code also as appropriate Resection of Lymph Nodes by Open approach by site			Code also as appropriate Resection of Thorax Muscle by Open approach	
		Axillary	Internal Mammary	Thorax	Right	Left
Breast, Right	ØHTTØZZ	07T50ZZ	07T80ZZ	07T70ZZ	ØKTHØZZ	—
Breast, Left	ØHTUØZZ	07T60ZZ	07T90ZZ	07T70ZZ	—	ØKTJØZZ
Breast, Bilateral	ØHTVØZZ	07T50ZZ and 07T60ZZ	07T80ZZ and 07T90ZZ	07T70ZZ	ØKTHØZZ	ØKTJØZZ

DRG 584-585 Breast Biopsy, Local Excision and Other Breast Procedures

Resection of Breast With Resection of Lymph Nodes and Thorax Muscle

Site	Resection by Open approach	Code also as appropriate Resection of Lymph Nodes by Open approach by site			Code also as appropriate Resection of Thorax Muscle by Open approach	
		Axillary	Internal Mammary	Thorax	Right	Left
Breast, Right	ØHTTØZZ	07T50ZZ	07T80ZZ	07T70ZZ	ØKTHØZZ	—
Breast, Left	ØHTUØZZ	07T60ZZ	07T90ZZ	07T70ZZ	—	ØKTJØZZ
Breast, Bilateral	ØHTVØZZ	07T50ZZ and 07T60ZZ	07T80ZZ and 07T90ZZ	07T70ZZ	ØKTHØZZ	ØKTJØZZ

Replacement of Breast Tissue

Site	Replacement by Percutaneous approach with Autologous Tissue	Code also as appropriate Extraction of Subcutaneous Tissue by Percutaneous approach					
		Abdomen	Back	Buttock	Chest	Leg, Upper, Right	Leg, Upper, Left
Breast, Right	ØHRT37Z	ØJD83ZZ	ØJD73ZZ	ØJD93ZZ	ØJD63ZZ	ØJDL3ZZ	ØJDM3ZZ
Breast, Left	ØHRU37Z	ØJD83ZZ	ØJD73ZZ	ØJD93ZZ	ØJD63ZZ	ØJDL3ZZ	ØJDM3ZZ
Breast, Bilateral	ØHRV37Z	ØJD83ZZ	ØJD73ZZ	ØJD93ZZ	ØJD63ZZ	ØJDL3ZZ	ØJDM3ZZ

DRG 628-63Ø Other Endocrine, Nutritional and Metabolic Procedures

Hip Procedures

Open Removal of Hip Spacer with Replacement

Removal of Spacer		Code also as appropriate Replacement by Device Type					
		Metal	Metal on Poly	Ceramic	Ceramic on Poly	Oxidized Zirc on Poly	Synthetic Substitute
Hip, RT	ØSP908Z	ØSR901[9,A,Z]	ØSR902[9,A,Z]	ØSR903[9,A,Z]	ØSR904[9,A,Z]	ØSR906[9,A,Z]	ØSR90J[9,A,Z]
Hip, LT	ØSPB08Z	ØSRB01[9,A,Z]	ØSRB02[9,A,Z]	ØSRB03[9,A,Z]	ØSRB04[9,A,Z]	ØSRB06[9,A,Z]	ØSRB0J[9,A,Z]

Open Removal of Hip Spacer with Replacement

Removal of Spacer		Code also as appropriate Replacement by Device Type						
		Acetabular Surface				Femoral Surface		
		Poly	Metal	Ceramic	Synthetic	Metal	Ceramic	Synthetic
Hip, RT	ØSP9Ø8Z	ØSRAØØ[9,A,Z]	ØSRAØ1[9,A,Z]	ØSRAØ3[9,A,Z]	ØSRAØJ[9,A,Z]	ØSRRØ1[9,A,Z]	ØSRRØ3[9,A,Z]	ØSRRØJ[9,A,Z]
Hip, LT	ØSPBØ8Z	ØSREØØ[9,A,Z]	ØSREØ1[9,A,Z]	ØSREØ3[9,A,Z]	ØSREØJ[9,A,Z]	ØSRSØ1[9,A,Z]	ØSRSØ3[9,A,Z]	ØSRSØJ[9,A,Z]

Open Removal of Hip Spacer with Liner Insertion (supplement)

Removal of Spacer		Code also as appropriate Supplement of Body Part by Site		
		Joint	Acetabular Surface	Femoral Surface
Hip, RT	ØSP9Ø8Z	ØSU9Ø9Z	ØSUAØ9Z	ØSURØ9Z
Hip, LT	ØSPBØ8Z	ØSUBØ9Z	ØSUEØ9Z	ØSUSØ9Z

Open Removal of Hip Liner with Replacement

Removal of Liner		Code also as appropriate Replacement by Device Type					
		Metal	Metal on Poly	Ceramic	Ceramic on Poly	Oxidized Zirc on Poly	Synthetic Substitute
Hip, RT	ØSP9Ø9Z	ØSR9Ø1[9,A,Z]	ØSR9Ø2[9,A,Z]	ØSR9Ø3[9,A,Z]	ØSR9Ø4[9,A,Z]	ØSR9Ø6[9,A,Z]	ØSR9ØJ[9,A,Z]
Hip, LT	ØSPBØ9Z	ØSRBØ1[9,A,Z]	ØSRBØ2[9,A,Z]	ØSRBØ3[9,A,Z]	ØSRBØ4[9,A,Z]	ØSRBØ6[9,A,Z]	ØSRBØJ[9,A,Z]

Open Removal of Hip Liner with Replacement

Removal of Liner		Code also as appropriate Replacement by Device Type						
		Acetabular Surface				Femoral Surface		
		Poly	Metal	Ceramic	Synthetic	Metal	Ceramic	Synthetic
Hip, RT	ØSP9Ø9Z	ØSRAØØ[9,A,Z]	ØSRAØ1[9,A,Z]	ØSRAØ3[9,A,Z]	ØSRAØJ[9,A,Z]	ØSRRØ1[9,A,Z]	ØSRRØ3[9,A,Z]	ØSRRØJ[9,A,Z]
Hip, LT	ØSPBØ9Z	ØSREØØ[9,A,Z]	ØSREØ1[9,A,Z]	ØSREØ3[9,A,Z]	ØSREØJ[9,A,Z]	ØSRSØ1[9,A,Z]	ØSRSØ3[9,A,Z]	ØSRSØJ[9,A,Z]

Open Removal of Hip Liner with Liner Insertion (supplement)

Removal of Liner		Code also as appropriate Supplement of Body Part by Site		
		Joint	Acetabular Surface	Femoral Surface
Hip, RT	ØSP9Ø9Z	ØSU9Ø9Z	ØSUAØ9Z	ØSURØ9Z
Hip, LT	ØSPBØ9Z	ØSUBØ9Z	ØSUEØ9Z	ØSUSØ9Z

Open Removal of Hip Resurfacing Device with Replacement

Removal of Resurfacing Device		Code also as appropriate Replacement by Device Type					
		Metal	Metal on Poly	Ceramic	Ceramic on Poly	Oxidized Zirc on Poly	Synthetic Substitute
Hip, RT	ØSP9ØBZ	ØSR9Ø1[9,A,Z]	ØSR9Ø2[9,A,Z]	ØSR9Ø3[9,A,Z]	ØSR9Ø4[9,A,Z]	ØSR9Ø6[9,A,Z]	ØSR9ØJ[9,A,Z]
Hip, LT	ØSPBØBZ	ØSRBØ1[9,A,Z]	ØSRBØ2[9,A,Z]	ØSRBØ3[9,A,Z]	ØSRBØ4[9,A,Z]	ØSRBØ6[9,A,Z]	ØSRBØJ[9,A,Z]

Open Removal of Hip Resurfacing Device with Replacement

Removal of Resurfacing Device		Code also as appropriate Replacement by Device Type						
		Acetabular Surface				Femoral Surface		
		Poly	Metal	Ceramic	Synthetic	Metal	Ceramic	Synthetic
Hip, RT	ØSP9ØBZ	ØSRAØØ[9,A,Z]	ØSRAØ1[9,A,Z]	ØSRAØ3[9,A,Z]	ØSRAØJ[9,A,Z]	ØSRRØ1[9,A,Z]	ØSRRØ3[9,A,Z]	ØSRRØJ[9,A,Z]
Hip, LT	ØSPBØBZ	ØSREØØ[9,A,Z]	ØSREØ1[9,A,Z]	ØSREØ3[9,A,Z]	ØSREØJ[9,A,Z]	ØSRSØ1[9,A,Z]	ØSRSØ3[9,A,Z]	ØSRSØJ[9,A,Z]

Open Removal of Hip Resurfacing Device with Liner Insertion (supplement)

Removal of Resurfacing Device		Code also as appropriate Supplement of Body Part by Site		
		Joint	Acetabular Surface	Femoral Surface
Hip, RT	ØSP9ØBZ	ØSU9Ø9Z	ØSUAØ9Z	ØSURØ9Z
Hip, LT	ØSPBØBZ	ØSUBØ9Z	ØSUEØ9Z	ØSUSØ9Z

Open Removal of Hip Synthetic Substitute with Replacement

Removal of Synthetic Substitute		Code also as appropriate Replacement by Device Type					
		Metal	Metal on Poly	Ceramic	Ceramic on Poly	Oxidized Zirc on Poly	Synthetic Substitute
Hip, RT	ØSP9ØJZ	ØSR9Ø1[9,A,Z]	ØSR9Ø2[9,A,Z]	ØSR9Ø3[9,A,Z]	ØSR9Ø4[9,A,Z]	ØSR9Ø6[9,A,Z]	ØSR9ØJ[9,A,Z]
Hip, LT	ØSPBØJZ	ØSRBØ1[9,A,Z]	ØSRBØ2[9,A,Z]	ØSRBØ3[9,A,Z]	ØSRBØ4[9,A,Z]	ØSRBØ6[9,A,Z]	ØSRBØJ[9,A,Z]

Open Removal of Hip Synthetic Substitute with Replacement

Removal of Synthetic Substitute		Code also as appropriate Replacement by Device Type						
		Acetabular Surface				Femoral Surface		
		Poly	Metal	Ceramic	Synthetic	Metal	Ceramic	Synthetic
Hip, RT	ØSP9ØJZ	ØSRAØØ[9,A,Z]	ØSRAØ1[9,A,Z]	ØSRAØ3[9,A,Z]	ØSRAØJ[9,A,Z]	ØSRRØ1[9,A,Z]	ØSRRØ3[9,A,Z]	ØSRRØJ[9,A,Z]
Hip, LT	ØSPBØJZ	ØSREØØ[9,A,Z]	ØSREØ1[9,A,Z]	ØSREØ3[9,A,Z]	ØSREØJ[9,A,Z]	ØSRSØ1[9,A,Z]	ØSRSØ3[9,A,Z]	ØSRSØJ[9,A,Z]

Open Removal of Hip Acetabular/Femoral Surface with Replacement

Removal of Acetabular/Femoral Surface		Code also as appropriate Replacement by Device Type					
		Metal	Metal on Poly	Ceramic	Ceramic on Poly	Oxidized Zirc on Poly	Synthetic Substitute
Hip, RT	ØSP[A,R]ØJZ	ØSR9Ø1[9,A,Z]	ØSR9Ø2[9,A,Z]	ØSR9Ø3[9,A,Z]	ØSR9Ø4[9,A,Z]	ØSR9Ø6[9,A,Z]	ØSR9ØJ[9,A,Z]
Hip, LT	ØSP[E,S]ØJZ	ØSRBØ1[9,A,Z]	ØSRBØ2[9,A,Z]	ØSRBØ3[9,A,Z]	ØSRBØ4[9,A,Z]	ØSRBØ6[9,A,Z]	ØSRBØJ[9,A,Z]

Open Removal of Hip Acetabular/Femoral Surface with Replacement

Removal of Acetabular/Femoral Surface		Code also as appropriate Replacement by Device Type						
		Acetabular Surface				Femoral Surface		
		Poly	Metal	Ceramic	Synthetic	Metal	Ceramic	Synthetic
Hip, RT	ØSP[A,R]ØJZ	ØSRAØØ[9,A,Z]	ØSRAØ1[9,A,Z]	ØSRAØ3[9,A,Z]	ØSRAØJ[9,A,Z]	ØSRRØ1[9,A,Z]	ØSRRØ3[9,A,Z]	ØSRRØJ[9,A,Z]
Hip, LT	ØSP[E,S]ØJZ	ØSREØØ[9,A,Z]	ØSREØ1[9,A,Z]	ØSREØ3[9,A,Z]	ØSREØJ[9,A,Z]	ØSRSØ1[9,A,Z]	ØSRSØ3[9,A,Z]	ØSRSØJ[9,A,Z]

Percutaneous Endoscopic Removal of Hip Spacer with Replacement

Removal of Spacer		Code also as appropriate Replacement by Device Type					
		Metal	Metal on Poly	Ceramic	Ceramic on Poly	Oxidized Zirc on Poly	Synthetic Substitute
Hip, RT	ØSP948Z	ØSR9Ø1[9,A,Z]	ØSR9Ø2[9,A,Z]	ØSR9Ø3[9,A,Z]	ØSR9Ø4[9,A,Z]	ØSR9Ø6[9,A,Z]	ØSR9ØJ[9,A,Z]
Hip, LT	ØSPB48Z	ØSRBØ1[9,A,Z]	ØSRBØ2[9,A,Z]	ØSRBØ3[9,A,Z]	ØSRBØ4[9,A,Z]	ØSRBØ6[9,A,Z]	ØSRBØJ[9,A,Z]

Percutaneous Endoscopic Removal of Hip Spacer with Replacement

Removal of Spacer		Code also as appropriate Replacement by Device Type						
		Acetabular Surface				Femoral Surface		
		Poly	Metal	Ceramic	Synthetic	Metal	Ceramic	Synthetic
Hip, RT	ØSP948Z	ØSRAØØ[9,A,Z]	ØSRAØ1[9,A,Z]	ØSRAØ3[9,A,Z]	ØSRAØJ[9,A,Z]	ØSRRØ1[9,A,Z]	ØSRRØ3[9,A,Z]	ØSRRØJ[9,A,Z]
Hip, LT	ØSPB48Z	ØSREØØ[9,A,Z]	ØSREØ1[9,A,Z]	ØSREØ3[9,A,Z]	ØSREØJ[9,A,Z]	ØSRSØ1[9,A,Z]	ØSRSØ3[9,A,Z]	ØSRSØJ[9,A,Z]

Percutaneous Endoscopic Removal of Hip Spacer with Liner Insertion (supplement)

Removal of Spacer		Code also as appropriate Supplement of Body Part by Site		
		Joint	Acetabular Surface	Femoral Surface
Hip, RT	ØSP948Z	ØSU9Ø9Z	ØSUAØ9Z	ØSURØ9Z
Hip, LT	ØSPB48Z	ØSUBØ9Z	ØSUEØ9Z	ØSUSØ9Z

Percutaneous Endoscopic Removal of Hip Synthetic Substitute with Replacement

Removal of Synthetic Substitute		Code also as appropriate Replacement by Device Type					
		Metal	Metal on Poly	Ceramic	Ceramic on Poly	Oxidized Zirc on Poly	Synthetic Substitute
Hip, RT	ØSP94JZ	ØSR9Ø1[9,A,Z]	ØSR9Ø2[9,A,Z]	ØSR9Ø3[9,A,Z]	ØSR9Ø4[9,A,Z]	ØSR9Ø6[9,A,Z]	ØSR9ØJ[9,A,Z]
Hip, LT	ØSPB4JZ	ØSRBØ1[9,A,Z]	ØSRBØ2[9,A,Z]	ØSRBØ3[9,A,Z]	ØSRBØ4[9,A,Z]	ØSRBØ6[9,A,Z]	ØSRBØJ[9,A,Z]

Percutaneous Endoscopic of Hip Synthetic Substitute with Replacement

Removal of Synthetic Substitute		Code also as appropriate Replacement by Device Type						
		Acetabular Surface				Femoral Surface		
		Poly	Metal	Ceramic	Synthetic	Metal	Ceramic	Synthetic
Hip, RT	ØSP94JZ	ØSRAØØ[9,A,Z]	ØSRAØ1[9,A,Z]	ØSRAØ3[9,A,Z]	ØSRAØJ[9,A,Z]	ØSRRØ1[9,A,Z]	ØSRRØ3[9,A,Z]	ØSRRØJ[9,A,Z]
Hip, LT	ØSPB4JZ	ØSREØØ[9,A,Z]	ØSREØ1[9,A,Z]	ØSREØ3[9,A,Z]	ØSREØJ[9,A,Z]	ØSRSØ1[9,A,Z]	ØSRSØ3[9,A,Z]	ØSRSØJ[9,A,Z]

Percutaneous Endoscopic Removal of Hip Synthetic Substitute with Liner Insertion (supplement)

Removal of Synthetic Substitute		Code also as appropriate Supplement of Body Part by Site		
		Joint	Acetabular Surface	Femoral Surface
Hip, RT	ØSP94JZ	ØSU9Ø9Z	ØSUAØ9Z	ØSURØ9Z
Hip, LT	ØSPB4JZ	ØSUBØ9Z	ØSUEØ9Z	ØSUSØ9Z

Percutaneous Endoscopic Removal of Hip Acetabular/Femoral Surface with Replacement

Removal of Acetabular/Femoral Surface		Code also as appropriate Replacement by Device Type					
		Metal	Metal on Poly	Ceramic	Ceramic on Poly	Oxidized Zirc on Poly	Synthetic Substitute
Hip, RT	ØSP[A,R]4JZ	ØSR9Ø1[9,A,Z]	ØSR9Ø2[9,A,Z]	ØSR9Ø3[9,A,Z]	ØSR9Ø4[9,A,Z]	ØSR9Ø6[9,A,Z]	ØSR9ØJ[9,A,Z]
Hip, LT	ØSP[E,S]4JZ	ØSRBØ1[9,A,Z]	ØSRBØ2[9,A,Z]	ØSRBØ3[9,A,Z]	ØSRBØ4[9,A,Z]	ØSRBØ6[9,A,Z]	ØSRBØJ[9,A,Z]

Percutaneous Endoscopic of Hip Acetabular/Femoral Surface with Replacement

Removal of Acetabular/Femoral Surface		Code also as appropriate Replacement by Device Type						
		Acetabular Surface				Femoral Surface		
		Poly	Metal	Ceramic	Synthetic	Metal	Ceramic	Synthetic
Hip, RT	ØSP[A,R]4JZ	ØSRAØØ[9,A,Z]	ØSRAØ1[9,A,Z]	ØSRAØ3[9,A,Z]	ØSRAØJ[9,A,Z]	ØSRRØ1[9,A,Z]	ØSRRØ3[9,A,Z]	ØSRRØJ[9,A,Z]
Hip, LT	ØSP[E,S]4JZ	ØSREØØ[9,A,Z]	ØSREØ1[9,A,Z]	ØSREØ3[9,A,Z]	ØSREØJ[9,A,Z]	ØSRSØ1[9,A,Z]	ØSRSØ3[9,A,Z]	ØSRSØJ[9,A,Z]

Percutaneous Endoscopic Removal of Hip Acetabular/Femoral Surface with Liner Insertion (supplement)

Removal of Acetabular/Femoral Surface		Code also as appropriate Supplement of Body Part by Site		
		Joint	Acetabular Surface	Femoral Surface
Hip, RT	ØSP[A,R]4JZ	ØSU9Ø9Z	ØSUAØ9Z	ØSURØ9Z
Hip, LT	ØSP[E,S]4JZ	ØSUBØ9Z	ØSUEØ9Z	ØSUSØ9Z

Knee Procedures

Open Removal of Knee Liner with Synthetic Substitute Replacement

Removal of Liner		Code also as appropriate Replacement by Type of Synthetic Substitute						
		Oxidized Zircon on Poly	Synthetic Substitute	Medial Unicondylar	Lateral Unicondylar	Patello-femoral	Femoral Surface	Tibial Surface
Knee, RT	ØSPCØ9Z	ØSRCØ6[9,A,Z]	ØSRCØJ[9,A,Z]	ØSRCØL[9,A,Z]	ØSRCØM[9,A,Z]	ØSRCØN[9,A,Z]	ØSRTØJ[9,A,Z]	ØSRVØJ[9,A,Z]
Knee, LT	ØSPDØ9Z	ØSRDØ6[9,A,Z]	ØSRDØJ[9,A,Z]	ØSRDØL[9,A,Z]	ØSRDØM[9,A,Z]	ØSRDØN[9,A,Z]	ØSRUØJ[9,A,Z]	ØSRWØJ[9,A,Z]

Open Removal of Patellar Surface of Knee with Synthetic Substitute Replacement

Removal of Patellar Surface		Code also as appropriate Replacement by Type of Synthetic Substitute	
		Femoral Surface	Tibial Surface
Knee, RT	ØSPCØJC	ØSRTØJ[9,A]	ØSRVØJ[9,A,Z]
Knee, LT	ØSPDØJC	ØSRUØJ[9,A]	ØSRWØJ[9,A,Z]

Open Removal of Knee Synthetic Substitute with Synthetic Substitute Replacement

Removal of Synthetic Substitute		Code also as appropriate Replacement by Type of Synthetic Substitute	
		Femoral Surface	Tibial Surface
Knee, RT	ØSPCØJZ	ØSRTØJ[9,A]	ØSRVØJ[9,A]
Knee, LT	ØSPDØJZ	ØSRUØJ[9,A]	ØSRWØJ[9,A,Z]

Open Removal of Knee Medial/Lateral Unicondylar Device with Synthetic Substitute Replacement

Removal of Medial/Lateral Unicondylar Device		Code also as appropriate Replacement by Type of Synthetic Substitute	
		Femoral Surface	Tibial Surface
Knee, Medial Unicondylar, RT	ØSPCØLZ	ØSRTØJ[9,A]	ØSRVØJ[9,A]
Knee, Medial Unicondylar, LT	ØSPDØLZ	ØSRUØJ[9,A]	ØSRWØJ[9,A,Z]
Knee, Lateral Unicondylar, RT	ØSPCØMZ	ØSRTØJ[9,A]	ØSRVØJ[9,A]
Knee, Lateral Unicondylar, LT	ØSPDØMZ	ØSRUØJ[9,A]	ØSRWØJ[9,A,Z]

Open Removal of Knee Patellofemoral Device with Synthetic Substitute Replacement

Removal of Patellofemoral Device		Code also as appropriate Replacement by Type of Synthetic Substitute	
		Femoral Surface	Tibial Surface
Knee, RT	ØSPCØNZ	ØSRTØJ[9,A]	ØSRVØJ[9,A]
Knee, LT	ØSPDØNZ	ØSRUØJ[9,A]	ØSRWØJ[9,A,Z]

Open Removal of Femoral/Tibial Surface of Knee with Synthetic Substitute Replacement

Removal of Femoral/Tibial Surface		Code also as appropriate Replacement by Type of Synthetic Substitute	
		Femoral Surface	Tibial Surface
Knee, RT	ØSP[T,V]ØJZ	ØSRTØJ[9,A]	ØSRVØJ[9,A]
Knee, LT	ØSP[U,W]ØJZ	ØSRUØJ[9,A]	ØSRWØJ[9,A,Z]

Percutaneous Endoscopic Removal of Patellar Surface of Knee with Synthetic Substitute Replacement

Removal of Patellar Surface		Code also as appropriate Replacement by Type of Synthetic Substitute	
		Femoral Surface	Tibial Surface
Knee, RT	ØSPC4JC	ØSRTØJ[9,A]	ØSRVØJ[9,A]
Knee, LT	ØSPD4JC	ØSRUØJ[9,A]	ØSRWØJ[9,A,Z]

Percutaneous Endoscopic Removal of Knee Synthetic Substitute with Synthetic Substitute Replacement

Removal of Synthetic Substitute		Code also as appropriate Replacement by Type of Synthetic Substitute	
		Femoral Surface	Tibial Surface
Knee, RT	ØSPC4JZ	ØSRTØJ[9,A]	ØSRVØJ[9,A,Z]
Knee, LT	ØSPD4JZ	ØSRUØJ[9,A]	ØSRWØJ[9,A,Z]

Percutaneous Endoscopic Removal of Knee Medial/Lateral Unicondylar Device with Synthetic Substitute Replacement

Removal of Medial/Lateral Unicondylar Device		Code also as appropriate Replacement by Type of Synthetic Substitute	
		Femoral Surface	Tibial Surface
Knee, Medial Unicondylar, RT	ØSPC4LZ	ØSRTØJ[9,A]	ØSRVØJ[9,A]
Knee, Medial Unicondylar, LT	ØSPD4LZ	ØSRUØJ[9,A]	ØSRWØJ[9,A,Z]
Knee, Lateral Unicondylar, RT	ØSPC4MZ	ØSRTØJ[9,A]	ØSRVØJ[9,A]
Knee, Lateral Unicondylar, LT	ØSPD4MZ	ØSRUØJ[9,A]	ØSRWØJ[9,A,Z]

Percutaneous Endoscopic Removal of Knee Patellofemoral Device with Synthetic Substitute Replacement

Removal of Patellofemoral Device		Code also as appropriate Replacement by Type of Synthetic Substitute	
		Femoral Surface	Tibial Surface
Knee, RT	ØSPC4NZ	ØSRTØJ[9,A]	ØSRVØJ[9,A]
Knee, LT	ØSPD4NZ	ØSRUØJ[9,A]	ØSRWØJ[9,A,Z]

Percutaneous Endoscopic Removal of Femoral/Tibial Surface of Knee with Synthetic Substitute Replacement

Removal of Femoral/Tibial Surface		Code also as appropriate Replacement by Type of Synthetic Substitute	
		Femoral Surface	Tibial Surface
Knee, RT	ØSP[T,V]4JZ	ØSRTØJ[9,A]	ØSRVØJ[9,A,Z]
Knee, LT	ØSP[U,W]4JZ	ØSRUØJ[9,A]	ØSRWØJ[9,A,Z]

DRG 662-664 Minor Bladder Procedure

Repair of Bladder	Code also as appropriate Repair of Abdominal Wall	
	with Stoma	without Stoma
ØTQB[Ø,3,4]ZZ	ØWQFXZ2	ØWQFXZZ

DRG 665-667 Prostatectomy

Site	Resection by approach				Code also as appropriate Resection of Seminal Vesicles, Bilateral by approach	
	Open	Percutaneous Endoscopic	Via Natural or Artificial Opening	Via Natural or Artificial Opening Endoscopic	Open	Percutaneous Endoscopic
Prostate	ØVT00ZZ	ØVT04ZZ	ØVT07ZZ	ØVT08ZZ	ØVT30ZZ	ØVT34ZZ

DRG 7Ø7-7Ø8 Major Male Pelvic Procedures

Site	Resection by approach				Code also as appropriate Resection of Seminal Vesicles, Bilateral by approach	
	Open	Percutaneous Endoscopic	Via Natural or Artificial Opening	Via Natural or Artificial Opening Endoscopic	Open	Percutaneous Endoscopic
Prostate	ØVT00ZZ	ØVT04ZZ	ØVT07ZZ	ØVT08ZZ	ØVT30ZZ	ØVT34ZZ

DRG 734-735 Pelvic Evisceration, Radical Hysterectomy and Radical Vulvectomy

Pelvic Evisceration

Resection by Site						
Bladder	Cervix	Fallopian Tubes, Bilateral	Ovaries, Bilateral	Urethra	Uterus	Vagina
ØTTBØZZ	ØUTCØZZ	ØUT7ØZZ	ØUT2ØZZ	ØTTDØZZ	ØUT9ØZZ	ØUTGØZZ

Radical Hysterectomy

Approach	Resection by Site		
	Cervix	Uterus	Uterine Support Structure
Vaginal	ØUTC[7,8]ZZ	ØUT9[7,8]ZZ	ØUT4[7,8]ZZ
Abdominal, Endoscopic	ØUTC4ZZ	ØUT9[4,F]ZZ	ØUT44ZZ
Abdominal, Open	ØUTCØZZ	ØUT9ØZZ	ØUT4ØZZ

Radical Vulvectomy

Resection by Site	Code also as appropriate Excision of Inguinal Lymph Nodes by Approach	
Vulva	Right	Left
ØUTM[Ø,X]ZZ	07BH[Ø,4]ZZ	07BJ[Ø,4]ZZ

Non-OR procedure combinations

Note: The following table identifies procedure combinations that are considered Non-OR even though one or more procedures of the combination are considered valid DRG OR procedures

Insertion With Removal of Intraluminal Device

Code as appropriate Insertion of Intraluminal Device into Hepatobiliary Duct	Code also as appropriate Removal of Intraluminal Device by Approach and Site			
	Via Natural or Artificial Opening		External	
	Hepatobiliary Duct	Pancreatic Duct	Hepatobiliary Duct	Pancreatic Duct
ØFHB7DZ	ØFPB[7,8]DZ	ØFPD[7,8]DZ	ØFPBXDZ	ØFPDXDZ

Appendix M: Coding Exercises and Answers

Using the ICD-10-PCS tables construct the code that accurately represents the procedure performed.

Medical Surgical Section

Procedure	Code
1. Excision of malignant melanoma from skin of right ear	
2. Laparoscopy with excision of endometrial implant from left ovary	
3. Percutaneous needle core biopsy of right kidney	
4. EGD with gastric biopsy	
5. Open endarterectomy of left common carotid artery	
6. Excision of basal cell carcinoma of lower lip	
7. Open excision of tail of pancreas	
8. Percutaneous biopsy of right gastrocnemius muscle	
9. Sigmoidoscopy with sigmoid polypectomy	
10. Open excision of lesion from right Achilles tendon	
11. Open resection of cecum	
12. Total excision of pituitary gland, open	
13. Explantation of left failed kidney, open	
14. Open left axillary total lymphadenectomy	
15. Laparoscopic-assisted vaginal hysterectomy	
16. Right total mastectomy, open	
17. Open resection of papillary muscle	
18. Total retropubic prostatectomy, open	
19. Laparoscopic cholecystectomy	
20. Endoscopic bilateral total maxillary sinusectomy	
21. Amputation at right elbow level	
22. Right below-knee amputation, proximal tibia/fibula	
23. Fifth ray carpometacarpal joint amputation, left hand	
24. Right leg and hip amputation through ischium	
25. DIP joint amputation of right thumb	
26. Right wrist joint amputation	
27. Trans-metatarsal amputation of foot at left big toe	
28. Mid-shaft amputation, right humerus	
29. Left fourth toe amputation, mid-proximal phalanx	
30. Right above-knee amputation, distal femur	
31. Cryotherapy of wart on left hand	
32. Percutaneous radiofrequency ablation of right vocal cord lesion	
33. Left heart catheterization with laser destruction of arrhythmogenic focus, A-V node	
34. Cautery of nosebleed	
35. Transurethral endoscopic laser ablation of prostate	
36. Percutaneous cautery of oozing varicose vein, left calf	
37. Laparoscopy with destruction of endometriosis, bilateral ovaries	
38. Laser coagulation of right retinal vessel, percutaneous	
39. Thoracoscopic pleurodesis, left side	
40. Percutaneous insertion of Greenfield IVC filter	
41. Forceps total mouth extraction, upper and lower teeth	

Procedure	Code
42. Removal of left thumbnail	
43. Extraction of right intraocular lens without replacement, percutaneous	
44. Laparoscopy with needle aspiration of ova for in vitro fertilization	
45. Nonexcisional debridement of skin ulcer, right foot	
46. Open stripping of abdominal fascia, right side	
47. Hysteroscopy with D&C, diagnostic	
48. Liposuction for medical purposes, left upper arm	
49. Removal of tattered right ear drum fragments with tweezers	
50. Microincisional phlebectomy of spider veins, right lower leg	
51. Routine Foley catheter placement	
52. Incision and drainage of external anal abscess	
53. Percutaneous drainage of ascites	
54. Laparoscopy with left ovarian cystotomy and drainage	
55. Laparotomy and drain placement for liver abscess, right lobe	
56. Right knee arthrotomy with drain placement	
57. Thoracentesis of left pleural effusion	
58. Phlebotomy of left median cubital vein for polycythemia vera	
59. Percutaneous chest tube placement for right pneumothorax	
60. Endoscopic drainage of left ethmoid sinus	
61. External ventricular CSF drainage catheter placement via burr hole	
62. Removal of foreign body, right cornea	
63. Percutaneous mechanical thrombectomy, left brachial artery	
64. Esophagogastroscopy with removal of bezoar from stomach	
65. Foreign body removal, skin of left thumb	
66. Transurethral cystoscopy with removal of bladder stone	
67. Forceps removal of foreign body in right nostril	
68. Laparoscopy with excision of old suture from mesentery	
69. Incision and removal of right lacrimal duct stone	
70. Nonincisional removal of intraluminal foreign body from vagina	
71. Right common carotid endarterectomy, open	
72. Open excision of retained sliver, subcutaneous tissue of left foot	
73. Extracorporeal shockwave lithotripsy (ESWL), bilateral ureters	
74. Endoscopic retrograde cholangiopancreatography (ERCP) with lithotripsy of common bile duct stone	
75. Thoracotomy with crushing of pericardial calcifications	
76. Transurethral cystoscopy with fragmentation of bladder calculus	
77. Hysteroscopy with intraluminal lithotripsy of left fallopian tube calcification	
78. Division of right foot tendon, percutaneous	

Procedure	Code
79. Left heart catheterization with division of bundle of HIS	
80. Open osteotomy of capitate, left hand	
81. EGD with esophagotomy of esophagogastric junction	
82. Sacral rhizotomy for pain control, percutaneous	
83. Laparotomy with exploration and adhesiolysis of right ureter	
84. Incision of scar contracture, right elbow	
85. Frenulotomy for treatment of tongue-tie syndrome	
86. Right shoulder arthroscopy with coracoacromial ligament release	
87. Mitral valvulotomy for release of fused leaflets, open approach	
88. Percutaneous left Achilles tendon release	
89. Laparoscopy with lysis of peritoneal adhesions	
90. Manual rupture of right shoulder joint adhesions under general anesthesia	
91. Open posterior tarsal tunnel release	
92. Laparoscopy with freeing of left ovary and fallopian tube	
93. Liver transplant with donor matched liver	
94. Orthotopic heart transplant using porcine heart	
95. Right lung transplant, open, using organ donor match	
96. Transplant of large intestine, organ donor match	
97. Left kidney/pancreas organ bank transplant	
98. Replantation of avulsed scalp	
99. Reattachment of severed right ear	
100. Reattachment of traumatic left gastrocnemius avulsion, open	
101. Closed replantation of three avulsed teeth, lower jaw	
102. Reattachment of severed left hand	
103. Right open palmaris longus tendon transfer	
104. Endoscopic radial to median nerve transfer	
105. Fasciocutaneous flap closure of left thigh, open	
106. Transfer left index finger to left thumb position, open	
107. Percutaneous fascia transfer to fill defect, right neck	
108. Trigeminal to facial nerve transfer, percutaneous endoscopic	
109. Endoscopic left leg flexor hallucis longus tendon transfer	
110. Right scalp advancement flap to right temple	
111. Bilateral TRAM pedicle flap reconstruction status post mastectomy, muscle only, open	
112. Skin transfer flap closure of complex open wound, left lower back	
113. Open fracture reduction, right tibia	
114. Laparoscopy with gastropexy for malrotation	
115. Left knee arthroscopy with reposition of anterior cruciate ligament	
116. Open transposition of ulnar nerve	
117. Closed reduction with percutaneous internal fixation of right femoral neck fracture	
118. Trans-vaginal intraluminal cervical cerclage	
119. Cervical cerclage using Shirodkar technique	
120. Thoracotomy with banding of left pulmonary artery using extraluminal device	
121. Restriction of thoracic duct with intraluminal stent, percutaneous	

Procedure	Code
122. Craniotomy with clipping of cerebral aneurysm	
123. Nonincisional, transnasal placement of restrictive stent in right lacrimal duct	
124. Catheter-based temporary restriction of blood flow in abdominal aorta for treatment of cerebral ischemia	
125. Percutaneous ligation of esophageal vein	
126. Percutaneous embolization of left internal carotid-cavernous fistula	
127. Laparoscopy with bilateral occlusion of fallopian tubes using Hulka extraluminal clips	
128. Open suture ligation of failed AV graft, left brachial artery	
129. Percutaneous embolization of vascular supply, intracranial meningioma	
130. Percutaneous embolization of right uterine artery, using coils	
131. Open occlusion of left atrial appendage, using extraluminal pressure clips	
132. Percutaneous suture exclusion of left atrial appendage, via femoral artery access	
133. ERCP with balloon dilation of common bile duct	
134. PTCA of two coronary arteries, LAD with stent placement, RCA with no stent	
135. Cystoscopy with intraluminal dilation of bladder neck stricture	
136. Open dilation of old anastomosis, left femoral artery	
137. Dilation of upper esophageal stricture, direct visualization, with Bougie sound	
138. PTA of right brachial artery stenosis	
139. Transnasal dilation and stent placement in right lacrimal duct	
140. Hysteroscopy with balloon dilation of bilateral fallopian tubes	
141. Tracheoscopy with intraluminal dilation of tracheal stenosis	
142. Cystoscopy with dilation of left ureteral stricture, with stent placement	
143. Open gastric bypass with Roux-en-Y limb to jejunum	
144. Right temporal artery to intracranial artery bypass using Gore-Tex graft, open	
145. Tracheostomy formation with tracheostomy tube placement, percutaneous	
146. PICVA (percutaneous in situ coronary venous arterialization) of single coronary artery	
147. Open left femoral-popliteal artery bypass using cadaver vein graft	
148. Shunting of intrathecal cerebrospinal fluid to peritoneal cavity using synthetic shunt	
149. Colostomy formation, open, transverse colon to abdominal wall	
150. Open urinary diversion, left ureter, using ileal conduit to skin	
151. CABG of LAD using pedicled left internal mammary artery, open off-bypass	
152. Open pleuroperitoneal shunt, right pleural cavity, using synthetic device	
153. Percutaneous placement of ventriculoperitoneal shunt for treatment of hydrocephalus	
154. End-of-life replacement of spinal neurostimulator generator, multiple array, in lower abdomen	
155. Percutaneous insertion of spinal neurostimulator lead, lumbar spinal cord	

Procedure	Code
156. Percutaneous replacement of broken pacemaker lead in left atrium	
157. Open placement of dual chamber pacemaker generator in chest wall	
158. Percutaneous placement of venous central line in right internal jugular, with tip in superior vena cava	
159. Open insertion of multiple channel cochlear implant, left ear	
160. Percutaneous placement of Swan-Ganz catheter in pulmonary trunk	
161. Bronchoscopy with insertion of Low Dose, Pd-103 brachytherapy seeds, right lung	
162. Open insertion of interspinous process device into lumbar vertebral joint	
163. Open placement of bone growth stimulator, left femoral shaft	
164. Cystoscopy with placement of brachytherapy seeds in prostate gland	
165. Percutaneous insertion of Greenfield IVC filter	
166. Full-thickness skin graft to right lower arm, autograft (do not code graft harvest for this exercise)	
167. Excision of necrosed left femoral head with bone bank bone graft to fill the defect, open	
168. Penetrating keratoplasty of right cornea with donor matched cornea, percutaneous approach	
169. Excision of abdominal aorta with Gore-Tex graft replacement, open	
170. Total right knee arthroplasty with insertion of total knee prosthesis	
171. Tenonectomy with graft to right ankle using cadaver graft, open	
172. Mitral valve replacement using porcine valve, open	
173. Percutaneous phacoemulsification of right eye cataract with prosthetic lens insertion	
174. Transcatheter replacement of pulmonary valve using of bovine jugular vein valve	
175. Total left hip replacement using ceramic on ceramic prosthesis, without bone cement	
176. Aortic valve annuloplasty using ring, open	
177. Laparoscopic repair of left inguinal hernia with marlex plug	
178. Autograft nerve graft to right median nerve, percutaneous endoscopic (do not code graft harvest for this exercise)	
179. Exchange of liner in femoral component of previous left hip replacement, open approach	
180. Anterior colporrhaphy with polypropylene mesh reinforcement, open approach	
181. Implantation of CorCap cardiac support device, open approach	
182. Abdominal wall herniorrhaphy, open, using synthetic mesh	
183. Tendon graft to strengthen injured left shoulder using autograft, open (do not code graft harvest for this exercise)	
184. Onlay lamellar keratoplasty of left cornea using autograft, external approach	
185. Resurfacing procedure on right femoral head, open approach	
186. Exchange of drainage tube from right hip joint	
187. Tracheostomy tube exchange	
188. Change chest tube for left pneumothorax	
189. Exchange of cerebral ventriculostomy drainage tube	

Procedure	Code
190. Foley urinary catheter exchange	
191. Open removal of lumbar sympathetic neurostimulator lead	
192. Nonincisional removal of Swan-Ganz catheter from right pulmonary artery	
193. Laparotomy with removal of pancreatic drain	
194. Extubation, endotracheal tube	
195. Nonincisional PEG tube removal	
196. Transvaginal removal of brachytherapy seeds	
197. Transvaginal removal of extraluminal cervical cerclage	
198. Incision with removal of K-wire fixation, right first metatarsal	
199. Cystoscopy with retrieval of left ureteral stent	
200. Removal of nasogastric drainage tube for decompression	
201. Removal of external fixator, left radial fracture	
202. Trimming and reanastomosis of stenosed femorofemoral synthetic bypass graft, open	
203. Open revision of right hip replacement, with readjustment of prosthesis	
204. Adjustment of position, pacemaker lead in left ventricle, percutaneous	
205. External repositioning of Foley catheter to bladder	
206. Taking out loose screw and putting larger screw in fracture repair plate, left tibia	
207. Revision of totally implantable VAD port placement in chest wall, causing patient discomfort, open	
208. Thoracotomy with exploration of right pleural cavity	
209. Diagnostic laryngoscopy	
210. Exploratory arthrotomy of left knee	
211. Colposcopy with diagnostic hysteroscopy	
212. Digital rectal exam	
213. Diagnostic arthroscopy of right shoulder	
214. Endoscopy of maxillary sinus	
215. Laparotomy with palpation of liver	
216. Transurethral diagnostic cystoscopy	
217. Colonoscopy, discontinued at sigmoid colon	
218. Percutaneous mapping of basal ganglia	
219. Heart catheterization with cardiac mapping	
220. Intraoperative whole brain mapping via craniotomy	
221. Mapping of left cerebral hemisphere, percutaneous endoscopic	
222. Intraoperative cardiac mapping during open heart surgery	
223. Hysteroscopy with cautery of post-hysterectomy oozing and evacuation of clot	
224. Open exploration and ligation of post-op arterial bleeder, left forearm	
225. Control of post-operative retroperitoneal bleeding via laparotomy	
226. Reopening of thoracotomy site with drainage and control of post-op hemopericardium	
227. Arthroscopy with drainage of hemarthrosis at previous operative site, right knee	
228. Radiocarpal fusion of left hand with internal fixation, open	
229. Posterior approach spinal fusion at L1-L3 level with BAK cage interbody fusion device, open	
230. Intercarpal fusion of right hand with bone bank bone graft, open	

Procedure	Code
231. Sacrococcygeal fusion with bone graft from same operative site, open	
232. Interphalangeal fusion of left great toe, percutaneous pin fixation	
233. Suture repair of left radial nerve laceration	
234. Laparotomy with suture repair of blunt force duodenal laceration	
235. Perineoplasty with repair of old obstetric laceration, open	
236. Suture repair of right biceps tendon (upper arm) laceration, open	
237. Closure of abdominal wall stab wound	
238. Cosmetic face lift, open, no other information available	
239. Bilateral breast augmentation with silicone implants, open	
240. Cosmetic rhinoplasty with septal reduction and tip elevation using local tissue graft, open	
241. Abdominoplasty (tummy tuck), open	
242. Liposuction of bilateral thighs	
243. Creation of penis in female patient using tissue bank donor graft	
244. Creation of vagina in male patient using synthetic material	
245. Laparoscopic vertical (sleeve) gastrectomy	
246. Left uterine artery embolization with intraluminal biosphere injection	

Obstetrics

Procedure	Code
1. Abortion by dilation and evacuation following laminaria insertion	
2. Manually assisted spontaneous abortion	
3. Abortion by abortifacient insertion	
4. Bimanual pregnancy examination	
5. Extraperitoneal C-section, low transverse incision	
6. Fetal spinal tap, percutaneous	
7. Fetal kidney transplant, laparoscopic	
8. Open in utero repair of congenital diaphragmatic hernia	
9. Laparoscopy with total excision of tubal pregnancy	
10. Transvaginal removal of fetal monitoring electrode	

Placement

Procedure	Code
1. Placement of packing material, right ear	
2. Mechanical traction of entire left leg	
3. Removal of splint, right shoulder	
4. Placement of neck brace	
5. Change of vaginal packing	
6. Packing of wound, chest wall	
7. Sterile dressing placement to left groin region	
8. Removal of packing material from pharynx	
9. Placement of intermittent pneumatic compression device, covering entire right arm	
10. Exchange of pressure dressing to left thigh	

Administration

Procedure	Code
1. Peritoneal dialysis via indwelling catheter	
2. Transvaginal artificial insemination	
3. Infusion of total parenteral nutrition via central venous catheter	
4. Esophagogastroscopy with Botox injection into esophageal sphincter	
5. Percutaneous irrigation of knee joint	
6. Systemic infusion of recombinant tissue plasminogen activator (r-tPA) via peripheral venous catheter	
7. Transabdominal in vitro fertilization, implantation of donor ovum	
8. Autologous bone marrow transplant via central venous line	
9. Implantation of anti-microbial envelope with cardiac defibrillator placement, open	
10. Sclerotherapy of brachial plexus lesion, alcohol injection	
11. Percutaneous peripheral vein injection, glucarpidase	
12. Introduction of anti-infective envelope into subcutaneous tissue, open	

Measurement and Monitoring

Procedure	Code
1. Cardiac stress test, single measurement	
2. EGD with biliary flow measurement	
3. Right and left heart cardiac catheterization with bilateral sampling and pressure measurements	
4. Temperature monitoring, rectal	
5. Peripheral venous pulse, external, single measurement	
6. Holter monitoring	
7. Respiratory rate, external, single measurement	
8. Fetal heart rate monitoring, transvaginal	
9. Visual mobility test, single measurement	
10. Left ventricular cardiac output monitoring from pulmonary artery wedge (Swan-Ganz) catheter	
11. Olfactory acuity test, single measurement	

Extracorporeal or Systemic Assistance and Performance

Procedure	Code
1. Intermittent mechanical ventilation, 16 hours	
2. Liver dialysis, single encounter	
3. Cardiac countershock with successful conversion to sinus rhythm	
4. IPPB (intermittent positive pressure breathing) for mobilization of secretions, 22 hours	
5. Renal dialysis, 12 hours	
6. IABP (intra-aortic balloon pump) continuous	
7. Intra-operative cardiac pacing, continuous	
8. Intraoperative ECMO (extracorporeal membrane oxygenation), central	
9. Controlled mechanical ventilation (CMV), 45 hours	
10. Pulsatile compression boot with intermittent inflation	

Extracorporeal or Systemic Therapies

Procedure	Code
1. Donor thrombocytapheresis, single encounter	
2. Bili-lite phototherapy, series treatment	
3. Whole body hypothermia, single treatment	
4. Circulatory phototherapy, single encounter	
5. Shock wave therapy of plantar fascia, single treatment	
6. Antigen-free air conditioning, series treatment	
7. TMS (transcranial magnetic stimulation), series treatment	
8. Therapeutic ultrasound of peripheral vessels, single treatment	
9. Plasmapheresis, series treatment	
10. Extracorporeal electromagnetic stimulation (EMS) for urinary incontinence, single treatment	

Osteopathic

Procedure	Code
1. Isotonic muscle energy treatment of right leg	
2. Low velocity-high amplitude osteopathic treatment of head	
3. Lymphatic pump osteopathic treatment of left axilla	
4. Indirect osteopathic treatment of sacrum	
5. Articulatory osteopathic treatment of cervical region	

Other Procedures

Procedure	Code
1. Near infrared spectroscopy of leg vessels	
2. CT computer assisted sinus surgery	
3. Suture removal, abdominal wall	
4. Isolation after infectious disease exposure	
5. Robotic assisted open prostatectomy	
6. In vitro fertilization	

Chiropractic

Procedure	Code
1. Chiropractic treatment of lumbar region using long lever specific contact	
2. Chiropractic manipulation of abdominal region, indirect visceral	
3. Chiropractic extra-articular treatment of hip region	
4. Chiropractic treatment of sacrum using long and short lever specific contact	
5. Mechanically-assisted chiropractic manipulation of head	

Imaging

Procedure	Code
1. Noncontrast CT of abdomen and pelvis	
2. Intravascular ultrasound, left subclavian artery	
3. Fluoroscopic guidance for insertion of central venous catheter in SVC, low osmolar contrast	
4. Chest x-ray, AP/PA and lateral views	
5. Endoluminal ultrasound of gallbladder and bile ducts	
6. MRI of thyroid gland, contrast unspecified	
7. Esophageal videofluoroscopy study with oral barium contrast	

Procedure	Code
8. Portable x-ray study of right radius/ulna shaft, standard series	
9. Routine fetal ultrasound, second trimester twin gestation	
10. CT scan of bilateral lungs, high osmolar contrast with densitometry	
11. Fluoroscopic guidance for percutaneous transluminal angioplasty (PTA) of left common femoral artery, low osmolar contrast	

Nuclear Medicine

Procedure	Code
1. Tomo scan of right and left heart, unspecified radiopharmaceutical, qualitative gated rest	
2. Technetium pentetate assay of kidneys, ureters, and bladder	
3. Uniplanar scan of spine using technetium oxidronate, with first-pass study	
4. Thallous chloride tomographic scan of bilateral breasts	
5. PET scan of myocardium using rubidium	
6. Gallium citrate scan of head and neck, single plane imaging	
7. Xenon gas nonimaging probe of brain	
8. Upper GI scan, radiopharmaceutical unspecified, for gastric emptying	
9. Carbon 11 PET scan of brain with quantification	
10. Iodinated albumin nuclear medicine assay, blood plasma volume study	

Radiation Therapy

Procedure	Code
1. Plaque radiation of left eye, single port	
2. 8 MeV photon beam radiation to brain	
3. IORT of colon, 3 ports	
4. HDR brachytherapy of prostate using low dose palladium-103, unidirectional source	
5. Electron radiation treatment of right breast, with custom device	
6. Hyperthermia oncology treatment of pelvic region	
7. Contact radiation of tongue	
8. Heavy particle radiation treatment of pancreas, four risk sites	
9. LDR brachytherapy to spinal cord using iodine	
10. Whole body Phosphorus 32 administration with risk to hematopoetic system	

Physical Rehabilitation and Diagnostic Audiology

Procedure	Code
1. Bekesy assessment using audiometer	
2. Individual fitting of left eye prosthesis	
3. Physical therapy for range of motion and mobility, patient right hip, no special equipment	
4. Bedside swallow assessment using assessment kit	
5. Caregiver training in airway clearance techniques	
6. Application of short arm cast in rehabilitation setting	
7. Verbal assessment of patient's pain level	
8. Caregiver training in communication skills using manual communication board	

Procedure	Code
9. Group musculoskeletal balance training exercises, whole body, no special equipment	
10. Individual therapy for auditory processing using tape recorder	

Mental Health

Procedure	Code
1. Cognitive-behavioral psychotherapy, individual	
2. Narcosynthesis	
3. Light therapy	
4. ECT (electroconvulsive therapy), unilateral, multiple seizure	
5. Crisis intervention	
6. Neuropsychological testing	
7. Hypnosis	
8. Developmental testing	
9. Vocational counseling	
10. Family psychotherapy	

Substance Abuse Treatment

Procedure	Code
1. Naltrexone treatment for drug dependency	
2. Substance abuse treatment family counseling	
3. Medication monitoring of patient on methadone maintenance	
4. Individual interpersonal psychotherapy for drug abuse	
5. Patient in for alcohol detoxification treatment	
6. Group motivational counseling	
7. Individual 12-step psychotherapy for substance abuse	
8. Post-test infectious disease counseling for IV drug abuser	
9. Psychodynamic psychotherapy for drug dependent patient	
10. Group cognitive-behavioral counseling for substance abuse	

New Technology

Procedure	Code
1. Infusion of terlipressin via peripheral venous catheter	
2. Transcatheter dilation of left peroneal artery with 2 SAVAL stents	

Answers to Coding Exercises

Medical Surgical Section

Procedure	Code
1. Excision of malignant melanoma from skin of right ear	ØHB2XZZ
2. Laparoscopy with excision of endometrial implant from left ovary	ØUB14ZZ
3. Percutaneous needle core biopsy of right kidney	ØTB03ZX
4. EGD with gastric biopsy	ØDB68ZX
5. Open endarterectomy of left common carotid artery	Ø3CJØZZ
6. Excision of basal cell carcinoma of lower lip	ØCB1XZZ
7. Open excision of tail of pancreas	ØFBGØZZ
8. Percutaneous biopsy of right gastrocnemius muscle	ØKBS3ZX
9. Sigmoidoscopy with sigmoid polypectomy	ØDBN8ZZ
10. Open excision of lesion from right Achilles tendon	ØLBNØZZ
11. Open resection of cecum	ØDTHØZZ
12. Total excision of pituitary gland, open	ØGTØØZZ
13. Explantation of left failed kidney, open	ØTT1ØZZ
14. Open left axillary total lymphadenectomy	Ø7T6ØZZ (RESECTION is coded for cutting out a chain of lymph nodes.)
15. Laparoscopic-assisted vaginal hysterectomy	ØUT9FZZ
16. Right total mastectomy, open	ØHTTØZZ
17. Open resection of papillary muscle	Ø2TDØZZ (The papillary muscle refers to the heart and is found in the *Heart and Great Vessels* body system.)
18. Total retropubic prostatectomy, open	ØVTØØZZ
19. Laparoscopic cholecystectomy	ØFT44ZZ
20. Endoscopic bilateral total maxillary sinusectomy	Ø9TQ8ZZ, Ø9TR8ZZ
21. Amputation at right elbow level	ØX6BØZZ
22. Right below-knee amputation, proximal tibia/fibula	ØY6HØZ1 (The qualifier *High* here means the portion of the tib/fib closest to the knee.)
23. Fifth ray carpometacarpal joint amputation, left hand	ØX6KØZ8 (A *complete* ray amputation is through the carpometacarpal joint.)
24. Right leg and hip amputation through ischium	ØY62ØZZ (The *Hindquarter* body part includes amputation along any part of the hip bone.)
25. DIP joint amputation of right thumb	ØX6LØZ3 (The qualifier *low* here means through the distal interphalangeal joint.)
26. Right wrist joint amputation	ØX6JØZØ (Amputation at the wrist joint is actually complete amputation of the hand.)
27. Trans-metatarsal amputation of foot at left big toe	ØY6NØZ9 (A *partial* amputation is through the shaft of the metatarsal bone.)
28. Mid-shaft amputation, right humerus	ØX68ØZ2
29. Left fourth toe amputation, mid-proximal phalanx	ØY6WØZ1 (The qualifier *High* here means anywhere along the proximal phalanx.)
30. Right above-knee amputation, distal femur	ØY6CØZ3

Procedure	Code
31. Cryotherapy of wart on left hand	ØH5GXZZ
32. Percutaneous radiofrequency ablation of right vocal cord lesion	ØC5T3ZZ
33. Left heart catheterization with laser destruction of arrhythmogenic focus, A-V node	Ø2583ZZ
34. Cautery of nosebleed	Ø93K7ZZ
35. Transurethral endoscopic laser ablation of prostate	ØV5Ø8ZZ
36. Percutaneous cautery of oozing varicose vein, left calf	ØY3J3ZZ
37. Laparoscopy with destruction of endometriosis, bilateral ovaries	ØU524ZZ
38. Laser coagulation of right retinal vessel, percutaneous	Ø85G3ZZ (The *Retinal Vessel* body-part values are in the *Eye* body system.)
39. Thoracoscopic pleurodesis, left side	ØB5P4ZZ
40. Percutaneous insertion of Greenfield IVC filter	Ø6HØ3DZ
41. Forceps total mouth extraction, upper and lower teeth	ØCDWXZ2, ØCDXXZ2
42. Removal of left thumbnail	ØHDQXZZ (No separate body-part value is given for thumbnail, so this is coded to *Fingernail*.)
43. Extraction of right intraocular lens without replacement, percutaneous	Ø8DJ3ZZ
44. Laparoscopy with needle aspiration of ova for in vitro fertilization	ØUDN4ZZ
45. Nonexcisional debridement of skin ulcer, right foot	ØHDMXZZ
46. Open stripping of abdominal fascia, right side	ØJD8ØZZ
47. Hysteroscopy with D&C, diagnostic	ØUDB8ZX
48. Liposuction for medical purposes, left upper arm	ØJDF3ZZ (The *Percutaneous* approach is inherent in the liposuction technique.)
49. Removal of tattered right ear drum fragments with tweezers	Ø9D77ZZ
50. Microincisional phlebectomy of spider veins, right lower leg	Ø6DY3ZZ
51. Routine Foley catheter placement	ØT9B7ØZ
52. Incision and drainage of external anal abscess	ØD9QXZZ
53. Percutaneous drainage of ascites	ØW9G3ZZ (This is drainage of the cavity and not the peritoneal membrane itself.)
54. Laparoscopy with left ovarian cystotomy and drainage	ØU914ZZ
55. Laparotomy and drain placement for liver abscess, right lobe	ØF91ØØZ
56. Right knee arthrotomy with drain placement	ØS9CØØZ
57. Thoracentesis of left pleural effusion	ØW9B3ZZ (This is drainage of the pleural cavity)
58. Phlebotomy of left median cubital vein for polycythemia vera	Ø59C3ZZ (The median cubital vein is a branch of the basilic vein)
59. Percutaneous chest tube placement for right pneumothorax	ØW993ØZ
60. Endoscopic drainage of left ethmoid sinus	Ø99V4ZZ
61. External ventricular CSF drainage catheter placement via burr hole	ØØ963ØZ
62. Removal of foreign body, right cornea	Ø8C8XZZ

Procedure	Code
63. Percutaneous mechanical thrombectomy, left brachial artery	03C83ZZ
64. Esophagogastroscopy with removal of bezoar from stomach	0DC68ZZ
65. Foreign body removal, skin of left thumb	0HCGXZZ (There is no specific value for thumb skin, so the procedure is coded to *Hand*.)
66. Transurethral cystoscopy with removal of bladder stone	0TCB8ZZ
67. Forceps removal of foreign body in right nostril	09CKXZZ (Nostril is coded to the *Nasal mucosa and soft tissue* body-part value.)
68. Laparoscopy with excision of old suture from mesentery	0DCV4ZZ
69. Incision and removal of right lacrimal duct stone	08CX0ZZ
70. Nonincisional removal of intraluminal foreign body from vagina	0UCG7ZZ (The approach *External* is also a possibility. It is assumed here that since the patient went to the doctor to have the object removed, that it was not in the vaginal orifice.)
71. Right common carotid endarterectomy, open	03CH0ZZ
72. Open excision of retained sliver, subcutaneous tissue of left foot	0JCR0ZZ
73. Extracorporeal shockwave lithotripsy (ESWL), bilateral ureters	0TF6XZZ, 0TF7XZZ (The *Bilateral Ureter* body-part value is not available for the root operation FRAGMENTATION, so the procedures are coded separately.)
74. Endoscopic retrograde cholangiopancreatography (ERCP) with lithotripsy of common bile duct stone	0FF98ZZ (ERCP is performed through the mouth to the biliary system via the duodenum, so the approach value is *Via Natural or Artificial Opening Endoscopic*.)
75. Thoracotomy with crushing of pericardial calcifications	02FN0ZZ
76. Transurethral cystoscopy with fragmentation of bladder calculus	0TFB8ZZ
77. Hysteroscopy with intraluminal lithotripsy of left fallopian tube calcification	0UF68ZZ
78. Division of right foot tendon, percutaneous	0L8V3ZZ
79. Left heart catheterization with division of bundle of HIS	02883ZZ
80. Open osteotomy of capitate, left hand	0P8N0ZZ (The capitate is one of the carpal bones of the hand.)
81. EGD with esophagotomy of esophagogastric junction	0D948ZZ
82. Sacral rhizotomy for pain control, percutaneous	018R3ZZ
83. Laparotomy with exploration and adhesiolysis of right ureter	0TN60ZZ
84. Incision of scar contracture, right elbow	0HNDXZZ (The skin of the elbow region is coded to *Lower Arm*.)
85. Frenulotomy for treatment of tongue-tie syndrome	0CN7XZZ (The frenulum is coded to the body-part value *Tongue*.)
86. Right shoulder arthroscopy with coracoacromial ligament release	0MN14ZZ

Procedure	Code
87. Mitral valvulotomy for release of fused leaflets, open approach	02NG0ZZ
88. Percutaneous left Achilles tendon release	0LNP3ZZ
89. Laparoscopy with lysis of peritoneal adhesions	0DNW4ZZ
90. Manual rupture of right shoulder joint adhesions under general anesthesia	0RNJXZZ
91. Open posterior tarsal tunnel release	01NG0ZZ (The nerve released in the posterior tarsal tunnel is the tibial nerve.)
92. Laparoscopy with freeing of left ovary and fallopian tube	0UN14ZZ, 0UN64ZZ
93. Liver transplant with donor matched liver	0FY00Z0
94. Orthotopic heart transplant using porcine heart	02YA0Z2 (The donor heart comes from an animal [pig], so the qualifier value is *Zooplastic*.)
95. Right lung transplant, open, using organ donor match	0BYK0Z0
96. Transplant of large intestine, organ donor match	0DYE0Z0
97. Left kidney/pancreas organ bank transplant	0FYG0Z0, 0TY10Z0
98. Replantation of avulsed scalp	0HM0XZZ
99. Reattachment of severed right ear	09M0XZZ
100. Reattachment of traumatic left gastrocnemius avulsion, open	0KMT0ZZ
101. Closed replantation of three avulsed teeth, lower jaw	0CMXXZ1
102. Reattachment of severed left hand	0XMK0ZZ
103. Right open palmaris longus tendon transfer	0LX50ZZ
104. Endoscopic radial to median nerve transfer	01X64Z5
105. Fasciocutaneous flap closure of left thigh, open	0JXM0ZC (The qualifier identifies the body layers in addition to fascia included in the procedure.)
106. Transfer left index finger to left thumb position, open	0XXP0ZM
107. Percutaneous fascia transfer to fill defect, right neck	0JX43ZZ
108. Trigeminal to facial nerve transfer, percutaneous endoscopic	00XK4ZM
109. Endoscopic left leg flexor hallucis longus tendon transfer	0LXP4ZZ
110. Right scalp advancement flap to right temple	0HX0XZZ
111. Bilateral TRAM pedicle flap reconstruction status post mastectomy, muscle only, open	0KXK0Z6, 0KXL0Z6 (The transverse rectus abdominus muscle (TRAM) flap is coded for each flap developed.)
112. Skin transfer flap closure of complex open wound, left lower back	0HX6XZZ
113. Open fracture reduction, right tibia	0QSG0ZZ
114. Laparoscopy with gastropexy for malrotation	0DS64ZZ
115. Left knee arthroscopy with reposition of anterior cruciate ligament	0MSP4ZZ
116. Open transposition of ulnar nerve	01S40ZZ
117. Closed reduction with percutaneous internal fixation of right femoral neck fracture	0QS634Z
118. Trans-vaginal intraluminal cervical cerclage	0UVC7DZ
119. Cervical cerclage using Shirodkar technique	0UVC7ZZ
120. Thoracotomy with banding of left pulmonary artery using extraluminal device	02VR0CZ
121. Restriction of thoracic duct with intraluminal stent, percutaneous	07VK3DZ

Procedure	Code
122. Craniotomy with clipping of cerebral aneurysm	03VG0CZ (The clip is placed lengthwise on the outside wall of the widened portion of the vessel.)
123. Nonincisional, transnasal placement of restrictive stent in right lacrimal duct	08VX7DZ
124. Catheter-based temporary restriction of blood flow in abdominal aorta for treatment of cerebral ischemia	04V03DJ
125. Percutaneous ligation of esophageal vein	06L33ZZ
126. Percutaneous embolization of left internal carotid-cavernous fistula	03LL3DZ
127. Laparoscopy with bilateral occlusion of fallopian tubes using Hulka extraluminal clips	0UL74CZ
128. Open suture ligation of failed AV graft, left brachial artery	03L80ZZ
129. Percutaneous embolization of vascular supply, intracranial meningioma	03LG3DZ
130. Percutaneous embolization of right uterine artery, using coils	04LE3DT
131. Open occlusion of left atrial appendage, using extraluminal pressure clips	02L70CK
132. Percutaneous suture exclusion of left atrial appendage, via femoral artery access	02L73ZK
133. ERCP with balloon dilation of common bile duct	0F798ZZ
134. PTCA of two coronary arteries, LAD with stent placement, RCA with no stent	02703DZ, 02703ZZ (A separate procedure is coded for each artery dilated, since the device value differs for each artery.)
135. Cystoscopy with intraluminal dilation of bladder neck stricture	0T7C8ZZ
136. Open dilation of old anastomosis, left femoral artery	047L0ZZ
137. Dilation of upper esophageal stricture, direct visualization, with Bougie sound	0D717ZZ
138. PTA of right brachial artery stenosis	03773ZZ
139. Transnasal dilation and stent placement in right lacrimal duct	087X7DZ
140. Hysteroscopy with balloon dilation of bilateral fallopian tubes	0U778ZZ
141. Tracheoscopy with intraluminal dilation of tracheal stenosis	0B718ZZ
142. Cystoscopy with dilation of left ureteral stricture, with stent placement	0T778DZ
143. Open gastric bypass with Roux-en-Y limb to jejunum	0D160ZA
144. Right temporal artery to intracranial artery bypass using Gore-Tex graft, open	031S0JG
145. Tracheostomy formation with tracheostomy tube placement, percutaneous	0B113F4
146. PICVA (percutaneous in situ coronary venous arterialization) of single coronary artery	02103D4
147. Open left femoral-popliteal artery bypass using cadaver vein graft	041L0KL
148. Shunting of intrathecal cerebrospinal fluid to peritoneal cavity using synthetic shunt	00160J6
149. Colostomy formation, open, transverse colon to abdominal wall	0D1L0Z4
150. Open urinary diversion, left ureter, using ileal conduit to skin	0T170ZC
151. CABG of LAD using pedicled left internal mammary artery, open off-bypass	02100Z9

Procedure	Code
152. Open pleuroperitoneal shunt, right pleural cavity, using synthetic device	0W190JG
153. Percutaneous placement of ventriculoperitoneal shunt for treatment of hydrocephalus	00163J6
154. End-of-life replacement of spinal neurostimulator generator, multiple array, in lower abdomen	0JH80DZ (Taking out of the old generator is coded separately to the root operation *Removal*)
155. Percutaneous insertion of spinal neurostimulator lead, lumbar spinal cord	00HV3MZ
156. Percutaneous replacement of broken pacemaker lead in left atrium	02H73JZ (Taking out the broken pacemaker lead is coded separately to the root operation *Removal*.)
157. Open placement of dual chamber pacemaker generator in chest wall	0JH606Z
158. Percutaneous placement of venous central line in right internal jugular, with tip in superior vena cava	02HV33Z
159. Open insertion of multiple channel cochlear implant, left ear	09HE06Z
160. Percutaneous placement of Swan-Ganz catheter in pulmonary trunk	02HP32Z (The Swan-Ganz catheter is coded to the device value *Monitoring Device* because it monitors pulmonary artery output.)
161. Bronchoscopy with insertion of Low Dose Pd-103 brachytherapy seeds, right lung	0BHK81Z, DB11BBZ
162. Open insertion of interspinous process device into lumbar vertebral joint	0SH00BZ
163. Open placement of bone growth stimulator, left femoral shaft	0QHY0MZ
164. Cystoscopy with placement of brachytherapy seeds in prostate gland	0VH081Z
165. Percutaneous insertion of Greenfield IVC filter	06H03DZ
166. Full-thickness skin graft to right lower arm, autograft (do not code graft harvest for this exercise)	0HRDX73
167. Excision of necrosed left femoral head with bone bank bone graft to fill the defect, open	0QR70KZ
168. Penetrating keratoplasty of right cornea with donor matched cornea, percutaneous approach	08R83KZ
169. Excision of abdominal aorta with Gore-Tex graft replacement, open	04R00JZ
170. Total right knee arthroplasty with insertion of total knee prosthesis	0SRC0JZ
171. Tenonectomy with graft to right ankle using cadaver graft, open	0LRS0KZ
172. Mitral valve replacement using porcine valve, open	02RG08Z
173. Percutaneous phacoemulsification of right eye cataract with prosthetic lens insertion	08RJ3JZ
174. Transcatheter replacement of pulmonary valve using of bovine jugular vein valve	02RH38Z
175. Total left hip replacement using ceramic on ceramic prosthesis, without bone cement	0SRB03A
176. Aortic valve annuloplasty using ring, open	02UF0JZ
177. Laparoscopic repair of left inguinal hernia with marlex plug	0YU64JZ
178. Autograft nerve graft to right median nerve, percutaneous endoscopic (do not code graft harvest for this exercise)	01U547Z
179. Exchange of liner in femoral component of previous left hip replacement, open approach	0SUS09Z (Taking out of the old liner is coded separately to the root operation *Removal*)

Procedure	Code
180. Anterior colporrhaphy with polypropylene mesh reinforcement, open approach	0JUC0JZ
181. Implantation of CorCap cardiac support device, open approach	02UA0JZ
182. Abdominal wall herniorrhaphy, open, using synthetic mesh	0WUF0JZ
183. Tendon graft to strengthen injured left shoulder using autograft, open (do not code graft harvest for this exercise)	0LU207Z
184. Onlay lamellar keratoplasty of left cornea using autograft, external approach	08U9X7Z
185. Resurfacing procedure on right femoral head, open approach	0SUR0BZ
186. Exchange of drainage tube from right hip joint	0S2YX0Z
187. Tracheostomy tube exchange	0B21XFZ
188. Change chest tube for left pneumothorax	0W2BX0Z
189. Exchange of cerebral ventriculostomy drainage tube	0020X0Z
190. Foley urinary catheter exchange	0T2BX0Z (This is coded to *Drainage Device* because urine is being drained.)
191. Open removal of lumbar sympathetic neurostimulator lead	01PY0MZ
192. Nonincisional removal of Swan-Ganz catheter from right pulmonary artery	02PYX2Z
193. Laparotomy with removal of pancreatic drain	0FPG00Z
194. Extubation, endotracheal tube	0BP1XDZ
195. Nonincisional PEG tube removal	0DP6XUZ
196. Transvaginal removal of brachytherapy seeds	0UPH71Z
197. Transvaginal removal of extraluminal cervical cerclage	0UPD7CZ
198. Incision with removal of K-wire fixation, right first metatarsal	0QPN04Z
199. Cystoscopy with retrieval of left ureteral stent	0TP98DZ
200. Removal of nasogastric drainage tube for decompression	0DP6X0Z
201. Removal of external fixator, left radial fracture	0PPJX5Z
202. Trimming and reanastomosis of stenosed femorofemoral synthetic bypass graft, open	04WY0JZ
203. Open revision of right hip replacement, with readjustment of prosthesis	0SW90JZ
204. Adjustment of position, pacemaker lead in left ventricle, percutaneous	02WA3MZ
205. External repositioning of Foley catheter to bladder	0TWBX0Z
206. Taking out loose screw and putting larger screw in fracture repair plate, left tibia	0QWH04Z
207. Revision of totally implantable VAD port placement in chest wall, causing patient discomfort, open	0JWT0WZ
208. Thoracotomy with exploration of right pleural cavity	0WJ90ZZ
209. Diagnostic laryngoscopy	0CJS8ZZ
210. Exploratory arthrotomy of left knee	0SJD0ZZ
211. Colposcopy with diagnostic hysteroscopy	0UJD8ZZ
212. Digital rectal exam	0DJD7ZZ
213. Diagnostic arthroscopy of right shoulder	0RJJ4ZZ
214. Endoscopy of maxillary sinus	09JY4ZZ
215. Laparotomy with palpation of liver	0FJ00ZZ
216. Transurethral diagnostic cystoscopy	0TJB8ZZ
217. Colonoscopy, discontinued at sigmoid colon	0DJD8ZZ
218. Percutaneous mapping of basal ganglia	00K83ZZ
219. Heart catheterization with cardiac mapping	02K83ZZ
220. Intraoperative whole brain mapping via craniotomy	00K00ZZ

Procedure	Code
221. Mapping of left cerebral hemisphere, percutaneous endoscopic	00K74ZZ
222. Intraoperative cardiac mapping during open heart surgery	02K80ZZ
223. Hysteroscopy with cautery of post-hysterectomy oozing and evacuation of clot	0W3R8ZZ
224. Open exploration and ligation of post-op arterial bleeder, left forearm	0X3F0ZZ
225. Control of post-operative retroperitoneal bleeding via laparotomy	0W3H0ZZ
226. Reopening of thoracotomy site with drainage and control of post-op hemopericardium	0W3D0ZZ
227. Arthroscopy with drainage of hemarthrosis at previous operative site, right knee	0Y3F4ZZ
228. Radiocarpal fusion of left hand with internal fixation, open	0RGP04Z
229. Posterior approach spinal fusion at L1-L3 level with BAK cage interbody fusion device, open	0SG10AJ
230. Intercarpal fusion of right hand with bone bank bone graft, open	0RGQ0KZ
231. Sacrococcygeal fusion with bone graft from same operative site, open	0SG507Z
232. Interphalangeal fusion of left great toe, percutaneous pin fixation	0SGQ34Z
233. Suture repair of left radial nerve laceration	01Q60ZZ (The approach value is *Open*, though the surgical exposure may have been created by the wound itself.)
234. Laparotomy with suture repair of blunt force duodenal laceration	0DQ90ZZ
235. Perineoplasty with repair of old obstetric laceration, open	0WQN0ZZ
236. Suture repair of right biceps tendon (upper arm) laceration, open	0LQ30ZZ
237. Closure of abdominal wall stab wound	0WQF0ZZ
238. Cosmetic face lift, open, no other information available	0W020ZZ
239. Bilateral breast augmentation with silicone implants, open	0H0V0JZ
240. Cosmetic rhinoplasty with septal reduction and tip elevation using local tissue graft, open	090K07Z
241. Abdominoplasty (tummy tuck), open	0W0F0ZZ
242. Liposuction of bilateral thighs	0J0L3ZZ, 0J0M3ZZ
243. Creation of penis in female patient using tissue bank donor graft	0W4N0K1
244. Creation of vagina in male patient using synthetic material	0W4M0J0
245. Laparoscopic vertical (sleeve) gastrectomy	0DB64Z3
246. Left uterine artery embolization with intraluminal biosphere injection	04LF3DU

Obstetrics

Procedure	Code
1. Abortion by dilation and evacuation following laminaria insertion	10A07ZW
2. Manually assisted spontaneous abortion	10E0XZZ (Since the pregnancy was not artificially terminated, this is coded *Delivery* because it captures the procedure objective. The fact that it was an abortion will be identified in the diagnosis code.)
3. Abortion by abortifacient insertion	10A07ZX

Procedure	Code
4. Bimanual pregnancy examination	10J07ZZ
5. Extraperitoneal C-section, low transverse incision	10D00Z1
6. Fetal spinal tap, percutaneous	109O3ZA
7. Fetal kidney transplant, laparoscopic	10Y04ZS
8. Open in utero repair of congenital diaphragmatic hernia	10Q00ZK (Diaphragm is classified to the *Respiratory* body system in the *Medical and Surgical* section.)
9. Laparoscopy with total excision of tubal pregnancy	10T24ZZ
10. Transvaginal removal of fetal monitoring electrode	10P073Z

Placement

Procedure	Code
1. Placement of packing material, right ear	2Y42X5Z
2. Mechanical traction of entire left leg	2W6MX0Z
3. Removal of splint, right shoulder	2W5AX1Z
4. Placement of neck brace	2W32X3Z
5. Change of vaginal packing	2Y04X5Z
6. Packing of wound, chest wall	2W44X5Z
7. Sterile dressing placement to left groin region	2W27X4Z
8. Removal of packing material from pharynx	2Y50X5Z
9. Placement of intermittent pneumatic compression device, covering entire right arm	2W18X7Z
10. Exchange of pressure dressing to left thigh	2W0PX6Z

Administration

Procedure	Code
1. Peritoneal dialysis via indwelling catheter	3E1M39Z
2. Transvaginal artificial insemination	3E0P7LZ
3. Infusion of total parenteral nutrition via central venous catheter	3E0436Z
4. Esophagogastroscopy with Botox injection into esophageal sphincter	3E0G8GC (Botulinum toxin is a paralyzing agent with temporary effects; it does not sclerose or destroy the nerve.)
5. Percutaneous irrigation of knee joint	3E1U38Z
6. Systemic infusion of recombinant tissue plasminogen activator (r-tPA) via peripheral venous catheter	3E03317
7. Transabdominal in vitro fertilization, implantation of donor ovum	3E0P3Q1
8. Autologous bone marrow transplant via central venous line	30243G0
9. Implantation of anti-microbial envelope with cardiac defibrillator placement, open	3E0102A
10. Sclerotherapy of brachial plexus lesion, alcohol injection	3E0T3TZ
11. Percutaneous peripheral vein injection, glucarpidase	3E033GQ
12. Introduction of anti-infective envelope into subcutaneous tissue, open	3E0102A

Measurement and Monitoring

Procedure	Code
1. Cardiac stress test, single measurement	4A02XM4
2. EGD with biliary flow measurement	4A0C85Z
3. Right and left heart cardiac catheterization with bilateral sampling and pressure measurements	4A023N8

Procedure	Code
4. Temperature monitoring, rectal	4A1Z7KZ
5. Peripheral venous pulse, external, single measurement	4A04XJ1
6. Holter monitoring	4A12X45
7. Respiratory rate, external, single measurement	4A09XCZ
8. Fetal heart rate monitoring, transvaginal	4A1H7CZ
9. Visual mobility test, single measurement	4A07X7Z
10. Left ventricular cardiac output monitoring from pulmonary artery wedge (Swan-Ganz) catheter	4A1239Z
11. Olfactory acuity test, single measurement	4A08X0Z

Extracorporeal or Systemic Assistance and Performance

Procedure	Code
1. Intermittent mechanical ventilation, 16 hours	5A1935Z
2. Liver dialysis, single encounter	5A1C00Z
3. Cardiac countershock with successful conversion to sinus rhythm	5A2204Z
4. IPPB (intermittent positive pressure breathing) for mobilization of secretions, 22 hours	5A09358
5. Renal dialysis, 12 hours	5A1D80Z
6. IABP (intra-aortic balloon pump) continuous	5A02210
7. Intra-operative cardiac pacing, continuous	5A1223Z
8. Intraoperative ECMO (extracorporeal membrane oxygenation), central	5A15A2F
9. Controlled mechanical ventilation (CMV), 45 hours	5A1945Z
10. Pulsatile compression boot with intermittent inflation	5A02115 (This is coded to the function value *Cardiac Output*, because the purpose of such compression devices is to return blood to the heart faster.)

Extracorporeal or Systemic Therapies

Procedure	Code
1. Donor thrombocytapheresis, single encounter	6A550Z2
2. Bili-lite phototherapy, series treatment	6A601ZZ
3. Whole body hypothermia, single treatment	6A4Z0ZZ
4. Circulatory phototherapy, single encounter	6A650ZZ
5. Shock wave therapy of plantar fascia, single treatment	6A930ZZ
6. Antigen-free air conditioning, series treatment	6A0Z1ZZ
7. TMS (transcranial magnetic stimulation), series treatment	6A221ZZ
8. Therapeutic ultrasound of peripheral vessels, single treatment	6A750Z6
9. Plasmapheresis, series treatment	6A551Z3
10. Extracorporeal electromagnetic stimulation (EMS) for urinary incontinence, single treatment	6A210ZZ

Osteopathic

	Procedure	Code
1.	Isotonic muscle energy treatment of right leg	7W06X8Z
2.	Low velocity-high amplitude osteopathic treatment of head	7W00X5Z
3.	Lymphatic pump osteopathic treatment of left axilla	7W07X6Z
4.	Indirect osteopathic treatment of sacrum	7W04X4Z
5.	Articulatory osteopathic treatment of cervical region	7W01X0Z

Other Procedures

	Procedure	Code
1.	Near infrared spectroscopy of leg vessels	8E023DZ
2.	CT computer assisted sinus surgery	8E09XBG (The primary procedure is coded separately.)
3.	Suture removal, abdominal wall	8E0WXY8
4.	Isolation after infectious disease exposure	8E0ZXY6
5.	Robotic assisted open prostatectomy	8E0W0CZ (The primary procedure is coded separately.)
6.	In vitro fertilization	8E0ZXY1

Chiropractic

	Procedure	Code
1.	Chiropractic treatment of lumbar region using long lever specific contact	9WB3XGZ
2.	Chiropractic manipulation of abdominal region, indirect visceral	9WB9XCZ
3.	Chiropractic extra-articular treatment of hip region	9WB6XDZ
4.	Chiropractic treatment of sacrum using long and short lever specific contact	9WB4XJZ
5.	Mechanically-assisted chiropractic manipulation of head	9WB0XKZ

Imaging

	Procedure	Code
1.	Noncontrast CT of abdomen and pelvis	BW21ZZZ
2.	Intravascular ultrasound, left subclavian artery	B342ZZ3
3.	Fluoroscopic guidance for insertion of central venous catheter in SVC, low osmolar contrast	B5181ZA
4.	Chest x-ray, AP/PA and lateral views	BW03ZZZ
5.	Endoluminal ultrasound of gallbladder and bile ducts	BF43ZZZ
6.	MRI of thyroid gland, contrast unspecified	BG34YZZ
7.	Esophageal videofluoroscopy study with oral barium contrast	BD11YZZ
8.	Portable x-ray study of right radius/ulna shaft, standard series	BP0JZZZ
9.	Routine fetal ultrasound, second trimester twin gestation	BY4DZZZ
10.	CT scan of bilateral lungs, high osmolar contrast with densitometry	BB240ZZ
11.	Fluoroscopic guidance for percutaneous transluminal angioplasty (PTA) of left common femoral artery, low osmolar contrast	B41G1ZZ

Nuclear Medicine

	Procedure	Code
1.	Tomo scan of right and left heart, unspecified radiopharmaceutical, qualitative gated rest	C226YZZ
2.	Technetium pentetate assay of kidneys, ureters, and bladder	CT631ZZ
3.	Uniplanar scan of spine using technetium oxidronate, with first-pass study	CP151ZZ
4.	Thallous chloride tomographic scan of bilateral breasts	CH22SZZ
5.	PET scan of myocardium using rubidium	C23GQZZ
6.	Gallium citrate scan of head and neck, single plane imaging	CW1BLZZ
7.	Xenon gas nonimaging probe of brain	C050VZZ
8.	Upper GI scan, radiopharmaceutical unspecified, for gastric emptying	CD15YZZ
9.	Carbon 11 PET scan of brain with quantification	C030BZZ
10.	Iodinated albumin nuclear medicine assay, blood plasma volume study	C763HZZ

Radiation Therapy

	Procedure	Code
1.	Plaque radiation of left eye, single port	D8Y0FZZ
2.	8 MeV photon beam radiation to brain	D0011ZZ
3.	IORT of colon, 3 ports	DDY5CZZ
4.	HDR brachytherapy of prostate using low dose palladium-103, unidirectional source	DV10BB1
5.	Electron radiation treatment of right breast, with custom device	DM013ZZ
6.	Hyperthermia oncology treatment of pelvic region	DWY68ZZ
7.	Contact radiation of tongue	D9Y57ZZ
8.	Heavy particle radiation treatment of pancreas, four risk sites	DF034ZZ
9.	LDR brachytherapy to spinal cord using iodine	D016B9Z
10.	Whole body Phosphorus 32 administration with risk to hematopoetic system	DWY5GFZ

Physical Rehabilitation and Diagnostic Audiology

	Procedure	Code
1.	Bekesy assessment using audiometer	F13Z31Z
2.	Individual fitting of left eye prosthesis	F0DZ8UZ
3.	Physical therapy for range of motion and mobility, patient right hip, no special equipment	F07L0ZZ
4.	Bedside swallow assessment using assessment kit	F00ZHYZ
5.	Caregiver training in airway clearance techniques	F0FZ8ZZ
6.	Application of short arm cast in rehabilitation setting	F0DZ7EZ (Inhibitory cast is listed in the equipment reference table under E, *Orthosis.*)
7.	Verbal assessment of patient's pain level	F02ZFZZ
8.	Caregiver training in communication skills using manual communication board	F0FZJMZ (Manual communication board is listed in the equipment reference table under M, *Augmentative/ Alternative Communication.*)

Procedure	Code
9. Group musculoskeletal balance training exercises, whole body, no special equipment	F07M6ZZ (Balance training is included in the motor treatment reference table under *Therapeutic Exercise*.)
10. Individual therapy for auditory processing using tape recorder	F09Z2KZ (Tape recorder is listed in the equipment reference table under *Audiovisual Equipment*.)

Mental Health

Procedure	Code
1. Cognitive-behavioral psychotherapy, individual	GZ58ZZZ
2. Narcosynthesis	GZGZZZZ
3. Light therapy	GZJZZZZ
4. ECT (electroconvulsive therapy), unilateral, multiple seizure	GZB1ZZZ
5. Crisis intervention	GZ2ZZZZ
6. Neuropsychological testing	GZ13ZZZ
7. Hypnosis	GZFZZZZ
8. Developmental testing	GZ10ZZZ
9. Vocational counseling	GZ61ZZZ
10. Family psychotherapy	GZ72ZZZ

Substance Abuse Treatment

Procedure	Code
1. Naltrexone treatment for drug dependency	HZ94ZZZ
2. Substance abuse treatment family counseling	HZ63ZZZ
3. Medication monitoring of patient on methadone maintenance	HZ81ZZZ
4. Individual interpersonal psychotherapy for drug abuse	HZ54ZZZ
5. Patient in for alcohol detoxification treatment	HZ2ZZZZ
6. Group motivational counseling	HZ47ZZZ
7. Individual 12-step psychotherapy for substance abuse	HZ53ZZZ
8. Post-test infectious disease counseling for IV drug abuser	HZ3CZZZ
9. Psychodynamic psychotherapy for drug dependent patient	HZ5CZZZ
10. Group cognitive-behavioral counseling for substance abuse	HZ42ZZZ

New Technology

Procedure	Code
1. Infusion of terlipressin via peripheral venous catheter	XW03367
2. Transcatheter dilation of left peroneal artery with 2 SAVAL stents	X27U395